CLINICAL HEMATOLOGY

EDITED BY

Cheryl A. Lotspeich-Steininger
MS, MBA, MT (ASCP), CLS (NCA)

Formerly Assistant Professor
Program in Medical Technology/Cytogenetics
School of Allied Health Sciences
The University of Texas Health Science Center
Houston, Texas

E. Anne Stiene-Martin
PhD, MT (ASCP)

Professor
Department of Clinical Sciences
Division of Clinical Laboratory Science
University of Kentucky
Lexington, Kentucky

John A. Koepke, MD

Professor of Pathology
Associate Professor of Medicine
Department of Pathology
Duke University Medical Center
Durham, North Carolina

WITH 61 CONTRIBUTORS

J. B. Lippincott Company
Philadelphia • New York • London • Hagerstown

CLINICAL HEMATOLOGY

PRINCIPLES

PROCEDURES

CORRELATIONS

Sponsoring Editor: Andrew Allen
Editorial Assistant: Miriam Benert
Project Editor: Melissa McGrath
Indexer: Barbara Littlewood
Design Coordinator: Kathy Kelley-Luedtke
Cover Design: Anita Curry
Production Manager: Helen Ewan
Production Coordinator: Maura C. Murphy
Compositor: TCSystems, Inc.
Printer/Binder: Courier Westford

6 5 4 3 2 1

Library of Congress Cataloging-in-Publication Data

Clinical hematology : principles, procedures, correlations / edited by
 Cheryl A. Lotspeich-Steininger, E. Anne Stiene-Martin, John A.
 Koepke : with 61 contributors.
      p.   cm.
   Includes bibliographical references.
   Includes index.
   ISBN 0-397-54806-0
   1. Hematology.   I. Lotspeich-Steininger, Cheryl A.   II. Stiene
-Martin, E. Anne.   III. Koepke, John A., 1929-
   [DNLM: 1. Hematologic Diseases.   WH   100   C6412]
 RB45.C57   1992
 616.1′5—dc20
 DNLM/DLC
 for Library of Congress   90-13631
                                                  CIP

Any procedure or practice described in this book should be applied by the
health-care practitioner under appropriate supervision in accordance with
professional standards of care used with regard to the unique
circumstances that apply in each practice situation. The authors and
publisher have exerted every effort to ensure that reference ranges, test
methodologies, and drug selection and dosage set forth in this text are in
accord with current recommendations and practice at the time of
publication. However, in view of ongoing research, changes in
government regulations, and the constant flow of information relating to
test methodologies and drug therapy and drug reactions, the reader is
urged to check the package insert for each analyte and drug for any
change in indications and dosage and for added warnings and precautions.
This is particularly important when the recommended agent is a new or
infrequently employed drug or test procedure.

To our spouses, John, Ken, and Evelyn, and our families, students, and colleagues who have continually inspired and encouraged us in our work; and to those who seek to understand the science and art of clinical hematology.

Contributors

F. Sue Allison, MA, MT (ASCP), CLS (NCA)
Associate Professor of Medical Technology
The University of Alabama, Tuscaloosa
University, Alabama

Geraldine L. Anderson, BS, MT (ASCP), CLS (NCA)
Flow Cytometry Consultant
FCM Specialists
Minneapolis, Minnesota

Robert L. Baglini, BS, MT (ASCP), CLS (NCA)
Formerly Supervisor, Coagulation Laboratory
Rhode Island Hospital
Providence, Rhode Island

Lee A. Barbieri, BS, MT (ASCP)
Operations Director
Hematology and Transfusion Services
Duke University Medical Center
Durham, North Carolina

Joyce A. Behrens, MS, MT (ASCP), CLS (NCA)
Assistant Professor
University of Washington
Department of Laboratory Medicine
Division of Medical Technology
University Hospital
Seattle, Washington

Ann Bell, MS, SH (ASCP), CLSpH (NCA)
Assistant Professor of Medicine
Professor of Clinical Laboratory Sciences
The University of Tennessee, Memphis
The Health Science Center
Division of Hematology/Oncology
Department of Medicine
Memphis, Tennessee

Pamela B. Bollinger, BS, MT (ASCP)
Laboratory Director
Northeast Medical Center Hospital
Humble, Texas

Marshall E. Bowman, BS, MT (ASCP), CLS (NCA)
Loma Linda University
School of Allied Health Professions
Department of Clinical Laboratory Science
Loma Linda, California

Carrie D. Brailas Ventura, BS, MT (ASCP)
Formerly Chief Technologist
The University of Texas at Houston
M.D. Anderson Hospital and Tumor Institute
Section of Laboratory Hematology
Division of Laboratory Medicine
Houston, Texas

Darlean Brown, BS, MT (ASCP)
  Manager
  Hematology Laboratory
  Department of Pathology and Laboratory Medicine
  Hermann Hospital
  Houston, Texas

Michael R. Buchanan, PhD
  Associate Professor of Pathology
  Director of Surgical Research
  McMaster University Health Science Centre
  Department of Pathology
  Hamilton, Ontario
  Canada

Cheryl S. Cook, BS, MT (ASCP)
  Supervisor
  Coagulation Department
  Riverside Methodist Hospital
  Columbus, Ohio

Gerald L. Davis, PhD, MT (ASCP)
  Director
  Michigan State University
  Medical Technology Program
  East Lansing, Michigan

Janis Schaeffer Dixon, MS, MT (ASCP)
  Formerly Coagulation Research Technologist
  Ball Memorial Hospital
  Special Hematology
  Muncie, Indiana

Mary Ann Dotson, BS, MT (ASCP), CLS (NCA)
  Analytical Specialist
  Duke University Medical Center
  Department of Hospital Laboratories
  Durham, North Carolina

Patricia Dow, BS
  Research Associate
  John Sealy Hospital
  Department of Internal Medicine
  Special Hematology Laboratory
  Galveston, Texas

Benjamin Drewinko, MD, PhD
  (Deceased)
  The University of Texas at Houston
  M.D. Anderson Hospital and Tumor Institute
  Section of Laboratory Hematology
  Division of Laboratory Medicine
  Houston, Texas

Rita C. East, MS, MT (ASCP)
  Chief Medical Technologist
  VA Medical Center
  Hematology–Oncology Section
  Lexington, Kentucky

Harriet J. Echternacht, BS, MT (ASCP)
  Program Associate
  University of Iowa Hospitals and Clinics
  Hematopathology Division
  Iowa City, Iowa

Gordon E. Ens, MT (ASCP), CLS (NCA)
  Laboratory Director
  Colorado Coagulation Consultants, Inc. Laboratory
  Denver, Colorado

Valerie J. Evans, BS, CLS (NCA)
  Manager
  Department of Clinical Pathology
  University of Arizona
  Arizona Health Sciences Center
  University Medical Center
  Tucson, Arizona

Judith K. Fincher, MS, MT (ASCP) SH
  Formerly Assistant Professor/Clinical Coordinator
  The University of Texas
  Health Science Center at Dallas
  School of Allied Health Sciences
  Department of Medical Laboratory Sciences
  Dallas, Texas

Vincent S. Gallicchio, PhD, MT (ASCP)
  Associate Professor and Associate Dean of Research
  Department of Clinical Sciences
  Division of Clinical Laboratory Science
  University of Kentucky
  Lexington, Kentucky

Cynthia A. Gauger, MS, MT (ASCP), CLS (NCA)
  Formerly Instructor
  The University of Texas
  Health Science Center at San Antonio
  School of Allied Health Sciences
  Program in Medical Technology
  San Antonio, Texas

Virginia Haight, BS
  Supervisor, Hematology
  Lawrence Memorial Hospital
  New London, Connecticut

Dianne M. Hansen, MT (ASCP)
  Formerly Instructor
  University of South Dakota
  Department of Medical Technology
  Vermillion, South Dakota

Ruth Ann Henriksen, PhD
  Department of Medicine
  East Carolina University School of Medicine
  Greenville, North Carolina

Anne S. Hobson, MA, MT (ASCP) SH
    Technical Director of Hematology
    University of Virginia Medical Center
    Clinical Laboratories
    Charlottesville, Virginia

Muriel I. Jobe, BS, MT (ASCP) SH, CLS (NCA)
    Supervisor
    Hematology Laboratories
    St. Louis University Hospital
    St. Louis, Missouri

Dona D. Knapp, PhD, MT (ASCP), CLS (NCA)
    Professor
    Director of Medical Technology
    University of South Dakota Medical School
    Department of Laboratory Medicine
    Vermillion, South Dakota

John A. Koepke, MD
    Professor of Pathology
    Associate Professor of Medicine
    Department of Pathology
    Duke University Medical Center
    Durham, North Carolina

Lynn A. LaBounty, PhD, CLS (NCA)
    Clinical Laboratory
    University of South Alabama Medical Center
    Mobile, Alabama

Louann W. Lawrence, MEd, CLSpH (NCA),
        MT (ASCP) SH
    Assistant Professor
    The University of Texas
    Health Science Center at Houston
    School of Allied Health Sciences
    Program in Medical Technology/Cytogenetics
    Houston, Texas

Susan J. Leclair, MS, CLS (NCA)
    Associate Professor
    University of Massachusetts/Dartmouth
    Department of Medical Laboratory Science
    North Dartmouth, Massachusetts

Carol N. LeCrone, MS, MT (ASCP)
    Assistant Professor
    Director, Division of Medical Technology
    Codirector, Hemolysis Laboratory
    University of Washington
    Department of Laboratory Medicine
    University Hospital
    Seattle, Washington

Karen G. Lofsness, MS
    Assistant Professor
    University of Minnesota
    Division of Medical Technology
    Department of Laboratory Medicine and Pathology
    Minneapolis, Minnesota

Cheryl A. Lotspeich-Steininger, MS, MBA, MT (ASCP),
        CLS (NCA)
    Formerly Assistant Professor
    The University of Texas
    Health Science Center at Houston
    School of Allied Health Sciences
    Program in Medical Technology/Cytogenetics
    Houston, Texas

F. Bernhard Ludvigsen, PhD
    Associate Professor
    University of South Alabama
    College of Allied Health Professions
    Department of Medical Technology
    Mobile, Alabama

Lynne H. Lyons, MS, MT (ASCP)
    Technologist
    University of Kentucky Medical Center
    Department of Pathology
    Clinical Hematology Laboratory
    Lexington, Kentucky

Joan C. McNeely, MA, CLSpH (NCA)
    Clinical Coordinator—Laboratory
    St. Joseph Hospital
    Houston, Texas

Charles E. Manner, MD
    Formerly Assistant Professor
    The University of Texas
    Health Science Center at Houston
    School of Medicine Department of Internal Medicine
    Division of Hematology–Oncology
    Houston, Texas

Barbara A. Smith Michael, MS, MT (ASCP), CLS (NCA)
    Assistant Professor and Educational Resources
        Coordinator
    The University of Texas
    Health Science Center at Houston
    School of Allied Health Sciences
    Program in Medical Technology/Cytogenetics
    Houston, Texas

Mary Ann Morris, CLS (NCA)
    Supervisor
    Cytochemistry/Hematology
    Mayo Clinic
    Department of Laboratory Medicine
    Rochester, Minnesota

Kim A. Musgrave, BS, MT (ASCP) H–SH
    Formerly Coagulation Research Technologist
    Ball Memorial Hospital
    Special Hematology
    Muncie, Indiana

Harlene S. Palkuti, BS, MT (ASCP)
    Hemostasis Consulting
    Alexandria, Virginia

Janice H. Parrish, MEd, MT (ASCP)
   Formerly Assistant Professor
   University of Florida
   Health Science Center
   College of Health Related Professions
   Department of Medical Laboratory Sciences
   Gainesville, Florida

Barbara A. Payne, BA, MT (ASCP), CLS (NCA)
   Hematology Supervisor
   Cell Counting Area
   Mayo Clinic
   Department of Laboratory Medicine
   Rochester, Minnesota

Carolyn J. Pearce, MS, MT (ASCP) SH
   Formerly Associate Professor
   The University of Texas
   Medical Branch at Galveston
   School of Allied Health Sciences
   Medical Technology Department
   Galveston, Texas

Irma T. Pereira, BA, MT (ASCP) SH
   Clinical Hematology Specialist and Consultant
   Stanford University Hospital and Medical Center
   Stanford, California

Robert V. Pierre, MD
   American Board of Internal Medicine
   Subspecialty Board in Hematology
   Professor of Internal Medicine and Laboratory
      Medicine Consultant
   Mayo Clinic
   Hematology Section
   Department of Laboratory Medicine
   Department of Pathology
   Rochester, Minnesota

Bernadette F. Rodak, MS, MT (ASCP) SH,
      CLSpH (NCA)
   Assistant Professor
   Indiana University—Purdue University at Indianapolis
   Medical Technology Program
   Indianapolis, Indiana

Margaret C. Schmidt, EdD, MAT, MT (ASCP) SH,
      CLS (NCA), CLSpH (NCA)
   Associate in Pathology
   Director
   Education Service
   Hospital Laboratories
   Duke University Medical Center
   Durham, North Carolina

Linda C. Schumacher, MPH, MT (ASCP), CLS (NCA)
   Hematology Manager
   Clinical Pathology
   Clinical Associate Professor
   Medical Laboratory Sciences
   The University of Illinois at Chicago
   Chicago, Illinois

Jean A. Shafer, MA, MT (ASCP)
   Associate Professor of Medicine and Pathology
   University of Rochester School of Medicine and
      Dentistry
   Department of Medicine
   Hematology Unit
   Rochester, New York

Reaner G. Shannon, PhD, MT (ASCP)
   Assistant Professor
   University of Missouri at Kansas City
   School of Medicine
   Kansas City, Missouri

Sister Catherine Sherry, MS, MPS, MT (ASCP)
   Associate Director
   Department of Laboratories
   St. Vincent's Hospital and Medical Center of
      New York
   New York, New York

Ella M. Spanjers, BS
   Laboratory Manager
   Special Hematology Laboratory
   Department of Laboratory Medicine and Pathology
   University of Minnesota Hospitals
   Minneapolis, Minnesota

Charles E. Stewart, BHS, MT (ASCP)
   Person County Memorial Hospital
   Department of Laboratory Medicine
   Roxboro, North Carolina

E. Anne Stiene-Martin, PhD, MT (ASCP)
   Professor
   Department of Clinical Sciences
   Division of Clinical Laboratory Science
   University of Kentucky
   Lexington, Kentucky

Martha T. Thomas, MS, MT (ASCP) SH, CLS (NCA)
   Professor Emeritus
   Michigan State University
   Medical Technology Program
   East Lansing, Michigan

Judith S. Watson, BS, MT (ASCP) SH
   Formerly Chief Supervisor
   University of North Carolina
   The North Carolina Memorial Hospital
   Hematology Laboratories
   Chapel Hill, North Carolina

Foreword

Of the sciences that constitute clinical laboratory science (medical technology), none has been more subject to advancements and to the influences of technologic innovation than clinical laboratory hematology. The expansion of knowledge and diagnostic methodology and the development of pharmacologic and immunologic treatment regimens have pushed the frontiers of the practice of clinical hematology to points considered impossible only a few decades ago. Clinical laboratory hematology has been transformed into something of a space age science with futuristic instruments capable of enhancing the investigation of disease processes.

These changes compel the laboratory professional to develop new approaches for the education of those who will deliver health services. Obviously new types of instructional materials are necessary. New kinds of texts, such as Clinical Hematology—Principles, Procedures, Correlations, are essential to integrate the understanding of disease processes and the knowledge of analytic technologies so that both practitioners and students can comprehend the impact of these advances.

Hematologists and clinicians have responded to these new technologies with an avalanche of articles, monographs, and books. Cheryl A. Lotspeich–Steininger, E. Anne Stiene–Martin, and John A. Koepke, editors of this book, have been productive authors in clinical laboratory hematology with many scholarly contributions to the literature. Each has been recognized by professional associations for highest achievement in hematopathology or instruction of clinical hematology.

Practitioners and students in clinical hematology have searched widely for a text that offers a clearly presented review of subjects in this field. The contributing authors to Clinical Hematology—Principles, Procedures, Correlations have responded to this challenge. For this significant and comprehensive text, the editors have organized all the major topics that represent laboratory hematology and hemostasis, from the collection and handling of specimens to advanced instrumentation and diagnostic techniques to theoretical and practical aspects of these areas of clinical science. Each subject is expertly covered by one of the 61 contributors to this text. The list of contributors reads like a "who's who" of the clinical hematology laboratory.

It has been my good fortune to know many of the contributors to this textbook. Several have been respected faculty colleagues, and most are recognized as authorities in the practice and teaching of hematology in medical and allied health professional schools. It was especially pleasing to observe the development of a former student, who is one of the editors of this book, and another who is a contributor.

The unique character and organization of Clinical Hematology—Principles, Procedures, Correlations promise to make it a standard text for clinical laboratory scientists and a valuable resource for other health professionals and clinicians. In 63 chapters, the authors deal with specific topics or areas of laboratory hematology practice in concise, easy-to-comprehend language. The chapters are well referenced and illustrated with several hundred drawings and photographs. The section of more than 60 color plates is extremely helpful for instructional purposes, and the many tables and case studies are excellent for highlighting important concepts and differential characteristics. Perhaps two of the more innovative contributions this textbook makes to the field include the presentation of appropriate algorithms for laboratory diagnosis of disease and the direct approach to the problem of knowledge and technology integration.

Those who use this book will find superb writing that deals with all aspects of the technical and scientific operation of the hematology and hemostasis laboratories. It is a stimulating text that should satisfy the needs of students and practitioners of clinical hematology.

Mary Stevenson Britt, MS, MT(ASCP), CLS(NCA)
Program Director and Associate Professor
Department of Medical Laboratory Sciences
College of Health Related Professions
University of Florida Health Science Center
Gainesville, Florida

Preface

The field of clinical hematology has become increasingly complex during the last decades of the 20th century. Fortunately, the understanding of this clinical science also has advanced dramatically. In this textbook, we have presented our knowledge of the disorders of hematology and hemostasis and the laboratory studies used in their diagnosis and treatment. It is organized in a manner that is conducive to logical teaching and study, and it is written in easy-to-understand language. It should be valuable to undergraduate and graduate students of clinical laboratory science and to practicing laboratory scientists, at both the bench and the management level. In addition, this text should be useful to nursing and medical students studying laboratory hematology and hemostasis and to residents and fellows in hematology/oncology or pathology.

When *Clinical Hematology—Principles, Procedures, Correlations* was first proposed, we wanted to develop a textbook that would contain many of the "tricks of the trade" that have been presented at professional seminars and workshops but not published in a textbook. The contributors have helped us meet this challenge. We have endeavored to provide students and practioners with valuable information regarding the various disease states and clinical laboratory procedures for their diagnosis. We have paid special attention to the sources of technical and physiologic error in procedures (and their possible solutions) in extensive "Comments and Sources of Error" sections. Another unique feature included in the chapters on disease processes is "Effects of Treatment on Laboratory Results," in which

the expected changes in laboratory values following treatment are addressed where appropriate.

Case studies are provided at the end of many chapters, which include study questions that challenge the reader's ability to apply what has been learned about the described disease process, particularly with respect to laboratory values, tests, and their sources of error. Answers to the questions are provided in an appendix at the end of the textbook. Most chapters have a summary that students will find useful to quickly review chapter content and to recall key points.

Other features of this textbook are the chapters dedicated to bone marrow evaluation, blood cell cytochemistry, body fluid evaluation, hematologic instrumentation (including routine analyzers, automated differential counters, and flow cytometers), and quality control and quality assurance for hematology and hemostasis laboratories. The final chapter on hematology laboratory management has been included as a result of the federal legislation and budgetary constraints under which laboratories must now function.

In this textbook, all special or unique laboratory procedures are integrated into the discussion of disease processes where appropriate. We believe that the diseases and the special procedures employed in their diagnosis should be studied together in a single chapter. The student should no longer think of laboratory analysis without correlating it to the disease process and recognizing the effects of diseases and their treatment on laboratory test results. For example, hemoglobinopathies and hemoglobin electrophoresis procedures are discussed in the same chapter so that the reader may easily understand the meaning of the abnormal results associated with the many hemoglobinopathies and how they are determined in the laboratory.

Current procedures and laboratory instrumentation used for the diagnosis of many different disorders are discussed in separate chapters placed at strategic points throughout the textbook. In some cases, procedures have not been delineated step-by-step because this information is available in original references, laboratory manuals, or even commercial package inserts. However, we have attempted to include sections on the testing principle, specimen and quality control requirements, a brief explanation of the critical steps, reference ranges, and comments and sources of error for all procedures where appropriate. References on most procedures are included to allow the reader to obtain further information.

We look forward to receiving comments and suggestions from interested readers. We hope to embark on a second edition of this textbook at some point in the future to incorporate readers' ideas and new clinical hematology principles, procedures, and correlations as they become available.

Cheryl A. Lotspeich-Steininger, MS, MBA, MT (ASCP), CLS (NCA)

E. Anne Stiene-Martin, PhD, MT (ASCP)

John A. Koepke, MD

Acknowledgments

The editors are very grateful to the 61 contributors for sharing their knowledge and insight in this textbook, and for their cooperation, patience, and endurance during the lengthy writing and editing process. Each contributor was selected based on his or her expertise in hematology or hemostasis. As evidenced by the preceding contributor list, the vast majority are laboratory scientists who are actively engaged in the practice of laboratory hematology or hemostasis or in education related to these fields. Two are medical doctors who, like the other contributors and the editors, have a keen interest in the education of clinical laboratory scientists and others studying clinical hematology and hemostasis.

We are also grateful to the staff at JB Lippincott Company who have worked diligently with us during this lengthy and complex project to make this textbook a reality. We wish to extend our personal thanks to Delois Patterson, Developmental Editor, Andrew Allen, Allied Health Editor, and Melissa McGrath, Project Editor, all of whom worked with us directly to assist with every aspect of this publication. We are most appreciative of them and of everyone who contributed to this endeavor.

Contents

CLINICAL HEMATOLOGY

PART I

INTRODUCTION

TO

HEMATOLOGY

Introduction

to

Clinical

Hematology

E. Anne Stiene–Martin

This introductory section provides a brief background on the development of clinical hematology. Hematologic vocabulary is introduced in terms of common prefixes and suffixes used to form the medical terms used in this discipline. The chapters in this text provide an overview of clinical hematology and hemostasis, with an emphasis on the laboratory aspects of hematologic and coagulation abnormalities.

HISTORY OF CLINICAL HEMATOLOGY

For centuries man has been aware that blood is necessary for life. Until the seventeenth century, blood could be examined only by its gross appearance, and little was understood about its composition or biologic functions, although many theories were proposed that have since been disproved. During the seventeenth century Leeuwenhoek and others studied blood with the aid of primitive microscopes, and the science of studying blood was born. The word "hematology" is derived from the Greek words *haima* meaning blood and *logos* meaning study or science. Thus, hematology is the science of blood. Blood consists of two main parts: (1) the liquid portion and (2) the "formed elements," which include the leukocytes or white blood cells, erythrocytes or red blood cells, and platelets.

Clinical hematology has a relatively short history in that until the 1920s, the study of diseases related to alterations in blood cell number or appearance was a branch of clinical medicine and pathology.[1] In the last 70 years, however, the science of clinical hematology has grown enormously and now is concerned with the study of normal and abnormal development, physiology, function, and death or destruction of the formed elements of blood. Additionally, because of a variety of factors, the modern hematology laboratory encompasses the study of hemostatic mechanisms, hemorrhagic disease, and thrombosis. These studies occur in both research and clinical laboratories and in a wide variety of settings.

Unlike other subdivisions of the clinical laboratory, clinical hematology does not have a single basic science as its foundation. Clinical chemistry is founded on the basic chemical sciences (inorganic, organic, analytical, biologic), clinical bacteriology is likewise based on one basic science—microbiology, and immunohematology (blood banking) depends largely on the basic science of immunology. Clinical hematology, on the other hand, draws from a wide range of basic sciences including biochemistry, cell biology, cytology, genetics, histology, immunology, pathology, physiology, and even, to some extent, radiation physics (nuclear medicine). In recent years the clinical science of hematology frequently has been linked with another relatively new clinical science: oncology—the study of malignant or neoplastic changes in cells.

The clinical hematology laboratory has evolved over the past half century from a place where small aliquots of blood cell suspensions were measured, counted, and examined visually with the aid of stains and microscopes to the present, where larger, statistically sound aliquots of blood cell suspensions are analyzed. For example, a manual leukocyte count performed with a hemocytometer and microscope routinely samples only 0.02 μL of blood, whereas many automated counters today sample at least one full microliter. Today's analyses are based on cellular resistance to electric current, the manner in which cells deflect a light beam, their ability to bind or incorporate dyes, their functions, or the ability of their surface receptors to bind marker ligands. Automation in the modern hematology laboratory has increased objectivity (or decreased bias) in the identification, classification, and counting of cells; it has decreased, to a considerable extent, the labor-intensive aspects (drudgery) of cell analysis; and it has increased the time available for other pursuits such as clinical investigations, research, and method development.

Laboratory investigation of hemostasis has also matured considerably. Forty years ago there were only a few routine determinations for evaluating the hemostatic mechanism: the platelet count, bleeding time, whole-blood clotting time, and the prothrombin time (which, before commercial preparations of thromboplastin were available, required the tedious preparation of home-made thromboplastin from rabbit brain extracts). Today with good commercially available reagents, automation has improved the precision and accuracy of coagulation testing. Coagulation enzymes are no longer regarded as mysterious and magical but can be evaluated functionally by use of synthetic substrates. The number of tests has grown exponentially to the point where many hemostasis laboratories have become bona fide independent operations in the clinical laboratory.

The extent of services provided by the modern clinical hematology laboratory differs considerably from one institution to another. Services that may be offered can be categorized as listed in Table 1.

To perform the services listed in Table 1 adequately, the student laboratorian will find it necessary to learn normal blood cell physiology and common pathologic alterations of the hematologic mechanism. The principles and procedures of both routine and special hematology tests must be studied, and a thorough understanding of the sources of error in each test must be gained to ensure that valid results are generated for the benefit of the patient. In addition to

TABLE 1. Primary Services Offered by the Hematology and Hemostasis Laboratory

Specimen collection and preparation for examination
Quantitative manual and instrumental measurements of cells
Measurements of cell volumes
Evaluation of cellular contents and components
Cellular identification according to various criteria:
   Morphologic
   Cytochemical markers
   Cell surface markers
Identification of reactive or neoplastic alterations in cell populations
Evaluation of leukocyte, erythrocyte, and platelet function
Evaluation of cellular development and formation (bone marrow)
Evaluation of hemostatic function

TABLE 2. Common Prefixes from Greek and Latin Used in the Vocabulary of Hematology

PREFIX	MEANING
a-/an-	Lack, without, absent, decreased
aniso-	Unequal, dissimilar
cyt-	Cell
dys-	Abnormal, difficult, bad
erythro-	Red
ferr-	Iron
hemo- (hemato-)	Pertaining to blood
hypo-	Beneath, under, deficient, decreased
hyper-	Above, beyond, extreme
iso-	Equal, alike, same
leuk(o)-	White
macro-	Large, long
mega-	Large, giant
meta-	(1) After, next; (2) change
micro-	Small
myel(o)-	(1) From bone marrow; (2) spinal cord
pan-	All, overall, all-inclusive
phleb-	Vein
phago-	Eat, ingest
poikilo-	Varied, irregular
poly-	Many
schis-	Split
scler-	Hard
splen-	Spleen
thromb(o)-	Clot, thrombus
xanth-	Yellow

TABLE 3. Common Suffixes from Greek and Latin Used in the Vocabulary of Hematology

SUFFIX	MEANING
-cyte	Cell
-emia	Blood
-itis	Inflammation
-lysis	Destruction or dissolving
-oma	Swelling, tumor
-opathy	Disease
-osis	(1) Abnormal increase; (2) disease
-penia	Deficiency, decreased
-phil(ic)	Attracted to, affinity for
-plasia (-plastic)	Cell production or repair
-poiesis	Cell production, formation, and development
-poietin	Stimulates production

TABLE 4. Examples of Hematologic Terms Formed by Combining Prefixes and Suffixes

PREFIX–SUFFIX COMBINATION	HEMATOLOGIC TERM	INTERPRETATION
an + iso + cyte + osis	= anisocytosis	Abnormal (osis) lack (an) of equality (iso) among cells (cyte): variation in cell size
a + plasia	= aplasia	Absent (a) cell production (plasia)
an + emia	= anemia	Decreased (an) blood (emia)
dys + myelo + poiesis	= dysmyelopoiesis	Abnormal (dys) development (poiesis) of marrow cells (myelo)
pan + myel(o) + osis	= panmyelosis	An abnormal increase (osis) in all (pan) marrow cells (myel)

learning hematologic theory and techniques it is important to understand the operation of the instruments used in the clinical hematology laboratory. These topics are addressed in the following chapters.

BASIC TERMINOLOGY IN HEMATOLOGY

Learning will be aided by an understanding of common terminology used in hematology and of the origin of some of these terms. Like any other science, hematology has accumulated a distinct vocabulary. A clinical chemist once observed, "The problem with hematology is that all words begin with *m*"—a humorous exaggeration that underscores the need to have a working knowledge of the common terms.

Most hematologic terms used in this text are defined when they are introduced. Nevertheless, it may be helpful to know the meanings of several prefixes and suffixes, generally derived from Greek and Latin, that are common in the hematologic vocabulary. (Medical schools once required a course in Latin, Greek, or both for admission.) For example, most people will recognize the suffix "cyte" as meaning cell and the prefix "micro" as meaning small. These two words form the term *microcyte*, which means small cell. This word is used most often in hematology to refer specifically to small erythrocytes (red cells). Table 2 is a list of commonly used prefixes; Table 3 provides commonly used suffixes. Table 4 demonstrates how prefixes and suffixes may be combined to form hematologic terms.

The many facets of hematology and hemostasis are both fascinating and perplexing. The story unfolds in the chapters that follow.

REFERENCE

1.   Wintrobe MM: Hematology: The Blossoming of a Science, p 1. Philadelphia, Lea & Febiger, 1985

Safety in the Clinical Hematology Laboratory

E. Anne Stiene-Martin

In this chapter the principal laboratory safety rules are introduced. Strict observance of safety practices is essential in the student as well as clinical laboratory. An understanding of safety rules therefore is an absolute necessity before beginning work in any laboratory. These rules must be strictly applied to avoid accidents that can cause illness and even death. Safe laboratory practice ensures the well-being of laboratory personnel as well as those who enter the laboratory for consultation and those responsible for cleaning the laboratory and discarding hazardous waste.

Books have been written on the topic of laboratory safety (see Suggested Readings). The intent of this chapter is not to be all-inclusive but to stress the safety hazards that are of particular concern in the hematology and hemostasis laboratories. These hazards may be classified as biologic, chemical, electrical, mechanical, and thermal (fire).

BIOLOGIC HAZARDS

Definition

Blood, urine, feces, spinal fluid, and all other body fluids present biologic safety hazards because they may contain highly infectious and potentially lethal organisms or viruses. Extreme caution should be used in collecting, handling, and processing of all body fluids. These materials are referred to collectively as "biohazards."

Safe Handling of Biohazards

Biohazards probably cause the greatest concern of all the hazards in the hematology laboratory because a primary function is the collection, analysis, and safe disposal of blood. Blood may contain many highly infectious agents, including the viral agents that cause infectious hepatitis and acquired immune deficiency syndrome (AIDS). Because the infectious agent may be present in the specimen long before the patient shows any signs or symptoms of disease, *all biologic specimens, regardless of source, should be considered biohazardous.* The next chapter on specimen collection will address the precautions that should be taken while collecting blood specimens. Recently, the National Committee for Clinical Laboratory Standards (NCCLS) published a tentative guideline for protection of laboratory workers from infectious diseases transmitted by biologic materials.[2] This document is a valuable guide to safe laboratory practices for the prevention of infectious disease transmission, and every laboratory worker should be familiar with it.

The following general rules should be strictly followed in the laboratory.

1. **Gloves must be worn when handling biologic specimens.** Gloves are an absolute necessity in all laboratories to prevent skin contamination with infectious agents. Latex, vinyl, or polyethylene gloves all provide adequate protection. However, gloves present a problem in hematology. They usually are packaged by the manufacturer with a liberal amount of powder or starch to make them easier to put on. Unfortunately, if these particles of powder get into the specimen or a dilution of the specimen, they may be counted as cells, causing a falsely elevated count. One possible solution is to rinse gloved hands in tap water and dry them with a lint-free towel before handling specimens. This rinsing process also permits detection of any leaks; obviously, leaking gloves do not provide appropriate protection to the laboratorian. However, some gloves become sticky if they are washed, in which case this practice is unacceptable. Also, gloves should *not* be washed with detergents or disinfectants; detergents may enhance penetration of liquids through undetected holes, and disinfectants may cause glove deterioration.

2. **Areas or equipment used by personnel who are not gloved should not be touched with contaminated gloves.** Nothing that personnel who are not gloved may touch, such as the telephone or door knob, should ever be touched with contaminated gloves. When gloves become contaminated, they should be discarded and a clean pair put on. As long as the hands are not contaminated, hand washing between glove changes is not required.[2] Gloves must be removed aseptically to prevent hand contamination. Some equipment, such as computer keyboards and certain telephones, may be specially labeled as biohazardous to be used only with gloved hands. In other words, personnel who are not gloved should not touch equipment labeled as biohazardous.

3. **Wash hands immediately if they become contaminated, with or without gloves on.** Always wash hands after removing gloves when work is completed and before leaving the laboratory. Handwashing facilities should be separate from those used for washing equipment or for waste disposal. Hands must be washed before eating, drinking, smoking, applying makeup, handling contact lenses, and before and after using lavatory facilities. They must also be washed before hand contact with mucous membranes, eyes, or breaks in the skin. Washing with soap and water is recommended. Hand towelettes and cleansing foams are not recommended except in field conditions where water is not available. No additional benefit has been established for washing with antiseptic soaps or antiseptics.[2]

4. **Do not remove specimen tube stoppers until necessary.**
   A. Tube centrifugation should be performed with stoppers in place to prevent aerosol contamination.
   B. Stoppers should be covered with absorbent material such as gauze before removing them to prevent spraying of the specimen.
   C. Some cell counting instruments may be purchased with blood sampling devices that automatically obtain an aliquot of blood specimen by piercing the stopper, thus avoiding stopper removal.
   D. A clear Plexiglas shield between laboratorian and blood sample being manipulated has been used successfully in many laboratories.

5. **Mouth pipeting is strictly prohibited.** There are numerous types of safety devices on the market for pipeting and measuring blood. There is even a suction device available for blood cell pipets, discussed in Chapters 9 and 25. This device may be used to aspirate small amounts of blood and diluent into blood cell pipets for manual blood cell counting.

6. **Replace clay slabs for microhematocrit tube sealing frequently.**[2] These clay slabs often become contaminated with blood. Therefore, they should be treated as biohazards and should not be recycled (*i.e.,* re-formed to extend their life). Rather, they should be replaced at appropriate intervals.

7. **Decontaminate sedimentation tube racks regularly** and do so immediately if a leak occurs.

8. **Unfixed or unstained slides should be considered infectious.**

9. **Do not handle needles.** Accidental needle sticks are one of the most common accidents that can transmit infectious diseases. Needles should be disposed of, without recapping, bending, or cutting, in rigid puncture-resistant containers clearly marked as biohazardous. These containers should be carried in the collection tray. Needles should not be removed from disposable syringes. Disposable needles that attach to adapters for use with evacuated tubes can be removed from the adapter without touching the needle with the aid of special devices. Inexpensive disposable single-use adapters are now available also. One-handed needle removal techniques are described by NCCLS[2] if needle removal from adapter is absolutely necessary.

10. **Obtain immediate treatment for accidental and inappropriate contact with biohazards.** Any accident that results in inappropriate contact with a patient specimen (*e.g.,* contamination of skin cuts or needle punctures of skin) must be reported immediately to the supervisor so that appropriate prophylactic precautions may be taken.

11. **Properly dispose of contaminated laboratory supplies.** All laboratory supplies, such as gauze, tissues, work mats, or Pasteur pipets, that come in contact with patient specimens must be disposed of properly as biohazardous waste. All contaminated supplies may be incinerated or autoclaved prior to being discarded. Nondisposable pipets used to measure or dilute blood should be disinfected using a solution such as a 1:100 dilution of household bleach before being washed with glassware detergent.

12. **Disinfect and clean biohazardous spills immediately.** Decontaminate all surfaces and devices where biologic materials are handled at completion of work. All spills should be cleaned immediately with appropriate disinfectant solutions, and materials used to wipe up spills should be disposed of as potentially biohazardous. NCCLS recommends the steps listed in Table 1-1 for spill decontamination.[2] Table 1-2 lists the dilutions of household bleach that may be used for decontamination. For example, a 1:10 dilution may

TABLE 1–1. Appropriate Steps for Decontamination and Disinfection of Spills Involving Biohazardous Materials

1. Put on heavyweight puncture-resistant utility gloves, a gown, and, if necessary, water-impermeable shoes.
2. Remove any sharp broken objects without touching them by using rigid sheets of cardboard to scrape them up. Discard cardboard with broken objects in puncture-resistant biohazard container.
3. Absorb the spill with disposable absorbent material (e.g., paper towels, gauze pads, or tissue paper wipes). Dispose of contaminated materials in biohazardous waste.
4. Clean spill site of all visible spilled material using any aqueous household detergent. This dilutes spilled material, lyses erythrocytes, and removes proteins.
5. Disinfect spill site using intermediate- to high-level hospital disinfectant such as a dilution of household bleach (see Table 1-2). Flood spill site or wipe down with disposable towels soaked in disinfectant to make site glistening wet. Phenolic disinfectants are acceptable for use on laboratory instruments, floors, or countertops.
6. Absorb disinfectant with disposable material or allow disinfectant to dry.
7. Rinse spill site with water to remove odors. Dry spill site to prevent slipping.
8. Dispose of all contaminated materials used in cleaning process in a biohazard container.

Adapted from National Committee for Clinical Laboratory Standards: Protection of Laboratory Workers from Infectious Disease Transmitted by Blood, Body Fluids, and Tissue: Tentative Guideline M29-T, vol 9, no 1. Villanova, PA, NCCLS, 1989, with permission.

be required if the contaminated surface is porous and cannot be cleaned adequately before disinfection. For hard, smooth surfaces that can be decontaminated adequately, disinfection with a 1:100 dilution of bleach may be sufficient. Time of exposure to diluted bleach may be brief; a 500 mg/L solution (1:100) inactivates hepatitis B virus (HBV) in 10 minutes and human immunodeficiency virus (HIV) in 2 minutes.[2] If the spill is decontaminated adequately before disinfection, diluted bleach may be blotted up with disposable absorbent towels immediately after spill area has been soaked with bleach.

Note that some metals may be corroded by bleach; therefore, alternative disinfectants must be considered, such as iodophors registered as hard-surface disinfectants (iodophors labeled as antiseptics should not be used) or phenolic disinfectants.[2]

Large spills of infectious agents should first be flooded and mixed with a concentrated disinfectant such as 1% (1:5 dilution) bleach and then allowed to stand for 20 minutes before being decontaminated.

13. **Protective clothing should always be worn in the laboratory but never outside the laboratory.** A laboratory coat that is worn while handling specimens may be contaminated with hazardous specimen droplets. Frequent laundering is mandatory unless the clothing is disposable. Contaminated clothing should be sent to the institutional laundry.

CHEMICAL HAZARDS

Definition

Solid, liquid, or gaseous chemicals may be hazardous if transported, handled, stored, or dispensed inappropriately. Chemicals may have toxic, flammable, or carcinogenic properties.

Safe Handling of Chemicals

Toxic or corrosive chemicals may adversely affect one or more body systems and should be used only under a fume hood. Flammable or explosive chemicals should be stored in a safety cabinet designed for such chemicals.

Carcinogenic chemicals are those capable of causing mutations in body cells that may lead to the development of cancer. A few reagents used for special staining of cells in hematology, as well as one or two reagents used for identification of variant hemoglobin types, are considered carcinogenic. These are specifically pointed out in the discussions of the appropriate procedures. Skin must not come into contact with these chemicals; therefore, gloves must be worn when performing procedures where no alternative reagent is available. When possible, substitute reagents are recommended.

Safety glasses should be used when working with acid or alkaline solutions to avoid chemical burns in the eyes. Mouth pipeting is not permissible. Bottles or flasks of chemicals should be carried by securely grasping the body of the container rather than the neck.

When preparing a reagent requiring the mixing of concentrated acid and water, the acid should be added very slowly to the water. *Never add water to concentrated acid.* Mixing of acid with water should be performed in a deep sink so that the area may be immediately flooded with water if necessary.

All reagents must be properly labeled with the name and concentration of the reagent, the initials of the person who prepared the reagent, and the date on which the reagent was prepared. Any special storage requirements and the expiration date should be included.

TABLE 1–2. Dilutions of Household Bleach Used for Decontamination of Biohazard Spills*

VOLUME OF BLEACH (PART)	VOLUME OF WATER (PART)	DILUTION RATIO	SODIUM HYPOCHLORITE (%)	AVAILABLE CHLORINE (MG/L)
Undiluted	0	1/1	5.25	50,000
1	9	1/10	0.5	5,000
1	99	1/100	0.05	500

* All dilutions should be made up daily with tap water to prevent loss of germicidal action during storage.
From National Committee for Clinical Laboratory Standards: Protection of Laboratory Workers from Infectious Disease Transmitted by Blood, Body Fluids, and Tissue: Tentative Guideline M29-T, vol 9, no 1. Villanova, PA, NCCLS, 1989, with permission.

Federal law now requires all chemical and reagent manufacturers to include a material safety data sheet (MSDS) in the packing carton describing all information necessary for the safe handling of the material. These publications should be kept in an accessible place for easy reference in case questions arise.

Safe Disposal of Chemicals

Federal standards are not available for all types of chemical waste disposal, although some municipalities have their own regulations. Most noncarcinogenic, dilute acidic or alkaline reagents used in the hematology and hemostasis laboratories may be flushed down the sink with copious amounts of water. An environmental safety specialist in the laboratory's institution or the community should be contacted for specific instructions on chemical disposal.

ELECTRICAL HAZARDS

Definition

Electrical hazards are caused by inappropriate use or maintenance of electrical instruments or equipment that can cause electrical shock, burns, or a fire or explosion.

Safe Use of Electrical Equipment

Proper equipment maintenance is mandatory for its safe use in the laboratory. This maintenance includes immediate replacement of frayed wires or electrical connections. In the hematology laboratory the electrical connections of microscopes, automated cell counters, spectrophotometers, centrifuges, and any other equipment should be inspected regularly. All equipment must be grounded by a three-pronged plug according to federal regulations stipulated by the Occupational Safety and Health Act (OSHA) of 1970. NCCLS strongly opposes the use of extension cords for any laboratory equipment.[3]

Electrical equipment should never be operated with wet hands.

MECHANICAL HAZARDS

Definition

Mechanical hazards may result from improper use, storage, or disposal of glassware, sharp instruments, compressed gases, or equipment.

Safe Handling of Mechanical Devices

Glassware must be treated carefully to avoid breakage that could cause injury or infection. Glass and sharp objects such as microcapillary pipets, Pasteur pipets, or needles that are contaminated with biologic specimens should be disposed of in puncture-proof containers to avoid injury to either laboratory personnel or those responsible for discarding hazardous waste.

Sharp instruments should be stored and used carefully to avoid skin puncture or cuts. This includes needles, which

should be disposed of in an appropriate container. The NCCLS now recommends that needles be left uncapped after venipuncture and simply discarded in a puncture-proof container that must be carried by the phlebotomist[2] to avoid needle stick accidents, which occur frequently when trying to recap needles.

Compressed gases are not used routinely in the hematology laboratory. Whenever they are used, the strict guidelines for their handling and storage should be observed because of the dangers of explosion, mechanical injury, and fire. These guidelines are outlined elsewhere.[1]

Safe handling of equipment dictates that the laboratorian be instructed, either by a knowledgeable colleague or by carefully reading the manufacturer's instruction manual, before operating any equipment. In the hematology laboratory, for example, the centrifuge for blood samples as well as microhematocrit tubes may be a source of injury if sample tubes are not balanced or if the lid is raised before the centrifuge rotor has stopped. Long hair should always be tied back to avoid catching in an instrument, which could result in serious injury.

FIRE HAZARDS

Definition

Fire or thermal hazards may result from the improper use or storage of either cryogenic substances (those stored at very low temperatures such as in liquid nitrogen) or substances capable of combustion (igniting into flames). Fires can obviously cause burns, and skin contact with cryogenic substances has essentially the same effect—it causes a thermal burn. Cryogenic and combustible substances may cause a fire, explosion, or asphyxiation.

Fire Safety

Prevention is the easiest way to deal with fire hazard. A fire extinguisher must be easily accessible from anywhere in the laboratory. A dry chemical extinguisher is popular because of its versatility. It can be used on many types of fires. A safety shower also is necessary in any laboratory in case the clothing catches fire or a laboratorian is exposed to a large chemical spill. A fire blanket for smothering small fires also should be readily available.

The National Fire Protection Association (NFPA) and OSHA publish standards on fire prevention that are useful in planning a good fire prevention and containment program.

Cryogenic substances are not routinely used in the clinical hematology laboratory; they have specific safety requirements for their use and storage, which are explained elsewhere.[1]

LABORATORY SAFETY SUMMARY

Table 1-3 provides a summary of the cardinal rules of laboratory safety. Observance of these rules and those discussed in detail in the sections above is in the best interest of each laboratorian as well as of those who enter the laboratory for

TABLE 1–3. Cardinal Safety Rules of the Clinical Laboratory

Good Personal Habits

Wear proper attire and protective clothing; do not wear protective clothing outside laboratory.

Tie back long hair.

Do not eat, drink, or smoke in the work area.

Wear gloves when working with biologic specimens or hazardous chemicals.

Never pipet by mouth.

Do not put any objects in mouth (*e.g.*, pens or pencils).

Wash hands frequently.

Keep hands away from mouth, nose, eyes, and any other mucous membranes.

Good Housekeeping Practices

Keep work areas free of chemicals and dirty glassware.

Store chemicals properly.

Label reagents and solutions.

Post warning signs.

Good Laboratory Technique

Be careful when transferring chemicals from container to container and always add acid to water slowly.

Do not operate new or unfamiliar equipment until you are trained and authorized.

Read all labels and instructions carefully.

Use the personal safety equipment that is provided.

For the safe handling, use, and disposal of chemicals, learn their properties and hazards.

Learn emergency procedures and become familiar with the location of fire exits, fire extinguishers, fire blankets, and eyewash stations.

Adapted from Michael BS, Chantly PDJ: Laboratory safety. In Bishop ML, Duben–Von Laufen JL, Fody EP (eds): Clinical Chemistry— Principles, Procedures, Correlations. Philadelphia, JB Lippincott, 1985, with permission.

business or custodial services. These rules are meant to help maintain a healthy and safe work environment for everyone.

CHAPTER SUMMARY

Clinical laboratory safety hazards may be classified as biologic, chemical, electrical, mechanical, and thermal (fire). Of these, probably the most common hazards in the hematology laboratory are biologic. Table 1-1 presents the steps required for appropriate decontamination and disinfection of biohazardous

spills. Table 1-2 provides information on commonly used dilutions of household bleach that are acceptable for disinfection of biohazardous spills.

Attention to safety practices is necessary to recognize all hazards and is essential to a safe work environment. Table 1-3 provides an important summary of the rules of laboratory safety.

REFERENCES

1. Michael BS, Chantly PDJ: Laboratory safety. In Bishop ML, Duben–Von Laufen JL, Fody EP (eds): Clinical Chemistry— Principles, Procedures, Correlations, p 34. Philadelphia, JB Lippincott, 1985

2. National Committee for Clinical Laboratory Standards: Protection of Laboratory Workers from Infectious Disease Transmitted by Blood, Body Fluids, and Tissue: Tentative Guideline M29-T, vol 9, no 1. Villanova, PA, NCCLS, 1989

3. National Committee for Clinical Laboratory Standards: Power Requirements for Clinical Laboratory Instruments and for Laboratory Power Sources: Approved Standard 15-A. Villanova, PA, NCCLS, 1980

SUGGESTED READINGS

College of American Pathologists: Summary of Recent Information: Acquired Immunodeficiency Syndrome. Traverse City, MI, College of American Pathologists, 1983

Evenson G, Krueger P: Setting up a lab safety program. In Fitzgibbon RJ (ed): Legal Guidelines for the Clinical Laboratory. Oradell, NJ, Medical Economics, 1981

Fisher Scientific Company: Fisher Safety Manual. Pittsburgh, Fisher Scientific Co, 1982

Hawk WA, Hoeltge GA: Safety in the medical laboratory. Clin Lab Med 3:467, 1983

Hicks RM: Basics of clinical laboratory safety. In Snyder JR, Larsen AL (eds): Administration and Supervision in Laboratory Medicine. Philadelphia, Harper & Row, 1983

National Committee For Clinical Laboratory Standards: Clinical Laboratory Hazardous Waste: Proposed Guideline GP5-P. Villanova, PA, NCCLS, 1986

Rose SL: Clinical Laboratory Safety. Philadelphia, JB Lippincott, 1984

2

Specimen

Collection

Cynthia A. Gauger

Proper patient specimen collection is vital, it is the laboratory's first step toward reporting accurate and reliable results. Blood specimens may be obtained for hematologic tests either by venipuncture or by skin puncture. Because venipuncture is the method of choice for routine hematology tests, it will be discussed in detail in this chapter. Important issues concerning skin puncture also will be addressed. Regardless of the method employed, specimen collection requires knowledge of the necessary equipment and supplies, technical skill, strict attention to patient and specimen identification, awareness of and adherence to institutional safety requirements, and proper specimen transport techniques.

In addition to blood specimens, the hematology laboratory may analyze cerebrospinal fluid (Chap. 31), bone marrow (Chap. 29), and several other body fluids. See Chapter 51 for the special techniques required for collection of specimens for hemostasis testing.

PROFESSIONALISM AND INTERPERSONAL SKILLS

The phlebotomist (person trained in blood collection) is essential to the health care team and provides the link between the patient and laboratory. Good interpersonal skills are necessary; the phlebotomist's professional attitude, neat appearance, and consideration and concern for the patient play an important role in determining how the patient perceives the laboratory and the quality of health care. Such skills also help to alleviate patient apprehension. The phlebotomist must ensure patient confidentiality. Laboratory results and personal information about a patient should not be discussed unless the information is directly relevant to the patient's care and even then should not be discussed in public places.

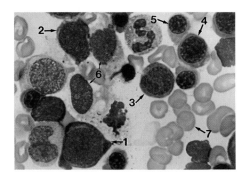

PLATE 1. Bone marrow erythrocyte precursors surrounding two histiocytes. (1) Rubriblast. (2, 3) Prorubricytes. (4) Early rubricyte. (5) Early metarubricyte. (6) Two histiocytes. (7) Mature erythrocyte (background). Erythroid precursors often are in contact with iron-containing histiocytes.

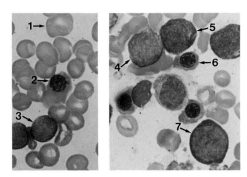

PLATE 2. Contrasting morphology between bone marrow erythrocyte precursors, lymphocytes, and a myeloblast. (1) Reticulocyte (polychromatophilic erythrocyte). (2) Metarubricyte. (3) Lymphocyte. (4) Myeloblast. (5) Prorubricyte. (6) Metarubricyte. (7) Rubriblast.

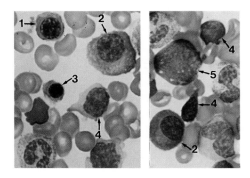

PLATE 3. Contrasting morphology between bone marrow erythroid precursors, plasma cells, and lymphocytes. (1) Rubricyte. (2) Plasma cell. (3) Metarubricytes. (4) Lymphocytes. (5) Rubriblast. Note that the three lymphocytes display slightly different morphologic characteristics.

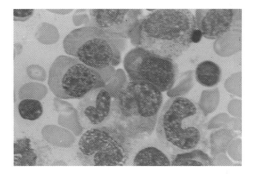

PLATE 4. Bone marrow (Wright stain × 1000) from a patient with pernicious anemia displaying a giant band (lower right), a giant metamyelocyte (left of band), a smaller metamyelocyte (left to giant metamyelocyte), and two orthochromic megaloblasts (directly above smaller metamyelocyte). The megaloblasts display nuclear–cytoplasmic asynchrony. The abundant cytoplasm is almost pink, which normally would be found with a fairly pyknotic nucleus, but these nuclei have a fine "particulate" chromatin structure. Above the large metamyelocyte is a myeloblast and above that, three myelocytes. Macroovalocytes are evident when comparing erythrocyte size to the lymphocyte at the right.

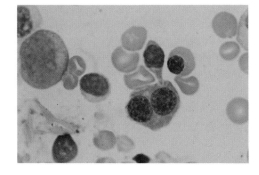

PLATE 5. Bone marrow (Wright stain) from patient with refractory anemia with excess blasts (RAEB), a myelodysplastic disorder. The two normoblasts (one cell in the orthochromic stage—a lymphocyte is to its left; and the other an abnormal binucleated cell in the polychromatophilic normoblast stage) show the typical megaloblastoid morphology with the coarser clumping of the nuclear chromatin. Macrocytic erythrocytes are obvious when their size is compared to the two lymphocytes present.

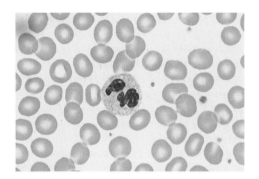

PLATE 6. A segmented neutrophil.

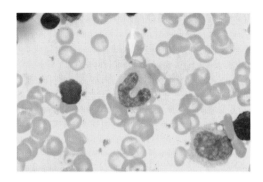

PLATE 7. Neutrophil band.

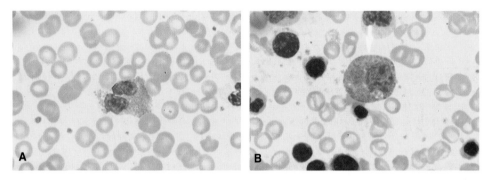

PLATE 8. Eosinophils. **(A)** a mature eosinophil in peripheral blood; **(B)** an eosinophilic myelocyte found in normal bone marrow.

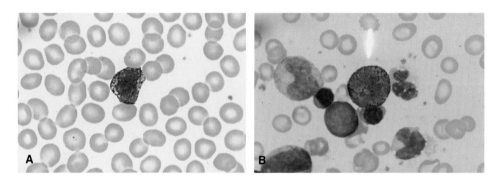

PLATE 9. Basophils. **(A)** a mature basophil found in peripheral blood; **(B)** an immature basophil found in normal bone marrow.

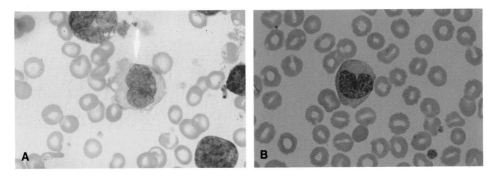

PLATE 10.   Monocytes. The monocytes in these two frames show how different Wright stains can affect the appearance of a cell. Both samples are of peripheral blood of healthy persons. **(A)** Wright stain at pH 6.4; **(B)** Wright stain at pH 6.8.

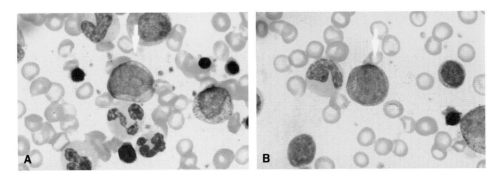

PLATE 11.   Myeloblasts. **(A)** agranular, type I, blast; **(B)** a blast with a few primary granules, a type II blast.

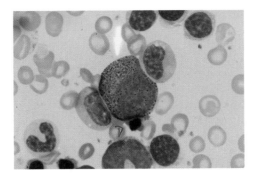

PLATE 12.   In this promyelocyte note the eccentric nucleus and the large number of primary (purple) granules in the cytoplasm.

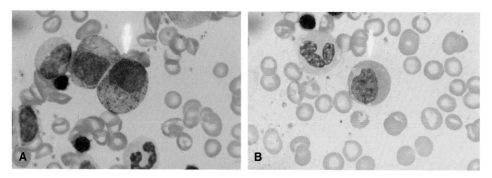

PLATE 13.   Neutrophilic myelocytes. **(A)** the *arrow* points to an early form; **(B)** a later form.

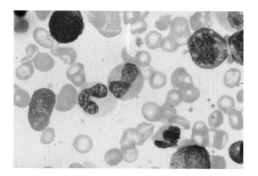

PLATE 14.   A neutrophilic metamyelocyte (arrow). The cell immediately adjacent to it is a neutrophilic band form.

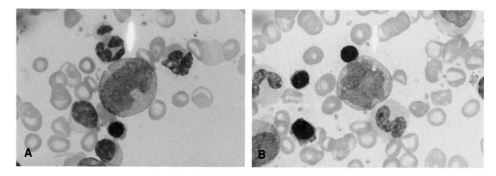

PLATE 15 **(A, B).**   Two examples of promonocytes found in nonneoplastic marrow.

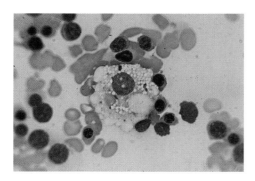

PLATE 16. In this macrophage note the small, eccentric nucleus, abundant foamy cytoplasm, and evidence of ingested cells (debris).

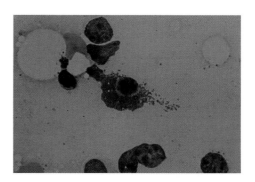

PLATE 17. A mast cell.

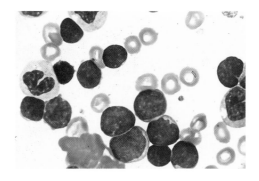

PLATE 18. Hematogones in bone marrow stained with Wright-Giemsa. Strikingly homogeneous nuclear chromatin without visible nucleoli and with extremely scant blue, agranular cytoplasm are observed. Nuclear cleavages appear in a few of the cells (courtesy Richard D. Brunning, MD).

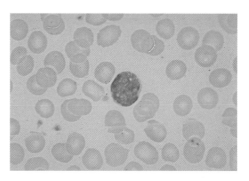

PLATE 19. Lymphoid cell from peripheral blood of premature infant is believed to represent a pre-B cell. Note scanty cytoplasm and homogeneous chromatin pattern.

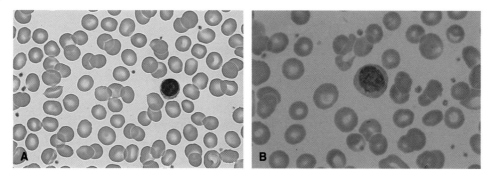

PLATE 20 (A, B). Two examples of normal small lymphocytes as demonstrated by different stains and magnifications. Note the sparse cytoplasm and the chromatin pattern.

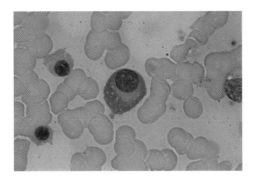

PLATE 21.   Normal bone marrow plasma cell and two rubricytes. The perinuclear chromophobic area in the cytoplasm is
striking in the deeply basophilic cytoplasm (courtesy Ann Bell,
MA).

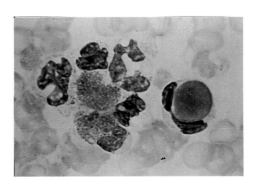

PLATE 22.   The lupus erythematosus cell. A neutrophil has
been attracted by an antinuclear antibody in the serum to engulf a
homogeneous mass. The homogeneous mass is an extruded cell
nucleus that has been transformed by the antinuclear antibody
through traumatization of the blood specimen.

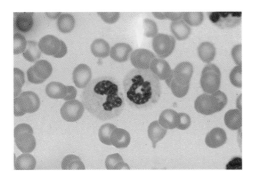

PLATE 23.   Döhle body. The neutrophil in the center of the
field (arrow) contains a Döhle body just inside the plasma membrane. The color of Döhle bodies varies from blue to gray, depending on the type of specimen.

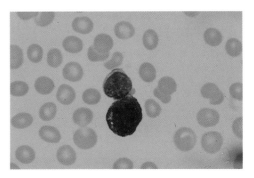

PLATE 24.   The smaller cell is a small normal lymphocyte.
The larger cell is a type I variant lymphocyte, also known as a
plasmacytoid lymphocyte or a Turk irritation cell. Note the extremely blue cytoplasm.

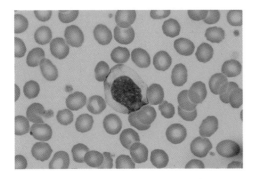

PLATE 25.   Type II variant lymphocyte. Note the abundant
clear cytoplasm with radiating basophilia, which gives it a flared-
skirt appearance. Also note the nuclear banding.

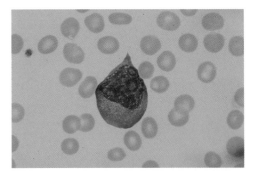

PLATE 26.   Type III variant lymphocyte. Note the immature-
looking nucleus with visible nucleoli. The cytoplasm is basophilic, indicating that this is probably a B-cell blast. Type III
variant lymphocytes also may have clear or pale cytoplasm.

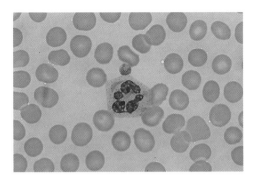

PLATE 27. Neutrophil from patient with May-Hegglin anomaly. Note large spindle-shaped basophilic inclusion in cytoplasm.

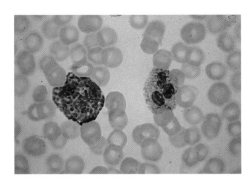

PLATE 28. Alder-Reilly syndrome. (Left) Neutrophil with large azurophilic granules. (Right) A basophil. (From American Society of Hematology Slide Bank, 1977, used with permission)

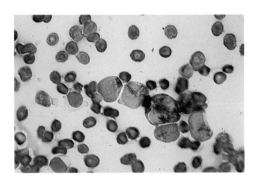

PLATE 29. Peroxidase stain. Note positive staining in blast forms. A lymphocyte in field is negative for peroxidase. Pseudoperoxidase is seen as dark brown staining in mature red cells.

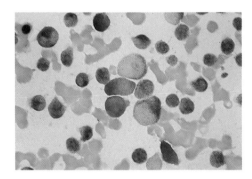

PLATE 30. Dual esterase stain. Blue reaction is chloroacetate esterase staining in neutrophils or their precursors. Red staining represents butyrate esterase within monocytes and their precursors.

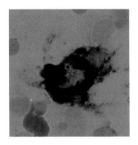

PLATE 31. Acid phosphatase in reticuloendothelial cell in normal bone marrow. Specimen has been treated with tartrate; hence, other cells are negative.

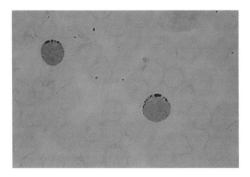

PLATE 32. PAS positivity in two lymphoblasts from patient wil L1 ALL. Note coarse, granular (chunky) appearance of reaction.

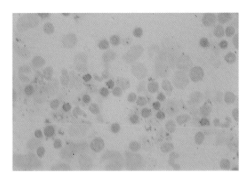

PLATE 33. Iron staining. Positive reaction is seen as green precipitate. This field contains ringed sideroblasts: green granules encircling red nucleus of red cell precursor.

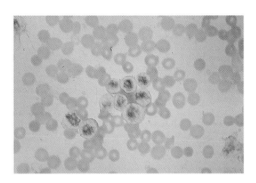

PLATE 34. Immunocytochemistry. Positive nuclear immunochemical staining with brown precipitate using TdT polyclonal antibovine reagent.

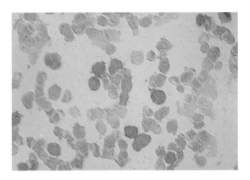

PLATE 35. Positive immunocytochemical staining with monoclonal anti-common ALL antigen (CALLA) in specimen from patient with suspected acute lymphocytic leukemia.

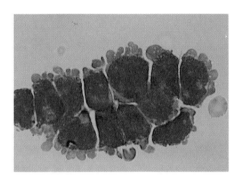

PLATE 36. Tumor cells in CSF. Note cytoplasmic tags on edges of cells. Slide made using cytocentrifuge (original magnification × 630; Wright stain).

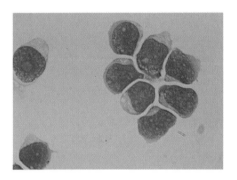

PLATE 37. Leukemic lymphoblasts in CSF. Slide made using cytocentrifuge (original magnification × 500; Wright stain).

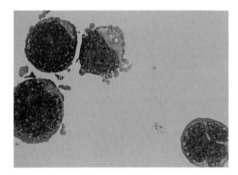

PLATE 38. Lymphoma cells in CSF. Slide made using cytocentrifuge (original magnification × 630; Wright stain).

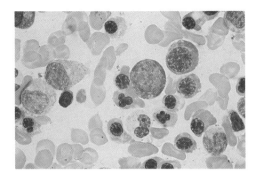

PLATE 39. Bone marrow from patient with refractory anemia. Note evidence of dyserythropoiesis, represented by multilobed nucleated red cells (Wright stain).

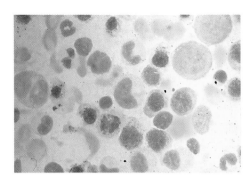

PLATE 40. Bone marrow from patient with refractory anemia with ringed sideroblasts (Prussian blue stain).

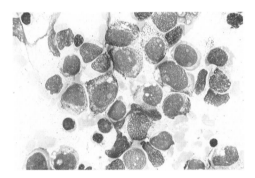

PLATE 41. Bone marrow from patient with refractory anemia with excess blasts in transformation. Note increased numbers of blast forms (Wright stain).

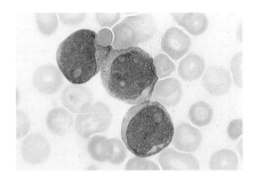

PLATE 42. M1 acute myelocytic leukemia without maturation. Blood film illustrates uniform population of type I blast cells. No cells with further granulocytic maturation are observed (original magnification × 500; Wright stain).

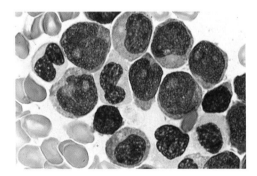

PLATE 43. M2 acute myelocytic leukemia with maturation. Bone marrow aspirate shows blasts and more differentiated granulocytic cells, including myelocytes, metamyelocyte, and neutrophil band cell (original magnification × 500; Wright stain).

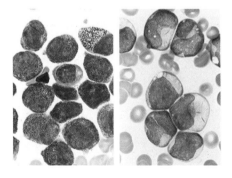

PLATE 44. M3 acute promyelocytic leukemia (A) Bone marrow of patient with hypergranular promyelocytic leukemia. Note heavy granulation, which fills cytoplasm of cells and sometimes obscures outline of nucleus. (B) Blood film of patient with microgranular variant of promyelocytic leukemia (M3m). Note that cells appear to be devoid of granules. Numerous Auer rods are present (original magnification × 500; Wright stain).

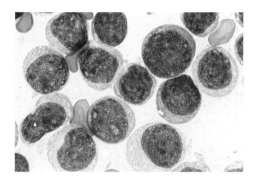

PLATE 45. M4 acute myelomonocytic leukemia. Bone marrow Romanowsky stained specimens such as this cannot differentiate adequately between abnormal granulocyte and monocyte precursors; esterase stains are necessary (original magnification × 500).

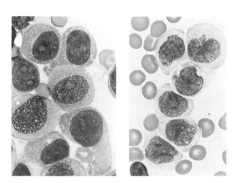

PLATE 46. M5 acute monocytic leukemia. (A) Bone marrow from patient with poorly differentiated monoblastic leukemia (M5a). (B) Peripheral blood from patient with differentiated monocytic leukemia (M5b) (original magnification × 500; Wright stain).

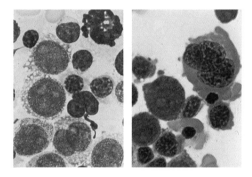

PLATE 47. M6 acute erythroleukemia. (A) Bone marrow field illustrating highly vacuolated red cell precursors seen in some cases. (B) This field is representative of bizarre, megaloblastoid red cell precursors characteristic of this leukemia (original magnification × 500; Wright stain).

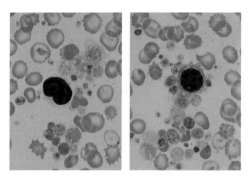

PLATE 48. M7 acute megakaryocytic leukemia. (A) Abnormal micro (dwarf) megakaryocyte. Note dense chromatin pattern. (B) Cytoplasmic blebbing (source of abnormal giant platelets) that is commonly seen (original magnification × 500; Wright stain).

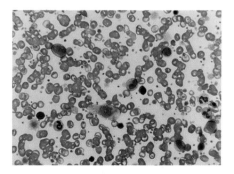

PLATE 49. Polycythemia vera in spent phase. Note micromegakaryoblasts, myeloblasts, nucleated red blood cells, and giant and bizarre platelets in this peripheral blood film (original magnification × 500).

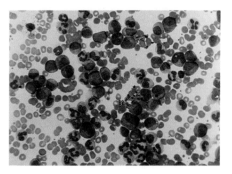

PLATE 50. Chronic myelogenous leukemia (CML). Note high leukocyte count and orderly left shift progression to blast in this peripheral blood film (original magnification × 500).

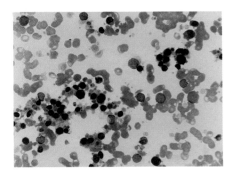

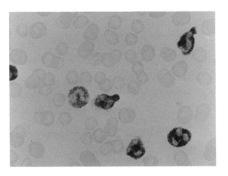

PLATE 51. Megakaryocytic leukemia. Blast transformation of patient with agnogenic myeloid metaplasia. Note multiple clumps of platelet producing micromegakaryocytes in this peripheral blood film (original magnification × 500).

PLATE 52. Chronic neutrophilic leukemia (CNL). Peripheral blood film stained for leukocyte alkaline phosphatase (LAP). Note markedly increased LAP in neutrophils (original magnification × 1000).

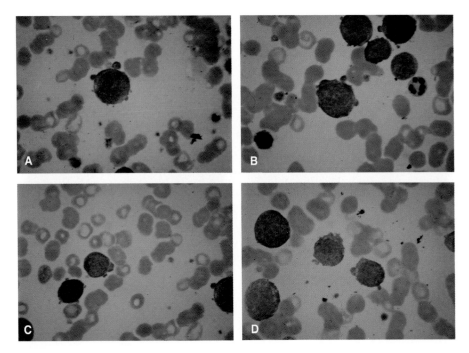

PLATE 53. Megakaryocytic blast transformation of CML. (A) Single micromegakaryocyte. (B) Three micromegakaryocytes, as evidenced by platelet blebs on cytoplasm. There also is a neutrophil; other two cells are blasts. (C) Two micromegakaryocytes and two giant platelets. (D) Two micromegakaryocytes, blast (upper left), and early promyelocyte (lower left) in this peripheral blood film (original magnification × 1000).

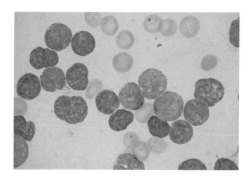

PLATE 54. L1 ALL. Homogeneous population of small cells with scanty cytoplasm (original magnification × 1000).

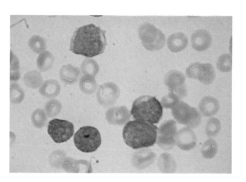

PLATE 55. L2 ALL. Heterogeneous population of large and small cells. Nucleoli are large; cytoplasm is moderately abundant (original magnification × 1000).

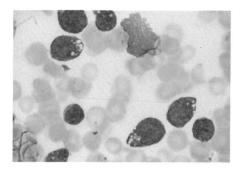

PLATE 56. L3 ALL. Primitive cells with abundant, very basophilic cytoplasm; highly vacuolated (original magnification × 1000).

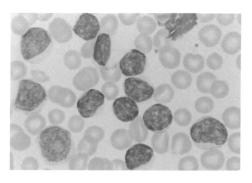

PLATE 57. Chronic lymphocytic leukemia. Note similarity of lymphocytes (monotonous picture). Also note smudge cell in upper part of field (original magnification × 1250).

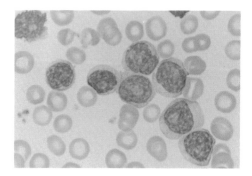

PLATE 58. Prolymphocytic leukemia. Note that nuclei of majority of lymphoid cells contain large vesicular nucleolus (original magnification × 1250).

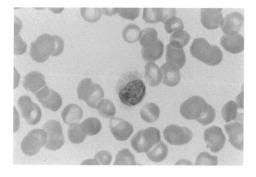

PLATE 59. Hairy cell leukemia. Presence of only one cell reflects fact that patient does not have increased leukocyte count. Note hairlike projections of cytoplasm (original magnification × 1250).

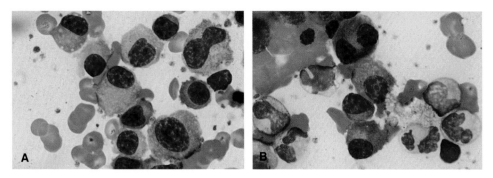

PLATE 60 **(A, B).** Bone marrow fields from two patients with multiple myeloma. Note marked difference in morphology of plasma cells in the two patients.

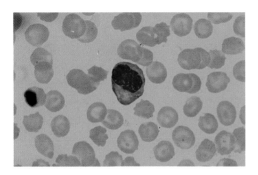

PLATE 61. Flame cell. Note pink areas in cytoplasm.

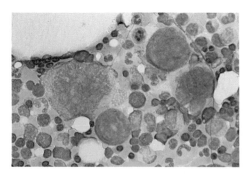

PLATE 62. Megakaryocytic maturation (bone marrow). Note large size of four megakaryocytic cells compared to other cells in the marrow. Two smaller cells are early forms, possibly megakaryoblasts; large intact cell on left is probably a promegakaryocyte; the large cell with multilobulated nucleus on right is probably a more mature form, but is too damaged to identify. Also refer to Plates 63 and 64. (From The American Society of Hematology Slide Bank, 2nd ed, 1977. Used with permission.)

MEGAKARYOBLAST*	PLASMA CELL*	TISSUE NEUTROPHIL (FERRATA CELL)*

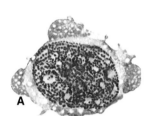

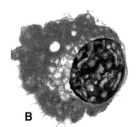

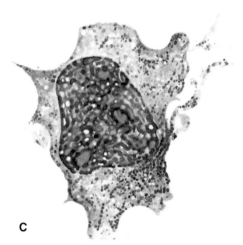

Single centrally-located nucleus with 1 or more nucleoli; nuclear chromatin strands distinct; marginal cytoplasmic extensions represent early platelet formation; N : C = 10 : 1; cytoplasm is blue and nongranular.

Single, round eccentric nucleus with nucleolus; cytoplasm is blue, "bubbly," and nongranular; cytoplasm is more abundant than megakaryoblast's; cytoplasm contains prominent light zone adjacent to the nucleus. Generally smaller than osteoblast.

Nuclear parachromatin more distinct than megakaryoblast's; nucleoli usually distinct; chromatin is more coarse and cytoplasm more abundant (N : C = 1 : 1) than megakaryoblast's; cytoplasm stains light blue; cytoplasmic granules vary in number and usually stain reddish-purple; cell is generally bizarre in shape with blunt cytoplasmic pseudopods.

OSTEOCLAST*	TUMOR CELLS	REED STERNBERG CELL

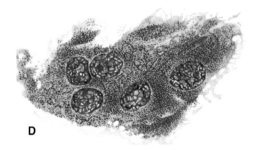

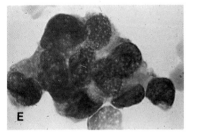

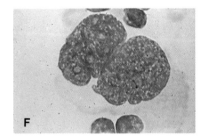

Very large cell; multinucleated; nuclei are separate and not visibly connected; number of nuclei may by uneven; cytoplasm has pink background with blue granules and frayed edges.

Nuclei have variable color and chromatin clumping; nucleoli common; cells are variable in size and shape; cytoplasmic borders may be difficult to distinguish; cells tend to clump; cytoplasm color is variable.

Nuclear lobes are often mirror images; nucleoli are more prominent than megakaryoblast's; cytoplasm color is variable

★ From: Diggs LW, Sturm D, Bell A: The Morphology of Human Blood Cells, 5th ed. Abbott Park, IL, Abbott Laboratories, 1985 with permission.

PROMEGAKARYOCYTE*	OSTEOBLAST*

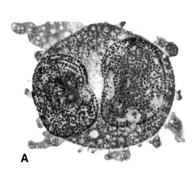

A

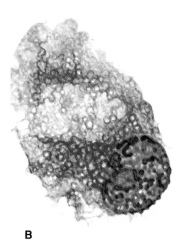

B

Double centrally-located nucleus; nuclei connected by strands or superimposed; cytoplasm is blue and scant but often has extensions that stain blue and have rounded contours with a homogeneous or bubbly appearance; bluish granules may appear near nucleus.

Single, round eccentric nucleus with nucleolus; cytoplasm is blue, "bubbly," and nongranular; cytoplasm contains prominent light zone separated from the nucleus. Generally larger than plasma cell.

MULTINUCLEATED RBC*	TUMOR CELL

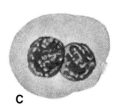

C

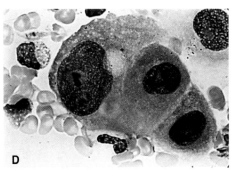

D

RBC cytoplasm polychromatophilic or pink and nongranular; nuclear chromatin clumpy; cell is smaller than pro- and meta-megakaryocyte.

Nuclei have variable color and chromatin clumping; nucleoli are common; cells are variable in size and shape; cytoplasmic borders may be difficult to distinguish; cells tend to clump; cytoplasm color is variable.

PLATE 64 A-H. (*continued*)

MULTINUCLEATED PLASMA CELL*

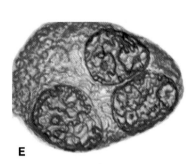

E

Foamy cytoplasm stains dark blue; nuclei may be double, or triple but never more.

OSTEOCLAST*

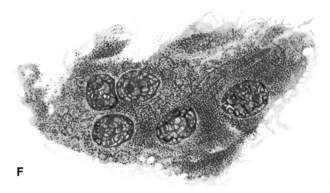

F

Very large cell; multinucleated; nuclei separate and not visibly connected; number of nuclei may be uneven; cytoplasm has pink background with blue granules and frayed edges.

MEGAKARYOCYTE*

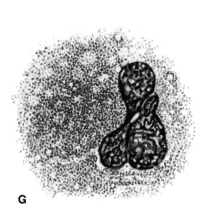

G

Very large cell with 2 or more nuclei; number of nuclei is always even; nuclei connected by strands or superimposed; cytoplasm reddish-blue with granules; very similar to metamegakaryocyte except that platelet budding is not yet detectable.

METAMEGAKARYOCYTE*

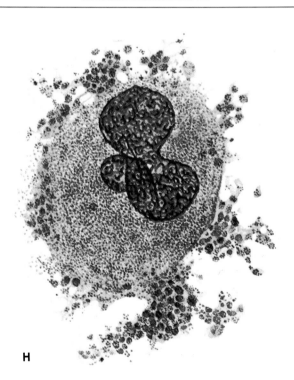

H

Very large cell with multiple (up to 32) nuclei; number of nuclei is always even; abundant granular cytoplasm (granules stain pinkish-red) with evident platelet budding.

---

* From: Diggs LW, Sturm D, Bell A: The Morphology of Human Blood Cells, 5th ed. Abbott Park, IL, Abbott Laboratories, 1985, with permission.

SPECIMEN COLLECTION BY VENIPUNCTURE

The most common technique used to obtain a blood specimen is venipuncture. Venipuncture requires skillful performance to ensure accurate laboratory values and preservation of patient vein integrity. Proper performance requires knowledge of the sequential steps listed in Table 2-1.

Initial Steps

Patient Identification

The first step in the reporting of accurate and reliable values is correct patient identification. Serious problems occur if results are reported for and subsequently documented on the wrong patient. In the hospital, the patient's name, identification number, and any additional information on the test requisition should initially be compared with, and found to be identical to, the information posted outside the patient's room or on the chart.

As the phlebotomist enters the room, he or she should greet the patient and identify himself or herself, explaining that it is necessary to collect a blood sample to aid in diagnosis and treatment.[21] The patient should be asked to state his or her full name and to spell any unusual name. The patient should never be asked a yes or no identity question such as, "Are you Mr. John Smith?" because an ill or semiconscious patient may mistakenly answer incorrectly. Finally, the requisition information should be compared with that found on the patient's wristband. If a patient is unconscious or does not have a wristband, ask the responsible nurse for positive identification. Age and sex should also be verified because hematology reference ranges are often age and sex dependent.

TABLE 2–1. Venipuncture Procedure

Patient Interaction
  Identify the patient
  Note patient isolation restrictions
  Note patient dietary restrictions
  Reassure patient
  Verify paperwork
  Position patient
Assemble Supplies and Equipment
Venipuncture
  Select general venipuncture location
  Apply the tourniquet
  Select exact venipuncture site
  Cleanse area
  Inspect needle
  Perform venipuncture
  Release tourniquet
  Position gauze over puncture site
  Remove needle and apply pressure
Specimen Preparation
  If syringe used, fill tubes
  Discard needle
  Label specimens
  Transport specimens promptly and properly

Adapted from National Committee for Clinical Laboratory Standards: Standard Procedures for the Collection of Diagnostic Blood Specimens by Venipuncture. Villanova, PA, NCCLS, 1977.

Note Isolation Restrictions

The phlebotomist should note any color-coded isolation sign on the patient's room door. Strict adherence to the posted precautions is required. Patients are placed in isolation either to prevent the spread of disease or to protect the patient from potential life-threatening infection by employees and visitors. Gowns, gloves, masks, and other supplies required for isolation procedures are located just outside the patient's room. After washing hands, appropriate protective clothing should be donned just before entering the room. Special clothing and accessories must also be discarded in or just outside the patient's room in appropriate receptacles for contaminated items.

Note Dietary Restrictions

If the ordered tests require patient fasting, make certain the patient has fasted for the required period of time. Failure to adhere to required dietary restrictions may cause inaccurate results. Fasting is not required for routine hematology procedures.

Reassure Patient

Procedures with needles induce stress and anxiety in many patients, and emotional stress can affect certain laboratory test values.[6] The phlebotomist therefore should do his or her best to relieve such apprehension. Communicate with the patient in a calm, professional, and reassuring manner. Gain the patient's confidence by soliciting his or her cooperation. Reassure the patient that although the puncture itself may be slightly painful, it will be over quickly. Never deceive the patient by saying the procedure will not hurt.

Position the Patient

The patient should be comfortable with his or her arm easily accessible and fully extended. Patients in bed should be instructed to lie on their backs, if possible. Attending personnel's assistance should be requested if patient movement is required. If additional support is needed, a pillow may be placed under the elbow of the arm from which the specimen is to be drawn. Ambulatory patients should be seated comfortably in a chair, preferably one with an interlocking armrest for firm support. The phlebotomist should position himself or herself in front of the chair to protect the patient from falling forward if fainting occurs. The arm should be extended downward below shoulder level, and the opposite fist should be placed under the elbow for support.

Patient position should be noted on the requisition because of the variation in blood count values depending on whether the patient is sitting up or lying down. For example, packed cell volume can decrease an average of 8% when a patient is lying down because of hemodilution.[18] Conversely, when a patient gets out of bed, hemoconcentration occurs. This same type of variation occurs with leukocyte counts.[17,22]

Assemble Supplies

Organization is important before initiating venipuncture. Select the appropriate supplies and equipment (Fig. 2-1) for each individual patient and place them in an easily accessible location. The following equipment should be

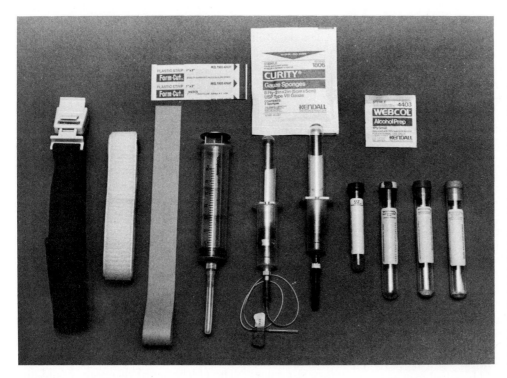

FIG. 2-1. Venipuncture supplies. (Bottom, left to right) Tourniquets—Seraket™, Velcro™, and rubber tubing; syringe with Luer-Lock needle; evacuated tube holder with Luer adapter connecting butterfly set; tube holder with evacuated tube and multisample needle; and other evacuated tubes. (Top) Adhesive bandage, gauze sponge, alcohol preparation pad. (From Lotspeich CA: Specimen collection and processing. In Bishop ML, Duben–Von Laufen JL, Fody ET (eds): Clinical Chemistry—Principles, Procedures, Correlations. Philadelphia, JB Lippincott, 1986, with permission. Photograph by J Bradley Perkins.)

available: collection devices—evacuated tubes and tube holder, syringes, and butterfly infusion sets; needles; tourniquet (or occasionally blood pressure cuff); alcohol pads; gauze pads; adhesive bandages or gauze bandage rolls; and protective gloves.

NEEDLES.   The most appropriate needle gauge and length depends on the size and depth of the patient's vein and the amount of blood to be drawn. Gauge number refers to the diameter, or bore, of the needle. The higher the gauge, the smaller the diameter. Routinely, 19-, 20-, and 21-gauge needles are used; the 20-gauge needle is most common. A 21-gauge needle is recommended for small, difficult veins to decrease the vacuum pressure and the likelihood of vein collapse. However, use of a smaller needle (higher gauge) has been reported as a cause of hemolysis in venipuncture,[15] and hemolyzed specimens are unacceptable for hematology and most other laboratory tests.

The needle length chosen is an individual preference. The most commonly used lengths are 1 and 1.5 inches. For the evacuated system, needles are available for single and multisample collection. When using the evacuated system, the multisample needle should be used if more than one tube of blood is to be collected in order to prevent leakage during tube changes. Single-sample needles manufactured specifically for syringes are generally used with the syringe method. Use of the appropriate needle is important.

EVACUATED TUBES.   Several sizes of tubes are available that may or may not contain an anticoagulant. The appropriate collection tube depends on the test ordered. When blood is removed from the body, coagulation or clotting normally takes place, allowing separation and collection of serum and cells. However, some laboratory tests, including those performed in hematology, require whole blood or plasma specimens, in which case an anticoagulant must be mixed immediately with the blood to prevent coagulation. The disodium or tripotassium salt of EDTA is the anticoagulant of choice for complete blood counts. In addition, other types of additives may be present either to preserve a specific blood constituent or to aid in the separation of serum from cells. The specific additive in the tube is indicated by the color of the rubber stopper (Table 2-2).

Evacuated tubes are marked with an expiration date. Tubes used past this date may have lost their vacuum or have an ineffective additive.[12] Vacuum tubes containing anticoagulant have the appropriate amount for the volume of blood drawn; thus, each tube must be filled to ensure a correct blood-to-anticoagulant ratio. Too much anticoagulant may cause significant changes in cell size and morphology. Too little anticoagulant results in clots, which artifactually decrease red and white cell and platelet counts, to say nothing of the nuisance they cause in automated blood analyzers.

Evacuated tubes for special procedures are also available (e.g., special tubes for Westergren sedimentation rate determination) (Chap. 9).

In most laboratories, 5- or 7-mL evacuated tubes are used for adult specimen collection. However, tubes of the size

TABLE 2–2. Evacuated Tubes Routinely Used in Blood Collection

STOPPER COLOR	ADDITIVE
Red	None
Red and gray	Inert polymer barrier material; no anticoagulant
Lavender	EDTA★ (K_3 or Na_2)
Blue	Citrate
Green	Heparin
Gray	Sodium fluoride

★ Ethylenediaminetetraacetic acid

used in pediatrics (2–3 mL) contain enough blood or serum to meet most requirements for testing and would reduce the amount of blood drawn from adults by 40% to 45%.[16] To reduce patient blood loss from phlebotomy, the use of smaller tubes should seriously be considered when the laboratory's analyzer is capable of analyzing small quantities.

Table 2-3 lists some of the tubes available for hematology specimens. Note that a final EDTA concentration of 1.5 mg/mL is recommended for complete anticoagulation without cellular damage or alteration. However, as noted in Table 2-3, there may be tubes on the market with a lower, unacceptable, EDTA concentration.

TOURNIQUETS.   Several forms of tourniquets are available. The most commonly used is a pliable piece of rubber tubing. Velcro, Seraket, and blood pressure cuffs are additional types. The Seraket is made of cloth, and is secured using a seatbeltlike apparatus, which is advantageous because the phlebotomist can partially release venous pressure, thus preventing hemoconcentration, without removing the tourniquet from the patient's arm. The tourniquet may easily be retightened if necessary.

Verify the Paperwork
When supplies are ready all paperwork should be reverified. Many laboratories use computer systems that assign accession numbers to each patient requisition. Accession numbers on the preprinted specimen labels and test requisitions must be identical.

Select General Venipuncture Location
Veins in the arm are the most commonly used for adult venipuncture. The three major veins of the arm are the median cubital, the cephalic, and the median basilic (Fig. 2-2). Generally, the median cubital is chosen for venipuncture because it is large, close to the skin surface, and usually well anchored by tissue so that it does not roll (move away) when punctured. The cephalic and median basilic veins may be used; however, these veins tend to bruise and roll more easily.

The inner aspect of the elbow is the best site for venipuncture. If this is not possible, alternate sites include the ventral forearm, wrist area, back of the hand, ankle, or foot. If the ankle or foot must be used, a nurse or physician should be consulted because these sites cannot be used in patients with certain clinical conditions[15] (*e.g.*, circulatory

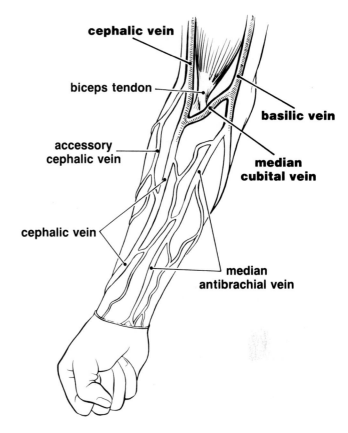

FIG. 2-2.   The veins of the arm.

problems in the lower extremity, diabetes in poor control, or hemoglobinopathies).

In selecting the site several factors should be considered. Avoid areas with hematomas, burns, scars, or edema (swelling). Avoid collection from the side on which a mastectomy was performed. If a patient is receiving an intravenous (IV) infusion, specimens should be drawn from the opposite arm. Certain situations may preclude collection from the opposite arm, or IV infusion may be running in both arms. Under these circumstances, blood should be drawn below the IV site from a vein other than the one with the IV line after the IV fluids have been stopped for 2 minutes.[15] A small amount of blood should be discarded before specimen collection; otherwise the specimen becomes diluted with IV fluid. The exact amount of blood to

TABLE 2-3. EDTA Vacuum Collection Tubes for Hematology Specimens*

TUBE			EDTA ANTICOAGULANT		
DRAW VOLUME	SIZE (MM)	FORM		MG/TUBE	FINAL CONCENTRATION (MG/ML)
2	10.25 × 47–50	K_3	(7.5% liquid)	3.0	1.5
3	10.25 × 64–65	K_3	(7.5% liquid)	3.75	1.25 (too low)
3.5	16 × 75	K_3	(15% liquid)	5.25	1.5
4	10.25 × 82	Na_2	(powder)	5.5	1.37 (too low)
7	13 × 100	K_3	(15% liquid)	10.5	1.5
10	16 × 100	K_3	(15% liquid)	15.0	1.5

* As marketed by Becton-Dickinson Vacutainer Systems, Rutherford, NJ 07070; Terumo Medical Corp., Elkton, MD 21921; or Jelco Laboratories, Raritan, NJ 08869. Other tubes are available that are not listed.

be discarded depends on the volume of the catheter lumen. A nurse or physician should always be asked to disconnect the IV line and restart it once the specimen has been collected. Recent evidence indicates that blood specimens acceptable for hematologic and serum biochemical profiles for all analytes except glucose and phosphorus may be drawn below the IV line during infusion or from the IV needle once the IV infusion has been stopped for 2 minutes. Again, a small amount of blood should first be discarded.[19] The phlebotomist should adhere to the procedure recommended by the individual laboratory.

Blood Collection Methods

Blood specimens for laboratory testing are collected by one of three methods: (1) evacuated tube system; (2) syringe; or (3) butterfly infusion set. The syringe method will simply be summarized; the other two methods will be discussed in some depth in the next section of this chapter.

Evacuated Tube System

The evacuated tube system is the most commonly used of the three systems.[15] The components of this system are a Vacutainer two-way needle, a plastic tube holder, and an evacuated glass tube (see Fig. 2-1). The tubes have been evacuated so that when the rubber stopper is pierced by the two-way needle, a predetermined amount of blood is drawn into the tube.

Vacuum tube equipment should be assembled before applying the tourniquet. The shorter end of the two-way needle screws securely into the plastic tube holder; the long end of the needle is sterile and should be kept covered until the phlebotomist is ready to enter the vein to avoid contamination. The vacuum tube is inserted into the plastic tube holder and pushed forward onto the needle to the level of the recessed guideline on the holder. This partially embeds the needle in the stopper but must not break the vacuum. Once the needle completely punctures the rubber stopper, the vacuum will draw blood into the tube.

Syringe Method

Although used less often, the syringe is the method of choice in some instances. The syringe consists of a barrel and plunger to which a needle is attached. The phlebotomist can control the vacuum by gently pulling back on the plunger while drawing blood. Small, fragile, or damaged veins require use of the syringe method because they may easily collapse under the vacuum pressure of evacuated tubes. Refer to a textbook of phlebotomy for further details on the syringe method.[13,15]

Butterfly Infusion Set

The butterfly set consists of a stainless steel beveled needle with attached plastic wings for the phlebotomist to grasp during the needle insertion (Fig. 2-3). A piece of plastic tubing connects the needle to an adapter that in turn is attached to a syringe or to a Luer adapter that screws into a tube holder, making a modified evacuated system. When a syringe is attached to a butterfly set, it is much easier to manipulate than in the conventional syringe method. For this reason the butterfly is commonly used for pediatric venipuncture, blood collection from patients with "difficult" veins, and special collections requiring more than one

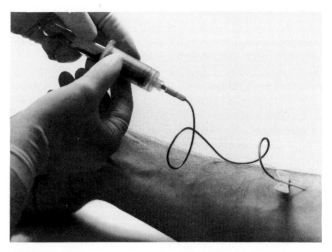

FIG. 2-3. Blood collection by modified evacuated system using a Luer adapter to attach the tube holder to butterfly set. (From Lotspeich CA: Specimen collection and processing. In Bishop ML, Duben–Engelkirk JL, Fody ET (eds): Clinical Chemistry—Principles, Procedures, Correlations, 2nd ed. Philadelphia, JB Lippincott, 1992, with permission. Photograph by J Bradley Perkins.)

syringe.[6,21] However, this equipment is more costly than that used for the routine evacuated tube system method.

Final Steps

The final steps of the venipuncture procedure are shown in Figure 2-4.

Apply the Tourniquet

The tourniquet should be securely wrapped around the unclothed arm about 7.5 to 10 cm (3–4 inches) above the selected site. The tourniquet will increase venous filling, making the veins prominent and easier to locate. Have the patient make a fist to aid in venous filling. Vigorous hand pumping will result in hemoconcentration and can cause erroneous test results. Although the phlebotomist should select the best vein carefully, the tourniquet should never be left on for longer than 2 minutes, because prolonged application may cause hemoconcentration.[14] This may lead to falsely increased red cell numbers and may activate certain blood components, causing inaccurate hemostasis results (Chap. 51).

Select Venipuncture Site

While the tourniquet is applied, and with protective gloves on, palpate the site using the tip of the index finger to find the best vein. Even if the vein is visible, palpate to determine the vein location and path. A vein should feel like an elastic tube, pliable and spongy. Thrombosed veins are not pliable and feel cordlike; they should not be punctured. Arteries may be detected by feeling a pulsating sensation and should not be punctured either. Once the vein has been chosen, decide on the best method of venipuncture: evacuated system or syringe method.

Cleanse the Site

The venipuncture site must be cleansed thoroughly with a commercial alcohol prep or a cotton ball or gauze pad soaked in 70% isopropanol. Cotton balls are recommended

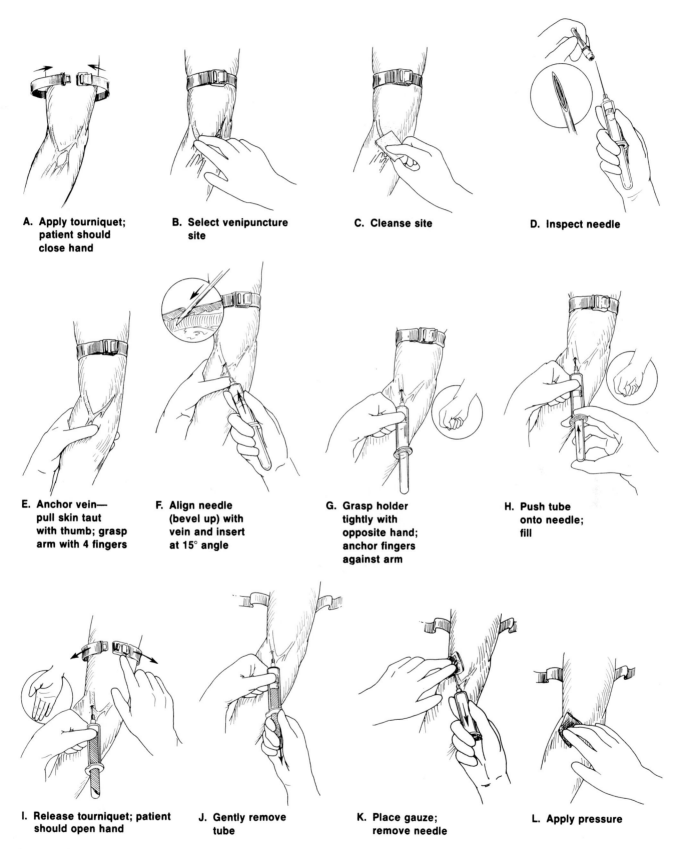

A. Apply tourniquet; patient should close hand

B. Select venipuncture site

C. Cleanse site

D. Inspect needle

E. Anchor vein— pull skin taut with thumb; grasp arm with 4 fingers

F. Align needle (bevel up) with vein and insert at 15° angle

G. Grasp holder tightly with opposite hand; anchor fingers against arm

H. Push tube onto needle; fill

I. Release tourniquet; patient should open hand

J. Gently remove tube

K. Place gauze; remove needle

L. Apply pressure

FIG. 2-4. Venipuncture procedure. (From Lotspeich CA: Specimen collection and processing. In Bishop ML, Duben–Engelkirk JL, Fody ET (eds): Clinical Chemistry—Principles, Procedures, Correlations, 2nd ed. Philadelphia, JB Lippincott, 1992, with permission.)

for patients with dermatitis, as gauze may irritate the skin. The site should be rubbed vigorously in a circular motion starting from the center moving outward. Allow the area to air dry or wipe off the alcohol with sterile gauze. Residual alcohol is painful to the patient at the puncture site and may cause hemolysis, invalidating certain test results, including those in hematology. If the cleansed area is touched, it must be cleansed again. Patients who are immunosuppressed (*e.g.*, transplant or chemotherapy patients) require a more thorough cleansing before venipuncture because alcohol does not sterilize the site.

Inspect the Needle

Remove the cover and examine the needle, especially the tip, to be certain there are no hooks or obstruction of the opening that would interfere with blood flow. If a syringe is used, inspect the needle in a similar manner and move the plunger back and forth to ensure free movement and to expel all air.

Perform Venipuncture—Evacuated System

Figure 2-4E through H illustrates the steps involved in venipuncture described here. Grasp the patient's arm firmly, placing the thumb 2 to 3 cm below the puncture site, and draw the skin taut. This anchors the vein and helps to prevent it from rolling. Hold the Vacutainer assembly in the opposite hand between the thumb, third, and fourth fingers. Place the index finger near base of needle to guide it as it enters the vein. Align the needle in the same direction as the vein, making sure the bevel of the needle faces up. Using one deliberate, smooth motion, insert the needle into the vein at approximately a 15° angle with the skin. Once the needle has entered the vein, carefully but firmly push the evacuated tube into the holder, being careful not to move the needle. The butt end of the needle should completely puncture the stopper, allowing blood to flow into the tube. Instruct the patient to open the fist. The tourniquet should also be loosened at this time. Allow the tube to fill until blood ceases to flow. Normally, the tube will not be completely full; an air space of 1 to 2 inches is common. Gently remove the tube from the holder. If multiple samples are to be drawn, immediately insert the next tube. Evacuated tubes containing anticoagulant should be mixed immediately by gentle inversion several times after removal from the needle. Do not mix vigorously because hemolysis may result.

When collecting multiple tubes it is important to do so in the correct order. One manufacturer recommends the following order: (1) sterile blood culture tubes; (2) nonadditive tubes; (3) coagulation tubes; and (4) other tubes with additive. Studies have suggested that the order of draw of multiple additive tubes is equally important because the additive in one tube may contaminate the specimen collected into the subsequent additive tube. The recommended order of draw for additive tubes is listed in Table 2-4.[5] Blood for coagulation testing (the citrate additive tube) should never be the first tube collected because tissue thromboplastin from the initial puncture may contaminate the specimen, invalidating the coagulation results (Chap. 51). Therefore, if only coagulation tests are ordered, first collect a small amount of blood in a nonadditive tube and discard that tube in biohazardous waste, then collect the citrate additive tube.

TABLE 2–4. Order of Draw for Specimen Collection into Additive-Containing Tubes

1. Citrate
2. Heparin
3. EDTA
4. Fluoride

Perform Venipuncture—Syringe Method

When using a syringe the same basic procedure should be followed. Refer to a phlebotomy textbook for procedural details.[13,15] Blood must be transferred from the syringe to appropriate evacuated tubes. The needle of the syringe is inserted through the tube stopper allowing the vacuum to draw blood slowly into the tube.[15] Blood must not be forced through the syringe needle—this can cause hemolysis. If nonevacuated tubes are used, the syringe needle and tube cap are removed and the blood is allowed to flow slowly down the side of the tube.

Release Tourniquet

The tourniquet should be released as blood begins to flow into the first tube or once the tube has filled, but always before removal of the needle. Prolonged tourniquet application causes hemoconcentration and erroneous test results.

Remove Needle and Apply Pressure

After the tourniquet is released and the required amount of blood drawn, a dry gauze or cotton ball is placed over the needle without applying pressure. Gently but quickly withdraw the needle and immediately apply pressure on the wound for several minutes until bleeding has stopped. Failure to apply pressure results in a hematoma (blood seeping into surrounding tissues). The patient's arm should be kept straight and fully extended and may be elevated above the heart. Do not bend the patient's arm at the elbow, as this reopens the wound and may result in hemorrhage into surrounding tissues. Before leaving the patient, be certain the bleeding has stopped. Application of an adhesive or gauze bandage over the wound may be necessary. If bleeding does not cease, attending personnel must be notified.

Discard Needle

Immediately after venipuncture, dispose of the needle properly in a container specifically made for this purpose. Do not discard needles into wastebaskets. In some institutions needles are clipped in two using a needle cutter box to prevent reuse, although there is some evidence that this procedure can create a blood aerosol. Never use a needle more than once—not even to perform a second venipuncture on the same patient. A sterile needle is required for every venipuncture.

Label Specimens

Tubes should *not* be labeled prior to blood collection. If for some reason blood was not obtained from the patient, the tubes may mistakenly be used for another patient. Label each specimen before leaving the patient with the patient's name, hospital number, date, time collected, the phlebotomist's initials, and any other information required by the institution.

Any unusual circumstances during the venipuncture should be noted on the requisition, such as excessive tourniquet time, crying (which can also alter blood counts), difficulty in venipuncture because of an obese arm, or repeated venipunctures. Also the puncture site should be noted, whether the antecubital fossa, indwelling line, or hand vein.

Discard gloves, wash hands, and thank the patient immediately before leaving the room. Check to ensure that all supplies and equipment brought in are removed.

Transport Specimens Promptly and Properly

Proper handling and timely transport of specimens to the laboratory are important for maintaining specimen integrity and the quality of test results. Some tests require the specimen to be placed on ice during transport; examples include those for acetone and CO_2.[15] Coagulation specimens were transported on ice in the past; however, this is no longer believed to be necessary.

Special Considerations

Pediatric Venipuncture

Although skin-puncture collection techniques may be preferred for infants and young children, venipuncture is essential for certain tests, such as blood cultures, most coagulation studies, and when there are combined test requisitions requiring more blood than is available from skin puncture.

Veins utilized in venipuncture should be superficial. Recommended sites include the antecubital veins and those on the back of the wrist. Avoid using veins needed for IV infusions. Ask attending personnel to hold and comfort the child while firmly securing the arm in an extended position. The National Committee for Clinical Laboratory Standards[11] recommends using either a 3-mL or a tuberculin syringe with a 21- or 23-gauge needle. A 23-gauge butterfly set is also suitable. Before leaving the infant, be sure the bleeding has stopped. Adhesive bandages are not recommended because the neonate's skin is often sensitive to adhesive and because of the potential hazard of the infant placing the bandage in the mouth and choking.

Extensive phlebotomy for diagnostic testing in neonates is a well documented cause of anemia and may even result in the need for blood transfusions.[16] For this reason special consideration must be given to the blood volume withdrawn. Documentation of each blood withdrawal, including the amount, date, and time, is usually recorded on the neonate's chart to help monitor blood loss from phlebotomy.

Infectious Disease Precautions

Most laboratories have specific policies regarding the collection, labeling, and processing of specimens from suspected or known cases of hepatitis, AIDS, or other infectious diseases. All laboratory personnel should be familiar with these policies and adhere to them strictly. It is recommended that gloves be worn for *all* phlebotomy procedures, regardless of the clinical diagnosis. In some cases, gowning may also be required. Wash the hands thoroughly before entering the room, when leaving the room, and any time they become contaminated with blood. Take only

needed equipment into the room, and be sure to dispose of all equipment in appropriate receptacles before leaving the room. It is important that all persons coming in contact with the blood specimen be aware of its special precautions; therefore, all blood specimens must be properly labeled. Place the blood specimens in a self-sealing polyethylene bag for transport, taking care not to contaminate the outside of the bag. Articles soiled with blood should be placed in a biohazard-labeled bag. These items must be autoclaved, as with all blood products, and then disposed of in the usual manner.[6,20]

Adverse Patient Reactions

Occasionally a patient becomes dizzy, faint, or nauseated during the venipuncture. The phlebotomist must be constantly aware of the patient's condition. If a patient feels faint, immediately remove the tourniquet and terminate the procedure. If the patient is sitting, lower the head between the legs and instruct him or her to breathe deeply. A cool wet towel may be applied to the forehead and back of the neck, and if necessary, ammonia inhalant may be applied briefly. If a patient remains unconscious, a physician should be notified immediately.

Sources of Error

There are many potential sources of error in venipuncture. Table 2-5 lists some of the more common errors.

SPECIMEN COLLECTION BY SKIN PUNCTURE

Indications

Venous blood is preferred to skin puncture specimens for most hematologic tests. However, there are several situations where skin puncture should be used to obtain the

---

TABLE 2–5. Sources of Error in Venipuncture

Errors in Venipuncture Preparation
  Improper patient identification
  Failure to check patient adherence to dietary restrictions
  Failure to calm patient prior to blood collection
  Use of improper equipment and supplies
  Inappropriate method of blood collection
Errors in Venipuncture Procedure
  Failure to dry the site completely after cleansing with alcohol
  Inserting needle bevel side down
  Use of needle that is too small, causing hemolysis of specimen
  Venipuncture in an unacceptable area (*e.g.,* above an IV line)
  Prolonged tourniquet application
  Wrong order of tube draw
  Failure to mix blood collected in additive-containing tubes
    immediately
  Pulling back on syringe plunger too forcefully
  Failure to release tourniquet prior to needle withdrawal
Errors after Venipuncture Completion
  Failure to apply pressure immediately to venipuncture site
  Vigorous shaking of anticoagulated blood specimens
  Forcing blood through a syringe needle into tube
  Mislabeling of tubes
  Failure to label appropriate specimens with infectious disease
    precaution
  Failure to put date, time, and initials on requisition
  Slow transport of specimens to laboratory

blood specimen. Infants, particularly newborns, have a much smaller total blood volume than adults; drawing blood by routine venipuncture on a daily basis can quickly result in hospital-induced anemia. Skin puncture is also a much safer means of blood collection. Venipuncture is often difficult and even dangerous when performed on very small children and infants.[2,7,9] For adults skin puncture may be required because of obesity, burns, or extremely small or severely damaged veins or when IV fluid is flowing into the only accessible veins. Skin puncture is also used to save the veins of patients receiving chemotherapy and in the elderly when possible.

Blood collected by skin puncture is a mixture of capillary, venous, and arterial blood and also contains interstitial and intracellular fluids. Therefore, the laboratory values obtained may be different from those obtained on venous specimens.[7] For example, the erythrocyte count, hematocrit, hemoglobin, and platelet count are lower in skin puncture blood than in venous blood.[4] Therefore, "skin puncture" should be noted on the test requisition.

The technique involves many of the same steps as for venipuncture. Refer to a textbook of phlebotomy for the exact procedure.[13,15]

Sources of Error

Hemolyzed specimens are a common source of error, especially in blood specimens obtained from skin puncture of newborns and infants.[10] Infants' erythrocytes are more fragile than those of adults, and their hematocrits are much higher; therefore, the risk of hemolysis is somewhat greater.[8] Other important sources of error include failure to dry the site completely after cleansing with alcohol, excessively deep skin puncture, failure to wipe away the first drop of blood, vigorous massaging or milking of area causing hemolysis, and accidental capturing of air bubbles in capillary tubes or Unopette pipets used for collection of exact specimen amounts.

SPECIAL HEMATOLOGY COLLECTION PROCEDURE—DEFIBRINATION

Certain special hematology tests, such as osmotic fragility, autohemolysis, and the acid serum test, require a defibrinated specimen. Defibrination involves the removal of fibrin from a whole blood specimen. The phlebotomist must prepare the defibrinated specimen at the patient's bedside before the blood is allowed to clot. Immediately after venipuncture, the whole blood is added to an Erlenmeyer flask containing glass beads or paper clips. After gauze or cotton is placed in the top of the flask to prevent specimen contamination, the flask is rotated for about 10 minutes until the beads (or clips) are covered with fibrin and no longer make a rattling noise. For some tests a sterile flask and beads are required.

ANTICOAGULANTS

Once blood leaves the body, a series of reactions involving platelets and plasma coagulation factors causes blood to clot within minutes. Most hematology tests are performed on whole blood. Therefore, as soon as blood is withdrawn, it must be mixed with an anticoagulant, a compound that irreversibly interrupts the coagulation process. Although several anticoagulants are available, the most commonly used for hematologic procedures are EDTA, citrate, and heparin. The choice of a particular anticoagulant depends on the test procedure. An appropriate concentration of the anticoagulant for the volume of blood drawn is critical; significant errors may result with an inappropriate anticoagulant concentration.

EDTA

The disodium or tripotassium salt of ethylenediaminetetraacetic acid (EDTA) is the most commonly used anticoagulant in hematology. Blood coagulation is inhibited by chelating or binding of calcium ions. The optimal anticoagulant concentration is 1.5 mg/mL of blood (see Table 2-3). This quantity has no adverse effects on routine cell counts and preserves cellular morphology when the blood smears are made within 2 hours of blood collection. However, excessive EDTA induces red cell shrinkage, causing the hematocrit value and erythrocyte sedimentation rate to be falsely decreased. EDTA prevents platelet aggregation and is therefore the preferred anticoagulant for platelet counts.

Citrate

Citrate inhibits blood clotting by binding calcium in a soluble complex and is used for many coagulation studies. Refer to Chapter 51 for information on the collection of coagulation specimens.

Heparin

Heparin is an acid mucopolysaccharide that inhibits coagulation by the inactivation of thrombin; the optimal concentration is 15 to 20 U/mL of blood. Heparin is the anticoagulant of choice for the osmotic fragility test if defibrinated blood is not used; other anticoagulants may alter the pH of the blood–saline mixture in the test procedure.[4] Heparin is not satisfactory for specimens to be used in blood film preparation because it causes morphologic distortion of platelets and leukocytes. It also causes a bluish coloration of the background on blood films stained with a Romanowsky stain because of its pH.[23] Heparinized blood should never be used for coagulation studies because of heparin's inhibitory effect on thrombin. Heparin may also cause errors in automated cell counting.

CHAPTER SUMMARY

As members of the health care team, phlebotomists must recognize that their primary responsibility is to the patient's health and well-being. It is important for the phlebotomist to maintain a professional attitude and neat appearance. Good interpersonal skills help establish patient trust and alleviate apprehension.

Specimen collection by venipuncture or skin puncture involves a series of steps that must receive careful consideration to ensure the best possible specimen for laboratory analysis. It is the responsibility of the phlebotomist to have a thorough understanding of and to abide by these guidelines to avoid the many potential sources of error.

EDTA is the most commonly used anticoagulant for hematology test specimens. It inhibits blood coagulation by binding calcium, thus preventing activation of the clotting mechanism and preserving the specimen in its fluid state for blood cell analysis.

REFERENCES

1. Becton Dickinson: Product Catalog: Becton Dickinson VACU-TAINER Systems. Rutherford, NJ, Becton Dickinson, 1981
2. Blumenfeld TA: Infant blood collection and chemical analysis. Diagn Med 1:58, 1978
3. Blumenfeld TA, Turi GK, Blanc WA: Recommended site and depth of newborn heel skin punctures based on anatomical measurements and histopathology. Lancet 1:230, 1979
4. Brown BA: Hematology: Principles and Procedures, 4th ed. Philadelphia, Lea & Febiger, 1984
5. Calam RR, Cooper MH: Recommended "order of draw" for collecting blood specimens into additive-containing tubes. Clin Chem 28:1399, 1982
6. Garza D, Becan–McBride K: Phlebotomy Handbook. Norwalk, Appleton-Century-Crofts, 1984
7. Hammond KB: Blood specimen collection from infants by skin puncture. Lab Med 11:9, 1980
8. Koepke JA: Specimen collection—cellular hematology. In Koepke JA (ed): Laboratory Hematology, vol 1, p 821. New York, Churchill Livingstone, 1984
9. Meites S, Levitt MJ: Skin-puncture and blood-collecting techniques for infants. Clin Chem 25:183 1979
10. Meites S, Lin SS, Thompson C: Studies on the quality of specimens obtained by skin puncture of children 1. Tendency to hemolysis, and hemoglobin and tissue fluid as contaminants. Clin Chem 27:875, 1981
11. National Committee for Clinical Laboratory Standards: Standard Procedures for the Collection of Diagnostic Blood Specimens by Venipuncture. Villanova, PA, NCCLS, 1977
12. National Committee for Clinical Laboratory Standards: Standard for Evacuated Tubes for Blood Specimen Collection, 2nd ed. Villanova, PA, NCCLS, 1980
13. Pendergraph GE: Handbook of Phlebotomy. Philadelphia, Lea & Febiger, 1984
14. Slockbower JM: Venipuncture procedures. Lab Med 10:74, 1979
15. Slockbower JM, Blumenfeld TA: Collection and Handling of Laboratory Specimens: A Practical Guide. Philadelphia, JB Lippincott, 1983
16. Smoller BR, Kruskall MS: Phlebotomy for diagnostic laboratory tests in adults: Pattern of use and effect on transfusion requirements. N Engl J Med 314:1233, 1986
17. Statland BE, Winkel P, Harris SC et al: Evaluation of biologic sources of variation of leukocyte counts and other hematologic quantities using very precise automated analyzers. Am J Clin Pathol 69:48, 1978
18. Tombridge TL: Effect of posture on hematology results. Am J Clin Pathol 49:491, 1968
19. Watson KR, O'Kell RT, Joyce JT: Data regarding blood drawing sites in patients receiving intravenous fluids. Am J Clin Pathol 79:119, 1983
20. Welsby PD: How to take blood from patients who have hepatitis. Br Med J 282:1052, 1981
21. Whitelaw A, Valman B: Taking blood and putting up a drip in young children. Br Med J 281:602, 1980
22. Winkel P, Statland PE, Saunders A et al: Within-day physiologic variation of the concentration of leukocyte types in healthy subjects as assayed by two automated leukocyte differential analyzers. Am J Clin Pathol 75:693, 1981
23. Wintrobe MM: Origin and development of the blood and blood-forming tissues. In Wintrobe MM (ed): Clinical Hematology, 8th ed, p 59. Philadelphia, Lea & Febiger, 1981

MANUAL BLOOD FILM PREPARATION

Coverslip Method

Innate difficulties in the spreading of a drop of blood between two glass coverslips have prevented the coverslip method from being popular for routine peripheral blood smears. However, the technique is utilized extensively for bone marrow preparations. The one significant advantage of the coverslip preparation is its superior leukocyte distribution. In other words a leukocyte differential count performed on a coverslip preparation is less likely to contain errors caused by poor distribution. The disadvantages are several. One is the difficulty in learning the technique. Second, to ensure an even distribution of blood, coverslips must be manually cleaned of dirt, dust, grease, and fingerprints just prior to use. Third, because of the difficulty in labeling, transporting, and staining the small and easily broken glass coverslips, they must be mounted on glass 3 × 1-inch slides for microscopic examination. The use of mounting media prevents immediate storage. Fourth, coverslip pairs must be kept matched for estimating platelet numbers because platelets may be unevenly distributed between the two coverslips. Finally, there is the lack of specific areas to examine for unusual cells.

Technique

1. Hold a clean No. 1.5 coverslip (22 × 22 mm) at two adjacent corners between the thumb and index finger of one hand (Fig. 3-1A).
2. Place a small drop of blood (approximately 2 mm in diameter) in the center of the top surface of the coverslip. Place another clean coverslip on top in a crisscross direction so that the two coverslips resemble an eight-pointed star (Fig. 3-1B and C). *Note:* If using finger stick (capil-

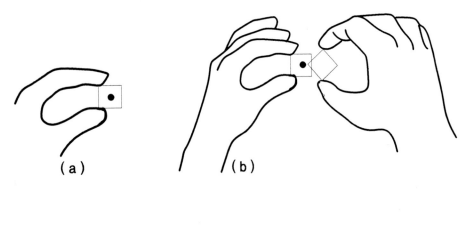

(a)   (b)

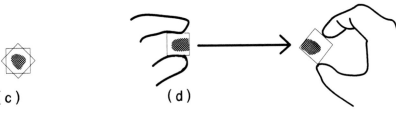

(c)   (d)

FIG. 3-1. Coverslip blood film preparation. (A) A drop of blood is placed on a clean 22-mm square coverslip. (B) A second coverslip is placed on top so that the two form (C) an eight-point star. (D) The two coverslips are pulled apart with a smooth, lateral, parallel sliding motion.

lary) blood, wipe away the first drop that emerges from the puncture and touch the undersurface of the coverslip to a fresh drop. Avoid touching the skin. Place this coverslip on top of another clean coverslip to form an eight-pointed star, as described above.
3. The drop of blood should begin to spread in all directions by capillary action. When its spread is almost complete, pull the two coverslips apart with a smooth, lateral, parallel sliding movement (Fig. 3-1D).
4. Keep coverslip pairs matched, and air dry them rapidly.
5. After staining, air dry and mount with the blood-film side down on a 1 × 3-inch glass slide. Label the slide.

A modification of the coverslip method is the substitution of two 1 × 3-inch glass slides for the coverslips. The top slide is placed directly over the slide containing a drop of blood in its center, with one end extending slightly (Fig. 3-2). The advantages of this modification are the larger examination area, the use of slides that are not as breakable as coverslips, and ease of labeling of the blood smears.

Troubleshooting
1. Assess the size of the drop of blood. Too large a drop may result in too thick a spread. Too small a drop may produce a thin spread or too small an examination area.
2. Timing and speed of separation of coverslips is important. Pulling the coverslips apart prematurely or too rapidly may create a thick or uneven spread. A delay in their separation may cause the coverslips to become stuck to each other, the platelets to clump, or the leukocytes to distribute unevenly.
3. Separation movement must be even. A jerky pulling movement or a variation in the horizontal level will cause uneven distribution of the cellular elements.
4. Assess the staining quality. The small surface area of coverslips makes it difficult to mix stain and buffer adequately, as well as to wash off the stain solution.

Wedge Type
Variations of the wedge technique are the most widely used for smear preparation. The smear may be termed a wedge, spreader-slide, or push smear.

Advantages
1. The technique is easier to master.
2. Commercially "precleaned" slides are generally ade-

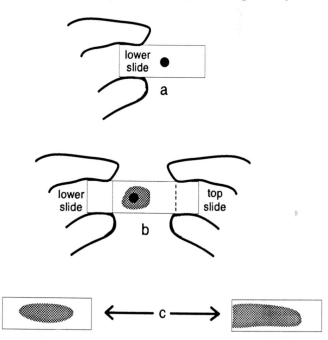

FIG. 3-2. Modification of the coverslip blood film technique using 3" x 1" slides. (A) A drop of blood is placed in the center of the lower slide. (B) The top slide is placed on the blood drop so that the ends of the two slides overlap slightly. (C) The two slides are pulled apart in a smooth, parallel motion.

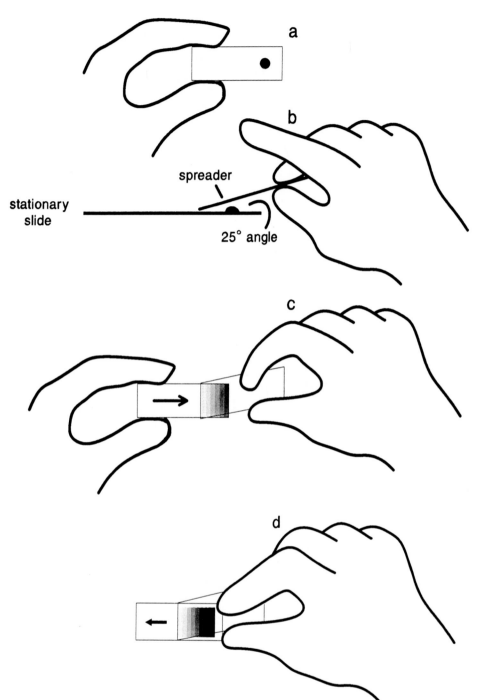

stationary
slide

spreader

25° angle

FIG. 3-3. Wedge type smear preparation. (A) A drop of blood is placed near one end of a clean 3" x 1" (stationary) glass slide. (B) A spreader slide is positioned at a 25° angle and backed into the blood drop. (C) The blood drop is allowed to spread along the edge of the spreader slide. (D) The spreader slide is pushed forward with a smooth rapid stroke.

quate. However, an occasional lot or batch may require further cleaning.
3. The slides are not easily broken.
4. Labeling, transporting, and staining are easier.
5. A coverslip is not necessary, and smears can be put in storage immediately.
6. The combination of above assets makes this the least expensive type of preparation.
7. The tendency of larger cells to settle at the slide edges and the feathered end makes it easier to find abnormal cells.

Disadvantages
1. There is an inherently poor distribution of nucleated cells. Neutrophils and monocytes have a greater ten-

dency to appear in the feathered end of the preparation rather than in the examination area, which may lead to artifactually increased lymphocyte counts when performing a leukocyte differential count.
2. There is greater trauma to the cells during the making of the blood film. This may lead to large numbers of "smudge" or "basket" cells, especially in lymphoproliferative disorders.

Technique
1. Place a clean 1 × 3-inch glass slide on a flat surface (stationary slide).
2. Transfer a drop of blood approximately 2 to 3 mm in diameter to the stationary slide about 0.25 inch from the

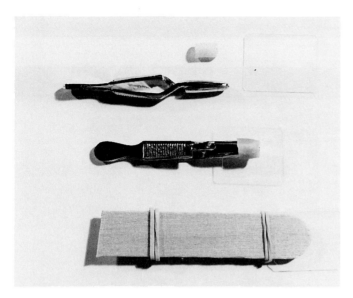

FIG. 3-4.   Use of hemocytometer coverslip as a spreader slide. The coverglass may be held by an artery clamp or between two applicator sticks.

end or frosted area on the same side as the writing hand (Fig. 3-3A). Anticoagulated blood should be well mixed before transfer.

3. Hold the end of the stationary slide that is without the drop of blood with the nonwriting hand (Fig. 3-3A).

4. Position a spreader slide at a 25° angle to the stationary slide and bring it back into the drop of blood (Fig. 3-3B and C).

5. Allow the blood drop to spread along the back edge of the spreader slide (Fig. 3-3C).

6. Immediately push the spreader slide forward with a smooth and rapid stroke, maintaining the same angle and exerting very little pressure. The blood will be pulled behind the spreader (Fig. 3-3D).

7. If the angle of the spreader slide is proper, the speed of the stroke is moderately fast, and the size of the drop of blood is as specified, the blood should feather into nothing somewhere between one-half and three-quarters of the way along the stationary slide.

8. Air dry the blood rapidly but thoroughly (several minutes) before staining. This can be done manually or with an electric fan or cool air blower.

9. Labeling with patient name, log number and date may be done on the frosted end of the slide or in the thicker end of the blood smear itself after it has dried.

The Spreader Slide

Certain properties of the spreader slide affect the distribution of the leukocytes and consequently the accuracy of the differential count.[8,17,28,44,49] This slide should be narrower than the glass slide on which the blood smear will be deposited (stationary slide). The spreading edge should be clean, smooth, polished, and thin, with no chips or scratches. A few companies manufacture beveled-edge microscope slides that meet these specifications.

An excellent spreader is a hemocytometer coverglass (20 × 26 × 0.4–0.6 mm) (Fig. 3-4). The 20-mm edge is the spreader edge. The coverglass may be held by a straight

artery clamp, one prong of which is enclosed in rubber tubing to prevent slipping.[48] A disadvantage of this type of spreader is the necessity to clean the edge of the spreader between patients.

Characteristics of a Proper Wedge Smear

The well prepared smear (Fig. 3-5) should have the following characteristics:

1. It should cover at least half the length of the glass slide. Smears to be stained in a platen-type automatic instrument (Ames Hema-Tek Stainer) should terminate at least 0.5 inch before the end of the slide.

2. It should be narrower than the slide on which it is made, so that the side edges may be examined with the microscope.

3. A smooth spread should be displayed with a gradual transition from thick to thin areas and with no waves, streaks, troughs, holes, or bubbles.

4. It should terminate in a straight feathered end (Fig. 3-6). Bullet-shaped preparations (see Fig. 3-6) tend to have higher accumulations of leukocytes along the side and tail edges of the smear than the straight-ended smear (Fig. 3-7). A bullet-shaped end results from spreading the blood before the drop has spread fully along the spreader slide.[49]

5. The smear should be thin enough to allow proper fixation during the staining procedure. Thick areas appear dark green or gray or are washed off during staining.

6. It should contain a least 10 low-power fields in which 50% of the erythrocytes do not overlap. The remainder may overlap slightly (a few doublets and triplets). Single erythrocytes should have a well preserved central pale area (see Fig. 3-5B).

Troubleshooting

1. Extremely thick smears are caused either by too large a drop of blood, by too fast a spread, or by too high an angle of the spreader slide (Figs. 3-5C and 3-8). In such preparations excess plasma causes nucleated cells to shrink and stain intensely, making identification difficult (see Fig. 3-5C). Red cells form more rouleaux in thick areas and cannot be evaluated.

2. Extremely thin smears (see Fig. 3-8) are caused by too small a drop of blood, too slow a spread, or too low an angle of the spreader slide. Smudge cells are increased, and red cells become artificially spheroid with a distorted shape (see Fig. 3-5A). There is a tendency for more nucleated cells to be carried out to the edges of smears that have been made with too slow a stroke, and this affects the accuracy of the differential count (see Fig. 3-7).

3. A gritty appearance of feathered or tail areas indicates an accumulation of nucleated cells, which may be attributable to a large number of leukocytes, to slow spreading or to a delay in spreading (Fig. 3-9). A related cause is using only a part of the drop of blood (Fig. 3-9B). A rough edge or dirty spreader may also produce a gritty or jagged end. With some anticoagulants, especially heparin, there is a tendency for leukocytes to accumulate at the tail end.

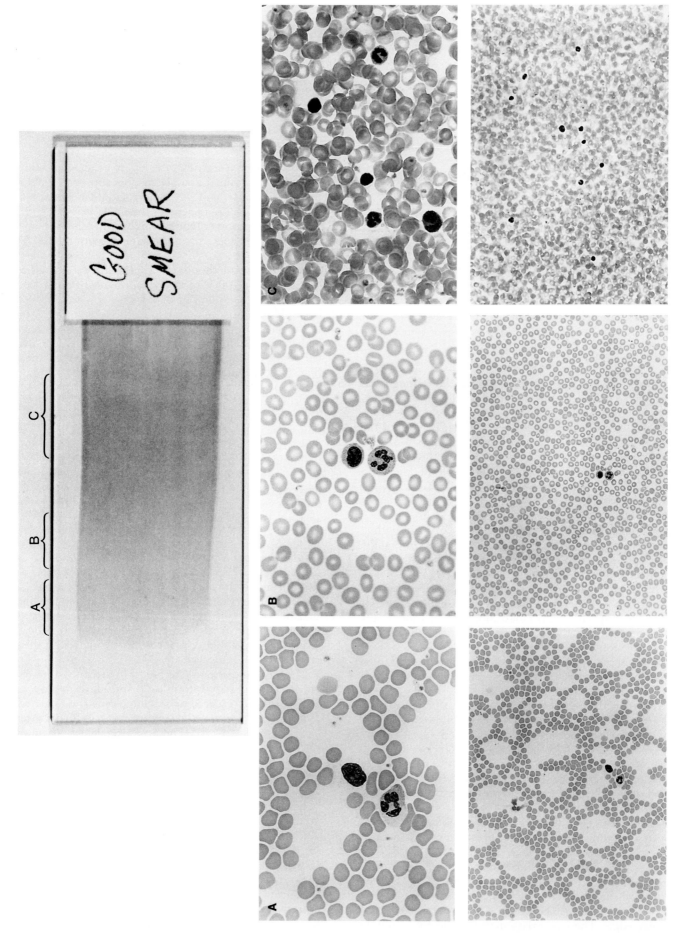

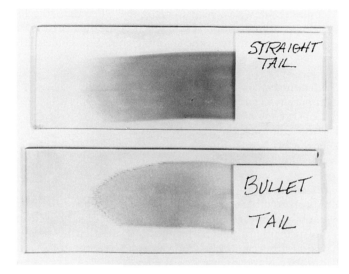

FIG. 3-6.   Straight *v* bullet feather edge or tail.

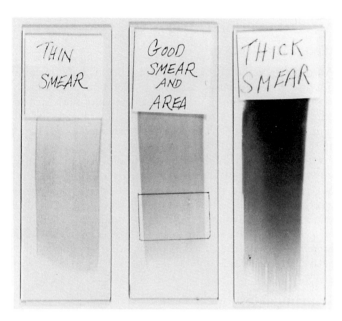

FIG. 3-8.   Excessively thin and thick smears compared with a "good" smear.

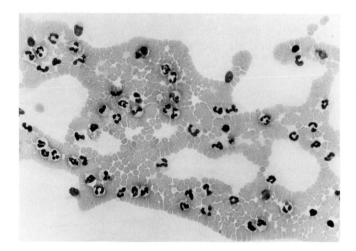

FIG. 3-7.   Accumulation of leukocytes in edges of blood film.

Because leukocytes may be poorly distributed with the wedge preparation, many hematology laboratories have instituted rules to govern procedures in certain instances. For example, if the leukocyte differential count reveals greater than 40% lymphocytes, the differential should be repeated on another slide. In another example if the numbers of monocytes, eosinophils, or basophils exceed the normal reference ranges, a second 100 cells are to be differentiated on the same slide. The most efficient check is a low-power inspection of the peripheral (side and feathered end) areas for a disproportionate number of neutrophils.

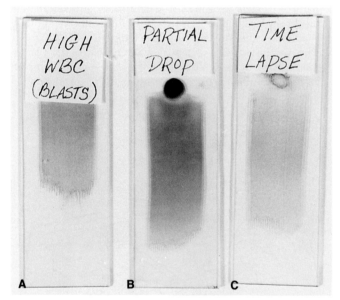

FIG. 3-9.   Causes of streaks in feathered edge. (A) Extremely high leukocyte count with blast forms. (B) Picking up only part of the blood drop. (C) Allowing too much time to elapse between placing blood on slide and spreading.

FIG. 3-5.   A good blood smear (see text for criteria). These areas of the blood smear are demarcated on low power (right row) and high power (left row). (A) Feather edge (tail)—blood film is too thin for examination. Note distribution of red cells and the fact that they have no central pallor. (B) Examination area. Note cell distribution, the fact that some red cell overlapping occurs, and central pallor of the red cells. (C) Body of smear—blood film is too thick for examination. Note that all red cells are overlapped and that leukocytes are smaller and appear thicker.

AUTOMATED BLOOD FILMS

Wedge (Push) Type

Automatic methods for smear preparations have become popular in recent years. Geometric Data Corporation developed the Miniprep,[14] a portable semiautomatic instrument that simulates the manual spreader-type technique (Fig. 3-10). It contains two spreader blades mounted at a set angle that are moved mechanically along the length of a 1 × 3 inch glass slide containing a drop of blood. The operator must place the slides in the machine, place a drop of blood on each slide, and press a lever to initiate the spreader's movement. The speed can be varied according to the hematocrit. The advantages and disadvantages of this automated wedge smear are the same as those of manual wedge preparation with the added advantage of more consistency between blood films.

Centrifugal (Spinner) Type

Automated instruments[6,14] can utilize centrifugation to spread a monolayer of whole blood on a 1 × 3 inch glass slide.

Technique

1. A clean 1 × 3 inch glass slide is placed on a horizontal platform within the instrument.
2. Approximately 0.2 mL of well mixed anticoagulated blood is placed in the center of the slide. Isotonic diluent is added to the blood in some instruments.
3. The instrument spins the platen at a high speed, causing the slide to become covered with a thin monolayer of cells. A beam of light passing through the smear during spinning allows a sensor to recognize when the red cells have separated properly, at which point the instrument stops. Adjustment of the spinning time is possible with some models.

Advantages

1. Superior, even (random) cell distribution
2. Consistency of preparations
3. Large examination area (monolayer)
4. Fewer broken (smudge) lymphoid cells in chronic lymphocytic leukemia.

Disadvantages

1. Automated blood films require longer preparation time per blood smear in addition to the time necessary to clean the instrument, which must be done several times a day.
2. Blood films cannot be made outside the laboratory, and capillary blood cannot be used.
3. A smaller number of leukocytes appears on the monolayer smear because of its thinness compared with the wedge-type preparation.
4. No specific location exists to search for immature, abnormal, or clustered cells.
5. Occasional cellular morphology is distorted by the centrifugal force.

SUMMARY OF BLOOD FILM PREPARATION

Most hematology laboratories in this country are still producing blood films using manual techniques. Of the two available manual techniques the wedge or spreader-slide is

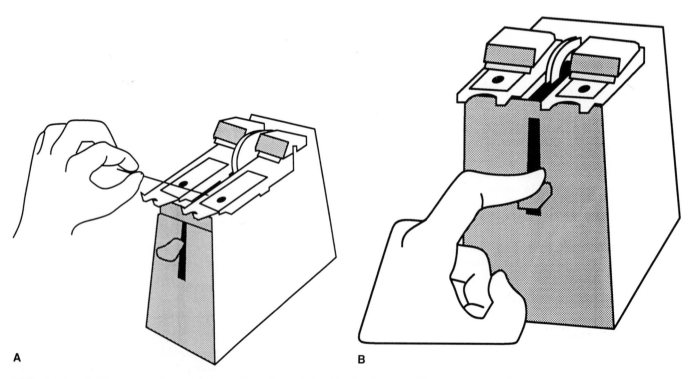

A   **B**

FIG. 3-10.   Automated wedge-type smear. (A) A drop of blood is placed at a specific spot on each of two slides. (B) By pressing a lever, the wedges are advanced, placed into the blood drops, and pulled back to spread the blood.

more popular. At the time of this writing only the Miniprep is available for purchase for automating the blood film technique, and it possesses the advantages and disadvantages of the manual wedge preparation. The chief inherent error of the wedge-type preparation (both manual and automated) is poor distribution of leukocytes, which is directly related to the speed and thinness of the preparation.

BUFFY COAT PREPARATION

Nucleated cells and platelets will layer above red cells during centrifugation (Fig 3-11). This fraction of nucleated cells is referred to as the "buffy coat" because of its tan color. A white top layer usually represents platelets accumulated above the nucleated cells. The buffy coat can be removed, mixed, and used to prepare smears.

The buffy coat preparation is a simple procedure that often provides diagnostic information and may reduce or eliminate the need for more complex, costly, and time-consuming tests. A buffy coat preparation may be indicated for the following:

1. Finding reactive, immature, or abnormal cells (*e.g.*, rare blasts) that are present in small numbers, especially with pancytopenic samples
2. Finding megaloblastic nucleated red cells or an increased number of hypersegmented neutrophils in megaloblastic anemias
3. Finding abnormal plasma cells
4. Detecting tumor cells circulating in the blood
5. It may be easier to locate bacteria or parasites. For example, mature red cells containing malarial parasites are concentrated at the top of the red cell layer. Study of this

layer may therefore be more fruitful than examining the "thick drop" preparation described in the early literature.

Technique
1. Fill a Wintrobe hematocrit tube with well mixed EDTA-anticoagulated blood.
2. Centrifuge for 6 minutes at $1000 \times$ g. The low relative centrifugal force will not cause cellular distortion.
3. With a capillary pipet, remove plasma from the tube until an amount slightly greater than the buffy coat layer remains (see Fig. 3-11).
4. Aspirate the remaining plasma, buffy coat layer, and the very top (about 1%) of the mature red cell layer and express this mixture onto a watch glass or clean glass slide.
5. Rinse the bore of the capillary pipet several times with the mixture to remove all the cells sticking to the glass.
6. Mix the sample well by stirring with a glass rod. Transfer drops of the mixture to clean glass slides or coverslips and make smears.
7. Air dry and stain.

A *double concentrate* may be helpful in situations where the leukocyte count is below 3×10^9/L. Several tubes are filled with the specimen and centrifuged as above. Two-thirds of the plasma is discarded from each. The remaining plasma, the buffy coat, and 0.25 inch of the red cell layer is removed from all tubes, mixed thoroughly, and placed in another tube for a second centrifugation followed by steps 3 through 7 of the original procedure.

Microhematocrit Technique

When only a small amount of blood is available, such as with finger stick samples, several microhematocrit tubes may be used to concentrate the nucleated cells.

1. Fill the tubes to at least three-fourths with blood.
2. Seal one end of the tubes and place them in a microhematocrit centrifuge. Centrifuge for 2 to 3 minutes (less than the normal full-packing time).
3. Score each tube just *below* the buffy coat layer (Fig. 3-12A) with a glass marking pencil or file.
4. Break the tube at scored mark. Wear gloves and be careful of glass fragments.
5. Hold the tube section containing the plasma, the buffy coat, and a small fraction of the red cell layer between the thumb and central finger with the index finger over the end of the tube to control fluid flow. A smallpox vaccination bulb may be used to control fluid flow.
6. Touch the tube to a clean glass slide and gently express the red cells and buffy coat and a small amount of the plasma (Fig. 3-12B). Mix thoroughly and make a wedge smear. Air dry, stain, and examine. Repeat for each capillary tube.

If the microhematocrit tube contains heparin anticoagulant, there will be a tendency for white cell and platelet agglutination, a more intense blue–purple staining quality of the white cells, and an orange–red coloration of the red cells.

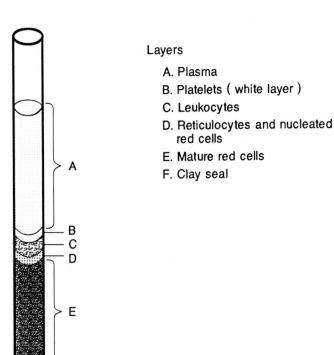

Layers

A. Plasma
B. Platelets (white layer)
C. Leukocytes
D. Reticulocytes and nucleated red cells
E. Mature red cells
F. Clay seal

FIG. 3-11.   Layers of blood components after centrifugation.

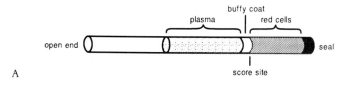

A

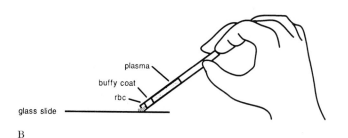

B

FIG. 3-12.   Microhematocrit technique for buffy coat preparation. (A) After centrifugation, the capillary tube is scored just below the buffy coat layer. (B) Gently express the remaining red cells, buffy coat, and a small amount of plasma onto a clean glass slide. Mix and spread.

Evaluation of a Preparation

The well prepared buffy coat smear should be representative of the general population of nucleated cells in that sample of blood. However, because of the manipulations of the specimen and centrifugation, an accurate differential count cannot be made. Likewise, mature red cell morphology cannot be evaluated, and platelets cannot be quantitated. A report of the buffy coat smear should describe the predominant populations of white cells and note the presence of any immature or abnormal white cells, nucleated red cells, megakaryocytic nuclei, or extraneous cellular findings. In cases of leukopenia or even with a normal leukocyte count, a few minutes of careful examination of a buffy coat smear allows one to review many times the number of nucleated cells seen in a routine examination of a direct blood film, and abnormalities are more likely to be discovered. When examining an ordinary wedge smear, it is advantageous to observe carefully the side edges and the feathered end, because immature and abnormal leukocytes and nucleated red cells may collect in these areas.

Rare young neutrophilic cells (metamyelocytes and myelocytes) and megakaryocyte nuclear fragments may be found in a buffy coat preparation of a healthy individual. Monocytes often are concentrated selectively. Nucleated red cells should not be present in normal adults.[12]

In a blood specimen anticoagulated with EDTA that is at least 1 hour old, morphologic distortions may be more pronounced than on direct smears. Smudge cells and necrotic (dead) cells may be more numerous.

Cytospin Buffy Coat

The cytocentrifuge[1,46] has been used primarily to concentrate nucleated cells in body fluid specimens, although there are at least two reports of its use for buffy coat preparations

or lupus erythematosus preparations.[11,13] Some laboratories are experimenting with the methodologies, but no evaluations have been published. One procedure[11] includes one or two concentrations in a Wintrobe tube, the addition of normal (0.86%) saline and 22% bovine albumin to the concentrated buffy coat, and cytocentrifugation. A balance between too much saline (too dilute) and too much albumin (dark cells with artifactual pseudopods) must be worked out for each sample. Another unpublished experimental technique entails incubation with erythrocyte-lysing agents before cytocentrifugation. As with the body fluid cytospin preparations, morphologic distortions (nuclear indentations and segmentation, localized or prominent cytoplasmic granulation, vacuolization) are introduced. Cytospin buffy coat methodology will undoubtedly become refined in the future.

ARTIFACTS OF SMEAR PREPARATION

Most blood smears are prepared from EDTA-anticoagulated samples. Cellular morphology in fresh samples is well preserved. Normal cells continue to demonstrate satisfactory morphology for at least 5 hours.[18,26] However, reactive and pathologic cells may assume changes within an hour that render them difficult to identify with certainty.[45] Storage at room temperature may accelerate these changes.[26]

Monocytes demonstrate immediate alteration in EDTA samples. Vacuolization is usual (Fig. 3-13). Reactive (variant) lymphocytes quickly develop vacuolated (Swiss cheese) cytoplasm and convoluted or clover leaf nuclei (see Fig. 3-13 E and F) similar to pathologic blast cells (see Fig. 3-13C). Toxic neutrophils may become vacuolated (autophagocytosis). Necrobiotic or dead leukocytes (see Fig. 3-13D) are more frequent in standing blood, especially in samples containing reactive and pathologic cells, and it is important not to mistake them for nucleated red cells. Red–purple cytoplasmic granulation in neutrophils is helpful in making the distinction. Some necrobiotic cells have multiple round nuclear fragments or prominent vacuoles.

Normal erythrocytes retain their size, color, and shape for at least 6 hours, after which a few may take on a spiculated or crenated appearance. In day-old blood crenated red cells are frequent, and spherocytes are conspicuous (see Fig. 3-13A). Abnormal erythrocytes may begin to manifest a spiculated appearance within an hour of blood collection, and within 2 to 4 hours this change may be significant. Coarse basophilic stippling and Dohle bodies may disappear on standing in EDTA-anticoagulated blood.[4]

Platelet distribution, size, and granules are affected by EDTA. Platelets are more uniformly distributed on an EDTA blood smear than on one made from capillary or needle point blood. However, they tend to swell and become spherical, and their granules spread, with consequent lighter staining than is usual on capillary blood smears. Platelet autoagglutinins have been reported to cause platelet clumping in the presence of EDTA.[19,29,47] Satellitism, the tendency for platelets to adhere to neutrophils in EDTA[3,20,40] (Fig. 3-14) is falsely interpreted as thrombocytopenia by particle counters and can be recognized only by visual smear evaluation.

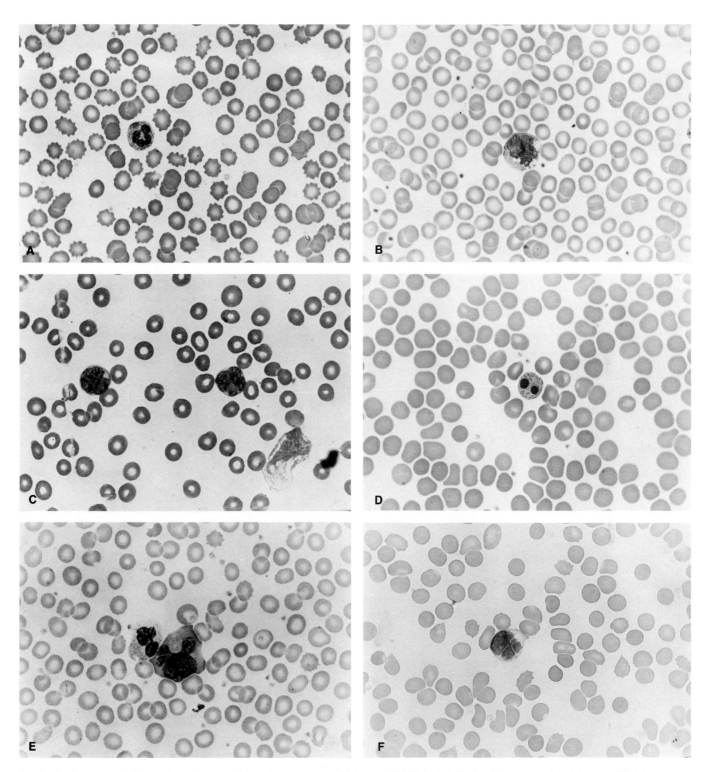

FIG. 3-13.   Morphologic alterations resulting from storage of blood in EDTA. (A) Red cells crenate after 6 hours. (B) Monocytes vacuolate within a few minutes. (C) Blast forms may acquire highly contorted nuclei. (D) Cells may die (necrotic neutrophil) after a few hours. (E) Variant (atypical) lymphocytes may become vacuolated. (F) Their nucleus may become contorted so that they might resemble blasts as depicted in C.

Wedge-type smears prepared from day-old EDTA-anticoagulated blood will show distribution defects, with many nucleated cells being carried to the tail area (Fig. 3-15). It is not possible to evaluate such samples accurately.

Slow air drying of a freshly prepared blood smear can cause drying or moisture red-cell artifact, a hairy appear-

ance of the cytoplasm of normal lymphocytes, and shrinkage of normal leukocytes. Drying artifact may render red cells falsely hypochromic; however, the sharp rather than gradual transition between the hemoglobinized rim and the clear center is helpful in identifying this artifact (Fig. 3-16). Sometimes the periphery of the cell has a crenated or moth-

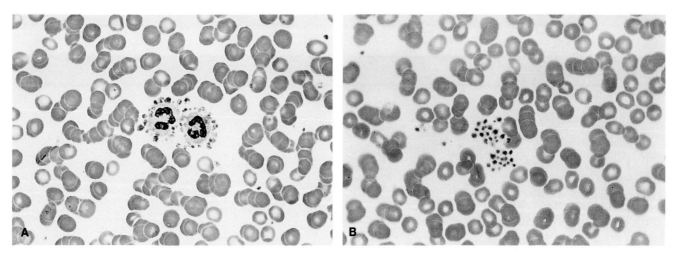

FIG. 3-14.   Artifacts of platelet smears. (A) Satellitism. (B) Clumping.

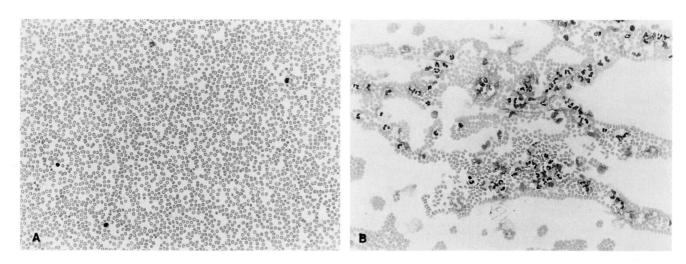

FIG. 3-15.   Day-old specimen with increased leukocyte count. (A) Examination area. Note that there are only three intact leukocytes and one broken leukocyte. (B) Feather edge. Note excessive accumulation of cells. Poor distribution such as this could lead to falsely low leukocyte estimates and to falsely high lymphocyte percentages in a differential count.

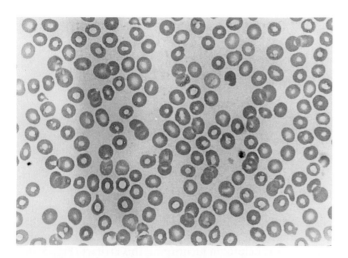

FIG. 3-16.   Red cells showing drying artifact.

eaten appearance. This drying artifact may have any of several causes:

1. Severe anemia, in which excessive amounts of plasma cause poor drying, regardless of the technique
2. A humid environment
3. An inadequate fixation period; may be avoided by pre-fixing the smears
4. Water contamination of the fixative or staining solution[5]
5. Excess buffer in the stain solution

The area of the smear may affect leukocyte morphology. In thin areas the glass effect enhances their spreading. In thick areas increased plasma causes shrinkage, and leuko-cytes remain three-dimensional with less cytoplasm.[7,45]

Even in a well prepared wedge-type smear, a few disinte-grated or smudge forms will be found. Smudge cells repre-sent leukocytes ruptured during preparation of the smear. Because these smudge cells were intact before smear preparation, their counterparts were included as leukocytes in the white cell count. When their number is noticeably increased (more than 25 per 100 leukocytes), they should be reported in the manual leukocyte differential count as the number per 100 leukocytes. The addition of one drop of 22% albumin to five drops of whole blood before smear preparation reduces the number of smudge cells on the smear.[10] Blood films made by centrifugal techniques are claimed to contain fewer smudge cells. Ruptured granulocytes often are surrounded by scattered granules, making their identification possible. Broken lymphocytes generally show only a smudged, amorphous nucleus with the cytoplasm dissolved in the background plasma. Smudge cells with an expanded nucleus having a loosely woven network appearance are sometimes called basket cells. Immature damaged cells may retain a blue-staining nucleolus.

STAINING THE BLOOD FILM

Romanowsky Stains

Romanowsky stains are composed of methylene blue, oxidative products of methylene blue (azures), and eosin dyes. Wright or Wright-Giemsa polychrome stains have been the most commonly used modifications of Romanowsky stains in this country. Other types that are more popular elsewhere are the Leishman, May-Grünwald, and Jenner stains, all named for their developers. Modifications differ in the ratios of dye components and the manufacturing methods used to oxidize the methylene blue.[24,25,27,30-32,35,36,38,41-43] Romanowsky stains may be used in combination with Giemsa, which contains azures, to intensify nuclear features or azurophilic and toxic granulation. Alone, Giemsa is inadequate for staining red cells, platelets, and leukocyte cytoplasm.

Cells must first be fixed to the slide with chemically pure, acetone-free methanol alone or in solution with the dye. After fixation, addition of a buffer solution changes the pH of the solution and ionizes the reactants to initiate the pH-dependent staining process. In general the acidic cellular elements such as nucleoproteins, nucleic acids, and certain cytoplasmic proteins react with the basic dye, methylene blue, and stain variations of blue. The term "basophilic" is used for these acidic elements and denotes their affinity or "love" (Greek *philic*) for basic dyes. Basic cellular elements such as hemoglobin molecules and some cytoplasmic constituents react with the acidic dye eosin, and stain a variation of orange–red. They may be called acidophilic or eosinophilic. The term "neutrophil" was coined to denote that cell's neutrality between vivid acidic (red) and basic (blue) colors. Some cellular organelles display blended shades of color, such as purple, representing combinations of acidic and basic molecular groups. Azures produce red–purple staining and are important for their ability to color primary or nonspecific granules in most myeloid cells, hence the term "azurophilic granules."

Romanowsky dyes have always been capricious. In the past, the best test for the quality of each stain lot was a trial run with different buffers and timings. Recent sophisticated analytic methods permit more exacting analysis of the constituent dye elements. As shown in Figure 3-17, demethyl-

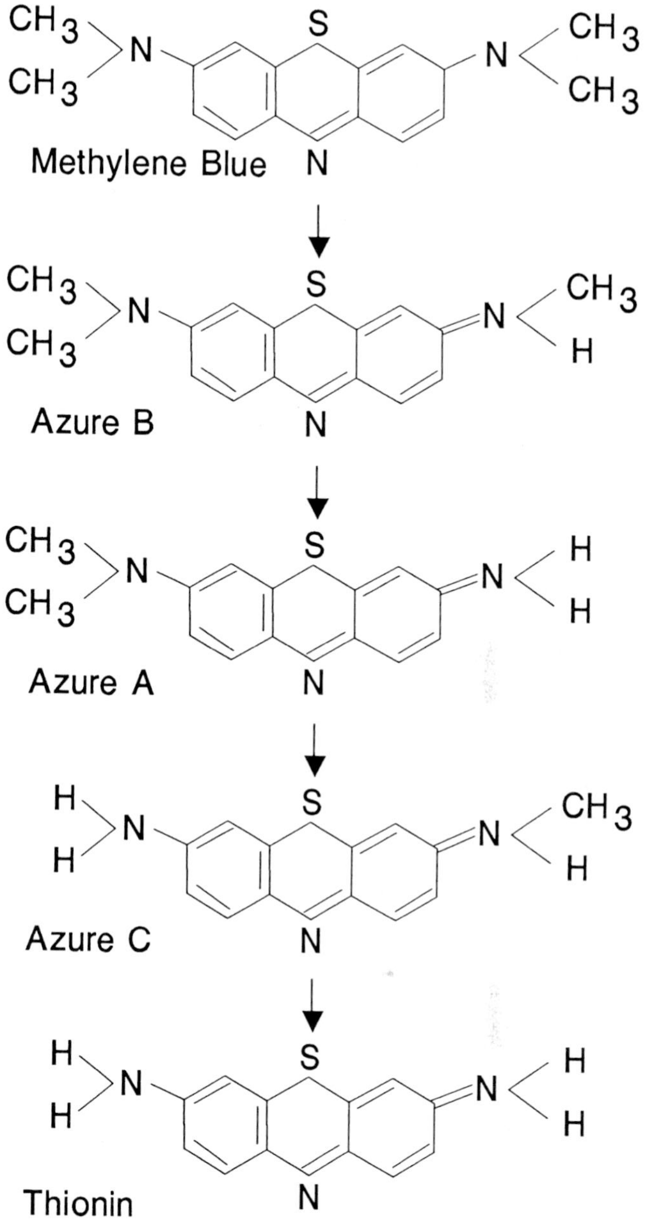

FIG. 3-17. Oxidation of methylene blue and the sequential oxidation products.

ation and deamination of methylene blue in alcoholic solution produces various oxidized products. This process continues as the Wright stain solution ages, causing variation in the stain quality. Refrigeration will inhibit this change,[9] and some manufacturers recommend 4°C storage. However, other blends of stains may be harmed by cold and should be stored at room temperature. Package inserts provide storage recommendations. Likewise, exposure to winter temperature during shipment may have adverse effects on stain solutions.[2,22] Some manufacturers add metallic elements to the solution[15,22,31] as stabilizers to extend the shelf life, but their presence may change the stain quality. The replacement of 50% of the methanol by glycerol will retard the oxidative process;[23-25] however, it produces a viscous stain solution that does not mix easily with the buffer and may lead to uneven staining.

Research on the "Romanowsky—Giemsa effect" by several investigators has provided an empiric basis for standardization of the Romanowsky-type stains. Methylene blue's prime function is to provide its oxidative products, the azures. Azure B is superior to the other azures. New polychrome stains composed of measured amounts of pure azure B and eosin Y have been developed.[21,33,34,36,37,39,51,52] Because oxidation is complete in these solutions and extraneous dyes and elements are eliminated, standardized stain quality is achieved.

Despite the advances in manufacturing and testing, it is still advisable to test-run every new stain solution.

Several fast or "quickie" stains have been developed for use in stat situations and small laboratories. Although adequate for assessing normal cell morphology, they generally are unsatisfactory for the evaluation of abnormal cells. The fixation period is short, which causes poor penetration of the stain, and the short stain exposure may produce unusual color tones. In addition, there is much variability from smear to smear.

Manual Staining Methods

Two types of manual methods are common: rack and dip.

Rack Method

The rack method uses rods overlying a sink or dish that hold glass slides or coverslips in a horizontal position during staining (see Fig. 3-18A). Small rubber corks set inside a dish can substitute when staining coverslip preparations (Fig. 3-18B).

Technique

1. Smears should be air dried for several minutes.
2. Wright stain solution is spread over the slide with a dropping bottle or pipet until the top surface is flooded. The edges of the slide should not touch other slides to

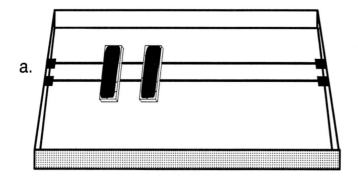

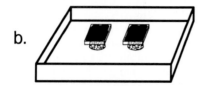

FIG. 3-18.   Rack method for manual staining of blood films. (A) Parallel rods to accommodate 3" x 1" glass slides or (B) rubber corks for staining coverslip preparations.

prevent stain runoff. Fixation of the cells to the slide takes place because of the alcoholic base of the stain solution. A *minimum* of 1 minute is required for proper fixation assuming a thin smear with normal or a decreased cell count. Specimens with greatly elevated leukocyte counts or bone marrow preparations require longer fixation times.

3. An equal amount of dilute phosphate buffer is added to each slide. The *p*H of the buffer will affect the quality of staining, the optimum being between *p*H 6.4 and 6.8. The buffer–stain solution is mixed gently by blowing on it. A greenish metallic sheen indicates the proper stain:buffer ratio. Stain for 4 to 6 minutes (depending on laboratory preference and experience with that particular stain).
4. The staining mixture is flushed thoroughly from the slide with a stream of distilled or deionized water until all stain is removed. Do not overwash. The *p*H of the wash water must be neutral so as not to affect the coloration of the stain.
5. The stain residue is cleaned off the back of the slide, and the specimen is air dried.

Although most laboratories buy commercially prepared Wright stain solution, it can be prepared manually by mixing 1 g of biologically certified Wright powder per 500 mL of chemically pure, acetone-free methanol. The stain is incubated for 1 week at 37°C and then at room or refrigerator temperature. Incubation can be shortened considerably by adding 0.1 g of Giemsa powder per 500 mL of stain. Polyethylene bottles may be more stable than glass for stain storage. Aging may cause lighter, less intense staining of cells, although the color balance generally remains the same. The stain should be filtered prior to use.

Buffer solutions may be made by dissolving commercially prepared buffer salts or tablets in distilled or deionized water. They may also be prepared by combining monobasic potassium phosphate and dibasic sodium phosphate according to the desired *p*H. Specific directions for making phosphate buffers are available in various chemistry manuals. The final solution should be checked with a *p*H meter.

The rack method is very cost effective for a small number of slides because it uses a minimum of stain solution per slide. One or several slides may be stained simultaneously. The disadvantages of the rack method include the time involved and the inconsistency in staining quality related to variances in the amounts of stain and buffer per slide and the timing per step.

Dip (Incubation) Method

Several dishes (large enough to contain a portable slide holder and an adequate amount of solution to cover the slides) are required. A method developed by this author has proved to be very satisfactory and reliable for more than 15 years.

Technique

1. The smears are fixed for 1 to 2 minutes in the dish with anhydrous methanol. The basket holding the slides should be completely dry to avoid water contamination.
2. The smear is transferred to a dish containing undiluted Wright stain for 4 minutes.

3. The smear is transferred to another dish with 75 mL of Wright stain and 325 mL of buffer (pH 6.4) for 4 minutes.
4. The smear is then transferred to a dish with 20 to 25 mL of Giemsa solution and 200 of mL deionized water for 4 minutes.
5. The slides are rinsed briefly in two dishes of distilled water and air dried.

The advantages of this method are greater consistency in staining quality, better penetration of the stain with more vivid colors and less precipitate, cost effectiveness for a large number of slides, and effective adaptability to an automated dip method. The disadvantages are the time necessary to prepare the stain solutions and transfer the slides from dish to dish and the limited stability (4 hours maximum) of the Wright–buffer and Giemsa stain solutions, making the method expensive for small numbers of smears.

Automated Staining Methods

Platen Type

The Ames Hema-Tek Slide Stainer[1] represents the platen type of stainer. Glass slides are placed on a platen and moved by a spiral conveyer through a polychrome methylene blue–eosin solution, a buffer solution, and a rinse solution, each of which is delivered from commercially prepared reagent packs through pump tubing (Fig. 3-19).

Carousel Type

Another instrument is the Aerospray Hematology Slide Stainer. This instrument sprays a measured amount of stain reagents onto the smears as they are transported in a rotating carousel.[50] Details of its operation are available from the manufacturer.

The advantages of the platen and carousel automated stainers include the following:

1. They are time saving. Once the slides are loaded into the instrument, the operator can walk away, and staining time is less than 10 minutes.
2. Stain quality is consistent from smear to smear.

3. Since small amounts of stain reagents are used compared with other staining techniques, the cost is lower.
4. Stat smears may be added and stained at any time with the Hema-Tek Slide Stainer.

The disadvantages include the following:

1. High maintenance is required. The platen must be kept clean to prevent precipitation of the dyes onto blood films. Tubing must be checked daily for precipitate and changed at least every 3 months.
2. The short fixation time often necessitates prefixation of smears in methanol, especially when leukocyte counts are markedly increased.
3. Stain reagents must be purchased and may be more expensive than "home-made." They are also subject to problems caused by shipping conditions such as freezing or heat that may affect the quality of staining.[2,9] In addition the manufacturing process is not reproducible from lot to lot, creating variances in color tones and the propensity for dye precipitation.
4. The instruments are not versatile relative to modifying the amount of stain delivered, the pH of the buffer, and the rinse and the timing for each step.
5. Incorporation of Giemsa stain to enhance coloration of the nucleus and granules is not possible unless a package with Giemsa is purchased. Toxic and basophil granules may not be stained if Giemsa is not added to the stain system.
6. Slides must be completely clean and not warped to obtain even staining on the platen-type instrument.
7. The Aerospray instrument expresses stain solutions for a full carousel (12 slides) regardless of the the number of slides present, which reduces its cost effectiveness.
8. Stat smears cannot be introduced into the Aerospray's carousel once it has begun the staining cycle.

Dip-Type Instruments

Several automated instruments use dip or immersion staining techniques similar to those of traditional histology staining. Batches of smears are moved from dish to dish at

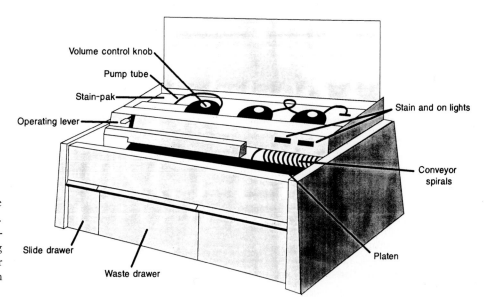

FIG. 3-19.   Automated, platen-type instrument for staining blood films. Slides are advanced by a conveyor spiral with the blood film side down along a platen. Stain, buffer, and rinse water are pumped up into the space between the blood film and platen.

Volume control knob
Pump tube
Stain-pak
Operating lever
Stain and on lights
Conveyor spirals
Slide drawer
Platen
Waste drawer

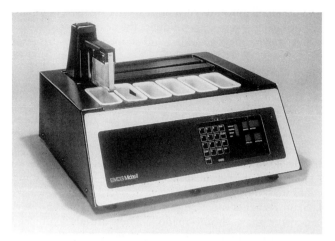

FIG. 3-20.   The Midas II stainer, an automated stainer that uses the dip technique. (Courtesy of EM Diagnostic Systems, Inc, Gibbstown, NJ; Subsidiary of E Merck, Darmstadt, Germany.)

programmed timed intervals (Fig. 3-20). The advantages include the following:

1. Walk-away instruments conserve operator time.
2. There is more versatility in the type and number of staining solutions, time per step, *p*H of the buffer and rinse solutions, and the ability to make stain reagents rather than purchasing them.
3. If staining solutions are replaced regularly, staining quality of smears is standardized.
4. Stain penetration is better and coloration of cellular elements is more intense, especially if Giemsa is added.
5. There is less chance of precipitate than on platen-type stainers.

The disadvantages of dip-type instruments include the following:

1. Staining of slides is lengthier than on platen-type instruments.
2. More time is required for preparing stain solutions daily or twice daily since stains have a limited working time.
3. More expense is incurred since large amounts of stain are required.
4. The instruments are unable to accept additional slides (*e.g.*, stats) if a staining cycle has begun.

Criteria for a Good Stain

The well stained smear should be reddish-brown. Microscopically, erythrocytes should be salmon pink, leukocyte nuclei should be purple–blue (depending on maturation), and platelets should have purple–blue to lilac cytoplasm containing red–purple granules. Additional criteria include distinct orange granules in eosinophils (an excellent *p*H meter), pinkish-tan cytoplasm in neutrophils, and gray ground-glass cytoplasm with many tiny red–purple granules in monocytes. Causes for deviations in color (the "red and blue stains") are listed in Table 3-1.

TABLE 3-1. Causes of Color Deviations

"RED STAIN"
  Too acid a buffer or stain solution (pH below 6.4)
  Excess buffer for stain solution
  Insufficient staining time
  Excessive washing
  Very thin smear
  Contaminants (*e.g.*, chlorine) in wash water
  Exposure of buffer or stain solution to acid fumes
  Old stain in which methanol has oxidized to fumic acid
"BLUE STAIN"
  Too alkaline a buffer or stain solution (pH above 6.8)
  Too little buffer for stain solution
  Excessive staining time
  Inadequate washing
  Short drying period
  Wash water too alkaline
  Thick smears
  Old smear (dried plasma produces blue background)
  Protein abnormality (*e.g.*, multiple myeloma)
  Heparin blood sample
  Very high leukocyte count with many blasts
  Low hematocrit

TROUBLESHOOTING STAIN PROBLEMS

Despite the advances in our knowledge of the action of Romanowsky-type stains and progress in their standardization, staining problems still occur. A few general hints to correct the more general problems are discussed below.

Fixation

Inadequate fixation may result in the blood smear being washed off the slide, indistinct nuclear detail, or poor staining of granules, especially in basophils. In addition, water contamination of the fixative may lead to the drying artifact.[5]

Freshly prepared smears should be air dried for at least 5 minutes to prevent drying artifact. Glass slides should be clean and clear before use. A haze on the slide may represent material that will interfere with proper fixation or disturb the acid–base relations needed for good-quality staining.

Methanol should be anhydrous and kept tightly stoppered away from moisture or chemical fumes. Moisture contamination of the Wright stain dissolved in the methanol may create problems. All staining dishes containing alcohol or alcoholic solutions should be kept covered to prevent evaporation and contamination and should be changed as necessary.

The fixation period should be a minimum of 1 minute.

Staining

Stain–buffer solutions have a limited working time, only a few hours. This becomes important in the dip methods. Some laboratories use interval timers to remind them to change the stain–buffer solution.

Tap water is *never* acceptable as a substitute for the buffer because it frequently is too alkaline or too acidic (depending on locale) and because it may contain chlorine. Distilled water often is unreliable because of contaminants in the system, and distilled or deionized water may absorb CO_2 on standing and become too acidic.[16]

For best results use a staining time at least twice the fixation period.

For the rack method the amount of buffer should be equal to or slightly greater than the amount of stain solution. Buffer and stain should be well mixed for uniform staining.

Rinse or Wash

Distilled water or a buffered rinse water should be used to wash off the stain. Too vigorous or prolonged washing may dislodge cells from underfixed smears or cause nuclear clumping or a lightly stained smear.

Underwashing may result in a blue smear or precipitate.

Drying

Air drying is most satisfactory. Forced rapid drying may alter the color intensities by shortening the exposure time to the wash water, because the red spectrum of colors continues to develop as long as the cellular elements are wet.

Stain Precipitate

Multiple blue–black granules or filamentous material overlying cellular and noncellular areas have several possible causes:

1. Precipitated stain powder may be in the stain solution. Filtration should remove this material.
2. A dirty or scratched platen with accumulated dried stain, precipitate in the stain pack, or too little stain expressed on the smear will result in precipitate on the blood film. Stain complexes may also precipitate within the instrument tubing. Replacement of tubing will alleviate this problem.
3. When using the rack method, evaporation or uneven spread of stain solution will result in precipitate on the slide. This may be caused by insufficient stain, unevenness of the rods on which the slides are placed, or placement of slides too close together, causing stain runoff.
4. The slides may be dirty.

Slides containing precipitate may be repaired in either of the following ways:

1. Redissolve the precipitate with additional stain by covering the smear with Wright stain for 5 to 10 seconds and flushing with distilled or deionized water.
2. Dip the slide three or four times in a solution of 30% ethanol in distilled water, air dry, and examine microscopically.

CHAPTER SUMMARY

A poorly made or poorly stained blood film, whether prepared manually or by automated instruments, is useless. It may, in fact, be the source of grave errors in diagnosis, patient monitoring, or quality control. A properly made and stained blood smear requires skill and practice. This chapter has described the proper procedures and techniques and has discussed the problems and their solutions.

REFERENCES

1. Ames Division, Miles Laboratories, Elkhart, IN 46515
2. Baer DM: Slide stainer problems. Med Lab Observ August 1986
3. Bauer HM: *In vitro* platelet–neutrophil adherence. Am J Clin Pathol 63:824, 1975
4. Ben-Bassat I, Brok–Simoni F, Kende G et al: A family with red cell pyrimidine 5'nucleotidase deficiency. Blood 47:919, 1976
5. Bettigole RE: Red cell staining artifacts and how to avoid them. N Engl J Med 271:1156, 1964
6. Coulter Electronics Inc, 601 West 20th Street, Hialeah, FL 33012
7. Cuadra M: The spreading of leukocytes released from their liquid environment. Blut 37:95, 1978
8. Dacie JV, Lewis SM: Practical Haematology, 6th ed. New York, Churchill Livingstone, 1984
9. Dean WW, Stastny M, Lubrano GJ: The degradation of Romanowsky-type blood stains in methanol. Stain Technol 52:35 1977
10. Densmore CM: Eliminating disintegrated cells on hematologic smears. Lab Med 12:640, 1981
11. DeNunzio J: Preparation of buffy coats from blood samples with extremely low white cell counts. Lab Med 16:497, 1985
12. Efrati P, Rosenszajn L: The morphology of buffy coat in normal human adults. Blood 16:1012, 1960
13. Garnet RF, Atkinson BF, Bonner H et al: Rapid screening for lupus erythematosus cells using cytocentrifuge-prepared buffy coat monolayers. Am J Clin Pathol 67:537, 1977
14. Geometric Data Corporation, 999 West Valley Road, Wayne, PA 19087
15. Gilliland JHW, Dean WW, Stastny M et al: Stabilized Romanowsky blood stain. Stain Technol 54:141, 1979
16. Green FJ: Getting more uniform results from biological stains. Lab Manage November 1969
17. Gyllensward C: Some sources of error at differential count of white corpuscles in blood-stained smears. Acta Paediatr (suppl II) 8:1, 1929
18. Kennedy JB, Machara KT, Baker AM: Cell and platelet stability in disodium and trisodium EDTA. Am J Med Technol 47:89, 1981
19. Kjeldsberg CR, Hershgold EJ: Spurious thrombocytopenia. JAMA 227:628, 1974
20. Kjeldsberg CR, Swanson J: Platelet satellitism. Blood 43:831, 1974
21. Lapen D: A standardized differential stain for hematology. Cytometry 2:309, 1982
22. Liao JC, Ponzo JL, Patel C: Improved stability of methanolic Wright's stain with additive reagents. Stain Technol 56:251, 1981
23. Lillie RD: Blood and malaria parasite staining with eosin azure methylene blue methods. Am J Public Health 33:948 1943
24. Lillie RD: Factors influencing the Romanowsky staining of blood films and the role of methylene violet. J Lab Clin Med 29:1181, 1944
25. Lillie RD: The deterioration of Romanowsky stain solutions in various organic solvents. Publ Health Rep (suppl) 178:1, 1944
26. Lloyd E: The deterioration of leukocyte morphology with time: Its effect on the differential count. Lab Perspect 1:13, 1982
27. Lubrano GJ, Dean WW, Heinsohn HG et al: The analysis of some commercial dyes and Romanowsky stains by high performance liquid chromatography. Stain Technol 52:13, 1977
28. MacGregor RGS, Richards W, Loh GL: The differential leukocyte count. J Pathol Bacteriol 51:337, 1940
29. Manthorpe R, Kofod B, Wiik A et al: Pseudothrombocytopenia: *In vitro* studies on the underlying mechanisms. Scand J Haematol 26:385, 1981

30. Marshall PN, Lewis SM: Batch variations in commercial dyes employed for Romanowsky-type staining: A thin layer chromatographic study. Stain Technol 49:351, 1974

31. Marshall PN, Lewis SM: Metal contaminants in commercial thiazine dyes. Stain Technol 50:143, 1975

32. Marshall PN, Bentley SA, Lewis SM: An evaluation of some commercial Romanowsky stains. J Clin Pathol 28:680, 1975

33. Marshall PN, Bentley SA, Lewis SM: A standardized Romanowsky stain prepared from purified dyes. J Clin Pathol 28:920, 1975

34. Marshall PN: Methylene blue–azure B–eosin as a substitute for May Grünwald–Giemsa and Jenner–Giemsa stains. Microsc Acta 79:153, 1977

35. Marshall PN: Romanowsky-type stains in haematology. Histochem J 10:1, 1978

36. Marshall PN, Bentley SA, Lewis SM: Standardization of Romanowsky stains: The relationship between stain composition and performance. Scand J Haematol 20:206, 1978

37. Marshall PN, Bentley SA, Lewis SM: Staining properties and stability of a standardized Romanowsky stain. J Clin Pathol 31:280, 1978

38. Marshall PN: Romanowsky staining: State of the art and "ideal" techniques. In Koepke JA (ed): Differential Leukocyte Counting. Skokie, IL, College of American Pathologists, 1979

39. Marshall PN, Galbraith WG, Navarro EF et al: Microspectrophotometric studies of Romanowsky stained blood cells. J Microscopy 124:197, 1981

40. Payne CM: Platelet satellitism: An ultrastructural study. Am J Pathol 103:116, 1981

41. Power KT: The Romanowsky stains: A review. Am J Med Technol 48:519, 1982

42. Roe MA, Lillie RD, Wilcox A: American azures in the preparation of satisfactory Giemsa stains for malarial parasites. Public Health Rep 55:1272, 1940

43. Scott BE, French RW: Standardization of biological stains. Military Surg 55:229, 1924

44. Shafer JA, Stein BL: Blood smear observations: Workshop manual. University of Rochester, NY, 1975

45. Shafer JA: Artifactual alterations in phagocytes in the blood smear. Am J Med Technol 48:507, 1982

46. Shandon Inc, Pittsburgh, PA 15275.

47. Shreiner DP, Bell WR: Pseudothrombocytopenia: Manifestation of a new type of platelet agglutinin. Blood 42:541, 1973

48. Stein BL, Shafer JA: A blood smear pusher. ESAMT Technol J 8:11, 1962

49. Stiene–Martin EA: Causes for poor leukocyte distribution in manual spreader-slide blood films. Am J Med Technol 46:624, 1980

50. Wescor, Inc, 459 South Main Street, Logan, UT 84321

51. Wittekind DH, Kretschmer V, Sohmer I: Azure B–eosin Y stain as the standard Romanowsky–Giemsa stain. Br J Haematol 51:391, 1982

52. Wittekind DH: On the nature of Romanowsky–Giemsa staining and its signficance for cytochemistry and histochemistry: An overall view. Histochem J 15:1029, 1983

4

Basic Microscopy in Hematology

Barbara A. Smith Michael

There are three basic requirements for accurate identification of blood cells and cellular changes that reflect disease processes: (1) properly collected and processed specimens; (2) an experienced hematologist; and (3) a high-quality optical system that is adjusted and maintained for optimum performance. Adjustment of the microscope's illumination system for optimum specimen contrast and resolution is a prerequisite for accurate image recognition and is crucial when using oil immersion microscopy. Proper adjustment requires that the technologist have a basic knowledge of image formation and of microscope structure, function, and components.

PRINCIPLES OF IMAGE FORMATION IN LIGHT MICROSCOPY

Light, which is the raw material of light microscopy, is a form of radiant energy. Although it is possible to describe some of light's properties and effects on matter, its true nature is still unclear. If a beam of white light, a mixture of all colors, is passed through a prism or lens, it is split into its component colors. These colors, which can be seen by the eye, comprise the visible spectrum or the wavelengths between 400 and 750 nm.

Light, which is proposed to travel in a manner analogous to waves, can be described by properties such as wavelength, frequency, amplitude, and phase. We can represent a light wave mathematically by a sine curve. Wavelength, or the distance between the corresponding points on adjacent waves, determines what the eye perceives as color. Frequency, or the number of vibrations per second of a given light wave, is closely related to wavelength: the shorter the wavelength, the higher the frequency and the greater the amount of radiant energy. Amplitude, the vertical displacement of a wave from the optical axis or equilibrium position, determines the intensity of an object as it is seen by the eye. These topics are discussed in greater detail elsewhere.[5,11,14,22]

Lenses

Types

A lens is an optical element composed of glass or other transparent material that is ground and polished to a specific shape.[21] Eyepieces, objectives, and condensers, the optical components of the microscope, are constructed of lenses in combinations. There are two basic lens types: (1) positive, convex lenses, which cause light rays passing through them to converge or collect to form a real image; and (2) negative, concave lenses, which cause parallel light rays to diverge or separate.

Optical Phenomena

Light rays passing from an optically light to an optically dense medium (i.e., a medium of higher refractive index) are changed in velocity and direction. The refractive index (RI) is the ratio of the speed of light in air to its velocity in another medium such as glass. Reflection, refraction, dispersion, diffraction, and interference are optical phenomena (effects) that can occur when light rays pass through lenses. For example, interference is the effect that two or more light rays from the same source have on one another, and refraction is the change in the direction of a ray of light that passes through a lens.

Resolution and Numerical Aperture

Resolution is the ability of a lens to delineate detail in a specimen.[3,5,11,20,22] It is expressed in micrometers (μm) as the distance between two structural elements that can still be distinguished from each other visually. Resolution is determined by two factors: the numerical aperture (NA), or the performance rating of a lens for gathering light, and the wavelength of the illuminating light. The relation of NA and wavelength (λ) to resolution (R) can be expressed mathematically as:

$$R = \frac{1.2\,\lambda}{2\,NA}$$

In optical microscopy the effect of wavelength can be largely ignored, because visible light between 400 and 700 nm is the primary source of illumination. However, NA is important in determining R. From the equation above it is apparent that the higher the NA, the lower the R (the greater the resolution). For example, an objective lens with an NA of 1.00 has the ability to resolve ten times the detail of an objective with an NA of 0.10.

The NA can also be expressed mathematically as n sin u. That is, NA is the product of n (the refractive index of the medium in the space between the object and the front lens of the objective) and sine u (the sine of half the angle of aperture or the cone of light admitted by the lens).

Dry objective lenses are designed to work with air in the "object space" and therefore do not have an NA greater than 1.00, the refractive index of air. Immersion objectives, which are used for most hematologic observations, must always have an immersion medium (oil) in the space between the objective and the specimen slide. If an air space exists, the NA of the immersion lens is reduced to no more than 1.00, and the effective NA and full resolving power of the objective cannot be achieved (Fig. 4-1).

Note that condensers also have NA ratings and should be matched with the objectives used. Keep in mind that dry objectives and condensers cannot be "oiled" to increase their NA; oil will ruin them. Only immersion lenses are designed for use with oil.

Magnification

Magnification is the visual enlargement of a specimen image by an optical instrument and is expressed in terms of diameters, power, times, or ×. In the compound light microscope the total magnification of an objective-eyepiece combination equals the product of the magnifying power of the objective lens and that of the eyepiece. If applicable, auxillary optics and tube factors must also be taken into account when calculating total magnification.

Relations of Microscope Features

Magnification, working distance, field diameter, depth of focus, and field brightness are interdependent.[11,21] Working distance, which decreases with increasing magnification, is the depth of space in millimeters between the top surface of the specimen slide and the front surface of the objective lens (Table 4-1). It is an important factor, particularly when using high-power objectives that have limited free working distances. With these objectives the optics or specimen can easily be damaged. This is why they usually have a spring-loaded front element that allows the lens to retract inside its housing if it comes into contact with a stationary surface.

Field diameter or field of view is the area of specimen that can be seen. It decreases with increasing magnification. Higher-power objectives thus show a smaller specimen area, but resolve more detail, than lower-power objectives. The actual diameter of the field of view in millimeters can

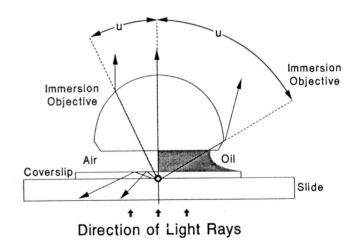

FIG. 4-1.   Principle of oil immersion microscopy. Note gain in numerical aperture and increase in cone of light admitted by lens when oil is used with an immersion objective. (Modified from Mollring FK: Microscopy from the Very Beginning. Thornwood, NY, Carl Zeiss, Inc, 1979, with permission.)

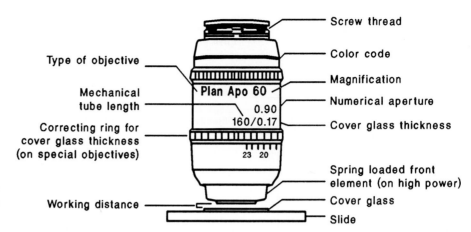

FIG. 4-2. Nomenclature of a microscope objective lens. (Courtesy of Nikon Inc, Garden City, NY.)

be calculated by dividing the field number of the eyepieces (oculars) by the objective magnification; check the manufacturer's technical specifications for the eyepiece field number. This calculation is important if different microscopes with different field diameters are used for peripheral blood-film cell counts in the same laboratory. A correction factor should then be used to maintain consistency when reporting results.

SAMPLE CALCULATION OF FIELD OF VIEW DIAMETER. For example, assume two microscopes are used for leukocyte and platelet count estimates in a hospital laboratory:

Microscope A: objective: 100×; eyepiece field number: 18;

$$\text{field of view diameter} = \frac{18}{100} = 0.18 \text{ mm}$$

Microscope B: objective: 100×; eyepiece field number: 20;

$$\text{field of view diameter} = \frac{20}{100} = 0.20 \text{ mm}$$

SAMPLE CALCULATION OF CORRECTION FACTOR. Compare the largest field of view with the smallest, and assume that the smallest field of view equals 100%. A ratio and proportion should be set up to solve for the correction factor:

$$0.18:100 = 0.20:x$$

The correction factor (x) equals 90% or 0.90. In this example all cell count estimates performed on microscope B must be multiplied by the correction factor 0.90 to adjust the counts to match those of microscope A.

Increasing magnification not only reduces the field of view but also reduces the depth of focus or the distance throughout which all parts of the specimen image are clearly in focus simultaneously. Also, with increasing magnification a greater amount of light is required to illuminate the field.

Lens Aberrations and Their Correction

Aberrations are optical system defects that degrade image quality.[11,14,20–22] In microscopy there are three important types of defects. *Chromatic aberrations* result in color fringes and poor image definition. *Spherical aberrations* result in poor image definition and loss of contrast. *Field curvature aberrations* result in a "curved" image of a flat specimen and create an out-of-focus edge while the center of the field is in focus or vice versa.

Correction or minimization of lens defects is achieved by using carefully selected combinations of lens shapes and different types of glass. *Achromats,* the most common and least expensive type of optics, are partially corrected for chromatic and spherical aberrations. *Apochromatic* objectives and condensers, required for critical microscopy and photomicrography, have superior chromatic correction (three-color) and spherical (two-color) correction. *Semiapochromats* have intermediate correction (and price).

Field curvature is a serious problem, particularly in photomicrography. Therefore, *plano* or *flatfield lenses* are recommended. In addition, the optimal correction of objective lenses is achieved when they are used with matched or compensating eyepieces. Refer to Figure 4-2 for objective nomenclature.

Compound Light Microscope

The compound light microscope is basically two sets of lenses mounted in tandem with one magnifying the image produced by the other and the final enlarged image appearing inverted and laterally reversed.[5,11,14,22] The objective lens projects a primary image of the specimen inside the focal length of the eyepiece, which, in turn, projects a secondary, further enlarged image of the object that appears to be located 250 mm (10 inches) from the eye at the level of the specimen stage. This is termed the virtual or "mind's

TABLE 4-1. Characteristics of Typical Objective Lenses

TYPE OF LENS	RESOLVING POWER (μm)	NUMERICAL APERTURE (NA)	MAGNIFYING POWER (x)	WORKING DISTANCE (mm)
Low power	1.34	0.25	10	7.20
High dry	0.52	0.65	40	0.60
Oil immersion	0.26	1.30	100	0.20

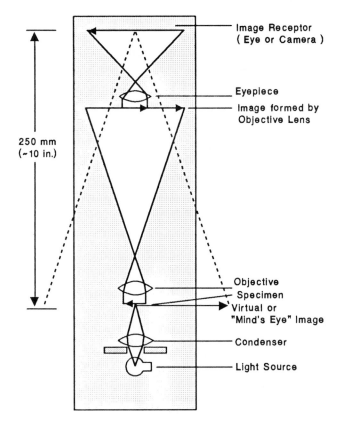

FIG. 4-3. Image formation in the compound light microscope. (Modified from Cormack D: Introduction to Histology. Philadelphia, JB Lippincott, 1984, with permission.)

eye" image, because it cannot be focused on a screen (Fig. 4-3).

The basic components of a standard microscope include oculars or eyepieces, body tube, objectives attached to a revolving nosepiece, mechanical stage, substage condenser, and illumination system (Fig. 4-4). The substage condenser directs and focuses light from the illumination source onto the specimen positioned on the stage. The specimen changes the light rays that illuminate it. The background light from the light source and the diffracted light from the specimen then combine to produce the specimen image.

BRIGHTFIELD MICROSCOPY

Application

Brightfield microscopy is the cornerstone of diagnostic hematology and the most common type of microscopy used in the clinical laboratory. In hematology brightfield microscopy is used to examine stained blood films.[5,11,15,22]

Principle

Brightfield microscopy is a method of examining specimens using transmitted light in which structural details of the object appear darker than the illuminated field of view. Brightfield microscopy depends on amplitude modulation to make the specimen visible. Specimens must be stained to enhance light absorption and contrast (Fig. 4-5).

KOEHLER METHOD OF ILLUMINATION

Principle

Koehler (or Köhler) illumination ensures optimum contrast and resolution for the maximum definition of specimen details by precisely focusing and centering the light path and spreading the light uniformly over the field of view. Whereas final specimen image definition is ultimately limited by the quality and maintenance of the optics, obtaining the best possible image depends on the microscopist's control of illumination. Table 4-2 lists the steps in the procedure.

Comments

The Koehler procedure must be performed daily before using the instrument, but with practice the procedure takes less than 20 seconds. Ideally it should be repeated when objectives are changed from one magnification to another, because objectives have different fields of view and require different illumination apertures depending on the magnifying power and NA. This is particularly important for critical microscopy and photomicrography.

Remember to adjust light intensity only with the brightness control, never by adjusting the field or aperture diaphragm. Once these are set during the Koehler illumination procedure, they should not be changed unless the objectives or operator are changed.

OIL IMMERSION MICROSCOPY

Application

Oil immersion microscopy is used extensively in hematology to observe erythrocyte morphology, estimate platelet counts, and differentiate leukocytes.[5,10,11] The procedure is as follows:

TABLE 4-2. Basic Steps of Koehler Illumination

1. Turn on microscope and adjust light intensity.
2. Switch to 10× objective, place specimen on stage, and focus using focus control knobs.
3. Close condenser aperture iris diaphragm and raise substage condenser with height adjustment knob to the top "stop." (Condenser aperture diaphragm controls angle of illumination and thus amount of light to objective lens.)
4. Close field iris diaphragm with field diaphragm control. (Field diaphragm limits area of illumination to image field.)
5. Move substage condenser until image of field diaphragm is in sharp focus. Refocus specimen image using focus control knobs if necessary.
6. Center field diaphragm image by adjusting condenser or field diaphragm centering screws; this depends on microscope type or model, and some microscopes have a preset light source and field diameter and do not have centering controls.
7. Enlarge field diaphragm image until it is just outside field of view and entire observation area is illuminated.
8. Remove one eyepiece; open and close substage condenser aperture diaphragm while looking down eyepiece tube and observe circular beam of light.
9. Adjust aperture diaphragm with aperture conrol until light beam fills approximately 75% of field.
10. Replace eyepiece.

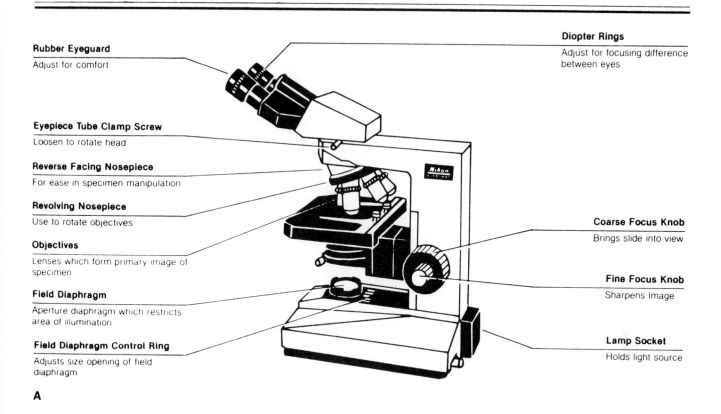

Rubber Eyeguard
Adjust for comfort

Diopter Rings
Adjust for focusing difference between eyes

Eyepiece Tube Clamp Screw
Loosen to rotate head

Reverse Facing Nosepiece
For ease in specimen manipulation

Revolving Nosepiece
Use to rotate objectives

Objectives
Lenses which form primary image of specimen

Field Diaphragm
Aperture diaphragm which restricts area of illumination

Field Diaphragm Control Ring
Adjusts size opening of field diaphragm

Coarse Focus Knob
Brings slide into view

Fine Focus Knob
Sharpens image

Lamp Socket
Holds light source

A

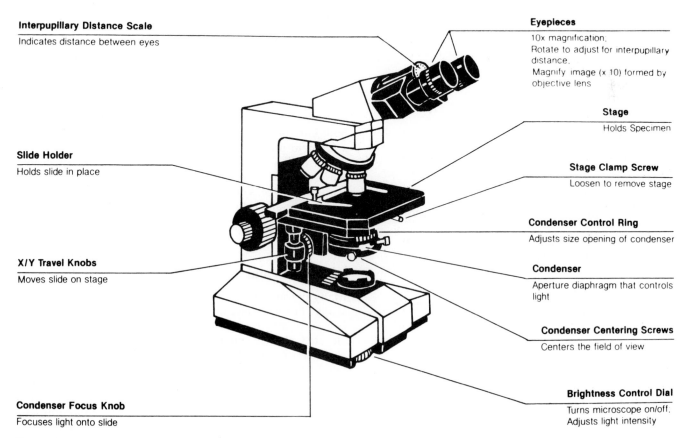

Interpupillary Distance Scale
Indicates distance between eyes

Eyepieces
10x magnification.
Rotate to adjust for interpupillary distance.
Magnify image (x 10) formed by objective lens

Stage
Holds Specimen

Slide Holder
Holds slide in place

Stage Clamp Screw
Loosen to remove stage

Condenser Control Ring
Adjusts size opening of condenser

Condenser
Aperture diaphragm that controls light

X/Y Travel Knobs
Moves slide on stage

Condenser Centering Screws
Centers the field of view

Brightness Control Dial
Turns microscope on/off.
Adjusts light intensity

Condenser Focus Knob
Focuses light onto slide

B

FIG. 4-4.   Basic components of the standard light microscope. (Courtesy of Nikon Inc, Garden City, NY.)

FOCUS UNDER LOW POWER

Oil immersion objectives cannot be focused just by switching to that lens. First, under low power (10×), focus and select viewing area. Rotate objective out of light path, and place a drop of immersion oil in center of specimen above beam of light. Refractive index of immersion medium should match that required by the particular immersion objective; check microscope manufacturer's specifications.

SWITCH TO OIL IMMERSION OBJECTIVE

Watching from side of microscope, rotate to oil immersion lens. Do not drag any dry objectives through oil. As oil objective is clicked into position, make sure it only glides into oil and does not crash into specimen slide; remember that there is minimum working distance at this high magnification (see Table 4-1). Focus carefully using fine adjustment knob only. (Note that immersion lens should be swung rather than lowered into oil to avoid trapping troublesome air bubbles between slide and objective).

ADJUST FINE FOCUS

Recenter and focus field diaphragm image if necessary using the condenser focus control. Enlarge field diaphragm image just outside field of view. Remove one eyepiece and adjust condenser aperture diaphragm. Adjust light intensity; more light is required at high magnification.

EXAMINE SPECIMEN

When observation is complete, rotate lens from the oil and clean excess oil from both lens and specimen slide. Check microscope instruction manual for recommended procedure.

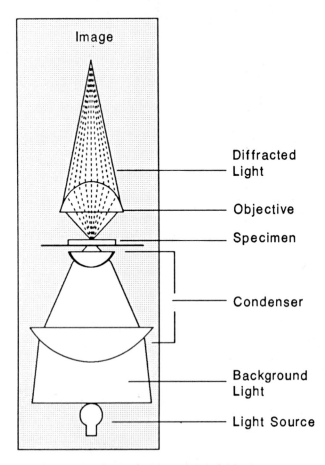

FIG. 4-5. Optical paths in brightfield microscopy.

COMMENTS

In high-precision microscopy and photomicrography, if the NA of the objective is higher than 1.00, use of an oil immersion condenser is recommended. In this case oil is also applied to the front lens of the condenser, and the condenser is raised until contact with the undersurface of the specimen slide is made to form a homogeneous oil immersion system.

PHASE-CONTRAST MICROSCOPY

Application

In hematology phase contrast is used to perform manual platelet counts in situations where the electronic count may be inaccurate (Chap. 59).

Principle

Phase contrast is an optical contrast enhancement technique that allows examination of unstained specimens that are invisible under ordinary brightfield microscopy.[4,5,19,22] This is accomplished by converting slight differences in thickness and refractive index (*i.e.,* phase differences) in the object into intensity or brightness differences that are detectable by the human eye. Depending on the type of phase optics used, the specimen appears brighter (bright contrast) or darker (dark contrast) than the surrounding area (Fig. 4-6).

Equipment

The equipment consists of a light microscope with special accessories: a phase condenser with an annular ring that controls the illumination and a phase-changing plate or ring built into the objective. This phase-shifting element creates a uniform phase change that increases the differences between the background light and the diffracted light from the specimen, thereby enhancing image contrast. A centering telescope, known as a Bertrand lens, is used to verify that the annular ring in the condenser and the phase plate in the objective are coincident (Fig. 4-7).

Comments and Sources of Error

Many precautions must be taken in phase-contrast microscopy. For example, debris may result in misleading data (*e.g.,* dust may be counted as platelets, resulting in a falsely elevated platelet count). Also the "halo effect," which is characteristic of phase, may conceal useful data, causing falsely decreased platelet counts. The exact centering of the annular diaphragm in the condenser is critical for achieving the desired contrast effect. Therefore, coincidence must be checked routinely. In critical microscopy and photomicrography the centering must be checked at each magnification used. Even a slight decentering of the diaphragm and phase plate can result in an image of low contrast and a shadowing effect that can cause inaccurate cell counts.

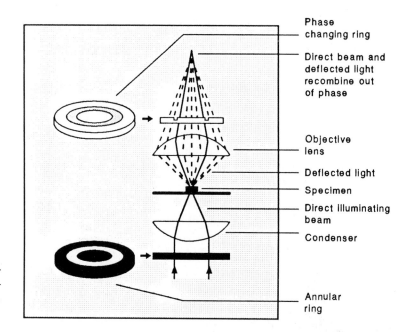

FIG. 4-6.   The optical path in phase-contrast micro-scopy. (From Special Contrast Enhancement Techniques [Transmitted Light Microscopy]. Cambridge, MA, Polaroid Corporation, 1981, with permission.)

FLUORESCENCE MICROSCOPY

Application

In hematology fluorescence microscopy is used primarily in antinuclear antibody (ANA) and T- and B-cell studies.

Principle

Fluorescence describes the emission by certain substances of radiation of a longer wavelength after absorption of light energy of a shorter wavelength[7,22] (Fig. 4-8). There are two basic types of fluorescence: primary or autofluorescence, when the object itself is fluorescent; and secondary or induced fluorescence, when the specimen is stained with a fluorochrome or fluorescent dye.

Equipment

A high-intensity light source (50 or 200 W mercury or high-power halogen lamp), exciter and barrier filters, darkfield condenser, and special optics free from auto-fluorescence are required. The exciter or light source filter transmits the required radiation and suppresses the other wavelengths. The barrier or secondary filter, located between the specimen and the observer, suppresses the exciting radiation from the light source and transmits the visible emitted radiation. This set-up applies to the transmitted technique.

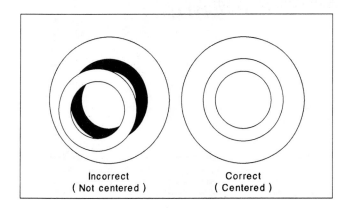

FIG. 4-7.   Quality control in phase microscopy. A Bertrand lens must be used for verification that the annular ring in the condenser and the phase plate in the objective are coincident. The rings will appear either not centered (left) or centered (right). Rings should be centered.

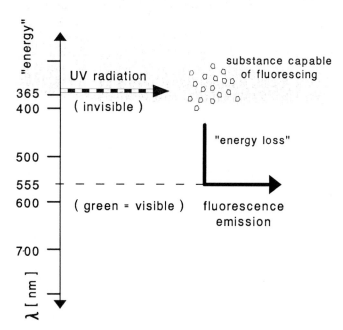

FIG. 4-8.   The origin of fluorescence radiation. (From Worthwhile Facts About Fluorescence Microscopy. Thornwood, NY, Carl Zeiss, Inc, 1975, with permission.)

Incident-light excitation, or epifluorescence, is a newer type of fluorescence microscopy in which a special dichroic mirror (presents one color in reflected light, another in transmitted light) functions as a dual-purpose filter (exciter and barrier). The objectives also double as a condenser. There are a number of advantages to this technique: brighter image intensity and better image quality; no problem with the critical condenser centering (as required in the transmitted technique) because the objective acts as a condenser; and the ability to combine other transmitted light techniques (*e.g.*, brightfield and phase) with fluorescence on the same microscope.

Comments and Sources of Error

Work should be done in a darkened room. Nonfluorescent immersion oil and mounting media must be used. Too much excitation light can cause a rapid fading of specimen fluorescence. Alignment of the light source is important. Also, the lamp housing should provide adequate ventilation and shield any high-intensity stray light, which could endanger the observer.

TROUBLESHOOTING PROBLEMS IN LIGHT MICROSCOPY

Although a microscope is not difficult to operate, occasionally there are problems.[10-12,15] Table 4-3 lists some common problems with their usual causes and corrective measures.

QUALITY CONTROL AND PREVENTIVE MAINTENANCE

The microscope is a precision optical instrument. Whereas more complex instruments often receive scheduled quality control and preventive maintenance, the microscope often receives little or no routine care. The microscope must be kept functional through adjustment and system checks, cleaning, and part replacement when required.[1,5,11,12,15]

The manufacturer's instruction manual is a valuable reference not only for the identification of components, operation, and optical data, but also for maintenance requirements and troubleshooting problems. The College of American Pathologists has published guidelines for microscope performance and function verification and for preventive maintenance (Table 4-4), including the performance of the Koehler illumination procedure.[1]

ELECTRON MICROSCOPY

Electron microscopes are expensive and complex. Although many applications for electron microscopy (EM) in medicine are still of a research nature,[13] the technique has been used increasingly in clinical studies and diagnosis. Whereas light microscopy provides a "macroscopic" view of cells and allows for their enumeration and classification based on morphology, EM permits observation of the fine

TABLE 4-3. Trouble Shooting in Light Microscopy

PROBLEM	PROBABLE CAUSE	CORRECTIVE ACTION
LIGHTING		
No light	Microscope not plugged in	Plug into outlet
	Brightness control dial turned off	Turn up light intensity
	Objective not clicked into position	Click objective into place
	Condenser image completely off center when field diaphragm is closed down	Adjust image with centering screws
	Bulb burned out	Replace bulb
	Bulb not inserted properly	Insert bulb correctly
	Fuse blown	Replace fuse
	Fuse not inserted properly	Insert fuse correctly
	No power from wall outlet	Test or try different outlet
Insufficient light	Brightness control dial set too low	Increase brightness
	Condenser diaphragm closed	Open condenser diaphragm
	Substage condenser lowered too far (not correctly focused)	Adjust height of substage condenser as per Koehler Method
Flickering	Loose power connection	Plug in microscope or try another wall outlet
	Corrosion on bulb pins	Clean pins on bulb
	Defective bulb socket	Replace socket
	Bulb not inserted properly	Insert bulb correctly
	Situation not covered above	Call for repair
Too bright	Light turned up too high	Adjust brightness
FOCUSING		
Won't focus on 40x or higher magnification	Specimen slide upside down	Turn glass slide over so that the specimen faces up
Nonparfocal	Set-up procedure not correctly followed	Repeat "Operation" steps
	Objective has come partially unscrewed	Tighten objective
MISCELLANEOUS		
Eyestrain	Illumination or field too intense	Reduce light intensity
	Eyepieces not focused for each eye	Adjust to correct
Floating spots	"Debris" in the vitreous humor of the retina noticeable at high magnifications	Taking a break and resting will often help
Field diaphragm noncenterable	Substage condenser seated improperly in condenser carrier	Loosen condenser clamp screw and reseat condenser
Bubbles or dark wave passes across the field of view when using immersion oil	Air bubbles in oil: contact between oil immersion objective and oil "broken"	Clean slide and/or add more oil

Courtesy Nikon Inc, Garden City, NY, and Health Sciences Consortium, Inc, Chapel Hill, NC.

TABLE 4-4. Guidelines for Verification and Maintenance of Microscopes

	DAILY OR MORE FREQUENTLY	OTHER
PERFORMANCE VERIFICATION		
Check light alignment	X	
Check visualization of slide material	X	
FUNCTION VERIFICATION		
Condenser height adjustment	X	
Center circular image of field diaphragm	X	
Field diaphragm aperture adjustment	X	
Condenser diaphragm aperture adjustment	X	
Check optical system for damage	X	
Check optical system for cleanliness		X
Check fine and coarse adjustments		X
Check condenser fork		X
Check mechanical stage		X
Check interpupillary distance		X
Check slide fingers		X
INSTRUMENT MAINTENANCE		
Cover instrument when not in use	X	
Thoroughly dust optical surfaces	X	
Thoroughly clean optical surfaces	X	
Thoroughly clean external surface		X
Clean and lubricate slide ways and gears		X
Complete general overhaul		X

Courtesy of College of American Pathologists, Skokie, IL.

structure of cells with a magnification of approximately ×100,000. Refer to appropriate references for further information on EM.[6,9]

CHAPTER SUMMARY

Knowledge of the microscope and its proper use and care are vital to accurate identification and counting of cells and to interpretation of special stains.

Light, the raw material of light microscopy, is a form of radiant energy. It is described in terms of wavelength, frequency, and amplitude.

Lenses are categorized as dry or immersion. When using oil immersion lenses, the space between the objective and slide must have oil for optimum specimen visibility.

Magnification is the visual enlargement of an image and is calculated by multiplying the magnifying power of the objective lens by that of the eyepiece. Higher-power objectives show a smaller field diameter but resolve more specimen detail.

All laboratories using microscopes with different field of view diameters for performing cell count estimates must calculate a correction factor to be used in adjusting the counts to maintain consistency in results.

The compound light microscope is the most commonly used microscope in hematology. Brightfield microscopy is the most frequently used type of microscopy in hematology. The Koehler illumination adjustment must be performed each time the microscope is used to ensure optimum specimen contrast and resolution for accurate cell identification. The proper technique for oil immersion examination must be mastered because cell examination requires it. The lens must be cleaned according to manufacturer's instructions, and dry objectives must not be exposed to oil.

Phase-contrast microscopy is used to perform manual platelet counts when automated counts are unreliable. For accurate counts the microscope must be checked periodically to be sure it is in phase. Fluorescence and electron microscopy are used mainly in research applications at present.

Troubleshooting microscope problems involves the identification of problems and taking appropriate corrective actions. Quality control and preventive maintenance are important to keep the microscope in top working condition.

REFERENCES

1. College of American Pathologists: Laboratory Instrument Verification and Maintenance Manual, 3rd ed. Skokie, IL, College of American Pathologists, 1982
2. Cormack DH: Introduction to Histology. Philadelphia, JB Lippincott, 1984
3. Culling CFA: Light microscopy—numerical aperture. Microscop Soc Can Bull 3(1):18, 1975
4. Culling CFA: Light microscopy—the phase contrast microscope. Microscop Soc Can Bull 3(2):11, 1975
5. Determann H, Lepusch F: The Microscope and Its Application. Rockleigh, NJ, E Leitz, Inc, Instrument Division, 1977
6. Hayat MA: Introduction to Biological Scanning Electron Microscopy. Baltimore, University Park Press, 1978
7. Holz HM: Worthwhile Facts about Fluorescence Microscopy. Thornwood, NY, Carl Zeiss, Inc, 1975
8. Klosevych S: Some observations at the back focal plane of microscope objectives. Microscop Soc Can Bull 14(3):13, 1986
9. Meek GA: Practical Electron Microscopy for Biologists, 2nd ed. New York, John Wiley & Sons, 1976
10. Michael BS, Lotspeich CA, Tryon CT: Introduction to the Microscope: Operation and Preventive Maintenance Using the Nikon Labophot. Guidebook accompanying 26-minute color videotape. Chapel Hill, Health Sciences Consortium, Inc, 1985
11. Mollring FK: Microscopy from the Very Beginning. Thornwood, NY, Carl Zeiss, Inc, 1981
12. Nikon Inc: Instruction Manual for the Labophot Biological Microscope. Garden City, NY, Nikon, Instrument Division, 1979
13. Olson JD, Moake JL, Collins MF et al: Adhesion of human platelets to purified solid-phase von Willebrand factor: Studies of normal and Bernard-Soulier platelets. Thrombosis Res 32:115, 1983
14. Olympus Corporation: Basics of the Optical Microscope. Lake Success, NY, Olympus, 1985
15. Olympus Corporation: Instruction Manual model BHTU Biological Microscope. Lake Success, NY, Olympus, 1989
16. Patzelt WJ: Polarized-Light Microscopy. Rochleigh, NJ, E Leitz, Inc, Instrument Division, 1977
17. Polaroid Corporation: The Effect of the Aperture Diaphragm Setting on the Image. Cambridge, MA, Polaroid, 1980
18. Polaroid Corporation: Koehler Illumination. Cambridge, MA, Polaroid, 1980
19. Polaroid Corporation: Special Contrast Enhancement Techniques—Transmitted Light Microscopy. Cambridge, MA, Polaroid, 1981
20. Schilling V: Basics concerning microscopy. Microscop Soc Can Bull 2(2):10, 1975
21. Wild–Heerbrugg Ltd: The Theory of Microscope Optics. Heerbrugg, Switzerland, Wild–Heerbrugg, 1972
22. Wilson MB: The Science and Art of Basic Microscopy. Washington, DC, American Society for Medical Technology, 1976

5

Hematopoiesis

and

Review

of Genetics

Vincent S. Gallicchio

HEMATOPOIETIC SYSTEM DEVELOPMENT

Blood cell production (hematopoiesis) encompasses the overall interactions of cellular proliferation, differentiation, morphogenesis, functional maturation, and death. Basically, the developmental pattern of embryogenesis that involves cellular differentiation is an orderly process of many morphologic and functional changes for which the regulatory mechanism is not understood. Many of the developmental patterns occur simultaneously in the embryo and fetus. Figure 5-1 provides a summary of the embryonic and fetal hematopoietic development process. The discussion below outlines three developmental periods—mesoblastic, hepatic, and myeloid.

Mesoblastic Period

Hematopoiesis begins during embryonic development in the blood islands of the yolk sac. These blood islands are first detected at approximately 19 to 20 days of gestation, and their appearance marks the beginning of the mesoblastic period of hematopoiesis. Most likely, blood islands develop from the mesodermal extraembryonic layer of the yolk sac. These blood islands remain active only through the 8 to the 12 week of gestation and are primarily responsible for red cell production (erythropoiesis), although areas of leukopoiesis and platelet production (megakaryocytopoiesis) have been identified. The immature red cells or erythroblasts produced by the yolk sac are unique in their morphology as well as the type of hemoglobin they produce. These cells constitute primitive hematopoietic cell lines and generally are not found after the third month of gestation. Primitive erythroblasts are large and cannot extrude their nucleus; erythroblasts of the later definitive series are smaller than the primitive series but still larger than the cells found in adults. The globin chains produced by primitive erythroblasts include epsilon (ε) and zeta (ζ), which are required for production of three embryonic forms of hemoglobin, Gower I, Gower II, and Portland (Chaps. 7 and 14).

Hepatic Period

Definitive morphologic hematopoiesis begins during the fifth and sixth weeks of gestation in the liver and marks the beginning of the hepatic period of hematopoiesis. At this point cells appear that are morphologically identifiable. The liver remains the primary site of blood cell production until the sixth month and may continue to produce blood cells, although to a much smaller degree, until the first or second week after birth. Because liver hemopoiesis is intravascular, infants normally have a few circulating nucleated red cells. At first the fetal liver is primarily an erythroid organ and produces red cells containing fetal hemoglobin (consisting of two alpha and two gamma globin chains) that is distinguishable from the embryonic hemoglobins. The production of granulocytes (granulopoiesis) and lymphocytes (lymphopoiesis) is minimal in the fetal liver. During the hepatic period, the spleen, thymus, and lymph nodes also become active in blood cell production. These other sites continue to produce lymphocytes throughout life.

The hematopoiesis of the fetal hepatic period is the counterpart of extramedullary hematopoiesis in the adult, which is blood cell production outside the bone marrow—mainly in the liver and spleen. Extramedullary hematopoiesis is rare, because adults normally have so much fatty marrow that can be reactivated if necessary. However, extramedullary hematopoiesis may be found in adults when the bone marrow fails to produce cells adequately.

Myeloid Period

During the fifth month of gestation, bone cavities begin to form, and bone marrow begins to assume responsibility as

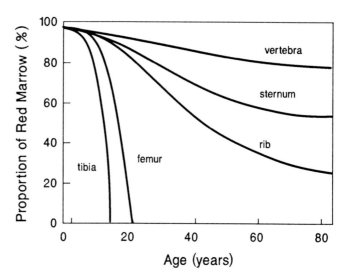

FIG. 5-2.   Sites of postnatal hematopoiesis.

the main site of blood cell production. This marks the beginning of the myeloid period. During this time hemoglobin A_1 (Hb A_1) consisting of two alpha and two beta globin chains, begins to appear and gradually increases in concentration. Most adult hemoglobin is Hb A_1 (Chap. 7).

After the first 3 weeks postpartum, the bone marrow becomes the only normal site of blood cell production and remains so throughout life. During the first few years of life, a delicate balance exists between developing bone marrow space and the developing infant's need for blood cells. Therefore, the hematopoietic capability of either the liver or spleen remains available. During the fourth year of life, the rate of bone marrow growth exceeds the need for blood cells. Therefore, active marrow sites are replaced with areas of fatty reserve.[52] Fat first develops in the shafts of long bones until the age of 18 years when the only active hematopoietic sites are in the pelvis, vertebrae, ribs, sternum, skull, and proximal extremities of the long bones (Fig. 5-2). If necessary fatty marrow may be reactivated for hematopoiesis in a relatively short time. Normally, however, there is a gradual increase in marrow fatty tissue throughout life.

BONE MARROW VOLUME AND ANATOMY

The volume of bone marrow increases from 1.5% of body weight at birth to about 4.5% in the adult. However, the blood volume actually decreases from 8% of total body weight at birth to 7% in the adult.

Anatomically, bone marrow consists of a pattern of vessels and nerves, differentiated and undifferentiated hematopoietic cells, reticuloendothelial cells, and fatty tissue, all of which are encased by the endosteum, which is a membrane lining the marrow cavity of the bone. The vascular system consists of a network of arterioles that empty into a complex system of venous sinusoids, which drain into a central collecting vein (Fig. 5-3).

The venous sinusoids are composed of an endothelial cell network with intermittent fat cells and adventitial cells (considered to be phagocytic) that support the sinusoidal walls (Fig. 5-4). The endothelium is a complete layer of

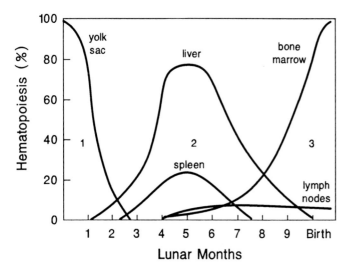

FIG. 5-1.   Sites of prenatal hematopoiesis. (1) Mesoblastic. (2) Hepatic. (3) Myeloid.

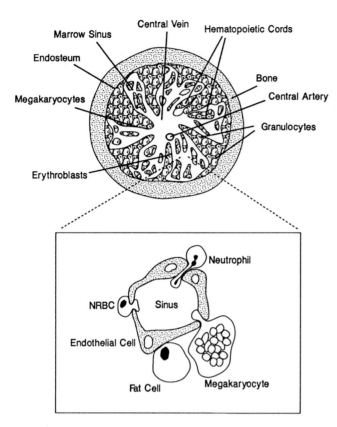

FIG. 5-3. Anatomy of bone marrow as a cross-section of bone with active marrow.

cells attached to one another at their edges. Usually the endothelium is one cell thick. The basement membrane is markedly deficient, being absent from large stretches of the sinusoidal wall and, when present, irregular in thickness and density. It is lacking in areas where cells are in direct passage. The elevated and rarefied adventitial cells of the sinus are phagocytic and form the outer portion of the sinus walls. They are classified as reticular cells—a form of connective tissue. The adventitial process is part of the adventitial layer that extends into the surrounding marrow parenchyma. Apertures are areas within endothelial cells where hematopoietic cells pass rather than through intracellular gaps. The trilaminar and unilaminar sinus walls form the lining of the marrow parenchyma and differ only in thickness.

Primary blood cell formation occurs outside the sinusoids in the hematopoietic cords, which have an intimate relation with the sinuses. Mature cells are capable of deforming such that they may pass through narrow sievelike openings in the endothelial vascular lining before entering the bone marrow sinuses and circulation (see Fig. 5-3). This structure of the marrow facilitates nuclear extrusion from the erythroblast and may also control the release of newly formed red cells.

The bone marrow system is also connected with an extensive nerve network. Many of these nerves are in close contact with hematopoietic blood cells. Pressure exerted by proliferative demands may produce signals transmitted by the nervous system, resulting in autoregulation of blood cell production.[13]

STEM CELL THEORIES AND CELL PRODUCTION

The replenishment of blood cells is dependent on the presence of undifferentiated hematopoietic cells termed stem cells. Such cells have a high degree of proliferative capability. Evidence from many studies has demonstrated that all hematopoietic cells originate from a common cell termed the pluripotential stem cell.

Pluripotential Stem Cells

A quantitative assay for pluripotential hematopoietic stem cells was developed in 1961.[50] Colony-forming unit–spleen (CFU-S) is the term applied to this stem cell, which may look like a lymphocyte.[3] The term was derived from the observation that bone marrow stem cells, after injection into lethally irradiated syngeneic recipient mice, form colonies in the animals' spleens after 7 to 9 days. The CFU-S colonies include erythrocytes, granulocytes, monocytes, and megakaryocytes.

The CFU-S has an extensive self-maintenance capability that does not appear to decline with age. The cell appears to proceed slowly through the cell cycle (Fig. 5-5) with a 1-week transit time, spending most of the time in the portion known as G_0.[2,29] Some cells move continuously around the cell cycle, whereas others leave the cycle temporarily to enter the limbo or resting state (G_0). The long G_0 phase allows time for DNA repair.[7] Other cells leave the cycle and die without dividing again. The population of pluripotential stem cells, often referred to as the stem cell pool, provides adequate numbers for differentiation into the various cell lines at different rates depending on the demand and the amount of stem cells in reserve.

Although a number of studies have not found a common stem cell for all cells, evidence indicates the existence of a cell called the "totipotent hematopoietic stem cell" (THSC) that gives rise to both a myeloid (CFU-S) and a lymphoid stem cell.[28] This leads to the current theory of stem cells and their progenitors (Fig. 5-6).

Committed Stem Cells

The CFU-S gives rise to descendants or progeny cells that eventually become restricted to a specific line of development. Under appropriate conditions, stem cells continue their differentiation only along a specific pathway—they lose their potential to develop as any other cell lineage. This loss is termed "commitment." Therefore, descendants of CFU-S committed to the granulocyte (G)–monocyte/macrophage (M) lineage are termed CFU-GM. They have limited proliferative capacity.[4,22,34,40] Erythroid progenitors, termed "burst-forming units–erythroid" (BFU-E), are the erythroid equivalent of the CFU-GM and are considered to be related closely to CFU-S.[1] The other erythroid progenitor, colony-forming unit–erythroid (CFU-E), is found late in the erythroid maturation sequence.

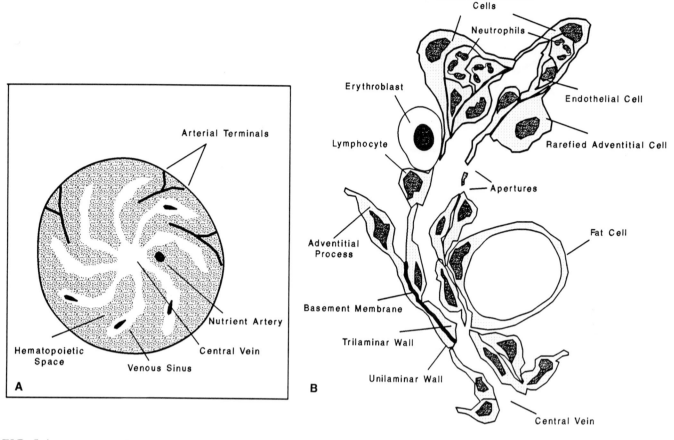

FIG. 5-4.   Anatomy of a bone marrow sinus. (*A*) Anatomy of the marrow as a cross-section of a marrow sinus into which various cell types pass through the endothelial cell network on their way to the circulation. (*B*) View of the sinus down the central vein.

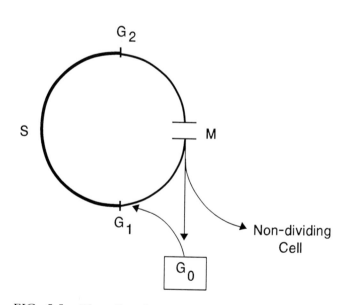

FIG. 5-5.   The cell cycle. G_0—limbo or resting stage; G_1—postmitotic, presynthetic stage; S—DNA synthesis stage; G_2—postsynthetic, premitotic stage; M—mitosis.

Less well defined but also considered to be committed stem cells are the megakaryocyte colony-forming unit (CFU-Meg) and eosinophil (and possibly basophil) colony-forming unit (CFU-Eo).[11] Likewise, the lymphoid stem cell is committed to lymphocyte production (Chap. 24).

REGULATION OF STEM CELL DEVELOPMENT—GROWTH FACTORS AND HORMONES

Pluripotential (CFU-S) Development

Many *in vitro* studies have demonstrated effects of humoral agents on CFU-S. Phytohemagglutinin (PHA),[8] cyclophosphamide,[17] and concanavalin A[47] all have positive effects on CFU-S. These effects are variable, including an increase in CFU-S number,[8,30] an increase in survival[3] or protection from death,[17] and an increase in proliferation.[17] Inhibitors of CFU-S proliferation have been demonstrated also, including hydroxyurea.[46] The physiologic significance of these inhibitors versus stimulators remains unclear.

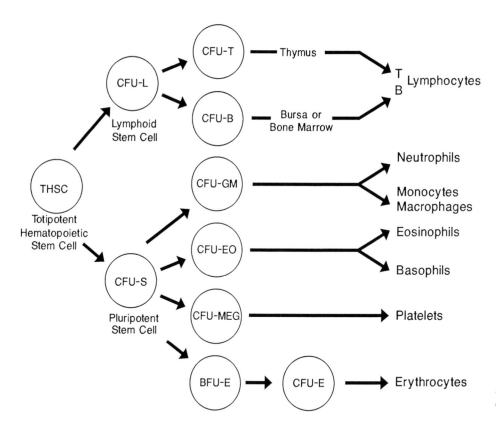

FIG. 5-6. The hematopoietic stem cell and progenitor systems.

Granulopoiesis

Granulopoiesis is the production of monocytes and granulocytes, including neutrophils, eosinophils, and basophils. Infection is the main stimulus for the generation of large numbers of neutrophils and monocytes in a short time and a restricted volume of tissue space. Neutrophils fight infection, as do eosinophils and basophils to a lesser degree. The response to microbial invasion entails at least three mechanisms. First, granulocytes and monocytes are recruited into and around the infected tissue by the release of chemotactic factors. Second, granulocytes and monocytes stored in the marrow are mobilized and released into the blood. Third, this response initiates accelerated cellular production to satisfy the increased demand (Chaps. 22, 23, and 26).

The processes that regulate granulocyte production, specifically that of neutrophils, are orderly, originating from the pluripotential stem cell, CFU-S, through to still cytologically unidentifiable committed stem cell precursors referred to as CFU-GM stem cells. These cells have the capability of expanding exponentially in total number and then developing into morphologically recognizable granulocyte–monocyte/macrophage progenitors with the capability for a few more mitotic divisions. Once the cell has made a commitment to the CFU-GM pathway, this process is irreversible, and it provides an adequate population of nondividing granulocytes, monocytes, and macrophages capable of eliminating and destroying potential pathogens.

Maintenance and sustained proliferation of the CFU-GM colony *in vitro* requires the continual presence of one of a number of molecules collectively termed colony-stimulating factors (CSF). Macrophages are an important source of CSF capable of promoting CFU-GM proliferation. The physiologic, biologic, and hematologic significance of CSF has been the subject of recent reviews[32,33] and studies.[21] The CSF may be responsible for regulation of granulopoiesis *in vivo*.[32,34] Negative feedback inhibitors of granulopoiesis may act *in vivo* and *in vitro*,[5,6] although more recent evidence concerning these proposed inhibitors brings their true physiologic significance into question.[12,45]

Eosinophils, and possibly basophils, are derived in granulopoiesis from a committed stem cell termed CFU-Eo. Eosinophils are bone marrow-derived cells that suppress the immunoinflammatory reaction and prevent its spread. Eosinophils also play a role in host defense because of their ability to phagocytize and kill invasive metazoan parasites. Basophils constitute a small fraction of the total body granulocyte pool and thus have been difficult to study (Chap. 23). They exhibit chemotaxis and some phagocytosis. Basophils contain all of the blood histamine and degranulate to release their contents in allergic reactions.

Erythropoiesis

The mature red cell is a highly specialized end-stage cell whose function is to maintain an adequate supply of oxygen in the tissues. It is eventually phagocytized by the reticuloendothelial system. Therefore, the production of new erythrocytes constantly needs to be regulated.

During the last several years, new information has focused on the dynamics of erythrocyte production. More primitive red cell precursors, not identifiable by light microscopy, have been detected by assays that measure the precursors' ability to produce new red cells.

Red cell production normally is dependent on a continual efflux of cells from the pluripotential stem cell compartment into the red cell pathway. During red cell differentiation, cells pass through at least 10 successive generations (Chap. 6). There is evidence that each sequential stage of red cell differentiation coincides with a decrease in proliferative capacity.

The process of producing mature cells from primitive erythroid precursors apparently involves the activation of certain genes that normally are not expressed in other cell types. An example is the genes responsible for the production of globin chains, which are confined to red cells. Red cell differentiation appears to be under a strict set of controls because at any given stage, the cells are phenotypically identical.

Erythropoiesis is regulated by the glycoprotein hormone erythropoietin, which is present in normal serum in concentrations that vary according to the oxygen-carrying capacity of the blood. Erythropoietin is a single-chain acidic glycoprotein with a molecular weight of 40,000 and a carbohydrate content of approximately 30%.[36] It augments erythropoiesis by stimulating the production of new erythroblastic cells synthesizing hemoglobin, whether in vivo or in vitro. These cells are unable to produce hemoglobin when erythropoietin is absent.

Culture systems exist to assay for the primitive erythropoietic precursor stem cells and usually require the recognition of erythroblast colonies or other more differentiated red cell types.[1,20,25] In vitro studies have demonstrated two types of erythroid progenitor stem cells capable of clonality, BFU-E[1] and CFU-E; the latter is also called colony-forming unit dependent on the hormone erythropoietin.[48] The BFU-E are more primitive than the CFU-E and have a number of phenotypic differences. Characteristically, BFU-E form large colonies after a long period of incubation with a high concentration of erythropoietin.[8] These colonies were described as "bursts" because of their appearance.[1] In contrast, CFU-E form small clusters consisting of 8 to 32 cells. CFU-E are the target cells for erythropoietin.[1]

Megakaryocytopoiesis

The blood platelet plays an important role in hemostasis and the development of thrombosis. Platelets originate from the megakaryocyte in the bone marrow.

Although many of the physiologic mechanisms that control both platelet and megakaryocyte production remain elusive, it appears that platelet production may be regulated by humoral factors.[14] Plasma harvested from severely thrombocytopenic animals (i.e., animals with very low platelet counts) contains a factor that significantly increases platelet production in recipient animals. This factor has been termed thrombopoietin or thrombopoiesis-stimulating factor.[16,23] The true physiologic role of thrombopoietin in megakaryocytopoiesis remains to be determined because of its inability to increase platelet counts when administered to normal animals, and to increase the size or protein content of individual platelets.

Much of the recent information on megakaryocytopoiesis has been obtained through in vitro clonal stem-cell assays

for the megakaryocyte precursor stem cell CFU-Meg.[26] Many in vitro investigations have clearly demonstrated the inability of erythropoietin, thrombopoietin, and CSF to induce CFU-Meg colony formation. This implies a regulatory molecule that may be important in the early events of megakaryocytopoiesis.[24] This molecule may be analogous to the action of the growth factors involved in erythropoiesis (Chap. 6).

More recently a factor that significantly increases CFU-Meg colony formation has been identified in the serum or plasma of patients having hypomegakaryocytic thrombocytopenia.[15,28] It appears that this factor, termed megakaryocyte colony-stimulating factor (Meg-CSF), responds to the number of bone marrow megakaryocytes rather than the peripheral blood platelet count. Meg-CSF has been purified from the plasma of a patient with selective hypomegakaryocytic thrombocytopenia[42] and proved to be a glycoprotein with a molecular weight of 46,000. Meg-CSF has no effect on other stem cells in vitro (e.g., BFU-E, CFU-E, or CFU-GM).

Lymphopoiesis

Lymphocytes provide for the immune defense of the body. There are two distinct classes, based on their functional characteristics, T lymphocytes and B lymphocytes. T lymphocytes mature in the thymus gland and then are distributed to the peripheral tissues, where they can react directly with antigens to become specific cells responsible for reactions that produce delayed-type hypersensitivity, graft rejection, tumor suppression, and resistance generally called cellular immunity. B lymphocytes originate in the bone marrow and then migrate to the peripheral tissues, where they can interact with antigens. This interaction produces plasma cells, which have the responsibility of producing immunoglobulins or antibodies. This line of resistance is generally referred to as humoral immunity. A third distinct class in the heterogeneous population of lymphocytes is the non-T, non-B cells, usually referred to as null cells (Chap. 24).

Current understanding of the regulatory mechanism of lymphocyte proliferation has resulted from laboratory studies of T and B lymphocytes in culture.

T Lymphocytes

Currently used T-cell clonal assays usually require a one-step method where the cell preparations are incubated in the presence of a mitogen (mitosis-stimulating plant protein), usually PHA. The ability of lymphocytes to clone in these in vitro assays was suggested to differ from that of other hematopoietic cell lines because it appeared that T cells were able to secrete their own necessary growth factor when plated in the presence of mitogen, whereas the other blood cells (with the exception of macrophages) require the addition of their specific growth hormone (e.g., erythropoietin, CSF, Meg-CSF, or BPA [burst-promoting activity—a growth factor associated with BFU-E]). Therefore, it appears that lymphocytes that have become blastlike because of mitogen exposure can release a growth factor and that production of this factor by T cells can be accelerated by monocytes or macrophages. More recent studies suggest that the T-cell growth factor is interleukin-2 (IL-2).[44]

B Lymphocytes

Understanding of the mechanism that regulates B-cell proliferation has come from the ability to clone B-cell precursors *in vitro*.[35] These clones require stimulation by a B-cell activator such as a bacterial lipopolysaccharide (LPS), a purified protein derivative, or dextran sulfate. Identification of B-cell progenitors has come from studies using inbred congenitally athymic (nude) mice, which are deficient in functional T cells. Stimulation of their lymphocytes by LPS induces the presence of colonies whose B-cell nature can be confirmed by the presence of cell surface-derived immunoglobulins. A B-cell growth factor is required, which usually can be provided by incubating mononuclear blood cells with mitogen for 72 hours. The requirement for B-cell growth factor is independent of the factor required for T-cell proliferation. IL-2 does not induce B-cell proliferation.

REVIEW OF GENETICS

Many genetic terms and definitions are important to understanding the origin of some hematologic disorders. The following discussion serves as a basic genetics reference for this text.

Genetics is the study of heredity, which is the transmission of physical traits from parents to offspring. The differences and resemblances among organisms related by descent are determined by the nuclear information in the gametes or sex cells of an organism. The nucleus houses genes, which are present on structures called chromosomes. Normal human cells contain 46 chromosomes, which may be divided into 22 different pairs of identical chromosomes (autosomes) and one pair of sex chromosomes (female: XX; male: XY). The chromosomes of each pair are referred to as homologous. One of each pair is derived from each of two parents.

Chromosomes make up the chromatin of the nucleus and provide information necessary for production of all substances and structures in the cell. The nucleic acid DNA is the primary constituent of chromosomes and allows for the passing on of inherited characteristics from generation to generation.

Mitosis and Meiosis

When the human sperm and egg meet for fertilization, a zygote is formed and begins development. This process requires two types of cell division: mitosis and meiosis.

Mitosis

Mitosis is the process of cell division that permits the number of cells in an organism to increase or be maintained as necessary. More specifically, mitosis provides for the production of two daughter cells having the same number and type of chromosomes as the parent cell.

Mitosis consists of four stages: prophase, metaphase, anaphase, and telophase. Between mitoses, a cell is in interphase or the resting phase (see Fig. 5-4). During mitotic division the cell cytoplasm simply cleaves into two approx-

imately equal halves, but the nucleus undergoes a complicated sequence of activities. Details on the stages of mitosis may be found in textbooks on genetics.

Meiosis

Meiosis is the cell division process whereby the daughter cells receive only half the chromosome number of the parent. This process manufactures the gametes or sex cells, which in humans require only 23 chromosomes (referred to as the haploid number). Fertilization of an egg by a spermatozoan restores the diploid (46 chromosome) number.

Formation of gametes by meiosis requires a two-phase process, meiosis I and II. Meiosis I is the pairing, replication, and subsequent separation of homologous pairs. Meiosis II involves four stages: prophase, metaphase, anaphase, and telophase. In humans, diploid cells going through meiosis I and II produce haploid cells with 23 single chromosomes—half the number found in cells produced by mitosis. Details on the stages of meiosis I and II may be found in textbooks on genetics.

The Genetic Code

The basic genetic material is DNA (deoxyribonucleic acid). It contains the plans for cellular protein synthesis and is composed of two polynucleotide chains formed in a double helix. The polynucleotide chains consist of a variable sequence of two purines, adenine (A) and guanine (G), and two pyrimidines, thymine (T) and cytosine (C). Purines and pyrimidines are matched in a sequence that is referred to as base pairing. For example, A binds with T and G binds with C. This pairing is obligatory and allows the DNA molecule to replicate itself precisely by separation of its strands and the formation of two new complementary strands.

The genetic code in its most basic form consists of sequences of three bases, each referred to as a *triplet* or *codon*, which directs the addition to a growing peptide or protein of a particular amino acid. For example, the codon CTC codes for glutamic acid, ATA codes for tyrosine, and AAA codes for phenylalanine. A gene is a sequence of codons that together encode the unique sequence of amino acids that create a particular protein.

The link between the DNA code and the cytoplasm where proteins are manufactured is messenger RNA (mRNA), a single strand of polynucleotides that is formed from the DNA template by an enzyme, RNA polymerase. mRNA migrates to the cytoplasm, where its message is read by ribosomal RNA (rRNA) and transfer RNA (tRNA), which collects and transfers the proper amino acids to the proper ribosome area.

Alterations or misreading of the DNA code may or may not produce mutations that result in disease. Examples of disorders in hematology include a mutation causing an amino acid substitution in the hemoglobin molecule producing hemoglobinopathies (*e.g.*, sickle cell anemia) (Chap. 14); mispairing of homologous chromosomes followed by nonhomologous crossing over of DNA segments between sister chromatids of a dyad during meiosis (*e.g.*, hemoglobin Lepore) (Chap. 15); mutation in the terminal codon of mRNA that permits abnormal addition of amino acids to a given sequence for protein production (*e.g.*, hemoglobin Constant Spring) (Chap. 14); unstable or defective mRNA or gene deletion (*e.g.*, thalassemias) (Chap. 15); mutation or defect of specific regulatory genes (*e.g.*, hereditary persistence of fetal hemoglobin) (Chap. 15); and disruption of postsynthetic modifications of proteins (*e.g.*, pyruvate kinase deficiency) (Chap. 17).

Genetic Terminology

All of the previously discussed disorders are hereditary. Thus a basic understanding of genetic terminology will be helpful in studying hematologic abnormalities.

A *hereditary* or *inherited* condition is always transmitted genetically but may or may not be detectable at birth. For example, pernicious anemia (Chap. 12) may be hereditary but is usually first detected in adult life.

A *congenital* condition is one that is present at birth although it may or may not be detectable then. It need not be hereditary. For example, a baby born deaf because of *in utero* exposure to rubella virus during the first trimester has a congenital condition that was not caused by genetic transmission and is thus not hereditary.

Although genes on a homologous chromosome pair code for the same trait, there are often alternate trait forms, such as blue or brown eyes or blood group A or B. Two genes in a homologous pair are referred to as *alleles* and may code for the same or alternate forms of a trait. An individual having two alleles for a particular genetic trait (*e.g.*, one allele for blue eyes, the other for brown) is said to be *heterozygous*. An individual with identical genes for a given homologous pair from each parent (e.g., both genes code for blue eyes) is *homozygous* for that trait.

Genotype is dependent on the type of alleles present on the chromosome pair. For example, for blood groups the genotype may be AA, AO, or AB. The *phenotype* of an individual is the morphologic, physiologic, or biochemical expression of the genotype. For example, a person will express blood group O only if both alleles coding for blood group are O. That is, the person must have the homozygous genotype OO to have the phenotype O. On the other hand, a person with the heterozygous genotype AO will have the phenotype A: the blood will type as group A just like the blood of a person with the homozygous genotype AA.

The phenotype concept becomes more clear with an understanding of the terms *dominant* and *recessive*. An allele is dominant (*e.g.*, blood group allele A) when it is expressed regardless of whether the genotype is homozygous or heterozygous. A recessive allele, on the other hand, is expressed phenotypically only when the genotype is homozygous (*e.g.*, blood group allele O).

Probability and Patterns of Gene Transmission

The genetic laws of probability determine the patterns of genetic transmission. Consider a hypothetical crossing of two parents who are each heterozygous for the trait T, making their genotypes Tt. Assume that T is dominant and associated with tall height and that t is recessive and represents short height. Figure 5-7 shows a Punnett square (developed by R. C. Punnett in the early 1900s), which helps to visualize the probable genetic composition. The genetic characteristics of one parent are placed at the top of the square and those of the other down the side. The possible

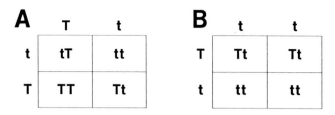

FIG. 5-7. Punnett square showing genetic probabilities. (*A*) Both parents are heterozygous for height (Tt). The resulting probability square indicates that most likely, 3/4 of the offspring will be tall (1/4 tT, 1/4 TT, 1/4 Tt) and 1/4 short (tt). (*B*) A heterozygous (Tt) and a homozygous (tt) parent; 1/2 of the offspring are expected to be tall and 1/2 short.

combinations for the zygote are then figured in the resulting squares. Note that the expected ratios are probabilities, not certainties; offspring of these two hypothetical parents could turn out to be all tall or all short.

There are four basic patterns of gene transmission important to understanding the inheritance of hematologic abnormalities: (1) autosomal dominant (*e.g.*, hereditary spherocytosis) (Chap. 17); (2) autosomal recessive (*e.g.*, pyruvate kinase deficiency) (Chap. 17); (3) X-linked or sex-linked dominant (no well-known hematologic disorders in this category); and (4) X-linked or sex-linked recessive (*e.g.*, hemophilia) (Chap. 55). Autosomal transmission refers to transmission by any of the 22 pairs of chromosomes not involved in the determination of sex. Sex-linked transmission is synonymous with X-linked (the X chromosome). That is, genes associated with the X chromosome are sex-linked. The Y chromosome has few if any proven loci other than those determining the male sex. Because the Y chromosome is basically inert, any allele present on the male's single X chromosome will be expressed phenotypically. Thus, X-linked traits are more commonly expressed in men than women. Each pattern is defined below. In the autosomal dominant pattern, the dominant trait generally appears in every generation without skipping and is transmitted by an affected person to at least half of his or her offspring. The trait is expressed whether the genotype is homozygous or heterozygous. A hypothetical case of a heterozygous Tt parent and a homozygous recessive (tt) parent is shown in Figure 5-7B. In the autosomal recessive pattern the zygote must receive two identical alleles for a trait, one from each parent, for expression of that trait to occur. In Figure 5-7B the offspring with the tt genotype provide an example of an autosomal recessive trait that would be exhibited phenotypically as short height because the genotype is homozygous recessive.

In the X-linked dominant pattern, the genetic abnormality is present on the X chromosome and is dominant. Consequently, both males and females will express the abnormality. As with any X-linked abnormality, a father with an abnormal X chromosome will transfer this abnormality to all of his daughters, but it is impossible to transmit the abnormality from father to son because the Y chromosome is normal. Affected heterozygous females are expected to transmit the trait to half of their children. Homozygous females transmit the trait to all of their children. In the X-linked recessive pattern, expression is far more common in males than females because males are affected by a single

X chromosome whereas female expression requires homozygosity. Hemophilia is a classic blood disorder in this category. The trait is passed from affected males by way of their single abnormal X chromosome to all daughters, who may transfer the abnormality to half of their offspring, male or female. X-linked recessive traits may never be passed directly from father to son because the Y chromosome is normal. The extent of expression of an X-linked disorder in a female heterozygote (carrier) can vary considerably because of random and fixed inactivation of one of the two X chromosomes during early embryonic life (Lyon hypothesis).

CYTOGENETICS

Cytogenetics is the structural analysis of chromosomes. The examination of chromosomes in blood cells can provide information important to the diagnosis and prognosis of leukemias, lymphomas, and related disorders. Figure 5-8 depicts a normal human male karyotype showing each of the 22 autosomal chromosome pairs with the sex chromosomes (XY) in the lower right corner. The chromosomes are matched according to their relative size and centromere location. Each pair has been assigned a unique number for karyotyping purposes.

The procedure for developing a karyotype involves culturing malignant hematopoietic tissue to obtain dividing cells in the metaphase stage, where the mitotic process is stopped and the cells are fixed. These cells are dropped onto a clean microscope slide where the chromosomes fall in a random pattern. The slides are then specially stained, usually with Giemsa or quinicrine, to allow for chromosome banding, which is necessary to identify any chromosomal abnormality. Giemsa colors certain discrete and unique bands (G bands); quinicrine likewise stains specific bands (Q bands). Whichever stain is used, the banding pattern is unique for every chromosome pair. Once stained the chromosomes may be photomicrographed. From this photograph the chromosomes are cut out and placed on the karyotype board for study. Figure 5-8 depicts normal G-banded chromosomes that have been placed in the correct positions on the board.

Karyotype study may reveal many types of abnormalities. For example, chromosomes may be totally deleted, or extra ones may be discovered. Parts of chromosomes may be added, deleted, inverted, or translocated (moved from one chromosome to another). Many abnormalities relate to the long (q) arm or the short (p) arm of a given chromosome.

The Philadelphia chromosome is a classic hematologic example of a diagnostic and prognostic karyotypic abnormality. It is found in chronic myelogenous leukemia and usually results from a translocation that is technically described as $t(9q^+ \cdot 22q^-)$, which means that the long (q) arm of chromosome 22 has translocated to the long (q) arm of

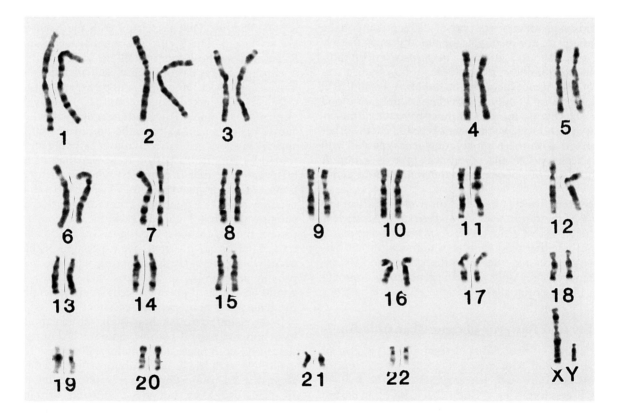

FIG. 5-8. Normal G-banded male karyotype. (With the permission of Ann Cork, Assistant Clinical Cytogeneticist, Section of Cytogenetics, and Dr. J M Trujillo, Head, Division of Laboratory Medicine and Chief, Section of Cytogenetics, The University of Texas System Cancer Center, MD Anderson Hospital and Tumor Institute, Houston, TX.)

chromosome 9 (Chap. 35). Note that the lower chromosome number is always written first, whether it has received or lost the arm. Another common translocation in leukemias and lymphomas is t($8q^-$;$14q^+$), which refers to translocation from the long arm of chromosome 8 to the long arm of chromosome 14. An abnormality receiving increasing attention in hematology is $5q^-$, which represents deletion of the long arm of chromosome 5.

CHAPTER SUMMARY

Development of the hematopoietic system has three defined periods: (1) the early, mesoblastic period; (2) the hepatic period (the counterpart of extramedullary hematopoiesis in the adult); and (3) the myeloid period, which continues throughout normal life.

The bone marrow is anatomically equipped for cellular development and for regulation of the release of mature cells. In the bone marrow the pluripotential stem cell is found. All blood cells except lymphocytes are believed to be derived from this cell. Lymphocytes are produced from the lymphoid stem cell. Both of these stem cells are thought to come from a primitive stem cell known as the totipotent stem cell.

Growth factors and hormones are necessary for pluripotential stem cell development, as well as for maturation of those committed stem cells involved in production of granulocytes, lymphocytes, erythrocytes, and megakaryocytes. Colony-stimulating factors may be responsible for regulating granulocyte production, although these factors are still poorly understood. Three classes of lymphocytes exist: B, T, and null cells. The T cell can produce its own growth factor, whereas B cells require outside stimulation. Erythrocyte production is regulated by the hormone erythropoietin. There are two types of erythroid progenitors that produce red cells: the burst-forming unit–erythroid (BFU-E) and the colony-forming unit–erythroid (CFU-E). Regulation of megakaryocyte production may be linked to a substance called thrombopoietin.

Concepts of genetics were reviewed in this chapter to provide a basis for understanding the inheritance of many hematologic abnormalities. The terms defined were genes, chromosomes, alleles, mitosis, meiosis, hereditary, congenital, heterozygous, homozygous, genotype, phenotype, dominant, and recessive. Probability and patterns of gene transmission were defined.

Cytogenetic study provides a useful tool in the diagnosis of leukemias, lymphomas, and related disorders. A normal human karyotype includes 22 autosomal chromosome pairs and the sex chromosomes. Chromosomes may be deleted, inverted, or translocated. Extra chromosomes may also be discovered in a karyotype study.

REFERENCES

1. Axelrad AA, McLeod DL, Shreeve MM et al: Properties of cells that produce erythrocytic colonies in vitro. In Robinson WA (ed): Hemopoiesis in Culture, p 226. Washington, DC, US Government Printing Office, 1974
2. Becker AJ, McCulloch EA, Siminovitch L et al: The effect of different demands for blood cell population in DNA synthesis by haemopoietic colony forming cells of mice. Blood 26:296, 1986
3. Blackburn MJ, Patt HM: Increased survival of haemopoietic pluripotent stem cells in vitro induced by a marrow fibroblast factor. Br J Haematol 37:337, 1977
4. Bradley TR, Metcalf D: The growth of mouse bone marrow cells in vitro. Aust J Exp Biol Med Sci 44:287, 1966
5. Broxmeyer HE: Inhibition in vivo of mouse granulopoiesis by cell-free activity derived from human polymorphonuclear neutrophils. Blood 51:899, 1978
6. Broxmeyer HE, Smithyman A, Egar RR et al: Identification of lactoferrin as the granulocyte-derived inhibitor of colony stimulating activity production. J Exp Med 148:1052, 1978
7. Cairns J: Mutation selection and the natural history of cancer. Nature 225:197, 1975
8. Cerny J: Stimulation of bone marrow haemopoietic stem cells by a factor from activated T-cells. Nature 249:63, 1974
9. Cronkite EP, Bond VP, Fliedner TM et al: The use of tritiated thymidine in the study of hemopoietic cell proliferation. In Wolsternholme GEW, O'Connor M (eds): Ciba Foundation Symposium on Hematopoiesis, p 92. London, J and A Churchill, 1960
10. Curry JL, Trentin JG: Hemopoietic spleen colony studies. I: Growth and differentiation. Dev Biol 15:395, 1967
11. Denburg JA, Telizyn S, Messner H et al: Heterogeneity of human peripheral blood eosinophil-type colonies: Evidence for a common basophil–eosinophil progenitor. Blood 66:312, 1985
12. Dezza L, Cazzola M, Piacibello W et al: Effect of acidic and basic isoferritins on in vitro growth of human granulocyte–monocyte progenitors. Blood 67:789, 1986
13. Drinker CK, Drinker KR, Lund CC: The circulation in the mammalian bone marrow. Am J Physiol 62:1, 1922
14. Ebbe S: Thrombopoietin. Blood 44:605, 1974
15. Enomoto K, Kawakita M, Koshimoto S et al: Thrombopoiesis and megakaryocytic colony stimulating factor in the serum of patients with aplastic anaemia. Br J Haematol 45:551, 1980
16. Evatt BL, Levin J: Measurement of thrombopoiesis in rabbits using ^{72}selenomethionine. J Clin Invest 48:1615, 1969
17. Fliedner TM, Cronkite EP, Robertson JS: Granulocytopoiesis. I: Senescence and random loss of neutrophilic granulocytes in human beings. Blood 24:402, 1964
18. Fliedner TM, Cronkite EP, Killman SA et al: Granulocytopoiesis. II: Emergence and pattern of labelling of neutrophilic granulocytes in human beings. Blood 24:402, 1964
19. Fried W, Barone–Varelas J, Helfgott M et al: Effect of plasma from cyclophosphamide-treated mice on CFU-S in an in vivo culture system. Blood 56:940, 1980
20. Gallicchio VS, Murphy MJ Jr: In vitro erythropoiesis II. Cytochemical enumeration of erythroid stem cells (CFU-E and BFU-E) from normal mouse and human hematopoietic tissues. Exp Hematol 7:219, 1979
21. Gough NM, Gough J, Metcalf D et al: Molecular cloning of cDNA encoding a murine haemopoietic growth regulator, granulocyte-macrophage colony stimulating factor. Nature 309:763, 1984
22. Gregory CG: Erythropoietin sensitivity as a differentiation marker in the hemopoietic system: Studies of three erythropoietic colony responses in culture. J Cell Physiol 89:289, 1976
23. Harker LA: Control of platelet production. Annu Rev Med 25:383, 1974
24. Hoffman R, Mazur E, Bruno E et al: Assay of an activity in the serum of patients with disorders of thrombopoiesis that stimulates formation of megakaryocytic colonies. N Engl J Med 305:533, 1981
25. Iscove NN: The role of erythropoietin in regulation of population size and cell cycling of early and late erythroid precursors in mouse bone marrow. Cell Tiss Kinet 10:323, 1977
26. Jackson CW: Cholinesterase as a possible marker for early cells of the megakaryocyte series. Blood 42:413, 1973
27. Kaplan J: Myeloid colony forming cells express human B-lymphocyte antigens. Nature 271:458, 1978
28. Kawakita M, Miyake T, Kishimoto S et al: Apparent heterogeneity of human megakaryocyte colony- and thrombopoiesis-

stimulating factors: Studies on urinary extracts from patients with aplastic anaemia and idiopathic thrombocytopenic purpura. Br J Haematol 52:429, 1982

29. Lajtha LG: Stem cell concepts. Differentiation 14:23, 1979

30. Lord BI, Mori KJ, Wright EG: A stimulation of stem cell proliferation in regenerating bone marrow. Biomedicine 27:223, 1977

31. Mazur EM, Hoffman R, Chasis J et al: Immunofluorescent identification of human megakaryocyte colonies using an antiplatelet glycoprotein antiserum. Blood 57:277, 1981

32. Metcalf D: The Hemopoietic Colony Stimulating Factors. Amsterdam, Elsevier, 1984

33. Metcalf D: The molecular biology and functions of the granulocyte–macrophage colony stimulating factors. Blood 67:257, 1986

34. Metcalf D, Burgess AW: Analysis of progenitor commitment to granulocyte or macrophage production. J Cell Physiol 111:275, 1982

35. Metcalf D, Warner NL, Nassal GJV et al: Growth of B-lymphocyte colonies in vitro from mouse lymphoid organs. Nature 255:630, 1975

36. Miyaki T, Kung CKH, Goldwasser E: Purification of human erythropoietin. J Biol Chem 252:5558, 1977

37. Moffatt DJ, Rosse C, Yoffey JM Jr: Identity of the hematopoietic stem cell. Lancet 2:547, 1967

38. Nakahata T, Gross AJ, Ogawa M: A stochastic model of self-renewal and commitment to differentiation of the primary hemopoietic stem cells in culture. J Cell Physiol 113:455, 1982

39. Nakahata T, Ogawa M: Identification in culture of a new class of hematopoietic colony-forming units with extensive capability to self-renew and generate multipotential colonies. Proc Natl Acad Sci USA 29:3843, 1982

40. Pluznik DH, Sach L: The cloning of normal mast cells in tissue culture. J Cell Comp Physiol 66:319, 1965

41. Rosendaal M, Hodgson GS, Bradley TR: Haemopoietic stem cells are organised for use on the basis of their generation-age. Nature 264:68, 1976

42. Rozenszajn LA, Shoham D, Kalechman I: Clonal proliferation of PHA-stimulated human lymphocytes in soft agar cultures. Immunology 29:1041, 1975

43. Rozenszajn LA, Zeevi A, Gopas J et al: Lymphocyte colony growth in vitro. ICN-UCLA Symp Mol Cell Biol 10:261, 1978

44. Ruscetti FW, Gallo RC: Human T-lymphocyte growth factor: Regulation of growth and function of T lymphocytes [review]. Blood 57:379, 1981

45. Sala G, Worwood M, Jacobs A: The effect of isoferritins on granulopoiesis. Blood 67:436, 1986

46. Schofield R: The relationship between the spleen colony-forming cell and the haematopoietic stem cell. Blood Cells 4:7, 1978

47. Schrader JW, Clark–Lewis I: A T cell derived factor stimulating multipotential hemopoietic stem cells: Molecular weight and distinction from T cell derived granulocyte–macrophage colony stimulating factor. J Immunol 139:30, 1982

48. Stephenson JR, Axelrad AA, McLeod DL et al: Induction of colonies of hemoglobin-synthesizing cells by erythropoietin in vitro. Proc Natl Acad Sci USA 68:1542, 1971

49. Till JE, McCulloch EA: A direct measurement of the radiation sensitivity of normal bone marrow cells. Radiat Res 14:213, 1961

50. Till JE, McCulloch EA, Siminovitch L: A stochastic model of stem cell proliferation, based on the growth of spleen colony forming cells. Proc Natl Acad Sci USA 78:29, 1964

51. VanZant G, Goldwasser E: Simultaneous effects of erythropoietin and colony-stimulating factor on bone marrow cells. Science 198:733, 1977

52. Weiss L: The histology of the bone marrow. In Gordon AS (ed): Regulation of Hematopoiesis, vol 1, p 79. New York, Appleton-Century-Crofts, 1970

53. Wong GG, Witek J, Temple PA et al: Human GM-CSF: Molecular cloning of the complementary DNA and purification of the natural and recombinant proteins. Science 228:810, 1985

54. Wright JH: The origin and nature of the blood platelets. Boston Med Surg J 154:643, 1906

55. Wu AM, Siminovitch L, Till JE et al: Evidence for a relationship between mouse hemopoietic stem cells and cells forming colonies in culture. Proc Natl Acad Sci USA 59:1209, 1968

PART II

THE

ERYTHROCYTES

6

Erythropoiesis and Erythrocyte Physiology

Harriet J. Echternacht

Erythrocytes play a vital role in human physiology. To appreciate this role and how it relates to disease states, a basic understanding of erythrocyte development is necessary. In this chapter, normal erythrocyte development and the factors that influence normal erythrocyte survival and function will be presented.

van Leeuwenhoek first viewed erythrocytes through his primitive microscope in 1673, describing them as "small round globules." At that time erythrocytes were thought to be insignificant. Today he would be amazed to learn of the intricacies of the erythrocyte's internal dynamics, the simple and yet complicated molecular membrane structure, and the numerous internal and morphologic changes that occur as the erythrocyte matures from a primitive cell. Even slight alterations in these complicated features can be associated with numerous disorders, some of which are life threatening.

Erythrocytes and their precursors can be thought of as a functioning organ called the erythron.[5] The primary function of the erythron is to deliver adequate oxygen (O_2) to the tissues. Oxygen, which is used by the cells for aerobic metabolism, is bound to hemoglobin (Hb) (Chap. 7) within the erythrocyte and carried from the lungs throughout the body. Removal of the waste product carbon dioxide (CO_2) is also a vital erythron function.

To function effectively, the body must maintain approximately 309×10^9/L circulating erythrocytes per kilogram of body weight.[11] Remarkable regulatory mechanisms keep the number of erythrocytes in balance. Normally, whenever there is blood loss or when old erythrocytes are destroyed after their normal 120-day life span,[3] they are quickly replaced from various production sites (Fig. 6-1). Erythrocyte production (erythropoiesis) is a constant process.

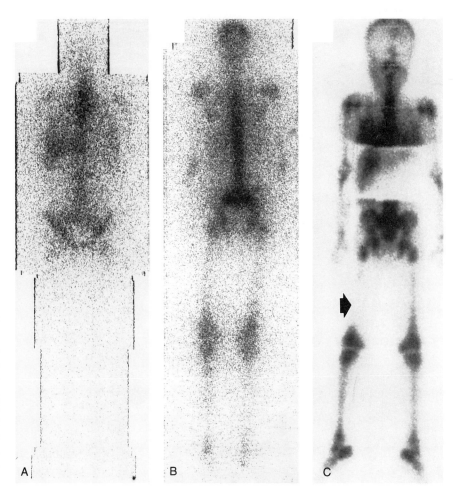

FIG. 6-1. Radionuclide images demonstrating erythrocyte production sites. (*A*) ^{52}Fe scan in normal man. (*B*) ^{52}Fe scan in adult with sickle cell disease. Note expansion of active marrow into the long bones and skull. (*C*) ^{99m}Tc-sulfur colloid scan in a child with sickle cell disease. Note finer detail of image. Active marrow is expanded into long bones. A "cold" defect secondary to an infarct is present in the right femur (*arrow*). (A and B courtesy of Dr. E W Fordham; C courtesy of Dr. P T Kirchner.)

ERYTHROCYTE PRODUCTION

Origin

Erythrocytes originate from a pluripotent stem cell (CFU-S) (Chap. 5). Maturation is gradual, because the cell becomes specialized and synthesizes proteins that will be needed later for function and survival. As proteins accumulate and various other changes occur, the morphology of the cell changes. These changes in the maturation process have been divided into stages (Fig. 6-2). The rubriblast, the earliest stage, and the stages that follow will be discussed later. These stages are found in the bone marrow and may be separated morphologically by light microscopy. The precursors between the pluripotent stem cell and the rubriblast are found in small numbers, however, and their presence has been postulated on the basis of the results of *in vitro* studies in the 1970s.

The burst forming unit–erythroid (BFU-E) is the earliest erythroid-committed cell thus far identified and is thought to be closely related to the CFU-S. The BFU-E is thought to mature gradually through several steps into the colony-forming unit–erythroid (CFU-E),[13,46] which is closely related to the rubriblast.

The terms BFU-E and CFU-E describe the cells' growth patterns in culture media. CFU-E was first to be identified. In 1971 Stephenson and associates[66] inoculated a plasma clot culture with bone marrow cells and added erythropoi-

etin (EPO), a glycoprotein long known as a stimulator of erythropoiesis.[30,56] After 1 to 2 days, pure colonies of maturing erythroid cells were detected. Those investigators postulated that primitive erythroid precursors in the bone marrow inoculum were stimulated by the EPO and that each precursor formed one colony of maturing erythroid precursors. These primitive cells were designated colony-forming units–erythroid or CFU-E.

Axelrad and coworkers[3] did a similar study in which a large amount of EPO was added. The expected CFU-E colonies grew and then diminished. After 7 days, another growth of colonies appeared. However, instead of the random colony formation of the first growth, the second growth was in clusters or "bursts" of colonies. Those investigators postulated that the high levels of EPO caused a CFU-E precursor to proliferate and produce CFU-Es, which then differentiated into colonies of maturing erythroid cells. The progenitor was designated burst forming unit–erythroid or BFU-E.

Only a few BFU-E normally are present in the bone marrow; therefore, BFU-E are difficult to identify morphologically. They are thought to be different from, although similar to, small to medium-sized lymphocytes. Circulating BFU-E have been grown from the peripheral blood[7] and are thought to reside in the null cell fraction of lymphocytes (*i.e.,* non-B, non-T lymphocytes) (Chaps. 5 and 24). Recent evidence suggests that they reside specifically in a subpopulation of null cells that lack the Fc frag-

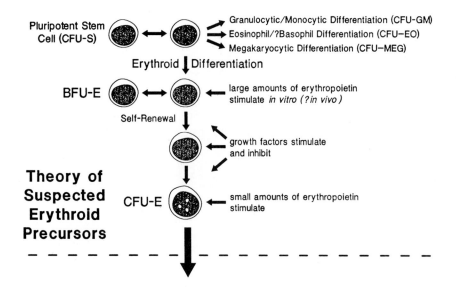

Theory of Suspected Erythroid Precursors

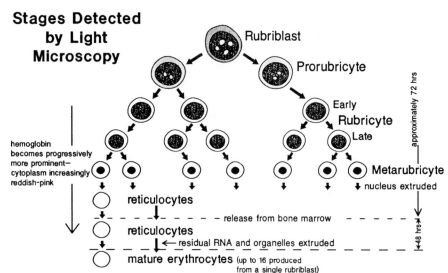

Stages Detected by Light Microscopy

FIG. 6-2. Steps in erythrocyte maturation.

ment of immunoglobulin G.[58] Increased numbers of circulating BFU-E have been demonstrated in some anemias.[49] The CFU-E (which may also be found in peripheral blood) may resemble early erythroid precursors by light microscopy but show much larger nucleoli and many more mitochondria by electron microscopy (EM).[48]

Growth Factors

The BFU-E and CFU-E can be viewed as a population of primitive erythroid-committed cells that respond as needed to both humoral and cellular growth factors to replenish the circulating erythrocyte pool. Identification of proliferation-enhancing and -inhibiting factors is the focus of many current studies.

The hormone EPO has a well documented role as a stimulator of erythropoiesis. The CFU-E are particularly sensitive to this hormone; only minute amounts are needed to stimulate growth. Primitive BFU-E appear to be insensitive to EPO, but cells become more sensitive as they mature into CFU-E.[13]

Other hormones also simulate erythropoiesis, including growth hormones,[22] various thyroid hormones,[37] an-

drogenic and nonandrogenic steroid hormones,[61] and insulin.[33] Monocytes or macrophages are strong enhancers.[24,71,72] In combination with other cells, they have also been reported as inhibitors.[12, 57] Likewise, different subsets of T lymphocytes identified by immunologic markers have stimulating[19,55,70] or inhibiting[40] effects. The inhibitory effect of T lymphocytes is evidenced by some disorders associated with increased T-cell activity and decreased erythropoiesis, such as some cases of B-cell chronic lymphocytic leukemia (CLL),[39] T-cell CLL,[45] and red cell aplasia.[28,36] Examples of other inhibitors of erythropoiesis identified through studies related to BFU-E and CFU-E include viruses[65] and interferon,[38] both of which may affect T-cell activity; uremic toxins produced in renal disease;[17,42] and alcohol.[21]

Production Sites

The main sites of adult hematopoiesis or blood cell production are the vertebrae, ribs, sternum, and skull and the proximal ends of the femur and humerus.[9] Figure 6-1A demonstrates these production sites as revealed by radioisotopes.

Radioisotopic Evaluation of Production Sites

Radioactive imaging is one technique used in nuclear medicine to identify sites of erythropoiesis as well as other physiologic characteristics and tumors. It involves the intravenous injection of a radioactive tracer element (radioisotope), which is carried by the circulation to the organs that normally metabolize or store that element. Studies of specific organs are performed by selecting the appropriate radioisotope. After radioisotope injection, total body surface counts are done with an external probe, which shows the locations of radioactivity in the body.

IRON-59 AND IRON-52. Historically, radioisotopes of iron (^{59}Fe and ^{52}Fe) have been used to image sites of erythropoiesis (see Fig. 6-1A). Ingested iron normally is bound to transferrin in the blood, carried to sites of erythrocyte production, and incorporated into the erythrocyte to be used in Hb formation. Thus, iron was the radioisotope of choice in the past to demonstrate both normal erythrocyte production sites and abnormal marrow space expansion into the long bones and extramedullary erythropoiesis in the spleen and liver (see Fig. 6-1B).

Many studies have been performed using radioiron to evaluate the production sites in anemias and myeloproliferative disorders and after radiation treatment.[10,32] The information gained from these studies has been correlated with other clinical and laboratory data, making it rarely necessary to use radioiron today. In addition, there are several drawbacks to its use. ^{59}Fe has a long half-life (45 days) and therefore exposes the patient to long-term radiation. It also emits photons with very high energies that do not permit good image production. ^{52}Fe, on the other hand, has an ideal half-life (8.2 hours) and is excellent for imaging, but it must be produced by a cyclotron, a highly sophisticated and expensive instrument not available to most institutions. The short half-life, which prohibits radioisotope transport over long distances, and the expense of production limit the clinical usefulness of ^{52}Fe.

TECHNETIUM-99m SULFUR COLLOID. Technetium-99m (^{99m}Tc) is the most widely used radioisotope in clinical imaging. It has a 6-hour half-life and has ideal physical characteristics to yield high-quality images with low patient radiation exposure. To be useful in imaging specific organs, ^{99m}Tc must be linked to particular molecules. For instance, ^{99m}Tc-labeled sulfur colloid particles will be phagocytized by histiocytes (macrophages) in the bone marrow, spleen, liver, and other tissues. Because regional histiocyte activity closely parallels regional erythropoiesis in most clinical settings, ^{99m}Tc sulfur colloid can detect increased erythropoiesis in the bone marrow space. Extramedullary erythropoiesis cannot be detected by this method, however, because histiocytes are normally found in the spleen and liver. ^{99m}Tc sulfur colloid studies also show regional areas of decreased radioactivity (cold defects), which are a valuable indicator of necrosis in such disorders as sickle cell disease (see Fig. 6-1C). In addition, they may indicate metastases, primary bone tumors, or regional fibrosis. These cold areas may also indicate disease progression. However, radioimaging should never be used diagnostically without supporting hematologic data.

ERYTHROCYTE MATURATION

Erythropoietin and other growth factors cause the early erythroid precursors (BFU-E and CFU-E) to differentiate to the rubriblast (pronormoblast) stage of development (see Fig. 6-2). The rubriblast is the first precursor that can be recognized by light microscopy. The rubriblast gives rise to 16 mature erythrocytes through four cell divisions (see Fig. 6-2) taking approximately 72 hours. Ultrastructural morphologic changes occur as the rubriblast differentiates from a primitive, nucleated cell to a mature, non-nucleated erythrocyte.

Ultrastructure

Organelles in early erythrocyte precursors are necessary for metabolism and synthesis of Hb, enzymes, and other proteins (Fig. 6-3). As proteins accumulate, the number of organelles gradually diminishes. These ultrastructural changes correlate with morphologic changes seen by light microscopy. The function and structure of the organelles are complex and not completely understood.

Nucleus

The nucleus is most important in the earliest stages of development, serving as the site for DNA and RNA synthesis and, as such, the center for the direction of cell development and maturation. Chromatin, composed of DNA, histones, and other proteins, is finely dispersed and appears either condensed or granular by EM. The more condensed areas of chromatin, called heterochromatin, are inactive. When the cells are stained with basic dyes, heterochromatin takes on a basophilic color (dark blue) when viewed by light microscopy. Euchromatin, which is active, appears more open by light microscopy and does not stain with basic dyes. It is not well demonstrated by EM. As the cell matures the chromatin becomes increasingly condensed and metabolic and synthetic activities decline until finally the nucleus becomes inactive and is extruded from the cell (Fig. 6-4).

Multiple nucleoli are present in the rubriblast, which stain intensely with basic dyes and are electron dense. They contain RNA, proteins, and small amounts of DNA.[20] Nucleoli are involved in the production and distribution of RNA.

Cytoplasm

Many free ribosomes and clusters of ribosomes called polyribosomes are present in the cytoplasm of the early erythrocyte precursors. They are the site of synthesis of globin (an Hb component) and other proteins. Polyribosomes may also be attached to the endoplasmic reticulum and are thought to form different proteins than those synthesized by free ribosomes. Ribosomes give stained early precursors a deep, dark blue cytoplasm by light microscopy. As Hb is formed the number of ribosomes gradually diminishes, and the dark blue color is gradually replaced with reddish pink.

The Golgi apparatus is located near the nucleus and appears by light microscopy as a pale or lightened area. By EM the Golgi apparatus appears as a cluster of vesicles and

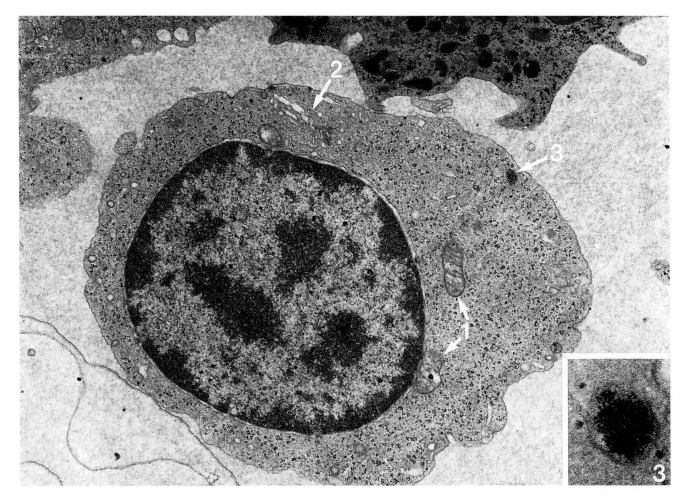

FIG. 6-3. Electron micrograph of early erythroid precursor (approximately at prorubricyte stage). (1) Mitochondria. (2) Golgi apparatus. (3) Vesicle containing ferritin. Note many ribosomes in cytoplasm, which appear as dark granules. The lighter areas of the nucleus are active (euchromatin); the darker areas are inactive (heterochromatin). Inset: magnified view of a vesicle containing ferritin. (Original magnification × 108,850.)

plates of different shapes. Glycoproteins enter the organelle to be modified, sorted, and sent to their appropriate destination within the cell. That is, the Golgi appears to act as "traffic director" for the thousands of protein molecules synthesized.[59]

Mitochondria, as seen by EM, are rod- or oval-shaped organelles that serve several functions in erythroid precursors. The most important are aerobic generation of energy for the maturing cell and insertion of ferrous iron into protoporphyrin IX during heme synthesis (Chap. 7). Mitochondria are not visible by light microscopy.

Iron is also present in the form of ferritin. It can be found freely dispersed in the cytoplasm or membrane bound in vesicles. Using light microscopy and an iron stain such as Prussian blue, ferritin can be demonstrated as small blue aggregates called siderotic granules.

Stages of Maturation as Seen by Light Microscopy

Staining a bone marrow sample with a modified Romanowsky stain such as Wright stain and observation by light microscopy allow the identification of six morphologic stages of erythrocyte maturation. Because maturation is a continuous process, there is some overlap between stages. However, the designation of stages is a helpful diagnostic tool, and these stages can be identified easily by the trained eye.

Normal morphology is dependent on adequate intake and metabolism of many nutrients necessary for maturation. Vitamin B_{12}, folate, and iron are particularly important. Abnormal morphology associated with deficiencies in these nutrients is discussed in Chapters 12 and 13.

Nomenclature

There are three nomenclatures used today to describe the six stages of erythrocyte maturation: rubri, normoblast, and erythroblast (Table 6-1). In the late 1800s Ehrlich used the term erythroblasts to describe nucleated erythrocyte precursors and divided them into two categories. Normal precursors he called normoblasts. Large, abnormal precursors, now known to be caused by impairment of DNA synthesis, he called megaloblasts (Chap. 12). Through the years, normoblasts and erythroblasts have been used with

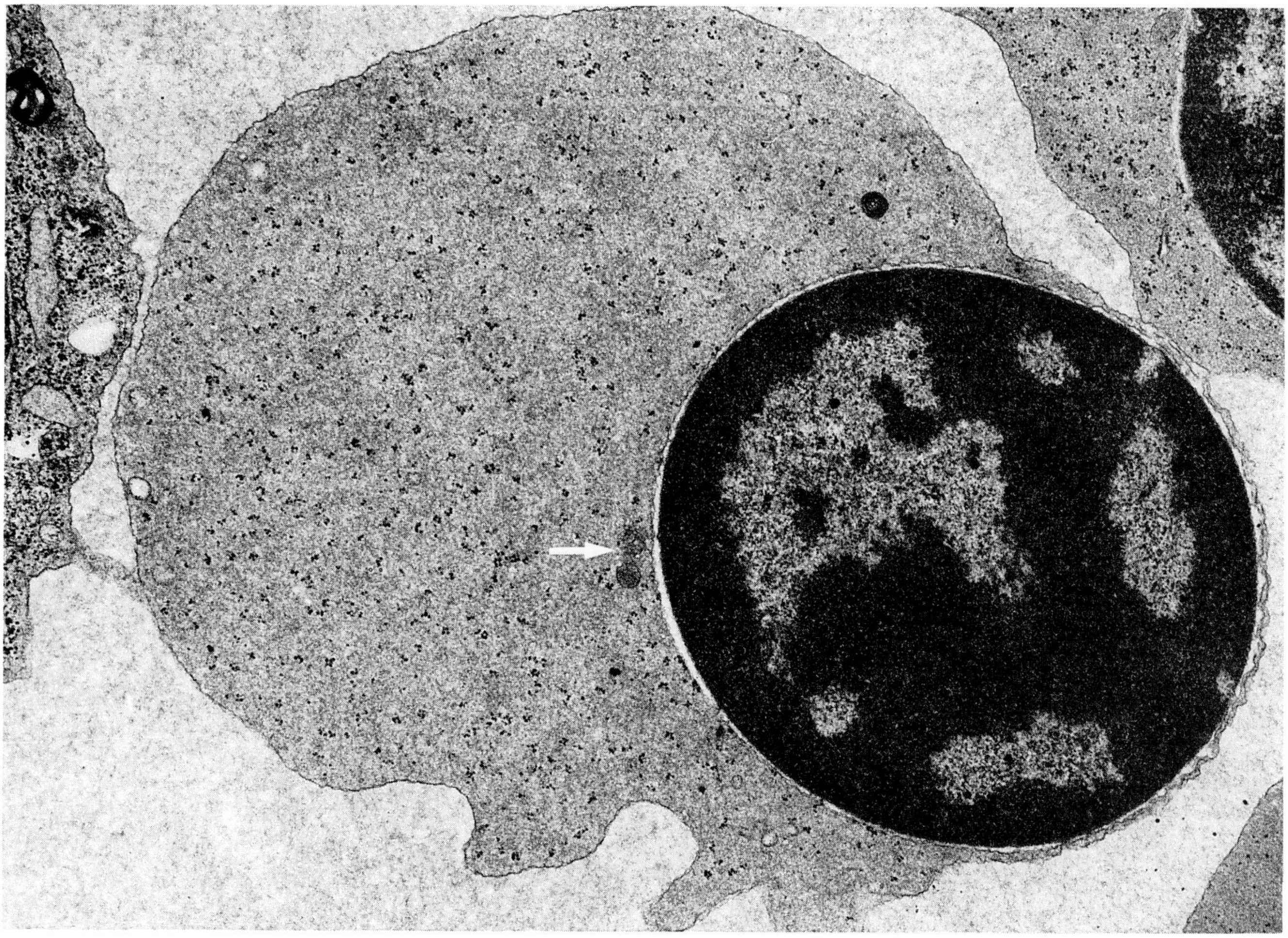

FIG. 6-4. Electron micrograph of metarubricyte extruding nucleus. Note residual mitochondria (*arrow*) and ribosomes (*dark granules*) in the cytoplasm and the irregular cytoplasmic borders. Most of the chromatin is condensed, inactive heterochromatin.

descriptive terms or prefixes to describe the first four stages of normal maturation. Use of the word "blast" has been confusing when referring to a cell beyond the blast stage of development. To solve this problem and to develop uniformity in classification, a new nomenclature was proposed by the American Society of Clinical Pathologists (ASCP).[8] Rubri, meaning red, was incorporated into the description

of four of the six stages of maturation. The rubri nomenclature has not been universally accepted, however, so it is necessary to be familiar with the older ones as well. The rubri and normoblast nomenclatures probably have the most usage.

General Guidelines

The College of American Pathologists[6] has set forth guidelines to promote uniformity in cell identification, which will be used, in part, in the following descriptions of erythrocyte precursors. The following are some general guidelines for the identification of erythroid precursors: they exhibit a progressive decrease in size as the cell matures; they exhibit a progressive decrease in the degree of cytoplasmic basophilia (blue color); their nuclei are round or oval in the blast stage, becoming very round thereafter; and there is a gradual increase in the coarseness and condensation of the chromatin, ranging from fine in the early stages to pyknotic (dense nuclear mass) in the stage just before nuclear extrusion.

Rubriblast (Pronormoblast, Erythroblast)

The rubriblast is the earliest erythrocyte precursor identifiable by light microscopy in the stained bone marrow

TABLE 6–1. Nomenclatures of Erythrocytic Stages of Maturation

RUBRI	NORMOBLAST	ERYTHROBLAST
Rubriblast	Pronormoblast	Proerythroblast
Prorubricyte	Basophilic normoblast	Basophilic erythroblast
Rubricyte	Polychromatophilic normoblast	Polychromatic erythroblast
Metarubricyte	Orthochromatic or orthochromatophilic normoblast	Orthochromatic erythroblast
Reticulocyte★	Reticulocyte★	Reticulocyte★
Erythrocyte	Erythrocyte	Erythrocyte

★ "Diffusely basophilic erythrocyte" and "polychromatophilic erythrocyte" are terms sometimes applied to the reticulocyte, particularly when seen on the peripheral blood film.

sample (Plates 1 through 3). Cell size is variable, ranging from 12 to 25 μm. The nucleus:cytoplasm ratio is high, with the nucleus usually occupying more than 80% of the cell. The cytoplasm is basophilic (intense dark blue) because of the high RNA content, which attracts the basic part of the stain (e.g., methylene blue). The Golgi apparatus may be visible as a pale area next to the nucleus. The nucleus is usually round to slightly oval, has dispersed fine clumps of chromatin, and contains nucleoli.

At times it is difficult to differentiate the rubriblast from a myeloblast (the earliest identifiable stage of granulopoiesis). However, a myeloblast usually has less cytoplasmic basophilia and a fine, lacy chromatin that stains less intensely than the rubriblast. At this stage of maturation the degree of basophilia probably is more helpful than nuclear characteristics in distinguishing between the two (see Plate 2). The rubriblast gives rise to two prorubricytes (see Fig. 6-2B).

Prorubricyte (Basophilic Normoblast)

The prorubricyte is slightly smaller (12–17 μm) than the rubriblast with the nucleus usually occupying 75% of the cell (see Plates 1 and 2). The cytoplasm is basophilic, and the Golgi apparatus is usually visible as a light area near the nucleus. The nucleus is round, and its chromatin is dark violet and definitely coarser and more clumped than that in the rubriblast. Parachromatin, the nonstaining or clear area of the nucleus, is slightly visible between the clumps of chromatin. Usually nucleoli are no longer visible. The coarser chromatin and the absence of nucleoli are the most helpful criteria in distinguishing the prorubricyte from the rubriblast.

The prorubricyte divides two times, giving rise to four rubricytes.

Rubricyte (Polychromatophilic Normoblast)

The rubricyte is usually smaller (12–15 μm) than the prorubricyte (see Plates 1 and 3). It has a round nucleus that may be eccentric. Throughout this stage of maturation, more cytoplasm becomes apparent as the nucleus becomes smaller. The cytoplasm shows a varied spectrum of blue color as Hb is synthesized. Blue RNA mixed with red Hb gives the cytoplasm an opaque, violet–blue color called polychromasia. Early rubricyte cytoplasm is moderately polychromatophilic, differing from the intensely dark blue cytoplasm of the prorubricyte. Late rubricytes have a paler blue-gray-violet to slightly pinkish color. The nuclear chromatin is very coarse and condensed. Distinct areas of parachromatin are visible amid clumps of chromatin. This cell may be confused with a lymphocyte (see Problems in Erythroid Cell Identification).

Each rubricyte gives rise to two metarubricytes. This is the last cell division during maturation.

Metarubricyte (Orthochromic Normoblast)

The metarubricyte is the last nucleated erythrocyte stage (see Plates 1 through 3). It is the same size as or slightly smaller than the rubricyte (8–12 μm). The distinguishing features of this cell are its paler, blue-gray-violet polychromatophilic to pinkish cytoplasm and dense nuclear chromatin pattern. The nucleus is pyknotic (dense mass of

degenerated chromatin), and Hb is the main constituent of the cytoplasm.

The nucleus is extruded at this stage (see Fig. 6-4), and the cell becomes a reticulocyte.

Reticulocyte (Diffusely Basophilic Erythrocyte, Polychromatophilic Erythrocyte)

The reticulocyte is slightly larger than the mature erythrocyte and may have irregular cytoplasmic borders (see Plate 2). The cytoplasm still contains small amounts of RNA, giving the cell various degrees of polychromasia (mixed pink and blue staining).

After nuclear expulsion reticulocytes are retained in the marrow for 2 to 3 days[15] before release into the marrow sinusoids to appear in the peripheral blood. The mechanism for their release is unknown, and many factors probably are involved. Perhaps as the erythrocyte matures, it loses its ability to adhere to fibronectin, a glycoprotein in the bone marrow matrix.[51]

The reticulocyte contains Golgi apparatus remnants and residual mitochondria that permit continued aerobic metabolism and Hb production, which decrease as the cell matures. Reticulocytes also contain residual RNA, which may be stained supravitally (in the living state) using stains such as new methylene blue or brilliant cresyl blue. Such staining causes the RNA to precipitate and aggregate into a network of strands or clumps visible by light microscopy. These stains permit laboratory performance of reticulocyte counts and calculation of the reticulocyte production index (RPI) (Chap. 9) for evaluation of the effectiveness of erythropoiesis in anemic states.

Within 24 to 48 hours, the cell loses the organelles and assumes a biconcave shape. It is then a mature erythrocyte.

Mature Erythrocyte

The mature erythrocyte is approximately 7.2 μm in diameter (see Plate 1). In a resting state it is a biconcave disc, thus the name discocyte. With Wright stain a central pale area is seen that fades gradually into reddish-pink cytoplasm. The central pallor corresponds to the indentation in the erythrocyte disc. The mature erythrocyte contains no mitochondria; therefore, neither proteins nor Hb is synthesized.

Problems in Erythroid Cell Identification

Problems in bone marrow erythroid cell identification may be encountered unless several precautions are taken. Proper identification requires selection of an area in the specimen where the cells are separated and thinly smeared (Chap. 29). Wright stain should be bright with good contrast between purple, blue, and pink. Granulocyte granules should be distinct. Even with good stain, however, it is difficult at times to distinguish erythroid precursors from plasma cells and lymphocytes.

Aside from early erythroid precursors, the only other normal cells in the bone marrow that usually display intense, dark blue cytoplasm are plasma cells. Plasma cells tend to have a low nuclear:cytoplasm ratio and a dense clumped chromatin pattern. Both the rubriblast and prorubricyte have a high nuclear:cytoplasm ratio. The chromatin is fine to coarse at these stages but not as coarse or condensed as in a mature plasma cell. The eccentric nucleus and perinuclear halo of the plasma cell also help in its identification (see Plate 3).

Lymphocytes are often confused with rubricytes and metarubricytes. The nucleus of the lymphocyte tends to be less round (slightly oval), with a dense homogeneous chromatin pattern. The chromatin pattern of the rubricyte and metarubricyte is more clumped with lightened areas (parachromatin). Small lymphocytes usually have scant cytoplasm in contrast to the more abundant cytoplasm of erythroid cells (see Plates 2 and 3). The polychromatophilic to pinkish appearance of the cytoplasm of rubricytes and particularly, metarubricytes is also a distinguishing feature because the lymphocyte cytoplasm should be a distinct light blue.

STRUCTURE AND PHYSIOLOGY OF THE MATURE ERYTHROCYTE

The mature erythrocyte is unique in that it lacks a nucleus and organelles. All components necessary for survival and function are present. Hemoglobin is the main cell component. The erythrocyte is surrounded by a specialized membrane that allows it to carry out O_2 and CO_2 transport and to survive travel in the circulation for 120 days.[2]

Many factors are involved in erythrocyte membrane and Hb maintenance. A source of energy is vital. Membrane shape and deformability are also important; they are influenced by the cell's composition and structure, internal Hb viscosity, and energy status.[25,26,44,60]

Shape and Deformability

The biconcave disc shape of the resting mature erythrocyte can be seen by scanning EM (Fig. 6-5). This shape facilitates its O_2–CO_2 transport function by maximizing the ratio of the surface area to the volume. To a degree it also allows cell flexibility. Flexibility, or deformability, allows the cell to adjust to small vessels in the microvasculature (some of which are smaller than the mean cell diameter) and still maintain a constant surface area:volume ratio. Significant alteration in this ratio causes the cell to be less deformable and subject to fragmentation and lysis. For example, a spheroid shape can be caused by membrane loss secondary to fragmentation (decreased surface area) or by increased uptake of cations and water (increased volume).

Membrane Composition and Structure

The erythrocyte membrane's composition and structure allow the membrane to perform three basic functions: (1) to separate the intracellular fluid environment of the cytoplasm from the extracellular fluid environment of the plasma; (2) to allow nutrient and ion passage selectively into and out of the cell; and (3) to allow the cell to deform when required. The membrane is composed of lipids and proteins in approximately equal proportions by weight. Lipids and proteins located on the cytoplasmic side are different from those in the membrane interior or from those on the plasma side of the cell (Fig. 6-6). This asymmetric arrangement allows selective passage of molecules into and out of the cell.

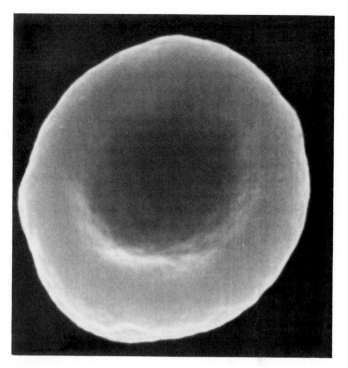

FIG. 6-5.   Scanning electron micrograph of a mature erythrocyte shows the normal discoid shape.

Lipids

Phospholipids and unesterified cholesterol predominate in the lipid fraction and are present in approximately equal proportions. Phospholipid molecules are arranged in a double layer called a lipid bilayer leaflet (see Fig. 6-6). As in other cell membranes, the phospholipid polar (head) groups are oriented toward the aqueous environment (cytoplasm and plasma), whereas the nonpolar fatty acid chains (tails) face the hydrophobic leaflet interior. This arrangement allows the membrane to act as a liquid sealer. Phospholipids are fluid because the fatty acid tails are free to move laterally within the membrane,[62,63] which allows lipids to interact with one another and with membrane proteins. Significant interactions between lipids and the membrane's structural or skeletal proteins are thought to take place.[60]

Cholesterol plays an important role in regulating membrane fluidity and also membrane permeability to electrolytes and nonelectrolytes, thus maintaining the surface area:volume ratio. Lipid exchange, most notably of cholesterol, occurs between the membrane and the plasma. Approximately 98% of the membrane cholesterol is unesterified, whereas 70% of plasma cholesterol is esterified.

Proteins

Proteins are bound to lipids throughout the membrane (see Fig. 6-6). Many membrane proteins have been characterized by the way they separate and form bands on polyacrylamide gel. They have been classified as peripheral or integral, depending on the extraction method and their location in the lipid bilayer. The peripheral protein fraction contains two important skeletal proteins, spectrin (bands 1 and 2) and actin (band 5). These are thought to underlie

Aqueous Plasma

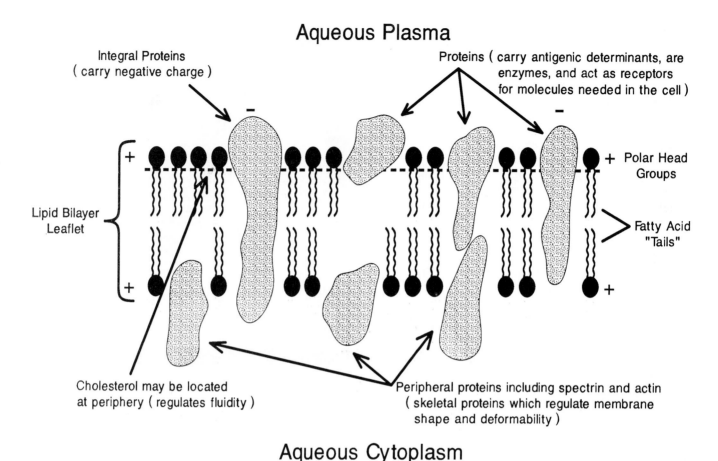

Integral Proteins (carry negative charge)

Proteins (carry antigenic determinants, are enzymes, and act as receptors for molecules needed in the cell)

Lipid Bilayer Leaflet

Polar Head Groups

Fatty Acid "Tails"

Cholesterol may be located at periphery (regulates fluidity)

Peripheral proteins including spectrin and actin (skeletal proteins which regulate membrane shape and deformability)

Aqueous Cytoplasm

FIG. 6-6.   Simplified diagram of erythrocyte membrane structure.

the lipid bilayer on the cytoplasmic side and to regulate membrane shape and deformability.[44] The presence of these proteins allows the membrane to have appropriate viscoelastic properties. Abnormalities in spectrin have been found in some anemias of abnormal shape, such as hereditary spherocytosis[60] and hereditary elliptocytosis[41] (Chap. 17).

The principal integral protein is the glycoprotein designated band 3 that spans the bilayer and is an inorganic anion transport protein. Integral proteins contain sialic acid, which gives erythrocytes a negative charge. This negativity between the cells, called the zeta potential, causes cells to repel one another as they move through the circulation. One cause of a decreased zeta potential is altered plasma proteins. This is reflected by an increase in the erythrocyte sedimentation rate (ESR) (Chaps. 9 and 39).

Membrane proteins are vital to erythrocyte function. In addition to making up the skeletal structure, many enzymes facilitate the movement of substrates and cofactors into and out of the cell. Two very important membrane enzyme systems are Na^+,K^+-ATPase and Ca^{+2},Mg^{+2}-ATPase. The former controls active transport of sodium and potassium. Increased sodium without loss of potassium causes the cell to gain water (increased volume) and subjects it to lysis, whereas increased potassium causes cell shrinkage. The second enzyme system, called the calcium pump, moves calcium out of the cell to the plasma against a high concentration gradient. Calcium is thought to be involved

in the regulation and stabilization of membrane phospholipid structure.[60] High intracellular calcium concentrations cause the cell to become less deformable and therefore abnormal in shape.

Membrane proteins also act as receptors for various molecules needed within the cell such as transferrin and EPO. Antigenic determinants for blood group identification are associated with erythrocyte membrane proteins.

Hemoglobin Viscosity

Normal erythrocyte Hb concentration has a low viscosity and is fluid. Cellular water loss and Hb that is precipitated, polymerized, or crystallized can all cause the cell to be less deformable and subject it to lysis. Precipitated Hb, called Heinz bodies, forms rigid cellular inclusions that are visible by light microscopy after special staining and are associated with various hematologic disorders (Chap. 8). Some hereditary Hb variants cause Hb to polymerize (*e.g.*, Hb S in sickle cell anemia) or crystallize (*e.g.*, Hb C disease) (Chap. 14).

Energy Metabolism

Energy Requirements

Energy is needed to maintain various components of the erythrocyte; preserving membrane shape, enzymatic reactions, and movement of calcium, sodium, and potassium all require energy. Energy also is required to reduce oxidized proteins. Hemoglobin must be maintained in its reduced state for proper function.

Two sites on the Hb molecule are particularly prone to oxidation: the iron atom in the heme ring and the sulfhydryl (–SH) groups on the globin chains (Chap. 7). Oxidation of the normal ferrous (Fe^{2+}) state to the ferric (Fe^{3+}) state results in the formation of methemoglobin, which has no O_2-carrying capacity. Normally, 1% to 3% is formed per day secondary to loss of an electron from ferrous iron to O_2 during deoxygenation when water is present in the heme pocket. Hereditary unstable hemoglobins (Chap. 14), methemoglobin reductase deficiency (Fig. 6-7), or exposure to oxidant drugs may cause large accumulations of methemo-

globin. Oxidation of sulfhydryl groups causes Hb precipitation (Heinz body formation).

Sources of Energy

Glucose is the principal energy source, although the erythrocyte can utilize other sugars such as galactose, fructose, and mannose. Pentoses and disaccharides are not metabolized. Glycogen is not normally metabolized as an energy source, but the cell does possess enzymes for its degradation if it accumulates. Membrane permeability differs for various sugars. Glucose can diffuse quickly without expense of energy, whereas the membrane is essentially impermeable to sucrose, lactose, and maltose.

Lacking mitochondria, mature erythrocytes depend on

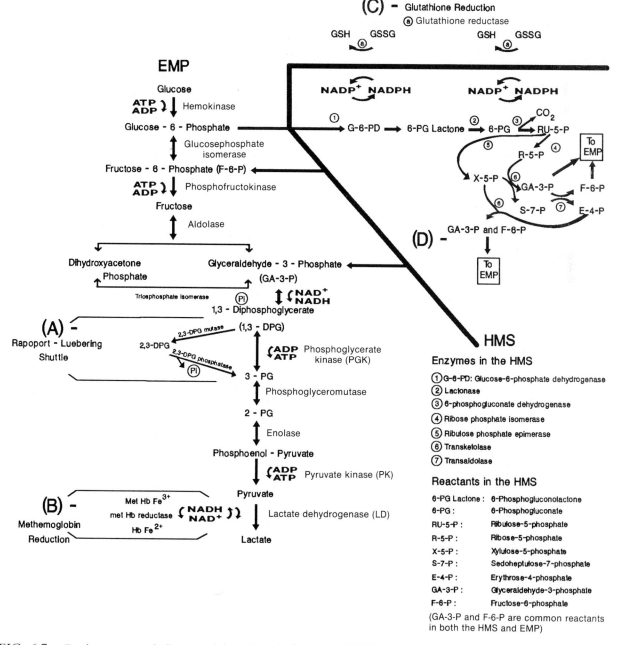

FIG. 6-7. Erythrocyte metabolism: Embden–Meyerhof pathway (EMP) and the hexose monophosphate shunt (HMS) (pentose phosphate shunt).

two much less efficient pathways for energy metabolism. Approximately 90% to 95% of the glucose used by the cell is normally metabolized by the anaerobic Embden–Meyerhof pathway (EMP). The cell utilizes the aerobic hexose monophosphate shunt (HMS) (also known as the pentose phosphate shunt [PPS]) for the remaining 5% to 10% (see Fig. 6-7).

EMBDEN–MEYERHOF PATHWAY. The EMP is an anaerobic method for energy generation through which glucose is catabolized to lactate. The erythrocyte EMP is similar to the EMP of other cells except for the formation of 2,3-diphosphoglycerate (2,3-DPG), which assists in modulating O_2 transport in the cell. At low O_2 tension, 2,3-DPG binds to the deoxyhemoglobin form. This causes Hb to resist oxygenation (*i.e.*, decreases its O_2 affinity and increases tissue O_2 delivery) (Chap. 7). In addition to 2,3-DPG, adenosine triphosphate (ATP) and nicotinamide adenine dinucleotide (NAD^+ and NADH) are important intermediates in the EMP, and each is discussed below.

2,3-Diphosphoglycerate is generated by the Rapoport–Luebering shuttle, a bypass pathway in the EMP (see Fig. 6-7A). Also 1,3-DPG can be catabolized to 3-phosphogluconate (3-PG) by using the shuttle, in which 2,3-DPG is an intermediate, or directly by a path in which high-energy ATP is generated. Because the erythrocyte needs both 2,3-DPG and ATP to function, intricate regulatory mechanisms direct the way 1,3-DPG will be catabolized. These mechanisms are not completely understood. One important factor is that hypoxia shifts catabolism through the shuttle, probably by increasing intracellular *p*H. On the other hand, decreased cellular ATP levels will cause direct metabolism of 1,3-DPG to increase ATP generation.

ATP, a high-energy phosphate, is used by the erythrocyte in three ways: (1) it maintains membrane shape and deformability, probably by phosphorylation of spectrin and perhaps by chelation of calcium[44]; (2) it provides energy for active transport of cations; and (3) it assists in modulating the amount of 2,3-DPG generated. Two molecules of ATP per molecule of glucose are utilized during the first three steps of the EMP, whereas four molecules may be generated—two from the 1,3-DPG to 3-PG step if the shuttle is not taken, and two at the pyruvate to lactate step (see Fig. 6-7). Thus, there is a net yield of two ATP molecules for each molecule of glucose catabolized in the EMP.

Oxidized NAD^+ and its reduced form NADH are involved in two steps along the pathway. First, NAD^+ is used as a coenzyme with glyceraldehyde-3-phosphate dehydrogenase in the formation of 1,3-DPG. Second, NADH acts as a coenzyme with lactate dehydrogenase (LDH) to reduce pyruvate to lactate. An important function of NADH is to act as a coenzyme with methemoglobin reductase and reduce methemoglobin to Hb. If this reaction occurs, pyruvate is the end product of the EMP (Fig. 6-7B). Pyruvate or lactate then diffuse out of the cell.

The rate of glycolysis is pH dependent. Hexokinase and phosphofructokinase, enzymes at the beginning of the EMP, both react optimally at a *p*H above 7.0. Glycolysis thus increases during hypoxia because of the increased intracellular pH. In addition, ATP affects the glycolysis rate. As ATP levels rise glycolysis is diminished. As small amounts of ATP are utilized, however, glycolysis will increase. Through these and other mechanisms, the cell can adjust its energy state as long as glucose is available and normal enzymes are present.

A number of hereditary enzyme deficiencies or mutants are known to occur in man, but because the EMP is the main energy-generating force in the cell, they are extremely rare. Pyruvate kinase deficiency is the most common (Chap. 17).

HEXOSE MONOPHOSPHATE SHUNT (PENTOSE PHOSPHATE SHUNT). The primary purpose of the HMS is to provide reducing potential for the cell by generating reduced nicotinamide adenine dinucleotide phosphate (NADPH). The HMS is an oxidative pathway in which glucose-6-phosphate, generated in the first step of the EMP, is catabolized to 6-phosphogluconate (6-PG) rather than passing though the EMP (see Fig. 6-7D). This reaction is driven by an important enzyme in the HMS, glucose-6-phosphate dehydrogenase (G6PD). Two HMS reactions involve reduction of $NADP^+$ to yield NADPH, which is important in the generation of reduced glutathione (see below).

The HMS also generates ribose-5-phosphate (R-5-P), which is used by nucleated cells during nucleic acid metabolism. Mature erythrocytes are capable of limited purine metabolism, and the R-5-P produced is usually recycled back into the EMP. The intermediates glyceraldehyde-3-phosphate and fructose-6-phosphate are common reactants in both pathways and are likewise fed back into the EMP (see Fig. 6-7D).

Reduced glutathione (GSH) is the principal reducing agent in the cell. It is used to reduce oxidized sulfhydryl groups in Hb and other proteins. The reducing reaction yields reduced sulfhydryl groups and oxidized glutathione (GSSG). Glutathione reductase and NADPH then reduce GSSG back to GSH, making it available for further reductions of sulfhydryl groups (see Fig. 6-7C).

The HMS is regulated largely by the $NADP^+$:NADPH ratio. As NADPH is utilized to reduce GSSG, $NADP^+$ is formed, which causes more glucose to be metabolized by the HMS. During oxidative insult this mechanism provides the cell with more reducing potential. NADPH also plays a minor role in methemoglobin reduction.[25]

REGULATION OF ERYTHROPOIESIS (ERYTHROKINETICS)

Erythropoiesis is regulated predominantly by renal O_2 tension, which, when decreased, causes the release of the erythroid growth factor EPO. The concept of erythropoiesis is best understood in the context of the erythron model.[5] The erythron is defined as the entire mass of mature and immature erythrocytes in both intravascular and extravascular locations. Included in the extravascular portion are all immature nucleated erythrocytes and reticulocytes in the marrow. The intravascular portion includes the circulating erythrocytes and the few reticulocytes normally found in the peripheral blood.

The erythron model relates the three phases of erythrocyte life: erythropoiesis or erythrocyte production, release from marrow to circulation, and destruction and death. A fine balance between production and destruction normally keeps the erythrocyte numbers fairly constant provided each of these phases is functioning normally. Production and maintenance of the erythron requires: a normally functioning, competent bone marrow; normal EPO production; and adequate nutrients such as iron, folate, and vitamin B_{12}. From these observations the two principal disturbances of the erythron become clear: (1) anemia, a condition characterized by a *decrease* in circulating erythrocytes (destruction exceeds production); and (2) erythrocytosis, a condition characterized by an *increase* in circulating erythrocytes (production exceeds destruction).

Erythrocyte Destruction

A variety of gradual changes occur as the erythrocyte ages that make it susceptible to destruction. Alterations in the membrane, in particular, loss of sialic acid[1] and lipids,[68] decreased ATP levels, and increased calcium,[4] all have been implicated in the aging process. Evidence also suggests a senescent antigen that appears as the cell ages, making it susceptible to destruction.[31] Whatever the reason, at approximately day 120, erythrocytes are recognized as abnormal and removed from the circulation by phagocytic cells in the reticuloendothelial system (RES).

Reticuloendothelial system is an antiquated term, which encompasses both intravascular and extravascular cells that make up the cellular and immunologic defense system in the body. Common use of the term usually refers to phagocytic cells, namely, the histiocytes, monocytes, and macrophages found primarily in the spleen, liver, lymph nodes, bone marrow, and to a lesser extent the lung and other tissues.

The spleen is the principal site of erythrocyte phagocytosis by tissue macrophages after damage by normal aging.[27,64] The liver, which has a greater blood flow, plays a more active role in the removal of severely damaged cells.[27]

Phagocytosis by Kupffer cells (fixed tissue macrophages) in the liver is known as extravascular hemolysis. Extremely damaged cells may lyse within the circulation before they reach the liver or spleen. This process is referred to as intravascular hemolysis (Chap. 16).

Erythropoietin Production and Regulation

Erythropoietin has a well established role in the regulation of erythropoiesis. It is a glycoprotein with a molecular weight of 34,000.[23,69]

Production Sites

Erythropoietin is produced primarily in the kidney, although the exact site within the organ remains controversial. It is well documented that EPO levels fall after kidney removal and at times rise above normal after transplantation.[67] The fact that some EPO remains after kidney removal points to another (minor) production site, presumably the liver.[18,47,52] Recent development of a technique to synthesize EPO by recombinant DNA has led to a commercial product to relieve anemia in patients with renal disease.[14,29,34,35]

It has been difficult to actually demonstrate EPO in the kidney. Possibly, the kidney produces a proerythropoietin molecule that is not activated until it is in the plasma.[54]

Regulation of Production

Production of EPO is regulated mainly by renal O_2 tension. Such factors as Hb O_2 saturation, 2,3-DPG levels, pO_2 of the plasma, Hb concentration, erythrocyte mass, basal metabolic rate, and blood flow all affect tissue O_2 tension. At low renal O_2 tension EPO levels rise; as hypoxia is reduced, EPO levels fall.

Prostaglandins are thought to help regulate EPO production and also to enhance its effect on the erythroid progenitor cells (CFU-E).[16,53] On the other hand, estrogen may

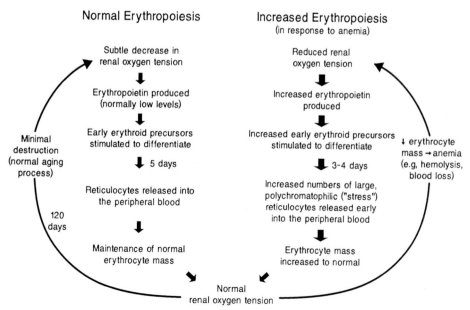

FIG. 6-8. Erythropoiesis regulation (erythrokinetics): normal vs response to anemia.

inhibit EPO production.[43] The action of estrogen probably helps account for the lower erythrocyte numbers normal for young women but not for men.

Erythropoietin Action in Normal and Anemic States

The BFU-E is much less sensitive to EPO and needs other growth factors to differentiate. From the CFU-E stage of maturation onward, EPO is necessary for cell maturation. Erythropoietin enters the cell through a specific membrane receptor. Once in the cell, it stimulates transcription of globin mRNA and may also be necessary for heme synthesis.[23]

If anemia is present, increased EPO produced in response to hypoxia stimulates more progenitors to differentiate. It also shortens the maturation time in the marrow. It was previously thought that this shortened maturation time was caused by cells skipping cell divisions. However, it is more likely that increased EPO simply causes increased Hb synthesis and early reticulocyte release.[50] These stress reticulocytes are larger than normal, contain more RNA (and are therefore more polychromatophilic), and retain Hb synthetic capability longer in the peripheral blood. It is thought that high plasma iron levels are necessary to cause increased cell proliferation and a shortened cell maturation time. Anemia attributable to blood loss is not associated with as great an erythroid response as that seen with hemolytic anemia, presumably because of the lower iron levels associated with blood loss (Hb iron is lost rather than recycled to the bone marrow).

Normal maturation takes approximately 5 days. During accelerated erythropoiesis, this time can be shortened to 3 to 4 days. Because this response to hypoxia is relatively slow, increased 2,3-DPG levels help reduce hypoxia by causing more O_2 to be released to the tissues until erythrocyte numbers are back in balance. As erythrocyte numbers increase, hypoxia is reduced, and EPO levels and the maturation cycle return to normal (Fig. 6-8).

CHAPTER SUMMARY

The erythrocyte's primary functions are transportation of O_2 from the lungs to the tissues to be used for aerobic metabolism and removal of the waste product CO_2.

Under normal circumstances erythrocyte production is in equilibrium with destruction. In addition, erythrocyte number is largely regulated by O_2 tension. Hypoxia stimulates production of erythropoietin (EPO), which in turn stimulates immature erythroid cells to mature more rapidly through the six normal morphologic stages of development—the rubriblast, prorubricyte, rubricyte, metarubricyte, reticulocyte, and mature erythrocyte (see Table 6-1).

2,3-Diphosphoglycerate regulates Hb affinity for O_2. In hypoxic states, an increase in 2,3-DPG concentration, generated through the Rapoport-Luebering shuttle in the Embden–Meyerhof pathway, and 2,3-DPG binding to Hb cause a decrease in Hb O_2 affinity. This permits release of O_2 to the tissues. As hypoxia is reduced by newly formed cells, EPO levels decrease. Normal structure and composition of the erythrocyte membrane (see Fig. 6-6) and Hb and efficient generation of energy through the aerobic Embden–Meyerhof pathway and anaerobic hexose monophosphate shunt (see Fig. 6-7) are necessary for the erythrocyte to function and survive.

Abnormalities in erythrocyte production, structure, composition, and energy metabolism are evidenced by erythrocyte-related disorders. These will be discussed in several chapters that follow (Part III: Erythrocyte Abnormalities).

REFERENCES

1. Aminoff D: Senescence and sequestration of RBC from circulation. Prog Clin Biol Res 195:279, 1985
2. Ashby W: The span of life of the red blood cell: A resume. Blood 3:486, 1948
3. Axelrad AA, McLeod DL, Shreeve MM et al: Properties of cells that produce erythrocytic colonies in vitro. In Robinson W (ed): Hemopoiesis in Culture, p 226. Washington, DHEW Publication No. (NIH) 74-205, 1973
4. Bookchin RM, Lew VL, Roth Jr EF: Elevated red cell calcium: Innocent bystander or kiss of death? Prog Clin Biol Res 195:369, 1985
5. Boycott AE: The blood as a tissue: Hypertrophy and atrophy of the red corpuscles. Proc R Soc Med 23:15, 1929
6. CAP Survey Manual, Section II, p 24. Skokie, IL, College of American Pathologists, 1986
7. Clarke BJ, Housman D: Characterization of an erythroid precursor cell of high proliferative capacity in normal human peripheral blood. Proc Natl Acad Sci USA 74:1105, 1977
8. Committee for Clarification of the Nomenclature of Cells and Diseases of the Blood and Blood Forming Organs: Second report. Am J Clin Pathol 19:56, 1949
9. Custer RP: Studies on the structure and function of the bone marrow. J Lab Clin Med 17:952, 1932
10. DeGowin RL, Chaudhuri TK, Christie JH et al: Marrow scanning in evaluation of hematopoiesis after radiotherapy. Arch Intern Med 134:297, 1974
11. Donahue DM, Reiff RH, Hanson ML et al: Quantitative measurement of the erythrocytic and granulocytic cells of the marrow and blood. J Clin Invest 37:1571, 1958
12. Eastman CE, Ruscetti FW: Regulation of erythropoiesis in long-term hamster marrow cultures: Role of bone marrow adherent cells. Blood 65:736, 1985
13. Eaves AC, Eaves CJ: Erythropoiesis in culture. Clin Haematol 13:373, 1984
14. Egrie JC, Browne J, Lai P et al: Characterization of recombinant monkey and human erythropoietin. Prog Clin Biol Res 191:339, 1985
15. Finch CA: Some qualitative aspects of erythropoiesis. Ann NY Acad Sci 77:410, 1959
16. Fisher JW, Hagiwara M: Effects of prostaglandins on erythropoiesis. Blood Cells 10:241, 1985
17. Freedman MH, Cattran DC, Saunders EF: Anemia of chronic renal failure: Inhibition by uremic serum. Nephron 35:15, 1983
18. Fried W: The liver as a source of extrarenal erythropoietin production. Blood 40:671, 1972
19. Froom P, Ramot B, Beniaminov M et al: Production of burst-promoting activity by monoclonal antibody defined malignant T lymphocytes from patients with lymphocytic leukemia and lymphoma. Blood 65:997, 1985
20. Ghadially FN: Ultrastructural Pathology of the Cell and Matrix, 2nd ed. London, Butterworths, 1982
21. Giglio MJ, Santoro RC, Bozzini CE: Effect of chronic ethanol administration on production of and response to erythropoietin in the mouse. Alcoholism 8:323, 1984
22. Golde DW, Bersch N, Li CH: Growth hormone: Species-specific stimulation of erythropoiesis in vitro. Science 196:1112, 1977
23. Goldwasser E: Erythropoietin and its mode of action. Blood Cells 10:147, 1984

24. Gordon LJ, Wesley JM, Branda RF et al: Regulation of erythroid colony formation by bone marrow macrophages. Blood 55:1047, 1980

25. Grimes AJ: Human Red Cell Metabolism. Oxford, Blackwell Scientific, 1980

26. Harrison PR: Molecular analysis of erythropoiesis: A current appraisal. Exp Cell Res 155:321, 1984

27. Jacob HS, Jandl JH: Effects of sulfhydryl inhibition on red blood cells II. Studies *in vivo*. J Clin Invest 41:1514, 1962

28. Jacobs AD, Champlin RE, Golde DW: Pure red cell aplasia characterized by erythropoietic maturation arrest: Response to anti-thymocyte globulin. Am J Med 78:515, 1985

29. Jacobs K, Shoemaker C, Rudersdorf R et al: Isolation and characterization of genetic and cDNA clones of human erythropoietin. Nature 313:806, 1985

30. Jacobson LO, Goldwasser E, Plzak LF et al: Studies on erythropoiesis IV. Reticulocyte response of hypophysectomized and polycythemic rodents to erythropoietin. Proc Soc Exp Biol Med 94:243, 1957

31. Kay MMB: Senescent cell differentiation antigen. Prog Clin Biol Res 195:251, 1985

32. Knospe WH, Rayuelu VMS, Cardello M et al: Bone marrow scanning with ^{52}iron (Fe). Cancer 37:1432, 1976

33. Kurtz A, Jelkmann W, Bauer C: Insulin stimulates erythroid colony formation independently of erythropoietin. Br J Haematol 53:311, 1983

34. Lee-Huang S: Cloning and expression of human erythropoietin cDNA in *Escherichia coli*. Proc Natl Acad Sci USA 81:2708, 1984

35. Lin FK, Suggs S, Lin CH et al: Cloning and expression of the human erythropoietin gene. Proc Natl Acad Sci USA 82:7580, 1985

36. Lynch DC, Cawley JC, MacDonald SM et al: Acquired pure red cell aplasia associated with an increase of T cells bearing receptors for the Fc of IgG. Acta Haematol 65:270, 1981

37. Malgor LA, Blanc CC, Klainer E et al: Direct effects of thyroid hormones on bone marrow erythroid cells of rats. Blood 45:671, 1975

38. Mamus SW, Beck-Schroeder S, Zanjani ED: Suppression of normal erythropoiesis by gamma interferon *in vitro*: Role of monocytes and T lymphocytes. J Clin Invest 75:1496, 1985

39. Mangan KF, D'Alessandro L: Hypoplastic anemia in B cell chronic lymphocytic leukemia: Evolution of T cell mediated suppression of erythropoiesis in early-stage and late-stage disease. Blood 66:533, 1985

40. Mangan KF, Hartnett ME, Matis SA et al: Natural killer cells suppress human erythroid stem cell proliferation in vitro. Blood 63:260, 1984

41. Marchesi SL, Knowles WJ, Morrow JS et al: Abnormal spectrin in hereditary elliptocytosis. Blood 67:141, 1986

42. McGonigle RJ, Wallin JD, Shadduck RK et al: Erythropoietin deficiency and inhibition of erythropoiesis in renal insufficiency. Kidney Int 25:437, 1984

43. Mirand EA, Gordon AS: Mechanism of estrogen action in erythropoiesis. Endocrinology 78:325, 1966

44. Mohandas N, Shohet SB: Control of red cell deformability and shape. In Piomelli S, Yachnin S (eds): Current Topics in Hematology, vol 1, p 71. New York, Alan R Liss, 1978

45. Nagasawa T, Abe T, Nakagawa T: Pure red cell aplasia and hypogammaglobulinemia associated with T-cell chronic lymphocytic leukemia. Blood 57:1025, 1981

46. Nathan DG, Sytkowski A: Editorial retrospective: Erythropoietin and regulation of erythropoiesis. N Engl J Med 308:520, 1983

47. Naughton GK, Naughton BA, Gordon AS: Erythropoietin production by macrophages in the regenerating liver. J Surg Oncol 30:184, 1985

48. Nijhof W, Wierenga PK: Isolation and characterization of the erythroid progenitor cell: CFU-E. J Cell Biol 96:386, 1983

49. Ogawa M, Grush OC, O'Dell RF et al: Circulating erythropoietic precursors in culture: Characterization in normal men and patients with hemoglobinopathies. Blood 50:1081, 1977

50. Papayannopoulou T, Finch CA: Radioiron measurements of red cell maturation. Blood Cells 1:535, 1975

51. Patel VP, Ciechanover A, Platt O et al: Loss of adhesion of erythrocyte precursors to fibronectin during erythroid differentiation. Prog Clin Biol Res 184:355, 1985

52. Paul P, Rothman SA, McMahon JT et al: Erythropoietin secretion by isolated rat Kupffer cells. Exp Hematol 12:825, 1984

53. Pavlovik-Kentera V, Susic D, Biljanovic-Paunovic et al: Prostaglandin synthesis inhibitors in erythropoiesis. Haematologia (Budap) 17:161, 1984

54. Peschle C, Condorelli M: Biogenesis of erythropoietin: Evidence for pro-erythropoietin in a subcellular fraction of kidney. Science 190:910, 1975

55. Pistoia V, Ghio R, Nocera A et al: Large granular lymphocytes have a promoting activity on human peripheral blood erythroid burst-forming units. Blood 65:464, 1985

56. Reissmann KR: Studies on the mechanism of erythropoietin stimulation in parabiotic rats during hypoxia. Blood 5:372, 1950

57. Roodman GD, Horadam VW, Wright TL: Inhibition of erythroid colony formation by autologous bone marrow adherent cells from patients with the anemia of chronic disease. Blood 62:406, 1983

58. Rosenthal CJ, Hassan M, Rieder RF et al: Identification of erythroid colony progenitors in a subset of human peripheral lymphocytes devoid of Fc receptors. Am J Hematol 19:109, 1985

59. Rothman JE: The compartment organization of the Golgi apparatus. Sci Am 253:74, 1985

60. Schwartz RS, Chiu DTS, Lubin B: Plasma membrane phospholipid organization in human erythrocytes. In Piomelli S, Yachnin S (eds): Current Topics in Hematology, vol 5, p 63. New York, Alan R Liss, 1985

61. Singer JW, Samuels AI, Adamson JW: Steroids and hematopoiesis I. The effect of steroids on *in vitro* erythroid colony growth: Structure/activity relationships. J Cell Physiol 88:127, 1976

62. Singer SJ: The molecular organization of membranes. Annu Rev Biochem 43:805, 1974

63. Singer SJ, Nicholson GL: The fluid mosaic model of the structure of cell membranes. Science 175:720, 1972

64. Smedsrød B, Aminoff D: Use of 75Se-labeled methione to study the sequestration of senescent red blood cells. Am J Hematol 18:31, 1985

65. Socinski MA, Ersler WB, Tosato G et al: Pure red cell aplasia associated with Epstein Barr virus infection: Evidence for T cell-mediated suppression of erythroid colony forming units. J Lab Clin Med 104:995, 1984

66. Stephenson JR, Axelrad AA, McLeod DL et al: Induction of colonies of hemoglobin-synthesizing cells by erythropoietin *in vitro*. Proc Natl Acad Sci USA 68:1542, 1971

67. Thevenod F, Radtke HW, Grutzmacher P et al: Deficient feedback regulation of erythropoiesis in kidney transplant patients with polycythemia. Kidney Int 24:227, 1983

68. Wagner G, Chiu DTY, Schwartz RS et al: Membrane phospholipid abnormalities in pathologic erythrocytes: A model for cell aging. Prog Clin Biol Res 195:237, 1985

69. Wang FF, Kung CKH, Goldwasser E: Some chemical properties of human erythropoietin (abstract). Fed Proc 42:1872, 1983

70. Wisniewski D, Strife A, Wachter M et al: Regulation of human peripheral blood erythroid burst-forming unit growth by T lymphocytes and T lymphocyte subpopulations defined by OKT4 and OKT8 monoclonal antibodies. Blood 65:456, 1985

71. Zuckerman KS: Human erythroid burst-forming units: Growth *in vitro* is dependent on monocytes, but not T lymphocytes. J Clin Invest 67:702, 1981

72. Zuckerman KS, Bagby GC Jr, McCall E et al: A monokine stimulates production of human erythroid burst-promoting activity by endothelial cells *in vitro*. J Clin Invest 75:722, 1985

7

Hemoglobin Synthesis and Function

F. Bernhard Ludvigsen

The single most common complex organic molecule in vertebrates is hemoglobin (Hb). In humans the weight of Hb represents a little more than 1% of total body weight. Nearly all of this metalloprotein is found in the erythrocytes. Hemoglobin is synthesized within maturing nucleated erythrocytes in the bone marrow. Upon the erythrocytes' release into the vascular system, Hb normally remains in the intracellular space of erythrocytes as they travel through the vascular system. Hemoglobin has several functions, most of which are effected on the adjacent extracellular fluid portion of the blood called plasma.

Body tissues and organs require oxygen (O_2) to function and survive. The primary functions of Hb are to deliver O_2 to these tissues and organs and to transport the waste product carbon dioxide (CO_2) away to the lungs, where it is exhaled from the body.

Hemoglobin is the primary biologic substance that permits adequate oxygenation of the body mass of man and other vertebrates. Oxygenation of plasma is not at all adequate to support the O_2 requirements of the large body mass of any vertebrate.

COMPONENTS OF HEMOGLOBIN

The complete adult Hb molecule consists of four significantly different constituents:

TABLE 7–1. Globin Chains in Hemoglobin

GREEK DESIGNATION	GREEK NAME	NO. OF AMINO ACIDS	COMMENTS
α	Alpha	141	
β	Beta	146	
δ	Delta	146	Differs from beta chain by 10 amino acids
γ	Gamma	146	Differs from beta chain by 39 amino acids
ε	Epsilon	146	Embryonic only★
ζ	Zeta	146	Embryonic only★

★ Found only in the first 3 mo of embryonic life.

1. A protein component called globin composed of two sets (dimers) of two different polypeptide chains
2. Four molecules of the nitrogenous substance protoporphyrin IX
3. Four iron atoms in the ferrous state (Fe^{+2}) that combine with protoporphyrin IX to form four heme molecules
4. One 2,3-diphosphoglycerate (2,3-DPG) molecule as a sometime resident in the center of the Hb unit.

Globin Chains

Globin chains consist of varied sequences of amino acids; thus they are polypeptide chains. The chains are designated by the Greek letters α, β, γ, δ, ϵ, and ζ. The difference in the globin chain designations relates both to the sequence and to the number of amino acids in the chain. Table 7-1 lists some characteristics of each of the chain types.

The amino acid sequences forming globin polypeptide chains and the proportions of these chains undergo a series of changes during fetal and early infant life. Soon after birth, however, the chains take on the proportions they will retain throughout life.

Protoporphyrin IX and Iron

Protoporphyrin IX is a nitrogenous substance synthesized partly inside the mitochondria and partly in the cytoplasm of the nucleated erythrocyte during maturation. When ferrous iron (Fe^{+2}) is added to the center of protoporphyrin IX, a substance called ferroprotoporphyrin IX, otherwise known as heme, is formed. The connection of heme and globin through chemical bonds forms the basis of the Hb molecule.

2,3-Diphosphoglycerate

2,3–DPG is a substance produced in the anaerobic glycolytic (Embden–Meyerhof) pathway. This pathway generates energy for the erythrocyte (Chap. 6). Specifically, 2,3-DPG is produced in the Rapoport–Luebering shunt. When Hb binds 2,3-DPG, O_2 affinity decreases. Conversely, when the plasma level of 2,3-DPG decreases, Hb 2,3-DPG is released, and the Hb affinity for O_2 increases. Thus, there is an inverse relation between the amount of 2,3-DPG available for binding by Hb and hemoglobin's affinity for O_2. Adequate tissue oxygenation requires, among other factors, adequate supplies of 2,3-DPG to encourage Hb to release O_2 to the tissues.

NORMAL HEMOGLOBIN VARIANTS

During the first 3 months after conception, the fetus produces three embryonic Hbs called Portland, Gower I, and Gower II, composed of different types of globin chains as well as heme and iron (Table 7-2). In the fourth month of embryonic development, α and γ globin chains are produced, which together form fetal hemoglobin, designated Hb F. This becomes the predominant variant at this point in fetal life, whereas the concentrations of the embryonic Hbs decrease so that none is detectable at birth. The molecular structure of Hb F is $\alpha_2\gamma_2$. In other words, Hb F consists of two α chains and two γ chains. At birth Hb F comprises about 80% of the total Hb, the remainder being Hb A_1 and Hb A_2 (see Table 7-2). By 1 year of age essentially all the child's Hb is in the adult forms: Hb A_1 ($\alpha_2\beta_2$), also called Hb A, accounts for approximately 97% of the Hb by this age and throughout life; Hb A_2 ($\alpha_2\delta_2$) accounts for approximately 2%; and the remainder, usually less than 1%, is Hb F.

Hemoglobin variants, normal and abnormal, may be identified by electrophoresis (Chap. 14). Special quantitative analyses of Hb A_2 and Hb F are useful in the diagnosis of some hematologic disorders (Chaps. 14 and 15).

HEMOGLOBIN STRUCTURE AND SYNTHESIS

Because so many factors are involved in the synthesis and final structure of Hb, it is not surprising that a multitude of

TABLE 7–2. Normal Human Hemoglobins

HEMOGLOBIN	MOLECULAR STRUCTURE	STAGE OF LIFE	PROPORTION (%) NEWBORNS	PROPORTION (%) ADULTS★
Portland	$\zeta_2\gamma_2$	Embryonic†	0	0
Gower I	$\zeta_2\varepsilon_2$	Embryonic†	0	0
Gower II	$\alpha_2\varepsilon_2$	Embryonic†	0	0
Fetal (F)	$\alpha_2\gamma_2$	Newborn and adult	80	<1
A_1	$\alpha_2\beta_2$	Newborn and adult	20	97
A_2	$\alpha_2\delta_2$	Newborn and adult	<0.5	2.5

★ Older than 1 yr.
† The Portland, Gower I, and Gower II Hbs are found only during embryonic life.

hematologic disorders are associated with both structural and synthetic defects in Hb. Structural defects (most commonly one or more substitutions of an incorrect amino acid[s] in a globin chain amino acid sequence) lead to abnormal variants that cause disorders called hemoglobinopathies (Chap. 14). Synthetic defects (most commonly decreased or nonexistent production of one or more globin chain types) cause thalassemic disorders (Chap. 15). It is therefore important to have knowledge of the intricate structure and complex synthetic process of Hb.

Three-Dimensional Structure

Like all proteins, Hb is species specific. However, the structural similarities between the Hbs of different species far outweigh the differences. As the name hemoglobin implies, the molecule has a globular shape. However, the locations and characteristic behaviors of the individual components of the molecule can easily be depicted in a two-dimensional simplification (Fig. 7-1).

Structural Relations of Globin, 2,3-DPG, and Heme

Figure 7-1 shows two Hb A molecules, each with four globin chains, two α and two β chains. There is a central cavity in which one molecule of 2,3-DPG is bonded to the β chains when the Hb molecule is in its nonoxygenated state (note that the term "reduced" is not appropriate in place of "nonoxygenated"). The 2,3-DPG is expelled when Hb A is in its oxygenated state. On each outside corner one heme group is contained in a pocket formed by a globin chain.

Hemoglobin $\alpha\beta$ Dimers

The α and β globin units on the left side of Figure 7-1 and the α and β units on the right each form a structure called a dimer. Thus, each Hb molecule contains two dimers. The bonds between the α and β units, indicated by an "a" for each dimer, are very strong, whereas the bonds between the two $\alpha\beta$ dimers, indicated by a "b," are of lesser strength. The two dimers can therefore move relative to each other, approaching and separating as well as twisting, thus allowing for the change between the tense and relaxed forms of Hb (see Fig. 7-1) as required by the body's tissue O_2 needs.

Nonoxygenated Hemoglobin Structure: Tense (T) Form

In its nonoxygenated state, Hb takes on its tense or T form. The β chains of the molecule move farther apart, and the molecule binds 2,3-DPG, with the formation of anionic salt bridges between the β chains. The presence of 2,3-DPG in the molecule encourages improved O_2 delivery to the tissues.

Oxygenated Hemoglobin Structure: Relaxed (R) Form

On partial oxygenation of Hb, 2,3-DPG is expelled, and Hb takes on its relaxed or R form. This permits further O_2 binding. The salt bridges are broken, and the β chains move closer together. This form of Hb has an increased affinity for O_2 binding.[30]

Genetic Coding for Globin Chains

The human chromosomes 11 and 16 contain all the genetic information necessary to direct the synthesis of the various globin chains required for normal Hb production. An illustration of these chromosomes is provided in Figure 15-2. Chapter 15 also provides details on the genetics of globin chain production in relation to thalassemia, which is caused by genetic defects leading to reduced globin chain production. The chromosome ends are designated as 3' and 5' to serve as points of reference. Note that chromosome 16 codes for α and ζ chains, whereas chromosome 11 codes for β, γ, δ, and ϵ chains.

Globin Chain Production

Globin chains are simple (nonconjugated) proteins consisting of amino acids (NH_2–$CH(R)$–$COOH$) only. The

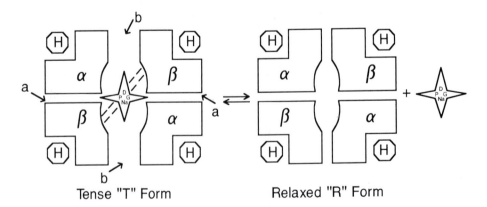

Tense "T" Form   Relaxed "R" Form

FIG. 7-1. Structure of the Hb A hemoglobin molecule. α and β indicate globin chains, H represents a heme molecule, DPG is 2,3-diphosphoglycerate, and a $\rightarrow$ represents the strong bonds inside each set of α and β chains. Each set forms a dimer; b $\rightarrow$ represents the weak bond between the two dimers. The dashed lines indicate anionic salt bridges between the β chains. The configuration to the left is the nonoxygenated state, also called the tense or T form. To the right is the relaxed or R form. It is formed after partial oxygenation of hemoglobin in which the central cavity of the molecule shrinks to expel the 2,3-DPG molecule, and the β chain salt bridges are broken. See text for details.

amino acids are connected by peptide bonds (–CO·NH–) in a specific sequence to form a given globin chain type. The genes along chromosomes 11 and 16 each provide a unique DNA code for each globin type.

Figure 7-2 illustrates the sequence of events involved in globin chain production beginning with the β gene on chromosome 11. Notice that the β gene has approximately 1900 bases. Not all base sequences are actually used to produce the β globin chain. Therefore, further processing must occur.

Globin production, like all protein synthesis, entails four basic phases: (1) transcription; (2) processing; (3) translation; and (4) transfer. DNA transcription produces a preliminary form of messenger RNA (mRNA) called pre-mRNA. Pre-mRNA undergoes processing in which certain bases are edited out to create the final mRNA molecule, which includes (1) a 5' region, not to be translated, with a cap (this area may help start the translation process); (2) the 444-base (3×148 codons) region, active in translation, which provides the instructions for globin chain production; (3) a 3' region, not to be translated, with an unknown function; and (4) a poly-A region that probably affects the stability or half-life of the molecule.[40]

During translation, mRNA leaves the nucleus for a ribosome in the cytoplasm, where proteins are manufactured under the direction of mRNA. In the transfer phase, transfer RNA (tRNA) is required to collect the amino acids from the cytoplasm and carry them to the appropriate site on the ribosome. Beginning with the initiator codon, AUG,

amino acid bonding continues until the terminator codon, UAA, is reached, at which time the completed globin chain is released from the ribosome, and the tRNA is released back into the cytoplasm.

Globin Chain Structure

Globin chains are best described by their primary and secondary structures.

Primary Structure

The primary globin structure is defined as a specified sequence of amino acid residues that together form a certain type of globin chain. Those of the α chain are numbered beginning with 1 at the N-terminal beginning of the chain to 141 at the C-terminal (the end) of the chain. Amino acid residues of the β, γ, and δ chains are similarly numbered from 1 through 146.

Secondary and Tertiary Structures

The secondary globin structure is defined by dividing the chain into eight separate helical segments. These segments are designated by the letters A through H (Fig. 7-3) and are structurally rigid. There are also seven nonhelical segments (NA, AB, CD, EF, FG, GH, and HC) that lie between the eight helical segments and provide the flexibility that allows physical bending of the globin chain to form the tertiary structure.[13] Figure 7-3 shows where such bending occurs.

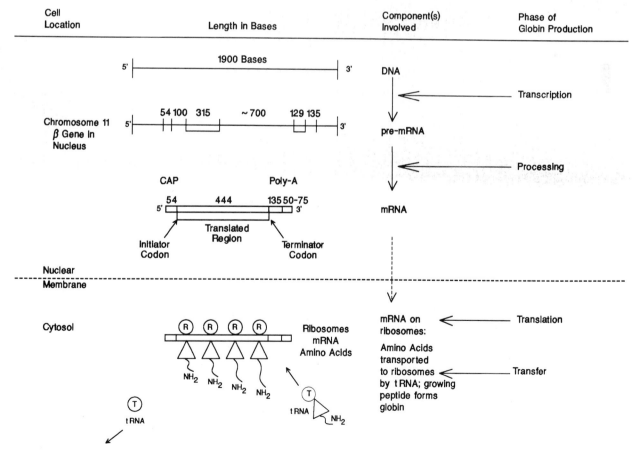

FIG. 7-2.   The events leading to biosynthesis of the β globin chain. See text for details.

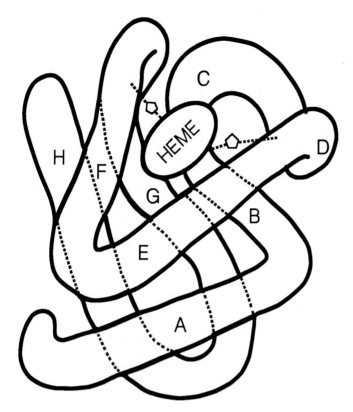

FIG. 7-3.   The tertiary structure of a β globin chain. Heme is contained in a pocket between the E and F helices. (Courtesy of C A Finch, MD.)

Heme Production and Structure

Heme production requires the formation of protoporphyrin IX and the availability of iron. Like all porphyrins, protoporphyrin is a derivative of porphin. This substance, also called tetramethenetetrapyrrole, is a cyclic compound consisting of four pyrrole rings connected with methene (=CH–) bridges at carbons 2 and 4 in the pyrrole rings. Figure 7-4 depicts porphin and names the individual rings and bridges. It also shows the eight hydrogen atoms where side chains may be substituted to form the various porphyrins. Heme protoporphyrin is named IX because it was the ninth of 15 possible isomers synthesized by Hans Fischer,[40] who was the first to study and describe porphyrins.

Formation of Protoporphyrin IX and Heme

Protoporphyrin IX is the last compound produced in a series of reactions leading to the formation of heme (Fig. 7-5). Four heme units ultimately bind with globin chains to create the Hb molecule.

MAIN EVENTS AND SIDE EVENTS.   The synthesis of heme requires a sequence of steps, all of which are enzymatically directed, as illustrated in Figure 7-5. Porphyrins may be formed from the intermediate compounds uroporphyrinogen and coproporphyrinogen; however, this will not take place to a significant degree unless the normal sequence of reactions is interrupted by inactivation or absence of the appropriate enzyme(s).

The porphyrins, including protoporphyrin IX, differ from the porphyrinogens in that the latter have methylene (–CH_2–) bridges (see Fig. 7-5) between the pyrrole rings. Porphyrins are very stable, are essentially flat, have a cavity in the center, and tend to stick together.

The raw materials for protoporphyrin formation are readily available inside the mitochondrion where heme production begins in the nucleated erythrocyte. Figure 7-5 details the chemistry of the reactions leading to heme synthesis. Upon formation of δ-aminolevulinic acid (ALA), heme synthesis is transferred to the cytoplasm outside the mitochondrion.

After the conversion of uroporphyrinogen III to coproporphyrinogen III, the remainder of heme synthesis takes place back inside the mitochondrion. Coproporphyrinogen III is oxidized to protoporphyrinogen IX by coproporphyrinogen oxidase, which causes oxidative decarboxylation of two of the four propionic acid (P) groups, resulting in formation of vinyl (V) groups (–CH=CH_2). Protoporphyrinogen IX is converted to protoporphyrin IX in the presence of protoporphyrinogen oxidase, which causes methene (=CH–) bridge formation and an internal rearrangement of the double bonds to the configuration of the porphin nucleus, where all double bonds are conjugated. Iron (Fe^{+2}) is then attached to the molecule in the presence of ferrochelatase, thus forming heme. Iron is transported in the ferric state to the forming erythrocyte by a specific transport protein called transferrin.

The rate of porphyrin synthesis is directly related to the rate of globin synthesis. Thus, synthesis of heme and globin are closely synchronized.[1]

REMNANTS OF HEME PRODUCTION.   Normally at the completion of heme synthesis, there is a small amount of

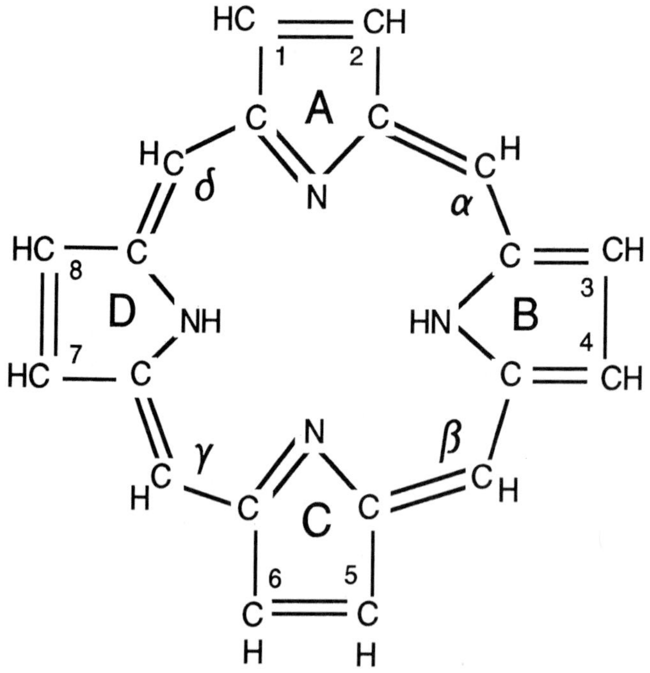

FIG. 7-4.   The porphin molecule, which forms the nucleus of porphyrins. Indicated letter and number codes are used consistently in porphyrin and porphyrinogen chemistry.

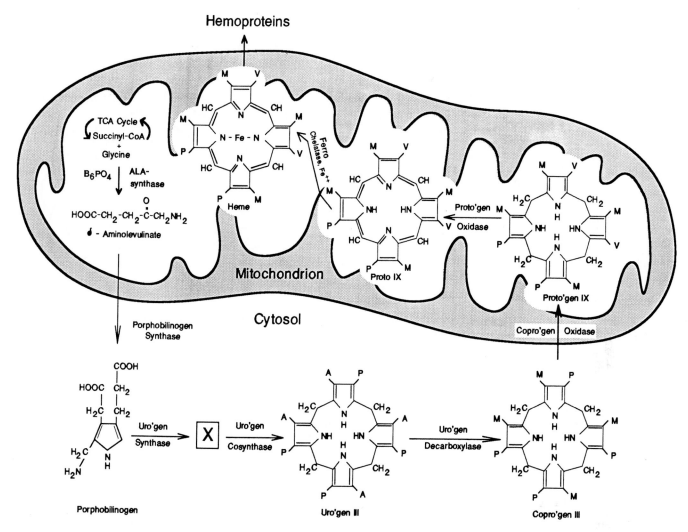

FIG. 7-5. The heme biosynthetic pathway showing the distribution of enzymes between the mitochondria and the cytoplasm. Intermediates between porphobilinogen and uroporphyrinogen III, designated by (X), remain unidentified. B_6PO_4 = pyridoxal phosphate. (From Labbe RF, Lamon JM: Porphyrins and disorders of porphyrin metabolism. In Tietz NW (ed): Fundamentals of Clinical Chemistry, 3rd ed. Philadelphia, WB Saunders, 1987, with permission.)

excess porphyrin in the mitochondrion that is complexed to zinc. This excess is called free erythrocyte protoporphyrin (FEP).[42] The amount of FEP in the erythrocyte is elevated when the iron supply is diminished. Free erythrocyte protoporphyrin can be measured in the laboratory, a useful test in the diagnosis of certain disorders (Chap. 13).

Ferritin aggregates are also found normally in the cytoplasm; such aggregates are visible microscopically after staining with Prussian blue. They represent storage iron that was not used in heme synthesis.[14]

Iron Metabolism for Heme Synthesis

Iron in the ferrous state (Fe^{+2}) is required to convert protoporphyrin to heme. Knowledge of the process by which iron is made available to the erythrocytes is necessary to understand some of the disorders of iron metabolism (Chap. 13).

Physiologic Locations of Iron

Iron is present throughout the body. Most is physiologically active, but some is stored for future use. Most of the stored iron is found in the intracellular space of the liver and bone marrow. Iron is stored for the most part in the form of ferritin, which is composed of iron and a protein called apoferritin. When apoferritin is unavailable, iron is stored as hemosiderin.

Sources, Recycling, and Loss of Iron

Proper nutrition provides the body with adequate iron. Dietary iron is ingested in both the ferric (Fe^{+3}) and ferrous (Fe^{+2}) states; however, only the ferrous (reduced) form is absorbed. Reduction is accomplished by the acid pH of the stomach and certain reducing substances. A small amount of iron is absorbed in the stomach, but most absorption occurs in the duodenum and jejunum. Only about 10% of the daily dietary iron intake is absorbed, because the body conserves iron so well by recycling it. Once the iron is absorbed, intestinal mucosal cells oxidize it to its ferric state, and the iron is stored temporarily in these cells as ferritin. When saturated, the mucosal cells will no longer absorb iron. Unabsorbed iron is then retained in the bowel and subsequently excreted in the feces.

An overwhelming amount of stored iron is derived from

the natural turnover of erythrocytes. On their natural destruction at approximately 120 days, erythrocyte iron is released for recycling. However, significant amounts of iron may be lost in episodes of chronic or acute blood loss.

Iron Transport

When iron is needed, Fe^{+3} is released from the mucosal cells. It then attaches to transferrin, the plasma iron transport protein, for circulation in the blood as ferric–transferrin. Transferrin can transport two atoms of iron simultaneously. It delivers iron for Hb, myoglobin, cytochrome, and other protein synthesis to the iron storage sites and to most body tissues. Developing erythrocyte precursors have transferrin–iron membrane receptors. When a ferric–transferrin complex binds to a receptor, the membrane invaginates, and a vacuole is formed that contains the iron-transferrin–receptor complex. Iron is then delivered either to the mitochondria for synthesis of heme or for storage as crystalline aggregates of ferritin. Special studies (e.g., electron microscopy) can reveal ferritin stores in nucleated and mature erythrocytes. Nucleated erythrocytes with stored ferritin are referred to as sideroblasts, and mature erythrocytes with ferritin are called siderocytes. Aggregated ferritin in sideroblasts or siderocytes can be seen microscopically in a bone marrow or peripheral blood sample after staining with Prussian blue.

After releasing iron the transferrin–receptor complex moves back to the cell membrane, and the transferrin is returned to the plasma for transport of more iron.

Assembly of the Hemoglobin Molecule

Formation of Hb requires iron (ferritin), globin chains, protoporphyrin IX, and the sometimes-resident 2,3-DPG. The source and synthesis of each of these components were described above.

To assemble the molecule, a ferric iron atom must be obtained from ferritin; it must be chemically reduced and then inserted as ferrous iron into the center of the protoporphyrin IX molecule. This process is aided by the enzyme ferrochelatase.

When a globin chain is completed on the ribosome, it is released to the cytoplasm. Individual α and β chains spontaneously and quickly form $\alpha\beta$ dimers, to which two heme molecules bind in the crevice between the E and F helices (see Fig. 7-3). Two of these dimers quickly form $\alpha_2\beta_2$ Hb tetramers and assume the final three-dimensional (quaternary) structure (Fig. 7-6). As a last step, one 2,3-DPG molecule is inserted in the central cavity of the Hb structure.

Assembly of Myoglobin

Myoglobin is discussed here because it is a molecule with many similarities to Hb, although there also are many differences. Myoglobin is a heme pigment found in striated muscle. It has a small molecular weight (17,000). Myoglobin production, like Hb production, requires amino acids, iron, and protoporphyrin IX as raw materials. Myoglobin has a single polypeptide chain very similar to a globin chain in hemoglobin. It has one heme molecule attached to the polypeptide chain, and the heme can bind O_2. A significant

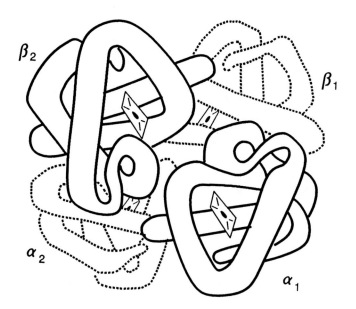

FIG. 7-6.   The three-dimensional Hb A (adult hemoglobin) molecule. It is comprised of two α and two β chains, each forming its own pocket containing a heme group (indicated by the four small rectangles). (Courtesy of Anne Stiene–Martin.)

difference between myoglobin and Hb is that the O_2 dissociation curve for the former is hyperbolic whereas that for the latter is sigmoid.[2] Thus, unlike Hb, myoglobin binds O_2 tightly and will release it only at very low values of tissue pO_2.

LOCATIONS OF HEMOGLOBIN DURING FUNCTION AND DEGRADATION

Except during fetal life, Hb is formed in the bone marrow. It is synthesized inside the developing erythrocytes from the stage of basophilic erythroblast (prorubricyte) until shortly after erythrocyte release into the circulation.

On erythrocyte destruction the cell remnants are captured by phagocytic cells of the reticuloendothelial system (RES), mostly the spleen[11] and liver,[36] but also the bone marrow. Hemoglobin degradation in the RES causes the release of iron, globin, and biliverdin, a noncyclic protoporphyrin derivative. Iron and globin chain amino acids are recycled for use in Hb synthesis, whereas biliverdin is degraded and excreted (Chap. 16).

PHYSIOLOGIC CHARACTERISTICS OF HEMOGLOBIN

Functions of Hemoglobin

Hemoglobin performs three functions, each of which is essential for life: (1) transport of molecular O_2 from the lungs to the tissues; (2) transport of CO_2 from the tissues to the lungs; (3) buffering of the blood to prevent changes in pH that are incompatible with life. The structure and composition of Hb make it eminently suited for such purposes.

Oxygen Transport

Heme–Heme Interaction

Oxygen affinity is affected by the phenomenon of heme–heme interaction. At any time the Hb molecule may be carrying one, two, three, or four O_2 molecules. Because of the nature of heme–heme interaction, the binding of one molecule causes an increased affinity of the other heme groups for O_2. In other words, the more O_2 bound by Hb, the greater Hb's affinity for O_2. This increase in affinity coincides with the expulsion of 2,3-DPG and conversion of Hb to the R form.

Oxygen Transport Mechanism

Each heme–polypeptide unit of the Hb molecule has the ability to bind one oxygen (O_2) molecule, so that a fully oxygenated Hb molecule should be represented by the symbol $Hb(O_2)_4$, rather than by the common form HbO_2. Hemoglobin acquisition of O_2 takes place in the alveolar capillaries of the lungs. The atmospheric air entering the lungs is approximately 20.93% O_2 at all altitudes on earth. At sea level the partial pressure of inspired O_2 is approximately 149 mm Hg. There is an average tension (pO_2) of slightly over 100 mm Hg in the air sacs. Because of the minute distance between the O_2 in the air sacs and the blood in the capillary network, the diffusion of O_2 is rapid. In the lung alveoli Hb becomes about 95% saturated with O_2 as a result of diffusion from alveolar O_2, which is at 100+ mm Hg partial pressure.

Hemoglobin is essential to the adequate oxygenation of body tissues because O_2 is only slightly soluble in water, the solvent for blood. Only about 3 mL of O_2 can be carried in solution by each liter of blood without the assistance of Hb, whereas an adult at rest needs about 250 mL of O_2 per minute. The Hb molecule solves this problem.

It is helpful to understand whole-blood O_2 content by comparing the content in plasma with the content in normal whole blood and anemic whole blood. Such a comparison shows that plasma supplies only 0.08 mmol of O_2 when 1 liter of blood passes through the capillary bed, whereas given a Hb of 16.0 g/dL, 2.41 mmol is supplied, and given a Hb of 8.0 g/dL, 1.22 mmol is supplied.

Hemoglobin and Oxygen Therapy

Breathing pure O_2 or hyperbaric (high pressure) O_2 is sometimes required to treat conditions such as carbon monoxide (CO) poisoning and infant respiratory distress syndrome. Hyperbaric therapy requires that the patient be put into a special chamber that provides O_2 at 2.5 to 3 times atmospheric pressure.

The goal of O_2 therapy is to increase the pO_2 *without* dependence on the Hb molecule. As pO_2 is increased, there is a significant increase in the plasma O_2 concentration without any significant change in the amount of O_2 bound to Hb. Breathing pure O_2 raises the pO_2 to more than 600 mm Hg and significantly elevates the available plasma O_2 content by 0.7 mmol/L. Breathing O_2 at a hyperbaric pressure may provide a pO_2 as high as 2400 mm Hg, at which the available plasma O_2 content will be 3.25 mmol/L more than that amount available when the pO_2 falls below 100 mm Hg, where Hb takes over the role of tissue O_2 supplier.

TABLE 7–3. Effects of Various Factors on Oxyhemoglobin Dissociation Curve

FACTOR	SHIFT CAUSED BY*	
	FACTOR INCREASE	FACTOR DECREASE
Blood temperature	R	L
pH	L	R
Erythrocyte 2,3-DPG	R	L
CO_2	R	L
Hb F admixture	L	NA†

* A shift to the left (L) is associated with an increased affinity for O_2.
 A shift to the right (R) is associated with a decreased affinity for O_2.
† Not applicable.

Oxyhemoglobin Dissociation Curve

Hemoglobin has the ability to bind large quantities of O_2; however, Hb must also be willing to release O_2 when needed. The Hb molecule can perform this feat because of its configuration (quaternary structure), which is altered with changes in the circulatory environment. These changes cause alterations in the chemical and physical characteristics of the molecule, particularly movement between the T and the R forms, both of which are related to O_2 affinity as previously discussed. Factors that affect Hb affinity for O_2 are listed in Table 7-3 and discussed in more detail later in this chapter.

It is common to represent the affinity of Hb for O_2 in a graph called the oxyhemoglobin dissociation curve. Figure 7-7 presents the curve (curve a) and the influences of environmental factors on Hb O_2 affinity (curves b and c). The y axis reflects the percentage of Hb saturated with oxygen, sO_2, for an Hb solution at pH 7.4. This is plotted against the

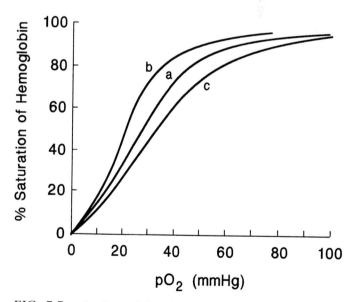

FIG. 7-7. Oxyhemoglobin dissociation curves under various influences: a = normal dissociation curve; b = "shift to the left," which can be associated with high pH, low erythrocyte 2,3-DPG concentration, or decreased blood temperature; c = "shift to the right," which can be associated with low pH, high erythrocyte 2,3-DPG concentration, or elevated blood temperature. See text for details.

partial pressure of oxygen at equilibrium, pO_2, on the x axis. Curve b represents a "shift to the left" from normal and curve c, a "shift to the right." Note the physiologically important sigmoidal (S) shape of the curves.

NORMAL CURVE (CURVE A).   The S shape reflects the following important points under normal conditions:

1. When the pO_2 is less than 20 mm Hg, Hb has a very low affinity for O_2.
2. When the pO_2 is between 20 and 60 mm Hg, the levels generally found in the tissues, Hb's affinity for O_2 increases substantially. Note that the curve in this range is steep, indicating that Hb can release O_2 rapidly. This steep slope also shows that, if necessary, the quantity of O_2 released may be large for a relatively small change in pO_2, thus permitting maximum O_2 delivery to the tissues when needed.
3. When the pO_2 is above 60 mm Hg, the curve begins to flatten rapidly toward the area of 100% Hb saturation, indicating an almost complete saturation of Hb with O_2. This situation is found in the alveoli of the lungs.

SHIFT TO THE LEFT (CURVE B).   When the curve is shifted to the left, Hb has an increased affinity for O_2 and does not readily release it to the tissues. Certain environmental conditions can cause this left shift (see Table 7-3), including a decrease in body temperature, a decrease in 2,3-DPG or carbon dioxide (CO_2) concentration, and an increase in blood pH, all of which increase the affinity of Hb for O_2, thus creating a potential for decreased delivery to the tissues.

One example of such a condition is hyperventilation, in which larger than normal amounts of CO_2 are lost as the individual breathes excessively, often because of severe anxiety. This CO_2 loss causes an increase in pH (*i.e.*, an excessively alkaline environment). Hemoglobin binding of O_2 causes it to release free hydrogen ions, which eventually reduce the pH to normal and shift the curve back to its normal position. Oxygenation of Hb also causes it to release 2,3-DPG, resulting in decreased levels of erythrocyte 2,3-DPG and allowing for further O_2 binding.

SHIFT TO THE RIGHT (CURVE C).   A shift to the right for the oxyhemoglobin dissociation curve represents a decreased affinity of Hb for O_2. This may result from increased body temperature, increased concentrations of 2,3-DPG or CO_2, or decreased blood pH, all of which necessitate increased delivery of O_2 to the tissues (see Table 7-3). Examples of such conditions are the physiologic state during exercise, in which the muscle tissue temperature rises, or the abnormal build-up of hydrogen ions in renal failure. An acidic state results from excess hydrogen ions (H^+) that are released into the blood. These ions can be bound by nonoxygenated Hb. As prescribed by the Bohr effect, which regulates the relation between pH and Hb oxygenation, Hb must release its O_2 to the tissues before it may bind H^+. By binding with these ions, the Hb plays its role as a buffer, and eventually, the pH is brought back to normal, thus shifting the dissociation curve in the direction of normal. In the deep tissues, the high concentrations of CO_2 encourage Hb to release O_2 as well.

Factors Affecting Hemoglobin Affinity for Oxygen

Six factors in the blood affect Hb affinity for O_2: (1) blood (body) temperature; (2) blood pH (the Bohr effect); (3) 2,3-DPG; (4) blood CO_2 levels: (5) the amount of Hb F; and (6) abnormal Hb variants.

Blood (Body) Temperature
Increased blood temperature causes Hb to release O_2 more readily because the oxyhemoglobin dissociation curve shifts to the right. The opposite is true for decreased blood temperature.

Blood pH (Bohr Effect)
The relation between blood pH and the O_2 affinity of Hb is referred to as the Bohr effect.[33] An increase in pH (decrease in acidity) shifts the dissociation curve to the left. Thus, the conditions in the lungs, where pH is at its highest, favor uptake of O_2 by Hb. Conversely, in the peripheral tissues where acidic metabolites are produced, the pH is lower, the curve shifts to the right, and O_2 is released readily.

Usually the arteriovenous pH difference is small (<0.04). Nevertheless, when local acidic conditions occur, the characteristics of the dissociation curve and the Bohr effect provide for a rapid increase in O_2 delivery and uptake of H^+.

2,3-Diphosphoglycerate
A similar shifting of the dissociation curve is seen as a result of variation in the erythrocytic 2,3-DPG concentration.[4] With increasing 2,3-DPG concentration the curve shifts to the right, the affinity for O_2 is diminished, and bound O_2 is released, while 2,3-DPG is bound by the salt bridges between the β chains. This is of specific importance in blood storage, in that some anticoagulants cause whole blood or packed cells to lose most of their native 2,3-DPG during storage. If blood with decreased 2,3-DPG levels is transfused to a patient, its Hb may not release O_2 when and where needed until adequate concentrations of 2,3-DPG have been built up from metabolic activities in the erythrocytes after transfusion.

Carbon Dioxide
Carbon dioxide exerts an effect on O_2 uptake and delivery similar to the Bohr effect. Increased blood CO_2 levels cause a shift to the right in the oxyhemoglobin dissociation curve, with a decreased Hb affinity for O_2, thus encouraging release of O_2 when CO_2 levels become elevated. Decreased CO_2 levels cause the opposite effect. These shifts are referred to as the Haldane effect.

Fetal Hemoglobin
Hemoglobin F, the normal Hb variant present in high concentrations at birth, has an oxyhemoglobin dissociation curve slightly to the left of normal. Although this usually causes a higher Hb O_2 affinity, Hb F does not react the same way with 2,3-DPG as does adult Hb. Therefore, its affinity for O_2 is not significantly affected. The slight increase in Hb F affinity for O_2 is helpful for the oxygenation of fetal blood, as the fetus exists in an environment with generally lower O_2 tension and slightly higher acidity.

Abnormal Hemoglobin Variants

A number of abnormal Hb variants show dissociation curve shifts, either right or left, compared with Hb A under identical environmental circumstances. This results from their structural abnormalities, often caused by globin chain amino acid substitutions (Chap. 14).

Hemoglobin Transport of Carbon Dioxide

Hemoglobin not only provides O_2 for tissues but also removes CO_2 from the tissues and transports it to the lungs for expiration. About 70% of CO_2 is carried to the lungs in the form of plasma bicarbonate (HCO_3^-) and 20% as erythrocyte bicarbonate. The reactions in this transport method not only remove CO_2 from the body but also buffer the blood.

About 5% of CO_2 transport by Hb is achieved by the binding of dissolved CO_2 with the N-terminal amino acids of the globin chains in nonoxygenated Hb to form carbaminohemoglobin (Hb–NH–COO$^-$). The final 5% of CO_2 is transported in solution.[31]

Hemoglobin Buffering Action in the Blood

As in any other protein, acidic groups (primarily –COOH) and basic groups (primarily –NH$_2$) on the surface of Hb cause it to act as an amphoteric substance; that is, one that may act both as an acid (proton donor) or as a base (proton acceptor). Although most carboxyl (–COOH) and amino (–NH$_2$) groups are tied up in peptide bonds, a sufficient number are available to play a significant role in acid–base balance in the blood. Because Hb is present in the blood stream in such a high concentration, it is effective as a buffer.

CO₂ Dissociation Curve: Haldane Effect

Blood containing nonoxygenated Hb (0% HbO$_2$) has a greater affinity for CO_2 than does oxygenated blood because of the Bohr effect. Further, a CO_2 dissociation curve (Fig. 7-8) reflects the relation between blood CO_2 content and the pCO_2 for 0% HbO$_2$, nonoxygenated blood, and 97.5% HbO$_2$, oxygenated blood. The difference in these curves demonstrates a phenomenon known as the Haldane effect, which facilitates CO_2 binding in the tissues, where pCO_2 is high, and excretion of CO_2 by means of expired air in the lungs, where pCO_2 is low. This mechanism provides the means whereby tissue CO_2 diffuses into the erythrocyte and allows Hb to play its role as a buffer, decreasing the acidity caused by the dissolved CO_2 in the blood.

Hemoglobin Acid–Base Balance

Nonoxygenated hemoglobin (Hb$^-$) is a stronger base than is oxyhemoglobin; therefore, it can more easily accept and neutralize H$^+$ ions formed as a result of increased blood CO_2 levels. The following two reactions are responsible for physiologic acid–base balance involving hemoglobin:

(1) $Hb(O_2)_4^- + H_2O + CO_2 \xrightleftharpoons{CA} Hb^- + H_2CO_3 + 4O_2$

(2) $Hb^- + HHCO_3 \rightleftharpoons HHb + HCO_3^-$

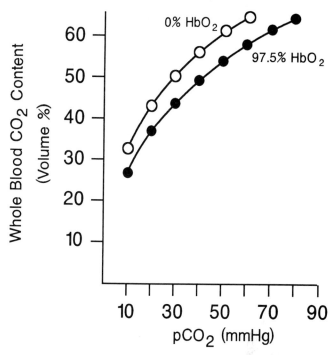

FIG. 7-8. The carbon dioxide dissociation curve of whole blood. The curve is relatively linear between pCO_2 40 and 60 torr (torr = 1/760 of normal atmospheric pressure). The Haldane effect is represented by the difference between the two curves, which reflect a comparison of oxygenated (97.5% HbO$_2$) and deoxygenated (0% HbO$_2$) blood.

The net result of these two reactions is that there is a very small difference in the arterial and venous pH. Figure 7-9 illustrates the interrelations of erythrocyte O_2 and CO_2 diffusion and transport.

In reaction 1, oxygenated Hb releases O_2 to the tissues while CO_2 diffuses into the erythrocyte and combines with H_2O to form carbonic acid. This reaction is accelerated by the enzyme carbonic anhydrase (CA). In reaction 2, nonoxygenated hemoglobin, Hb$^-$, acts as a base and accepts the proton (H$^+$) to form HHb and to reduce carbonic acid content. The buildup of bicarbonate ions in the erythrocyte eventually causes a concentration gradient between the cell and plasma, and bicarbonate begins to diffuse into the plasma. This loss of negative ions causes chloride ions (Cl$^-$) to diffuse into the cell to maintain electroneutrality. This is called the chloride shift.

The erythrocyte then travels back to the lungs, where the reactions go in the opposite direction. Hemoglobin again becomes oxygenated, making it a stronger acid, causing carbonic acid to convert back to water and CO_2, which is expelled.

HEMOGLOBIN DERIVATIVES AND THEIR ASSOCIATED DISORDERS

Hemoglobin derivatives are abnormal forms in which the heme is altered in some way but the globin chains are unaffected. These derivatives are nonfunctional and may or may not be reversible to a normal variant.

Hemoglobin and Erythrocyte Function

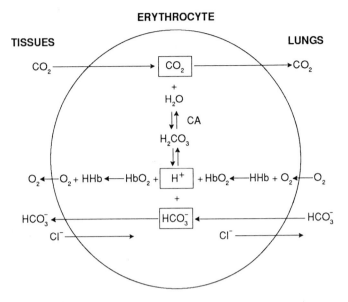

FIG. 7-9. The interrelations of oxygen and carbon dioxide transport in the erythrocyte that affect the whole blood acid–base balance. Arrows to the left indicate the direction of reactions taking place in the tissues; those to the right, in the lungs. In the tissue, CO_2 diffuses into the red cell, and its hydration is catalyzed by carbonic anhydrase (CA). Dissociation of the resulting carbonic acid produces bicarbonate and a proton (H^+). The bicarbonate is exchanged for chloride in the plasma. The proton is accepted by oxyhemoglobin (HbO_2), a reaction that by means of the Bohr effect, facilitates the dissociation of HbO_2. These reactions are reversed in the lungs because of the low pCO_2 and high pO_2. (From Wintrobe MM: The mature erythrocyte. In Wintrobe MM et al [eds]: Clinical Hematology. Philadelphia, Lea & Febiger, 1981, with permission.)

Hemoglobin is a very stable protein and functions during the full 120-day life span of the erythrocyte. It might function even longer if it were not dependent on the erythrocyte for its transportation. During the 120-day period, Hb passes through an incomprehensible number of metabolic cycles, each time without showing signs of aging. Nevertheless, the substance is not immune to reversible and irreversible conversions to the nonfunctional derivative states, which include methemoglobin, sulfhemoglobin, and carboxyhemoglobin. Each of these can cause an abnormal clinical state of varying severity.

Methemoglobin and Methemoglobinemia

Methemoglobin (also referred to as hemiglobin or Hi) is well known in the laboratory for its use as an intermediary in the cyanmethemoglobin method for quantitation of whole blood Hb. It is formed by gentle oxidation in which the iron in the heme groups is oxidized to its ferric state, Fe^{+3}. In this form, heme cannot bind O_2.[18]

Normal endogenous production is a continuing event. Approximately 0.5% to 3% of the total body Hb is spontaneously converted to methemoglobin daily.[18] However, this seldom causes any problems because of an enzyme,

NADH-methemoglobin reductase (diaphorase) (Chap. 6), which is present in the erythrocytes at a level sufficient to counter methemoglobin produced at rates many times those normally encountered. Methemoglobin reduction also requires a properly functioning Embden–Meyerhof pathway to produce NADH, which is the main source for electron donation in the reduction process. The electron is transferred from NADH to the enzyme and then to an erythrocyte cytochrome before being used in the actual heme reduction. Simplified, the basic reaction is:

$$Hb^{+3} \longrightarrow Hb^{+2}$$

$$\begin{array}{c} NADH \xrightarrow{e^-} Met\ Hb\ reductase \longrightarrow Cytochrome \\ NAD^+ \end{array}$$

Heme is thus reduced to its ferrous and functional form. Methemoglobin levels are rarely above 1% of the total hemoglobin.[35]

Methemoglobinemia is characterized by elevated erythrocyte methemoglobin concentrations. The clinical manifestations are few and generally mild. Rarely, the disorder is inherited; more often, it is acquired. Five inherited Hb variants, each a form of Hb M (M for methemoglobin) (Chap. 14), also cause methemoglobinemia.

Pathophysiology

Whether acquired or inherited, methemoglobinemia stems from the inability to adequately reduce methemoglobin that builds up in the circulation, thus causing cyanosis. Characteristically, the patient responds to therapeutic doses of methylene blue (except patients with a Hb M disorder), as evidenced by the return of normal skin color shortly after therapy is initiated.

INHERITED METHEMOGLOBINEMIA. When inherited, methemoglobinemia is most commonly attributed to inheritance of an NADH-methemoglobin reductase enzyme deficiency. This is also called diaphorase deficiency. Without this enzyme, even with sufficient NADH produced in the Embden–Meyerhof pathway, methemoglobin is not adequately reduced, causing increased circulating levels of methemoglobin. These patients respond to methylene blue treatment.[9]

ACQUIRED METHEMOGLOBINEMIA. Abnormal and toxic methemoglobin production may be caused by a variety of substances, either ingested or absorbed. These include oxidants from a plethora of sources, including antimalarial drugs, therapeutic drugs such as sulfonamides (among others), drugs of abuse, aniline dyes (e.g., fresh dye on shoes), nitrate-rich water and foodstuffs, and many common aromatic chemicals. These patients also respond to methylene blue treatment.

INHERITED HEMOGLOBIN M METHEMOGLOBINEMIA. The five Hb M variants are the result of various amino acid substitutions in the globin chains that directly affect the heme group, causing it to enter the ferric or oxidized state, which leads to a methemoglobin buildup in the blood. Patients with these disorders characteristically do not respond to methylene blue treatment. Treatment is actually not possible, nor is it necessary, because the patients show no clinical abnormalities other than their cyanotic appearance (Chap. 14).

Demographics and Genetics

Diaphorase deficiency is rare and inherited as an autosomal recessive trait. It was first described in Europe;[9] however, it is now found practically worldwide. Most cases involve inbreeding among siblings or other close relatives.

Symptoms and Physical Findings

Cyanosis (a bluish skin discoloration) appears when the methemoglobin level exceeds 10%. This is mainly a cosmetic problem, and affected patients do not report any specific symptoms. Although the cyanosis affects the skin color of the entire body, it is particularly evident on the lips, mucous membranes of the mouth, ears, cheeks, and nail beds. If the methemoglobin level exceeds 35%, symptoms of hypoxia such as shortness of breath, dizziness, headaches, or tachycardia may occur. Levels of 60% to 70% or even greater are rare and are usually fatal.[23]

Laboratory Findings and Correlations with Disease

PERIPHERAL BLOOD FILM. Heinz bodies (Chap. 8), which reflect denatured Hb, may be demonstrated in the erythrocytes of cells affected by ingested toxins. This requires the use of special stains (Chap. 15).

DIAPHORASE ENZYME SCREENING TESTS. Diaphorase screening tests are rapid.[24, 34] Specific enzyme assays for use with prepared hemolysates are also available.[17]

METHEMOGLOBIN QUANTITATION. This test is based on methemoglobin's small but characteristic absorbance peak at 630 to 635 nm. The addition of potassium cyanide (KCN) to a prepared hemolysate causes conversion of methemoglobin to cyanmethemoglobin, which does not absorb at 632 nm.[6] The difference in the absorbance at 632 nm of hemolysates containing methemoglobin and methemoglobin converted to cyanmethemoglobin is proportional to the methemoglobin concentration.

Any methemoglobin level above 1.5% of the total Hb concentration is considered abnormal. Levels in individuals with acquired methemoglobinemia secondary to toxic substances may range from 10% to greater than 70%, depending on the circumstances. Levels in untreated individuals with diaphorase deficiency usually stay between 15% and 30%.[41]

OTHER FINDINGS. As with normal Hb, the oxygenation of one heme group increases the affinity of the other three groups for O_2. In patients with methemoglobinemia, however, this can cause a slight compensatory erythrocytosis[21, 22] and a slight left shift in the O_2 dissociation curve. Erythrocyte survival is normal.[23]

Laboratory investigation of the Hb M disorders is discussed in Chap. 14.

Effects of Treatment on Laboratory Results

Whether the disorder is acquired or inherited, therapy is rarely required. Other than the bluish skin color, the patients are normal and live a normal life span.[23] For cosmetic purposes, oral administration of methylene blue will generally maintain the methemoglobin level below 10%, thus avoiding the cyanotic appearance. For toxic situations, intravenous infusion of methylene blue is suggested for rapid methemoglobin clearance from the circulation. Methylene blue is very effective as an electron donor when diaphorase levels are insufficient or overwhelmed in toxic situations. The electron is donated in the presence of NADPH to the enzyme NADPH-methemoglobin reductase, and methylene blue is subsequently reduced to leukomethylene blue. Leukomethylene blue can then nonenzymatically reduce methemoglobin, thus turning the skin back to a normal color. Treatment with methylene blue causes the urine to turn blue, which made one member of a "blue family" in the Kentucky mountains undergoing such treatment exclaim, "I can see that old blue running out of my skin." Members of that family with blue skin had been recognized for more than 160 years.[38]

Sulfhemoglobin and Sulfhemoglobinemia

Sulfhemoglobin formation is another oxidation derivative of Hb that cannot carry O_2. It does not form as a result of normal metabolic activities, and it probably is always an acquired condition. Patients may have a significantly cyanotic appearance.

In vitro, sulfhemoglobin forms when hydrogen sulfide (H_2S) is added to Hb; thus the name sulfhemoglobin. In vivo, sulfhemoglobin forms in the occasional patient as a result of Hb oxidation by certain drugs and chemicals (e.g., acetanilid, phenacetin, and sulfonamides).[8, 27, 32] It is unclear why some patients, on the same drug exposure, form sulfhemoglobin whereas others form methemoglobin, and still others develop erythrocyte globin precipitates.

Sulfhemoglobinemia results from excessive sulfhemoglobin concentrations in the blood, although they hardly ever exceed 20% of the total hemoglobin. Such levels are not life threatening, and the only significant effect is cyanosis. The condition generally is benign. Once formed, sulfhemoglobin stays in the erythrocyte during its entire 120-day life span. Sulfhemoglobin cannot be converted back to normal, functional Hb.

Sulfhemoglobin quantitation may be performed by examination of a prepared hemolysate for a distinct, broad increase in the absorption curve in the range of 600 to 620 nm.[15]

Treatment of the patient consists of removal of the offending agent.

Carboxyhemoglobin and Carboxyhemoglobinemia

Carboxyhemoglobin is a carbon monoxide (CO) derivative of Hb normally found in blood at levels of less than 1% of the total hemoglobin.

Pathophysiology

Hemoglobin has more than 200 times the affinity for CO that it has for O_2. Exposure to even small percentages of CO in the inspired air therefore prevents a substantial amount of Hb from carrying out its function in O_2 transport. This can lead to asphyxiation. Automobile exhaust is a well-known source of toxicity,[3] and exposure to this exhaust is a common method in attempted suicides. Industrial wastes such as coal gas (e.g., gas from burning charcoal) and water gas are also recognized sources of toxicity.[26]

Symptoms and Physical Findings

Carbon monoxide poisoning may be insidious, with the effects of hypoxia suddenly overwhelming an individual, particularly because the gas is colorless and odorless. The skin turns a bright cherry red with increasing levels of carboxyhemoglobin. With lower levels of exposure, symptoms such as dizziness, nausea, headache, vomiting, and confusion may occur. At high levels (approximately 50% to 70% of total Hb), an individual can be asphyxiated.

Laboratory Findings and Correlations with Disease

A proportion of 0.5% carboxyhemoglobin is typical in nonsmokers, whereas 5% is common among smokers. With only 0.04% (v/v) CO in air, the carboxyhemoglobin proportion can increase to 10%, which is associated with shortness of breath on exertion. Long exposure at this level impairs judgment. With exposure to a CO level of 0.1% (v/v), carboxyhemoglobin levels can reach 50% to 70%, resulting in unconsciousness, respiratory failure, and death. Levels of 0.4% (v/v) are immediately fatal, causing the carboxyhemoglobin level to rise quickly to 80%.[39]

Laboratory screening tests for carboxyhemoglobin are available. One spot test calls for hemolyzing 0.5 mL of whole blood with 20 mL of distilled water, then adding 1 mL of NaOH, 1.0 mol/L. Blood containing more than 20% carboxyhemoglobin will cause the appearance of a light cherry-red color; normal blood will turn the mixture brown.[12]

Quantitation of CO can be performed by gas chromatography,[10] spectrophotometry,[37] and other techniques.[7] Dedicated spectrophotometric instruments now yield instantaneous highly accurate readings of Hb, carboxyhemoglobin, and oxygen saturation of Hb.

Effects of Treatment on Laboratory Results

Therapeutic measures in CO poisoning consist of removing the source of toxicity and administration of high levels of O_2, including, in some cases, hyperbaric O_2 therapy and maintaining proper ventilation. The carboxyhemoglobin level should then return to normal. Unless brain damage occurs, there are no long-term effects from such a toxic exposure as long as the patient receives proper and prompt treatment.

ABNORMAL HEME SYNTHESIS: THE PORPHYRIAS

Disorders of heme synthesis known as porphyrias will be addressed in this chapter. Addressed elsewhere are disorders of globin synthesis, both qualitative (Chap. 14) and quantitative (Chap. 15).

The laboratory analysis of aberrations in heme synthesis is necessary to detect the deficiency of, or a defect in, one or more of the hematopoietic enzymes involved in heme production. Such deficiencies or defects constitute a group of disorders, commonly known as porphyrias, which may be inherited or acquired.

Pathophysiology

The porphyrias lead to the accumulation of porphyrin precursors or of one or more of the porphyrin(ogen)s in the bone marrow (erythropoietic porphyrias) or the liver (hepatic porphyrias). Decreased Hb production is the result. With the exception of ALA synthase, deficiencies of all other enzymes have been described.

Primary porphyrias are inherited disorders. Table 7-4 lists characteristics of the enzymatic defects of porphyrias that are associated with erythropoietic abnormalities. All other enzyme abnormalities of the heme synthesis pathway are associated with hepatic porphyrias that show no hematologic abnormalities.

Secondary porphyrias are acquired disorders stimulated by certain drugs or chemicals through various mechanisms. The secondary porphyrias mainly affect the liver and seldom affect the bone marrow. The most important exception to this is the secondary porphyria caused by lead poisoning (Chap. 13). Lead poisoning causes the formation of

TABLE 7-4. The Primary Erythropoietic Porphyrias

PORPHYRIA	ENZYME DEFECT	INHERITANCE	CLINICAL PRESENTATION	LABORATORY FINDINGS AND COMMENTS
Hereditary PBG synthase deficiency	Porphobilinogen synthase*	Autosomal dominant	Not well known; possible neurologic abnormalities	Only decreased enzyme activity
Congenital erythropoietic porphyria (CEP)	Uroporphyrinogen III cosynthase	Autosomal recessive	Severe photocutaneous lesions; teeth fluoresce red under UV light; patients rarely survive past middle age	Rarest porphyria; hemolytic anemia; marked increase in RBC coproporphyrin; marked increase in urine uroporphyrin, causing red urine; marrow morphology shows normoblastic hyperplasia; possible anisocytosis, poikilocytosis, polychromasia
Protoporphyria (PP)	Ferrochelatase	Autosomal dominant	Photocutaneous lesions; mild to severe hepatobiliary disease	Possibly second most common porphyria; marked increase in FEP†; marrow morphology normal

* Porphobilinogen synthase = ALA dehydrase.
† Free erythrocyte protoporphyrin.

ringed sideroblasts (nucleated erythrocytes with a ring of mitochondria surrounding the nucleus) in the bone marrow similar to those seen in sideroblastic anemia.[5] The mitochondria have an abnormal accumulation of iron. The ringed sideroblasts reflect defective heme synthesis because of lead interference with several enzymes, particularly ALA dehydrase and ferrochelatase. Basophilic stippling in erythrocytes on the blood film is also a classic finding in cases of lead poisoning.

Symptoms and Physical Findings

Patients with primary porphyrias are generally either (1) asymptomatic; (2) suffering from characteristic skin lesions easily recognized by a physician; or (3) suffering from neurologic disturbances (see Table 7-4). The skin lesions, referred to as photocutaneous lesions, are formed on exposure to sunlight either indoors or outdoors because of the patient's increased porphyrin level; porphyrins strongly absorb Soret band wavelengths (400–430 nm; see below) from the sunlight through the skin, even from light coming through windows. Symptoms of anemia may be reported in cases of congenital erythropoietic porphyria (CEP), where hemolytic anemia may be involved.

Laboratory Findings and Correlations with Disease

Laboratory findings for the inherited erythropoietic porphyrias are summarized in Table 7-4. Note the characteristic increase in FEP in protoporphyria. This increase is caused by the lack of metal chelation secondary to the ferrochelatase enzyme deficiency. The FEP cannot be used in Hb synthesis and thus does not bind to globin. Elevated FEP also is found in iron deficiency anemia and anemia of chronic disease because of insufficiency of iron available to the erythron for Hb synthesis (Chap. 13).

Effects of Treatment on Laboratory Results

A variety of therapeutic measures have been used to alleviate the skin lesions, some of which have no effect on laboratory results, whereas others are said to reduce porphyrin levels. Hemolysis in CEP, as well as porphyrin levels, can sometimes be reduced by transfusions, splenectomy, or steroids, although these measures do not prevent the recurrence of hemolysis. The reader is referred to a textbook of clinical chemistry for more details on the porphyrias, both erythropoietic and hepatic.

LABORATORY EVALUATION OF HEMOGLOBIN

Hemoglobin analysis has played an important role in clinical diagnosis since early times. Of the many techniques proposed or used in the past to quantitate Hb, essentially only two analytical principles remain in use: the cyanmethemoglobin method for measurement of total Hb in whole blood and analysis of oxyhemoglobin to measure plasma Hb.

Cyanmethemoglobin Method for Measurement of Whole Blood Hemoglobin

The cyanmethemoglobin method is the recommended method for measurement of Hb in whole blood.[19,20,28] This method is advantageous because it can be used to measure all forms of peripheral blood Hb—nonoxygenated (Hb$^-$), oxygenated (HbO$_2$), carboxyhemoglobin (HbCO), and methemoglobin (Hi)—except sulfhemoglobin. The reaction mixture forms a color that has an absorption band at a wavelength of 540 nm that is broad and relatively flat. This procedure is presented in Chapter 9.

Oxyhemoglobin Method for Measurement of Plasma Hemoglobin

Plasma Hb measurements may be required in the diagnosis of acute hemolytic episodes (e.g., hemolytic transfusion reactions) or to determine the amount of hemolysis during extracorporeal treatment of blood. Plasma Hb, unlike total Hb, is best measured as oxyhemoglobin, because plasma Hb levels are too low to be detected by the cyanmethemoglobin method.

Each heme compound, including oxyhemoglobin, and in fact all porphyrins and porphyrin-containing compounds, have one characteristic sharp, narrow, and pronounced absorption peak somewhere in the lower part of the visible range, between 400 and 430 nm. The absorbance bands in this region are referred to as Soret bands. For example, the absorption maximum for oxyhemoglobin is in the narrow interval of 412 to 415 nm;[25] for carboxyhemoglobin, it is in the 417- to 418-nm interval. The absorbance in the Soret bands region is about 10-fold greater than the absorbance in the 500- to 650-nm interval.

The plasma Hb assay method of Harboe[16] is recommended in preference to methods that use benzidine derivatives,[15] such as that of Naumann.[29] In the method of Harboe, plasma Hb is measured as oxyhemoglobin at 415 nm, the Soret band of maximal absorbance for oxyhemoglobin. In the method of Naumann, benzidine derivatives are used in which Hb catalyzes the rapid oxidation of benzidine by hydrogen peroxide. Although the benzidine method is much more sensitive than the oxyhemoglobin method, the benzidine method is inaccurate because normal plasma contains a hydrogen peroxide inhibitor. Therefore, the benzidine method may underestimate the plasma Hb concentration by about 50%.[15] Also, from a practical standpoint, benzidine is considered carcinogenic and so is not recommended for laboratory use.

Because of the narrow absorption peak of oxyhemoglobin, the spectrophotometer must have a very narrow bandpass; that is, a 1-nm spectral resolution is required. The spectrophotometer must also be accurately calibrated for wavelength. In contrast, the cyanmethemoglobin method requires only a 10-nm spectral resolution because of the broader nature of the absorption peak at 540 nm.

LABORATORY EVALUATION OF IRON AVAILABILITY

Because Hb synthesis requires iron, the laboratory measurement of iron availability has long been a useful tool in the evaluation of anemias secondary to disorders of iron metabolism (Chap. 13). There are a number of chemical analyses for the evaluation of iron availability to the erythron. Most of these tests are performed in the chemistry laboratory, and a brief description of each may be found in Chapter 13.

CHAPTER SUMMARY

Hemoglobin is necessary for adequate tissue oxygenation in vertebrates because O_2 is minimally soluble in plasma. Hemoglobin also removes CO_2 from the tissues. Hemoglobin is synthesized in maturing nucleated red cells in the bone marrow and consists of globin, heme, and sometimes, 2,3-DPG (see Fig. 7-1). Globin chain composition (*i.e.*, amino acid sequence and number) determines the Hb variant, such as Hb A, which constitutes most adult Hb and consists of two α and two β chains ($\alpha_2\beta_2$). Heme consists of iron and protoporphyrin IX. The latter is synthesized partly inside and partly outside the red cell mitochondria (see Fig. 7-5). Excess porphyrin produced during heme synthesis in the mitochondria is called free erythrocyte protoporphyrin (FEP). It can be measured in the laboratory; when elevated, it often indicates some form of iron metabolism disorder. 2,3-DPG is synthesized in the Embden–Meyerhof pathway. When Hb binds 2,3-DPG, the former's affinity for O_2 decreases; on release of 2,3-DPG, affinity for O_2 increases.

Heme–heme interaction increases Hb's O_2 affinity. Hemoglobin can bind four O_2 molecules.

The oxyhemoglobin dissociation curve (see Fig. 7-7) is sigmoidal or S-shaped. Normally, when pO_2 is below 20 mm Hg, Hb has a low O_2 affinity; when pO_2 is 20 to 60 mm Hg (normal tissue levels), Hb can readily bind or release O_2 responding quickly to small changes in pO_2. When the curve shifts to the left, Hb O_2 affinity is increased; when it shifts to the right, affinity is decreased (see Table 7-3). In general, body temperature, blood pH (Bohr effect), 2,3-DPG, blood CO_2 levels, amount of fetal Hb, and abnormal hemoglobin variants all affect Hb O_2 affinity.

Hemoglobin derivatives contain an abnormal heme component (but normal globin chains), making them unable to carry O_2. They are: methemoglobin, in which iron is in its ferric state; sulfhemoglobin, in which Hb is permanently oxidized by certain drugs and chemicals; and carboxyhemoglobin, formed by CO binding to Hb. Clinical disorders, some hereditary, some acquired, are caused by these derivatives, and a number of laboratory tests exist for their diagnosis.

The porphyrias are inherited or acquired disorders of heme synthesis that lead to porphyrin or porphyrinogen precursor accumulation in the bone marrow or liver. Laboratory features are presented in Table 7-4. Lead poisoning is a well-known acquired porphyria associated with ringed sideroblasts in the bone marrow.

REFERENCES

1. Adamson SD, Herbert E, Godchaux W: Factors affecting the rate of protein synthesis in lysate systems from reticulocytes. Arch Biochem 125:671, 1968
2. Bauer JD: Hemoglobin. In Kaplan LA, Pesce AJ (eds): Clinical Chemistry: Theory, Analysis and Correlation, 2nd ed, p 514. St Louis, CV Mosby, 1989
3. Beck HG, Schulze WH, Suter GM: Carbon monoxide—a domestic hazard. JAMA 115:1, 1940
4. Benesch R, Benesch RE: Effect of organic phosphate from human erythrocytes on allosteric properties of hemoglobin. Biochem Biophys Res Commun 26:162, 1967
5. Berk PD, Tschudy DP, Shepley LA et al: Hematological and biochemical studies in a case of lead poisoning. Am J Med 48:137, 1970
6. Betke K, Steim H, Tonz O: A family with congenital methaemoglobinaemia due to reductase deficiency. Germ Med Month, 7:217, 1962
7. Blanke RV, Decker WJ: Analysis of toxic substances. In Tietz NW (ed): Fundamentals of Clinical Chemistry, p 885. Philadelphia, WB Saunders, 1987
8. Brandenburg RO, Smith HL: Sulfhemoglobinemia: Study of 62 clinical cases. Am Heart J 42:582, 1951
9. Codounis A et al: Hereditary methaemoglobinaemic cyanosis. Acta Genet Statist Med 7:131, 1957
10. Collison HA, Rodkey FL, O'Neal JD: Determination of carbon monoxide in blood by gas chromatography. Clin Chem 14:162, 1968
11. Cooper RA, Shattil SJ: Mechanisms of hemolysis: The minimal red cell defect. N Engl J Med 285:1514, 1971
12. Decker WJ, Treuting JJ: Spot tests for rapid diagnosis of poisoning. Clin Toxicol 4:89, 1971
13. Dickerson RE: X-ray analysis and protein structure. In Neurath H (ed): The Proteins: Composition, Structure and Function, vol 2, pp 603–778. New York, Academic Press, 1964
14. Douglas AS, Dacie JV: The incidence and significance of iron containing granules in human erythrocytes and their precursors. J Clin Pathol 6:307, 1953
15. Fairbanks VF, Klee GG: Biochemical aspects of hematology. In Tietz NW (ed): Fundamentals of Clinical Chemistry, 3rd ed, pp 805, 806. Philadelphia, WB Saunders, 1987
16. Harboe M: A method for determination of hemoglobin in plasma by near-ultraviolet spectrophotometry. Scand J Clin Lab Invest 11:66, 1959
17. Hegesh E, Calmanovici N, Avron M: New method for determining ferrihemoglobin reductase (NADH-methemoglobin reductase) in erythrocytes. J Lab Clin Med 72:339, 1968
18. Hsieh H-S, Jaffe ER: The metabolism of methemoglobin in human erythrocytes. In Surgenor DM (ed): The Red Blood Cell, 2nd ed, p 799. New York, Academic Press, 1975
19. International Committee for Standardization in Haematology: Recommendations for haemoglobinometry in human blood. Br J Haematol (suppl) 13:71, 1967
20. International Committee for Standardization in Haematology: Recommendations for reference method for haemoglobinometry in human blood (ICSH Standard EP 6/2:1977) and specifications for international haemiglobincyanide reference preparation (ICSH Standard EP 6/3:1977). J Clin Pathol 31:139, 1978
21. Jaffe ER: Hereditary methemoglobinemia associated with abnormalities in the metabolism of erythrocytes. Am J Med 41:786, 1966
22. Jaffe ER, Neumann G, Rothberg H et al: Hereditary methemoglobinemia with and without mental retardation. Am J Med 41:42, 1966
23. Jaffe ER, Heller P: Methemoglobinemia in man. In Moore CV, Brown EB (eds): Progress in Hematology, vol 4, p 48. New York, Grune & Stratton, 1964
24. Kaplan JC, Nicolas AM, Hanzlickova-Leroux A et al: A simple spot screening test for fast detection of red cell NADH-diaphorase deficiency. Blood 36:330, 1970
25. Lemberg P, Legge JW: Hematin Compounds and Bile Pigments, p 228. New York, Interscience, 1949
26. Mayers MR: Carbon monoxide poisoning in industry and its prevention. NY State Dept of Labor, Albany, NY, Special Bull 194, 1938
27. McCutcheon AD: Sulphaemoglobinaemia and glutathione. Lancet 2:240, 1960

28. National Committee for Clinical Laboratory Standards: Reference procedure for the quantitative determination of hemoglobin in blood, vol 4, no 3. Villanova, PA, NCCLS, 1984

29. Naumann HN: The measurement of hemoglobin in plasma. In Sunderman FW, Sunderman FW Jr (eds): Hemoglobin, Its Precursors and Metabolites. Philadelphia, JB Lippincott, 1964

30. Perutz MF: Hemoglobin structure and respiratory transport. Sci Am 239:92, 1978

31. Pruden EL, Siggaard–Andersen O, Tietz NW: Blood gases and pH. In Tietz NW (ed): Textbook of Clinical Chemistry, p 1195. Philadelphia, WB Saunders, 1986

32. Reynolds TB, Ware AGL: Sulfhemoglobinemia following habitual use of acetanilid. JAMA 149:1538, 1952

33. Riggs A: Functional properties of hemoglobins. Physiol Rev 45:619, 1965

34. Rogers LE: Rapid method for detection of erythrocyte NADH-methemoglobin reductase deficiency. Am J Clin Pathol 57:186, 1972

35. Scott EM: Congenital methemoglobinemia due to DPNH-diaphorase deficiency. In Beutler E (ed): Hereditary Disorders of Erythrocyte Metabolism, p 102. New York, Grune & Stratton, 1968

36. Singer K, Weisz L: The life cycle of the erythrocyte after splenectomy and the problems of splenic hemolysis and target cell formation. Am J Med Sci 210:301, 1945

37. Tietz NW, Fiereck EA: The spectrophotometric measurement of carboxyhemoglobin. Ann Clin Lab Sci 3:36, 1973

38. Trost C: The blue people of Troublesome Creek. Science 82, 3(9):24, 1982

39. Winter PM, Miller JN: Carbon monoxide poisoning. JAMA 236:1502, 1976

40. Wintrobe M: Erythropoiesis. In Wintrobe MM (ed): Clinical Hematology, 8th ed, pp 118, 119. Philadelphia, Lea & Febiger, 1981

41. Wintrobe M: Methemoglobinemia and other disorders usually accompanied by cyanosis. In Wintrobe MM (ed): Clinical Hematology, 8th ed, p 1013. Philadelphia, Lea & Febiger, 1981

42. Wranne L: Free erythrocyte copro- and protoporphyrin. Acta Paediatr Scand 49:1, 1960

8

Morphologic

Evaluation

of

Erythrocytes

Ann Bell

A careful and thorough examination of erythrocytes by light microscopy in the optimal area on a well-made, well-stained peripheral blood film provides an experienced observer with valuable information about morphology, normal or abnormal. Erythrocytes should be examined for deviation in size, shape, distribution, concentration of hemoglobin (Hb), and inclusions. A systematic manner of reporting abnormal findings should be established in each laboratory. The morphologist should also be aware of artifacts that hinder proper evaluation of erythrocytes.

Some features of erythrocytes will be diagnostic, whereas others may provide clues to suggest a particular disease state. Certain characteristics may indicate the necessity for additional procedures to confirm a diagnosis. A thorough examination of red cell morphology serves as a check on red cell indices and other hematologic procedures.

DISTRIBUTION

Normal Distribution

An ideal normal blood film has an even distribution of erythrocytes in the thin portion adjacent to the feather end of the film. In this thin area red cells should be slightly separated from one another or barely touching without overlapping. The thin area should represent at least one-third of the entire film. Normal red cells should be circular with a smooth edge and a central pale area that gradually fades into reddish-pink cytoplasm (Fig. 8-1).

At the feather end of the film and often at the edges, the red cell distribution is irregular with artifactual shapes and colors and size distortions. In the thicker portions of the film red cells may overlap or lie on top of one another, making them unsuitable for evaluation.

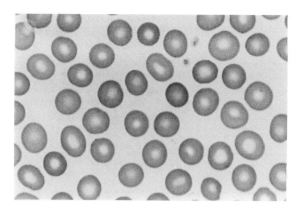

FIG. 8-1.   Normal adult peripheral blood film showing normocytic, normochromic cells. ×1000.

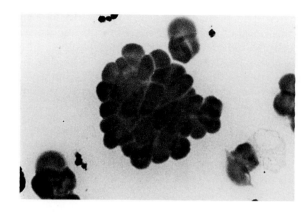

FIG. 8-3.   Autoagglutination. ×1000.

Abnormal Distribution

Rouleaux

Formation of rouleaux is reflected by erythrocytes in the usual observation area that are not separated from one another; rather, they appear in short or long stacks (rouleaux) resembling coins or flat plates. The entire outline of each cell is not visible. Rouleaux is the arrangement of red cells with their biconcave surfaces in apposition (Fig. 8-2).

Rouleaux is characteristic of hyperproteinemia and multiple myeloma (Chap. 39) because of an increased amount of plasma gamma globulin. In macroglobulinemia, rouleaux formation is often pronounced and creates lengthy chains. The first clue to the presence of a paraprotein or protein abnormality is rouleaux along with an increased erythrocyte sedimentation rate. Making satisfactory blood films in protein dyscrasias may be impossible. Cell size and shape cannot always be evaluated in the presence of rouleaux formation.

When fibrinogen is significantly increased (*e.g.,* in infections, tissue necrosis, and pregnancy), rouleaux forms long stacks. Even normal red cells may form rouleaux in a thick moist preparation of blood under a coverslip. Spherocytes, on the other hand, cannot form rouleaux.

Agglutination

Erythrocyte agglutination occurs as cells aggregate into random clusters or masses (Fig. 8-3) when exposed to various red cell antibodies. Thus, the outline of each individual cell is not seen. Rouleaux does *not* form in the presence of red cell antibodies.

Autoagglutination occurs when an individual's red cells agglutinate in his own plasma or serum that contains no known specific agglutinins. Sometimes, autoagglutination is seen in the blood of apparently normal individuals but is more likely to be observed in certain hemolytic anemias, atypical pneumonia, staphylococcal infections, and trypanosomiasis.[7,68,69] Autoagglutination may be observed in the tube of anticoagulated blood as it is being rotated at room temperature.

A common form of autoagglutination is seen in cold agglutinin disease. Here clumps of red cells may be noted on a blood film when the temperature is below 31°C and particularly below 25°C, which enhances autoantibody activity.[52] Blood film preparation and red cell description are almost impossible without warming of the blood and the glass slide. The clumps of agglutinated cells disintegrate on warming of the tube. Evaluation of red cells on films made from warmed samples does not correlate with red cell indices performed on electronic counters because cell clumping interferes with accurate automated red cell evaluation. The mean corpuscular volume (MCV) (Chap. 9) is artifactually elevated by clumps of red cells being counted as single large cells.

NORMAL MORPHOLOGY

A normal red cell *in vivo* is a biconcave disc and thus has been named a discocyte. This shape is well suited for the erythrocyte's task of gas transport and its survival in the circulation.[49] On the slide the cell has been flattened and thus has a round appearance with an area of central pallor representing the indented region of the disc. Normal red cells are almost uniform in size, shape, and Hb concentration. They stain a light red to pink with Wright stain and have a relatively clear central area that gradually leads to a more deeply stained periphery. The diameter of the central clear area should not be more than one-third of the cell

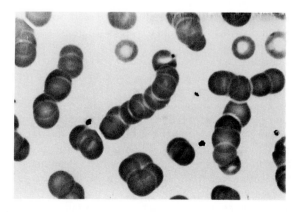

FIG. 8-2.   Rouleaux formation by erythrocytes. ×1000. (From Bell A, Lofsness KG: A photo essay on red cell morphology. J Med Technol 3:85, 1986, with permission.)

diameter. The gradual transition to deeper stain is an important morphologic feature because it distinguishes normal cells from those with artifactual morphologic changes. There are no inclusions in normal red cells (see Fig. 8-1).

The diameter of a normal red cell varies slightly, with a mean of 7 to 8 μm,[6,50] and is approximately the same as or slightly smaller than the nucleus of a small lymphocyte. Other characteristics include an average thickness of 2.5 μm,[7] an average volume of 90 fL[26] (1 fL = 10^{-15} L), and an average surface area of 160 μm^2.[7]

The relation between the limited metabolic factors within the non-nucleated erythrocyte and the cell membrane, as well as the external environment, help to maintain the disc shape throughout the cell's life. If any of these factors is altered, the cell usually becomes spherical.

HEMOGLOBIN CONTENT

Erythrocytes with a normal Hb content have a clear central pallor that occupies about one-third of the cell diameter. Such cells are described as *normochromic*. There may be slight variations in the amount of central pallor in different areas of the normal blood film.

With decreasing Hb concentration, there is increasing central pallor, and the cells are then described as *hypochromic*. Hypochromia is caused by impaired Hb synthesis and ranges from slight pallor to marked pallor, in which there may be only a thin rim of Hb. The changes in Hb content in severe iron deficiency anemia (Chap. 13) are evident in the mean corpuscular hemoglobin (MCH) and mean corpuscular hemoglobin concentration (MCHC) (Chap. 9). Hypochromia is associated most often with microcytosis. Examples of hypochromic, microcytic anemias include iron deficiency anemia, thalassemia, and sideroblastic anemia. Hypochromia is sometimes associated with normocytic (normal-size) red cells in disorders such as rheumatoid arthritis, chronic infections, or inflammation. These conditions result from defective macrophage iron release, which prevents iron from reaching the normoblasts for proper red cell maturation.

Anisochromia is the term used to describe the variation in Hb content when both hypochromic and normochromic cells are present. In sideroblastic anemia, hypochromic and normochromic cells are seen, indicating the marrow production of two populations of red cells. After transfusions for hypochromic anemia, anisochromia is often present because the patient's hypochromic cells are visible along with the transfused normal cells. Although hematologists may use this term, it is rarely used in reporting red cell morphology.

Macrocytic cells usually do not have an area of central pallor because of their increased thickness. Spherocytes have reduced central concavity and no central pallor because of their increased thickness.[7] Sickled red cells do not show normal central pallor. Hemoglobin is concentrated within a crystal in the abnormal Hb genotypes CC and SC. Technically, these erythrocytes are *hyperchromic* because of their lack of central pallor even though they lie in a desirable area for morphologic observation. Erythrocytes along the extreme feather edge often appear hyperchromic; however, this is an artifact. True hyperchromia exists when the MCHC is elevated. Hyperchromia is common on films from patients with hemolytic anemias, including hemolysis caused by burns resulting in microspherocytes with a reduced surface:volume ratio, causing the increased MCHC. Although cells may be hyperchromic, hyperchromia is almost never reported by the laboratory. By convention, reporting the type of hyperchromic cell present is, *de facto*, an indication of hyperchromia.

SIZE

Average Size Correlated with MCV

Normocytic

Automated complete blood counts usually include measurement of the MCV, which is important because this value indicates the average size of erythrocytes. Observation of red cell morphology on the blood film provides a quality control check on the electronic MCV, as well as the other two red cell indices, MCH and MCHC. An MCV in the normal range suggests that the red cells are generally of normal size (normocytic); however, the film may demonstrate a minor population of smaller or larger cells, which may not significantly alter the MCV. There may be a mixture of different populations of erythrocytes on the film, in which case the MCV should be in the normal range because of the averaging of large and small cell sizes.

Macrocytic

Erythrocytes are generally described as macrocytic if the diameter exceeds 8.5 to 9.0 μm and the MCV exceeds 100 fL.[7] Automated blood counts have led to increasing awareness of macrocytosis with or without anemia.[25] A slight macrocytosis is observed frequently in hospital patients and probably does not warrant investigation. Although low vitamin B_{12} or folate levels cause macrocytosis, tests for B_{12} or folate are not necessary unless the MCV is at least 10% above the laboratory's established reference range.[42]

Common causes of a slight to moderate increase in MCV and of round macrocytes are alcoholism (Fig. 8-4A) with or without hepatic disease; cancer chemotherapy because it interferes with DNA synthesis; chronic hemolytic anemia with reticulocytosis; myeloma; leukemia; lymphoma; metastatic carcinoma; hypothyroidism; and hemolytic disease of the newborn.[7,25] Large red cells are seen occasionally in stem cell disorders, particularly aplastic anemia, refractory anemia, pure red cell aplasia, myelofibrosis, and sideroblastic anemia.[25] Occasionally, macrocytes are found in chronic obstructive pulmonary disease. However, a cause for macrocytosis often is not apparent.

Patients with liver disease may have macrocytosis; however, this concept is debatable.[25] Excess plasma cholesterol may be taken up by the red cell membrane, increasing the surface area of the cell. When the erythrocyte is spread on the slide, a thin macrocyte is formed. True macrocytes with MCV exceeding 100 fL probably are rare in liver disease without folate deficiency.[25]

The presence of oval macrocytes (usually also lacking central pallor), increased MCV, and low levels of vitamin B_{12} or folate suggest a nuclear maturation defect, which may be observed in the megaloblastic red cells in the bone

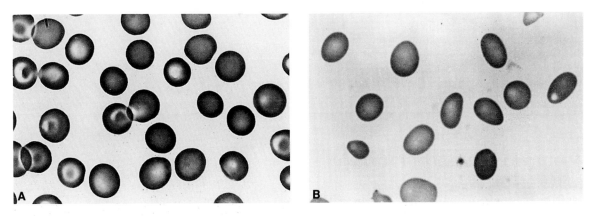

FIG. 8-4.   Types of macrocytosis. (A) Macrocytes in film of patient with alcoholism and liver disease. (From Bell A, Lofsness KG: A photo essay on red cell morphology. J Med Technol 3:85, 1986, with permission.) (B) Oval macrocytes in film of patient with vitamin B_{12} deficiency. Both ×1000.

marrow (Chap. 12). The developmental abnormality of oval macrocytic cells (Fig. 8-4B) is discussed later in this chapter.

Normal non–nucleated erythrocytes that have just left the bone marrow sinusoids are slightly macrocytic and appear in stained peripheral blood films as diffusely basophilic (polychromatophilic) cells. Prematurely released red cells, called "shift" cells, occur as a result of stimulated erythropoiesis in acute hemolytic anemia. These polychromatophilic cells have an increased MCV, suggesting a macrocytosis.[13]

When the blood glucose is above 600 mg/dL, the high intracellular osmolarity causes fluid to be taken into the cell when it is placed in isotonic diluent. The result is a spurious macrocytosis if the count is performed before equilibration.[39]

With *Mycoplasma pneumonia* infection or high titers of cold agglutinins, the MCV may be artifactually high because red cells in doublets or triplets may pass the aperture of an electronic counter.

Microcytic

Small erythrocytes with reduced volume are termed microcytes. Microcytes have normal or decreased Hb content and reduced, normal, or increased diameters. These electronic and visual changes in morphology are not apparent until iron stores have been completely exhausted and additional iron depletion restricts iron to the erythron. Iron deficiency is first apparent in biochemical iron studies. As anemia develops, Hb concentration is depressed, and red cells become more hypochromic and microcytic.

Microcytes occur on the blood film when the MCV is below 80 fL. However, only a few microcytic cells may not cause a decreased MCV. Significant numbers of microcytes are not produced until storage iron has been depleted for many weeks.

Microcytes with a diameter of 6 μm or less are characteristic of iron deficiency anemia (Fig. 8-5; Chap. 13). Inflammation may also cause a slight microcytosis.

Decreased globin synthesis in β-thalassemia results in a variable number of microcytic, hypochromic red cells along with target cells (Chap. 15). Because some blood films in iron deficiency and thalassemia are similar, special Hb determinations and family studies are needed for differential diagnosis.

Erythrocytes that are small, lack central pallor, and appear to have an increased Hb concentration are seen in some hemolytic anemias. Such cells are called spherocytes.

Erythrocytes that are thinner than normal and have a colorless center are designated leptocytes (Gr. *lepto*: thin). A leptocyte has an increased surface area that is out of proportion to the volume. Leptocytes may be normocytic or microcytic. Microcytic leptocytes are formed because of a lack of Hb, as seen in severe iron deficiency. Small leptocytes may be seen in thalassemia, hemoglobinopathies such as Hb C, occasionally sideroblastic anemia, obstruction of the bile ducts, and sometimes cirrhosis and steatorrhea (fatty feces).[7]

Variation in Size (Anisocytosis) Correlated with Distribution Width

Variation in red cell population size or diameter is termed anisocytosis. To report anisocytosis the examiner should see a mixture of normal cells with small or large cells or both. Anisocytosis should be estimated in a semiquantitative manner: slight, moderate, or marked. If the variation is

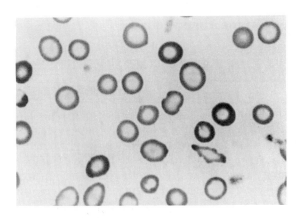

FIG. 8-5.   Microcytic, hypochromic red cells in a patient with iron deficiency anemia. ×1000.

primarily microcytes or macrocytes or both, this should be reported also.

Some automated cell counters generate the red cell distribution width (RDW), which is reported to quantitate anisocytosis. The RDW is said to identify minor populations of microcytic or macrocytic cells[10] that are not apparent from the MCV, although the clinical significance of the RDW requires further study (Chap. 10).[26]

SHAPE VARIATION–POIKILOCYTOSIS

Normal erythrocytes show little or no shape variation. Variation only on the edges of films primarily is an artifact of preparation.

The term used for variation in red cell shape is poikilocytosis. Recognition of various shapes or poikilocytes on the film is helpful in the differentiation of anemias. Examples of poikilocytes characteristic of certain anemias include elliptical, sickled, fragmented, and spherical forms. Generally a descriptive term of Greek (Gr.) origin is used to identify the poikilocyte. Poikilocyte shapes can sometimes be explained by structural and biochemical changes in the membrane, a metabolic state in the cell, hemoglobin molecule abnormalities, an abnormal microenvironment, changes in the red cell's ability to deform, or red cell age. Electron microscopy has greatly advanced our understanding of the mechanism of poikilocyte production.

Poikilocytes Secondary to Developmental Macrocytosis (Oval Macrocytes)

A markedly increased MCV (more than 125 fL) strongly implicates megaloblastic erythropoiesis caused by vitamin B_{12} or folate deficiency. A nuclear maturation defect in the early nucleated red cells of the bone marrow leads to development of macrocytes, which are mostly oval (oval macrocytes or macroovalocytes) (see Fig. 8-4B). Even a few oval macrocytes are significant and suggest megaloblastic anemia. The cells appear well filled with Hb because of their increased thickness. Hemoglobin content increases as the cell increases in size, thus forming a macrocyte that no longer has a central pale area.

Poikilocytes Secondary to Membrane Abnormalities

Certain poikilocytes suggest hemolytic disorders and hereditary or acquired conditions involving the red cell membrane.[37,38,63,64,67]

Spherocytes

Spherocytes are round red cells lacking central pallor, showing increased staining intensity, and having a smaller volume than a normal cell (Fig. 8-6). However, every spherocyte may not be truly spherical *in vivo,* and a slight concavity may be revealed with stereoscan microscopy. Spherocyte diameter is approximately 6.2 to 7.0 μm, and the thickness is greater than 2.2 up to 3.4 μm.[30,60]

Spherocytes may be caused by a hereditary or acquired condition. Several molecular defects in membrane proteins have been identified in hereditary spherocytosis (Chap. 17);

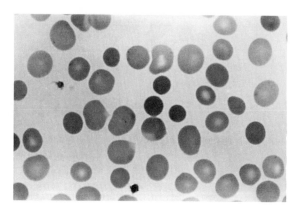

FIG. 8-6. Spherocytes in film of patient with hereditary spherocytosis. ×1000.

spectrin deficiency has been found in many patients.[34,41,67] Spherocytes are not easily deformed and therefore may lose membrane by fragmentation during passage through the circulation. These cells become smaller and denser with increased Hb content and become less deformable with age. When the cell is deprived of membrane as it ages, it assumes the spherical shape. Spherocytes have a shortened survival time because they can be sequestered in the spleen and destroyed.[65]

The presence of spherocytes indicates a hemolytic process because hemolysis results from a membrane abnormality. The hallmark of hereditary spherocytosis is a spherocyte that is fairly uniform in size and density with a decreased membrane surface:volume ratio. The MCV may be normal or slightly decreased; the MCHC is often increased. Spherocytes show increased fragility when placed in increasing dilutions of hypotonic saline in the osmotic fragility test. After splenectomy in patients with hereditary spherocytosis, spherocytes persist,[16] indicating that the abnormality involves the red cell membrane itself rather than splenic damage to the cells.

Frequent causes of acquired spherocytosis are immunohemolytic anemia secondary to autoimmune or isoimmune antibodies, Heinz body hemolytic anemia, microangiopathic hemolytic anemia, and hemolysis secondary to water dilution.[67] Banked blood stored for a long time develops spherocytes. Transfused cells are often spherical when viewed on a blood film and can be differentiated from the patient's cells.

Elliptocytes and Ovalocytes

Elliptocytes or ovalocytes are erythrocytes that have an elliptical or oval shape (Fig. 8-7). These cells result from hereditary or acquired conditions and range from egg-shaped or slightly oval to sausage, rod, or pencil forms.[24] With electron microscopy, Hb appears to be concentrated at the two ends of the cell, leaving a normal central area of pallor.[43]

Late nucleated red cells in the bone marrow of patients with elliptocytosis are not elliptical except in rare cases of hereditary elliptocytosis.[43]

Usually no more than 1% of the red cells in normal individuals are slightly elliptical.[28] Ovalocytes or elliptocytes may be acquired in iron deficiency anemia, megalo-

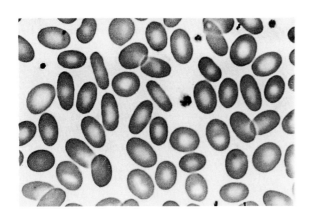

FIG. 8-7. Elliptocytes in film of patient with hereditary ellipto-cytosis. ×1000.

blastic anemia, and myelophthisic anemia, where as many as 10% of the cells may be oval. Megaloblastic anemia is characterized by oval macrocytes, which may be 9 μm or more in diameter and lack central pallor. Elliptocytes are also observed in thalassemia and sickle cell anemia.

Hereditary elliptocytosis (Chap. 17) is characterized on the blood film by 25% to 90% elliptocytes, but it is not typically associated with hemolysis.[20] The principal defect is considered to be in the cytoskeleton, with a decrease in the skeletal membrane protein band 4.1.[1] An increased heat sensitivity of spectrin in some families with hereditary elliptocytosis has been reported.[57] The life span of elliptocytes may be somewhat shortened in a few individuals; however, elliptocytes usually function normally. The osmotic fragility is normal.

Echinocytes and Burr Cells

Echinocytes (Gr. *echinos*: sea urchin) have evenly distributed, uniform-size blunt spicules or bumps on their surfaces (Fig. 8-8A). Echinocytes or crenated red cells may be seen on films made from anticoagulated blood several hours old, but such cells are artifacts not normally present *in vivo*. Bessis[7] states that crenation is caused by release of basic substances from glass slides that change the *p*H and transform the cells into echinocytes. In stored blood echinocytes may be numerous because of depletion of ATP and

biochemical abnormalities in plasma. Echinocytes formed *in vitro* can be reversed to normal shape, whereas those formed *in vivo* cannot.[7] Transformation of discocytes to echinocytes can be observed on a glass slide using a moist saline preparation of red cells in the presence of an elevated *p*H.[7]

In anemia associated with renal insufficiency, some red cells acquire a membrane abnormality with irregularly sized and unevenly spaced spicules.[53] Such red cells are named burr cells (see Fig. 8-8B). The number of burr cells often increases as blood urea nitrogen increases. This membrane alteration is probably related to plasma chemical abnormalities. The spicules of burr cells are usually reversible, as the cells can be induced to revert to normal shape.

The differences between crenated cells (echinocytes) and burr cells may be minimal and not always recognizable. Crenated cells with uniform blunt spicules represent an artifact that is evident in practically every cell in the thin portion of the film and should not be reported. Burr cells may be distinguished by their irregularly sized spicules and variable number in different microscopic fields and should be reported. A burr cell has also been called an echinocyte by several hematologists because of its membrane irregularities.

Acanthocytes

Acanthocytes (Gr. *acantho*: thorn or spike) are small, densely stained red cells that are no longer disc shaped and have a few irregularly spaced, pointed spicules or thornlike projections of various lengths and widths over the surface (Fig. 8-9). The spicules may appear clublike. Acanthocytes may be acquired or inherited and are smaller than normal red cells because they are becoming spheroidal. Generally acanthocytes have fewer, more irregular, and more blunted points than burr cells. Also, unlike burr cells, acanthocytes cannot be induced to regain a normal shape. Acanthocytes may be caused by changes in the ratio of plasma lipids (lecithins and sphingomyelins).[62]

Acanthocytes have been observed in alcoholic cirrhosis with hemolytic anemia, malabsorption states, postsplenectomy states, hepatitis of newborns, pyruvate kinase deficiency, and disorders of lipid metabolism.[7] Cells similar to acanthocytes have been named *spur cells* in severe hemo-

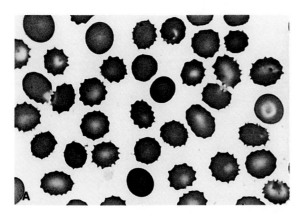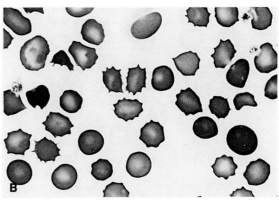

FIG. 8-8. (*A*) Echinocytes or crenated cells in film of normal peripheral blood. (*B*) Burr cells in film of patient with uremia. Note resemblance to echinocytes. Both ×1000.

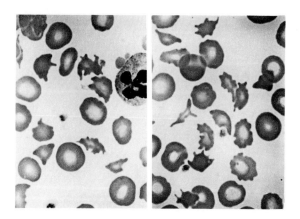

FIG. 8-9.   Acanthocytes. As seen in film of patient with micro-angiopathic hemolytic anemia. ×1000.

lytic anemia associated with cirrhosis and in metastatic liver disease because of their sharp points.[43]

Increased numbers of acanthocytes have been reported in a rare congenital syndrome called abetalipoproteinemia, which is characterized by mild hemolytic anemia, retinal degeneration, and steatorrhea.[3,32]

Stomatocytes

Stomatocytyes on a fixed and stained film have an elongated or slitlike area of central pallor (Fig. 8-10) instead of the usual circular form. These cells may be hereditary or acquired. The Greek word *stoma* means mouth. Stomatocytes are so named for their mouth-shaped central pallor. These cells appear bowl shaped in a moist preparation and by stereoscan microscope.[6]

Blood films from normal individuals may demonstrate a few stomatocytes, but stomatocytes are usually observed in patients with alcoholism, cirrhosis, obstructive liver disease,[67] and Rh null disease.[56] These cells also may occur as artifacts of blood film preparation.

Hereditary stomatocytosis is characterized by numerous stomatocytes, but anemia is usually mild.[40] One of the suggested consequences involves a membrane defect that results in high cellular sodium and low potassium content (Chap. 17). The heterogeneous clinical picture results from an abnormal sodium:potassium transport ratio and a greatly increased rate of active cation transport.[70] Because of the shape of the red cell and the somewhat impaired deformability, stomatocytes may be retained in the spleen.

Codocytes (Target Cells)

Codocytes or target cells have a central area of Hb surrounded by a relatively colorless ring and a peripheral ring of Hb (Fig. 8-11). By scanning electron microscopy the codocyte has a bell or tall hat shape and appears to be thin walled and concave. A codocyte (Gr. *kodon:* bell) is also called a Mexican hat cell. This shape is always acquired. Codocytes appear when the membrane surface is increased after loading of the membrane with cholesterol and phospholipids.[18] In other words, a target cell is similar to a bag too large for its contents. Its greater osmotic resistance (or decrease in osmotic fragility) is explained by the increase in surface:volume ratio.

Finding target cells in only one portion of the film suggests an artifact of film preparation. Fixing slides in methanol may help avoid this. In pathologic states, target cells are observed throughout the usual examination area. Target cells do not appear at the ends of a film where cells are flattened nor in thick portions of the film.

Codocytes are characteristic of thalassemia; hemoglobinopathies SS, CC, DD, EE, and S-thalassemia; obstructive liver disease; postsplenectomy state; and iron deficiency anemia.[18,20,67,68]

Poikilocytes Secondary to Trauma

Erythrocytes may fragment and lyse when subjected to excessive physical trauma in the cardiovascular system. Intravascular hemolysis and shortened red cell survival may result with severe trauma. The hallmark of hemolytic anemia secondary to red cell fragmentation is the schistocyte, which takes several forms. Other cells caused by trauma are included in this section.

Schistocytes

When a red cell attempts to pass through fibrin strands,[14] altered vessels, or damaged heart valve prosthesis,[51,54] it undergoes cleavage and fragmentation and becomes a

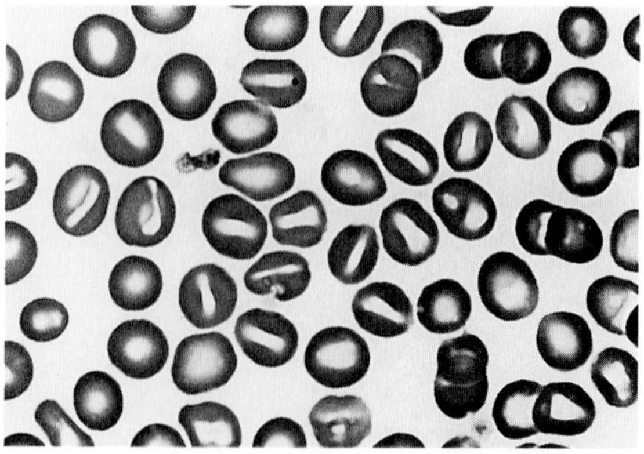

FIG. 8-10.   Stomatocytes in film of patient with hereditary stomatocytosis. ×1000.

FIG. 8-11.   Codocytes (target cells) in film of patient with liver disease. ×1000.

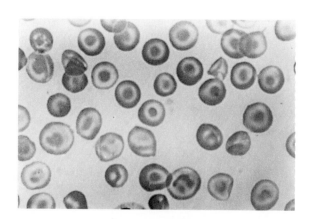

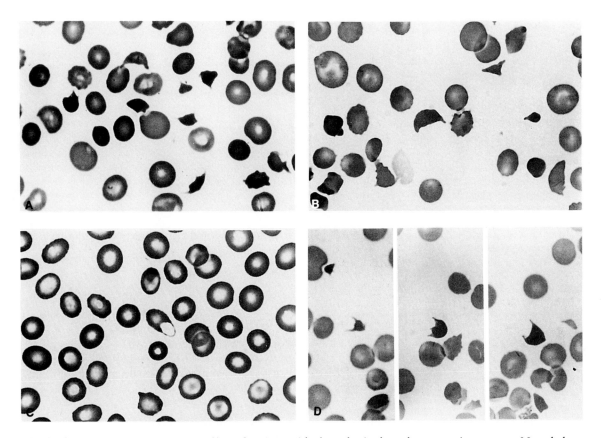

FIG. 8-12.   Schistocytes. *(A, B)* In film of patient with thrombotic thrombocytopenic purpura. Note helmet, triangular, fragmented, and bizarre shapes. *(C)* Blister cell in film of patient with probable microangiopathic hemolytic anemia. *(D)* Keratocytes (horn cells) in film of patient with microangiopathic hemolytic anemia. All ×1000.

schistocyte (Fig. 8-12A and B). The erythrocyte, trying to squeeze through an opening one-half its diameter, becomes stretched and develops a blister (Fig. 8-12C) because of the shear stress of the flowing blood. When this cell passes through the spleen, it is fragmented into two pieces, and the membrane is less deformable. Fragmented red cells do not survive long in the circulation.[65]

Schistocytes (Gr. *schistos*: cloven) or *schizocytes* (Gr. *schizo*: split) result from membrane damage; they are not hereditary. Schistocytes include helmet, triangular, and a variety of small, irregular shapes with a few pointed extremities. The finding of helmet and fragmented cells is strongly suggestive of a microangiopathic hemolytic anemia or traumatic hemolytic anemia.[12] Schistocytes occur in patients with severe burns, renal graft rejection, glomerulonephritis, vasculitis, thrombotic thrombocytopenic purpura, and diffuse intravascular coagulation.[7,67] Schistocytes accompanying march hemoglobinuria most likely are attributable to mechanical damage to the cells in the feet of individuals on long walking expeditions.

Keratocytes

A schistocyte with one or more hornlike projections has been identified as a keratocyte (Gr. *keras*: horn) (Fig. 8-12D). These cells have a relatively normal volume and usually an area of central pallor. A keratocyte is the result of an erythrocyte being caught on a fibrin strand, which could

cut the cell in two. As the sides of the erythrocyte are pushed against the fibrin strand, they tend to fuse together. When this cell escapes from the fibrin strand, it may have a vacuolelike area in the fused portion (this is known as a blister cell; Fig. 8-12C). This vacuole ruptures to form the keratocyte—a damaged red cell with horns. Keratocytes do not remain in circulation for more than a few hours, as they are fragile.[7] A keratocyte is a rare and interesting phenomenon and should be reported as a schistocyte.

Dacrocytes (Teardrops)

Dacryocytes (teardrops) have been so labeled because of their shape (Gr. *dakry*: tear) (Fig. 8-13). They may also be pear shaped with a blunt pointed projection and may be normal sized, small, or large.[6,58] If a red cell contains a rigid inclusion, such as a Heinz body, the portion with the inclusion cannot pass through small openings of splenic sinuses and thus remains behind. As the red cell squeezes through the small opening, it is stretched beyond its ability to regain its original shape. Thus, a teardrop or pear shape is created.[6]

Teardrop cells typically are observed in myelofibrosis with myeloid metaplasia because of the large size of the spleen. Other conditions with dacryocytes include myelophthisic anemia, pernicious anemia, β-thalassemia, after Heinz body formation induced by drug ingestion, tuberculosis, and tumor metastasized to the marrow.[7,58,68]

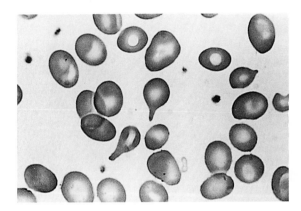

FIG. 8-13.   Dacryocytes (teardrop cells) in film of patient with vitamin B_{12} deficiency. ×1000.

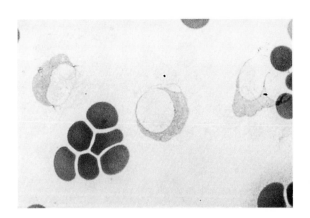

FIG. 8-15.   Semilunar bodies (red cell ghosts) in film of patient with malaria. ×1000.

Microspherocytes and Pyropoikilocytes

Microspherocytes (Fig. 8-14A) occur in severe burns as small, round cells. They are the result of thermal damage to the cell membrane.[55]

A rare hereditary hemolytic anemia designated pyropoikilocytosis presents a striking picture of microspherocytes (Fig. 8-14B) associated with heat sensitivity. The red cell abnormality probably is in the membrane protein spectrin (Chap. 17). These tiny, round, fragmented cells are greatly increased when blood cells are heated *in vitro* to 45°C in contrast to normal red cells, which fragment around 49°C.[70] The mean diameter of the spherical fragments is approximately 2 to 3 μm, and the MCV is extremely low (less than 60 fL).[15,66]

Semilunar Bodies

A semilunar body (half-moon cell; crescent cell) is the large, pale-pink staining ghost of the red cell—the membrane remaining after the contents have been released (Fig. 8-15). Semilunar bodies are as large as leukocytes and are always acquired. They are frequently seen in malaria and in other conditions causing overt hemolysis.

Poikilocytes Secondary to Abnormal Hemoglobin Content

Poikilocytes can be diagnostic of a chronic hereditary hemolytic anemia. Three types of poikilocytes are characteristic of three abnormal Hbs: drepanocytes, Hb CC crystals, and Hb SC crystals.

Drepanocytes (Sickle Cells)

Drepanocytes (sickle cells) (Gr. *drepane*: sickle) have been changed from the normal disc shape by the long rod-shaped polymers of the inherited abnormal Hb S (Chap. 14). A red cell does not appear sickled until it has lost its nucleus and has been fully hemoglobinized. Sickle cells are thin and elongated, with pointed ends and are well filled with Hb (Fig. 8-16). They may be curved or straight or have S, V, or L shapes.[23] This change is striking and irreversible secondary to permanent membrane damage by the polymerization of Hb S.[5,46]

Typical sickle cells are observed in films from patients with homozygous Hb S disease (Hb SS) but are not often seen in heterozygous Hb S (Hb AS) (sickle trait) except

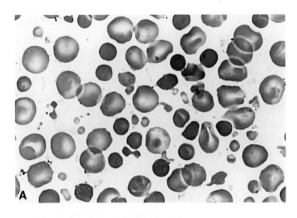

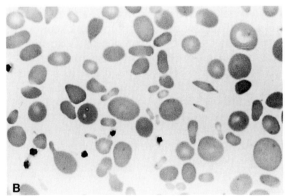

FIG. 8-14.   Microspherocytes. (A) As a result of thermal damage in film of patient with severe burns. (B) As a result of heat sensitivity in film from patient with hereditary pyropoikilocytosis. (From Bell A, Lofsness KG: A photo essay on red cell morphology. J Med Technol 3:85, 1986, with permission.)

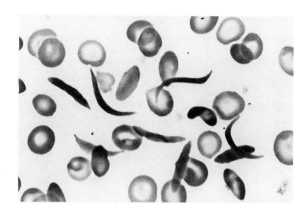

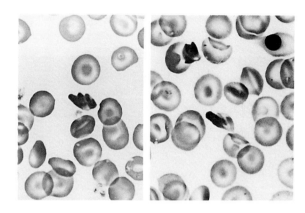

FIG. 8-16.   Drepanocytes (sickled red cells) in film of patient homozygous for Hb S (sickle cell anemia). ×1000. (From Bell A, Lofsness KG: A photo essay on red cell morphology. J Med Technol 3:85, 1986, with permission.)

FIG. 8-18.   Hemoglobin SC crystals in film of patient with Hb SC disease. ×1000. (From Bell A, Lofsness KG. A photo essay on red cell morphology. J Med Technol 1986; 3:85; with permission.)

under unusual situations when there is low *in vivo* oxygen tension. Therefore, morphology is not very helpful in the diagnosis of Hb AS. A few sickled cells may be seen in the abnormal Hb SC, Hb S-β-thalassemia, Hb C-Harlem, and Hb S-Memphis disorders.

Hemoglobin CC Crystals

Intraerythrocytic Hb CC crystals in homozygous C (Hb CC) disease tend to be hexagonal with blunt ends and stain darkly (Fig. 8-17). These angular crystals form within the cell membrane when Hb C crystallizes, often leaving the remainder of the cell relatively Hb free and colorless. Frequently, the cell membrane is not visible, and the crystal appears to be free. At times, several smaller CC crystals form within the red cell.[22]

Crystals of Hb CC are not observed in every patient with electrophoretically proven Hb CC and in most instances are seen only after searching. Actually, the crystals are more frequent after splenectomy. Crystals are not seen in Hb C trait (Hb AC).

Hemoglobin SC Crystals

Hemoglobin SC crystals within erythrocytes in Hb SC disease can be seen on searching. These dark-hued crystals of condensed Hb distort the red cell membrane (Fig. 8-18). The characteristic type of crystalline projection is often straight with parallel sides and one blunt, pointed, protruding end ("Washington monument" shape).[21] Another erythrocyte typical in Hb SC disease contains multiple crystals that protrude in different directions as fingerlike projections from a common crystalline center.

Hemoglobin condensed in one portion of the cell often is accompanied by relative pallor in the opposite portion. In occasional elongated cells, crystals form at opposite poles, leaving a hypochromic area in the center. Another feature is the bent or curved cellular shape caused by polymers of soluble Hb consisting of Hb S tactoids mixed with Hb C crystals.

Diggs and Bell[21] reported intraerythrocytic crystals in 70% of the blood films from 60 cases of electrophoretically proven Hb SC disease. The incidence of intracellular Hb SC crystals was found to be 0 to 23 per 1000 red cells, with an average of 3.2 per 1000. No correlation between the number of crystals and the clinical findings was apparent. The Hb SC erythrocytic abnormalities have not been observed with other abnormal Hbs.

Crystals of Hb SC are distinguished by the one or more fingerlike, blunt-pointed projections that protrude from the cell membrane in Hb SC disease, leaving a pale area at the opposite end, and by the fact that the SC crystal is not hexagonal. On the other hand, Hb CC crystals are hexagonal, form within the membrane, and have blunt ends. Suspected Hb SC or CC crystals on the blood film should always be confirmed by Hb electrophoresis.

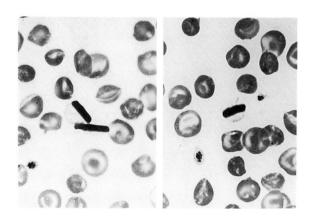

FIG. 8-17.   Hemoglobin CC crystals in film of patient with homozygous Hb C disease. ×1000. (From Bell A, Lofsness KG: A photo essay on red cell morphology. J Med Technol 3:85, 1986, with permission.)

INCLUSIONS

Normally erythrocytes contain no inclusions. However, many different inclusions may be seen because of hematologic disorders.

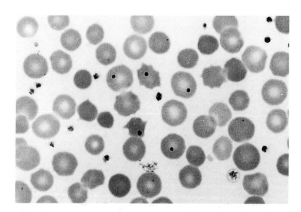

FIG. 8-19.   Howell-Jolly bodies in film of patient after splenectomy. ×1000.

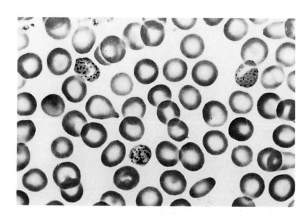

FIG. 8-20.   Stippled red blood cells in film of patient with lead poisoning. ×1000.

Developmental Organelles

Howell-Jolly Bodies

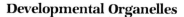

Howell-Jolly bodies are small, round fragments of the nucleus (resulting from karyorrhexis or nuclear disintegration) of a late nucleated red cell or metarubricyte and stain reddish-blue with Wright stain (Fig. 8-19). These inclusions may also result from incomplete extrusion of the nucleus or from chromosomes that were separated from the spindle during abnormal mitotic division. Howell-Jolly bodies give a positive Feulgen reaction and thus are presumed to contain DNA. A Howell-Jolly body usually appears singly in a cell and is ordinarily less than 1 μm in diameter; however, two or more may be noted in a cell in severe anemias and alcoholism.[36]

Normally as the immature erythrocyte passes through the endothelial slits in the splenic sinus, the Howell-Jolly body is pitted from the cell. Thus, after splenectomy, increased numbers of these inclusions are noted on the blood film. Howell-Jolly bodies are seen in sickle cell anemia (secondary to splenic fibrosis), other hemolytic anemias, megaloblastic anemia, congenital absence of the spleen, or splenic atrophy after multiple infarctions.[36]

Basophilic Stippling

Basophilic stippling is the fine or coarse, deep blue to purple staining inclusion that appears in erythrocytes on a dried Wright-stained film (Fig. 8-20). They are much smaller than Howell-Jolly bodies, are usually irregularly shaped, and appear homogeneously throughout the Hb portion of the erythrocyte. Bessis[6] states that these inclusions do not exist in the living cell, but they can be observed in well-made preparations for electron microscopic study.[35] Stippling represents aggregates of ribosomes that appear during the drying and staining of films.[6,35] Punctate basophilia may be found in nucleated red cells or diffusely basophilic cells.

Whenever there is alteration in the biosynthesis of Hb, such as in thalassemia, stippling in erythrocytes may be seen frequently. Stippling also is found in megaloblastic anemias and alcoholism. Marked basophilic stippling occurs in a deficiency of erythrocyte pyrimidine-5'-nucleotidase.[4] Stippling is likewise prominent in lead and

arsenic intoxication, but it may not always be observed, because formation is dependent on the manner in which the film is dried.

Basophilic stippling is an inclusion that may be confused, even by experienced observers, with Pappenheimer bodies (see below). The main differentiating factors are that stippling appears homogeneously over the cell, whereas Pappenheimer bodies tend to appear in groups at the cell periphery; and Pappenheimer bodies stain positively with an iron stain (Prussian blue), whereas stippling does not.

Pappenheimer Bodies

Pappenheimer bodies (siderotic granules) are small, irregular, dark-staining granules[47] that appear near the periphery of a young erythrocyte in a film stained with Wright or supravital stain (Fig. 8-21). With Perls' Prussian blue stain, these bodies stain positively, indicating their iron content. An erythrocyte that is positive for siderotic (iron) granules in a Prussian blue stain is designated a *sidero-cyte;* a normoblast (nucleated erythrocyte) with siderotic granules is called a *sideroblast.* Normally no more than three small iron particles are noted in developing nucleated red cells in bone marrow. Siderotic granules in normal sideroblasts and siderocytes represent, not only dispersed ferritin (a storage form of iron) molecules, but also aggregates of

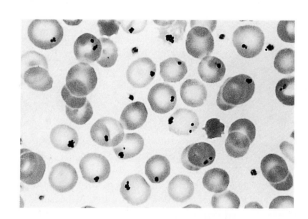

FIG. 8-21.   Pappenheimer bodies in film of patient with sideroblastic anemia. ×1000.

one to seven or eight particles of ferritin. Tiny particles are readily revealed in electron micrographs, but only aggregates may be seen by light microscopy.[8]

The spleen normally removes these inclusions without destroying the cell. The term *pitting* was introduced by Crosby[19] to describe this action by the spleen. However, after splenectomy Pappenheimer bodies are visible on the blood film. The spleen is thus responsible for removing excess iron-containing granules from young red cells in which Hb synthesis is complete. These granules are also found in hyposplenism, in which the spleen does not function normally.

With severe disturbance of Hb synthesis, pathologic sideroblasts and siderocytes are present in the bone marrow and peripheral blood. Siderotic granules may be present in sideroblastic anemia, thalassemia, refractory anemias, and dyserythropoietic anemias.

In sideroblastic anemia (a myelodysplastic disorder; Chap. 33), numerous siderotic granules are found within the mitochondria and form a ring around at least one-third of the nucleus. Such cells are called *pathologic ringed sideroblasts*.[9,11,44]

Iron overload in hemosiderosis and hemochromatosis (Chap. 13) is associated with an increase in the number of siderotic granules (approximately 20 per cell) and an increase in the size of the siderotic granules.

On a Wright-stained film it is possible to misidentify Pappenheimer bodies as basophilic stippling when the iron overload is severe. Therefore, when disorders of Hb synthesis or iron overload are suspected and there is doubt concerning the red cell inclusions observed, a Prussian blue stain should be performed for confirmation.

Polychromatophilic Red Cells

Diffusely basophilic red cells or polychromatophilic cells[48] are young red cells that no longer have a nucleus but still contain some RNA. As the name implies this RNA stains diffusely blue with Wright stain (see Plate 2). Such cells are slightly larger than mature red cells and contain ribosomes, mitochondria, and other organelles.

When polychromatophilic cells are stained supravitally with new methylene blue, they are identified as reticulocytes because of their granulofilamentous pattern. The supravital dye precipitates the ribosomes and other organelles in the living state to give this reticulated appearance. Thus, a diffusely basophilic cell is called a reticulocyte when a supravital dye is used.[31]

Normally these cells are seen in only an occasional oil immersion (× 1000 magnification) field. If more are seen, increased erythrocyte production is indicated secondary to increased erythropoietin stimulation of the marrow. Depending on the pH of the Romanowsky stain or buffer, basophilia may be more or less prominent. More acidic solutions tend to obscure basophilia.

Very large diffusely basophilic cells are known as *shift* cells and indicate premature release from the marrow during intense erythrocyte production.

Cabot Rings

A thin ringlike structure called a *Cabot ring* (Fig. 8-22) may appear in erythrocytes in megaloblastic anemia or other severe anemias, in lead poisoning, and in dyseryth-

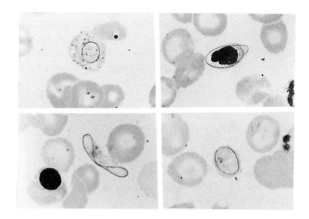

FIG. 8-22.   Cabot rings in film of patient with vitamin B_{12} deficiency. ×1000.

ropoiesis, in which erythrocytes are destroyed before being released form the marrow. A Cabot ring stains reddish violet in Wright stain. It may be circular or appear at the cell periphery, or it may form a figure eight, incomplete rings, or other configurations.[23] More than one ring may be present in a single cell.

A Cabot ring may be observed in a nucleated red cell or be associated with stippling or a Howell-Jolly body in the same erythrocyte. This threadlike structure may represent a part of the mitotic spindle, remnants of microtubules, or a fragment of the nuclear membrane. However, its origin is still unclear.[59]

Abnormal Hemoglobin Precipitation

Heinz Bodies

Heinz bodies are round, refractile inclusions not visible on a Wright-stained film. They range in size from about 1 to 3 μm and are attached to the erythrocyte membrane (Fig. 8-23). When appearing singly, a Heinz body is large, but when several are present in one cell, they are small. They are best identified by supravital staining with basic dyes

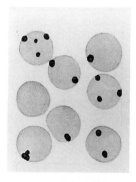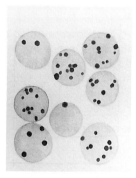

FIG. 8-23.   Heinz bodies in erythrocytes after 4-hour incubation with acetylphenylhydrazine followed by staining with crystal violet. (Left) Normal blood with one to four Heinz bodies in most cells. (Right) Five or more Heinz bodies per cell from a patient with G6PD deficiency. (From Diggs LW, Sturm D, Bell A: Morphology of Human Blood Cells, 5th ed. N. Chicago, IL: Abbott Laboratories, 1985, with permission.)

such as crystal violet, methylene blue, or brilliant cresyl blue. A Heinz body in a supravital preparation might be confused with a reticulocyte. A Heinz body is a round, discrete inclusion in contrast to the reticular filamented material in a reticulocyte. Multiple Heinz bodies may give a cell the appearance of a pitted golf ball.

Heinz bodies consist of denatured globin derived from destruction of the Hb molecule. These inclusions are not seen in normal individuals (unless the person is acutely poisoned) because they are pitted out by the spleen. When a Heinz body is pitted from an erythrocyte, the resulting cell may resemble a "bite cell" in which a portion of the cell has been removed. However, if the spleen has been removed or is atrophic or infarcted, these inclusions can be noted frequently.[33]

Heinz bodies are produced in the blood of normal persons who have been poisoned by aromatic nitro-compounds, amino-compounds, and inorganic oxidizing agents used in treatment protocols. With large doses of the drugs that cause Heinz bodies, hemolysis is present. Heinz bodies also occur in individuals with a hereditary deficiency of the enzymes glucose-6-phosphate dehydrogenase (G6PD) or glutathione as a result of exposure to drugs containing the above compounds and agents (Chaps. 6 and 17). In rare hereditary hemolytic anemias secondary to instability of the Hb molecule (*e.g.*, Hb Zurich and Hb Köln) (Chap. 14), such bodies are formed spontaneously in young and mature erythrocytes and also after exposure to sulfonamides or similar drugs. A patient with an unstable Hb reveals at least one large Heinz body in almost every cell after splenectomy.[33]

Hemoglobin H Inclusions

In patients with Hb H disease, an α-thalassemia with a moderate hemolytic anemia (Chap. 15), small greenish-blue inclusion bodies appear in many erythrocytes after four drops of blood is incubated with 0.5 mL of 1% brilliant cresyl blue for 20 minutes at 37°C. These inclusions represent precipitated Hb H (Fig. 8-24). They must be differentiated from reticulocytes, which also stain with brilliant cresyl blue. A reticulocyte has a granulofilamentous appearance, whereas an Hb H inclusion is a single body.

The Hb H inclusions also can be seen in early nucleated red cells in the bone marrow of patients with Hb H disease.[27] The disease is caused by a hereditary defect leading to a failure of synthesis of three of the four α globin genes, leaving an excess of β chains. Tetramers of β chains (Hb H) are unstable and easily oxidized and precipitate as inclusions with cell aging.[68]

Protozoan Inclusions

Malaria

There are four species of human malarial parasites that invade erythrocytes. They are transmitted to man by the bite of the *Anopheles* mosquito.

Plasmodium vivax is characterized by four maturation stages (from least to most mature): rings, trophozoites, schizonts, and gametocytes (all of which appear in infected red cells). An important feature of *P. vivax* infection is the enlarged red cell, which is usually first noted in the tropho-

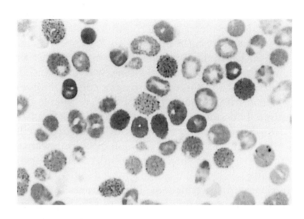

FIG. 8-24.   Hemoglobin H inclusions in film stained with brilliant cresyl blue from patient with hemoglobin H. ×1000. (Courtesy of the Hemoglobinopathy Laboratory, US Centers for Disease Control, Atlanta.)

zoite stage. Schüffner's stippling (or granules) is present in all stages beyond the early ring (Fig. 8-25). Pigment generally becomes visible in the trophozoite stage. Large amoeboid trophozoites, which almost fill the enlarged red cell and contain larger amounts of brown pigment and often a vacuole, are common. Maturing schizonts begin to show division of the chromatin and contain 12 to 24 merozoites and aggregates of pigment granules. Each merozoite is composed of a red chromatin dot and a ring of blue cytoplasm. Gametocytes practically fill the enlarged cell, contain a reddish chromatin mass, and show pigment grains scattered over the cytoplasm.[2]

Plasmodium malariae is characterized by the same stages as *P. vivax*. Erythrocytes invaded by *P. malariae* are normal in size and do not enlarge, as do the cells with *P. vivax*. The ring forms cannot be distinguished from those of *P. vivax*. As the trophozoite grows the cytoplasm often forms a narrow compact band across the cell and contains dark, coarse pigment. This feature is diagnostic of *P. malariae*.

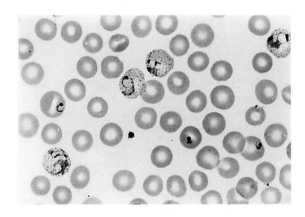

FIG. 8-25.   Malarial ring and trophozoite stages in enlarged erythrocytes in film from patient with *Plasmodium vivax*. Note Schüffner's granules. ×1000.

The mature schizont has 6 to 12 merozoites in the form of a rosette with coarse pigment, often in the central area of the parasite. The gametocytes are usually few in number and smaller than those of *P. vivax*, but pigment is less obvious than in *P. malariae*.[2]

Plasmodium falciparum has small delicate ring forms. Occasionally the ring has double chromatin dots. There may be more than one ring per erythrocyte. Rings are observed at the margin of the red cell. Intermediate trophozoites and schizonts are rarely seen in peripheral films but are present in visceral organs such as the liver. Gametocytes are crescent- or banana-shaped with coarse pigment and have a red staining chromatin mass near the center.[2]

The erythrocyte in *P. falciparum* infection is not enlarged. There may be a few reddish staining dots, but Schüffner's stippling is not present. If many rings are present and there are no other stages observed, *P. falciparum* is strongly indicated.

A malarial ring may be mistakenly identified as a platelet. The observer should note that a malarial ring has a central area that lacks color, whereas the platelet stains completely and has a surrounding halo under light microscopy.

Plasmodium ovale is found in large red cells that are oval and sometimes fringed. Red staining granules (Schüffner's stippling) are present. Ring forms and trophozoites are difficult to distinguish from those of *P. vivax* unless the cell is oval, its membrane is fringed, and it contains a fairly compact parasite. The schizont is also in oval cells, which often have a fringed outline. Pigment is present in all stages after the ring form but may be lighter and not as coarse as in *P. malariae*. Gametocytes and schizonts of *P. ovale* are not easily distinguished from those of *P. malariae* except for the fact that the red cells invaded by *P. ovale* are large and mostly oval.[2]

For information on geographic distribution, life cycle, and host location of the malaria stages, a publication by Ash and Orihel[2] is recommended. To examine color drawings of the four stages, the atlas by Diggs, Sturm, and Bell[23] is suggested.

Babesia

Babesia organisms are rarely transmitted to humans by a tick bite. *Babesia* in a red cell forms ringlike structures resembling the ring stages of malarial parasites.[2] *Babesia* rings may be round, oval, elongated, amoeboid, or pear shaped and are often tiny, ranging in size from 1 to 5 μm (Fig. 8-26). *Babesia microti* appears as tiny rings (usually less than 2 μm) with minimal cytoplasm and a little dot of chromatin. Reproduction occurs asexually by a division that results in a tetrad of organisms that somewhat resembles a cross. One or two chromatin dots with little evidence of cytoplasm is sometimes seen.

Red cells infected with *Babesia* are not enlarged, and pigment is not present. Schüffner's stippling is not observed. Babesiosis, rather than malaria, may be suspected when there are small (or tiny) rings and the tetrad form without other stages. A helpful distinguishing feature is to observe *Babesia* in groups outside the erythrocyte.[23] The patient's clinical presentation and travel history may aid in the differentiation of *Babesia* and *Malaria*.

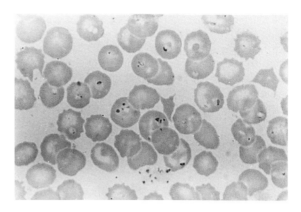

FIG. 8-26.   Rings in erythrocytes in film of patient infected with *Babesia microti*. ×1000. (Courtesy of the Parasitology Unit, US Centers for Disease Control, Atlanta.)

ARTIFACTS

Erythrocyte artifacts occasionally occur in a blood film. When blood is spread on slides, cells are mechanically traumatized, and artifacts occur as cells dry, are fixed with methanol, and stained. A peripheral film should not be fixed or stained until it is totally dry. Methanol fixative should be fresh daily and have the proper *pH* (8.4) to avoid creating refractile artifacts in cells.

Allowing Wright stain to remain longer than usual on the film leads to evaporation of the methanol in the stain and may cause precipitation of the dye granules, which interferes with red cell description.

Refractile artifacts must be identified if present. They may be caused by water contamination of the methanol or Wright stain. Under light microscopy, focusing up and down with the fine adjustment knob will cause these artifacts to refract rather than disappear, and use of this technique will help in their identification. Refractile artifacts must not be confused with red cell inclusions and should not be reported.

When examining a film several areas should be studied. For example, codocytes may be observed in some areas but not others. Therefore, codocytes should not be reported unless they appear in every acceptable area examined. On the sides and at the pushed-out end of the film, erythrocytes lack normal central pallor and appear solid. Evaluation of Hb content should be avoided in such areas. Near the sides of a film, there may be shape distortion with elongated cells arranged in the same direction, much like a school of fish swimming in the same direction; this formation is an artifact of spreading.

Echinocytes or crenated cells may also be artifacts if practically every cell in the thin portion of the film has a uniformly spiculed membrane. These features should not be reported.

Schistocytes may be an artifact of physical damage to the film. This most often results from removing oil from the slide using laboratory tissue, thereby slicing the cells on the film. Slides should be dabbed rather than wiped. These artifacts generally appear in a long regular line on the film.

A cell with a distinct colorless center and a well-defined inner ring of Hb, giving the appearance of a doughnut, is produced during preparation. This artifact should not be mistaken for hypochromia. True hypochromia is evidenced by a gradual transition from the central pallor to the hemoglobinated cytoplasm.

Additional artifacts may be produced by particles of fat or detergent on the glass itself.

MORPHOLOGY REPORTING

The purpose of reporting red cell morphology is to inform the physician of abnormal findings in an understandable, concise manner that will enable judgment concerning their clinical significance.[37] To achieve a level of reproducibility between observers in the same laboratory, it is necessary to have set criteria that everyone must uniformly follow.[61]

Appropriate oil immersion fields composed of approximately 200 red cells should be examined with 1000× magnification. The overall impression of size, shape, and Hb content should be expressed in a semiquantitative way. Emphasis should be placed on the abnormalities that seem significant. Specific size, variation, and shape changes should be reported. If rouleaux formation or agglutination are truly present, a statement to this effect should be made. The presence of inclusions should always be reported. Likewise, schistocytes and spherocytes should always be reported, even if they are rare because they may indicate a hemolytic process. Sickle cells must also be reported whenever seen.

Fifteen large hematology laboratories in different areas of the United States responded to a request for information regarding their method of reporting erythrocyte morphology on peripheral blood films. There were similarities and differences for each method, and it was evident that each laboratory was attempting to evaluate red cell morphology in a manner suitable to its particular instrumentation and personnel, as every laboratory should. One example of a method in current use is given in abbreviated form in Table 8-1. Several semiquantitative methods for evaluation of erythrocyte morphology have been published.[17,29,37,45,61]

This author's laboratory employs the following descriptive terms: slight (less than 5%), moderate (5%–15%), and marked (more than 15%) to denote variation in size, shape, or color content per average oil immersion field. If there is a particular size variation, such as macrocytes, or a poikiloycte, such as schistocytes, the terms occasional (less than 1%), few (1%–5%), frequent (5%–10%), and many (more than 10%) are used.

Semiquantitative reports on abnormalities in erythrocyte morphology should be formatted to promote both effective communication with the physician and laboratory reproducibility.

APPROACHING ERYTHROCYTE ABNORMALITIES ON THE UNKNOWN FILM

To aid in comparing particular erythrocyte abnormalities on an unknown film, several decision trees are presented.

TABLE 8-1. Sample Criteria for Erythrocyte Morphology Evaluation*

MORPHOLOGIC CHARACTERISTIC	WNL†	1+	2+	3+	4+
Macrocytes > 9 μm diameter	0–5	5–10	10–20	20–50	> 50
Microcytes < 6 μm diameter	0–5	5–10	10–20	20–50	> 50
Hypochromia	0–2	3–10	10–50	50–75	> 75
Poikilocytosis (generalized variations in shape)	0–2	3–10	10–20	20–50	> 50
Burr cells	0–2	3–10	10–20	20–50	> 50
Acanthocytes	< 1	2–5	5–10	10–20	> 20
Schistocytes	< 1	2–5	5–10	10–20	> 20
Teardrop poikilocytes (dacryocytes)	0–2	2–5	5–10	10–20	> 20
Target cells (codocytes)	0–2	2–10	10–20	20–50	> 50
Spherocytes	0–2	2–10	10–20	20–50	> 50
Ovalocytes	0–2	2–10	10–20	20–50	> 50
Stomatocytes	0–2	2–10	10–20	20–50	> 50
Sickle cells (drepanocytes)	Absent	Report as 1+ to indicate presence; do not quantitate			
Polychromatophilia					
Adult	< 1	2–5	5–10	10–20	> 20
Newborn	1–6	7–15	15–20	20–50	> 50
Basophilic stippling	0–1	1–5	5–10	10–20	> 20
Howell-Jolly bodies	Absent	1–2	3–5	5–10	> 10
Siderocytes (Pappenheimer bodies)	Absent	1–2	3–5	5–10	> 10

* Guidelines for semiquantitation are expressed in numbers of occurrences per oil immersion field (applies to fields of approximately 200 to 250 cells per 100× oil objective).
† Within normal limits
From University of California Medical Center, San Diego, Hematology Laboratory, with permission.

These trees should help the observer differentiate red cell inclusions by Wright stain (Fig. 8-27), supravital stain (Fig. 8-28), and Prussian blue stain for iron (Fig. 8-29). They should also help to differentiate cells with membrane irregularities (Fig. 8-30) and red cells containing Hb crystals (Fig. 8-31).

CHAPTER SUMMARY

Careful evaluation of red cell morphology on blood films can provide useful diagnostic information. The examiner should describe any inclusion and any variation in red cell size, shape, or Hb content. Red cells may be normocytic, microcytic, or macrocytic in size. Many abnormal shapes were described in this chapter, both hereditary and acquired, and the reasons for their appearance were summarized. Red cells may be normochromic, hypochromic, or hyperchromic, indicating their Hb content. Acquired and hereditary inclusions may also be seen in red cells on the peripheral blood film.

Red cell abnormalities must be recognized by the examiner to ensure accurate morphology reports. Using specific criteria to present important findings intelligently is essential for high-quality patient care.

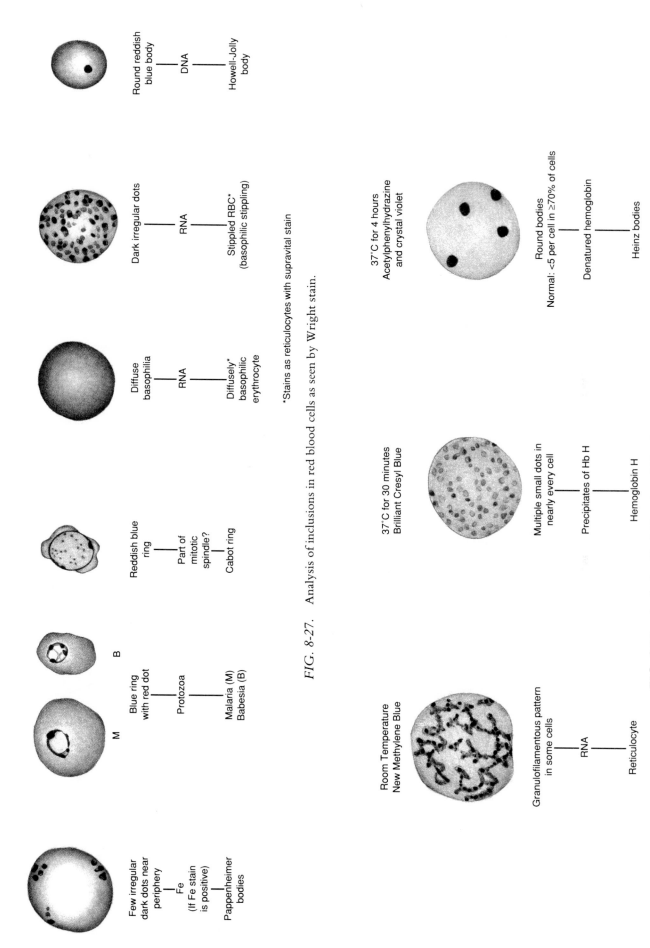

Round reddish blue body ── DNA ── Howell-Jolly body

Dark irregular dots ── RNA ── Stippled RBC* (basophilic stippling)

Diffuse basophilia ── RNA ── Diffusely* basophilic erythrocyte

Reddish blue ring ── Part of mitotic spindle? ── Cabot ring

Blue ring with red dot ── Protozoa ── Malaria (M) Babesia (B)

M

B

Few irregular dark dots near periphery ── Fe (If Fe stain is positive) ── Pappenheimer bodies

*Stains as reticulocytes with supravital stain

FIG. 8-27. Analysis of inclusions in red blood cells as seen by Wright stain.

37°C for 4 hours
Acetylphenylhydrazine and crystal violet

Round bodies
Normal: <5 per cell in ≥70% of cells ── Denatured hemoglobin ── Heinz bodies

37°C for 30 minutes
Brilliant Cresyl Blue

Multiple small dots in nearly every cell ── Precipitates of Hb H ── Hemoglobin H

Room Temperature
New Methylene Blue

Granulofilamentous pattern in some cells ── RNA ── Reticulocyte

FIG. 8-28. Analysis of inclusions in red blood cells as seen by supravital stains.

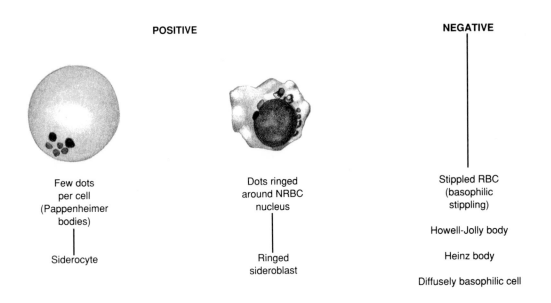

FIG. 8-29. Analysis of findings with Prussian blue stain for iron.

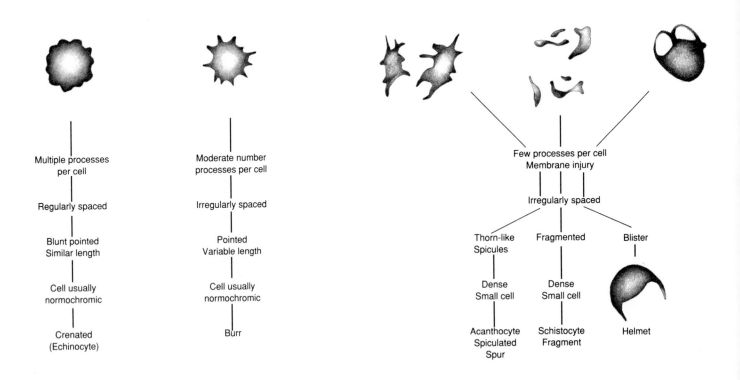

FIG. 8-30. Analysis of membrane irregularities in red blood cells.

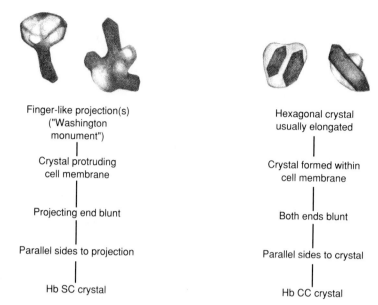

Finger-like projection(s)
("Washington
monument")

|

Crystal protruding
cell membrane

|

Projecting end blunt

|

Parallel sides to projection

|

Hb SC crystal

Hexagonal crystal
usually elongated

|

Crystal formed within
cell membrane

|

Both ends blunt

|

Parallel sides to crystal

|

Hb CC crystal

FIG. 8-31.   Analysis of hemoglobin crystals in red blood cells.

REFERENCES

1. Alloisio N, Dorleac E, Girot R et al: Analysis of the red cell membrane in a family with hereditary elliptocytosis: Total or partial absence of protein 4.1. Hum Genet 59:68, 1981
2. Ash LR, Orihel TC: Atlas of Human Parasitology, 2nd ed. Chicago, American Society of Clinical Pathology Press, 1984
3. Bassen FA, Kornzweig AL: Malformation of the erythrocytes in a case of atypical retinitis pigmentosa. Blood 5:381, 1950
4. Ben–Bassat I, Brok–Simoni F, Kende G et al: A family with red cell pyrimidine-5'-nucleotidase deficiency. Blood 47:919, 1976
5. Bertles JF, Milner PFA: Irreversibly sickled erythrocytes: A consequence of heterogenous distribution of hemoglobin types in sickle cell anemia. J Clin Invest 47:1731, 1968
6. Bessis M: Living Blood Cells and Their Ultrastructure. New York, Springer-Verlag, 1973
7. Bessis M: Blood Smears Reinterpreted. G Brecher (trans). New York, Springer International, 1977
8. Bessis M, Breton–Gorious J: Ferritin and ferruginous micelles in normal erythroblasts and hypochromic hypersideremic anemias. Blood 14:423, 1959
9. Bessis M, Jensen WN: Sideroblastic anaemia, mitochondria and erythroblastic iron. Br J Haematol 11:49, 1965
10. Bessman JD: Automated Blood Counts and Differentials: A Practical Guide. Baltimore, Johns Hopkins University Press, 1986
11. Bowman WD Jr: Abnormal (ringed) sideroblasts in various hematologic and nonhematologic disorders. Blood 18:662, 1961
12. Brain MC, Dacie JV, Hourihane D: Microangiopathic haemolytic anaemia: The possible role of vascular lesions in pathogenesis. Br J Haematol 8:358, 1962
13. Brecher G, Haley JE, Prenant M et al: Macronormoblasts, macroreticulocytes and macrocytes. Blood Cells 1:547, 1975
14. Bull BS, Kuhn IN: The production of schistocytes by fibrin strands (a scanning electron microscope study). Blood 35:104, 1970
15. Chang K, Williamson JR, Zarkhowsky HS: Effect of heat on the circular dichroism of spectrin in hereditary pyropoikilocytosis. J Clin Invest 64:326, 1979
16. Chapman RG: Red cell life span after splenectomy in hereditary spherocytosis. J Clin Invest 47:2263, 1968
17. Connors DM, Wilson MK: A new approach to the reporting of red cell morphology. J Med Technol 3:94, 1986
18. Cooper RA, Jandl JH: Bile salts and cholesterol in the pathogenesis of target cells in obstructive jaundice. J Clin Invest 47:809, 1968
19. Crosby WH: Siderocytes and the spleen. Blood 12:165, 1956
20. Dacie V: The Haemolytic Anaemias, 3rd ed, vol 1. Edinburgh, Churchill Livingstone, 1985
21. Diggs LW, Bell A: Intraerythrocytic hemoglobin crystals in sickle cell–hemoglobin C disease. Blood 25:218, 1965
22. Diggs LW, Kraus AP, Morrison DB et al: Intraerythrocytic crystals in a white patient with hemoglobin C in the absence of other types of hemoglobin. Blood 9:1172, 1954
23. Diggs LW, Sturm D, Bell A: Morphology of Human Blood Cells, 5th ed. Abbott Park, IL, Abbott Laboratories, 1985
24. Dresbach M: Elliptical human red corpuscles. Science 19:469, 1904
25. Eichner ER: Macrocytic anemia. In Spivak JL (ed): Fundamentals of Clinical Hematology, 2nd ed. Philadelphia, Harper & Row, 1985
26. England JM, Down MC: Red cell volume distribution curves and the measurement of anisocytosis. Lancet 1:701, 1974
27. Fessas P, Yataghanas X: Intraerythroblastic instability of hemoglobin β4 (Hgb H). Blood 31:323, 1968
28. Florman AL, Wintrobe MM: Human elliptical red corpuscles. Bull Johns Hopkins Hosp 63:209, 1938
29. Glasser L: Grading red cell morphology. Diag Med 3:15, 1980
30. Haden RL: The mechanism of the increased fragility of the erythrocytes in congenital hemolytic jaundice. Am J Med Sci 188:441, 1934
31. Hillman RS: Characteristics of marrow production and reticulocyte maturation in normal man in response to anemia. J Clin Invest 48:443, 1969
32. Isselbacher KJ, Scheif R, Plotkin GR et al: Congenital β-lipoprotein deficiency: A hereditary disorder involving a defect in the absorption and transport of lipids. Medicine 43:347, 1964
33. Jacob HS: Mechanism of Heinz body formation and attachment to red cell membrane. Semin Hematol 7:341, 1970
34. Jacob HS, Ruby A, Overland ES et al: Abnormal membrane protein of red blood cells in hereditary spherocytosis. J Clin Invest 50:1800, 1971
35. Jensen WN, Moreno GD, Bessis M: An electron microscopic description of basophilic stippling in red cells. Blood 25:933, 1965
36. Koyama S: Studies on Howell-Jolly body. Acta Haematol Jpn 23:20, 1960

37. Krause JR: Red cell abnormalities in the blood smear: Disease correlations. Lab Management 23:29, 1985

38. Lessin L, Klug P, Jensen W: Clinical implications of red cell shape. Adv Intern Med 21:451, 1976

39. Lindenbaum J: Brief review: Status of laboratory testing in the diagnosis of megaloblastic anaemia. Blood 61:684, 1983

40. Lock SP, Smith RS, Hardisty RM: Stomatocytosis: A hereditary red cell anomaly associated with haemolytic anaemia. Br J Haematol 7:303, 1961

41. Lux SE: Spectrin–actin membrane skeleton of normal and abnormal red cells. Semin Hematol 16:21, 1979

42. McPhedran P, Barnes MG, Weinstein JS et al: Interpretation of electronically determined macrocytosis. Ann Intern Med 78:677, 1973

43. Miale JB: Laboratory Medicine: Hematology, 6th ed. St Louis, CV Mosby, 1982

44. Mollin DL: Sideroblasts and sideroblastic anaemia. Br J Haematol 11:41, 1965

45. Napoli VM, Nichols CW, Cleck S: A semiquantitative estimate method for reporting abnormal RBC morphology. Lab Med 11:111, 1980

46. Padilla F, Bromberg PA, Jensen WN: The sickle–unsickle cycle: A cause of cell fragmentation leading to permanently deformed cells. Blood 41:653, 1973

47. Pappenheimer AM, Thompson WP, Parker DD et al: Anaemia associated with unidentified erythrocytic inclusions. Q J Med Sci 14:75, 1945

48. Perrotta AL, Finch CA: The polychromatophilic erythrocyte. Am J Clin Pathol 57:471, 1972

49. Ponder E: Hemolysis and Related Phenomena. New York, Grune & Stratton, 1948

50. Price–Jones C: Red Blood Cell Diameters. London, Oxford Medical Publications, 1933

51. Sayed HN, Dacie JV, Handley DA et al: Haemolytic anaemia of mechanical origin after open heart surgery. Thorax 16:356, 1961

52. Schubothe H: The cold hemagglutinin disease. Semin Hematol 3:27, 1966

53. Schwartz SO, Motto SA: The diagnostic significance of "burr" red blood cells. Am J Med Sci 218:563, 1949

54. Sears DA, Crosby WH: Intravascular hemolysis due to intracardiac prosthetic devices. Am J Med 39:341, 1965

55. Shen SC, Ham TH, Fleming EM: Studies on the destruction of red blood cells III. Mechanism and complications of hemoglobinuria in patients with thermal burns: Spherocytosis and increased osmotic fragility of red blood cells. N Engl J Med 229:701, 1943

56. Sturgeon P: Hematological observations on the anemia associated with blood type Rh null. Blood 36:310, 1970

57. Tomaselli MB, John KM, Lux SE: Elliptical erythrocyte membrane skeletons and heat-sensitive spectrin in hereditary elliptocytosis. Proc Natl Acad Sci USA 78:1911, 1981

58. van Assendelft O: Anemia and polycythemia: Interpretation of laboratory tests and differential diagnosis. In Koepke JA (ed): Laboratory Hematology, vol 2. New York, Churchill Livingstone, 1984

59. Van Oye E: L'origine des anneaux de Cabot. Rev Hematol 9:173, 1954

60. Vaughan JM: Red cell characteristics in acholuric jaundice. J Pathol Bacteriol 45:461, 1937

61. Walton JR: Uniform grading of hematologic abnormalities. Am J Med Technol 39:517, 1973

62. Ways P, Reed CF, Hanahan DJ: Red-cell and plasma lipids in acanthocytosis. J Clin Invest 42:1248, 1963

63. Weed RI: The importance of erythrocyte deformability. Am J Med 49:147, 1970

64. Weed RI, Reed C: Membrane alterations and red cell destruction. Am J Med 41:681, 1966

65. Weiss L, Tavassoli M: Anatomical hazards to the passage of erythrocytes through the spleen. Semin Hematol 7:372, 1970

66. Wiley JS, Gill FM: Red cell calcium leak in congenital hemolytic anemia with extreme microcytosis. Blood 47:197, 1976

67. Williams WJ, Beutler E, Erslev AJ et al: Hematology, 4th ed. New York, McGraw-Hill, 1990

68. Wintrobe MM, Lee GR, Boggs DR et al: Clinical Hematology, 8th ed. Philadelphia, Lea & Febiger, 1981

69. Woodruff AW, Topley E, Knight R et al: The anaemia of kala azar. Br J Haematol 22:319, 1972

70. Zarkowsky HS, Mohandas N, Speaker CB et al: A congenital haemolytic anaemia with thermal sensitivity of the erythrocyte membrane. Br J Haematol 29:537, 1975

Routine

Laboratory

Evaluation

of Erythrocytes

Bernadette F. Rodak

The evaluation of erythrocytes is an important part of the complete blood count (CBC), which is performed routinely in most clinical laboratories. This chapter discusses all the basic laboratory procedures relating to the qualitative and quantitative evaluation of erythrocytes and their composition. Although many of these tests are now performed by automated methods, every laboratory maintains procedures and equipment for manual performance of these tests, because some specimens have abnormalities that interfere with accurate automated hematologic testing.

The manual erythrocyte count is no longer performed because of its lack of accuracy and reliability. It used to be performed using a Thoma pipet for specimen dilution in isotonic saline, Hayem's solution, or Gower's solution. The diluted specimen was loaded on a hemocytometer and the cells counted under the microscope. Now this task is reserved for single or multiparameter instruments discussed in Chapters 42 and 43, respectively.

Other erythrocyte evaluation procedures are routinely performed manually, including the reticulocyte count and the erythrocyte sedimentation rate (ESR). Skill in performing these tests, as well as those performed manually on occasion, is essential for hematology laboratory personnel.

For all procedures in this chapter a whole blood specimen, anticoagulated with EDTA and less than 24 hours old, is required unless otherwise noted.

Table 9-1 presents a sample reference range for the peripheral blood erythrocyte count and other related erythrocyte measurements presented in this chapter. Note that these ranges are meant to give only general guidelines: every laboratory should endeavor to determine the reference range for each of these measurements based on its own patient population.

TABLE 9-1. Hematology References Ranges (Mean ± 2 SD)★

AGE (YEARS)	ERYTHROCYTE COUNT (× 10^{12} /L)†	HB (g/dL)†‡	HEMATOCRIT (L/L)†	MCV (fL)	MCH (pg)	MCHC (g/dL)
Birth (cord blood)	3.9–5.5	13.5–19.5	0.42–0.60	98–118	31–37	30–36
1 to 3 days (capillary blood)	4.0–6.6	14.5–22.5	0.45–0.67	95–121	31–37	29–37
0.5 to 2	3.7–5.3	10.5–13.5	0.33–0.39	70–86	23–31	30–36
2 to 6	3.9–5.3	11.5–13.5	0.34–0.40	75–87	24–30	31–37
6 to 12	4.0–5.2	11.5–15.5	0.35–0.45	77–95	25–33	31–37
12 to 18 (male)	4.5–5.3	13.0–16.0	0.37–0.49	78–98	25–35	31–37
12 to 18 (female)	4.1–5.1	12.0–16.0	0.36–0.46	78–102	25–35	31–37
18 to 49 (male)	4.5–5.9	13.5–17.5	0.41–0.53	80–100	26–34	31–37
18 to 49 (female)	4.0–5.2	12.0–16.0	0.36–0.46	80–100	26–34	31–37

Data from Dallman PR: Blood and blood forming tissues. In Rudolph A (ed): Pediatrics, 16th ed, p 1111. New York, Appleton-Century-Crofts, 1977; with permission. Compiled from the following sources: Dutcher: Lab Med 2:32, 1971; Koerper et al: J Paediatr 89:580, 1976; Marner: Acta Paediatr Scand 58:363, 1969; Matoth et al: Acta Paediatr Scand 60:317, 1971; Moe: Acta Paediatr Scand 54:69, 1965; Okuno: J Clin Pathol 25:599, 1972; Oski and Naiman: Hematological Problems in the Newborn. Philadelphia, WB Saunders, 1972, p 11; Penttila et al: Suomen Laakarilehti 26:2173, 1973; and Viteria et al: Br J Haematol 23:189, 1972.
★ Emphasis was given to studies employing electronic counters and to the selection of populations that are likely to exclude individuals with iron deficiency. The mean ± 2 SD can be expected to include 95% of the observations in a normal population.
† Erythrocyte count, Hb, and hematocrit are slightly lower in three significant situations: (1) after age 50; (2) in recumbency (i.e., a blood sample is taken when the patient is lying down); and (3) after meals (as much as 10% lower). Values may be significantly lower in runners than in nonrunners but seldom reflect true anemia.[5]
‡ Hemoglobin may be elevated in heavy smokers because of the increase in carboxyhemoglobin, which is not capable of carrying oxygen to tissues.

SPECTROPHOTOMETRIC DETERMINATION OF HEMOGLOBIN CONCENTRATION (HEMOGLOBINOMETRY)

Review of Spectrophotometry

The manual procedure for determining hemoglobin (Hb) concentration in whole blood requires the use of a spectrophotometer. This instrument measures monochromatic light transmitted through a solution to determine the concentration of the light-absorbing substance in that solution.

Spectrophotometer Components

A basic spectrophotometer has five components: (1) a stable source of radiant energy (lamp); (2) a wavelength selector or monochromator (prism, diffraction grating); (3) a container to hold the substance to be measured (cuvette); (4) a radiant energy detector (photomultiplier tube); and (5) a device to provide readout of the electronic signal generated by detector (e.g., galvanometer). Light from the lamp passes through the diffraction grating or prism, which allows light of only a chosen wavelength to pass through the cuvette. This transmitted light strikes a detector, where it is converted into electrical energy and presented to the readout device.

Beer's Law

The principle of spectrophotometry follows Beer's law, which states that the concentration of a substance is directly proportional to the amount of light absorbed and to the length of the light path through the solution. It also states that the concentration of a substance is inversely proportional to the logarithm of transmitted light. For example, plotting concentration versus absorbance of a 1% solution with an absorbance of 0.1, a 2% solution with an absorbance of 0.2, and a 3% solution with an absorbance of 0.3 would yield a straight line, thus demonstrating Beer's law, as each solution has a concentration directly proportional to its absorbance.

Percent transmittance (%T) is the term used for the amount of light transmitted, and absorbance (A) is the term for the amount of light absorbed. Absorbance is also known as optical density (O.D.), a term now obsolete. Many spectrophotometers have both an A and a %T scale. If absorbance cannot be measured directly by a spectrophotometer, it is derived mathematically from %T:

$$A = 2 - \log \%T$$

(refer to Appendix B for %T to A conversion chart).

Because absorbance is directly proportional to the concentration, it is easier to use than the %T relation. Because of this relation, the concentration (C) of an unknown may be determined by the following ratio:

$$\frac{C_{unknown}}{A_{unknown}} = \frac{C_{standard}}{A_{standard}}$$

or

$$C_{unknown} = \frac{C_{standard}}{A_{standard}} \times A_{unknown}$$

This formula may be applied to calculation of a specimen's Hb concentration based on a cyanmethemoglobin standard (discussed below).

Spectrophotometer Quality Control

To ensure accuracy, function verification should include checks on wavelength accuracy, stray light, and linearity of the detector response for any spectrophotometer used in the laboratory.[6] Details on such function verification may be found in standard textbooks of clinical chemistry.

Hemoglobin Concentration Determination

Hemoglobin concentration provides an estimate of the oxygen-carrying capacity of blood. The International Committee for Standardization in Haematology[16,18] and the National Committee for Clinical Laboratory Standards (NCCLS)[24] recommend the cyanmethemoglobin (hemiglobincyanide) method for Hb determination. Another method, formerly popular, is the oxyhemoglobin procedure, in which Hb is converted to oxyhemoglobin by shaking with aqueous NH₄OH, the solution being read on a colorimeter. Oxyhemoglobin concentration is then calculated from a standard curve. This method has the advantage of measuring oxygen-carrying capacity directly, but it is imprecise and requires meticulously clean, copper-free glassware.

Hemoglobin Standard Curve

A standard curve must be set up before testing patient specimens. Cyanmethemoglobin standard, available commercially, is used for this purpose. The cyanmethemoglobin standard is the only commercially available *standard* used in routine hematology; all other products for quality control maintenance are known as *controls* (Chap. 47).

The curve is set up by diluting Cyanmethemoglobin Certified Standard with cyanmethemoglobin reagent and measuring the absorbance of each dilution at 540 nm.

STANDARD CURVE PREPARATION
Procedure

1. For instruments that require cuvette volumes of 5.0 mL or less, make dilutions to achieve certain concentrations (Table 9-2). The amount of dilution will depend on the concentration of the standard and the total volume required by the cuvette. For further information on setting up standard curve dilutions, see standard package insert.
2. Transfer these solutions to matched cuvettes and read absorbance of each dilution against the blank on a spectrophotometer at 540 nm. Use same instrument and wavelength for standards and unknowns.
3. On linear graph paper plot absorbance of each standard against its concentration. Alternatively, on Semilogarithmic paper, plot %T against concentration (Fig. 9-1). This curve may be used to read Hb concentration of controls and unknowns.

Comments

1. Set up a new standard curve with each new lot of reagent prepared. Note that "curve" should be linear.
2. It is recommended that the standard curve be checked whenever repairs, relocations, or other alterations are made in the instrument (*e.g.*, whenever bulb is changed).[15]

CYANMETHEMOGLOBIN METHOD
FOR HEMOGLOBIN DETERMINATION
Principle

In the cyanmethemoglobin method whole blood is mixed with potassium ferricyanide and potassium cyanide to convert Hb to cyanmethemoglobin, which is very stable. The reaction is

$$Hb(Fe^{++}) \xrightarrow{K_3Fe(CN)_6} Methemoglobin(Fe^{+++}) \xrightarrow{KCN} cyanmethemoglobin$$

The absorbance of the solution is directly proportional to the amount of Hb present. All forms of Hb except sulfhemoglobin are measured completely.

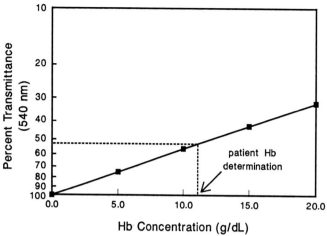

FIG. 9-1. Cyanmethemoglobin standard curve developed on the basis of the following percent transmission (T) readings obtained after preparing the hemoglobin concentrations as illustrated in Table 9-2: 0 g/dL = 100% T, 5 g/dL = 75% T, 10 g/dL = 56% T, 15 g/dL = 42.5% T, 20 g/dL = 32% T. This curve is presented for illustrative purposes only; every laboratory should develop its own standard curve using its own reagents and equipment. With the aid of the curve developed specifically for any given laboratory, any patient's hemoglobin concentration can be determined manually by finding the sample percent T on the y axis and then point of intersection with the x axis along the standard curve. For example, using this graph, if a patient's sample gave a T of 52%, the hemoglobin concentration (using these reagents and equipment) would be approximately 11 g/dL.

Specimen Requirements
Either venous blood collected with EDTA or capillary blood may be used.

Reagents
Cyanmethemoglobin reagent is available commercially as modified Drabkin's solution.

Quality Control
Commercial controls are available to determine accuracy of equipment and procedure. Proficiency testing also serves as a check (Chap. 47). A control should be run with each batch of specimens.

Procedure
1. Using Sahli or disposable "to contain" pipets, make a 1:301 dilution by adding 0.02 mL (20 μL) of venous or capillary blood to 6.0 mL of cyanmethemoglobin reagent and rinse pipet in specimen mixture several times to ensure accurate dilution. Cover and invert the tube to mix. Let stand for 10 minutes to allow full conversion to cyanmethemoglobin.
2. Set spectrophotometer wavelength to 540 nm. Blank spectrophotometer with Drabkin's reagent in one of two matched cuvettes.
3. Read absorbance (A_u) of specimen on spectrophotometer using other matched cuvette. Alternatively, %T may be read using a colorimeter and a green filter (540 nm).
4. Convert reading into grams of Hb per dL (g/dL) using a standard curve set up with same equipment and reagents used for specimen or calculate specimen concentration (C_u) based on Beer's law as follows:[9]

$$C_u \text{ (g/dL)} = 301 \frac{(A_u \times C_s)}{A_s} \times \frac{1}{1000} = \frac{0.301 (A_u \times C_s)}{A_s}$$

TABLE 9-2. Dilutions and Resulting Concentrations for Cyanmethemoglobin Standard Curve*

Hemoglobin concentration (g/dL)	Blank	5	10	15	20
Cyanmethemoglobin standard (mL)	0.0	1.5	3.0	4.5	6.0
Cyanmethemoglobin reagent (mL)	6.0	4.5	3.0	1.5	0.0

* This is an example using a standard containing 80 mg/dL hemoglobin.

where A_u is the absorbance of the unknown, C_s is the concentration of the standard (usually 80 mg/dL) and A_s is the absorbance of the standard run most recently under the same conditions as the patient specimen.

SEMIAUTOMATED MEASUREMENT OF HEMOGLOBIN CONCENTRATION

The cyanmethemoglobin method is also employed when using semiautomated instruments such as the hemoglobinometer (Coulter Diagnostics, Hialeah, FL).

Procedure

1. Make a 1:501 dilution by adding 20 μL of blood to a 10-mL volumetric flask. Dilute to volume with isotonic saline.
2. Add three drops of lysing and hemoglobin reagent. This reagent contains a cationic surfactant (that lyses erythrocytes) and potassium ferricyanide, which converts Hb to cyanmethemoglobin. Invert tube to mix. Let stand for 2 minutes for complete chemical reaction.
3. Introduce dilution into instrument (instrument blanks itself). Instrument provides a direct readout of Hb in g/dL.

Comments

1. Readings of duplicate dilutions should agree within 0.2 g/dL.
2. Waste should be treated as any blood-contaminated product.

Hemoglobin Reference Ranges

Refer to Table 9-1 for reference ranges at various ages.

Comments and Sources of Technical Error in Hemoglobin Measurement

Sources of technical error include pipeting error; use of dirty, scratched, or unmatched cuvettes; and use of deteriorated reagents. All instruments and pipets must be properly standardized. Drabkin's reagent deteriorates on long exposure to light and must therefore be kept in a dark cabinet, a container covered with foil, or a dark bottle. The reagent should be tightly capped.

Drabkin's reagent contains cyanide and is considered dangerous; it must be used with caution. However, a lethal dose would require ingestion of 4 to 16 L of reagent. Because hydrogen cyanide gas is liberated on acidification of the reagent, samples and spent reagents should be discarded into running water in a sink (free of acids) followed by copious flushing with water.[9]

Comments and Sources of Physiologic Error in Hemoglobin Measurement

Several patient conditions can cause erroneous Hb values. Turbidity in the mixture will cause falsely elevated values. Turbidity may be the result of the following:

1. Lipemia. Correct by adding 0.02 mL of patient's plasma to 6.0 mL of cyanmethemoglobin reagent and use this mixture as a patient blank.
2. Extremely high leukocyte counts (greater than 30.0 × 10^9/L). Correct by centrifuging mixture and determining the Hb in supernatant fluid.
3. Hb S and Hb C. Turbidity is caused by relative resistance of cells containing these variants to hemolysis. It is corrected by diluting hemoglobin mixture 1:2 by taking one part of sample and mixing it with one part distilled water. The absorbance result must be multiplied by the dilution factor, which is 2.
4. Easily precipitated globulins (e.g., those found in Waldenstrom's macroglobulinemia or multiple myeloma). This was a problem in the past; however, because Drabkin's reagent has been modified to contain KH_2PO_4 salt, this problem is not likely to occur. Using original Drabkin's reagent, this problem was corrected by adding 0.1 g of potassium carbonate to 1 L of Drabkin's before use. This increased the alkalinity of the reagent, causing globulins to remain in solution and thus prevented interference with absorbance reading.

In heavy smokers carboxyhemoglobin may represent as much as 10% of the total Hb. Carboxyhemoglobin takes 1 hour to convert completely to cyanmethemoglobin. Readings taken at the usual 10-minute development time may be erroneous; however, the degree of error probably is not clinically significant.

CENTRIFUGED MICROHEMATOCRIT

The term "hematocrit" (HCT) actually refers to the instrument used to determine packed cell volume (PCV). However, HCT is commonly used synonymously with PCV to denote the percentage of erythrocytes in a known volume of whole blood.

When performed manually, HCT is usually determined using the microhematocrit method. Historically a macrohematocrit technique was used in which the HCT was determined by filling a Wintrobe tube (see Wintrobe ESR Method section; Fig. 9-9) with whole blood and centrifuging it for 30 minutes, after which the PCV was read from a scale on the tube. However, this method has been abandoned for the most part because of the large amount of time and specimen required. The method is also inaccurate because of the amount of plasma trapped by platelets and leukocytes, which is greater than that found in the microhematocrit technique. This chapter presents only the microhematocrit technique.

MICROHEMATOCRIT TECHNIQUE

Principle

A small amount of whole blood is centrifuged to determine maximum packing of erythrocytes, expressed as PCV or HCT.

Specimen Requirements

Whole blood anticoagulated with EDTA (2 mg/mL of blood) or heparin is acceptable. Capillary blood collected in heparinized capillary tubes may also be used. Note that if blood from a vacuum tube containing EDTA requires a manual HCT, nonanticoagulated capillary tubes must be used to avoid overanticoagulation of specimen.

Reagents and Equipment

1. Capillary hematocrit tubes containing heparin (for skin puncture collection) or plain (for blood already anticoagulated)
2. Nonabsorbent sealing clay
3. Microhematocrit reader device (Figs. 9-2 and 9-3)
4. Microhematocrit centrifuge capable of sustaining a relative centrifugal force (RCF) of 10,000 to 15,000 × g (number of times greater than gravity) without exceeding a temperature of 45°C. Calculation of RCF is explained in Appendix B. The calculation requires measurement of centrifuge rotating speed in revolutions per minute (rpm), which may be obtained using a tachometer. RCF calculation also requires the centrifuge rotating radius, which should be listed in manufacturer's instrument operation manual. Standard American microhematocrit centrifuges develop the required force when rotating at 10,000 to 12,000 rpm.

Quality Control

1. Accuracy and reproducibility of centrifuge timer should be checked periodically with a stopwatch.
2. RCF or rpm must be verified periodically using a calibrated tachometer.

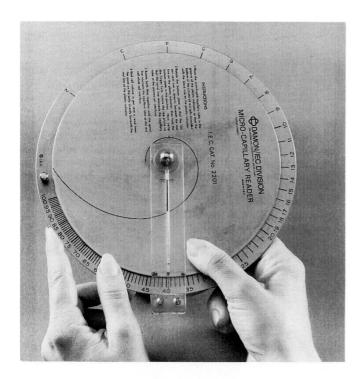

FIG. 9-2. Hematocrit sample prepared for reading on Micro-Capillary Reader. Hematocrit for this sample is 39.5% or 0.395 L/L. Caution: hematocrits may be misread by the untrained eye. Note that this value would mistakenly be read as 40.5% or 0.405 L/L if the scale were read in the wrong direction. The hematocrit numbers ascend from right to left.

3. Minimum time to achieve maximum cell packing should be determined for each instrument, both when it is new and on a periodic basis. This is determined as follows:
   A. Fill 10 to 14 microhematocrit tubes with EDTA-anticoagulated blood. Repeat this procedure for a second specimen. One of the two specimens should have an HCT greater than 0.50 L/L.
   B. Using two capillary tubes from each specimen, perform microhematocrits with a spin time of 2 minutes. Record results of all four tubes. Repeat this procedure a number of times, each time increasing spin time by 30 seconds. When HCT has remained at same value for two consecutive spins, minimum time for maximum packing has been determined.
   C. The second time interval where the HCT value has remained the same is the spin time used for all future specimens to ensure that enough time is allowed for optimal packing of RBCs. Specimens with HCTs greater than 0.50 L/L may take longer to pack; using the second time interval allows for this possibility without spinning any longer than necessary to obtain an accurate result on all specimens.[23]
4. Controls must be performed periodically at intervals specified by each laboratory. For example, a control sample may be run after every 20 specimens.
5. Centrifuge brushes should be checked and replaced whenever they are less than half their original size.
6. Centrifuge should be cleaned immediately if blood is spilled using an effective germicidal agent such as 5% bleach.

Procedure

1. Fill at least two capillary tubes approximately two-thirds full. If using tubes with a colored ring at one end, fill from opposite end.

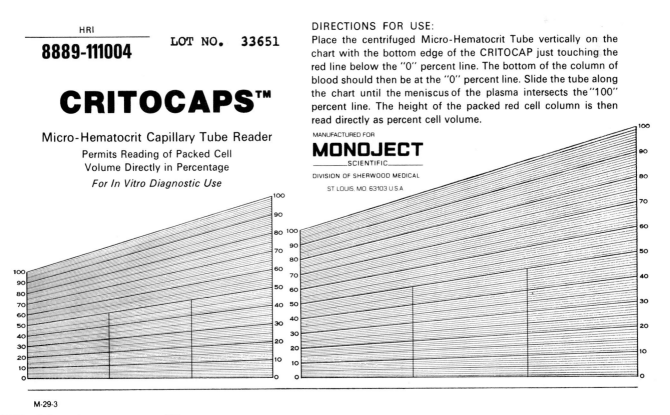

FIG. 9-3. The CRITOCAPS™ Micro-hematocrit Capillary Tube Reader provides an alternative to the Micro-Capillary Reader wheel. The lower RBC column in the tube is matched up with the 0 mark and the plasma meniscus is lined up with 100%. The hematocrit is then read at the top of the RBC column from the scale on either side.

2. Seal unfilled end (end with colored ring) with nonabsorbent material (*e.g.*, clay).

3. Place capillary tubes in opposite slots of microhematocrit centrifuge with their clay-filled ends against gasket. Be sure to note position number if spinning specimens from more than one patient.

4. Place head cover on centrifuge; tighten securely and close top. Centrifuge for 5 minutes or the minimum time determined for maximum cell packing on that centrifuge. Open lid, remove cover, and remove capillary tubes one at a time for reading HCT.

5. Using a microhematocrit reading device (see Figs. 9-2 and 9-3), determine HCT. Buffy coat (leukocytes and platelets) should *not* be included in the reading, which should be taken below the buffy coat.

8. Note presence of a buffy coat (Fig. 9-4) and plasma color (normal, icteric, lipemic, or hemolyzed) on patient requisition.

9. Results should agree within ± 0.02 L/L for the two patient samples run.

Microhematocrit Reference Ranges

Refer to Table 9-1 for ranges at various ages.[7]

Comments and Sources of Technical Error

The HCT may be falsely increased or decreased for many reasons relating to technical laboratory errors as outlined below.

1. Excess anticoagulant decreases HCT value because of shrinkage of erythrocytes.

2. Insufficient mixing of blood prior to obtaining HCT sample may decrease or increase HCT, depending on which part of specimen (plasma or cells) is drawn principally into microhematocrit tube.

3. Improper sealing of capillary tube decreases HCT because of leakage of specimen; erythrocyte loss is greater than plasma loss.

4. Inadequate centrifugation or allowing tubes to stand too long after centrifugation increases HCT. Results should be read within 10 minutes of centrifugation.

5. Including a large buffy coat in the reading increases HCT.

6. Improper use of HCT reader may increase or decrease HCT.

Comments and Sources of Physiologic Error

1. Trapped plasma may cause the HCT to be falsely increased by as much as 0.02 L/L. (Trapped plasma is the small amount of plasma that remains in the erythrocyte portion of the spun HCT even when proper centrifugation is used.) More plasma is trapped in sickle cell anemia, hypochromic anemia, spherocytosis, macrocytosis, and thalassemia. The amount of plasma trapped increases with the HCT. When determined by fully automated methods, the HCT may be 0.01 to 0.03 L/L lower than the microhematocrit method because it is electronically calculated and therefore is unaffected by trapped plasma.

2. Certain abnormal erythrocyte shapes (*e.g.*, spherocytes and sickle cells) inhibit complete packing.

3. Immediately after a blood loss, the HCT is not a reliable estimate of the degree of anemia because plasma volume is replaced faster than erythrocyte volume, causing a temporarily lower HCT.

4. Dehydration can falsely increase HCT because of fluid loss, which causes a decrease in plasma volume.

5. Specimen collection errors may alter HCT. Leaving the tourniquet on the arm too long causes hemoconcentration, which falsely increases HCT. Difficult venipuncture or skin puncture may introduce interstitial fluid to the sample, caus-

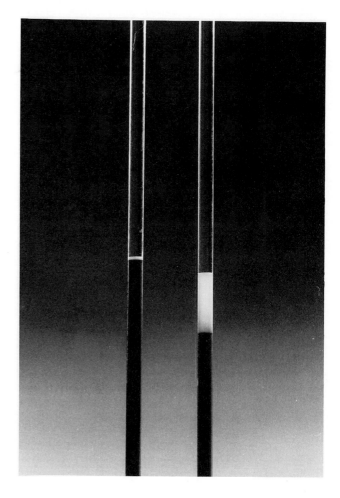

FIG. 9-4. Comparison of a small (left) and large (right) buffy coat in hematocrit samples from two patients. Large buffy coat results from increased WBC and platelet counts.

ing a falsely decreased HCT. Hemolysis also causes a false decrease in HCT.

AUTOMATED METHODS FOR ERYTHROCYTE, HEMOGLOBIN, AND HEMATOCRIT DETERMINATION

All of the erythrocyte measurements may be made using automated equipment. Refer to Chapter 43 for details.

CORRELATIONS AND CALCULATIONS BASED ON ERYTHROCYTE MEASUREMENTS

Rule of Three

Under ordinary circumstances, it is possible to check the accuracy of the erythrocyte count, Hb, and HCT values (manually or by automated instruments) by quick visual inspection of the values. This is accomplished by applying the "rule of three," as shown in Table 9-3. The rule of three

TABLE 9.3. The Rule of Three

BASIC EQUATIONS
$$3 \times RBC = Hb$$
$$3 \times Hb = HCT \pm 3\ (\%)$$

CASE A: ACCURATE SPECIMEN

Patient Results	Accuracy Check	Confirmation
RBC = 3.0×10^{12}/L	$3 \times 3.0 = 9.0$	RBC checks with Hb
Hb = 9.2 g/dL	$3 \times 9.2 = 27.6$	Hb checks with HCT (26 ± 3)
HCT = 26% (0.26 L/L)		

CASE B: INACCURATE SPECIMEN

Patient Results	Accuracy Check	Confirmation
RBC = 4.0×10^{12}/L	$3 \times 4.0 = 12.0$	RBC does not check with Hb
Hb = 3.5 g/dL	$3 \times 3.5 = 10.5$	Hb does not check with HCT (37 ± 3)
HCT = 37% (0.37 L/L)		

The most commonly used rule is $3 \times Hb = HCT \pm 3$. These rules apply only to red cells of normal size and color (normocytic, normochromic). The example in Case A shows specimen results that comply with the Rule of Three. In case B, applying the Rule of Three demonstrates an apparent problem with the Hb which appears too low. Problems such as a malfunctioning instrument reading device should be investigated. This Hb value should not be reported until the problem is resolved, and the Hb measurement should be performed again when the instrument is back in control. See text for more details.

applies only to normocytic, normochromic erythrocytes, which can be verified by visual inspection of the blood film. If the erythrocytes are found to be abnormal, the automated values cannot be expected to conform to these rules. On the other hand, if the erythrocytes on the blood film appear normal but the automated values do not conform to the rule of three, laboratory personnel should check to ensure that a random error has not occurred (Chap. 48). Random error is an error that occurs by chance. An example is sample or blood film misidentification. The possibility of a systematic error should also be considered. Such errors affect all samples equally in a proportionate or constant manner and often involve an instrument malfunction (Chap. 47).

Table 9-3 provides an example of two blood counts. In case A the assay conforms to the rule of three. In case B there appears to be a problem with the Hb: it is unrealistically low because it does not conform to the rules of matching with the erythrocyte count or HCT. In this case, because the problem seems to be isolated with the Hb and the error seems so great, a systematic error should be considered. Reports from specimens run before and after this one should also be checked to see if the Hb was unrealistically low compared with the erythrocyte count and HCT. Problems such as a malfunctioning Hb reading device should be investigated. A control blood sample could also be run at this time if no instrument malfunction can be detected to ensure that the Hb procedure is in control.

Consider an automated report in which the Hb appears to be too high when compared with the erythrocyte count and HCT. If erythrocyte morphology appears normal and the Hb was valid on the samples run before and after this specimen, a common problem to consider is a markedly elevated leukocyte count. In such cases the Hb concentra-

tion must be obtained manually to avoid interference by the leukocytes with the spectrophotometric reading of Hb concentration.

Whenever the rule of three indicates a problem with any specimen, a systematic approach to investigation of the discrepancy must be undertaken until the nature of the problem is determined. If necessary, corrective action should be taken, whether it involves the specimen or the instrument.

Erythrocyte Indices

In addition to serving as quality control checks on one another, the erythrocyte count, Hb, and HCT can be utilized in calculations to determine the erythrocyte indices: mean corpuscular volume (MCV), mean corpuscular Hb (MCH), and mean corpuscular Hb concentration (MCHC). The indices are used both in quality control (Chap. 47) and in classifying and differentiating anemias (Chap. 10). The diagnostic interpretation of the indices should always be combined with a careful examination of the blood film because indices are *average* values for many cells examined either manually or electronically.

MEAN CORPUSCULAR VOLUME

MCV indicates the average volume of a single erythrocyte in a given blood sample. It is expressed in SI units (see below) as femtoliters (fL; $1\ fL = 10^{-15}\ L$). Formerly, MCV was expressed in μm^3 (see Table 9-6).

Calculation and Reference Ranges

$$MCV = \frac{HCT(\%) \times 10}{RBC\ (10^{12}/L)}$$

For example, if HCT equals 36% (0.36 L/L) and RBC equals 4.0×10^{12}/L, then

$$MCV = \frac{36 \times 10}{4.0} = 90\ fL$$

Refer to Table 9-1 for reference ranges at various ages.[7]

Terminology

Values of 80 to 100 fL are described as normocytic, those of <80 as microcytic, and those >100 as macrocytic.

Interpretation

MCV will be discussed in relation to all anemias and hematologic disorders in appropriate chapters in this text. In general MCV is increased in megaloblastic anemias such as folate or vitamin B_{12} deficiencies. It may also be elevated in nonmegaloblastic macrocytic anemias, which are sometimes caused by chronic hemolytic anemias, liver disease, and hypothyroidism. A decreased MCV is associated with such conditions as iron deficiency, defective iron utilization (chronic disease), and thalassemia.

Comments and Sources of Error

Because the MCV is, as it says, a mean or average value for many cells examined, a dimorphic population of microcytes and macrocytes, which may be observed on a peripheral blood film, yields an average normal calculated MCV value. This normal MCV is misleading without the blood film comments. An increased number of reticulocytes, which are larger in volume, may elevate the MCV. However, if the patient's normal MCV is at the low end of the reference range, the elevation may not be significant enough to put the MCV above the reference range.

MEAN CORPUSCULAR HEMOGLOBIN

MCH indicates the average weight of Hb per erythrocyte, expressed in SI units as picograms (pg; 1 pg = 10^{-12} g). Formerly, MCH was expressed in $\mu\mu$g (see Table 9-6).

Calculation and Reference Ranges

$$MCH = \frac{Hb\ (g/dL) \times 10}{RBC\ (10^{12}/L)}$$

For example, if Hb equals 12.0 g/dL and RBC equals 4.0 × 10^{12}/L, then

$$MCH = \frac{12.0 \times 10}{4.0} = 30\ pg$$

Refer to Table 9-1 for reference ranges at various ages.[7]

Terminology

Values of 26 to 34 pg are considered normal, those <26 decreased, and those >34 increased.

Interpretation

MCH should correlate with the MCV and MCHC. There is a higher MCH in macrocytic anemias because the erythrocytes are larger and carry more Hb. A lower MCH is found in hypochromic anemias and in microcytic anemias unless the erythrocytes are also spherocytic.

Comments

When describing anemias, MCH is rarely used; the MCV and MCHC are more commonly used.

MEAN CORPUSCULAR HEMOGLOBIN CONCENTRATION

MCHC indicates the average concentration of Hb in the erythrocytes of any specimen. It is expressed in SI units as g/dL. Formerly, MCHC was expressed in percent (see Table 9-6).

Calculation and Reference Ranges

$$MCHC = \frac{Hb\ (g/dL)}{HCT\%} \times 100$$

For example, if Hb equals 12.0 g/dL and HCT equals 36% (0.36 L/L), then

$$MCHC = \frac{12.0 \times 100}{36} = 33.3\ g/dL$$

Refer to Table 9-1 for reference ranges at various ages.[7]

Terminology

Values of 31 to 37 g/dL are considered normochromic, those <31 are hypochromic, and those >37 are hyperchromic.

Interpretation

Hypochromic erythrocytes occur commonly in iron deficiency, thalassemias, and defective iron utilization.

Hyperchromic erythrocytes are actually caused by a shape change such as that found in spherocytes. "Hyperchromia" is not used in actual descriptions of erythrocyte morphology in the laboratory (Chap. 8). Erythrocytes cannot accommodate more Hb than 37 g/dL; therefore, a result above 37 g/dL should be recalculated, ensuring that all values were correctly measured and no interfering substances are present (see Sources of Error in Hb and HCT Determinations).

Problem Solving for Erythrocyte Indices

To obtain accurate erythrocyte indices, the values used in the calculations must be accurate. All of the fully automated cell counters either calculate indices automatically or measure the MCV directly and calculate the HCT and other indices. The erythrocyte count may be falsely decreased in the presence of strong cold agglutinins (Chap. 19), thus falsely elevating the MCV and also causing an abnormal MCH and MCHC. This problem may be eliminated by warming the specimen just before running it on an automated counter.

RETICULOCYTE COUNTS

A reticulocyte is an immature erythrocyte that has lost its nucleus but retains aggregates of ribonucleic acid (RNA) within its ribosomes (Chap. 6). The amount of RNA decreases as the erythrocyte matures. After the normoblast loses its nucleus, the reticulocyte usually remains 2 days in the bone marrow and 1 day in the peripheral blood before becoming a mature erythrocyte. The reticulocyte count, with its associated corrections, can be used to assess bone marrow erythropoietic activity.

ROUTINE RETICULOCYTE COUNT
Principle

The ribosomal RNA of reticulocytes must be stained supravitally; that is, with the erythrocytes in the living state. A reticulocyte (Fig. 9-5) is defined as any nonnucleated erythrocyte that contains two or more particles of blue-stained, granulofilamentous material after new methylene blue (supravital) staining.[19]

Specimen Requirements

Whole blood anticoagulated with EDTA is recommended, but any common anticoagulant may be used. Capillary blood is also acceptable.

Reagents and Equipment

No special equipment is required, but enumeration may be facilitated by use of a calibrated disk placed in the ocular of the microscope (see procedure below).

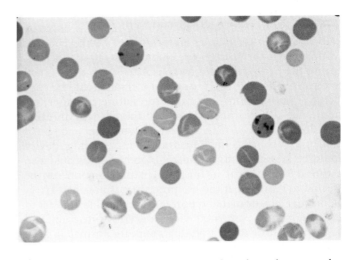

FIG. 9-5. Reticulocytes are nonnucleated erythrocytes that contain two or more particles of blue-stained, granulofilamentous material after new methylene blue (supravital) staining.

Supravital stains in common use include new methylene blue and brilliant cresyl blue. New methylene blue is recommended by the NCCLS.[22] The stain should be filtered before use.

Quality Control

There is no adequate method of quality control for reticulocyte counts. There are four important reasons for discrepancies in reticulocyte counting: (1) interobserver variation in the definition of a reticulocyte (at least two ribosomal remnants should be seen); (2) size of sample evaluated (at least 1000 erythrocytes should be examined); (3) type of film examined (wedge versus spun); and (4) lack of standardized area if a calibrated disk is not used. Until uniformity of these variables can be achieved, there are several ways to increase the accuracy of reticulocyte counts. One technologist can count 500 cells on each of two slides, or two technologists can each count 500 or 1000 cells independently. Precision limits between slides should be established. It has been suggested that results obtained by two technologists should agree within ± 20%.[4]

On high reticulocyte counts the percentage of reticulocytes should correlate roughly with the number of polychromatophilic erythrocytes seen on the peripheral blood film. The higher the reticulocyte count, the less error is involved in the procedure.

Procedure and Calculations

Specimen Preparation

1. Mix equal amounts of whole blood and stain in a small tube.
2. Incubate mixture at room temperature. NOTE: Although many references state that the mixture should incubate for no less than 10 minutes[4] to as much as 15 minutes,[3] a recent report notes that staining is rapid and need not be done for more than 2 minutes.[19]
3. After incubation, thoroughly mix the blood and stain solution and immediately prepare two or three films. Allow films to air dry.

Reticulocyte Counting

There are several methods of counting reticulocytes.[4] The methods presented here are the routine light microscope method and the calibrated Miller disk method.

Routine Light Microscope Method

1. Switch to 100× oil immersion objective (oculars should be standard 10×).
2. Select an area where erythrocytes are close but not overlapping and reticulocytes appear to be well stained.
3. Count the reticulocytes and erythrocytes in each field using the same pattern normally used for performing a leukocyte differential count (Chap. 25). Reticulocytes should also be counted as erythrocytes.
4. Continue counting until 1000 erythrocytes have been observed.
5. Calculate reticulocytes using this formula:

$$\text{Retic (\%)} = \frac{\text{\# of Retics}}{1000 \text{ RBC observed}} \times 100$$

For example, if 10 reticulocytes were seen among 1000 RBCs, the reticulocyte percentage would be calculated as:

$$\text{Retic (\%)} = \frac{10}{1000} \times 100 = 1.0\%$$

Calibrated Miller Disk Method

A calibrated Miller disk may be placed in one microscope ocular to aid in the counting process. The Miller disk appears in

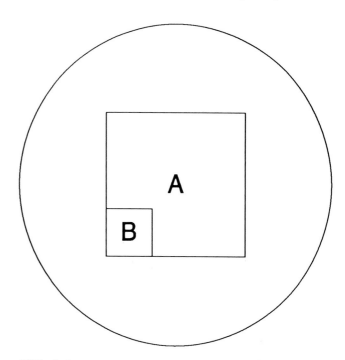

FIG. 9-6. Miller disk for microscopic reticulocyte counting.

the field of view with two squares, one inside the other (Fig. 9-6), the smaller square (B) being one-ninth the size of the larger square (A).

1. Place calibrated Miller disk in one ocular. Locate an acceptable area to begin count, as in standard reticulocyte count method.
2. Count the erythrocytes in square B and the reticulocytes in square A in successive fields on the film until 500 erythrocytes have been counted. A reticulocyte in square B is counted as both an erythrocyte and a reticulocyte. At this point, theoretically, the number of reticulocytes in 4500 erythrocytes has been counted.
3. Compute reticulocyte count as:

$$\text{Retic (\%)} = \frac{\text{Total retics in square A}}{\text{Total RBCs in square B} \times 9} \times 100$$

For example, if five successive fields were examined, and a total of 150 reticulocytes was seen in square A after counting 500 RBCs in the five observations of square B, the reticulocyte (%) would be calculated as:

$$\text{Retic (\%)} = \frac{150}{500 \times 9} \times 100 = 3.3\%$$

Any calibrated disk may be used in the same manner by determining the areas of the large and small squares.

Reticulocyte Reference Ranges

Reticulocyte counts are expressed as a percentage, as shown in the calculations above, or in absolute numbers per liter. The reference range for adults in some laboratories is 0.5% to 1.5%, whereas in others, a broader range of 0.5% to 2.0% is used. The range may be slightly higher in women[8] and persons living at an altitude higher than 6000 feet above sea level.[22] It is higher in newborns (2.0%–6.0%) but drops to adult levels in 1 to 2 weeks.[21] In absolute numbers the reference value is approximately 50×10^9/L.[22]

Comments and Sources of Technical Error

1. The use of a counterstain with Romanowsky dyes is no longer advised because it may obscure the supravitally stained granulofilamentous material of the reticulocyte.[22]
2. Refractive artifacts in erythrocytes caused by moisture in the air and poor drying of the blood film must not be confused with RNA filaments, which do not appear refractory when adjusting the fine focus on the microscope. The RNA filaments simply disappear when out of focus.
3. Blood and stain must be well mixed before making films because reticulocytes have a lower specific gravity than mature erythrocytes and thus settle at the top of the mixture during incubation.
4. Increased levels of glucose in the blood may inhibit staining of reticulocytes.[4]
5. Pappenheimer, Howell-Jolly, and Heinz bodies will also stain supravitally. (See Figs. 8-28 and 8-29 for a summary of the differentiating factors among and between these inclusions and those of the reticulocyte.) If Pappenheimer or Howell-Jolly bodies are suspected, examination of the Romanowsky-stained peripheral blood film will confirm their presence, because these inclusions will stain, whereas reticulocyte granulofilamentous material will not. Pappenheimer bodies must also be confirmed by an iron stain. Heinz bodies do not stain with Romanowsky stain. However, on supravitally stained films, they may be differentiated from reticulocytes because they usually cling to the erythrocyte membrane and are usually larger than ribosomal RNA. Heinz bodies often make the cell look like a pitted golf ball (see Figs. 8-28 and 17-10).

Comments and Sources of Physiologic Error

The reticulocyte percentage may be misleading if one does not consider the degree of anemia or of intense erythropoietic stimulation. The reticulocyte count may be truly elevated, indicating increased effective erythropoiesis, or it may only appear elevated because the total number of erythrocytes is decreased. Therefore, reticulocyte counts should be corrected for anemia. Several corrections may be made to this percentage taking into consideration total erythrocyte count, HCT, and early release of reticulocytes from the bone marrow. These corrections are considered below.

ABSOLUTE RETICULOCYTE COUNT
Principle
The absolute reticulocyte count (ARC) reflects the actual number of reticulocytes in one liter of whole blood. The value is not commonly used in the clinical laboratory.

Calculation and Reference Range

$$ARC = \frac{Reticulocytes\ (\%)}{100} \times \frac{red\ cell}{count}\ (\times 10^{12}/L) \times 1000$$

For example, if a patient's reticulocyte count is 4% and the RBC count is $3.30 \times 10^{12}/L$, the ARC would be:

$$ARC = \frac{(4) \times (3.30 \times 10^{12}/L)}{100} \times 1000 = 132 \times 10^9/L$$

Values between 25 and $75 \times 10^9/L$ are considered to fall within the reference range.[19]

CORRECTED RETICULOCYTE COUNT
The corrected reticulocyte count (CRC) is sometimes referred to as a reticulocyte index (RI) or hematocrit correction.

Principle
The percentage of reticulocytes may appear increased because of early reticulocyte release into the circulation or because of a decrease in the number of mature cells in circulation. The CRC corrects the observed reticulocyte count to a normal HCT of 0.45 L/L to allow correction for the degree of patient anemia.

Calculation

$$CRC = Reticulocytes\ (\%) \times \frac{HCT\ (L/L)}{0.45\ L/L}$$

For example, if a patient's reticulocyte count is 4.5% and the HCT is 0.30 L/L, the CRC would be:

$$CRC = 4.5 \times \frac{0.30}{0.45} = 3.0\%$$

Reference Range
The expected value of CRC depends on the degree of anemia. Normally, CRC should be approximately 1%. Patients with an HCT of 0.35 L/L are expected to have a CRC of 2% to 3%; those at or below 0.25 L/L, CRC should increase to 3% to 5%.

Comments
CRC is most often used as part of the reticulocyte production index (RPI) calculation (discussed below). RPI is clinically more useful than CRC.

RETICULOCYTE PRODUCTION INDEX
RPI (also known as shift correction) provides a further refinement of the CRC. It is a general indicator of the rate of erythrocyte production increase above normal in anemias.

Principle
During intense erythropoietic stress the maturation time in the bone marrow may be shortened from the usual 3.5 days to as little as 1 day, allowing the reticulocytes to circulate longer than usual in the peripheral blood (Fig. 9-7). Cells released early to the peripheral blood are referred to as shift cells and have a polychromatophilic appearance (see Plate 2).

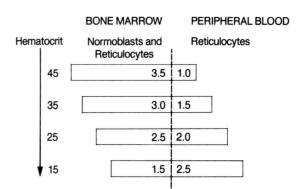

FIG. 9-7. Correlation of hematocrit with marrow and blood reticulocyte maturation times. Ordinarily, erythropoietin increases in proportion to the degree of anemia present. With increasing erythropoietin stimulation, the maturation time of the erythroid marrow normoblasts and marrow reticulocytes shortens progressively from a normal of 3.5 days to as little as 1.5 to 1.0 day. Much of this shortening is secondary to a shift of marrow reticulocytes into the circulation. This results in a prolongation of the maturation time of circulating blood reticulocytes from a normal of 1 day to as much as 2.5 to 3.0 days with severe anemia. This needs to be taken into account when calculating the reticulocyte production index. The maturation time values shown for the blood reticulocytes can be used as a correction factor in this calculation (see text). (From Hillman RS, Finch CA: Red Cell Manual. Philadelphia, FA Davis, 1985, with permission.)

Under such intense erythropoietic stress the number of reticulocytes in the peripheral blood may be markedly increased without a corresponding increase in the bone marrow. Because the life span of the reticulocyte in the peripheral blood corresponds to the degree of anemia, the RPI is corrected for both the HCT and maturation time in the peripheral blood.

Calculation

$$RPI = \frac{Retic\ (\%) \times \dfrac{HCT\ (L/L)}{0.45\ L/L}}{Maturation\ time\ in\ peripheral\ blood}$$

or

$$RPI = \frac{CRC}{Maturation\ time\ in\ peripheral\ blood}$$

The approximate maturation time varies with HCT as follows (see Fig. 9-7), and these figures are to be used in RPI calculation:[14]

HCT (L/L)	MATURATION TIME (DAYS)
0.45 ± 0.05	1.0
0.35 ± 0.05	1.5
0.25 ± 0.05	2.0
0.15 ± 0.05	2.5

For example, if a patient has a reticulocyte count of 5.0% and an HCT of 0.28 L/L, the maturation time correction factor is 2.0. The RPI calculation is:

$$RPI = \frac{5.0 \times \dfrac{0.28}{0.45}}{2.0} = 1.6$$

This RPI indicates that erythrocyte production is increased to 1.6 times the normal level, which is not an effective erythropoietic response to this degree of anemia (see below).

Reference Range

The reference range for the RPI is 1 when the hematocrit is 0.45 L/L (which is in the reference range) because the normal maturation time of reticulocytes in the peripheral blood is 1 day.[19] Guidelines have been set to interpret the RPI. An RPI greater than three generally indicates an adequate bone marrow response to anemia, whereas an RPI less than two represents an inadequate response.[13,19] An elevated RPI is associated with chronic hemolysis, recent hemorrhage, and response to therapy. A decreased RPI may be found in bone marrow failure (*e.g.*, aplastic anemia) and in ineffective erythropoiesis (*e.g.*, vitamin B_{12} or folate deficiency) causing megaloblastic anemia.

The RPI will be addressed in each chapter on the various anemias.

Problem Solving in Reticulocyte Count Corrections

To illustrate the utility of reticulocyte corrections, consider the example in Table 9-4. At first glance the 4.0% uncorrected reticulocyte count seems to indicate an adequate marrow response, but after appropriate corrections, the RPI of 0.64 indicates that there is an inadequate response for the degree of anemia.

Comments

There are several other methods of reticulocyte counting, some of which involve automated instruments that identify reticulocytes utilizing pattern recognition.[12,27] Pattern recognition instruments are not available for purchase at this time; however, many of these instruments are still in use in the United States. Flow cytometry, combined with fluorescent staining techniques, increases the possibility of a more accurate assessment of effective erythrocyte production.[28–30] These methods count large numbers of cells, reducing statistical error, and are capable of assessing the degree of maturation of the reticulocyte population. Both pattern recognition and flow cytometry have been found to be acceptable alternatives to manual reticulocyte counts.[12] (The reader is referred to Chapter 10 for further discussion of reticulocytes and RPI in anemia.)

ERYTHROCYTE SEDIMENTATION RATE

Two principal methods have been used for the ESR: the Westergren and the Wintrobe methods. The Westergren method is recommended by the NCCLS.[26] Both will be discussed below, as will a disposable ESR method that has gained popularity but may be slightly more expensive. The zeta sedimentation ratio (ZSR) for ESR determination will also be discussed.

ESR
Principle

The ESR is a measure of the degree of settling of erythrocytes in plasma in an anticoagulated whole-blood specimen during a specified period of time. Erythrocyte rouleaux formation is enhanced by increased concentrations of fibrinogen or of alpha or beta globulins, all of which increase the ESR. ESR is directly proportional to red cell mass and inversely proportional to plasma viscosity. Normally erythrocytes settle slowly because of a small red cell mass and because normal red cells do not form rouleaux.

TABLE 9-4. Sample Calculations of Absolute Reticulocyte Count, Corrected Reticulocyte Count, and Reticulocyte Production Index from Sample Patient Results

	CALCULATION/RESULT	COMMENTS
Patient RBC	$2.1 \times 10^{12}/L$	Anemic
HCT	0.18 L/L	Anemic
Reticulocyte	4.0%	Increased
ARC	$\dfrac{(4.0 \times 2.1 \times 10^{12}/L)}{100} \times 1000 = 84.0 \times 10^9/L$	Inadequate for 0.18 L/L HCT
CRC	$\dfrac{4.0 \times 0.18}{0.45} = 1.6\%$	Inadequate for 0.18 L/L HCT
RPI	$\dfrac{4.0 \times \left(\dfrac{0.18}{0.45}\right)}{2.5} = 0.64$	Inadequate for 0.18 L/L HCT

Specimen Requirements

Whole blood anticoagulated with EDTA drawn atraumatically within no more than 30 seconds is the recommended specimen for performance of the modified Westergren method,[26] as EDTA blood is readily available in most laboratories. Some laboratories prefer the original Westergren method, which calls for drawing blood into 3.8% sodium citrate as the anticoagulant. A special vacuum collection tube is available that allows for the automatic collection of four parts blood into one part 3.8% sodium citrate.

No matter which anticoagulant is used, the specimen must be mixed immediately after drawing. Blood kept at room temperature must be set up within 2 hours; at 4°C specimens have been reported by one source to be stable for 6 hours[17] and by another, up to 12 hours.[10] In any case a specimen should be brought to room temperature before testing.

WESTERGREN ESR METHOD

The Westergren pipet, as specified by the NCCLS,[26] must be made of thick-walled glass or hard plastic with an overall length of 300 mm ± 0.5 mm, length of blood column of 200 mm, external diameter of 5.5 ± 0.5 mm, tube bore of 2.65 ± 0.15 mm, and uniformity of tube bore of ±0.05 mm. Markings on the tube should extend over the lower 200 ± 0.35 mm of the pipet, numbered from 0 at the top of the scale to at least 180, no less than 20 mm from the lower end of the pipet, in increments of 10 mm or less.

The rack to hold the Westergren tubes must not allow leakage from the pipets and must be held motionless in a vertical position. Racks equipped with a leveling bubble ensure this vertical position to within ± 2°.

Quality Control

A reference ESR method involves adjusting the hematocrit of a specimen to 0.35 L/L by adding or removing autologous plasma. It is recommended that on a daily basis (if ESRs are run daily) each laboratory select a specimen to perform simultaneously the reference ESR and the procedure routinely used in the laboratory on the specimen with the adjusted hematocrit. Further discussion may be found in the NCCLS ESR reference procedure.[26] It explains how to convert the reference ESR reading to the equivalent routine method reading and how to compare the converted reading with the results obtained on the specimen tested using the routine method to ensure accurate results.

Procedure

The original and modified Westergren methods differ only in the anticoagulant used and the time at which the blood is diluted; both methods will be discussed in this section.

1. Specimen Preparation
   A. Original Westergren Method. Whole blood is drawn into 3.8% sodium citrate (one volume of sodium citrate to four volumes of blood) using a specially prepared vacuum collection tube (also available commercially). No further dilution is performed when using this type of specimen.
   B. Modified Westergren Method. Combine 2.0 mL of well mixed EDTA-anticoagulated whole blood with 0.5 mL of 0.85% NaCl or 0.5 mL 3.8% sodium citrate. This method is much more convenient in most laboratories, because EDTA-anticoagulated blood is readily available.
2. Place blood containers in pipet rack directly under each hole. Insert a Westergren pipet through each hole into the blood mixture.
3. Firmly press a safety bulb or hand pump on top of the Westergren pipet and watch the blood being aspirated to the "0" mark. If using a plugged pipet (Ulster Scientific, High-

land, NY), the plug should be well soaked with blood. Repeat for all specimens to be tested.
4. After exactly 60 minutes, record the distance, in millimeters, from the bottom of plasma meniscus (at 0 mark) to the top of the column of sedimented erythrocytes. Do not include the buffy coat (leukocytes and platelets) in the reading.
5. Report results as "ESR (Westergren, 1 hour) = _____mm." Note that this test does not measure a rate (i.e., distance per time interval (mm/h). Rather, it measures distance after a specified time.[26]
6. Dispose of all Westergren tubes containing blood carefully in biohazardous puncture-proof waste containers.

Disposable Westergren ESR System

A completely disposable system is available for performing ESRs (Ulster Scientific, Highland, New York) (Fig. 9-8). The disposable Westergren tube, referred to as a Dispette, has a safety plug made of nonwettable, and therefore nonabsorbent, material that provides automatic zeroing (at the 0-mm mark) of the specimen, as any excess blood adheres to the plug, which also holds the column of blood in place. The procedure for this system is shown in Figure 9-8.

Westergren ESR Reference Range

Each laboratory should establish its own Westergren ESR reference range. Approximate values are as follows (1 h = 1 hour):

Males[1]	< 50 years	1 h = 0–15 mm
	> 50 years	1 h = 0–20 mm
Females[1]	< 50 years	1 h = 0–20 mm
	> 50 years	1 h = 0–30 mm
Children[31]		1 h = 0–10 mm

Among people older than 65 years, the reference range may be even higher; the reason is not apparent.[2,11]

WINTROBE ESR METHOD
Specimen Requirements

Whole blood anticoagulated with EDTA or ammonium–potassium oxalate is used.

Equipment

The Wintrobe tube (Fig. 9-9) is 115 mm long with an internal bore of 3 mm. It has two series of graduations from 0 to 100, one ascending and one descending. For the sedimentation rate, the scale on the left side of the tube is used (0 is at the top). The scale on the right (100 at the top) was historically used to read a macrohematocrit, which is no longer considered a valuable test.

The rack that holds the Wintrobe tubes must be level and in an area free from vibration, direct sunlight, or drafts.

General Procedure

1. Fill a Wintrobe tube to 0 mark using a Pasteur pipet with a 15-cm stem. The column of blood must be bubble free.
2. Place tube in the rack and set timer for 60 minutes.
3. After 60 minutes read the level of sedimented erythrocytes from the scale on the left side of tube and record as ESR (Wintrobe, 1 hour) = _____mm.

Wintrobe ESR Reference Range

The range for males is 1 hour equals 0 to 9 mm; that for females is 1 hour equals 0 to 20 mm. The range for children is 1 hour equals 0 to 13 mm.[32]

Comments and Sources of Error

1. ESR is considered a nonspecific indicator of tissue damage, and it is increased in a number of disorders. Some of the more significant conditions are listed in Table 9-5.
2. Because the ESR depends on the ability of erythrocytes to form rouleaux, conditions in which rouleaux formation is

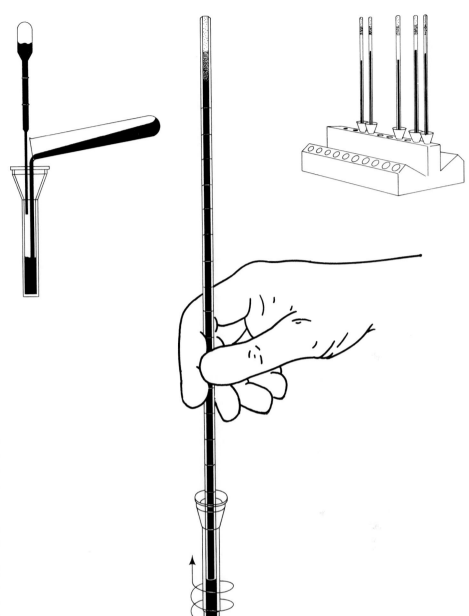

FIG. 9-8. Westergren Dispette System for erythrocyte sedimentation rate (ESR) determination. (Left) After mixing 4 parts EDTA-anticoagulated whole blood with 1 part 0.85% saline, mixture is poured into vial. (Center) Dispette is placed in vial using a twisting motion until blood reaches bottom of safety autozeroing plug. (Right) Vial and Dispette are placed vertically in a special rack for 60 minutes before reading the ESR. (Courtesy of Ulster Scientific, Inc., Highland, NY)

inhibited, such as sickle cell anemia, Hb CC, and spherocytosis, may be accompanied by normal sedimentation rates (*i.e.*, the ESR will not be as elevated as expected for the degree of anemia in these specimens).

3. Leaving the specimen for more than 2 hours at room temperature will cause erythrocytes to become spherical and inhibit rouleaux formation.

4. Overanticoagulation causes lower values.

5. Even slight tilting of the tube increases the ESR.

6. If area of RBC–plasma separation is hazy, read the level where the full RBC density is apparent.

7. Marked changes in room temperature will increase (in high temperatures) or decrease (in low temperatures) the ESR.

8. The presence of anemia invalidates the ESR as a tool to detect rouleaux (as an indication of some disease process).

Zeta Sedimentation Ratio

A ZSR test is performed using a Zetafuge (Coulter Diagnostics, Inc., Hialeah, FL) and special capillary tubes. The Zetafuge applies controlled centrifugation to blood, producing alternating compaction and dispersion of erythrocytes to measure how closely the erythrocytes approach one another under a specific, standardized gravitational force. As in the other sedimentation procedures, the ZSR result is dependent on the concentration of fibrinogen and gamma globulins.

ZSR METHOD
Specimen Requirements
EDTA-anticoagulated venous or capillary blood is required.

Equipment
Zetafuge and special capillary tubes, 75 mm long, outer diameter 2.3 mm, inner diameter 2.0 mm, are needed.

General Procedure
1. Place well mixed specimen in a Zetafuge capillary tube. Plug end of tube with clay, and place tubes vertically in Zetafuge,

TABLE 9-5. Expected ESR in Various Conditions

CONDITION	COMMENTS
ESR INCREASED	
Inflammatory conditions	Associated with elevated plasma proteins, in particular, fibrinogen and alpha and beta globulins
Acute and chronic infections	
Rheumatic fever	
Rheumatoid arthritis	
Myocardial infarction	
Nephrosis	
Tuberculosis	
Multiple myeloma	
Waldenstrom's macroglobulinemia	
Subacute bacterial endocarditis	
Hepatitis	
Menstruation	
Pregnancy	After the third month
ESR NORMAL	
Polycythemia	
Spherocytes	When large numbers present in peripheral blood
Sickle cells	When large numbers present in peripheral blood
Sickle cell anemia	
Hemoglobin CC disease	
Hereditary spherocytosis	

assuring that they are balanced, and allow them to spin for 4 minutes.

2. Read zetacrit percent at "knee" of curve that forms as a result of centrifugation (Fig. 9-10). An HCT reader is acceptable for this determination.

Calculation and Reference Range

The zetacrit represents the percentage of sedimented erythrocytes. This value is compared with the patient's HCT to obtain the ZSR.

$$ZSR(\%) = \frac{HCT(\%)}{Zetacrit(\%)} \times 100$$

For example, given that HCT equals 45% (0.45 L/L) and zetacrit equals 87%, the ZSR equals 52%.

The reference range for males and females is 40% to 51%. Values of 51% to 54% are considered borderline normal, 55% to 59% is mildly elevated, 60% to 64% is moderately elevated, and greater than 65% is markedly elevated.

Comparison of Sedimentation Rate Methods

The Westergren method is the most sensitive of the sedimentation rate methods because of the longer tube, but it requires more blood.

The Wintrobe method requires a smaller amount of blood and involves no dilution. In addition, once the ESR has been read, the Wintrobe tube can be centrifuged to obtain a macrohematocrit, and blood films can be made from the buffy coat. However, because of the shorter column of blood, the Wintrobe method is not as sensitive as the Westergren.

The ZSR requires a small amount of specimen, is not affected by anemia, and is faster than the other methods. Moreover, the reference range is the same for both sexes. However, it does require special equipment.

The disposable ESR method has the advantage of disposable equipment and ease of set up.

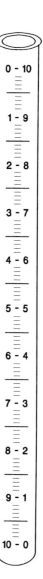

FIG. 9-9. Wintrobe tube for erythrocyte sedimentation rate determination.

UNITS OF HEMATOLOGIC MEASUREMENT

In recent years the hematology community has been steered away from using conventional units for hematologic measurements to the International System of Units (SI; from the French *Système International d'Unités*) to promote worldwide communication in laboratory measurements.[20,25] Throughout this text SI units are used for measurement of leukocytes, erythrocytes, platelets, and hematocrit, all of which are easy to translate from conventional units. In addition, the SI unit of measurement will be used for erythrocyte indices where possible.

Conventional units of measure used in hematology and their SI equivalents are listed in Table 9-6. Table 9-6 also presents an overview of all common hematologic measurements with examples in their conventional format and their SI unit equivalents. It is easy to see that conversions are simple, requiring no calculation—just a change in unit format (with the exception of Hb, which requires multiplication by 0.155 to obtain the SI unit equivalent). Fortunately, the International Committee for Standardization in Haematology has recommended that the convention g/dL be used instead of SI units for Hb. The NCCLS has published

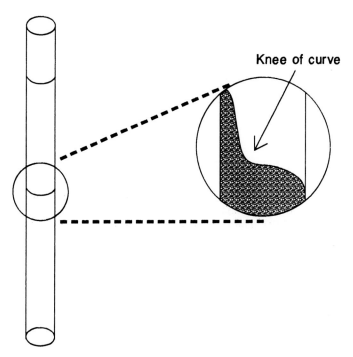

Knee of curve

FIG. 9-10.   Knee of the curve represents Zetacrit%; *i.e.,* sedimented RBC% used in determination of zeta sedimentation ratio.

a report summarizing many laboratory measurements according to their conventional units of expression and the proposed SI units.[25]

CHAPTER SUMMARY

Laboratory tests to assess the qualitative and quantitative adequacy of erythrocytes include hemoglobin (Hb), hematocrit (HCT), erythrocyte count, erythrocyte indices, reticulocyte count, and sedimentation rate.

The Hb concentration provides an estimate of the oxygen-carrying capacity of the blood. The standard method for manual and automated quantitation is based on the cyanmethemoglobin reaction. When quantitated manually, Hb concentration must be determined on the basis of a standard curve generated by each laboratory using the cyanmethemoglobin standard, available commercially. This is the only standard available in hematology.

Errors in Hb determination may be caused by poor technique, spectrophotometer malfunction, reagent deterioration, or abnormal specimens. Specimens may be turbid because of lipemia or elevated leukocyte counts. Turbidity may cause false increases in Hb readings; however, these problems may be overcome by using special manual techniques.

Hematocrit refers to the packed cell volume of whole blood. The timer, rpm indicator, brushes, and minimum time to achieve maximum packing must be checked periodically for each microhematocrit centrifuge to ensure accurate results. When reading an HCT a number of errors may be made. For example, the buffy coat, which contains leukocytes and platelets, must not be included in the HCT value.

The rule of three demonstrates the correlation of Hb, HCT, and the erythrocyte count to check the accuracy of manual or automated methods (see Table 9-3). Only normochromic, normocytic erythrocytes can be expected to conform to this rule.

Erythrocyte indices aid in the diagnosis of anemias. They include mean corpuscular volume (MCV), calculated as HCT × 10/RBC; mean corpuscular Hb (MCH), calculated as Hb × 10/RBC; and mean corpuscular Hb concentration (MCHC) calculated as Hb × 100/HCT. The MCV indicates that the average erythrocyte is either normocytic, macrocytic, or microcytic. The MCH indicates the average weight of Hb per erythrocyte. The MCHC determines whether erythrocytes are normochromic, hypochromic, or hyperchromic (the last condition is not normally reported). Indices are also useful in quality control (Chap. 47).

TABLE 9-6. Common Prefixes Indicating Multiples and Their Equivalents and Conventional Unit with SI Unit Report Format for Hematologic Measurements

PREFIX		MULTIPLE	EQUIVALENTS
deci (d)	=	10^{-1}	1 dL = 1 × 10^{-1} L = 0.1 L
milli (m)	=	10^{-3}	1 mL = 1 × 10^{-3} L = 0.001 L
micro (μ)	=	10^{-6}	1 μL = 1 × 10^{-6} L = 0.000001 L
pico (p)	=	10^{-12}	1 pg = 1 × 10^{-12} g = 0.000000000001 g
femto (f)	=	10^{-15}	1 fL = 1 × 10^{-15} L = 0.000000000000001 L

$$1 \text{ mm}^3 = 1.00003 \ \mu\text{L} \star$$

	CONVENTIONAL UNITS REPORT FORMAT	EXAMPLE (CONVENTIONAL)	SI UNITS REPORT FORMAT	EXAMPLE (SI)
WBC	× 10^3/mm^3 or × 10^3/uL	4.5 × 10^3/μL	× 10^9/L	4.5 × 10^9/L
RBC	× 10^6/mm^3 or × 10^6/uL	5.21 × 10^6/μL	× 10^{12}/L	5.21 × 10^{12}/L
Hb†	g/dL	15.4 g/dL	mM/L	2.39 mM/L
HCT	%	45.1%	L/L	0.451 L/L
MCV	μ^3 or μm^3	88 μ^3 or μm^3	fL	88 fL
MCH	$\mu\mu$g	29 $\mu\mu$g	pg	29 pg
MCHC	%	33%	g/dL	33 g/dL
PLT	× 10^3/mm^3 or × 10^3/μL	182 × 10^3/μL	× 10^9/L	182 × 10^9/L

★ The difference between 1 mm^3 and 1 μL is so insignificant that the two volumes are considered equivalent. Therefore, conventionally, cells have been reported using either cells/mm^3 or cells/μL as indicated for WBC, RBC, and PLT.

† Hb will be reported in g/dL in this text because the conversion from conventional to SI units is not easily translated or compared with RBC or HCT values using the Rule of Three, as can be seen from the SI unit example. The multiplication factor to convert conventional Hb to SI units is 0.155 (in the example above, 15.4 g/dL × 0.155 = 2.39 mM/L).

The reticulocyte count provides a measure of bone marrow erythropoietic activity. It can be refined further by calculating the absolute reticulocyte count (ARC), corrected reticulocyte count (CRC), or the reticulocyte production index (RPI) (see Table 9-4). The RPI is often the most useful in assessing the bone marrow response to anemia because it is corrected for both the degree of anemia and the maturation time of reticulocytes in the peripheral blood.

A nonspecific indicator of inflammation or tissue damage is provided by the erythrocyte sedimentation rate (ESR) (see Table 9-5). In this test anticoagulated whole blood is placed in a standardized tube and allowed to settle for exactly 60 minutes. At that time the erythrocyte level is recorded. Test conditions must be carefully controlled to avoid vibrations, drafts, or excessive heat or cold. Of the available methods, including the Westergren, Wintrobe, and zeta sedimentation ratio, the Westergren is clinically the most sensitive.

SI units, rather than conventional units, are now popular for expression of the HCT, erythrocyte and leukocyte counts, and erythrocyte indices. Conversion of all measures (except Hb) is easy and results in numbers related to commonly accepted reference ranges (see Table 9-6).

CASE STUDY 9-1

A technologist obtained an Hb of 15 g/dL and an HCT of 0.36 L/L on the same specimen.
1. What is the discrepancy indicated in these results?
2. Other than technical error, what four sources of error could cause this discrepancy?
3. How could each of these problems be resolved?

CASE STUDY 9-2

A woman severely burned in a house fire had blood drawn in the trauma center. Her Hb was 18.0 g/dL, and the HCT was 0.54 L/L.
1. Are these values normal for a woman? Explain why or why not.
2. Are the Hb and HCT technically and physiologically accurate? Why or why not?

CASE STUDY 9-3

A technologist received a STAT order for a manual Hb and HCT on three specimens. To save time, while centrifuging the HCT specimens, the technologist read the Hbs on the three patients 2 minutes after making the test dilutions. The Hb levels are all lower than expected compared with the HCTs.
1. List two possible explanations for this discrepancy.

CASE STUDY 9-4

Because of lack of space in the laboratory, the rack for sedimentation rate tubes was placed directly on top of a small refrigerator.
1. List three ways in which the results could be adversely affected.

CASE STUDY 9-5

A technologist consistently reads HCTs higher than other coworkers.
1. What could cause a technologist consistently to read such higher HCTS?

CASE STUDY 9-6

A leukemia patient with an elevated leukocyte count (200.0×10^9/L) had the following results on erythrocyte measurements performed manually: RBC 2.60×10^{12}/L; Hb 12.0 g/dL; and HCT 0.41 L/L.
1. Which result(s) should be questioned?
2. What is the most likely reason for these abnormalities?
3. How could the discrepancies be resolved or verified?

REFERENCES

1. Böttiger LE, Svedberg CA: Normal erythrocyte sedimentation rate and age. Br Med J 2:85, 1967
2. Boyd RD, Hoffbrand BI: Erythrocyte sedimentation rate in elderly hospital in-patients. Br Med J 1:901, 1966
3. Brecher G: New methylene blue as a reticulocyte stain. Am J Pathol 19:895, 1949
4. Brown BA: Hematology Principles and Procedures, 5th ed. Philadelphia, Lea & Febiger, 1988
5. Bunch TW: Blood test abnormalities in runners. Mayo Clin Proc 55:113, 1980
6. Coiner D: Analytical techniques and instrumentation. In Bishop ML, Duben–Von Laufen JL, Fody EP (eds): Clinical Chemistry—Principles, Procedures, Correlations, p 94. Philadelphia, JB Lippincott, 1985
7. Dallman PR: Blood and blood forming tissues. In Rudolph A (ed): Pediatrics, 16th ed, p 1111. New York, Appleton-Century-Crofts, 1977
8. Deiss A, Kurth D: Circulating reticulocytes in normal adults as determined by the new methylene blue method. Am J Clin Pathol 53:481, 1970
9. Fairbanks VF, Klee GG: Biochemical aspects of hematology. In Tietz NW (ed): Fundamentals of Clinical Chemistry, p 804. Philadelphia, WB Saunders, 1987
10. Gambino SR, DiRe JJ, Monteleone M et al: The Westergren sedimentation rate using K_3EDTA. Am J Clin Pathol 43:173, 1965
11. Gilbertsen VA: Erythrocyte sedimentation rate in older patients: A study of 4,341 cases. Postgrad Med 38:A44, 1965
12. Hackney JR, Cembrowsi GS, Prystowsky MB et al: Automated reticulocyte counting by image analysis and flow cytometry. Lab Med 20:551, 1989
13. Hillman RS, Finch CA: Red Cell Manual, 5th ed. Philadelphia, FA Davis, 1985
14. Hillman RS, Finch CA: Erythropoiesis: Normal and abnormal. Semin Hematol 4:327, 1967
15. Hycel Cyanmethemoglobin Certified Standard Package Insert. Houston, TX, Hycel, Inc. (a Boehringer Mannheim Company), 1980
16. International Committee for Standardization in Haematology: Recommendations for reference method for haemoglobinometry in human blood (ICSH Standard EP 6/2:1977) and specifications for international haemiglobincyanide reference preparation (ICSH Standard EP 6/3:1977). J Clin Pathol 31:139, 1978
17. International Committee for Standardization in Haematology: Reference method for the erythrocyte sedimentation rate (ESR) test on human blood. J Clin Pathol 26:301, 1973
18. International Committee for Standardization in Haematology: Recommendations for haemoglobinometry in human blood. Br J Haematol 13 (suppl):71, 1967
19. Koepke JF, Koepke JA: Reticulocytes. Clin Lab Haematol 8:169, 1986
20. Lehmann HP: Metrication of clinical laboratory data in SI units. Am J Clin Pathol 65:2, 1976

21. Lowenstein L: The mammalian reticulocyte. Int Rev Cytol 8:135, 1959
22. National Committee for Clinical Laboratory Standards, H16-P: Method for Reticulocyte Counting, vol 5, no 10. Villanova, PA, NCCLS, 1985
23. National Committee for Clinical Laboratory Standards: Procedure for Determining Packed Cell Volume by the Microhematocrit Method, vol 5, no 5. Villanova, PA, NCCLS, 1985
24. National Committee for Clinical Laboratory Standards: Reference Procedure for the Quantitative Determination of Hemoglobin in Blood, vol 4, no 3. Villanova, PA, NCCLS, 1984
25. National Committee for Clinical Laboratory Standards, C11-CR: Quantities and Units, SI, vol 3, no 3. Villanova, PA, NCCLS, 1983
26. National Committee for Clinical Laboratory Standards, H2-A2: Reference Procedure for the Erythrocyte Sedimentation Rate (ESR) Test, vol 8, no 3. Villanova, PA, NCCLS, 1988
27. Perel I, Hermann N, Watson L: Automated differential leukocyte counting by the Geometric Data Hematrak system: Eighteen months' experience in a private pathology laboratory. Pathology 12:449, 1980
28. Sage B, O'Connell J, Mercolino T: A rapid, vital staining procedure for flow cytometric analysis of human reticulocytes. Cytometry 4:222, 1983
29. Tanke H, Rothbarth P, Vossen J et al: Flow cytometry of reticulocytes applied to clinical hematology. Blood 61:1091, 1983
30. Tanke H, Nieuwenhuis I, Koper G et al: Flow cytometry of human reticulocytes based on RNA fluorescence. Cytometry 1:313, 1980
31. Westergren A: Die Senkungsreaction. Ergeb Inn Med Inderheild 26:577, 1924
32. Wintrobe MM, Landsberg JW: A standardized technique for blood sedimentation test. Am J Med Sci 189:102, 1935

PART *III*

ERYTHROCYTE ABNORMALITIES (NONMALIGNANT)

10

Introduction

to

Erythrocyte

Abnormalities

Dona D. Knapp

This chapter is an introduction to hematologic disorders involving quantitative changes in erythrocytes and how those disorders are classified. Under normal conditions, red cell production and the circulating red cell mass (RCM) remain at a constant level regulated by the erythropoietic mechanism, which functions to meet the body's oxygen requirement. If the RCM is excessively either decreased or increased, significant clinical problems occur. *Anemia* is the term used to denote conditions associated with decreased red cells; *erythrocytosis* and *polycythemia* designate conditions involving the presence of too many red cells in the circulation.

Assisting in the diagnosis of red cell disorders is a significant challenge in the hematology laboratory. The goal is prompt detection and recognition of anemic or polycythemic states so that a definitive diagnosis can be sought and proper treatment given. Anemia or erythrocytosis is only a sign that points to the existence of an underlying pathophysiologic process.

ABSOLUTE VERSUS RELATIVE RED CELL ABNORMALITIES

Conditions associated with anemia and erythrocytosis can be subdivided into two groups on the basis of whether the change in RCM is absolute or only relative (*i.e.*, secondary to a change in the plasma volume). In absolute anemia or polycythemia there is a true decrease or increase in the RCM, respectively. In relative anemia there is a fluid shift from the extravascular to the intravascular compartment, expanding plasma volume and diluting RCM. This is most often seen in association with pregnancy and in individuals with diseases associated with hyperproteinemia. Relative erythrocytosis, on the other hand, is the result of a decrease in the plasma volume. The RCM is normal. This most commonly occurs in conditions associated with dehydration. Although relative anemia or erythrocytosis are not true hematologic disorders, they must be differentiated from conditions involving an absolute change in RCM.

LABORATORY DEFINITION OF RED CELL ABNORMALITIES

Anemic and polycythemic conditions are detected by red cell measurements that are outside the established reference range. Anemia is best defined in reference to a decreased hemoglobin (Hb) level, as the physiologic consequences and symptoms are the direct result of the decreased oxygen-carrying capacity of the blood. Polycythemia or erythrocytosis is best defined in relation to hematocrit (packed red cell volume) levels above the established reference range. The primary clinical consequences include hypervolemia and hyperviscosity.

Reference ranges for red cell measurements (Chap. 9) vary with test methodology, environmental factors, sex, and age. They are based on statistical studies of a representative sample of a healthy population. Each determined range encompasses 95% of the results (*i.e.*, ± 2 standard deviations from the mean); in other words, 5% of healthy individuals are expected to have values above or below the reference range.

Even accurately determined reference ranges are of limited value when used to define quantitative erythrocyte abnormalities. Each laboratory value must be interpreted by the physician, taking into account the patient's baseline physiologic state. An occasional patient will have a red cell measurement that is within the population reference range yet physiologically inadequate for him or her as an individual. The converse is also true.

DISORDERS CHARACTERIZED BY DECREASED RED CELL CONCENTRATION

The detection of anemia suggests the presence of an underlying disease process. However, establishing a definitive diagnosis is complicated by the fact that there are many possible causative mechanisms. Basically, anemias can be categorized into four groups: (1) hypoproliferative; (2) maturation disorders; (3) hemolytic disorders; and (4) blood loss. The first two groups are characterized by decreased or ineffective bone marrow erythrocyte production, whereas the last two are the result of increased red cell destruction or blood loss.

Physiologic Response to Anemia

Chemical and Physical Response

Anemia results in a reduction in the oxygen-carrying capacity of the blood and subsequent hypoxia. The body normally attempts to compensate. The first adjustments involve a shift to the right in the oxyhemoglobin dissociation curve and an increase in red cell 2,3-diphosphoglycerate (2,3-DPG), both of which increase release of oxygen to the tissues by Hb (Chap. 7). A second re-

sponse involves the selective redistribution of blood flow to areas of highest oxygen demand. Finally, cardiac output is increased. In mild to moderate anemic states these three mechanisms together are effective in maintaining the oxygen pressure at close to normal levels, and the patient remains asymptomatic. More severe anemia leads to increasing cardiac output and greater cardiac stress; at this point, signs such as tachycardia are manifested.

Hematologic Response

A slower but more effective response to anemia involves the triggering of increased red cell production. Tissue hypoxia resulting from anemia normally leads to increased erythropoietic marrow stimulation. Receptors in the kidney are sensitive to the decreased oxygen tension and trigger increased production of erythropoietin. Erythropoietin acts on the marrow to increase the number of erythroid precursors, increase their rate of proliferation and maturation, and accelerate their release from the bone marrow (Chap. 6, Fig. 6-8). As a result, "shift reticulocytes" or immature red cells are seen in the peripheral blood, causing an increased reticulocyte count and reticulocyte production index (RPI). The RPI indicates whether or not the bone marrow is responding adequately to anemia (Chap. 9). A normal bone marrow is capable of increasing erythropoiesis approximately six- to eight-fold; however, it takes at least 1 week for a full response to be manifested. The marrow may fail to respond because of intrinsic disease, lack of essential hematopoietic factors, or a failure in the erythropoietic mechanism itself.

Clinical Manifestations

Mild anemic states often cause no symptoms because of the body's ability to compensate. Palpitations and dyspnea may be manifested during exercise. With increasing severity, the increased cardiac stress may cause tachycardia, shortness of breath, and headaches. Pallor is the result of dermal vasoconstriction and blood redistribution. Leg cramps, dizziness, fatigue, and insomnia, all of which are common as anemia progresses, are secondary to tissue hypoxia. In its most severe form, anemia may lead to coma and death.

Classification of Anemia

Once anemia has been detected, classifying it is usually beneficial, as it assists in the establishment of a definitive diagnosis. Three basic formats are used: etiologic, morphologic, and physiologic.

Etiologic Classification

The etiologic classification approach focuses on the principal underlying pathophysiologic mechanisms. Table 10-1 lists six groups of anemias, and each group is expanded to list the types of anemias in each category and their primary causative mechanism.

It often is difficult to classify anemias by etiology because they are often caused by multiple factors. For example, iron deficiency may coexist with folate deficiency. Anemia also frequently involves more than one underlying pathophysiologic mechanism. Megaloblastic anemias may display both disordered maturation and decreased red cell sur-

TABLE 10–1. Etiologic Classification of Anemia

TYPE	CAUSES
RELATIVE ANEMIA	
Pregnancy	Increased plasma volume
Hyperproteinemia	
Intravenous fluids	
ANEMIA ASSOCIATED WITH DEFECTIVE HEMOGLOBIN SYNTHESIS	
Iron deficiency	Excessive loss
	Increased requirements
	Deficient intake
	Defective absorption
Sideroblastic anemia	Enzymatic defect in heme synthesis
Primary	
Secondary	
Anemia of chronic disease	Defective iron utilization
	Infection
	Inflammation
	Neoplasm
Thalassemia syndromes	Imbalanced globin synthesis
ANEMIA ASSOCIATED WITH VITAMIN B_{12} OR FOLATE DEFICIENCY	
Vitamin B_{12} deficiency	Inadequate dietary intake
	Defective absorption
	Increased requirements
	Defective production of intrinsic factor
Folate deficiency	Inadequate dietary intake
	Defective absorption
	Increased requirements
	Impaired utilization—folate antagonists
ANEMIA ASSOCIATED WITH IMPAIRED BONE MARROW OR STEM CELL FUNCTION	
Bone marrow injury	Reduced hematopoietic tissue
Primary aplastic anemia	Idiopathic defect
Secondary aplastic anemia	Injury by drugs, radiation, chemicals, infectious agents
Bone marrow replacement	Infiltration with abnormal tissue
Myelophthisic anemia	Myelofibrosis, leukemia, lymphoma, myeloma, metastatic neoplasm, storage disease
Ineffective hematopoiesis	Hematopoietic stem cell disorder: abnormal proliferation and maturation
Myelodysplastic anemias	Refractory anemia
	Refractory anemia with ringed sideroblasts
	Refractory anemia with excess blasts
	Refractory anemia with excess blasts in transformation
	Chronic myelomonocytic leukemia
Decreased marrow stimulation	Reduced secretion of erythropoietin
Anemia of renal failure	
Anemia of endocrine disorders	
Anemia of chronic disease	
Constitutional anemia	Congenital or genetic predisposition to bone marrow failure
Diamond-Blackfan anemia	
Faconi anemia	
Familial aplastic anemia	
Acquired pure red cell aplasia	Erythroid marrow suppression
Acute self-limited	Associated with viral agents
Thymoma	Immunologic suppression
Paroxysmal noctural hemoglobinuria	Acquired stem cell disorder
ANEMIAS ASSOCIATED WITH DECREASED RED CELL SURVIVAL AND INCREASED RED CELL DESTRUCTION	
Intrinsic red cell defect	
Membrane defect	Defect in membrane resulting in shortened survival
Hereditary spherocytosis	Structural defect
Hereditary elliptocytosis	Structural defect
Hereditary stomatocytosis	Structural defect
Hereditary pyropoikilocytosis	Structural defect
Hereditary acanthocytosis	Abetalipoproteinemia/abnormal lipid content
Lecithin–cholesterol acyltransferase deficiency	Decreased membrane cholesterol esters
Paroxysmal nocturnal hemoglobinuria	Membrane sensitive to complement lysis
Enzyme defect	Enzyme defect resulting in shortened RBC survival
G6PD deficiency	Oxidative damage
Pyruvate kinase deficiency	Failure to generate normal ATP levels
Others	

(continued)

TABLE 10–1. Etiologic Classification of Anemia (*continued*)

TYPE	CAUSES
Hemoglobinopathies	Defective globin chain synthesis
Qualitative defects	Structural abnormality in globin chain
Sickle cell disease	
Hemoglobin C disease	
Unstable hemoglobins	
Other	
Quantitative defects	Imbalanced globin chain synthesis
Beta-thalassemia	Beta-chain defect
Alpha-thalassemia	Alpha-chain defect
Other	
Qualitative and quantitative defect	Structural abnormality and defective globin chain synthesis combined
Hb S/Beta-thalassemia	
Others	
Extrinsic red cell defect	
Immune	Immune destruction
Isoimmune hemolytic anemia	
Hemolytic disease of the newborn	
Hemolytic transfusion reactions	
Autoimmune hemolytic anemia	
Warm antibodies	
Cold antibodies	
Drug-induced immune hemolytic anemia	
Nonimmune	
Microangiopathic hemolytic anemia	Destruction secondary to fibrin deposition
Disseminated intravascular coagulation	
Thrombotic thrombocytopenic purpura	
Hemolytic uremic syndrome	
Hemolytic anemia associated with infection (bacterial, viral, protozoal)	Premature destruction secondary to interaction with infectious agent
Hemolytic anemia associated with toxic agents, chemicals, drugs	Toxic damage
Hemolytic anemia associated with physical agents (vascular prosthesis, march hemoglobinuria, burns)	Physical damage
Hypersplenism	Premature destruction in spleen
ANEMIA SECONDARY TO BLOOD LOSS	
Acute	Decreased blood volume
Chronic	

vival. Because anemia often is also complicated by another process such as chronic disease, clear cut etiologic classification is sometimes difficult.

Morphologic Classification

The morphologic classification of anemia can be established using red cell indices and direct examination of morphology. Red cell morphology is observed and described using a properly prepared and stained blood film (Chap. 8). Anemia can be classified according to erythrocyte size and Hb content. Although widely utilized and accepted, this approach has been criticized for lack of sensitivity and standardization.[11] In recent years standardized procedures and reporting formats have been presented in the literature,[5,18,20] and morphology review remains important in the classification of anemias.

The definition and procedure for determining red cell indices is described in Chapter 9. As early as 1934, Wintrobe presented a scheme for classifying anemias morphologically based on indices calculated from manually determined red cell measurements.[25] The indices, including the MCV, MCH, and MCHC, became the basis for classifying anemias into four categories: (1) normocytic, normochromic; (2) microcytic, hypochromic; (3) microcytic, normochromic; and (4) macrocytic, normochromic. Although this format has been widely used for many years, problems sometimes occur.[1] In prior years indices derived

from manually determined red cell measurements were questioned because of the high level of procedural variability and error, especially in the manual red cell count.[4] Today red cell indices are computed automatically by sophisticated electronic cell counters (Chaps. 42 and 43). Although results are now more reliable, the reported indices are still only as good as the instrumentation and data used to calculate them. Table 10-2 provides a general morphologic classification of anemia based on the MCV that differentiates microcytic, macrocytic, and normocytic anemias.

Electronic determination of red cell indices has increased the clinical value and usefulness of the MCV and decreased that of the MCH and MCHC. The MCV is now derived directly from red cell size distribution data. Most instruments now calculate the hematocrit (MCV × RBC count) in addition to the MCH and MCHC. The MCH varies in a linear relation to the MCV and provides no additional diagnostic information. Also, it is now recognized that calculated hematocrits are low in comparison with spun microhematocrits because of plasma trapping in the latter. The MCHC derived from a calculated hematocrit is, in turn, artifactually high and loses its sensitivity as an indicator of iron deficiency; it is decreased only in severe microcytic anemias. Although the MCH and MCHC have lost some clinical value, all red cell indices are useful quality control tools and aid in the detection of instrument malfunctions (Chap. 47).

TABLE 10–2. Morphologic Classification of Anemias

MICROCYTIC (MCV <80 fL)
  Commonly microcytic
    Iron deficiency
    Thalassemias
    Hereditary sideroblastic anemia
  Occasionally microcytic
    Anemia of chronic disease
    Hemoglobinopathies
MACROCYTIC (MCV >100 fL)
  Commonly macrocytic
    Folic acid deficiency
    Vitamin B_{12} deficiency
  Occasionally macrocytic
    Hypoproliferative anemia
    Refractory anemia
    Liver disease
    Hemolytic anemia
    Blood loss anemia
NORMOCYTIC (MCV 80–100 fL)
  Commonly normocytic
    Hypoproliferative anemia
    Myelophthisic anemia
    Refractory dysmyelopoietic anemia
    Hemolytic anemia
    Hemoglobinopathies
    Blood loss anemia
    Anemia of chronic disease
    Acquired sideroblastic anemia
  Occasionally normocytic
    Early iron deficiency
    Refractory anemia

TABLE 10–3. Classification of Anemia Using the MCV and RDW

	MCV LOW	MCV NORMAL	MCV HIGH
RDW NORMAL	Microcytic Homogeneous	Normocytic Homogeneous	Macrocytic Homogeneous
RDW HIGH	Microcytic Heterogeneous	Normocytic Heterogeneous	Macrocytic Heterogeneous

The MCV also has limitations. It represents the mean size of a given heterogeneous red cell population and does not reflect size variation (anisocytosis) within the population. This shortcoming has been overcome somewhat with the development of a new hematologic parameter that provides a measure of red cell size variation. This parameter, most commonly known as the *red cell distribution width* (RDW), is a size distribution measurement generated from a red cell histogram. It functions as an index of red cell population heterogeneity and can reflect anisocytosis on the peripheral blood film. It is expressed as the ratio of standard deviation (width of histogram) to the MCV or the coefficient of variation of red cell size within a given red cell population.[2] Many automated hematology instruments, both electrical impedance and light scatter systems, now provide RDW-type measurements. Each instrument derives this parameter differently, and data must be carefully interpreted in light of each laboratory's established reference ranges.

Investigators have performed retrospective studies on the application of the RDW in anemia classification, finding that RDW can be used in conjunction with the MCV to make classification more accurate.[3,16] The proposed classification scheme in Table 10–3 separates anemias into six categories on the basis of MCV and RDW. The RDW provides a measure of homogeneity (normal RDW) or heterogeneity (high RDW) within the red cell population. The RDW may be useful in the differential diagnosis of microcytic anemias. This is significant because the most common anemias are microcytic, and they often are difficult to differentiate. The RDW is reported to be increased in iron deficiency but normal in heterozygous thalassemias and anemias associated with chronic disease. The RDW may be more sensitive than other indicators in detecting early iron deficiency anemia.[19]

The RDW parameter is not without critics. Investigators warn that when complicating conditions are present, the RDW is not reliable. Others report that the RDW is a poor discriminator among microcytic anemias and state that it must be used with caution and should not replace other diagnostic tests such as iron studies and Hb electrophoresis.[7,13] Further research is needed to clarify the diagnostic value of the RDW. Also, published studies assessing use of the RDW in classifying anemias have been done primarily with only one hematology instrument system; studies using other systems await confirmation.

Physiologic Classification

The physiologic classification system is based on the ability of the bone marrow to respond to anemia with increased erythropoiesis. It involves assessing erythrocyte production using the reticulocyte count and calculated RPI. When anemia occurs, if the bone marrow is capable of responding, increased numbers of young, nonnucleated red cells enter the circulation. These young polychromatophilic red cells, released prematurely from the marrow because of erythropoietin stimulation, are called *shift reticulocytes,* a term reflecting their shift from the bone marrow to the peripheral blood at an earlier than usual stage of development. Thus, reticulocytes may be significantly increased in the circulation without an actual increase in marrow red cell production.

In order to use the reticulocyte count as an index of marrow red cell production effectiveness, it must be converted to the RPI using two mathematical corrections (Chap. 9). The first correction determines the absolute number of circulating reticulocytes, and the second compensates for the reticulocytes being shifted out of the marrow early and spending a longer time in the circulation.[15]

The accuracy and reliability of the manually determined reticulocyte count (and thus the RPI) have been questioned. Studies suggest unacceptable interlaboratory and intralaboratory variability.[14,21,22] However, greater attention is being given to standardization of the procedure. Furthermore, great accuracy is not absolutely necessary for the RPI to be of value. Significantly increased RPIs, whether four or five, for example, indicate an increased and effective marrow response to anemia. On the other hand, accuracy does become more critical at the cutoff point between effective and ineffective marrow production, where RPI interpretation is more difficult.

Table 10-4 demonstrates how the RPI can be used to classify anemia into two principal groups based on the marrow response. An RPI greater than 3.0 indicates an effective bone marrow response, whereas an RPI of less

TABLE 10–4. Physiologic Classification of Anemia

RPI <2.0 (INEFFECTIVE ERYTHROPOIESIS)		RPI >3.0 (EFFECTIVE ERYTHROPOIESIS)	
Hypoproliferative anemias	Maturation disorders	Hemolytic anemia	Blood loss anemia

than 2.0 suggests an ineffective bone marrow response.[15] Each group can be subdivided into two categories. An ineffective response is associated with hypoproliferative anemias and anemias resulting from maturation disorders. An effective response is characteristic of hemolytic anemias and anemias secondary to blood loss. In the case of effective erythropoiesis the bone marrow is intact, the hematopoietic mechanism is functional, and the components necessary for red cell production are available. In the presence of a significant anemia, an effective bone marrow response will be seen after a sufficient span of time. However, the bone marrow of an occasional individual with hemolytic anemia or blood loss will fail to respond because of an underlying defect in the marrow or the erythropoietic mechanism.

Combined Morphologic and Physiologic Classification

The schematics in Figures 10-1 and 10-2 integrate the physiologic and morphologic classification formats and provide a systematic approach to classifying anemias. Anemias are divided into the four major groups shown in Table 10-4 on the basis of the RPI.

INEFFECTIVE ERYTHROPOIESIS. The two groups demonstrating ineffective erythropoiesis (RPI < 2.0) are hypoproliferative anemias and anemias secondary to maturation disorders (Fig. 10-1). Hypoproliferative anemias tend to be normocytic, normochromic (N/N). This group encompasses a wide variety of anemias, including hypoplastic anemias, both idiopathic and those associated with drugs, chemicals, and infectious agents; myelophthisic anemia secondary to marrow infiltration and replacement (*e.g.*, leukemia); and refractory myelodysplastic anemia caused by a failure in stem cell maturation and characterized by dysplasia of developing precursor cells in the marrow; and finally a group of moderate anemias seen in association with diseases causing decreased marrow stimulation. Differentiation of anemias in this group often requires a bone marrow examination. Depending on the anemia, the marrow appearance ranges from normal to neoplastic.

Anemias associated with maturation disorders can be further separated into two groups based on the MCV. Microcytic anemias have a decreased MCV; macrocytic anemias, an increased MCV. Macrocytic anemias must be differentiated into those that are true megaloblastic anemias associated with B_{12} or folate deficiency (MCV may exceed 115 fL) and those that are nonmegaloblastic (MCV usually less than 115 fL), including hemolytic anemia with reticulocytosis and liver disease. Red cell morphology also is helpful in differentiating macrocytic anemias (see Fig. 10-1). Microcytic anemias include, in order of prevalence, iron deficiency, anemia of chronic disease, heterozygous thalassemia, and some sideroblastic anemias. Iron studies and Hb electrophoresis are often required in their differential diagnosis. Red cell morphology provides useful clues.

The RDW may be helpful in differentation (see Fig. 10-1); however, this awaits substantiation.

EFFECTIVE ERYTHROPOIESIS. The two groups of anemias usually demonstrating effective erythropoiesis (RPI > 3.0) are hemolytic anemias and those associated with chronic or acute blood loss (Chap. 20). These anemias tend to be normocytic and normochromic with a normal to slightly elevated MCV (see Fig. 10-2).

Hemolytic anemias are a diverse group that are caused by hereditary and acquired red cell defects. Red cell morphology is useful in differentiating hemolytic anemias into four groups (see Fig. 10-2). The presence of a predominant red cell morphologic variant is suggestive of a hereditary defect involving the red cell membrane. Predominant target cells suggest a hemoglobinopathy. Fragmented red cells may suggest a microangiopathic hemolytic process (Chap. 18). Normal morphology or only minor changes, including spherocytes and spiculated red cells, are seen in many types of hemolytic anemia, including immune hemolytic types (Chap. 19) and red cell enzyme deficiencies (Chap. 17).

After initial classification a definitive diagnosis may require additional laboratory testing, as discussed in appropriate chapters. Periodic referral to Figures 10-1 and 10-2 as subsequent chapters are read may be helpful during the initially complex study of this subject.

DISORDERS CHARACTERIZED BY INCREASED RED CELL CONCENTRATION

Disorders involving an increased number of circulating red cells and thus an increased RCM are described as erythrocytosis or polycythemia. Erythrocytosis is associated with an increased red cell number, Hb content, hematocrit, or some combination thereof. A hematocrit of greater than 0.52 L/L (52%) in men and 0.50 L/L (50%) in women is often used as the diagnostic criterion. Erythrocytosis may be classified as relative or absolute (Table 10-5). In relative erythrocytosis there is not a true increase in RCM but rather an apparent

(text continues on page 134)

TABLE 10–5. Classification of Erythrocytosis

RELATIVE ERYTHROCYTOSIS
  Dehydration
  Gaisböck's syndrome
  Stress/spurious
  Tobacco
ABSOLUTE ERYTHROCYTOSIS
  Primary
    Polycythemia vera
    Erythremia
  Secondary
    Appropriate
      High altitude
      Pulmonary disease
      Cardiovascular disease
      Alveolar hypoventilation
      Hemoglobinopathy
      Tobacco/carboxyhemoglobin
      Essential (idiopathic)
    Inappropriate
      Renal disease
      Extrarenal tumors

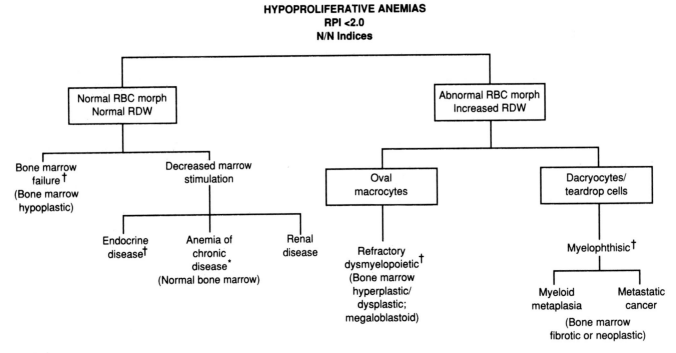

* May be microcytic.
† May be macrocytic.

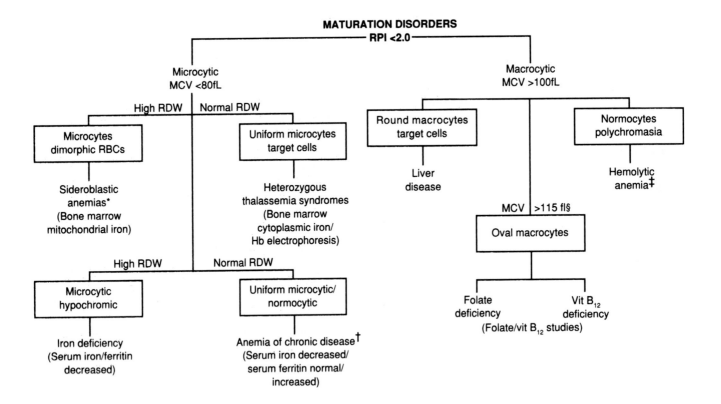

* May be normocytic or macrocytic.
†May be normocytic, normochromic.
‡ May have RPI >2.0.
§ MCV not always >115.

FIG. 10-1.   Systematic approach to the classification of anemias with ineffective erythropoiesis: hypoproliferative anemias (above) and disorders of maturation (below). Laboratory tests in parentheses are used to differentiate the disorders in that category.

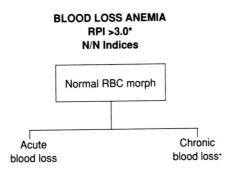

BLOOD LOSS ANEMIA
RPI >3.0*
N/N Indices

Normal RBC morph

Acute
blood loss

Chronic
blood loss⁺

*Given adequate response time.
⁺Without treatment, becomes microcytic, hypochromic

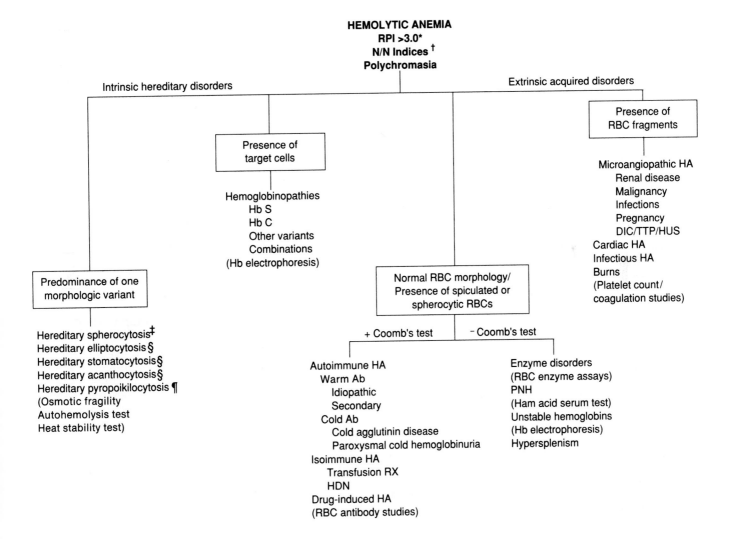

HEMOLYTIC ANEMIA
RPI >3.0*
N/N Indices †
Polychromasia

Intrinsic hereditary disorders   Extrinsic acquired disorders

Presence of
RBC fragments

Presence of
target cells

Microangiopathic HA
Renal disease
Malignancy
Infections
Pregnancy
DIC/TTP/HUS
Cardiac HA
Infectious HA
Burns
(Platelet count/
coagulation studies)

Hemoglobinopathies
Hb S
Hb C
Other variants
Combinations
(Hb electrophoresis)

Predominance of one
morphologic variant

Normal RBC morphology/
Presence of spiculated or
spherocytic RBCs

Hereditary spherocytosis‡
Hereditary elliptocytosis§
Hereditary stomatocytosis§
Hereditary acanthocytosis§
Hereditary pyropoikilocytosis ¶
(Osmotic fragility
Autohemolysis test
Heat stability test)

+ Coomb's test   − Coomb's test

Autoimmune HA
  Warm Ab
    Idiopathic
    Secondary
  Cold Ab
    Cold agglutinin disease
    Paroxysmal cold hemoglobinuria
Isoimmune HA
    Transfusion RX
    HDN
Drug-induced HA
(RBC antibody studies)

Enzyme disorders
(RBC enzyme assays)
PNH
(Ham acid serum test)
Unstable hemoglobins
(Hb electrophoresis)
Hypersplenism

* In the presence of a significant anemia and after a sufficient response time.
† May be macrocytic with extreme polychromasia.
‡ Microcytic, hyperchromic.
§ Anemia often not exhibited because of bone marrow compensation.
¶ Microcytic red cells displaying extreme morphologic variability.

FIG. 10-2.   Systematic approach to the classification of anemias with effective erythropoiesis: blood loss anemia (above) and hemolytic anemias (below). Laboratory tests in parentheses are used to differentiate the disorders in that category.

increase attributable to a decrease in plasma volume. Absolute erythrocytosis refers to a true increase in RCM and is associated with various causes.

Pathophysiology

Relative erythrocytosis is caused by a decrease in plasma volume that gives the appearance of an increased RCM in relation to total blood volume rather than a true increase in RCM.

Absolute erythrocytosis may be primary or secondary (Table 10-5). Primary erythrocytosis refers to a true increase in RCM associated with a myeloproliferative disorder known as polycythemia vera (Chap. 35). The increased RCM is the result of unregulated red cell production. Absolute secondary erythrocytosis is caused by two mechanisms, termed appropriate and inappropriate (Table 10-5). In an appropriate response, more erythropoietin is generated in an attempt to alleviate hypoxia through stimulation of red cell production. In an inappropriate response, increased generation of erythropoietin is the result of localized renal hypoxia or tumor generation of a substance that mimics the action of erythropoietin.

Absolute erythrocytosis has both a positive and a negative physiologic impact. The associated hypervolemia and vasodilation enhance perfusion of the blood and oxygenation; however, when the red cell volume exceeds a certain limit, the resulting hyperviscosity decreases blood flow and tissue oxygenation and increases the risk of thrombosis. When this critical point is exceeded, the benefits of enhanced oxygen delivery are outweighed by the potential negative impact of increased blood viscosity and the accompanying cardiac stress. Fortunately, the kidney and erythropoietic mechanism do not respond to hypoxia when excessive blood viscosity is detected, thus preventing a damaging spiral of further increases in red cell production and blood viscosity.[8]

Clinical Manifestations

The general symptoms of absolute and relative erythrocytosis are vague and depend on the severity and underlying pathologic mechanism. Symptoms include general malaise, dizziness, and headaches. A full feeling in the head, tinnitus, and sometimes, bleeding and thrombosis are also found in cases of absolute erythrocytosis. Some individuals may appear plethoric with bloodshot eyes secondary to vessel dilation needed to accommodate the increased blood volume.

Management of erythrocytosis depends on whether the increase in RCM is an appropriate response to hypoxia or unrelated to it, the severity of hypoxia, the extent of erythrocytosis, and the individual's clinical state. At times, phlebotomy is used to lower the RCM. It usually is effective in controlling the symptoms associated with erythrocytosis. It lowers the risk of thromboembolic complications while maintaining adequate blood flow to the brain and other organs.

Classification of Erythrocytosis

Table 10-5 summarizes the classification of erythrocytosis defined below.

Relative Erythrocytosis

The decreased plasma volume causing relative erythrocytosis may be the result of dehydration secondary to diarrhea, vomiting, excessive sweating, increased vascular permeability (burns or anaphylaxis), or the use of diuretics. Relative erythrocytosis also has been associated with a condition seen in individuals experiencing anxiety and stress. This condition has been called stress syndrome, spurious erythrocytosis, or Gaisböck's syndrome.[24] Affected individuals are usually middle-aged, overweight men complaining of headaches, dizziness, and fatigue. It has been suggested that smoking is a critical causative factor and that this syndrome should be recognized as "tobacco polycythemia." In most cases it has been suggested that there probably was an absolute increase in RCM accompanied by a decrease in plasma volume.[23]

Relative erythrocytosis is not a hematologic disorder; however, it must be differentiated from absolute erythrocytosis. This will be discussed in the Differential Diagnosis section later in this chapter.

Absolute Primary Erythrocytosis

An absolute increase in RCM resulting from a clonal, pluripotent stem cell disorder is seen in polycythemia vera (PV), which is one of a group of chronic myeloproliferative disorders (Chap. 35) characterized by uncontrolled proliferation of bone marrow elements. In the case of PV, erythrocyte production is not controlled by erythropoietin levels as reflected by the fact that erythropoietin is decreased in PV. Clinical and laboratory criteria for diagnosis of PV have been established[1] as detailed in Chapter 35. A subgroup of PV called erythremia has been described as a clonal disorder that affects autonomous bone marrow production of red cells only.[9] (PV may affect leukocytes or platelets as well). In erythremia the erythropoietin level is decreased, as in PV; however, all of the other diagnostic criteria for PV are absent.

Absolute Secondary Erythrocytosis (Appropriate)

The absolute secondary erythrocytosis disorders associated with an appropriate response to hypoxia may be caused by high altitude adjustment, pulmonary disease, cardiovascular disease, alveolar hypoventilation, or defective oxygen transport. Secondary erythrocytosis is appropriate for individuals living at high altitudes because of the low pO_2 of the air, which reduces arterial oxygen saturation. Except at very high altitudes, physiologic adjustments are normally made to compensate and satisfy unusual oxygen needs. Such adjustments include increased blood volume, increased oxygen-carrying capacity of blood, increased levels of 2,3-DPG to reduce Hb affinity for oxygen, and increased cardiac output and pulmonary function. Chronic mountain sickness (Monge's disease) is seen in individuals who fail to adapt to living at high altitudes. The causative factor appears to be alveolar hypoventilation secondary to an impaired respiratory response to hypoxia.

Chronic obstructive pulmonary diseases with decreased arterial oxygen tension occasionally cause erythrocytosis; however, the erythropoietic response usually is not as great as expected. Cardiac diseases, both congenital and acquired, occasionally are recognized as causing erythrocytosis. Alveolar hypoventilation, especially in association with extreme obesity, is associated with erythrocytosis. Hypoventilation with erythrocytosis may also be secondary to mechanical interference such as in poliomyelitis and muscle dystrophies or to an impaired respiratory center in cerebral thrombosis, encephalitis, or barbituate intoxication.

Hemoglobin variants are rare causes of secondary erythrocytosis. Structural changes in the Hb molecule may cause a shift to the left in the oxyhemoglobin dissociation curve, resulting in increased Hb affinity for oxygen, tissue hypoxia and increased erythropoietin production, and hence secondary erythrocytosis. Examples of such conditions are Hb Chesapeake and some Hb M disorders (Chap. 14).

It is now recognized that carbon monoxide exposure from excessive smoking is the most common cause of secondary erythrocytosis. It is estimated that 3% of cigarette smokers have elevated hematocrits.[23] Hemoglobin binds preferentially with CO when that gas is present, resulting in the formation of nonfunctional carboxyhemoglobin. As carboxyhemoglobin levels increase, there is also a shift to the left in the oxyhemoglobin dissociation curve and a decrease in P_{50}. This increases Hb oxygen affinity, reduces oxygen delivery to the tissues, and triggers erythrocytosis. In addition, smoking often causes a decrease in the plasma volume. In some individuals there is a low plasma volume but a normal RCM. Therefore, changes in the red cell volume and plasma volume among smokers may result in an absolute erythrocytosis in some individuals and a relative erythrocytosis in others.

Absolute Secondary Erythrocytosis (Inappropriate)

Secondary erythrocytosis not associated with generalized hypoxia and therefore considered an inappropriate response is seen most often in association with a variety of urologic disorders, including tumors, renal artery stenosis, pyelonephritis, urethral obstruction, and renal cystic disease.[12] Renal tumors and disease may interfere with renal blood flow, causing localized hypoxia, which in turn triggers erythropoietin production. Also, it is suggested that some tumors, involving the kidneys, themselves secrete an erythropoietinlike substance capable of stimulating erythropoiesis. Erythrocytosis is seen in about 10% of kidney transplant recipients.[26] A variety of extrarenal tumors can also inappropriately trigger increased erythropoiesis through secretion of humoral substances with an erythropoietinlike activity. Such tumors include those of the brain, liver, ovary, uterus, prostate, thymus, and adrenal glands.[12] Rarely an idiopathic overproduction of erythropoietin occurs. It has

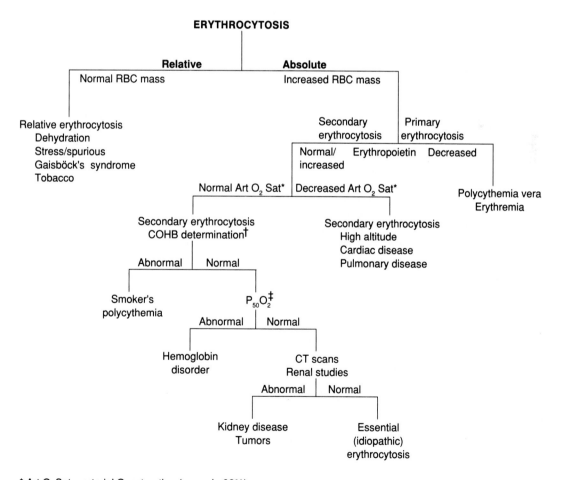

* Art O_2 Sat = arterial O_2 saturation (normal >92%).
† COHB = carboxyhemoglobin.
‡ $P_{50}O_2$ = oxygen pressure at which hemoglobin is half saturated.

FIG. 10-3.   Differential diagnosis of erythrocytosis.

been suggested that this disorder be designated as a sub-group of secondary erythrocytosis called "essential erythrocytosis."[9]

Differential Diagnosis of Erythrocytosis

Figure 10-3 provides a model for the differential diagnosis of erythrocytosis. Relative and absolute erythrocytosis are differentiated on the basis of blood volume studies from which the RCM may be determined. This is accomplished using isotope dilution techniques (Chap. 35). Values in excess of 36 mL/kg of body weight for males and 32 mL/kg for females are considered excessive. If the erythrocytosis is absolute, it must be determined whether it is primary (Chap. 35) or secondary. Erythropoietin levels measured by radioimmunoassay[17] tend to be decreased in primary conditions, but normal or increased in secondary conditions. However, some investigators have reported conflicting data, suggesting that the erythropoietin level is a poor discriminator of primary versus secondary erythrocytosis.[6]

Arterial blood gas measurements also aid in the differential diagnosis. Arterial oxygen saturation is normal (> 92%) in primary erythrocytosis. Appropriate and inappropriate secondary erythrocytosis usually can be differentiated on the basis of arterial oxygen saturation. Normal saturation values exclude cardiac and pulmonary erythrocytosis. However, not all conditions involving appropriate erythrocytosis cause a decrease in arterial oxygen saturation. Erythrocytosis attributable to the presence of an abnormal Hb with high oxygen affinity often demonstrates normal arterial oxygen saturation. The definitive diagnosis for this abnormal Hb usually requires studies of the oxyhemoglobin dissociation curve and determination of the partial pressure of oxygen at which Hb is 50% saturated (P_{50}). A decreased P_{50} value documents a shift to the left in the dissociation curve and confirms a nonfunctional Hb. Electrophoresis can detect some of these abnormal Hb (Chap. 14). Increased carboxyhemoglobin is useful in confirming tobacco-related erythrocytosis. Erythrocytosis associated with carboxyhemoglobin may be accompanied by an abnormal P_{50}. Inappropriate erythrocytosis associated with renal disease or tumors requires CT scanning and other renal studies.

CHAPTER SUMMARY

The diagnosis of disorders involving red cells provides a challenge to the laboratory. Anemias are disorders characterized by decreased red cell counts, whereas polycythemias or erythrocytoses are characterized by increased red cell counts. Both conditions can be relative, secondary to a change in the plasma volume, or absolute, with a quantitative increase or decrease in the RCM.

Classification of these disorders facilitates diagnostic evaluation. Several anemia classification schemes, including etiologic (Tables 10-1), morphologic (Table 10-2), and physiologic (Table 10-4) have been presented. A combined morphologic and physiologic classification scheme based on routine laboratory procedures, including red cell morphologic evaluation and reticulocyte count and calculated RPI, also has been offered (Figs. 10-1 and 10-2).

Classification and diagnostic schemes for polycythemia and erythrocytosis are presented in Table 10-5 and Figure 10-3, respectively. A diagnostic evaluation involves separating relative and absolute disorders and further differentiating primary and secondary absolute conditions. A number of laboratory tests, many complex, may be required to establish a definitive diagnosis.

REFERENCES

1. Berk PD, Goldberg JD, Donovan PB et al: Therapeutic recommendations in Polycythemia Vera Study Group protocols. Semin Hematol 23:132, 1986
2. Bessman JD: Automated Blood Counts and Differentials: A Practical Guide, p 9. Baltimore, The Johns Hopkins University Press, 1986
3. Bessman JD, Gilmer PR, Gardner FH: Improved classification of anemias by MCV and RDW. Am J Clin Pathol 80:31, 1983
4. Beutler E: The red cell indices in the diagnosis of iron deficiency anemia. Ann Intern Med 50:313, 1959
5. Connors DM, Wilson MK: A new approach to the reporting of red cell morphology. J Am Med Technol 3:94, 1986
6. Cotes PM, Dore CJ, Liu Yin JA et al: Determination of serum immunoreactive erythropoietin in the investigation of erythrocytosis. N Engl J Med 315:283, 1986
7. England JM: Future needs and expected trends in peripheral blood cell analysis: Erythrocyte histograms. Blood Cells 11:61, 1985
8. Erslev AJ, Caro J: Secondary polycythemias: A boon or a burden? Blood Cells 10:177, 1984
9. Erslev AJ, Caro J: Pure erythrocytosis classified according to erythropoietin titers. Am J Med 76:57, 1984
10. Fairbanks VF: Is the peripheral blood film reliable for the diagnosis of iron deficiency anemia? Am J Clin Pathol 55:447, 1971
11. Fairbanks VF: Nonequivalence of automated and manual hematocrit and erythrocytic indices. Am J Clin Pathol 73:55, 1980
12. Figueroa WG: Hematology. New York, John Wiley & Sons, 1981
13. Flynn MM, Reppun TS, Bhagavan NV: Limitations of red blood cell distribution width (RDW) in evaluation of microcytosis. Am J Clin Pathol 85:445, 1986
14. Gilmer PR, Koepke JA: The reticulocyte: An approach to definition. Am J Clin Pathol 66:262, 1976
15. Hillman RS, Finch CA: The Red Cell Manual, 5th ed. Philadelphia, FA Davis. 1985
16. Johnson CS, Tegos C, Beutler E: Thalassemia minor: Routine erythrocyte measurements and differentiation from iron deficiency. Am J Clin Pathol 80:31, 1983
17. Koeffler HP, Goldwasser E: Erythropoietin radioimmunoassay in evaluating patients with polycythemia. Ann Intern Med 94:44, 1981
18. Lloyd EM: How flowcharts improve RBC morphology reporting. MLO 14:49, 1982
19. McClure S, Custer E, Bessman D: Improved detection of early iron deficiency in nonanemic subjects. JAMA 253:1021, 1985
20. Napoli VM, Nichols CW, Fleck SH: A semiquantitative estimate method for reporting abnormal RBC morphology. Lab Med 11:111, 1980
21. Peebles DA, Hochberg A, Clarke TD: Analysis of manual reticulocyte counting. Am J Clin Pathol 76:713, 1981
22. Savage RA, Skoog DP, Rabinovitch A: Analytic inaccuracy and imprecision in reticulocyte counting: A preliminary report from the College of American Pathologists Reticulocyte Project. Blood Cells 11:97, 1985

23. Smith JR, Landaw SA: Smoker's polycythemia. N Engl J Med 298:6, 1978

24. Stefanini M, Urbas JV, Urbas JE: Gaisböck's syndrome: Its hematologic, biochemical and hormonal parameters. Angiology 29:520, 1978

25. Wintrobe MM: Anemia: Classification and treatment on the basis of differences in the average volume and hemoglobin content of red corpuscles. Arch Intern Med 54:256, 1934

26. Wu KK, Gibson TP, Freeman RM et al: Erythrocytosis after renal transplantation. Arch Intern Med 132:898, 1973

Anemia of Bone Marrow Failure and Systemic Disorders

Joyce A. Behrens

Anemia can be the result of an absolute failure of the bone marrow to replace those erythrocytes that are normally destroyed after 120 days or those that are prematurely destroyed, such as by hemolysis. This failure may be the result of a primary defect in the marrow itself, which occurs in *aplastic anemia* and *pure red cell aplasia* (PRCA). Normal bone marrow myeloid cells may also be replaced by metastatic tumor (a space-occupying lesion). The resulting anemia is called myelophthisic anemia and obviously represents altered hematopoiesis. There also are a number of systemic diseases, including those that affect the renal and endocrine systems, that can result directly in a secondary decrease in the absolute number of erythroid precursors in the marrow. Here, a factor, usually hormonal, is decreased or absent; this factor normally has some erythropoietic stimulatory effect. The bone marrow in these cases is functionally normal; however, anemia may develop.

ANEMIA OF BONE MARROW FAILURE

Aplastic Anemia

Definition

Aplastic anemia is a condition in which there is a peripheral blood *pancytopenia*, which is defined as a decrease in all cellular constituents: leukocytes, erythrocytes, and platelets. The bone marrow in aplastic anemia is, by definition, severely hypoplastic or aplastic.[10,12,24] The name of this disorder is misleading, as it implies that anemia is the primary problem experienced by these patients; however, their most serious clinical problems relate to neutropenia and thrombocytopenia. The criteria for laboratory diagnosis of severe aplastic anemia are listed in Table 11-1. There are milder forms of aplastic anemia that do not meet these

TABLE 11–1. Diagnostic Criteria for Severe Aplastic Anemia

BONE MARROW

Cellularity	<25% of normal
	or
	<50% of normal cellularity with <30% hematopoietic cells

Plus Any Two of the Following:

PERIPHERAL BLOOD

Granulocytes	$<0.5 \times 10^9$/L
Platelets	$<20 \times 10^9$/L
Anemia with	<1% reticulocytes (corrected for hematocrit)

From Camitta BM, Thomas ED, Nathan DG et al: A prospective study of androgens and bone marrow transplantation for treatment of severe aplastic anemia. Blood 53:504, 1979

strict criteria and are thus not diagnosed as frank aplastic anemia, such as hypoplastic anemia secondary to drug toxicity. In aplastic anemia there are no immature myeloid cells in the peripheral blood. This finding, along with the aplastic or hypoplastic marrow (where hematopoietic cells are replaced by fat) and the lack of splenomegaly in these patients, helps to differentiate aplastic anemia from a number of other pancytopenic conditions.

Age Incidence and Demographics

The incidence of aplastic anemia is low before the age of 1 year, then increases at an intermediate rate until the age of 50, after which the incidence is highest. Marrow aplasia is two to five times more frequent in the Far East than in either North America or Europe.[10]

Classification

Aplastic anemias can be divided into primary and secondary types (Table 11-2). The primary group contains congenital or hereditary Fanconi's anemia (which is rare) and idiopathic aplastic anemia for which there is no known precipitating factor. Forty to seventy percent of the cases in the United States and more than 90% of the cases in Japan[10] are idiopathic. In contrast, secondary aplastic anemias have a number of identified causative factors and agents (Table 11-3). These secondary types are discussed first in this chapter because they are more easily understood.

Several mechanisms have been implicated as the underlying defect in all forms of aplastic anemia. These include a deficiency in the number of bone marrow stem cells, immune suppression of stem cells, or a defect in the stem cells themselves, making them unresponsive to differentiation

TABLE 11–2. Classification of Aplastic Anemia

PRIMARY
Congenital Fanconi anemia
Acquired idiopathic
SECONDARY
Drugs (Table 11–3)
Chemicals (Table 11–3)
Radiation
Immune mechanism
Infection
  Non-A, non-B hepatitis
  Other viral infections
  Miliary tuberculosis
  Brucellosis
  Parasites

TABLE 11–3. Drugs for which Association with Aplastic Anemia, as an Idiosyncratic Reaction, Has Been Well Established on Clinical Grounds

ANTIBACTERIALS
Chloramphenicol
Sulfonamides
ANTI-INFLAMMATORY/ANTIRHEUMATIC AGENTS
Phenylbutazone
Oxyphenbutazone
Gold salts
Indomethacin
ANTICONVULSANTS
Phenytoin
Methoin
DIURETICS
Chlorothiazide and other thiazides
ANTITHYROID DRUGS
Propylthiouracil
Methylthiouracil
Carbimazole
Potassium perchlorate
Thiocyanate
ORAL HYPOGLYCEMIC AGENTS
Chlorpropamide and other sulfonylureas
ANTIMALARIALS
Amodiaquine
Chloroquine
Mepacrine (quinacrine)

From Vincent PC: Drug-induced aplastic anemia and agranulocytosis: Incidence and mechanisms. Drugs 31:52, 1986. Auckland, New Zealand, ADIS Press Limited, with permission.

or mitotic stimuli. Damage to the bone marrow microenvironment has also been implicated; however, this seems less likely today because bone marrow transplants have become more successful, showing that donor stem cells are capable of thriving in the recipient's microenvironment. Whatever the etiology or mechanism, the end result is the same—failure of hematopoietic stem cell growth, resulting in a hypoplastic marrow and pancytopenia.

Secondary Aplastic Anemia

Etiology and Pathophysiology

There is extensive literature implicating drugs (see Table 11-3), chemicals, radiation, abnormal immune mechanisms, and various other factors as causes of secondary aplastic anemia. Data from each of these areas are summarized briefly in the following paragraphs.

DRUGS AND CHEMICALS. Chloramphenicol is the classic drug associated with marrow aplasia. The incidence of aplastic anemia is 5- to 40-fold higher in persons who have taken the drugs than in persons not so exposed.[10] Transient marrow hypoplasia after treatment with chloramphenicol is fairly common.[10,21,24] This is associated with the appearance of vacuolated cells in the bone marrow, especially among the erythroid series.[21] Sometimes a more serious persistent marrow aplasia follows chloramphenicol therapy.

Other drugs and chemicals associated with development of aplastic anemia include benzene and benzene derivatives, hydantoins, sulfonamides, and gold preparations.[21,24] Insecticides such as chlordane, chlorophenothane (DDT), and gamma benzene hexachloride (Lindane) have also been cited.[76] Table 11-3 lists drugs associated with idiosyncratic development of aplastic anemia. Many other drugs, including "innocent" drugs such as aspirin, may be etiologic in an occasional patient.

RADIATION.   Individuals exposed to long-term low-dose irradiation have an increased incidence of aplastic anemia. For example, patients receiving radiation for ankylosing spondylitis have a 40-fold increase in the incidence of aplastic anemia. American radiologists have a 20-fold increase in incidence.[10]

Radiation may damage the stem cells[21] or the hematopoietic microenvironment; in other words, those elements within hematopoietic tissue that provide mechanical support for developing hematopoietic cells.[7] An in vitro study has shown that low-dose irradiation damages bone marrow stromal cells and that this damage affects cell-to-cell interactions, resulting in a decrease in the growth response of bone marrow cells in culture.[32] However, it is likely that damage to the microenvironment is reversible, as indicated by successful marrow transplants in aplastic patients.

High-dose radiation associated with acute exposure—radiotherapy, radioactive isotope administration, or work in unsafe nuclear power plants—can result in rapidly developing bone marrow aplasia and death.[21] After the 1986 Chernobyl (USSR) nuclear accident, 35 individuals who were exposed to doses exceeding 800 rads were in grave condition with severe marrow aplasia; 11 of these died within 3 weeks of the accident.[72] Bone marrow transplants performed on a number of these patients were largely unsuccessful because of complications linked to the severe burns they had suffered in the accident.[28]

IMMUNE MECHANISM.   There is some support for an autoimmune mechanism as the cause of aplasia, either directly by lymphocytes or by some humoral factor. In 11 of 22 patients with aplastic anemia who received syngeneic (identical twin) transplants (where theoretically there should be no rejection of the graft), rejection was experienced. Six of these 11 patients were then conditioned with cyclophosphamide, an immunosuppressive agent, prior to receiving a second infusion of identical twin marrow. In all of these cases engraftment was then successful and permanent, suggesting an immunologic mechanism for aplastic anemia.[67]

Occasionally, lymphocytes from patients with aplastic anemia suppress growth of normal marrow cells in vitro. To suppress this process in vivo, patients have been given antithymocyte globulin (ATG). Thereafter, lymphocytes from the patients no longer suppress in vitro growth of their own marrow colony-forming units culture (CFU-C).[10,69]

Human natural killer (HNK) cells (null cell lymphocytes capable of killing a target cell directly without prior sensitization) inhibit growth of hematopoietic cells in vitro. Therefore, it has been proposed that HNK cells are responsible for lymphocyte-mediated aplasia. However, in one study 76% of 43 patients with aplastic anemia were shown to have deficient HNK activity,[29] a finding that does not support this hypothesis.

Another study demonstrated that in vitro inhibition of erythropoiesis was the result of an abnormal composition of T cell subsets in the bone marrow (an excess of activated Tac+ T3+ and T11+ lymphocytes). After successful engraftment of bone marrow, these abnormalities disappeared, and the patients' T cells no longer suppressed erythroid colony growth in vitro.[51]

Humoral inhibitors of stem cell growth have been reported in a few patients whose aplastic anemia was either idiopathic or associated with systemic lupus erythematosus, quinidine, or cryoglobulinemia.[10]

MISCELLANEOUS ETIOLOGIES.   Numerous other associations with aplastic anemia have been observed, most quite rare. Occasionally, infection precedes the syndrome. Most commonly, this infection is non-A, non-B hepatitis; 0.3% to 0.5% of aplastic anemia cases follow overt hepatitis. These patients usually have not had severe hepatitis, and the infection usually has resolved by the time the aplasia develops several months later.[10] This situation is predominantly seen in young adults, and these patients have a poor prognosis, with the disease often being rapidly fatal.[64] Other reported cases have been associated with miliary tuberculosis, brucellosis, and parasitic infestation.[10] In other infections where pancytopenia has been reported, there is usually increased peripheral destruction of all blood cells, often as a result of hypersplenism, in which the spleen may destroy or simply pool cells from all blood cell lines.

Aplastic anemia is also related to other myeloid disorders. Twenty-five percent of patients with paroxysmal nocturnal hemoglobinuria (PNH), an acquired clonal disorder (Chap. 18), develop aplastic anemia. Conversely, 5% to 10% of patients with aplastic anemia develop PNH. In addition, 1% to 5% of patients who present with aplastic anemia actually have leukemia. The leukemic cells may release one or more factors that suppress hematopoiesis, causing hypoplastic marrow with peripheral blood pancytopenia. On the other hand, aplastic anemia sometimes progresses to acute leukemia (Chap. 34).

On rare occasions aplasia has occurred during pregnancy, with recovery after conclusion of the pregnancy.[10]

Clinical Presentation

The symptoms are directly related to pancytopenia.[21,24] If anemia is severe enough, the typical symptoms occur, such as pallor, weakness, and easy fatigability. Decreased neutrophils result in an increased incidence of bacterial infections; there is no increase in viral infections. Hemorrhage may be seen as a consequence of thrombocytopenia. The lack of a palpable spleen (i.e., a normal spleen) is significant in the diagnosis, because these patients do not generally demonstrate splenomegaly.

Laboratory Findings and Correlations with Disease

PERIPHERAL BLOOD.   The patient is anemic, neutropenic, and thrombocytopenic (Fig. 11-1). The total leukocyte count also is decreased.[11,21,24] Table 11-1 summarizes the laboratory criteria for the diagnosis of aplastic anemia. Lymphocytes are normal to slightly decreased, unless the patient has been on immunosuppressive therapy, in which case lymphocytes may be significantly decreased. The anemia is usually normocytic, normochromic, although occasionally, slight macrocytosis is observed. The morphology of the red cells is normal; the reticulocyte

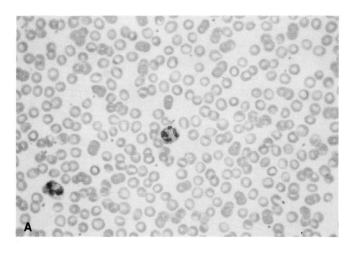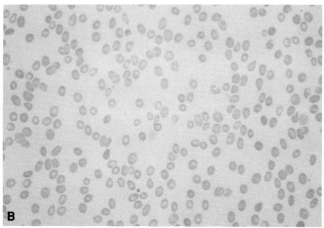

FIG. 11-1. Normal peripheral blood (A) compared with peripheral blood pancytopenia (B). Note the lack of leukocytes in (B) and obvious scarcity of both red cells and platelets compared with the normal picture.

count is decreased, and the calculated reticulocyte production index (RPI) is significantly decreased (Chap. 9). Of great significance is that there are no immature cells in the peripheral blood.

BONE MARROW. Both a bone marrow aspirate for observation of cell morphology and cell differentiation and a bone marrow biopsy for observation of overall marrow structure and cellularity should be performed. The marrow biopsy specimen is usually hypoplastic or aplastic, with increased fat and decreased hematopoietic cells (Fig. 11-2).

The principal cells present are lymphocytes and plasma cells; megakaryocytes generally are notably absent. There are no increased numbers of immature cells observed in the marrow, as would be seen for example in a pancytopenic patient with acute leukemia as the etiology. However, it should be noted that the bone marrow in patients with aplastic anemia has patchy areas of cellularity. Thus, occasionally a bone marrow sample indicates some cellularity rather than the hypoplastic state defined for aplastic anemia.

SPECIAL HEMATOLOGY TESTS. Hemoglobin F (Hb F) is elevated in some patients with aplastic anemia[8,11] and is distributed unevenly in red cells when a Kleihauer-Betke acid elution test is performed. In the past it was believed that a high Hb F was associated with a better prognosis,[8] but this view has not been substantiated.[56] Scores for leukocyte alkaline phosphatase (LAP) are often increased. The Ham acid-serum test, the confirmatory test for PNH, also may be positive in aplastic anemia. (See Differential Diagnosis for an explanation of laboratory differentiation of the two disorders.)

CHEMISTRY. Serum iron generally is elevated and plasma iron clearance delayed because the patient has adequate iron stores but decreased uptake of iron by developing red cells.[11] These abnormalities are a reflection of decreased erythropoiesis. Humoral stimulators of hematopoiesis such as erythropoietin are usually normal or elevated.[10]

CYTOGENETICS. Marrow chromosomes are normal in most patients. When abnormalities are found, the diagnosis of a myelodysplastic syndrome should be considered (Chap. 33).[11]

Differential Diagnosis

Because a number of disorders cause peripheral blood pancytopenia, acquired aplastic anemia must be differentiated from them, often by exclusion of all other possibilities, to ensure proper therapy. Table 11-4 lists the disorders most commonly associated with pancytopenia (although they do not always cause pancytopenia) and their distinguishing laboratory characteristics. None of the disorders in Table 11-4 causes a strikingly hypocellular marrow like that of aplastic anemia. Therefore, the differential diagnosis based on examination of a marrow biopsy usually is not difficult. Figure 11-2 shows a marrow biopsy from a normal individual, termed normocellular, contrasted with marrows that are hypocellular (as seen in aplastic anemia), fibrotic, and hypercellular.

Physical findings that generally rule out aplastic anemia include splenomegaly or lymphadenopathy. Radiographic studies of the bone may be necessary to rule out primary or metastatic bone tumors or other focal lesions.

The significant finding of immature erythrocytes or leukocytes in the peripheral blood usually rules out aplastic anemia and indicates any number of disorders including leukemia, lymphoma, myelofibrosis, and myelodysplastic syndromes (see Table 11-4). Usually, the marrow in these disorders is hypercellular.

Table 11-5 summarizes the tests recommended to assist in the diagnosis of aplastic anemia. Note that the tests most frequently used are most commonly performed to make the initial diagnosis. However, it is not necessary to perform these tests frequently on a patient with aplastic anemia unless the patient is undergoing treatment to which the response must be verified.

Effects of Treatment on Laboratory Results

Occasionally, a spontaneous remission occurs in aplastic anemia. For most patients, however, the only cure is bone

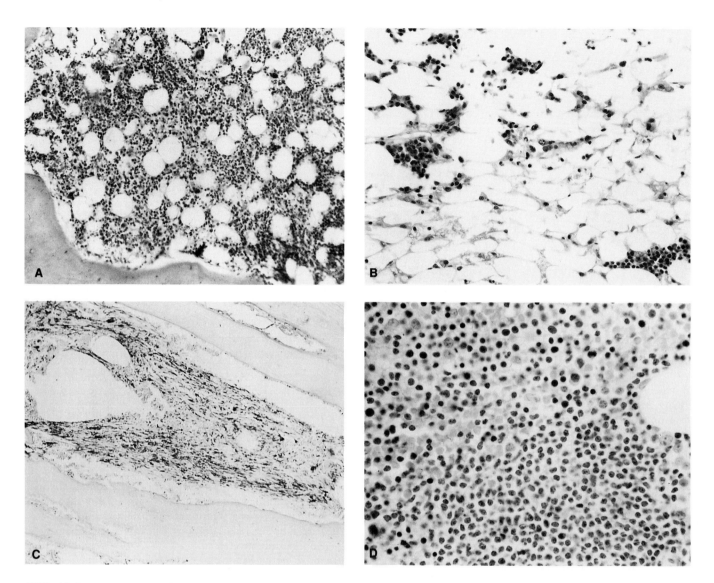

FIG. 11-2. Comparison of marrow biopsies from (A) a normal individual with a normocellular marrow, showing a 1:1 fat : cell ratio; (B) an individual with aplastic anemia, showing a hypocellular marrow where fat has replaced normal hematopoietic cells. The remaining cells are primarily lymphocytes and plasma cells; (C) a fibrotic marrow, which is associated with a number of disorders, such as agnogenic myeloid metaplasia; and (D) a hypercellular marrow, which is associated with a number of disorders, including leukemia. Note the striking difference among the abnormal marrow structures even though each may cause pancytopenia in the peripheral blood.

marrow transplantation from a compatible donor. The ideal donor is syngeneic (an identical twin). Other acceptable donors are allogeneic, with the donor being a human leukocyte antigen (HLA)-matched, mixed lymphocyte culture (MLC)-nonreactive family member, usually a sibling; or allogeneic, with the donor being an HLA-matched, MLC-nonreactive unrelated donor. Patients who undergo bone marrow transplantation have a much more favorable prognosis and survival rate than those for whom no donor can be found, especially in the first 6 months after diagnosis.[12]

The principal problems associated with bone marrow transplantation are failure of sustained marrow engraftment (*i.e.*, rejection) and the development of graft versus host disease (GVHD).[67,68] Successful Nand maintained engraftment is greatly improved if patients receive the trans-

plant early in their disease, prior to any blood product transfusions. If transfusions are necessary because of a life threatening event, the blood should not come from potential donors to avoid sensitization of the patient to minor histocompatibility antigens (for which no immunohematologic typing is available) that may be present in the donor but not in the recipient.[67] When this rule was followed, engraftment was achieved in 90% of the patients. Of these successes, 83% were surviving from 9 to 84 months following transplantation. In contrast, engraftment in multiply transfused patients studied during the same period was 69%, with a survival rate of 54%.[68]

Patients receiving allogeneic transplants require previous conditioning with cyclophosphamide to decrease the risk of rejection;[68] some groups condition with cyclophosphamide plus a reduced dose of total-body irradiation, total lymphoid irradiation, or thoracicoabdominal irradiation,[67] in which radiation is restricted to the chest and abdominal areas. The use of radiation in a patient with a nonmalignant disease carries the risk of future development of malignancy.[11] However, in a recent study, engraftment in previously transfused patients (considered at high risk for rejections) was reported to be significantly improved (55 of 58 patients, or 95%) when total lymphoid irradiation was added to cyclophosphamide in the conditioning regime.[53] Most grafts now are successful with complete hematologic recovery,[67] as evidenced by increasing marrow cellularity, followed by a rise in peripheral blood counts within 2 to 4 weeks after grafting.

Acute and chronic GVHD are still a significant concern. GVHD is understood to be an immune reaction triggered by an incompatibility between the donor and recipient HLA antigens. As its name implies, it is mediated by donor lymphocytes acting against host tissues.[67,68] In the past, methotrexate (MTX) was the agent most frequently used to prevent acute GVHD. In spite of this treatment, acute GVHD was seen in 25% to 30% of patients who had successful engraftment. The overall mortality rate from acute GVHD after transplantation has been reported as 8%.[11,67]

In the last few years a new immunosuppressive agent, cyclosporin A (CyA), has been reported to be effective in the treatment of acute GVHD, particularly after kidney transplantation. However, it is difficult to interpret the data with respect to patients receiving bone marrow transplants. Although some studies indicate promise,[6,40] more data are needed to prove the effectiveness of CyA in the treatment of acute GVHD after bone marrow transplantation. Also, there are indications that the long-term effects of CyA will present problems.

If acute GVHD does appear, it is usually anywhere from day 10 to day 70 after grafting. Organs attacked include the gut, skin, and liver. Chronic GVHD occurs between 3 to 15 months after grafting, ranging from mild to severe forms, and is responsible for a 12% mortality rate in long-term survivors. It is treated with prednisone, sometimes in combination with azathioprine. Both of these drugs are immunosuppressants. The clinical features of chronic GVHD include a persistent immune deficiency, impaired granulocyte chemotaxis, recurrent bacterial infections, disfiguring skin lesions, and liver dysfunction.[11,67,68] Infectious complications can also be seen in patients who have received a bone marrow transplant. The most serious of these is interstitial pneumonia, the frequency of which is much greater (40%–50%) in patients conditioned with total-body irradiation than in those receiving cyclophosphamide alone (around 16%).[11]

For patients who do not have a suitable donor, other modes of therapy for aplastic anemia are attempted. Most important is blood product support as needed, including both red cell and platelet transfusions. Immunosuppressive therapy is the next mode of treatment usually attempted. This includes the use of either antithymocyte globulin (ATG) or antilymphocyte globulin (ALG). The mechanism of the response in some patients is not clear,[10] but theoreti-

TABLE 11–4. Differential Diagnosis of Pancytopenias

CONDITION	PERIPHERAL BLOOD	BONE MARROW	SPLENOMEGALY	ADDITIONAL COMMENTS*
Aplastic anemia	No immature leukocytes or erythrocytes; MCV usually normal	Hypoplastic to aplastic (Fig. 11–1)	Absent	LAP score N to ↑ ; Ham's acid serum test ±
Acute leukemia	Blasts usually present	Hyperplastic to neoplastic (Fig. 11–1) with immature cells dominant	May be present	
Myelofibrosis	Leukoerythroblastosis often seen; tear drop RBCs prominent	Increased reticulin (Fig. 11–1); may be hypoplastic	Prominent	LAP score variable; usually N to ↑
Megaloblastic anemia	Anemia most prominent MCV >110 fL	Hypercellular with megaloblastic features	Absent	Serum folate &/or B_{12} ↓
Hairy cell leukemia	Hairy cells usually present	Increased reticulin; characteristic "fried egg" appearance on biopsy because of cells' abundant cytoplasm with hairline projections	Present	Marrow aspirate usually dry tap; malignant cells TRAP+
Paroxysmal nocturnal hemoglobinuria	Anemia most prominent feature; mild to moderate reticulocytosis	Erythroid hyperplasia; may be hypoplastic to aplastic	Absent	Sucrose hemolysis test +; Ham acid serum test +; LAP score ↓ ; hemosiderinuria present
Multiple myeloma	Rouleaux present; anemia most prominent	Plasmacytosis (clonal)	Usually absent	Monoclonal protein in serum; monoclonal light chains in urine
Waldenstrom's macroglobulinemia	Rouleaux present; anemia most prominent	Increased B lymphocytes ("plasmacytoid lymphs")	Often present	IgM monoclonal protein in serum; monoclonal light chains in urine
Lymphoma	Pancytopenia rare	(See Chap. 38)	Usually absent	Lymphadenopathy
Myelodysplastic syndromes	Pancytopenia variable; evidence of dyspoiesis (see Chap. 33)	Hypercellular; dyspoiesis in one or more cell lines	Absent	

* LAP = leukocyte alkaline phosphatase; N = normal; TRAP = tartrate-resistant acid phosphatase.

TABLE 11–5. Tests Recommended to Assist in Differential Diagnosis of Aplastic Anemia

Most frequently required (These tests usually do not need to be repeated frequently)	Complete blood count Platelet count Reticulocyte count (with RPI) Differential Bone marrow biopsy Bone marrow aspirate
Required occasionally	Sucrose hemolysis test Ham acid serum test (if sucrose hemolysis test is positive)
Required rarely	Haptoglobin Bilirubin (unconjugated) Serum B_{12} Serum erythropoietin LAP Urine urobilinogen (quantitative) Ferrokinetic studies

cally, these agents are useful when an immune mechanism is the etiology for the aplasia.

Androgens stimulate erythropoiesis and, to a lesser degree, granulopoiesis and thrombopoiesis. In spite of a multi-institutional study that showed no benefit to patients receiving androgens compared with patients who did not,[12] some patients do respond, and therefore androgens continue to be used in the hope of improvement.

Recently CyA has been used to treat patients with severe aplastic anemia who have no suitable marrow donor and are refractory to ATG.[9,59] The results were mixed, and more data are needed to determine its effectiveness.

Because of the current success of bone marrow transplantation in aplastic anemia, it is the recommended therapy if a suitable donor is available, especially for patients less than 40 years of age. For patients over age 40, immunosuppressive therapy is recommended.[67]

Prognosis

Prognosis is dependent on the mode of therapy used. Bone marrow transplants in nontransfused patients result in long-term survival rates as high as 83%; many of these patients have now been followed for more than 12 years and are hematologically normal.[11,67] The prognosis is much poorer for patients for whom a suitable donor cannot be found.[12]

Regardless of the mode of therapy, the survival curves in aplastic anemia are biphasic, with considerable early mortality rates followed by a much slower decline[11] for those who survive the initial period. Children have a somewhat better prognosis than adults. Long-term survivors of bone marrow transplants can be considered cured, but those receiving other modes of therapy probably are never truly cured.[11]

Fanconi Anemia (Congenital Aplastic Anemia)

Pathophysiology

Fanconi anemia is a rare, inherited form of aplastic anemia, first reported in three brothers by Fanconi, after whom the disease was named. More than 100 cases have now been reported,[17] and inheritance appears to be autosomal recessive.[17,34,37,52] It is defined as a pancytopenic disorder with a hypoplastic to aplastic bone marrow.

Clinical Presentation

Prominent congenital abnormalities in this disorder include microencephaly (abnormally small brain), brown skin pigmentation, short stature, malformations of the thumbs, internal strabismus (crossed eyes), malformations of the kidney, genital hypoplasia, and mental retardation.[57]

There apparently are variants of the disorder. For example, there is one report of two brothers with Fanconi anemia with no accompanying congenital abnormalities.[34] In this family, a culture of fibroblasts from both the mother and a sister showed increased susceptibility to malignant transformation in vitro; this feature may be useful in diagnosis of the carrier state.

Laboratory Findings and Correlations with Disease

HEMATOLOGY.   Peripheral blood abnormalities generally do not manifest themselves until 5 to 10 years after birth[37,52] when anemia, neutropenia, and thrombocytopenia may occur. Both anisocytosis and poikilocytosis are seen. There is a marked increase in Hb F, with a resultant marked decrease in Hb A. Osmotic fragility is increased, as is the erythrocyte sedimentation rate (although this may be simply a reflection of the anemia).[37,52] Occasionally the bone marrow in these patients is initially described as normocellular if the condition is diagnosed early, but invariably, it becomes hypoplastic and eventually aplastic.[52]

CYTOGENETICS.   These patients may have multiple chromosomal abnormalities, including ring chromosomes, translocations, dicentric forms, and spontaneous breaks.[17,34,37,52] In contrast to the late appearance of peripheral blood abnormalities years after birth, chromosomal abnormalities can be demonstrated at birth in lymphocytes, myeloid cells, fibroblasts, and other body tissues.[37,52]

Effects of Treatment on Laboratory Results and Prognosis

Before the advent of androgen therapy, the prognosis of patients with Fanconi anemia was poor, with a life expectancy of 2 to 4 years after the appearance of hematologic symptoms.[34,37,52] The use of androgens to stimulate erythropoiesis, accompanied by corticosteroids, has made it possible to maintain a reasonable Hb level for a period of time,[37] but the disease nevertheless progresses to bone marrow aplasia. Death is most often secondary to hemorrhage or infection and only rarely to the results of severe anemia.[34]

Bone marrow transplantation is a possibility. However, the widespread chromosomal damage in all body tissues still leaves the patient vulnerable to malignant disease.[37] The multiple chromosomal defects, particularly the translocations, are believed to predispose these patients to the development of acute myeloid leukemia (and rarely, other malignancies).[17,34,37] The patient's family also is at increased risk of leukemia because Fanconi anemia is hereditary.[17]

Acquired Pure Red Cell Aplasia

Pure red cell aplasia (PRCA) is a rare condition that may be inherited or acquired as a primary or secondary disorder (Table 11-6). The inherited form of PRCA is known as Diamond-Blackfan anemia and will be discussed later in this chapter. The acquired form is seen primarily in individuals older than 40 years of age[43] and is characterized by a severe anemia with normal to slightly decreased peripheral blood leukocyte and platelet counts. In the bone marrow overall cellularity is normal, as are granulopoiesis and thrombopoiesis. However, there is a severe decrease in erythroid elements; sometimes almost no erythroid elements are seen.

Pathophysiology

The etiology of primary PRCA involves either an idiopathic or an immune mechanism. Some patients have an immunoglobulin inhibitor of erythroid precursors such that *in vitro* incubation of a patient's own serum and marrow cells inhibits erythroid growth. In the absence of the patient's serum the patient's erythroid cells do grow. Patients have increased erythropoietin levels. Much less common with respect to an immune etiology is an inhibitor of erythropoietin; such individuals have little or no erythropoietin.[43,44,70]

Pure red cell aplasia may also be secondary to a variety of etiologic agents (see Table 11-6). Probably the most significant association is that with benign thymomas (tumors of the thymus gland).[43,44] Twenty nine percent of these patients have a remission of their anemia when the thymoma is resected, suggesting a primary relation between the two. The frequencies of primary PRCA and PRCA associated with thymoma are about the same.

There are a variety of other immunologic associations with PRCA, including the fact that some patients have antinuclear antibodies, some a spike on protein electrophoresis, and some hypogammaglobulinemia. Other etiologic agents are drugs, chemicals, and infections, and the aplastic crisis of hemolytic anemia. In contrast to the first three etiologies, the aplastic crisis of hemolytic anemia is usually acute and self-limited, requiring no therapy unless the degree of anemia warrants transfusion.[43]

Clinical Presentation

The anemia develops insidiously, and the onset is so gradual that the patient effectively compensates. Thus, by the time a patient presents with symptoms, the anemia usually is severe.[70] The only constant clinical finding is extreme pallor; a significant number of patients have splenomegaly, hepatomegaly, or both, but this may be a consequence of the hemosiderosis that follows the multiple red cell transfusions required for treatment.[43]

Laboratory Findings and Correlations with Disease

HEMATOLOGY.   In symptomatic patients there is a severe normocytic, normochromic anemia with the reticulocyte count greatly depressed or even 0%. The leukocyte and platelet counts are usually normal, although they may be mildly depressed. The leukocyte differential usually is normal. The bone marrow is normal except for the extreme decrease in or even absence of erythroid precursors.[43,44]

CHEMISTRY.   Serum iron and percent transferrin saturation are increased because of the multiple red cell transfusions. Erythropoietin levels are increased in most patients as the erythropoietic control mechanism attempts to stimulate erythrocyte production, which is impossible without erythroid precursors.

Effects of Treatment on Laboratory Results

A significant number of patients undergo a spontaneous remission, in which hematologic measurements return to normal, sometimes after years of therapy. The mainstay of therapy is red cell transfusion to maintain a reasonable erythrocyte mass. Because of the high incidence of thymomas, the clinician usually searches for a thymoma, and if possible, this tumor is removed, which often results in improved clinical and laboratory conditions. Immunosuppressive therapy has proven beneficial in some patients; therefore, a clinical trial is justified. Androgens have also been effective in some patients in stimulating erythropoiesis.[43,44]

If patients do not respond to therapy, such that long-term maintenance with transfusions is necessary, they may eventually succumb to either hepatitis or hemosiderosis.[44]

Diamond-Blackfan Anemia (Congenital Pure Red Cell Aplasia)

Diamond-Blackfan anemia (congenital hypoplastic anemia or PRCA) is a rare congenital disorder that was first described in 1938. It is defined as a normochromic, normocytic anemia with normal leukocyte and platelet counts and a marked decrease in marrow erythroblasts. The diagnosis is usually made in infancy or early childhood.[1,16,56]

The etiology of Diamond-Blackfan anemia is unknown, partly because there are so few patients available for study. However, one *in vitro* study, in culture, demonstrated a lack of responsiveness of the patient's marrow sample to added erythropoietin. In other words, the few colony-forming units–erythroid (CFU-E) in the culture were insensitive to erythropoietin stimulation.[56] Another study showed that patient lymphocytes were able to inhibit *in vitro* erythropoiesis of normal bone marrow, even in the presence of added erythropoietin.[35] Serum from the patients did not inhibit erythropoiesis. Therefore, in at least some patients there may be an immunologic etiology.

TABLE 11-6. Classification of Pure Red Cell Aplasias

Acquired
  Primary
    Idiopathic
    Immune mechanism
      Immunoglobulin inhibitor to RBC precursors
      Erythropoietin inhibitor
  Secondary
    Benign thymomas
    Drugs
    Chemicals
    Infections
    Hemolytic anemia—aplastic crisis
Congenital
  Diamond-Blackfan anemia

Genetics

Whether this anemia is congenital (simply present at birth because of some unknown cause) or truly inherited is not clear. However, there is growing evidence that it may be inherited because of reports of a few family members who have the disorder, and the fact that the disorder becomes evident at such an early age.

Clinical Presentation

There rarely are any significant symptoms or physical findings in this disorder. Pallor may be evident at birth and is almost always evident by the age of 1 year.

A study of 200 cases of Diamond-Blackfan anemia revealed 17 patients with abnormal thumbs.[5] In another study all patients with Diamond-Blackfan anemia who were more than 14 years of age demonstrated retarded growth, bone age retardation, and failure of secondary sexual maturation.[16] Osteoporosis has also been reported. Marked growth retardation may be the result of both intermittent anemia and hemosiderosis; the latter eventually interferes with liver function and endocrine maturation. Characteristically, Diamond-Blackfan patients do not demonstrate renal abnormalities.[16]

Laboratory Findings and Correlations with Disease

The diagnosis is usually made in infancy, with Hb values ranging from as low as 1.7 g/dL to 9.4 g/dL in a newborn. The expected increase in nucleated red blood cells is not found on the peripheral blood film. The anemia is usually normocytic, normochromic with normal red cell morphology, although occasional poikilocytes have been reported; reticulocytes are less than 1%, and often less than 0.2%. Similarly, the RPI is extremely low, indicating a poor erythropoietic response to the anemia. Platelet counts are normal for the age of the patient, as are the leukocyte count and differential.[16] The bone marrow is cellular with a marked decrease in red cell precursors.[16,35] Those erythroid precursors present are primarily pronormoblasts,[56] with no megaloblastic changes seen. Myeloid cells, megakaryocytes, and lymphocytes are normal in the marrow. Erythropoietin levels have been reported to be elevated;[42] however, red cell survival is normal.[16] The percentage of Hb F is elevated.

Clinical and Laboratory Differentiation of Diamond-Blackfan and Fanconi Anemias

The reader may find differentiation of the two hereditary forms of bone marrow failure somewhat difficult. Table 11-7 is provided to summarize and clarify the principal differentiating factors.

Effects of Treatment on Laboratory Results and Prognosis

Red cell transfusions are one of the mainstays of therapy and may be necessary every 3 to 6 weeks to prevent the symptoms of anemia. Occasionally, after months to years of red cell transfusions, patients undergo a spontaneous remission, which may or may not be maintained.[16] Forty to fifty percent of patients respond to corticosteroid therapy,[16,35] supporting a lymphocyte abnormality as the basis for the disorder in some patients.

TABLE 11-7. Principal Clinical and Laboratory Factors for Differentiation of Congenital Disorders Causing Bone Marrow Failure

CLINICAL/LABORATORY FEATURES	FANCONI ANEMIA	DIAMOND-BLACKFAN ANEMIA
Hematologic classification	Aplastic anemia	Pure red cell aplasia
Brown skin pigmentation	Common	Uncommon
Thumb abnormalities	Common	Uncommon
Renal abnormalities	Common	Uncommon
Onset of hematologic abnormalities (years of age)	5 to 10	<1
Bone marrow biopsy	Hypoplastic to aplastic	Cellular
Bone marrow aspirate	Pancytopenia	Marked decrease only in erythroid precursors
Peripheral blood	Pancytopenia	Decrease in RBC; normal WBC and platelets
Cytogenetics	Multiple chromosomal abnormalities in many tissues	No associated abnormalities

Occasionally splenectomy may be appropriate if hypersplenism develops secondary to congestive heart failure. However, a number of patients have succumbed to overwhelming infections after splenectomy. Other possible complications of treatment with multiple transfusions are hepatitis and hemosiderosis, both of which contribute to liver failure.[16]

Recently bone marrow transplantation has been successful in four patients with congenital PRCA, and this is now seen as a potential curative therapy.[47] However, the overall prognosis remains poor,[1,16] with most of the complications being related to the anemia itself or secondary to hemosiderosis.

Myelophthisic Anemia

Myelophthisic anemia is a common finding in patients with carcinoma; it is present in as many as 94% of these patients.[14] It is most often a hypoproliferative anemia classified as the anemia of chronic inflammation (chronic disease) (Chap. 13).[14,26] In some patients the degree of anemia correlates with the tumor burden. The greater the tumor load, the more severe the anemia.[26] In others, however, there is no good correlation between tumor burden and the degree of anemia.[78]

Pathophysiology

Myelophthisic anemia results when the bone marrow is replaced by abnormal cells;[26,46,74] most often, this term refers to replacement by metastatic carcinoma, although some authors include the hematologic malignancies (leukemia and lymphoma) (see Parts VII and VIII of this text) and myelofibrosis (Chap. 35). There also are nonmalignant conditions that can invade the marrow and cause the same picture, including miliary tuberculosis and granulomas.[74,78]

The term *myelophthisic anemia* is sometimes used interchangeably with leukoerythroblastic reaction[14,33,74,78]; however, they are not synonymous. The leukoerythroblastic reaction is the presence of circulating nucleated red blood cells (NRBC) and immature leukocytes in the peripheral blood. This reaction may not be associated with anemia. If anemia is present, the quantity of NRBC is much greater than expected for the degree of anemia. Stippled or polychromatophilic red cells or both may also be present. The peripheral blood granulocytic shift to the left is most frequently associated with the appearance of bands, metamyelocytes, and myelocytes; only rarely are more immature granulocytes encountered.[26,64,78] The release of immature granulocytes to the peripheral blood is also inappropriate; that is, there generally is no evident infection to explain it. The mechanism for inappropriate release of immature erythroid and myeloid cells is not understood but may be related to damage to the underlying marrow stroma by invasion of abnormal cells (myelophthisis).

Historically, a leukoerythroblastic reaction was associated with metastatic carcinoma.[2,14,74] Conversely, it was accepted that if a patient had carcinoma metastatic to the bone marrow, a leukoerythroblastic reaction would invariably occur.[13,14,46] However, neither of these assumptions is necessarily true. In patients with proven bone marrow metastases, only 24% to 58% had a blood picture of leukoerythroblastosis.[14,46] Another study of 340 carcinoma patients with known marrow metastases showed that only 0.9% had a leukoerythroblastic reaction.[2] This was true even when a large part of the marrow had been replaced by tumor. Most studies do show patients with known marrow metastases to be anemic, with variable leukocyte and platelet counts, although most often, a mild thrombocytopenia is seen. However, leukoerythroblastosis *per se* is not a common finding. If leukoerythroblastosis is found in a patient with known metastases, it is likely that marrow metastases are present.[14,74] Leukoerythroblastosis is often found among patients in whom the disease is far advanced, thus forecasting a grave prognosis.

In contrast, leukoerythroblastosis may be found in patients with no evidence of malignancy. In a study of 215 patients showing a leukoerythroblastic reaction in the peripheral blood, 37% had no malignancy. Diagnoses in these patients ranged from hemolytic anemia, immune thrombocytopenic purpura, and iron deficiency anemia to infectious mononucleosis. The 63% with malignancy included cases of leukemia and lymphoma.[74] Thus, a leukoerythroblastic reaction is not synonymous with myelophthisic anemia, as was once thought.

Differential Diagnosis

The carcinomas most likely to metastasize to bone marrow are those of the breast, prostate, lung (especially the small cell or oat cell types), neuroblastoma (children), adrenal cortex, thyroid, kidney, gastrointestinal tract, and genitourinary tract and malignant melanoma.[14,26,33,46,78] However, carcinoma at any site has the potential of metastasizing to the marrow, possibly causing marrow failure. Marrow biopsy is the best method of demonstrating metastatic tumor[14,26,46,78] (Chap. 29), as a biopsy provides an overall view of marrow structure, cellularity, and any for-eign infiltrates. From 70% to 94% of patients with known marrow involvement will be positive with a biopsy, whereas only 45% are positive with an aspirate.[14] In one study most false-negative biopsies were attributed to an inadequate specimen.[46] However, because there may be false-negative biopsies, it is important to do both a biopsy and an aspirate when searching for metastatic carcinoma in the marrow.

Effects of Treatment on Laboratory Results and Prognosis

Treatment and prognosis depend on the underlying cause of the myelophthisic anemia. See the chapters in Parts VII and VIII of this text for more information.

ANEMIA OF SYSTEMIC DISORDERS

A variety of systemic disorders may be associated with anemia. In this section, the anemia of chronic renal disease and the anemia of several endocrine disorders (hypothyroidism, hypopituitarism, adrenal abnormalities, and hypogonadism) will be considered, along with the anemia of pregnancy, all of which may be associated with temporary hormonal variations.

Anemia of Chronic Renal Disease

A hypoproliferative anemia that can be severe almost invariably occurs in patients with chronic renal failure (CRF).[15,20,73] Indeed, anemia is almost as frequent a finding as an elevated blood urea nitrogen (BUN) concentration.

Pathophysiology

The etiology of anemia in CRF is complex. It is related to the etiology of the renal disease itself; the failure of the renal excretory function, with resultant accumulation of waste products in plasma; and failure of renal production and release of erythropoietin.[20,39,62] The principal cause is the inadequate marrow response to anemia because of decreased production of erythropoietin.[15,20,22] In fact, if the marrow were stimulated with adequate levels of erythropoietin, very few uremic patients would be anemic, for the marrow could easily compensate with increased production for the slight shortening of red cell survival and the modest blood loss.[15,20] However, there is some evidence that the marrow of these patients may not be able to respond normally to any form of erythropoietin,[20,73] suggesting a possible erythropoietin toxin,[73] adding to the complexity of the anemia.

Clinical Presentation

The patient may have all the signs and symptoms of anemia, depending on its severity. These symptoms may be the patient's chief complaint because development of renal disease is slow. One third to one half of patients with CRF experience gastrointestinal or gynecologic bleeding, with resultant blood loss, because of abnormal platelet function, and this loss contributes to the anemia.[20]

Laboratory Findings and Correlations with Disease

HEMATOLOGY.   Uremia, the accumulation of waste products, is associated with shortened red cell survival and a resultant mild hemolytic anemia[26,39] in as many as 70% of patients with renal failure.[15] The hematocrit usually falls between 0.15 and 0.30 L/L[4] and the anemia is generally normocytic, normochromic[19] with normal indices.[39] Because of the diseased kidneys, plasma volume is increased,[20] resulting in an artifactually decreased hematocrit. Thus, Hb and hematocrit levels are difficult to use as accurate measures of anemia.

Although erythrocyte morphology usually is normal, the uremic condition occasionally results in abnormal erythrocyte forms, particularly burr cells and possibly some helmet cells and fragments.[15,20] The reticulocyte count usually is normal unless the serum creatinine is significantly elevated, with a corresponding higher degree of anemia.[66] Leukocyte counts usually are normal, and platelet counts are normal to slightly elevated. Accumulated waste products may coat platelets, causing abnormal tests of platelet function (Chaps. 59 and 61).

BONE MARROW.   The marrow generally is moderately hypercellular, and erythroid hyperplasia may be present. However, erythroid hypoplasia has been associated with acute renal failure.[54]

CHEMISTRY.   There is a rough correlation between the degree of renal insufficiency, as measured by the creatinine level, and the hematocrit. The higher the serum creatinine, the lower the hematocrit and the more severe the anemia.[20,22,39,62] The degree of shortening of red cell survival is directly proportional to the creatinine level.

Renal disease is associated with low serum iron but normal total iron binding capacity (TIBC).[20,39] Administration of radiolabeled iron reveals a rapid clearance of iron from the plasma.[39] Iron is believed to be stored preferentially in the liver and spleen rather than in the marrow. This is likely to contribute to the low serum iron. There is depressed marrow utilization of the labeled iron,[15,39] as it does not reappear, as expected, in circulating red cells. Also contributing to low serum iron is the routine loss of blood and iron along with folate in the disposable hemodialysis coils during treatments.[39]

Effects of Treatment on Laboratory Results

Transfusions are not indicated for most patients with this disorder because of the risks of hepatitis, acquired immune deficiency syndrome, and volume overload, which increases the risk of pulmonary edema.[39] With good dialysis therapy, erythropoiesis does improve slightly, although it takes several months or even years of treatment for the hematocrit to rise to reasonable levels.[22] Uremia causes considerable fatigue, but this is relieved by dialysis. These patients tolerate hematocrits just above 0.15 L/L fairly well.[22,39]

After successful allotransplantation of a kidney, erythropoietin levels rise to normal with progressive normalization of the hematocrit.[55] Just prior to rejection of a renal graft, should this occur, erythropoietin levels increase, and NRBCs may appear in the circulation. This change is probably useful in the diagnosis of chronic renal graft rejection.[55]

A recent report has indicated that recombinant human erythropoietin (r-HuEPO) is valuable in the treatment of the anemia of chronic renal disease.[23] Soon after infusion, there is a reticulocytosis, followed by a gradual elevation of the Hb level. More clinical trials are necessary to evaluate this innovative therapy.

Anemia of Endocrine Disorders

It is well known that hormones play a role in hemopoiesis (Fig. 11-3). Thus, patients with various endocrine abnormalities may be anemic, although the incidence is low. Anemia may develop secondary to interference with the normal action of hormones on red cell production. Hormones normally stimulate erythropoiesis by exerting a direct effect on marrow stem cells; a stimulatory action on erythropoietin production; an augmenting effect on erythropoietin; or an indirect influence on the release of erythropoietin consequent to the changes in general metabolic rate induced by various hormones.[71]

Most commonly the anemia seen in endocrine disorders is mild, and red cells are usually normocytic, normochromic, with the marrow showing only decreased erythroid production with normal myeloid and megakaryocyte production.[3,36,45,71] Thus, these conditions are classified as hypoproliferative disorders.

Hypothyroidism

Oxygen requirements are influenced by a number of factors, including thyroid function.[71,77] As the body's metabolic rate decreases with diminished thyroid function, its needs for O_2 decrease. Thus, one third to one half of untreated hypothyroid patients are anemic.[71] Anemia seems more likely to occur in hypothyroid males than females.[36] The incidence of anemia in hypothyroidism may even be underestimated, because there is a decrease in plasma volume, which may mask a mild anemia.[3,71]

Anemia, when found, is most often a result of the thyroid deficiency alone but can be seen in combination with other disorders that can result in anemia, such as iron deficiency and pernicious anemia. Hypothyroidism and pernicious anemia are both thought to be autoimmune disorders. Thyroid antibodies occur in a high proportion of patients with pernicious anemia, and a significant number of patients with thyroid disease have antibodies to stomach gastric mucosa,[71] suggesting pernicious anemia.

LABORATORY FINDINGS AND CORRELATIONS WITH DISEASE.   In patients with hypothyroidism in whom the etiology of anemia is thyroid deficiency alone, the red cells tend to be large. Patients may have a macrocytic anemia in spite of normal B_{12} and folate levels.[36] The erythrocytes are normochromic.

Acanthocytes may be seen, but they usually are rare and can easily be missed on routine inspection of the blood film. Although acanthocytes have increased cholesterol in their cell membranes, there is no correlation between the presence of acanthocytes and serum cholesterol levels,[36] as these cells are found in association with both high and low

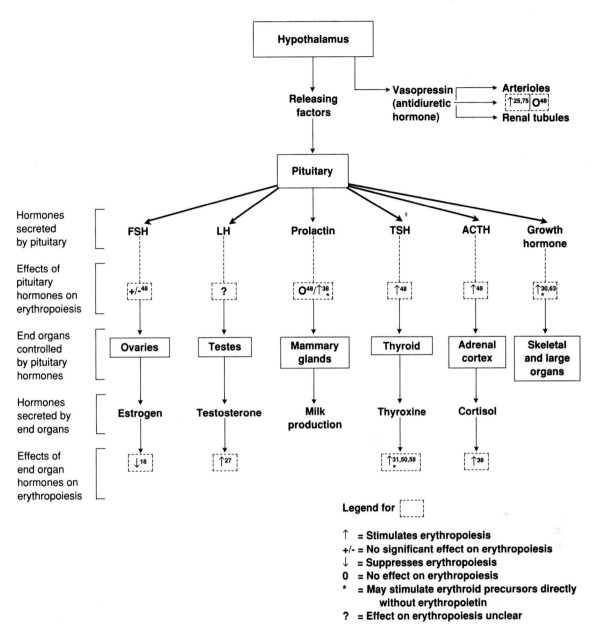

FIG. 11-3. Normal hormonal effects on erythropoiesis. FSH = follicle-stimulating hormone; LH = luteinizing hormone; TSH = thyroid-stimulating hormone, ACTH = adrenocorticotropin.

serum cholesterol. Patients with thyroid deficiency characteristically have elevated cholesterol levels.

In most anemias, red cell 2,3-diphosphoglycerate (2,3-DPG) levels are increased, which permits increased delivery of O_2 to the tissues. However, in the anemia of thyroid deficiency, red cell 2,3-DPG levels, as well as the P_{50}, are normal. Thus, there is no shift in the oxyhemoglobin dissociation curve, which supports the hypothesis that there is a diminished need for O_2 in these patients and that this may be the etiology of the anemia.

EFFECTS OF TREATMENT ON LABORATORY RE-SULTS. When these patients are treated with thyroxin, their MCV falls and stabilizes at a more normal value,[36] whereas their Hb slowly rises.[45] With therapy the Hb may

initially fall because of plasma volume normalization, thus creating a relative anemia. Complete hematologic recovery may take as long as 6 months.[3]

Hypopituitarism

The anemia frequently seen in patients with decreased pituitary function may be a result of the deficiency of pituitary hormones, which normally control the thyroid, gonads, or adrenals,[71] among other organ systems (see Fig. 11-3). The anemia is caused by reduced metabolic demands and a resultant decrease in stimulation of erythropoietin production[3] and is mild to moderate, with normocytic, normochromic red cell morphology.

The hypothalamus secretes vasopressin, which stimulates erythropoiesis (see Fig. 11-3).[25] Releasing factors from the hypothalamus act on the pituitary gland, which in turn releases a number of hormones that may or may not affect erythropoiesis and also act on end-organs of the pituitary. These organs secrete hormones that may also have effects on erythropoiesis (see Fig. 11-3).

Note that growth hormone,[30] thyroxine,[31,50] and prolactin[38] have been reported to stimulate erythropoiesis directly (i.e., independent of erythropoietin). Other hormones may stimulate erythropoiesis by stimulating endogenous erythropoietin production. Thus, the anemia of hypopituitarism is believed to result from a dysfunction in the normal conditioning role that pituitary hormones exert on the secretion of testosterone by the testes, thyroxine by the thyroid gland, and cortisol by the adrenal cortex because these are the three main hormones produced by pituitary gland end-organs that stimulate erythropoiesis,[27,38,58,63] as indicated in the last section of Figure 11-3. Pituitary dysfunction results in a deficiency of these three hormones and consequently anemia. In addition, a deficiency of the pituitary hormones themselves may contribute to the anemia.

Treatment of anemia in hypopituitarism has included administration of various combinations of pituitary hormones, hormones from the adrenal and thyroid glands, and sex hormones.

Adrenal Abnormalities

Abnormalities in the secretion of adrenocortical steroids, such as cortisol, have multiple effects on blood cells, most markedly on circulating lymphocytes and eosinophils. Adrenal hormones also have an effect on red cell production, although the mechanism is not understood. The effects are dependent on the type of adrenal abnormality.

Hypoadrenalism results in Addison disease, and hyperadrenalism results in Cushing disease. Patients with Addison disease, where there is a decrease in adrenal production of cortisol, are characteristically anemic. However, with the adrenal insufficiency, there is a reduction in plasma volume,[3,71] and this may mask a mild anemia in these patients. Often, there is also a granulocytopenia and lymphocytosis.[65]

In contrast, patients with Cushing disease have an increased secretion of cortisol accompanied by normal to high normal erythrocyte counts. Rarely, these patients are polycythemic.[71] Generally, neutrophils and platelets are increased in Cushing disease, whereas lymphocytes and eosinophils demonstrate absolute decreases in their number.[3,71]

Hypogonadism

Hypogonadism is characterized by retarded growth and sexual development secondary to a deficiency of the male sex hormone testosterone, which exerts significant influence over the male genital tract. Testosterone is an androgen (male sex hormone) produced primarily by the testes. In the endocrine disorder of hypogonadism, the reduction in testosterone secretion causes erythrocyte values to fall within the female reference range.

When normal boys reach puberty, the red cell mass increases to levels approximately 10% to 13% higher than those of women. This is attributed to testicular secretion of testosterone. Androgens, most notably testosterone, have the ability to increase erythropoiesis.[3,71] The primary mechanism for this seems to be increased stimulation of renal erythropoietin production.[3] In contrast to androgens, the female sex hormone estrogen has been shown to cause suppression of erythropoiesis in female rats.[18]

Therapeutic administration of androgens increases urinary excretion of erythropoietin and increases reticulocyte production, with a subsequent increase in red cell mass. This finding has led to the therapeutic use of androgens in anemia; occasional remissions in both children and adults with aplastic anemia and various other refractory anemias are documented.[3,12,71]

Anemia of Pregnancy

Anemia in pregnancy is most often a result of iron deficiency because of the significant increase in iron demand, or, much less commonly, of folate deficiency. However, even in a woman who is well maintained during pregnancy, a relative anemia usually develops around the 8th week and increases slowly until the 32nd to 34th week, when it becomes stable, although anemia is commonly present at the time of delivery. There is an expansion of both red cell mass and plasma volume during pregnancy, the mechanisms for which are poorly understood. The increased plasma volume is more pronounced[49] so the anemia may be caused by dilutional effects.[49,60] The anemia is moderate in severity, with Hb concentrations seldom going below 10 g/dL. The life span of the red cells is normal, with increased production of red cells leading to an increased red cell mass.[61] The expansion of total blood volume may be a physiologic protective mechanism against the effects of excessive blood loss at the time of delivery (average 450 mL)[49] and in the immediate postpartum period.[49,60]

CHAPTER SUMMARY

Aplastic anemia is associated with an absolute failure of the bone marrow. It may be inherited or acquired, either for unknown reasons (idiopathic) or secondary to drugs, chemicals, radiation, or other mechanisms. It is diagnosed by a hypocellular bone marrow in which hematopoietic tissue is replaced by fat. The peripheral blood is pancytopenic with granulocytes below 0.5×10^9/L, platelets below 20×10^9/L, and anemia with less than 1% reticulocytes. Classically, no immature leukocytes or erythrocytes are found on the blood film. Many other hematologic disorders may be associated with pancytopenia; however, usually the marrow in these conditions is hyperplastic or displays some other distinguishing characteristic (see Table 11-4).

Patients with aplastic anemia are at great risk for infection, bleeding, and signs and symptoms of anemia. The treatment of choice is a bone marrow transplantation. Antithymocyte globulin and cyclosporin A are alternatives.

Congenital aplastic anemia is called Fanconi anemia. The laboratory findings are similar to those in acquired aplastic anemia except that chromosome abnormalities that predispose these patients to the development of acute myeloid leukemia are common in Fanconi anemia but uncommon in acquired aplastic anemia. The onset of abnormal hematologic findings is usually between 5 and 10 years of age.

Pure red cell aplasia (PRCA) is an acquired or inherited disorder, generally affecting only the erythroid cell line, which results in anemia. The marrow is normocellular; however, erythroid elements are severely decreased. The reticulocyte count may be 0%. Acquired PRCA is classified as either primary (immune related or idiopathic) or secondary (benign thymomas, drugs, chemicals, infections, or hemolytic crisis). Red cell transfusions are a mainstay of therapy, and androgens to stimulate erythropoiesis have been used effectively.

Congenital PRCA is known as Diamond-Blackfan anemia. It usually is diagnosed in infancy or early childhood. Laboratory findings are similar to those of acquired PRCA. This disorder has many characteristics that differentiate it from Fanconi anemia (see Table 11-7).

Myelophthisic anemia results when the bone marrow is replaced by abnormal cells in conditions such as leukemia or metastatic carcinoma. Myelophthisic anemia and leukoerythroblastic reaction are not synonymous. Leukoerythroblastosis refers to the presence of immature red and white cells in the peripheral blood. Leukoerythroblastosis is not common in patients with metastatic carcinoma to the marrow.

Systemic diseases can also cause anemia. Chronic renal disease may cause anemia secondary to decreased erythropoietin production by the kidney, resulting in lack of marrow erythroid production. Uremia in renal disease may cause poikilocytes, including burr cells, helmet cells, or fragments.

Endocrine disorders may also cause anemia because endocrine hormones play an important role in hemopoiesis. Figure 11-3 summarizes this role. Pregnancy may cause anemia, even with adequate nutritional support, as a result of changes in the circulating red cell mass and plasma volume.

CASE STUDY 11-1

A 25-year-old man was admitted to the hospital in obvious distress. He had multiple, deep soft-tissue abscesses, which were cultured and later grew *Bacillus* spp. A blood culture taken at the same time was likewise positive for *Bacillus*. He had a fever of 99.8°F but no hepatosplenomegaly or lymphadenopathy. He had had a physical and laboratory evaluation 6 months previously, both of which were normal. At the time of presentation, results of his CBC were as follows: WBC 1.8 × 10^9/L; RBC 3.07 × 10^12/L; Hb 9.0 g/dL; HCT 0.27 L/L; MCV 88 fL; MCH 29 pg; MCHC 33 g/dL; RDW 13.6; platelets 19 × 10^9/L; reticulocytes: none seen; manual differential: neutrophils 5% (0.08 × 10^9/L); lymphocytes 94% (1.7 × 10^9/L); monocytes 1% (0.02 × 10^9/L); RBC normocytic, normochromic; platelets markedly decreased; buffy coat preparation: no immature cells seen.

His bone marrow aspirate was markedly hypocellular, consisting primarily of fat cells with a few stromal cells, lymphocytes, and plasma cells. The bone marrow biopsy demonstrated less than 5% cellularity.

1. Given the peripheral blood pancytopenia, which of the following diagnoses is most likely and why: megaloblastic anemia, aplastic anemia, Fanconi anemia, acute leukemia, or myelodysplastic syndrome?
2. Which of the following would be the preferred method of treatment if available: chemotherapy, red cell transfusions, red cell and platelet transfusions, bone marrow transplantation, or irradiation? Why?
3. Are the results of the marrow aspirate sufficient to make the diagnosis, or is it important to have the biopsy results also? Explain briefly.
4. List a minimum of two questions that would be helpful to ask concerning the patient's history. These questions should be helpful in elucidating the etiology of the condition.
5. The patient was given two courses of antithymocyte globulin but showed no response. Does this result support an immune etiology for his condition? Explain briefly.

CASE STUDY 11-2

A 25-year-old man was normal hematologically until the age of 10 years, when he was found to have "aplastic anemia." At that time, cytogenetic studies on peripheral blood lymphocytes showed a single chromosomal abnormality. He was treated for 3 years with androgens and corticosteroids but remained pancytopenic.

At the time of this admission, he complained of acute abdominal pain. Abdominal ultrasound showed a mass behind the right kidney. A laparotomy was performed, an abscess found, and a 30-cm segment of the small bowel was resected. The patient did well on antibiotics for 2 weeks but suddenly developed a fever with no leukocytosis. Hematologic studies revealed: WBC 1.3 × 10^9/L; RBC 3.27 × 10^12/L; Hb 11.0 g/dL; HCT 0.33 L/L; MCV 101 fL; MCH 34 pg; MCHC 33 g/dL; platelets 32 × 10^9/L; manual differential: neutrophils 62% (0.8 × 10^9/L); lymphocytes 23% (0.3 × 10^9/L): monocytes 15% (0.2 × 10^9/L); RBC normocytic, normochromic; and platelets markedly decreased.

A bone marrow aspirate and biopsy were performed. The marrow was markedly hypoplastic with patchy cellularity; there appeared to be a slight increase in myeloblasts. In contrast, his marrow 6 months before this was essentially aplastic. Cytogenetic studies showed additional chromosomal abnormalities, all translocations or deletions. Thus, it was speculated that the patient was developing an acute leukemia.

1. What is the most likely diagnosis: megaloblastic anemia, aplastic anemia, Fanconi anemia, or a myelodysplastic syndrome?
2. Is this an inherited or acquired disorder? If inherited, what is the probable genetic pattern of inheritance?
3. Name two other body systems that would be expected to show abnormalities in this patient.
4. What is the prognosis for patients with this disease? Is progression to an acute leukemia an unexpected event?

REFERENCES

1. Aase JM, Smith DW: Congenital anemia and triphalangeal thumbs: A new syndrome. J Pediatr 74:471, 1969
2. Abasov IT: The state of peripheral blood in cancer metastases to bone marrow. Haematologica 2:381, 1968
3. Adamson JW: Anemia of endocrine disorders. In Lichtman MA (ed): Hematology and Oncology, pp 44. New York, Grune & Stratton, 1980.
4. Adamson JW, Eschbach J, Finch CA: The kidney and erythropoiesis. Am J Med 44:725, 1968
5. Alter BP: Thumbs and anemia. Pediatrics 62:613, 1978
6. Bacigalupo A, Frassoni F, van Lint MT et al: Cyclosporin A in marrow transplantation for leukemia and aplastic anemia. Exp Hematol 13:244, 1985
7. Bentley SA: Bone marrow connective tissue and the haemopoietic microenvironment. Br J Haematol 50:1, 1982
8. Bloom GE, Diamond LK: Prognostic value of fetal hemoglobin levels in acquired aplastic anemia. N Engl J Med 278:304, 1968
9. Bridges R, Pineo G, Blahey W: Cyclosporin A for the treatment of aplastic anemia refractory to antithymocyte globulin. Am J Hematol 26:83, 1987
10. Camitta BM, Storb R, Thomas ED: Aplastic anemia: Pathogenesis, diagnosis, treatment, and prognosis. N Engl J Med 306:645, 1982
11. Camitta BM, Storb R, Thomas ED: Aplastic anemia: Pathogenesis, diagnosis, treatment, and prognosis. N Engl J Med 306:712, 1982
12. Camitta BM, Thomas ED, Nathan DG et al: A prospective study of androgens and bone marrow transplantation for treatment of severe aplastic anemia. Blood 53:504, 1979
13. Chen HP, Walz DV: Leukemoid reaction in the bone marrow, associated with malignant neoplasms. Am J Clin Pathol 29:345, 1979
14. Contreras E, Ellis LD, Lee RE: Value of the bone marrow biopsy in the diagnosis of metastatic carcinoma. Cancer 29:778, 1972
15. Desforges JF: Anemia in uremia. Arch Intern Med 126:808, 1970
16. Diamond LK, Allen DM, Magill FB: Congenital (erythroid)

hypoplastic anemia, a 25 year study. Am J Dis Child 102:403, 1961; Adv Pediatr 22:349, 1976

17. Dosik H, Hsu LY, Todaro GJ et al: Leukemia in Fanconi's anemia: Cytogenetic and tumor virus susceptibility studies. Blood 36:341, 1970

18. Dukes PP, Goldwasser E: Inhibition of erythropoiesis by estrogens. Endocrinology 69:21, 1961

19. Eklund SG, Johansson SV, Strandberg O: Anemia in uremia. Acta Med Scand 190:435, 1971

20. Erslev AJ: Anemia of chronic renal disease. Arch Intern Med 126:774, 1970

21. Erslev AJ: Aplastic anemia. In Williams WJ, Beutler E, Erslev AJ et al (eds): Hematology, 3rd ed. New York, McGraw-Hill, 1983

22. Eschbach JW, Adamson JW, Cook JD: Disorders of red blood cell production in uremia. Arch Intern Med 126:812, 1970

23. Eschbach JW, Egrie JL, Downing MR et al: Correction of the anemia of end-stage renal disease with recombinant human erythropoietin. N Engl J Med 316:73, 1987

24. Feig SA: Aplastic pancytopenia. In Lichtman MA (ed): Hematology and Oncology, pp 156. New York, Grune & Stratton, 1980

25. Fisher JW: Erythropoietin: Pharmacology, biogenesis and control of production. Pharmacol Rev 24:459, 1972

26. Frei E: Hematologic complications of cancer. In Holland JF, Frie E (eds): Cancer Medicine, pp 1085. Philadelphia, Lea & Febiger, 1973

27. Fried W, Gurney CW: The erythropoietic-stimulating effects of androgens. Ann NY Acad Sci 149:356, 1978

28. Gale RP, Reisner Y: The role of bone marrow transplants after nuclear accidents. Lancet 1:923, 1988

29. Gascon P, Zoumbos N, Young N: Analysis of natural killer cells in patients with aplastic anemia. Blood 67:1349, 1986

30. Golde DW, Bersch N, Li CH: Growth hormone: Species-specific stimulation of erythropoiesis in vitro. Science 196:1112, 1977

31. Golde DW, Bersch N, Chopra IJ et al: Thyroid hormones stimulate erythropoiesis in vitro. Br J Haematol 37:173, 1977

32. Greenberger JS, Klassen V, Kae K et al: Effects of low dose rate irradiation on plateau phase bone marrow stromal cells in vitro: Demonstration of a new form of non-lethal, physiologic damage to support of hematopoietic stem cells. Int J Radiat Oncol Biol Phys 10:1027, 1984

33. Hansen HH, Muggia FM, Selawry OS: Bone-marrow examination in 100 consecutive patients with bronchogenic carcinoma. Lancet 2:443, 1971

34. Hirschman RJ, Shulman RR, Abuelo JG et al: Chromosomal aberrations in two cases of inherited aplastic anemia with unusual clinical features. Ann Intern Med 71:107 1969

35. Hoffman R, Zanjani ED, Vila J et al: Diamond-Blackfan syndrome: Lymphocyte-mediated suppression of erythropoiesis. Science 193:899, 1976

36. Horton L, Coburn RJ, England JM et al: The haematology of hypothyroidism. Q J Med 45:101, 1976

37. Jacobs P, Karabus C: Fanconi's anemia: A family study with 20-year follow-up including associated breast pathology. Cancer 54:1850, 1984

38. Jepson JH, Lowenstein L: The effect of testosterone, adrenal steroids and prolactin on erythropoiesis. Acta Haematol 38:292, 1967; Blood 24:726, 1964; Proc Soc Exp Biol Med 121:1077, 1966; ibid 122:457, 1966; Br J Haematol 15:465, 1968, Arch Intern Med 122:265, 1968

39. Kaye M: The anemia associated with renal disease. J Lab Clin Med 52:83, 1958

40. Kennedy MS, Deeg HJ, Storb R et al: Treatment of acute graft-versus-host disease after allogeneic marrow transplantation. Am J Med 78:978, 1985

41. Knospe WH: Aplastic anaemia: A disorder of the bone-marrow sinusoidal microcirculation rather than stem-cell failure? Lancet 1:20, 1971

42. Krantz SB: Annotation: Pure red cell aplasia. Br J Haematol 25:11, 1973; N Engl J Med 291:345, 1974

43. Krantz SB: Diagnosis and treatment of pure red cell aplasia. Med Clin North Am 60:945, 1976

44. Krantz SB: Pure red cell aplasia. In Lichtman MA (ed): Hematology and Oncology, pp 45. New York, Grune & Stratton, 1980

45. Larsson SO: Anemia and iron metabolism in hypothyroidism. Acta Med Scand 157:349, 1957

46. Leland J, Macpherson B: Hematologic findings in cases of mammary cancer metastatic to bone marrow. Am J Clin Pathol 71:31, 1979

47. Lenarsky C, Weinberg K, Guinan E et al: Bone marrow transplantation for constitutional pure red cell aplasia. Blood 71:226, 1988

48. Lindemann R, Trygstad O, Halvorsen S: Pituitary control of erythropoiesis. Scand J Haematol 6:77, 1969

49. Low JA, Johnston EE, McBride RL: Blood volume adjustments in the normal obstetric patient with particular reference to the third trimester of pregnancy. Am J Obstet Gynecol 9:356, 1965

50. Malgor LA, Blanc CC, Klainer E et al: Direct effects of thyroid hormones on bone marrow erythroid cells of rats. Blood 45:671, 1975

51. Mangan KF, Mullaney MT, Rosenfeld CS et al: In vitro evidence for disappearance of erythroid progenitor T suppressor cells following allogeneic bone marrow transplantation for severe aplastic anemia. Blood 71:144, 1988

52. McDonald R, Goldschmidt B: Pancytopenia with congenital defects (Fanconi's anaemia). Arch Dis Child 35:367, 1960

53. McGlave PB, Haake R, Miller W et al: Therapy of severe aplastic anemia in young adults and children with allogeneic bone marrow transplantation. Blood 70:1325, 1987

54. Morgan T, Innes M, Ribush N: The management of the anaemia of patients on chronic haemodialysis. Med J Aust 1:848, 1972

55. Murphy GP, Mirand EZ, Grace JT: Erythropoietin activity in anephric or renal allotransplanted man. Ann Surg 170:581, 1969

56. Nathan DG, Clarke BJ, Hillman DG et al: Erythroid precursors in congenital hypoplastic (Diamond-Blackfan) anemia. J Clin Invest 61:489, 1978

57. Nilsson LR: Chronic pancytopenia with multiple congenital abnormalities. Acta Paediatr 49:518, 1960

58. Popovic WJ, Brown JE, Adamson JW: Thyroid hormone (TH)-stimulated erythropoiesis: Mediation by a β-adrenergic receptor (abstract). Blood 48:979, 1976

59. Porwit A, Panayotides P, Mansson E et al: Cyclosporine A treatment in four cases of aplastic anemia. Blut 54:73, 1987

60. Pritchard JA: Changes in the blood volume during pregnancy and delivery. Anesthesiology 26:393, 1965

61. Pritchard JA, Adams RH: Erythrocyte production and destruction during pregnancy. Am J Obstet Gynecol 79:750, 1960

62. Radtke HW, Claussner A, Erbes PM et al: Serum erythropoietin concentration in chronic renal failure: Relationship to degree of anemia and excretory renal function. Blood 54:877, 1979

63. Rodriguez JM, Shahidi NT: Erythrocyte 2,3-DPG in adaptive red cell volume deficiency. Blood 36:383, 1970

64. Sandberg T, Lindquist O, Norkrans G: Fatal aplastic anemia associated with non-A, non-B hepatitis. Scand J Infect Dis 16:403, 1984

65. Saphir R: Addison's disease presenting as a lymphocyte dyscrasia. Am J Med 42:855, 1967

66. Shaw AB, Scholes MC: Reticulocytosis in renal failure. Lancet 1:799, 1967

67. Storb R, Thomas ED, Buckner CD et al: Marrow transplantation for aplastic anemia. Semin Hematol 21:27, 1984

68. Storb R, Thomas ED, Buckner CD et al: Marrow transplantation in thirty "untransfused" patients with severe aplastic anemia. Ann Intern Med 92:30, 1980

69. Torok–Storb B, Doney K, Sale G et al: Subsets of patients with aplastic anemia identified by flow microfluorometry. N Engl J Med 312:1015, 1985

70. Tsai SY, Levin WC: Chronic erythrocytic hypoplasia in adults. Am J Med 22:322, 1957

71. Tudhope GR: Endocrine diseases. Clin Haematol 1:475, 1972

72. Waldrop MM: The UCLA-Occidental-Gorbachev connection. Science 233:19, 1986

73. Wallner SF, Kurnick JE, Ward HP et al: The anemia of chronic renal failure and chronic diseases: In vitro studies of erythropoiesis. Blood 47:561, 1976

74. Weick JK, Hagedorn AB, Linman JW: Leukoerythroblastosis: Diagnostic and prognostic significance. Mayo Clin Proc 49:110, 1974

75. Wintrobe MM: The normocytic, normochromic anemias. In Wintrobe MM, Lee GR, Boggs DR et al (eds): Clinical Hematology, p 683. Philadelphia, Lea & Febiger, 1981

76. Wintrobe MM: Pancytopenia, aplastic anemia, and pure red cell aplasia. In Wintrobe MM, Lee GR, Boggs DR et al (eds): Clinical Hematology, p. 698. Philadelphia, Lea & Febiger, 1981

77. Zaroulis CG, Kourides IA, Valeri CR: Red cell 2,3-diphosphoglycerate and oxygen affinity of hemoglobin in patients with thyroid disorders. Blood 52:181, 1978

78. Zucker S: Anemia associated with foreign cells in the marrow (myelophthisis). In Lichtman MA (ed): Hematology and Oncology, p 42. New York, Grune & Stratton, 1980

Anemia

of Abnormal

Nuclear

Development

Cheryl A. Lotspeich-Steininger

The anemias of abnormal nuclear development are a group of disorders in which cell maturation in the bone marrow is abnormal as a result of abnormal development of cellular nuclei. Abnormalities, reflected in both nucleus and cytoplasm, may be seen in cells in the bone marrow and peripheral blood. Characteristic changes in overall cell size, shape, and color are often easily identifiable, as are nuclear abnormalities in size, shape, and chromatin clumping.

The megaloblastic anemias represent a major subgroup of anemias caused by abnormal nuclear development. Classically, these anemias are associated with very large, oval erythrocytes, which most often are detected by the finding of increased mean cell volume (MCV) on electronic cell analysis. Megaloblastic anemias are caused by vitamin B_{12} or folate deficiency and are usually acquired disorders, but a rare case may be inherited. Less common causes include rare inherited defects of deoxyribonucleic acid (DNA) synthesis and drug-induced disorders of DNA synthesis. These anemias are characteristically classified as macrocytic, normochromic (so-called megaloblastic) anemias. Leukocytes, erythrocytes, and platelets may each be abnormal.

The congenital dyserythropoietic anemias (CDAs) are a rare subgroup of anemias of abnormal nuclear development that are demonstrated in the laboratory as abnormalities of bone marrow erythrocyte precursors. The CDAs, unlike megaloblastic anemias, virtually always are inherited and are not associated with leukocyte or platelet abnormalities.

VITAMIN B_{12} AND FOLATE

Since vitamin B_{12} and folate deficiency are the most common causes of megaloblastic anemia, a review of the biochemistry of these compounds, their dietary requirements, and their metabolism is presented.

Biochemistry

Vitamin B_{12}

Vitamin B_{12} belongs to a family of vitamins called cobalamins that have a corrin ring that contains cobalt (Fig. 12–1). This ring is attached to the nucleotide 5,6-dimethylbenzimidazole, a structure similar to riboflavin. The corrin nucleus contains four substituted pyrrole rings and is similar to the porphyrin nucleus of heme (Chap. 7). Vitamin B_{12} is required for a single critical reaction during normal DNA synthesis.

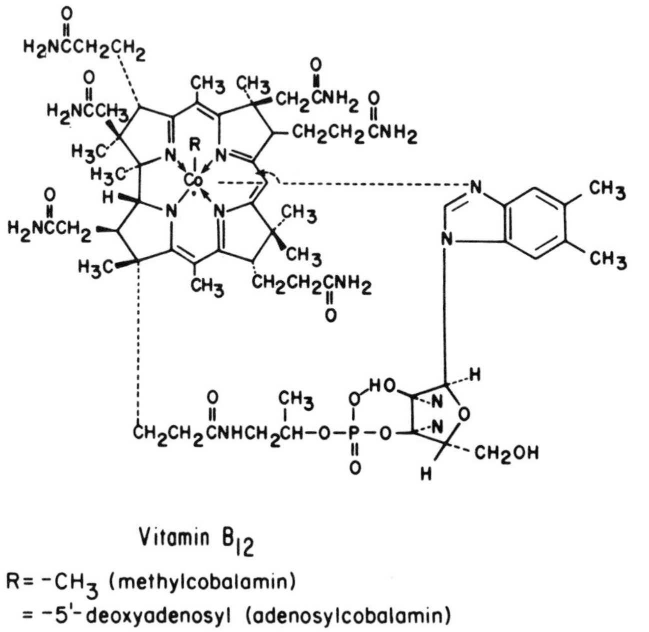

Adenosylcobalamin and methylcobalamin are B_{12} coenzyme forms.[17] The former is produced by covalent linkage of 5'-deoxyadenosine to the cobalt atom and the latter by linkage of a methyl group to the cobalt.[101] Methylcobalamin represents approximately 75% of the B_{12} in the plasma. Adenosylcobalamin represents about 75% of the B_{12} in the liver and most of the B_{12} in erythrocytes and kidneys.

When cyanide anion is covalently linked to the cobalt atom, cyanocobalamin is formed. This form is used to treat B_{12} deficiency.

Folate

The folates represent a family of compounds derived from folic acid, also called pteroylglutamic acid (Fig. 12–2). The parent compound is pteroic acid, which has a double-ring pteridine (2-amino-4-hydroxy-6-methylpterin) joined by a methylene bridge to para-aminobenzoic acid (PABA). Pteroic acid is linked by a peptide bond to one molecule of glutamic acid to form the complete folic acid structure. Multiple glutamic acid residues may be conjugated to the folic acid compound. A number of folate analogs, such as tetrahydrofolate (THF or FH_4), are formed by certain structural changes to the parent compound during folic acid metabolism. Folacin and folate are the terms used to refer to folic acid and its analogs. Folates participate in carbon transfers and are required for three reactions that lead to DNA synthesis, two involving purine synthesis and the third, pyrimidine synthesis.

Nutritional Requirements and Absorption

Vitamin B_{12}

Vitamin B_{12} is produced by microorganisms and certain molds. Its dietary sources include animal protein products such as meat, fish, eggs, and milk. It is not found in vegetables or fruit. The recommended daily allowance (RDA) is 3 μg,[97] much less than that for folic acid. During pregnancy, the RDA is 4 μg/day. Normally 3 to 5 μg are absorbed daily. The normal liver stores approximately 1 to 10 mg of vitamin B_{12}, an amount adequate for several years if no more is ingested.

Absorption of vitamin B_{12} in the gastrointestinal (GI)

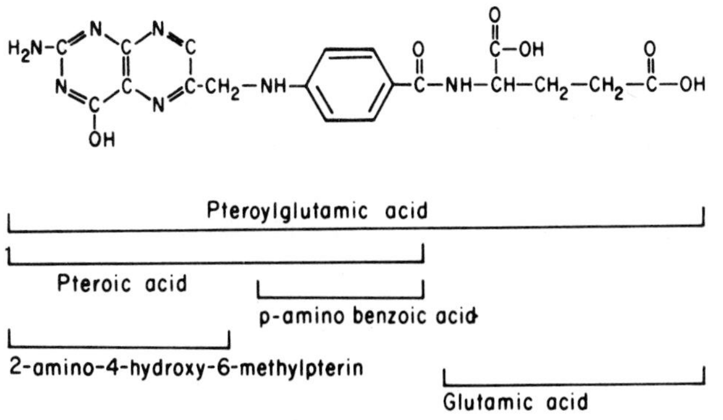

FIG. 12–1. The structure of vitamin B_{12}. (From Miller SM: Vitamins. In Bishop ML, Duben–Von Laufen JL, Fody EP (eds): Clinical Chemistry—Principles, Procedures, Correlations. Philadelphia, J.B. Lippincott, 1985, with permission.)

FIG. 12–2. The structure of folic acid. (From Miller SM: Vitamins. In Bishop ML, Duben–Von Laufen JL, Fody EP (eds): Clinical Chemistry—Principles, Procedures, Correlations. Philadelphia, J.B. Lippincott, 1985, with permission.)

tract requires several factors. First, the vitamin must be released from foods by peptic digestion in the stomach, which is facilitated by hydrochloric acid released from the gastric parietal cells. These cells also secrete an important protein called *intrinsic factor* (IF). In the stomach, IF forms a protective complex with vitamin B_{12} that is transported down the GI tract. Upon reaching the ileum (the section of the small intestine most distal from the stomach), the complex attaches to mucosal receptors, B_{12} is released from IF, and absorption takes place. Once in the plasma, vitamin B_{12} is bound by carrier proteins called transcobalamins I, II, and III (TC I, II, III). TC II, the most important of the transcobalamins, is a β globulin synthesized in the liver. TC II transports some B_{12} to storage sites in the liver and tissues and some to the bone marrow. TC II is necessary for transport of cobalamin through cell membranes.

The TC I and III vitamin B_{12}–binding proteins are present in gastric fluid, plasma, amniotic fluid, milk, saliva, and granulocytes. They are called R (rapid) proteins, or R binders, since they migrate faster than IF on zone electrophoresis. R proteins bind biologically active cobalamins and inactive analogs. The physiologic role of the R proteins is not clear, but it is known that they do not assist in ileal B_{12} absorption.[116] TC I binds most B_{12} in the plasma, and this B_{12} is not transported to the marrow. TC I is believed to be synthesized principally by granulocytes. Deficiency of TC II leads to megaloblastic anemia, whereas deficiencies of TC I and III apparently are harmless.

Folate

The dietary sources of folate are green leafy vegetables, liver, kidney, whole grain cereals, yeast, and fruit (especially oranges).[50] The RDA is either 50 μg folic acid or 400 μg food folate[97] (most food folate is present in the form of polyglutamates, which are more difficult to digest). For pregnant women the RDA is approximately doubled.

At any given time the body stores approximately 5 mg of folate, an amount that is adequate for several months if no additional folate is ingested. Note that folate body stores are consumed much more quickly than B_{12} stores (adequate for several years). Once in the small intestine, conjugases remove the excess glutamic acid residues from dietary polyglutamates to produce monoglutamates called methyl-tetrahydrofolates (methyl-THF). Such conversion allows folate absorption in the jejunum (the central segment of the small intestine), followed by transport to the liver and bone marrow. Folate is transported in the circulation as the monoglutamate 5-methyltetrahydrofolate (N^5-methyl-FH_4). Two thirds of plasma folate circulates loosely bound to proteins, including albumin, α_2-macroglobulin, and possibly transferrin. About half the body folate is stored in the liver. Much is also found in the kidneys and erythrocytes. Folate uptake by erythrocytes has been shown to require vitamin B_{12} as a cofactor.[50]

Vitamin B_{12} and Folate Metabolism

Vitamin B_{12} and folate are integral components in DNA synthesis. Without normal DNA synthesis, megaloblastic erythropoiesis results. Figure 12–3 shows the relationship of folate and B_{12} in DNA synthesis. Initially, the plasma folate monoglutamate N^5-methyl-FH_4 donates a methyl group to cobalamin (B_{12}) in the presence of methyl transferase to form methylcobalamin, which transfers the methyl group to homocysteine, forming the amino acid methionine. In the process, FH_4, a polyglutamate, is produced. FH_4 is the primary intracellular form of folate. As serine is converted to glycine, FH_4 is converted to the folate coenzyme N^5N^{10}-methylene FH_4, also a polyglutamate, which is part of the rate-limiting reaction in DNA synthesis. As N^5N^{10}-methylene FH_4 is converted to dihydrofolate (FH_2), deoxyuridylate (dUMP) is converted to thymidylate (dTTP), a pyrimidine nucleotide, in the presence of the enzyme thymidylate synthetase. Thymidylate is one of sev-

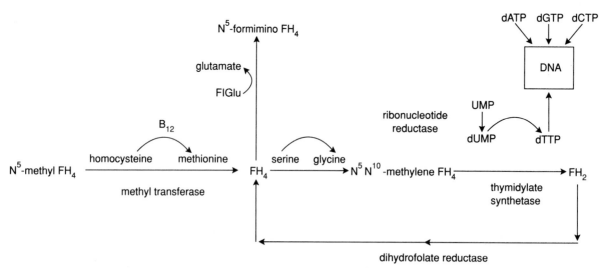

FIG. 12–3.   The interaction of vitamin B_{12} and folate in DNA synthesis. Synthesis of DNA requires vitamin B_{12} and the conversion of folates in the monoglutamate form to the polyglutamate N^5N^{10}-methylene FH_4 which is a cofactor in the rate-limiting reaction involving the conversion of dUMP to dTTP. The dTTP is needed for normal DNA synthesis, along with dATP, dGTP, and dCTP. Key: d, deoxyribose; A, adenine; G, guanine; C, cytosine; T, thymine; U, uracil; TP, triphosphate; MP, monophosphate; FH_4, tetrahydrofolate; FH_2, dihydrofolate; FIGlu, formiminoglutamic acid.

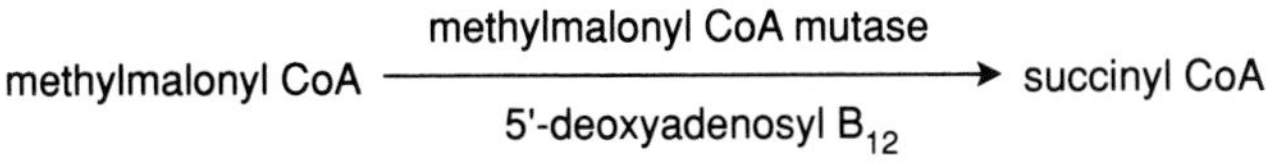

$$methylmalonyl\ CoA \xrightarrow[\text{5'-deoxyadenosyl } B_{12}]{\text{methylmalonyl CoA mutase}} succinyl\ CoA$$

FIG. 12–4. Vitamin B_{12} is required for propionate catabolism.

eral components required for DNA synthesis (see Fig. 12–3). FH_2 is reduced to FH_4 by the enzyme dihydrofolate reductase, thus conserving the supply of FH_4.

A second vitamin B_{12}–dependent reaction involves a step in the process of propionate catabolism (Fig. 12–4). In this reaction, methylmalonyl coenzyme A (CoA) is converted to succinyl CoA in the presence of vitamin B_{12} and methylmalonyl CoA mutase. This reaction provides the basis for a laboratory test discussed later in this chapter.

THE MEGALOBLASTIC ANEMIAS

Pathophysiology

Vitamin B_{12} deficiency causes defective DNA synthesis that results in a megaloblastic anemia. An explanation for this mechanism was first proposed in the early 1960s as the "methylfolate trap" hypothesis, which involves the interrelation between B_{12} and folate.[60]

When B_{12} is deficient, homocysteine cannot be converted to methionine, folate becomes "trapped" in the N^5-methyl FH_4 form, and cannot be converted to FH_4. FH_4 is necessary for the formation of N^5N^{10}-methylene FH_4, the folate coenzyme required for conversion of dUMP to dTTP (see Fig. 12–3). Also, if folate is trapped as N^5-methyl FH_4, formiminoglutamate (FIGlu) cannot be converted to glutamate, and urinary FIGlu excretion is greatly increased. Quantitation of urine FIGlu was used in the past to detect folate deficiency. However, urine FIGlu is seldom quantitated today, because it is not specific for folate deficiency since some patients with B_{12} deficiency also have increased urine FIGlu.

In addition, if vitamin B_{12} is deficient, propionate catabolism cannot take place. This causes increased urinary excretion of methylmalonic acid (MMA), which can be measured in the laboratory. The MMA level provides a sensitive test for B_{12} deficiency that is not affected by folic acid deficiency.

Because folate is a necessary component for DNA synthesis, a deficiency of folate, no matter what the source, produces defective DNA synthesis and megaloblastic anemia.

Peripheral Blood Megaloblastic Changes

Peripheral blood changes in the megaloblastic anemias are very similar no matter what the cause. With mild to moderate anemia, the MCV may increase to 110 fL. In severe anemia, it can range from 110 to 130 fL, although values up to 160 fL may be found.[143] Typically, the mean cell hemoglobin (MCH) value is also increased (from 33 to 38 pg), because hemoglobin content is increased in proportion to cell size. This may reduce or obliterate the normal central pallor of the cells, but the mean cell hemoglobin concentration (MCHC) usually remains normal.

As the megaloblastic anemia becomes more severe, the peripheral blood gradually reflects pancytopenia and a decreased reticulocyte count, even though the bone marrow is generally hypercellular, as a result of ineffective erythropoiesis and intramarrow erythrocyte destruction.

Erythrocyte Counts

The degree of anemia ranges from very mild to severe, depending on when the diagnosis is made. In the early 1900s, an erythrocyte count as low as $0.086 \times 10^{12}/L$ was reported for a patient with pernicious anemia (PA)[146] then the most common form of vitamin B_{12} deficiency in adults. Today, because patients are usually diagnosed much earlier in the course of the disease, severe anemia can be prevented.

Leukocyte and Platelet Counts

In the early stages, leukocyte counts are usually normal, but they gradually decline as the disorder progresses. With severe anemia, the leukocyte count has been reported to range between 1.0 and $3.0 \times 10^9/L$.[21] The leukopenia is generally attributable to absolute neutropenia. The platelet count generally declines with the erythrocyte count. It may fall below $100 \times 10^9/L$.[103]

Erythrocyte Morphology

Blood film examination often reveals macroovalocytes with little or no central pallor (Fig. 12–5). Anisocytosis is also common; usually it leads to an increase in the red cell distribution width (RDW). Macroovalocytes are the most prominent poikilocytes, but tear drops and fragments also may be seen. If anemia is severe, extremely bizarre poikilocytes may be observed (see Fig. 12–5) including dumbbell, anvil, cocked hat, and hand mirror forms, among others.[143] These cells may be smaller than normal erythrocytes. In advanced anemia, red cell inclusions may appear, including

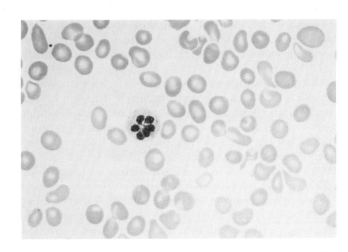

FIG. 12–5. Peripheral blood film from a patient with PA. The neutrophil displays the hypersegmentation typical of this disorder. Red cell morphology displays anisocytosis with some microcytic-looking cells and macroovalocytes that have a characteristic lack of central pallor. A few teardrops and a bizarre red cell are also present. Electronic cell analysis of this sample revealed an MCV of 119 FL. This field of view indicates a platelet deficiency (Wright stain; original magnification ×400).

Howell-Jolly bodies, Cabot rings (rare), and basophilic stippling. Megaloblasts (large, abnormal, nucleated red cells) in the basophilic, orthochromic, and polychromatophilic stages of maturation may also be present, some of which may be binucleated. Megaloblasts have an unusually fine nuclear chromatin structure typical of megaloblastic maturation. Nuclear-cytoplasmic asynchrony—a mature-looking cytoplasm (pink) surrounding an immature nucleus (delicate, fine chromatin)—is characteristic.

Reticulocytes

Reticulocytes are larger than normal, and the reticulocyte production index (RPI) (Chap. 9) often is less than 2, indicating inadequate marrow response to anemia.

Leukocyte Morphology

Giant neutrophils and bands are common. Nuclear hypersegmentation is a classic (although nonspecific) indicator of megaloblastic anemia. Neutrophils with five to ten lobes (see Fig. 12–5) may be detected in megaloblatic anemia (normal neutrophils have fewer than five lobes).

Platelets

Platelets may be granule deficient, in which case they stain poorly with Wright stain.

Bone Marrow Megaloblastic Changes

The marrow is usually hypercellular with erythrocyte precursors predominating (Plate 4). The ratio of megaloblasts to normoblasts in the marrow increases with the severity of the disease. Megaloblasts are not found in normal bone marrow. They are very large and have characteristically fine chromatin, which is reflected at all stages of maturation. The chromatin has been described as "particulate," in contrast to the clumped chromatin of normal marrow normoblasts. Early megaloblastic stages have an extremely basophilic cytoplasm. An increased number of mitotic forms is common.

The orthochromic megaloblast, with its distinct nuclear-cytoplasmic asynchrony, is particularly characteristic of megaloblastic anemias. It has an abundant, mature-looking pink cytoplasm similar to that of orthochromic normoblasts, but its nucleus resembles that seen in polychromatophilic normoblasts.

Giant metamyelocytes are characteristic, although giant leukocyte precursors at all maturation stages are common. A giant metamyelocyte contains a nucleus that is enlarged both absolutely and in relation to cell size. Because of the problems in DNA synthesis, its nuclear shape, chromatin structure, and staining characteristics may be bizarre. It is likely that these cells are arrested in a premitotic developmental stage.[141] They probably die in the marrow and are not precursors of peripheral blood hypersegmented neutrophils.

Megakaryocytes are the least affected of the three cell lines, but in severe anemia, they may be reduced in number and display abnormal nuclear shape (extreme lobulation) and immature chromatin patterns.[37]

PERNICIOUS ANEMIA

Since pernicious anemia (PA) of adults is the most representative form of megaloblastic anemia, it will be discussed in detail. Other forms of megaloblastic anemia have many features similar to those of PA and are discussed briefly later in the chapter.

Definition

PA is associated with vitamin B_{12} deficiency that results from an acquired atrophy of the stomach lining. Secretion of IF by the gastric parietal cells is thus reduced and sometimes eliminated. Without protection by IF, vitamin B_{12} is destroyed in the GI tract before it can be absorbed in the ileum. Gastric atrophy also causes reduction of hydrochloric acid secretion, which results in achlorhydria.

History

PA was probably first described in the early 1800s,[1,25] although its cause was poorly understood. It was not until the early 1900s that Whipple and his coinvestigators, and in separate studies Minot and his student William Castle, finally began to unravel the cause of this mysterious anemia.[14] It was Castle who first described the gastric protein IF (often called Castle's intrinsic factor) that is vital to vitamin B_{12} absorption.[13,15]

Demographics

PA is most common in Scandinavian, British, and Irish people,[43] although fewer than 1% of these populations are affected.[104] Caucasian Greeks and Italians are affected even less often.[43] PA occurs in blacks, although at only one third to one half the rate in Caucasians.[54]

In the United States, men and women are equally affected,[143] however in Europe, women seem to be diagnosed more often than men.[21] Onset generally is late in adult life; the peak age of occurrence is 60 years.[27]

It has been noted that patients with PA often have prematurely gray hair and light blue or gray eyes.[12] PA is also somewhat more common in people with blood group A.

Genetics

Congenital PA is rare and probably is inherited as an autosomal recessive trait.[92,125] The possible genetic origin of PA is suggested by studies that show relatives of PA patients are at significantly higher risk of developing PA than the general population.[21,121] For PA patients' relatives one study reported an incidence 20 times greater than that in families where no one has PA.[95] Autoantibodies to gastric parietal cells have been found in a significant number of relatives of PA patients when compared to the normal population.[21]

The exact defect inherited in PA remains unclear, however, two possibilities have been proposed. One is a defect in immunologic tolerance to some stomach, thyroid, skin, and pancreatic antigens. The other is a defect in a metabolic or enzyme system common to these tissues.[139]

Pathophysiology

The gastritis associated with PA that suppresses or arrests IF secretion and thus produces B_{12} deficiency may be caused by mucosal damage (mechanical, thermal, or chemical); nutritional deficiency (folate, ascorbate, or iron); endocrine disorders (thyroid, adrenal, or pancreatic); genetic disorders; or autoimmune mechanisms.[46] Autoimmune disorders have been demonstrated to have an increased incidence among patients with PA, including thyroid disease,[4] myxedema,[21] vitiligo (associated with patches of depigmented skin),[59] diabetes,[21] and hypogammaglobulinemia.[131] It is clear that autoimmune mechanisms are involved in most cases of PA, but the stimulus for the autoimmune changes that lead to PA is still unclear.

Although gastritis usually occurs late in adult life, it does rarely occur in children, in one of two forms—congenital or juvenile. Congenital PA usually presents around 2 years of age when vitamin B_{12} stores acquired *in utero* become depleted. Vitamin B_{12} malabsorption in these cases is due either to a congenital arrest of IF production or an abnormality of IF structure. Unlike the adult form, the stomach lining and secretion of hydrochloric acid are usually normal in congenital PA.

Juvenile PA, probably an acquired disorder involving autoimmune mechanisms, usually is identified in the second decade of life. Affected children show evidence of gastric atrophy, and the disorder is probably an early form of adult PA.

Clinical Findings

Symptoms often do not appear until the anemia is profound, and they do not necessarily reflect the degree of anemia unless the patient is suffering from the neurologic effects that may occur in PA. When the nervous system is affected, symptoms appear early and progress more rapidly than the developing anemia.

About half of PA patients develop a sore tongue (glossitis) early in the course of the disease. Severe glossitis is very painful, and the tongue appears "beefy red." Reappearance of a sore tongue during therapy indicates inadequate treatment. Typically, the tongue becomes very smooth and glazed between attacks of glossitis.

Complaints of weakness stem from anemia. At varying stages of the disorder other symptoms include gastrointestinal discomfort, weight loss due to anorexia, and difficulty walking.[27] Often, symptoms may suggest other disorders until peripheral blood examination reveals the characteristic megaloblastic changes.

Fever may be a feature of profound anemia. The skin may have a delicate lemon-yellow color caused by pallor and mild icterus, and blotchy, brownish pigmentation with patches of vitiligo may appear.[5]

Nervous System Findings

Abnormal nervous system findings are much less common today, because of earlier diagnosis and treatment of vitamin B_{12} deficiency. Approximately 30% of patients with PA may demonstrate neurologic disturbances, particularly paresthesias (see below), but only 7% have spinal cord involvement.[21]

The severity of the anemia generally is not an indicator of the severity of nervous system involvement.[27,35] The neurologic disturbances, including myelin degeneration and peripheral nerve degeneration, are caused mostly by the effects of B_{12} deficiency on the white matter of the cerebral cortex and of the spinal cord's dorsal and lateral columns. One cause of myelin degeneration may be defective lipid metabolism: the enzyme methylmalonyl CoA mutase cannot oxidize certain fatty acids in the absence of B_{12} (see Fig. 12-4).[101] Also, unlike neurons, the glial cells, which synthesize myelin, are dividing cells and are therefore vulnerable to the effects of poor DNA synthesis. Degeneration of myelin and peripheral nerves produces paresthesias, described as a prickling, tingling, "pins and needles" sensation in the hands and feet.[133] It also causes weakness, unsteady gait, clumsiness, and in severe degeneration, spasticity. Impaired memory is common at this stage.[118] Because multiple nerve pathways are involved this neurologic disorder is called "subacute combined degeneration." Psychiatric symptoms referred to as *megaloblastic madness* are infrequent but include hallucinations, maniacal outbursts, paranoia, and schizophrenia.[54a] Prompt therapy usually reverses them.

Laboratory Findings and Correlations with Disease

In addition to the hematologic and chemical findings described earlier for the megaloblastic anemias, PA has several other distinguishing laboratory features.

Special Hematology Tests

Erythrocyte survival is moderately decreased[41] partly because of intramarrow destruction of megaloblasts. Even normal cells are destroyed early when transfused into these patients,[53] probably in the extravascular system (Chap. 16). Haptoglobin may be decreased and methemalbumin may be increased, suggesting an intravascular component of hemolysis as well.[102]

Cytogenetics

There are a number of reports of cytogenetic abnormalities in the bone marrow cells.[75,82] These include chromosome elongation and abnormal gaps or breaks. These abnormalities are only temporary, however, and disappear with appropriate treatment of the disorder.

Chemistry

The serum level of vitamin B_{12} has been reported to range from less than 10 to 110 ng/L (reference range 160 to 1000 ng/L).[21] Erythrocyte folate is usually reduced, be-

TABLE 12-1 Biochemical Differentiation of Vitamin B_{12} and Folic Acid Deficiency

CONDITION	SERUM B_{12}	SERUM FOLIC ACID	ERYTHROCYTE FOLATE
Vitamin B_{12} deficiency	Marked decrease	Normal or increased	Moderate decrease
Folic acid deficiency	Normal or decreased	Marked decrease	Marked decrease
B_{12} and folic acid deficiency	Decreased	Decreased	Decreased

cause red cells need B_{12} to absorb folate. The serum folate value is usually normal or elevated (Table 12-1).

In progressive stages of PA, serum iron is usually moderately increased,[21] as are macrophage iron stores and marrow sideroblasts. Plasma total iron-binding capacity may be slightly reduced. Autopsy may reveal a large concentration of iron in the liver, spleen, and kidneys. Such iron overload is caused by ineffective erythropoiesis, which leads to a decrease in iron uptake in red cells. Early destruction of erythrocytes in the bone marrow also increases the level of serum lactate dehydrogenase (LD) in proportion to the degree of anemia. The LD value is usually much higher in PA than in other hemolytic anemias, when it is slightly increased. In PA, the serum LD-1 isoenzyme value is the highest of the five LD isoenzymes, whereas LD-2 has the greatest serum activity in the other hemolytic anemias.[36] Urine urobilinogen may be elevated, but unconjugated serum bilirubin usually is increased only in severe untreated PA.

Immunology

Because of the simultaneous occurrence of PA and autoimmune disorders in many patients, tests to evaluate both humoral and cell-mediated immunity in patients with PA may reveal a number of abnormalities. In tests of *humoral immunity,* patients may demonstrate serum IgG autoantibodies, including those to IF, parietal cells, and thyroid.

Approximately 56% of patients with PA produce IF antibodies.[21,32,70,107,129,132] Since they are rare in normal subjects, they are a more specific marker for the diagnosis of PA than parietal cell antibodies, which may be found in some healthy people.[62,85,107]

There are three types of IF antibodies, blocking antibodies and two types of binding antibodies. Both binding and blocking antibodies may be detected in the laboratory by radioimmunoassay techniques,[110] in which radioactive vitamin B_{12} is used to measure the ability of IF to bind B_{12}.

Blocking IF antibodies are believed to bind with IF and block its vitamin B_{12}–binding site. The test for IF-blocking antibodies is probably the immunologic test of choice in the diagnostic work-up for PA patients.

Binding IF antibodies are usually found in conjunction with blocking antibodies. The first type of binding antibody attaches to an antigenic site on IF that is distant from the actual B_{12}-binding site, and binding is not dependent on whether or not IF has complexed with B_{12}. The second type binds to both IF and its complexed B_{12}.

Parietal cell antibodies occur in approximately 84% of all patients with PA.[21,32,71,107,129,132] Laboratory detection is possible by complement fixation[67,89] or immunofluorescence[67,128] techniques. Tests for parietal cell antibodies are not very useful for diagnosing PA because of low specificity. These antibodies may be found in some healthy persons and in patients with other types of autoimmune diseases. Parietal cell and IF antibodies can be distinguished by gel filtration techniques.[70]

Thyroid antibodies are common in patients with PA and their relatives.[21,32,71,107,129,132] Laboratory detection techniques include complement fixation, immunofluorescence, and tanned red cell agglutination techniques.

Cell-mediated immunity may also play a role in PA, as evidenced by the transformation of lymphocytes from some patients with PA in the presence of human gastric juice.[23,127] The fact that human and hog IF concentrates can inhibit leukocyte migration in some PA patients is evidence of cell-mediated immunity to IF.[23,42,107]

Laboratory Tests for Vitamin B_{12} and Folate Deficiency

Measurement of serum vitamin B_{12}, serum folate, and erythrocyte folate values is essential to the diagnosis of megaloblastic anemia. The serum B_{12} level is considered a relatively accurate reflection of tissue stores. The erythrocyte folate level indicates tissue folate stores much more accurately than the serum folate value, which is sensitive to recent folate consumption.

In addition, testing for serum-blocking IF antibodies is very useful for diagnosing PA. The test is rapid, easy to perform, and cost effective.[85] Interested readers are referred to Chanarin[19] for a description of IF antibody testing.

SERUM MICROBIOLOGIC ASSAYS

Prior to the 1970s, microbiologic assays were the most common method of measuring serum vitamin B_{12}[3,91,120] and folic acid,[61] and they are still considered to be the reference methods with which all commerical kit methods must be compared. Microorganisms that require either B_{12} (*Euglena gracilis* or *Lactobacillus leichmannii*[45]) or folic acid (*Lactobacillus casei*) for growth are incubated with patient serum for 48 to 72 hours, after which serum turbidity is measured spectrophotometrically. The results are compared to standards of sera with known concentrations of B_{12} or folic acid to determine the patient's serum concentrations. Although these methods are accurate, sensitive, and specific, they are time consuming and inaccurate if the patient is taking antibiotics.

COMPETITIVE PROTEIN-BINDING RADIOASSAY FOR B_{12} AND FOLATE

Today, competitive protein-binding radioassays are the methods of choice for quantitation of B_{12} and folate because of their technical simplicity and lack of interference from antibiotics or antineoplastic drugs.[38] Only the highlights of these radioassays are presented here. Commercial kits are available for individual[115] and simultaneous[24] measurement of serum B_{12} and serum or erythrocyte folate. The individual kits contain exact procedures. The simultaneous method is described below.

Principle

Patient vitamin B_{12} and folate in serum compete for binding sites in the test system with ^{57}Co-labeled cobalamin and ^{125}I-labeled folic acid derivative, respectively. The B_{12} binder is usually nonhuman IF from hog stomach. The folate binder is β-lactoglobulin, a protein that occurs naturally in milk. After incubation and subsequent washing to remove unbound radioactive labels, the sample radioactivity level is measured with a γ-scintillation counter. The lower the patient's serum B_{12} or serum (or erythrocyte) folate value, the more radioactivity remains in the sample. Quantitation is accomplished by comparison with a standard curve.

Specimen and Patient Requirements

Serum B_{12} and Folate

Serum is preferred, but EDTA-anticoagulated plasma is acceptable. The patient should fast before any folic acid testing, because recent food intake may increase the serum level of folic acid (but not B_{12}). For serum folate measurement, serum should not be contaminated by cells or hemolysis, since erythrocytes contain about 40 times more folate than the serum. Serum must be protected from light to prevent folate deterioration. Store at 2 to 8° C for up to 3 hours or frozen (−20° C) for longer periods. The specimen must be either boiled or exposed to an alkaline agent to release the cobalamin and folate from endogenous binding proteins.

Erythrocyte Folate

Whole blood hemolysates for erythrocyte folate assay require EDTA-anticoagulated blood. After the hematocrit is measured, the hemolysate is prepared in ascorbic acid solution (to 100 μL whole blood, add 2 mL ascorbic acid solution, 0.2 g/dL) and incubated 90 minutes to hydrolyze folate polyglutamates. It must be protected from light. Storage is the same as for serum samples.

Reference Ranges

For fasting adults, serum vitamin B_{12} is 140 to 700 ng/L; serum folate, 3 to 16 μg/L; and RBC folate, 150 to 800 μg/L. For some procedures, reticulocytes have higher folate levels than mature red cells.[18] Vitamin B_{12} levels decline significantly with age in healthy adult males.

Comments and Sources of Error

This procedure is generally very sensitive and capable of measuring very low concentrations of B_{12}. B_{12} levels in patients with untreated PA are usually less than 100 ng/L. In folate-deficient patients, serum folate is usually less than 1.0 μg/L and erythrocyte folate, less than 100 μg/L. If results are indeterminate (i.e., B_{12}, 100 to 400 ng/L; serum folate, 2.0 to 3.0 μg/L), other laboratory or clinical findings may be helpful. Otherwise, serum levels should be checked again in a few months.

The nonhuman IF used in this test system must be as nearly pure as possible; otherwise it may contain R binders (transcobalamins I and III), which also bind B_{12} and metabolically inactive B_{12} analogs, causing falsely elevated B_{12} levels.[80] One report states that although claims have been made that large numbers of patients with B_{12} deficiency have gone undetected because of R binders, these claims are exaggerated as a result of badly designed and poorly executed assays, rather than the R binders.[16]

In procedures where the binding protein includes both IF and R binders, the R binders are saturated with cobinamide, a B_{12} analog that does not bind to IF. This facilitates blocking of all non-IF vitamin B_{12}–binding sites.

Another procedure that is very specific for cobalamin calls for the use of chicken serum-binding protein with a magnetizable solid-phase separation system.[66] In this procedure, no boiling or pretreatment of the patient sample is required.

Using reliable commercial assays, particularly those with purified IF as the binder or with IF and the nonspecific R-protein sites blocked with "cobinamide," it is reported that the results of B_{12} radioassays are comparable to those obtained by microbiologic assay and that they allow for appropriate diagnosis.[80] Reliable serum and erythrocyte folate radioassays can also provide valuable diagnostic information.[24] However, laboratories should evaluate any kit carefully before it is put into service for reporting patient results.[85]

THE SCHILLING TEST[19,117]
Principle

The Schilling test provides a measure of the body's ability to secrete viable IF and absorb orally administered ^{57}Co-labeled B_{12} in the ileum. Along with the ^{57}Co B_{12}, excessive amounts of unlabeled B_{12} are administered to the patient to fill all tissue binding sites. Normal absorption of vitamin B_{12} under such circumstances is reflected by a minimum level of urinary excretion of radiolabeled B_{12}.

Specimen and Patient Requirements

The patient should fast overnight. A 24-hour urine collection is begun immediately upon administration of the labeled B_{12} by mouth.

General Procedure

A physiologic dose of ^{57}Co-labeled vitamin B_{12} (0.5 to 2.0 μg) is given by mouth, followed by a "flushing dose" of 1000 μg unlabelled B_{12} injected intramuscularly within the next 1 to 2 hours. This dose is given to saturate the liver and tissue binding sites so that, if the labeled B_{12} is absorbed it will not be completely bound in B_{12}-depleted tissues and some will be excreted in the urine.

If results of the initial test are abnormal, the test is repeated 2 to 3 days later. In this phase, IF is administered *with* the ^{57}Co B_{12}, to eliminate IF as a variable and to determine whether provision of IF allows for normal B_{12} absorption. The results allow for distinguishing between a deficiency of or a defect in IF and a malabsorption syndrome such as that caused by ileal disease or fish tapeworm.

Reference Range

Normally more than 7% of the administered dose of ^{57}Co B_{12} is excreted in the initial 24-hour urine specimen. Patients with PA secrete less than 7%, usually about 3%.

Interpretation

Figure 12-6 provides a summary of the possible indications for the various results that may be obtained from this test.

If less than 7% of the labeled B_{12} is excreted in the first 24 hours, absorption is abnormal. If administering IF with the B_{12} corrects the malabsorption, then the cause of the deficiency is most likely IF deficiency or a defective IF molecule. If B_{12} still is not absorbed when IF is given, the cause of B_{12} deficiency may be small bowel bacterial consumption of B_{12}, fish tapeworm disease, congenital B_{12} malabsorption, ileal disease, or drug-induced malabsorption.

Comments and Sources of Error

Incomplete urine collection is a major source of error.[20] It can lead to false positive results (that indicate failure to absorb B_{12}) by reducing the level of radioactivity measured in the 24-hour urine sample. Chanarin[16] recommends assessing absorption by measuring the radioactivity in plasma 8 to 12 hours after the test is begun; this indicator is as reliable or more so than 24-hour urine collection.

Approximately 25% of patients with PA have a secondary intestinal malabsorption disorder that distorts results of the Schilling test performed with IF so it does not show the typical "correction."[38] Thus, lack of test correction after IF administration does not absolutely exclude PA.

If the patient is suffering from renal disease, excretion of labeled B_{12} may be decreased in the first 24-hour urine sample, as excretion may be delayed as long as 72 hours.[143]

DEOXYURIDINE SUPPRESSION TEST

The deoxyuridine (dU) suppression test is performed in some specialized laboratories to detect vitamin B_{12} or folate deficiency.[58] A highly sensitive test, it is particularly useful for detecting and identifying deficiency in patients with borderline or nonexistent hematologic changes, or when both serum B_{12} and folate levels are either low or normal.[85] It measures the degree to which unlabeled dU (a dUMP precursor) in the patient's plasma suppresses uptake of radioactive thymidine (added to the test system) into the DNA of bone marrow cells in culture. If the DNA takes up a significant amount of radioactive

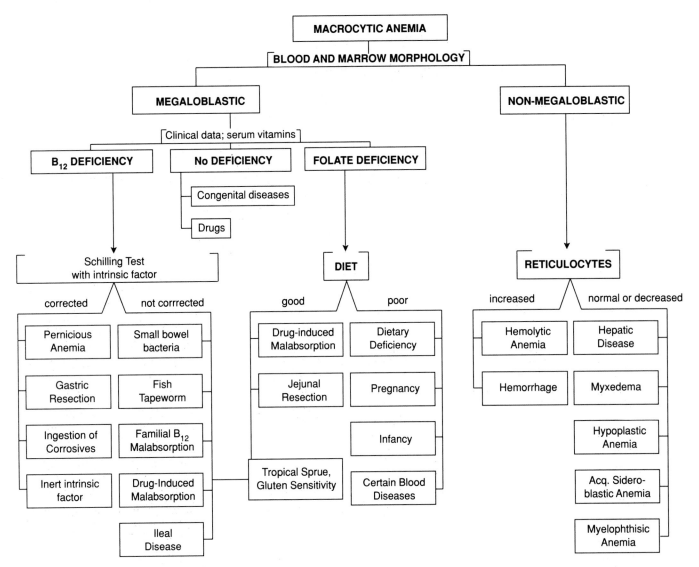

FIG. 12–6. The approach to a diagnostic problem in macrocytic anemia. Closed boxes indicate findings and open boxes, procedures. (From Wintrobe MM: Megaloblastic and nonmegaloblastic anemias. In Wintrobe MM et al (eds): Clinical Hematology, 8th ed. Philadelphia, Lea & Febiger, 1981, with permission.)

thymidine, then deficient patient thymidylate synthesis is indicated as a result of either folate or B_{12} deficiency. Either deficiency can result in failure to convert dU to thymidylate (see Fig. 12-3). Isolation of folate or B_{12} deficiency is achieved by adding each individually to the marrow culture and detecting whether thymidylate synthesis is corrected.

URINARY EXCRETION OF METHYLMALONIC ACID

Vitamin B_{12} and the enzyme methylmalonyl-CoA mutase are both necessary for conversion of methylmalonyl-coenzyme A to succinyl-CoA (see Fig. 12-4). Without B_{12}, urinary excretion of methylmalonic acid (MMA) is increased. Thus, a test for MMA provides a specific test for B_{12} deficiency.[26]

The most recently introduced procedure for MMA measurement is mass spectrometry.[99] It is said to provide a rapid, sensitive, and reproducible assay for urinary MMA,[98] and most medical center hospitals have a mass spectrometer. Techniques used less frequently today include ion exchange chromatography, gas chromatography,[27,47] and thin layer chromatography.[34,47] These techniques are laborious, time consuming, and not very sensitive.

Based on tests of over 1000 random urine samples by mass spectrometry, the reported reference value for MMA was less than 5.0 μg/mL urine.[98] In this same study, an MMA value greater than 20μg/mL urine was defined to be "clearly elevated." The researchers concluded that an abnormal urinary MMA value was a more reliable diagnostic indicator of cobalamin deficiency than was a serum cobalamin level. Excretion of elevated MMA has been reported to be the first indication of cobalamin deficiency, because it reflects the availability of B_{12} to tissue.[63]

X-RAY OR ENDOSCOPIC STUDIES

In cases of suspected PA, x-ray studies or endoscopy is usually performed to verify gastric atrophy and exclude stomach carcinoma. This ensures appropriate therapy.

Effects of Treatment on Laboratory Results and Prognosis

Treatment most often involves intramuscular or subcutaneous injections of vitamin B_{12} (in the hydroxycobalamin form), which if continued as needed throughout life can provide complete recovery for persons who are not severely affected by neurologic disturbances. Therapy with the correct agent is very important. If folate is given to treat B_{12} deficiency, the patient's hematologic abnormalities may improve temporarily but not as would be expected with appropriate therapy. Incorrect treatment may actually induce or exacerbate the neurologic abnormalities of a B_{12}-deficient patient.[69]

Peripheral Blood

With appropriate therapy the reticulocyte count should increase dramatically within a week, and the RPI should indicate an adequate response to the patient's degree of anemia. Normoblasts may also appear as a positive sign of effective erythropoiesis. The hematocrit value should begin to rise within 5 to 7 days and should rise fastest in patients who are severely anemic. Within 1 to 2 months, the hematocrit should be within the reference range, no matter how severe the anemia was at initiation of therapy.[68] In that same period, anisocytosis and poikilocytosis gradually disappear and the MCV should return to normal, although it may rise before it drops, because of reticulocytosis.

The number of neutrophilic leukocytes increases to normal within 7 days. Immature leukocytes may appear in the peripheral blood, causing a temporary left shift which gradually disappears. Usually hypersegmented neutrophils disappear within 2 weeks.[21,96] The platelet count increases and generally is within the reference range within 7 days of initiating therapy.[105]

Transfusion is rarely necessary except in cases of severe anemia, which may lead to, or may already have caused, a potentially fatal cardiac arrest.

Bone Marrow

It is not necessary to perform a bone marrow examination to determine response to therapy. Marrow abnormalities are remarkably reduced within 24 hours.[112] Within 6 to 10 hours after initiation of therapy, a significant reduction in megaloblasts is common.[29] Within 1 to 2 days, erythrocyte maturation is normoblastic.[122] The giant metamyelocytes, however, usually do not disappear for at least 7 days.[21]

Chemistry

Serum LD levels should decrease to normal within 1 to 2 weeks after treatment is initiated. Plasma bilirubin declines to normal within 3 to 4 weeks. Urinary urobilinogen begins to decrease as erythropoiesis levels off to a normal rate.[40]

Plasma iron usually declines within 24 to 48 hours and may even fall below the reference range[55] as accelerated erythropoiesis compensates for the anemia. The serum ferritin level decreases more slowly.

Neurologic Disorders

Neurologic disorders may or may not be reversible with therapy, depending on how long they were present before therapy was instituted. Disturbances present less than 3 months usually are reversible.[6] Improvement may take months, and any residual manifestations after a year of therapy are most likely irreversible. Spinal cord damage is also usually irreversible.

Prior to the early 1900s, PA was a fatal disease.[124] Today, when appropriate therapy is available fatalities occur only among patients who refuse to take or continue therapy.

OTHER CAUSES OF ACQUIRED VITAMIN B_{12} DEFICIENCY

Dietary Deficiency

Dietary deficiency is a rare cause of B_{12} deficiency particularly since normal body stores are sufficient to prevent megaloblastic anemia for several years if no more B_{12} is ingested. Strict vegetarians who avoid meat, eggs, and milk can eventually develop B_{12} deficiency, but this is rare. Infants breast fed by mothers who are vegans (and asymptomatic) may develop severe anemia.[63]

Castle's Intrinsic Factor Deficiency

Castle's IF deficiency may also result from total or partial gastrectomy if supplemental parenteral vitamin B_{12} is not provided. In one study, after total gastrectomy without B_{12} therapy, an average of 5 years elapsed before onset of anemia.[21] Vitamin B_{12} malabsorption occurs less often with partial gastrectomy and is less severe than that associated with PA or with total gastrectomy.[30]

Intrinsic Factor Molecular Defect

A molecular defect in IF is a rare cause of B_{12} deficiency. The IF in gastric secretions is inert but immunologically normal, it appears normal on chromatography, and its B_{12}-binding affinity is normal; however, it is incapable of facilitating ileal B_{12} absorption.[74]

Small Bowel Bacterial Overgrowth

Healthy persons have either a sterile proximal small bowel or a low concentration of bacterial growth.[48] Two factors normally prevent bacterial overgrowth: (1) normal intestinal peristalsis,[31] which prevents stasis and encourages recirculation of intestinal contents and (2) gastric acid secretion. Conditions that promote bacterial overgrowth include small bowel diverticulosis, fistulae, blind loops and pouches, strictures, scleroderma, and achlorhydria. Excessive bacterial growth successfully competes for ingested B_{12}, making it unavailable for ileal absorption. Patients may experience weight loss, steatorrhea, and diarrhea. Laboratory findings are similar to those in PA, except that correction of absorption is not demonstrated in the Schilling tests by administration of IF (see Fig. 12-6). Treatment with antibiotics, particularly tetracyclines,[52,94] usually corrects the problem.

Fish Tapeworm Disease

Diphyllobothrium latum, a common parasite of freshwater fish, especially pike, causes disease in humans. Most often found in Finland, it also occurs in the lakes of north central North America. Fish tapeworm infection is acquired by eating raw or under cooked fish. *D. latum* interferes with

B_{12} absorption by competing with IF for binding B_{12}.[100] Over time, this results in B_{12} deficiency. Treatment consists of B_{12} administration and eradication of the worms.

Ileal Disease

Because most B_{12} is absorbed in the ileum, ileal resection, bypass, or disease often leads to B_{12} malabsorption.[9,11] Crohn's disease, also called regional enteritis, is one of the better-known diseases that affects the ileum. Patients with Crohn's disease sometimes develop megaloblastic anemia. Vitamin B_{12} and folate deficiency may occur together in Crohn's disease.

Other Causes

Certain drugs or substances have been noted to cause vitamin B_{12} malabsorption, such as neomycin[72] and ethanol,[86] among others. This abnormality is usually reversible on removal of the offending agent. Hemodialysis has also been cited as a cause of decreased serum B_{12}.[109] Patients who are near term in normal pregnancy, have iron deficiency, have had a partial gastrectomy, or are being treated with certain drugs can also develop B_{12} deficiency.

HEREDITARY VITAMIN B_{12} DEFICIENCY— IMMERSLUND SYNDROME

Immerslund syndrome is a rare hereditary disorder that causes B_{12} malabsorption. It usually affects homozygous children during the first 2 years of life causing a megaloblastic anemia and proteinuria. Heterozygotes have decreased B_{12} absorption but are not anemic.[93] Inheritance is probably autosomal recessive.[143]

In this disorder B_{12} malabsorption is unrelated to IF deficiency or defect: the vitamin cannot be absorbed, with or without IF. Gastric secretion is normal. The exact defect is not clear, but it is thought to be related to the mechanism of absorption in the ileal mucosa that *follows* the binding of IF with B_{12} to ileal receptors.[143]

Anemia is corrected by B_{12} therapy, but proteinuria persists, perhaps because of an associated renal tubule defect.

FOLATE DEFICIENCY ANEMIA

With the exception of neurologic manifestations, folate deficiency is associated with the same general clinical findings as vitamin B_{12} deficiency. In the unusual case in which neurologic disturbances occur in association with folate deficiency, there is most likely a concurrent B_{12} deficiency or some other disorder.

Laboratory Findings and Correlations with Disease

The hematologic laboratory characteristics are generally the same as those described earlier in this chapter for any megaloblastic anemia.

Biochemical results help to differentiate folate deficiency from B_{12} deficiency (see Table 12-1). The serum B_{12} value is usually normal or decreased, the serum folate value is significantly decreased, and erythrocyte folate is also significantly decreased. The following values were reported in studies of folate-deficient patients and normal subjects: serum B_{12}, 50 to 500 ng/L, mean 190 (reference range 160 to 1000 ng/L, mean 450)[21]; serum folate, less than 3 μg/L (reference range 6 to 21 μg/L, mean 10)[138]; RBC folate, less than 100 μg/L (reference range 166 to 640 μg/L, mean 316).[65]

Other biochemical results are similar to those described for pernicious anemia because both folate deficiency and PA cause premature erythrocyte destruction in the bone marrow.

Urine Formiminoglutamic Acid[22]

In severe folic acid deficiency, the concentration in the urine of a degradation product of normal histidine metabolism called formiminoglutamic acid (FIGlu) is significantly increased because of the lack of tetrahydrofolate (FH_4), which normally reacts with FIGlu to form glutamate and N^5-formimino-FH_4 (see Fig. 12-3). When folate-deficient subjects are given histidine, urinary excretion of FIGlu is dramatically increased.[144] Excretion of FIGlu is also increased in vitamin B_{12} deficiency; thus, it cannot be used to differentiate B_{12} from folate deficiency.

Causes of Acquired Folate Deficiency

Folate deficiency may be acquired in many ways; only rarely is it inherited.[81,113]

Dietary Deficiency

Dietary folate deficiency occurs much more readily than dietary vitamin B_{12} deficiency, because body stores of folate are smaller. Significant deficiency is indicated by levels of serum folate below 3 μg/dL and of erythrocyte folate below 140 μg/L.[114] Deficiency may occur within 2 to 4 months if no folate is ingested. Dietary folate deficiency is most common in Southeast Asia and Africa, where diets often consist mostly of starch and grains and are low in animal protein and green leafy vegetables. Destruction of food folate by excessive heat during steaming and boiling can also lead to dietary deficiency.

Alcoholic Cirrhosis

Alcoholic cirrhosis has been reported to cause megaloblastic anemia in about 20% of those afflicted.[76,77,79] The MCV is generally greater than 120 fL, which is usually greater than that associated with *nonmegaloblastic* macrocytic anemia caused by liver disease.[8,73] Serum folate is reduced, but vitamin B_{12} is normal or increased. Both dietary deficiency and excess alcohol lead to folate deficiency. Alcohol interferes with folate metabolism.[64,123]

Pregnancy

Pregnancy may also bring about folate deficiency and megaloblastic anemia because of the developing fetus' requirement for large quantities of folate.

Infant Malnutrition

Infants in developed countries seldom have folate deficiency, in contrast to those in countries plagued with malnutrition.[84,87,137] Infants require about 50 μg folate per day, four to ten times the adult requirement by weight basis.[126] One liter of human or cow's milk contains about 50 μg folate.[44,90] Normal milk intake provides infants with adequate folate, but boiling the milk reduces the folate content by 40% to 80%. Goat's milk is very low in folate and inadequate for an infant's diet.[44,90] Rarely, megaloblastic anemia in infants may be caused by congenital folate malabsorption.

Folate Antagonists

A number of folate antagonists can impair DNA synthesis. Examples include the antimalarial drug pyrimethamine and chemotherapeutic agent methotrexate.[106] These antagonists inhibit the enzyme dihydrofolate reductase (see Fig. 12-3), which is part of the metabolic process of thymidylate and DNA synthesis. Taking drugs that inhibit DNA synthesis by inhibiting purine or pyrimidine synthesis—hydroxyurea, cytosine arabinoside, and 6-mercaptopurine, among others—may cause megaloblastic anemia.

CONDITIONS THAT CAUSE BOTH FOLATE AND B_{12} DEFICIENCY

Tropical Sprue and Gluten-Sensitive Enteropathy

Tropical sprue and gluten-sensitive enteropathy both can cause B_{12} and folate malabsorption as a result of intestinal atrophy. Patients suffer from steatorrhea, weight loss, weakness, and a wide-ranging nutritional deficiency caused by a general lack of nutrient absorption. Tropical sprue affects the entire small intestine[78] and so causes both B_{12} and folate deficiency; it appears to be caused by some infectious agent and responds to antibiotics[78] and folate therapy.

Gluten-sensitive enteropathy principally affects the proximal intestine.[111] Its two forms are childhood celiac disease and adult nontropical sprue. Affected people react abnormally to gluten, a protein in wheat and other grains,[39] possibly because they lack an intestinal peptidase that usually detoxifies a gluten peptide.[2]

In childhood celiac disease, anemia usually results from iron deficiency,[33] but sometimes the cause is folate deficiency, and rarely it is vitamin B_{12} deficiency. In adult nontropical sprue, most patients experience folate malabsorption and deficiency,[51] but less than half of those diagnosed demonstrate B_{12} deficiency.[21] Iron, folate, and in some cases B_{12} therapy is required to restore blood components to normal. The patient should eat a gluten-free diet to avoid future episodes of the disorder.

INHERITED DISORDERS THAT AFFECT DNA SYNTHESIS

Purines and pyrimidines, vitamin B_{12} and folate, several enzymes, and a number of other substances are necessary for normal DNA synthesis.

Orotic Aciduria

Orotic aciduria is a rare hereditary disorder of pyrimidine metabolism resulting in abnormal DNA synthesis, excessive urinary excretion of orotic acid, and a megaloblastic anemia[119] identical in appearance to the anemias of vitamin B_{12} and folate deficiency. Most patients exhibit physical and mental retardation. The mode of inheritance is probably autosomal recessive. Treatment with uridine is required to normalize anemia and growth.

Lesch-Nyhan Syndrome

The Lesch-Nyhan syndrome is a rare X-linked disorder of purine metabolism caused by lack of the enzyme xanthine-guanine phosphoribosyl-transferase. Features include hyperuricemia, self-mutilation, and mental and neurologic defects. Megaloblastic anemia has been reported in at least one case; it was corrected by administration of adenine.[134]

Other inherited disorders that cause defective DNA synthesis include abnormal or defective transcobalamin II and enzyme deficiencies, including methyl transferase, formiminotransferase, and dihydrofolate reductase (see Fig. 12-3), among others.

DIFFERENTIAL LABORATORY DIAGNOSIS OF THE MEGALOBLASTIC ANEMIAS

Differential diagnosis of the megaloblastic anemias in the laboratory can be somewhat perplexing at times. The most basic differentiation required is usually the cause, whether it be vitamin B_{12} or folate deficiency, or some other, because that informs the choice of appropriate therapy. A second source of confusion involves distinguishing between megaloblast*ic* and megaloblast*oid* anemias, which have some similar features. Third, megaloblastic anemias must be differentiated from normoblastic, macrocytic anemias. The sections below provide differentiating features in each of these areas.

Biochemical Differentiation of Deficiencies of Vitamin B_{12} and Folic Acid

While abnormalities in the hematologic measurements in these two types of anemia are very similar, serum B_{12} and serum and erythrocyte folate values usually help to identify the cause. Table 12-1 summarizes the results of these three assays in the different disorders. Note that serum folate is often increased in B_{12} deficiency and erythrocyte folate is moderately reduced. This is probably because B_{12} is necessary to act as a cofactor in the transfer of folate into erythrocytes.[130]

Differentiation of Megaloblastic and Megaloblastoid Cell Maturation

Megaloblastoid (literally, "resembling megaloblastic") erythrocyte maturation is an abnormal process that is *not* caused by B_{12} or folate deficiency. It is common in malignancies of the myeloid cell lines such as the myeloproliferative disorders (Chaps. 34 and 35) and the dysmyelopoietic or myelodysplastic syndromes (MDS) (Chap. 33). Megaloblastoid morphology generally displays a coarser clumping of the nuclear chromatin in nucleated red cells that makes the parachromatin more prominent than in megaloblastic red cell precursors (Plate 12-2). Recall that the chromatin structure in megaloblastic cells is very delicate in appearance (see Plate 5).

Sometimes, abnormal red cell maturation in the MDS may nonetheless be difficult to distinguish from that seen in megaloblastic anemias. Both may exhibit a macrocytic anemia with oval macrocytes, basophilic stippling, Howell-Jolly bodies, nucleated red cells, and giant platelets in the peripheral blood. Platelet granulation may be decreased in either disorder as well.

Distinguishing features include B₁₂ and folate levels that are usually normal or increased in the MDS. Also, the MDS generally demonstrate abnormal development in other myeloid cell lines such as neutrophils with prominent hypolobulation referred to as pseudo-Pelger-Huet cells, and reflect a left shift on the leukocyte differential, neither of which is typical of megaloblastic anemia. On the other hand, hypersegmentation may occur in both the MDS and megaloblastic anemias. Also the finding of micromegakaryocytes or megakaryoblasts in the peripheral blood would indicate a megaloblastoid rather than a megaloblastic anemia.

Differentiation of Macrocytic Anemias— Megaloblastic versus Normoblastic

Megaloblastic, macrocytic anemias must be distinguished from normoblastic, macrocytic anemias. In the latter, the red cells show an increase in MCV without the characteristic megaloblastic changes in cell maturation in the bone marrow or peripheral blood.

The oval shape of megaloblastic, macrocytic erythrocytes often distinguishes them from nonmegaloblastic, macrocytic erythrocytes, which are usually round and often thin. Polychromatophilia and reticulocytosis may also occur in the macrocytic, normoblastic anemias but seldom in the megaloblastic anemias. Figure 12-6 provides a flow chart that is useful in the differential diagnosis.

The normoblastic, macrocytic anemias may be caused by reticulocytosis resulting from blood loss or hemolysis. Other normoblastic, macrocytic anemias do not cause reticulocytosis, including those due to liver disease, hypoplastic anemia, acquired sideroblastic anemia and other myelodysplastic syndromes, myelophthisic anemia, and myxedema. Normoblastic macrocytes may also be seen in normal pregnancy and in neonates. Many cytotoxic drugs may also induce normoblastic macrocytosis, including among others, chlorambucil, mephelan, and azathioprine.

In hepatic disease, the macrocytes may appear as target cells or cells with increased central pallor; either feature differentiates the disorder from a megaloblastic anemia.

CONGENITAL DYSERYTHROPOIETIC ANEMIAS

The congenital dyserythropoietic anemias (CDA) are also anemias of abnormal nuclear development. They are rare, hereditary disorders characterized by refractory anemia that varies in severity, and by abnormalities of bone marrow erythrocyte precursors, including nuclear abnormalities such as karyorrhexis (inability of chromosomes to reform into a nucleus after mitosis resulting in disintegrated, structureless chromatin fragments), multinuclearity, and other bizarre changes. Peripheral blood and bone marrow leukocytes and platelets are not affected in CDA.

Based on cellular morphology, three types of CDA have been defined, types I, II, and III (Table 12-2).[56] Not all the laboratory findings for a given patient may fulfill the criteria for a single category. The disease may first be diagnosed in infancy,[83] in early adult life,[10] or later.[88] In all three types, the bone marrow generally shows significant erythroid hyperplasia while the peripheral blood reticulocyte count usually remains normal.

Type I

Type I CDA is a rare disorder that may cause neonatal jaundice[83] but patients usually have a normal life span. It has been diagnosed in older patients.[7,88] Clinically, patients may present with splenomegaly.[57]

Morphologic findings include mild macrocytosis, anisocytosis, and poikilocytosis. Basophilic stippling and Cabot rings may be seen regardless of whether the patient has a spleen.[57] The bone marrow demonstrates binucleated cells (Fig. 12-7), cells with incompletely separated or multilobulated nuclei, megaloblastic nuclear chromatin structure, and erythrophagocytosis. A diagnostic feature is the finding of thin, Feulgen-positive, internuclear chromatin bridges joining two normoblasts.[57]

Type II

Type II CDA is also referred to as hereditary erythroblast multinuclearity with positive acidified serum test (HEMPAS).[28,136] Of the three CDAs, type II is the most common, although it is also rare. Its major laboratory diagnostic finding is the abnormal erythrocyte sensitivity to

---

TABLE 12-2. Differentiating Features of Congenital Dyserythropoietic Anemias

TYPE	ANEMIA CLASSIFICATION	BINUCLEARITY	NRBC MULTINUCLEARITY	NRBC CHROMATIN STRUCTURE	MODE OF INHERITANCE	ACIDIFIED SERUM TEST
I	Slightly macrocytic (MCV 93–115 fL)	Yes	No	Megaloblastic	Autosomal recessive	Negative
II	Normocytic	Yes	Yes	Normoblastic	Autosomal recessive	Positive
III	Normocytic or slightly macrocytic	Occasional	Yes	Normoblastic	Autosomal dominant	Negative

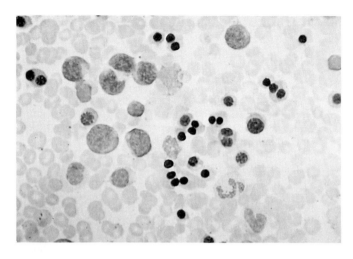

FIG. 12–7. Bone marrow from patient with type I CDA shows binucleated normoblasts associated with the dyserythropoiesis that characterizes this disorder.

acidified normal serum, which is similar to that seen in paroxysmal nocturnal hemoglobinuria (PNH) (Chap. 18).

Clinical findings include hepatosplenomegaly and varying degrees of jaundice. Anemia may appear early in life or not until adulthood.

The peripheral blood film commonly reveals anisocytosis, poikilocytosis, and basophilic stippling. Using phase-contrast microscopy, one may detect ghost red cells that reveal irregular dark stretches of thickened membrane believed to represent membrane doubling.[135] This is a significant diagnostic feature. Unlike type I, megaloblastic bone marrow morphology is not characteristic of type II CDA.

The positive acidified serum test in type II is attributed to the unique HEMPAS antigen found on the red cell surface in this disorder[135] and to a high concentration of fetal i antigens on type II cells. Certain common IgM antibodies bind with HEMPAS antigens and activate the classic complement pathway, causing hemolysis (Chap. 19).[108] Usually this is only an *in vitro* phenomenon, since intravascular hemolysis is not common in type II CDA.

HEMPAS cells, unlike PNH cells, do not lyse in the sugar water test (Chap. 18) because of the difference in complement activation pathways for these disorders (in PNH, hemolysis is caused by activation of the alternate complement pathway).

These patients usually have a normal life span. Splenectomy sometimes improves quality of life.[142]

Type III

Type III CDA, probably the first to be reported,[145] is known to have affected about 23 persons in four families.[10,49] The most noteworthy feature is the pronounced multinuclearity (up to 12 nuclei per cell) of bone marrow normoblasts (NRBCs) in these subjects. As many as 30% of the red cell precursors may be affected, and they may be gigantic—up to 50 to 60 μm in diameter. Thus their name, gigantoblasts.[142] Maturation of neutrophilic promyelo-

cytes and myelocytes does not appear to be abnormal.[140] Table 12-2 provides further details on type III CDA.

Other Laboratory Findings in CDA

Other findings common to CDA types I, II, and III include markedly increased plasma iron transport and increased levels of indirect serum bilirubin and fecal urobilinogen. Red cell survival is normal or only slightly decreased. These patients may develop a secondary hemosiderosis.

CHAPTER SUMMARY

The anemias of abnormal nuclear development, including the megaloblastic anemias and the congenital dyserythropoietic anemias (CDAs), are characterized by abnormal bone marrow cell maturation. Cells in the bone marrow and peripheral blood (and their nuclei) may be abnormal in size, shape, and color. Laboratory features of the megaloblastic anemias include peripheral blood macroovalocytes and hypersegmented neutrophils. The blood count reflects an increased MCV and a decreased hemoglobin, hematocrit, and erythrocyte count. Leukocyte and platelet counts are usually within the reference range.

Most often, megaloblastic anemia is caused by vitamin B_{12} or folate deficiency. Vitamin B_{12} is available in meat, fish, eggs, and milk, and the normal body tissue supply is enough to sustain a person for several years. Folate is available in green leafy vegetables, liver, kidney, whole grain cereals, yeast, and fruit, but body stores are adequate for only a few months.

Without adequate vitamin B_{12} or folate, normal DNA synthesis is interrupted (see Fig. 12-3) and megaloblastic erythropoiesis occurs in the bone marrow. This is reflected by hypercellular marrow containing megaloblasts (very large erythrocyte precursors) that have extremely basophilic cytoplasm and very fine particulate chromatin unlike the clumped chromatin of normal marrow normoblasts. Megaloblasts often display asynchrony of nuclear–cytoplasmic maturation (an immature nucleus and mature cytoplasm).

Most often, vitamin B_{12} deficiency is caused by an acquired gastric atrophy that causes a decrease or total shutdown of intrinsic factor (IF) secretion from gastric parietal cells. The resulting megaloblastic anemia is called pernicious anemia (PA). Without the protection of IF, vitamin B_{12} cannot withstand the long journey to the ileum, where it is normally absorbed.

Laboratory tests most useful for the diagnosis of PA include the IF-blocking antibody test (positive in PA), serum B_{12} assay (decreased in PA) as measured by competitive protein-binding radioassay, a peripheral blood count and review of peripheral blood morphology, and a Schilling test, first with oral administration of [57]Co-labeled vitamin B_{12} but without IF, then, if B_{12} absorption is abnormal (if less than 7% is excreted in the 24 hour urine), a second Schilling test with oral IF. Figure 12-6 summarizes the interpretation of the test results. Increased urine methylmalonic acid (MMA), measured by mass spectrometry, is also very specific for B_{12} deficiency. The deoxyuridine suppression test is useful for differentiating borderline cases of B_{12} and folate deficiency and cases where deficiency of neither component is clearly indicated.

Some other causes of B_{12} deficiency are *Diphyllobothrium latum* (fish tapeworm disease), ileal disease (e.g., Crohn's disease), certain drugs, and rarely, inadequate diet. Immerslund syndrome is a rare hereditary cause that may be related to a defect in ileal B_{12} absorption. For most patients with B_{12} deficiency, lifelong cyanocobalamin supplementation corrects the anemia.

Folate deficiency is characterized by the typical peripheral blood and bone marrow megaloblastic changes, by a decreased erythrocyte folate level (a more accurate reflection of tissue folate stores than serum folate) as measured by competitive protein-binding radioassay (see Table 12-1), and by increased urinary excretion of formiminoglutamic acid. Causes include dietary deficiency (which occurs more readily than B_{12} deficiency), alcoholic cirrhosis, pregnancy, infant malnutrition, and folate antagonists.

Orotic aciduria and Lesch-Nyhan syndrome are rare hereditary disorders that interfere with DNA synthesis, causing megaloblastic anemia.

Megaloblastoid cell maturation (observed in myeloproliferative and myelodysplastic disorders) can be differentiated from megaloblastic maturation by the pseudo-Pelger-Huet cells (hypolobulated neutrophils), the left shift in the differential cell count, and the normal or increased B_{12} and folate levels, all characteristic of megaloblastoid maturation.

The rare CDAs are classified as types, I, II, and III. Each displays some form of abnormality that affects bone marrow erythrocyte precursors (see Table 12-2).

CASE STUDY 12-1

A 63-year-old man, with a 20-year history of non-insulin-dependent diabetes mellitus, reported a recent 27-pound weight loss. His tongue was red and fissured. On neurologic examination, he had decreased fibratory sensation, and his thyroid appeared diffusely enlarged. His complete blood count results were as follows: WBC 8.1 × 10^9/L; RBC 2.49 × 10^{12}/L; Hb 10.1 g/dL; HCT 30.9 L/L; MCV 124 fL; MCH 40.5 pg; MCHC 32.7 g/dL; platelets 173 × 10^9/L.

His electronic leukocyte and platelet histograms appeared normal. The red cell distribution width was normal, 14.3. The red cell histogram was shifted to the right, indicating an increased MCV.

The peripheral blood film showed moderate macroovalocytes and hypersegmented neutrophils. Anisocytosis and poikilocytosis were moderate and elliptocytes and target cells were slight. The serum B_{12} value was less than 50 ng/L and serum folate, 10.3 ug/L. A Schilling test was performed without intrinsic factor, and 1% ^{57}Co-labeled B_{12} was excreted in the 24 hour urine collection. Upon repeat of the test with IF, 8% was excreted in the 24 hour urine. The result of the IF-blocking antibodies test was positive.

1. Which of the blood count results are abnormal? What do they indicate initially?
2. Is either the serum B_{12} or folate level abnormal?
3. Was it appropriate to order the Schilling test in this case? How might the test results be interpreted?
4. Is there a possible relationship between the patient's diabetes mellitus and the hematologic abnormality?
5. What are IF-blocking antibodies? What does the positive result on the IF-blocking antibodies test indicate?
6. Do the hypersegmented neutrophils or macroovalocytes allow for differentiation between B_{12} and folate deficiency? Are they specific for megaloblastic anemia? What is the minimum number of nuclear lobes necessary for a neutrophil to be considered hypersegmented?
7. What is the most likely diagnosis in this case? Explain.

This case study is reprinted with permission from Pierre R: Seminar and Case Studies The Automated Differential. Rochester, MN, Mayo Foundation, Medical Education Program. © Coulter Electronics, Inc. Presented as a service by Coulter Electronics, Inc., Hialeah, FL, 1985

REFERENCES

1. Addison T: On the Constitutional and Local Effects of Disease of the Suprarenal Capsules. London, S Highly, 1855
2. Alarcon-Segovia D, Herskovic T, Wakim KG et al: Presence of circulating antibodies to gluten and milk fractions in patients with nontropical sprue. Am J Med 36:485, 1964
3. Anderson BB: Investigations into the Euglena method for the assay of the vitamin B_{12} in serum. J Clin Pathol 17:14, 1964
4. Andrus EC, Wintrobe MM: Hyperthyroidism and pernicious anemia. Johns Hopkins Med J 59:291, 1936
5. Baker SJ, Ignatius M, Johnson S et al: Hyperpigmentation of skin. A sign of vitamin B_{12} deficiency. Br Med J 1:1713, 1963
6. Bethell FH, Sturgis CC: The relation of therapy in pernicious anemia to changes in the nervous system. Blood 3:57, 1948
7. Bethlenfalvay NC: CDA type I (letter). Blood 43:155, 1974
8. Bingham J: The macrocytosis of liver disease, I, II. Blood 14:694, 1959; 15:244, 1960
9. Booth CC: Absorption from the small intestine. Sci Basis Med Ann Rev 171, 1963
10. Bright M, Cobb J, Evans B et al: Congenital dyserythropoietic anaemia with erythroblastic multinuclearity. J Clin Pathol 25:561, 1972
11. Buchwald H: Vitamin B_{12} absorption deficiency following bypass of the ileum. Am J Dig Dis 9:755, 1964
12. Callender ST, Denborough MA, Sneath J: Blood groups and other inherited characters in pernicious anaemia. Br J Haematol 3:107, 1957
13. Castle WB: The conquest of pernicious anemia. In Wintrobe MM (ed): Blood, Pure and Eloquent. New York, McGraw–Hill, 1979
14. Castle WB: Current concepts of pernicious anemia. Am J Med 48:541, 1970
15. Castle WB, Heath CW, Strauss MB et al: Observations on the etiologic relationship of achylia gastrica to pernicious anemia. Am J Med Sci 194: 618, 1937
16. Chanarin I: Megaloblastic anaemia, cobalamin, and folate. J Clin Pathol 40:978, 1987
17. Chanarin I: The cobalamins (vitamin B_{12}). In Barker BM, Bender DA (eds): Vitamins in Medicine, 4th ed. London, William Heinemann, 1980
18. Chanarin I: The folates. In Barker BM, Bender DA (eds): Vitamins in Medicine 4th ed. London, William Heinemann, 1980
19. Chanarin I: The Megaloblastic Anaemias, 2nd ed, p 44. Oxford, England, Blackwell Scientific Publications, 1979
20. Chanarin I, Waters DAW: Failed Schilling tests. Scand J Haematol 12:245, 1974
21. Chanarin I: The Megaloblastic Anemias. Philadelphia, FA Davis, 1969
22. Chanarin I, Bennett MC: A spectrophotometric method for estimating formimino-glutamic and urocanic acid. Br Med J 1:27, 1962. Nature 196:271, 1962; Proc R Soc Med 57:384, 1964
23. Chanarin I, James D: Humoral and cell-mediated intrinsic factor antibody in pernicious anaemia. Lancet 1:1078, 1974
24. Chen I-W, Silberstein EB, Maxon HR et al: Semiautomated system for simultaneous assays of serum vitamin B_{12} and folic acid in serum evaluated. Clin Chem 28:2161, 1982
25. Cornell BS: Pernicious Anemia (bibliography). Durham, NC, Duke University Press, 1927
26. Cox EV, White AM: Methylmalonic acid excretion: An index of vitamin B_{12} deficiency. Lancet 2:853, 1962
27. Cox EV: The clinical manifestations of vitamin B_{12} deficiency in Addisonian pernicious anemia. In Heinrich HC (ed): Vitamin B_{12} und Intrisic Factor, 2nd Europäisches Symposon. Stuttgart, Enke, 1962

28. Crookston JH, Crookston MC, Burnie KL et al: Hereditary erythroblastic multinuclearity associated with a positive acidified serum test: A type of congenital dyserythropoietic anaemia. Br J Haematol 17:11, 1969

29. Davidson LSP, Davis LJ, Innes J: The effect of liver therapy on erythropoiesis as observed by serial sternal punctures in twelve cases of pernicious anaemia. Q J Med 11:19, 1942

30. Deller DJ, Richards WC, Witts LJ: Changes in the blood after partial gastrectomy with special reference to vitamin B_{12}. Q J Med 31:71, 89, 1962; Lancet 2:162, 1963

31. Donaldson RM: Small bowel bacterial overgrowth. Adv Intern Med 16:191, 1970

32. Doniach D, Roitt IM: An evaluation of gastric and thyroid autoimmunity in relation to hematologic disorders. Semin Hematol 1:313, 1964

33. Dormandy KM, Waters AH, Mollin DL: Folic acid deficiency in coeliac disease. Lancet 1:632, 1963

34. Dreyfus PM, Dube VE: The rapid detection of methylmalonic acid in urine—a sensitive index of vitamin B_{12} deficiency. Clin Chim Acta 15:525, 1967

35. Ellison ABC: Pernicious anemia masked by multivitamins containing folic acid. JAMA 173:240, 1960

36. Emerson PM, Wilkinson JH: Lactate dehydrogenase in the diagnosis and assessment of response to treatment of megaloblastic anaemia. Br J Haematol 12:678, 1966

37. Epstein RD: Cells of the megakaryocyte series in pernicious anemia. Am J Pathol 25:239, 1949

38. Fairbanks VF, Klee GG: Biochemical aspects of hematology. In Tietz NW (ed): Fundamentals of Clinical Chemistry, ed 3, pp 816–818. Philadelphia, WB Saunders, 1987

39. Falchuk ZM, Gebhard RL, Sessoms C et al: An *in vitro* model of gluten-sensitive enteropathy. J Clin Invest 53:487, 1974

40. Farquharson RF, Borsook H, Goulding AM: Pigment metabolism and destruction of blood in Addison's (pernicious) anemia. Arch Intern Med 48:1156, 1931

41. Finch CA: Erythrokinetics in pernicious anemia. Blood 9:807, 1956

42. Finlayson NDC, Fauconnet MH, Krohn K: *In vitro* demonstration of delayed hypersensitivity to gastric antigens in pernicious anemia. Am J Dig Dis 17:631, 1972

43. Friedlander RD: The racial factor in pernicious anemia: A study of five hundred cases. Am J Med Sci 187:634, 1934

44. Ghitis J: The labile folate of milk. Am J Clin Nutr 18:452, 1966

45. Gijzen AHJ, deKock HW, Meulendijk PN et al: The need for a sufficient number of low level sera in comparisons of different serum vitamin B_{12} assays. Clin Chim Acta 127:185, 1983

46. Glass GBJ: Antitrophic effects of gastric autoantibodies on parietal and peptic cells. In Glass GBJ (ed): Progress in Gastroenterology, vol 3, p 73. New York, Grune & Stratton, 1977

47. Gompertz D, Jones JH, Knowles JP: The measurement of urinary methylmalonic acid by a combination of thin-layer and gas chromatography. Clin Chim Acta 19:477, 1968

48. Gorbach SL: Population control in the small bowel. Gut 8:530, 1967

49. Goudsmit R, Beckers D, De Bruijne JI et al: Congenital dyserythropoietic anaemia, type III. Br J Haematol 23:97, 1972

50. Grant JP: Handbook of Total Parenteral Nutrition. Philadelphia, WB Saunders, 1980

51. Halsted CH, Reisenauer AM, Romero JJ et al: Jejunal perfusion of simple and conjugated folates in celiac sprue. J Clin Invest 59:933, 1977

52. Halsted JA, Lewis PM, Gasster M: Absorption of radioactive vitamin B_{12} in the syndrome of megaloblastic anemia associated with intestinal stricture or anastomosis. Am J Med 20:42, 1956

53. Hamilton HE, Sheets RF, DeGowin EL: Studies with inagglutinable erythrocyte counts. J Lab Clin Med 51:942, 1958

54. Hart RJ, McCurdy PR: Pernicious anemia in Negroes (letter). Ann Intern Med 74:448, 1971

54a. Hart RJ, McCurdy PR: Psychosis in vitamin B_{12} deficiency. Arch Intern Med 128:596, 1971

55. Hawkins CF: Value of serum iron levels in assessing effect of haematinics in the macrocytic anaemias. Br Med J 1:383, 1955

56. Heimpel H, Wendt F: Congenital dyserythropoietic anemia with karyorrhexis and multinuclearity of erythroblasts. Blut 31:261, 1976

57. Heimpel H: Congenital dyserythropoietic anemia type I: Clinical and experimental aspects. In Congenital Disorders of Erythropoiesis (Proceedings—Ciba Symposium), p 135. Amsterdam, Elsevier, 1976

58. Herbert V, Tisman G, Le-Teng-Go et al: The dU suppression test using ^{125}I-UdR to define biochemical megaloblastosis. Br J Haematol 24:713, 1973

59. Herbert V, Streiff RR, Sullivan LW: Notes on vitamin B_{12} absorption; autoimmunity and childhood pernicious anemia; relation of intrinsic factor to blood group substance. Medicine 43:679, 1964

60. Herbert V, Zalusky R: Interrelations of vitamin B_{12} and folic acid metabolism: Folic acid clearance studies. J Clin Invest 41:1263, 1962

61. Herbert V, Baker H, Frank O et al: The measurement of folic acid activity in serum: A diagnostic aid in the differentiation of the megaloblastic anemias. Blood 15:228, 1960

62. Hift W, Moshal MG, Pillay K: Megaloblastic anaemia, achlorhydria, low intrinsic factor, and intrinsic factor antibodies in the absence of pernicious anaemia. Lancet 1:570, 1973

63. Higginbottom MC, Sweetman L, Nyhan WL: A syndrome of methylmalonic aciduria, homocystinuria, megaloblastic anemia and neurologic abnormalities in a vitamin B_{12}–deficient breast-fed infant of a strict vegetarian. N Engl J Med 299:317, 1978

64. Hillman RS, McGuffin R, Campbell C: Alcohol interference with the folate enterohepatic cycle. Trans Assoc Am Physicians 90:145, 1977

65. Hoffbrand AV, Newcombe FA, Mollin DL: Method of assay of red cell folate activity and the value of the assay as a test for folate deficiency. J Clin Pathol 19:17, 1966

66. Houts TM, Carney JA: Radioassay for cobalamin (vitamin B_{12}) requiring no pretreatment of serum. Clin Chem 27:263, 1981

67. Irvine WJ: Gastric antibodies studied by fluorescence microscopy. Q J Exp Physiol 48:427, 1963

68. Isaacs R, Bethell FH, Riddle MC et al: Standards for red blood cell increase after liver and stomach therapy in pernicious anemia. JAMA 111:2291, 1938

69. Israels MCG, Wilkinson JF: Risk of neurological complication in pernicious anaemia treated with folic acid. Br Med J 2:1072, 1949

70. Jacob E, Glass GBJ: Separation of intrinsic factor antibodies from parietal cell antibodies in pernicious anemia serum by gel filtration. Proc Soc Exp Biol Med 137:243, 1971

71. Jacob E, Glass GBJ: The participation of complement in the parietal cell antigen-antibody reaction in pernicious anemia and atrophic gastritis. Clin Exp Immunol 5:141, 1969

72. Jacobson ED, Chodos RB, Faloon WW: An experimental malabsorption syndrome induced by neomycin. Am J Med 28:524, 1960

73. Jandl JH: The anemia of liver disease: Observations on its mechanism. J Clin Invest 34:390, 1955

74. Katz M, Lee SK, Cooper BA: Vitamin B_{12} malabsorption due to a biologically inert intrinsic factor. N Engl J Med 287:425, 1972

75. Keller R, Lindstrand K, Norden A: Disappearance of chromosomal abnormalities in megaloblastic anaemia after treatment. Scand J Haematol 7:478, 1970

76. Kilbridge TM, Heller P: Determinants of erythrocyte size in chronic liver disease. Blood 34:739, 1969

77. Kimber CL, Deller DJ, Ibbotson RN et al: The mechanism of anemia in chronic liver disease. Q J Med 34:33, 1965

78. Klipstein FA: Tropical sprue. Gastroenterology 54:275, 1968; 68:239, 1975; Blood 45:577, 1975

79. Krasnow SE, Walsh JR, Zimmerman HJ et al: Megaloblastic anemia in "alcoholic" cirrhosis. Arch Intern Med 100:870, 1957

80. Kubasic NP, Ricotta M, Sine HE: Commercially supplied binders for plasma cobalamin (vitamin B_{12}), analysis—"purified" intrinsic factor, "cobinamide"-blocked R protein binder, and nonpurified intrinsic factor R protein binder—compared to microbiological assay. Clin Chem 26:598, 1980

81. Lanzkowsky P: Congenital malabsorption of folate. Am J Med 48:580, 1970

82. Lawler SD, Roberts PD, Hoffbrand AV: Chromosome studies in megaloblastic anaemia before and after treatment. Scand J Haematol 8:309, 1971

83. Lay HN, Pemberton PJ, Hilton HB: Congenital dyserythropoietic anaemia type I in two brothers presenting with neonatal jaundice. Arch Dis Child 53:753, 1978

84. Lien-Keng K, Odang O: Megaloblastic anemia in infancy and childhood in Djakarta. Am J Dis Child 97:209, 1959

85. Lindenbaum J: Status of laboratory testing in the diagnosis of megaloblastic anemia. Blood 61:624, 1983

86. Lindenbaum J, Lieber CS: Alcohol-induced malabsorption of vitamin B_{12} in man. Nature 224:806, 1969

87. MacIver JE, Back EH: Megaloblastic anaemia of infancy in Jamaica. Arch Dis Child 35:134, 1960

88. Maldonado JE, Taswell HF: Type I dyserythropoietic anemia in an elderly patient. Blood 44:495, 1974

89. Markson JL, Moore JM: Autoimmunity in pernicious anaemia and iron deficiency anaemia. Lancet 2:1240, 1962

90. Matoth Y, Pinkas A, Sroka C: Studies on folic acid in infancy. III. Folates in breast fed infants and their mothers. Am J Clin Nutr 16:356, 1965

91. Matthews DM: Observations on the estimation of serum vitamin B_{12} using *Lactobacillus leichmannii*. Clin Sci 22:101, 1962

92. McIntyre OR, Sullivan LW, Jeffries GH et al: Pernicious anemia in childhood. N Engl J Med 272:981, 1965

93. Mohamed SD, McKay E, Galloway WH: Juvenile familial megaloblastic anaemia due to selective malabsorption of vitamin B_{12}. A family study and a review of the literature. Q J Med 35:433, 1966

94. Mollin DL: Vitamin B_{12} metabolism in man using cobalt-58 (^{58}Co) as a tracer. Proc R Soc Med 55:141, 1962

95. Mosbech J: Heredity in Pernicious Anemia. Copenhagen, Munksgaard, 1953

96. Nath BJ, Lindenbaum J: Persistence of neutrophil hypersegmentation during recovery from megaloblastic granulopoiesis. Ann Intern Med 90:757, 1979

97. National Academy of Sciences: Recommended Dietary Allowances, ed 9, rev. Washington, DC, Food and Nutrition Board of the National Research Council, 1980

98. Norman EJ, Martelo OJ, Denton MD: Cobalamin (vitamin B_{12}) deficiency detection by urinary methylmalonic acid quantitation. Blood 59:1128, 1982

99. Norman EJ, Berry HK, Denton MD: Identification and quantitation of urinary dicarboxylic acids as their dicyclohexyl esters in disease states by gas chromatography mass spectrometry. Biomed Mass Spectrom 6:546, 1979

100. Nyberg W, Gräsbeck R, Saarni M et al: Serum vitamin B_{12} levels and incidence of tapeworm anemia in a population heavily infected with *Diphyllobothrium latum*. Am J Clin Nutr 9:606, 1961

101. Orten JM, Neuhaus OW: Human Biochemistry. St Louis, CV Mosby, 1982

102. Owen JA, Carew JP, Cowling DC et al: Serum haptoglobins in megaloblastic anaemia. Br J Haematol 6:242, 1960

103. Paddock FK, Smith KE: The platelets in pernicious anemia. Am J Med Sci 198:372, 1939

104. Pedersen AB, Mosbeck J: Morbidity of pernicious anaemia. Acta Med Scand 185:449, 1969

105. Rak VK, Varga L, Krizsa F et al: Untersuchung der Thrombocytopoese bei Perniciosa-Kranken. Acta Haematol 34:175, 1965

106. Roe DA: Drug-Induced Nutritional Deficiencies. Westport, CT, AVI, 1976

107. Rose MS, Doniach D, Chanarin I et al: Intrinsic factor antibodies in absence of pernicious anaemia. Lancet 2:9, 1970

108. Rosse WF, Logue GL, Adams J et al: Mechanisms of immune lysis of the red cells in hereditary erythroblastic multinuclearity with a positive acidified serum test and paroxysmal nocturnal hemoglobinuria. J Clin Invest 53:31, 1974

109. Rostand SG: Vitamin B_{12} levels and nerve conduction velocities in patients undergoing maintenance hemodialysis. Am J Clin Nutr 29:691, 1976

110. Rothenberg SP, Kantha KR, Ficarra A: Autoantibodies to intrinsic factor: Their determination and clinical usefulness. J Lab Clin Med 77:476, 1971

111. Rubin CE et al: Biopsy studies on the pathogenesis of coeliac sprue. In Wolstenholme GEW, Cameron MP (eds): Intestinal Biopsy, p 67. Boston Little, Brown & Co, 1962

112. Samson D, Halliday D, Chanarin I: Reversal of ineffective erythropoiesis in pernicious anaemia following vitamin B_{12} therapy. Br J Haematol 35:217, 1977

113. Santiago-Borrero PJ, Santini R Jr, Perez Santiago E et al: Congenital isolated defect of folic acid absorption. J Pediatr 82:450, 1973

114. Sauberlich HF, Skala JH, Dowdy RP: Laboratory Tests for the Assessment of Nutritional Status. Cleveland, CRC Press, 1974

115. Schilling RF, Fairbanks VF, Miller R et al: "Improved" vitamin B_{12} assays: A report on two commercial kits. Clin Chem 29:582, 1983

116. Schilling RF: Vitamin B_{12}: Assay and absorption testing. Lab Management 20:31, 1982

117. Schilling RF: Intrinsic factor studies. II. The effect of gastric juice on the urinary excretion of radioactivity after the oral administration of radioactive vitamin B_{12}. J Lab Clin Med 42:860, 1953

118. Shulman R: Psychiatric aspects of pernicious anaemia. A prospective controlled investigation. Br Med J 3:266, 1967

119. Smith LH: Hereditary orotic aciduria and pyrimidine auxotrophism in man. Am J Med 38:1, 1965

120. Spray GH: An improved method for the rapid estimation of vitamin B_{12} in serum. Clin Sci 14:661, 1955

121. Stamos HF: Heredity in pernicious anemia. Am J Med Sci 200:586, 1940

122. Stasney J, Pizzolato P: Serial bone marrow studies in pernicious anemia. I. Fluctuation in number and volume of nucleated cells. Proc Soc Exp Biol Med 51:335, 1942

123. Steinberg SE, Campbell CL, Hillman RS et al: Kinetics of the normal folate enterohepatic cycle. J Clin Invest 64:83, 1979

124. Sturgis CC: An analysis of the causes of death in 150 fatal cases of pernicious anemia observed since 1927. Trans Assoc Am Physicians 54:46, 1939

125. Sullivan LW: Vitamin B_{12} metabolism and megaloblastic anemia. Semin Hematol 7:6, 1970

126. Sullivan LW, Luhby AL, Streiff RR: Studies of the daily requirement for folic acid in infants and the etiology of folate deficiency in goat's milk megaloblastic anemia. Am J Clin Nutr 18:311, 1966

127. Tai C, McGuigan JE: Immunologic studies in pernicious anemia. Blood 34:63, 1969

128. Taylor KB, Roitt IM, Doniach D et al: Autoimmune phenom-

ena in pernicious anaemia: Gastric antibodies. Br Med J 2:1347, 1962

129. teVelde K, Abels J, Anders GJPA et al: A family study of pernicious anemia by an immunologic method. J Lab Clin Med 64:177, 1964

130. Tisman G, Herbert V: B$_{12}$ dependence of cell uptake of serum folate: An explanation for high serum folate and cell folate depletion in B$_{12}$ deficiency. Blood 41:465, 1973

131. Twomey JJ, Jordan PH, Jarrold T et al: The syndrome of immunoglobulin deficiency and pernicious anemia. A study of 10 cases. Am J Med 47:340, 1969

132. Ungar B: Antibody to gastric intrinsic factor in blood donors and hospital patients. Aust Ann Med 17:107, 1968

133. van der Scheer WM, Koek HC: Peripheral nerve lesions in cases of pernicious anaemia. Acta Psychiatr Neurol 13:61, 1938

134. van der Zee SPM, Schretten EDAM, Monnens LAH: Megaloblastic anaemia in the Lesch-Nyhan syndrome (letter). Lancet 1:1427, 1968

135. Verwilghen RL: Congenital dyserythropoietic anaemia type II (HEMPAS) In Congenital Disorders of Erythropoiesis (Proceedings Ciba Symposium), p 151. Amsterdam, Elsevier, 1976

136. Verwilghen RL, Lewis SM, Dacie JV et al: HEMPAS: Congenital dyserythropoietic anaemia (type II). Q J Med 42:257, 1973

137. Walt F, Holman S, Hendrickse RG: Megaloblastic anaemia of infancy in kwashiorkor and other diseases. Br Med J 1:1199, 1956

138. Waters AH, Mollin DL: Observations on the metabolism of folic acid in pernicious anaemia. Br J Haematol 9:319, 1963

139. Whittingham S, Ungar B, Mackay IR et al: The genetic factor in pernicious anaemia. Lancet 1:951, 1969

140. Wickramasinghe SN, Goudsmit R: Some aspects of the biology of multinucleate and giant mononucleate erythroblasts in a patient with CDA, type III. Br J Haematol 41:485, 1979

141. Wickramasinghe SN, Pratt JR: Myelocyte proliferation in pernicious anaemia. Acta Haematol 44:37, 1970

142. Wintrobe MM: The normocytic, normochromic anemias. In Wintrobe MM, Lee GR, Boggs DR et al: Clinical Hematology, 8th ed, p 677. Philadelphia, Lea & Febiger, 1981

143. Wintrobe MM: Megaloblastic and nonmegaloblastic macrocytic anemias. In Wintrobe MM, Lee GR, Boggs DR et al: Clinical Hematology, 8th ed, p 559. Philadelphia, Lea & Febiger, 1981

144. Wintrobe MM: Nutritional factors in the production and function of erythrocytes. In Wintrobe MM, Lee GR, Boggs DR et al, (eds): Clinical Hematology, ed 8. Philadelphia, Lea & Febiger, 1981

145. Wolff JA, von Hofe FH: Familial erythroid multinuclearity. Blood 6:1274, 1951

146. Zadek I: Pathogenesis of pernicious anemia: Result of postmortem examination of patients who died during remission. Klin Wochenschr 9:1527, 1929

Iron is necessary for the synthesis of normal, oxygen-carrying hemoglobin (Hb) (Chap. 7). Circumstances that cause reduction in the iron available for Hb synthesis or failure to incorporate iron into heme will cause anemia to develop, with the usual range of signs and symptoms related to reduced oxygen-carrying capacity. Among the anemias of abnormal iron metabolism is iron deficiency anemia, the most common form of anemia in the United States[25] and worldwide.[94] Another form of anemia related to iron metabolism, anemia of chronic disorders, is also common, probably second only to iron deficiency.[75] These two anemias, plus two other disorders of iron metabolism, sideroblastic anemia and anemia associated with lead intoxication, will be considered in this chapter.

Synthesis of normally functioning Hb requires that developing erythrocytes have adequate supplies, including the polypeptide chains (*e.g.*, α, β), protoporphyrin IX rings, and iron. In this chapter anemias that occur secondary to low availability of the raw material iron will be presented. Three general etiologic mechanisms appear to be involved: (1) deficiency of the raw material (iron deficiency anemia); (2) defective release of stored iron from macrophages (anemia of chronic disorders); and (3) defective utilization of iron within the erythroblast (sideroblastic anemia, lead intoxication). These disorders differ in their clinical presentations and laboratory features.

CHEMICAL LABORATORY TESTS USEFUL IN DIFFERENTIATING DISORDERS OF IRON METABOLISM

Five chemical tests are particularly useful in the differential diagnosis of iron metabolism disorders: ferritin, free eryth-

TABLE 13-1. Differentiation Among Anemias of Abnormal Iron Metabolism Including Microcytic, Hypochromic Anemias*

	MARROW IRON†	SERUM FERRITIN	MARROW SIDEROBLASTS	SERUM IRON	TOTAL IRON BINDING CAPACITY	TRANSFERRIN SATURATION	FREE ERYTHROCYTE PROTOPORPHYRIN
Ref. range‡	Normal	30–250 µg/L (varies w/age, sex)	25%–30%	50–150 µg/dL (varies w/age, sex)	250–450 µg/dL (adult)	20%–55%	<50 µg/dL RBC
Iron deficiency anemia	Absent	↓	0	↓	↑	↓	↑
Thalassemia§	↑/N	↑/N	N (may be ringed)	↑/N	N	↑/N	N
Anemia of chronic disorders	N/↑	↑	0–few	↓	↓	N/↓	↑
Sideroblastic anemias	↑	↑	↑ (ringed)	↑	↓/N	↑	Mixed
Lead poisoning	N	N	N (may be ringed)	N–↑ (adults) N–↓ (children)	N	↑	↑↑

N = normal.
* Modified from Miale JB: Laboratory Medicine Hematology, 6th ed. St. Louis, CV Mosby, 1982, with permission.
† Based on evaluation of Prussian blue-stained marrow, estimate of iron in RE cells.
‡ From Tietz NW: Textbook of Clinical Chemistry. Philadelphia , WB Saunders, 1986.
§Increased marrow iron, serum fereritin, serum iron, and transferrin saturation = thalassemia major; these values are generally normal in thalassemia minor.

rocyte protoporphyrin (FEP), serum iron, total iron binding capacity (TIBC), and percent transferrin saturation. Table 13-1 provides an overview of the laboratory procedure results in the four disorders of iron metabolism and in thalassemia (Chap. 15), which may be confused with iron deficiency because both are microcytic, hypochromic anemias. This table should be referred to throughout the chapter for a summary of the laboratory findings in each disorder discussed.

A brief definition of these tests and their reference ranges is provided here. Procedural details for these chemical tests are beyond the scope of this text but may be found in textbooks of clinical chemistry.

SERUM FERRITIN

Serum ferritin reflects the body's tissue iron stores and thus is a good indicator of iron storage status. It is valuable in diagnosing iron deficiency because it is generally the first laboratory test to become abnormal when iron stores begin to decrease. It also becomes abnormal before erythrocyte morphology shows any signs of abnormality. Note in Table 13-1 that, among the disorders listed, serum ferritin is decreased only in iron deficiency anemia.

Principle

Serum ferritin is measured using radioimmunoassays.

Reference Range

The reference range in men is 15 to 200 µg/L and in women, 12 to 150 µg/L. Serum ferritin levels generally increase in women who have reached menopause. Each 1 µg/L of ferritin represents approximately 8 mg of tissue iron storage.[21] Children generally have low ferritin levels (approximately 30 µg/L); however, boys generally show an increase in their late teens. For children, ferritin is more accurately expressed as amount per kilogram of body weight; 1 µg of ferritin per liter is equal to approximately 120 µg of iron/kg.

FREE ERYTHROCYTE PROTOPORPHYRIN

Protoporphyrin is the compound to which ferrous iron is added to form heme needed for red cell Hb synthesis (Fig. 13-1).

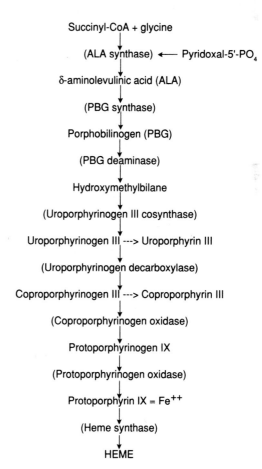

FIG. 13-1. Heme synthesis. Enzymes in this pathway are denoted by parentheses. PBG synthase is also known as δ-amino levulinic acid dehydratase; heme synthase is also known as ferrochelatase. (Modified from Gillen LAF: Hemoglobins, myoglobin, and porphyrins. In Bishop ML, Von Laufen JL, Fody E (eds): Clinical Chemistry—Principles, Procedures, Correlations. Philadelphia: JB Lippincott, 1985, with permission.)

Normally, red cells produce slightly more protoporphyrin than is needed; however, when iron is deficient, protoporphyrin levels build up in erythrocytes to several times the normal level.

Although FEP generally is a valuable early indicator of an iron metabolism disorder, it is not very helpful in differentiating iron deficiency and anemia of chronic disorders, as it is increased in both (see Table 13-1). It is mixed (i.e., increased and decreased) in the various types of sideroblastic anemia, and therefore FEP is not helpful in diagnosing these disorders. However, it generally is normal in thalassemias[52,81]; therefore, FEP is helpful in differentiating thalassemia from iron deficiency and anemia of chronic disorders.

There is disagreement about which laboratory test provides the first indicator of the onset of a decrease in iron stores. Some believe it is the ferritin level,[31] whereas others believe that tests of FEP detect falling iron stores before ferritin tests can.[53,83]

Principle

Free erythrocyte protoporphyrin may be measured directly by a hematofluorometer[67] or by an extraction and fluorescence method.[85]

Reference Range

The reference range depends on the method used. An approximate reference range is less than 50 μg/dL of RBC.[84]

SERUM IRON

Although serum iron assay may not always be necessary to the differential diagnosis of disorders of iron metabolism, it is still used for this purpose. It is particularly helpful in cases where the diagnosis is not obvious from other laboratory tests (see Table 13-1).

Principle

Serum ferric iron is first removed from attachment to transferrin by the addition of a chemical such as 0.05N hydrochloric acid. All iron is then chemically transformed to the reduced ferrous (Fe^{+2}) state by addition of a chromogenic reagent such as acid–ferrozine, which results in the formation of a colored complex that can be measured spectrophotometrically at 562 nm. The results are compared with a standard curve to obtain a quantitative serum iron measurement.

Specimen Requirements

A nonhemolyzed serum sample is required. Use of anticoagulated samples may cause erroneous results because of addition of iron by the anticoagulant (e.g., heparin) or because of iron chelation (e.g., EDTA). Samples should be drawn in the morning because serum iron levels may be approximately 25% lower in the evening.[11] The patient should have been fasting for 12 hours and should not take any iron-containing medication for 12 to 24 hours before the test.

Reference Range

The reference range is 50 to 150 μg/dL, with an average of 125 μg/dL for men and 100 μg/dL for women. Serum iron in the elderly is much lower, with a reference range of approximately 40 to 80 μg/dL.

TOTAL IRON BINDING CAPACITY

The total iron binding capacity (TIBC) occasionally is required to diagnose an iron metabolism disorder. It is helpful in cases where other laboratory data do not pinpoint the diagnosis (see Table 13-1).

Principle

In the TIBC test the concentration of transferrin is measured indirectly (i.e., the actual transferrin protein concentration is not measured) by measuring the ability of serum transferrin to bind iron. Transferrin is saturated by the addition of ferric (Fe^{+3}) iron to the serum sample. All excess, unbound iron is chemically removed from the specimen, and the remaining sample is then analyzed for iron content using the serum iron method described above. In measuring this iron, the total capacity of transferrin to bind iron is determined.

Specimen Requirements

The requirements are the same as for serum iron determination. However, unlike serum iron, TIBC values are not dependent on the time of day the sample is drawn.

Reference Range

The TIBC reference range for adults is approximately 250 to 450 μg/dL. This tends to decrease with age, and persons 70 years of age or older generally have a TIBC around 250 μg/dL.

TRANSFERRIN SATURATION

Transferrin saturation may be calculated only if serum iron and TIBC values are available. It is only occasionally required to diagnose disorders of iron metabolism but is frequently used for this purpose (see Table 13-1).

Principle

Transferrin saturation values are obtained through the following calculation based on measurements of serum iron and TIBC:

$$\% \text{ Transferrin Saturation} = \frac{\text{Serum Iron}}{\text{TIBC}} \times 100$$

Reference Range

The reference range is 20% to 55% saturation.

IRON DEFICIENCY ANEMIA

Pathophysiology and Populations Affected

Iron deficiency may occur by any one or a combination of mechanisms (Table 13-2). During infancy and childhood an individual needs an adequate supply of iron to increase the erythrocyte mass 30-fold from infant to adult levels. During the first year of life alone, the total Hb nearly doubles to meet the needs of a body that triples in size.[79] In children, because of the high demand for iron, iron reserves are usually low and would be considered depleted by adult standards.[71] The combination of high physiologic demand and low reserves makes infants, in particular, susceptible to iron deficiency anemia. This situation is combined with the low natural availability of iron in the infant's primary source of nutrition, milk. Cow's milk contains only about

---

TABLE 13-2. Mechanisms of Iron Deficiency

Increased physiologic demand
  Rapid growth: infants, children
  Pregnancy, lactation
Inadequate intake
  Iron-deficient diet
  Inadequate absorption (achlorhydria, decreased absorptive surface)
Chronic blood loss
  Menstrual flow
  Gastrointestinal bleeding
  Regular blood donation
  Chronic hemolysis

0.07 mg of iron per deciliter, and human milk supplies only slightly more. Neither of these, unsupplemented, is an adequate source of iron for a growing infant.[70]

Pregnancy presents a special physiologic need for additional iron. The pregnant woman requires about 30 to 75 mg of dietary iron per day (assuming the usual 10% absorption) to provide for the needs of the fetus as well as her own expanded blood volume. Even in the best of circumstances, this is too large an amount of iron to absorb from dietary sources. Hence, iron supplementation is required at least during the last half of pregnancy.[20] In addition, the loss of iron during lactation is approximately the same as iron loss during menstruation. Because menstruation is usually inhibited during lactation, the demand for iron is about the same in lactating women and nonlactating premenopausal women.[93]

The second important cause of iron deficiency anemia is inadequate intake of iron, which may result from a diet low in iron or from inability to absorb iron (see Table 13-2). The normal American diet provides adequate iron for a man or a postmenopausal woman. However, the amount of available iron in the normal diet of a woman of childbearing age is marginal. A variety of factors, including food selection and cooking methods, affect dietary iron levels. For example, iron in the form of heme, from red meats, is more readily absorbed than is nonheme iron from vegetables and iron-enriched grain foods.[65] Food cooked in iron utensils contains more iron than food cooked in Teflon-coated, aluminum, or glass utensils. Even typically iron-rich vegetables, when grown in iron-depleted soil, contribute to iron deficiency.[75]

Another factor contributing to iron deficiency is achlorhydria (reduced gastric acidity), which may cause inadequate absorption and thus reduced iron stores. Ingested Fe^{+3} in vegetables and grains must be reduced to Fe^{+2}, the absorbable form. This is dependent on proper gastric acidity, although the role of gastric acid in iron absorption is not entirely clear. In addition, malabsorptive syndromes that reduce the available intestinal absorptive surface may cause iron deficiency.[70]

A final important cause of iron deficiency is chronic blood loss (see Table 13-2). Iron deficiency anemia is prevalent in women ages 18 to 44,[25] presumably because of menstrual loss, which is the largest single contributor to iron deficiency anemia.[59] The recommended daily allowance (RDA) for men is approximately 10 mg, whereas the RDA for the typical premenopausal woman is 20 mg.[70] Iron typically is conserved by the body in reticuloendothelial (RE) cell stores. Thus, when iron deficiency anemia occurs in a man or a postmenopausal woman, it usually is the result of some form of chronic blood loss, most frequently gastrointestinal bleeding. Other possible causes are esophageal varices, peptic ulcer disease, neoplastic disease anywhere in the gastrointestinal tract (especially the colon), and hemorrhoids.[9]

Two other situations may cause chronic iron loss. Regular blood donation may cause iron deficiency in the otherwise healthy individual.[80] Chronic intravascular hemolytic disease causes excess loss in the urine in the form of hemoglobinuria, with iron losses of as much as 7.8 mg/d.[40] An example is the rare disorder paroxysmal nocturnal hemoglobinuria (PNH).

The development of iron deficiency anemia is gradual (Table 13-3). An individual with adequate iron stores, as tissue ferritin, is said to be *iron replete*. As the demand for iron increases, for whatever reason, or as iron is lost, the stored iron will be utilized. In this stage an individual is said to have *depleted* iron stores. If conditions continue to pro-

TABLE 13-3. Sequential Changes in Development of Iron Deficiency

IRON STATUS	IRON REPLETE (NORMAL)	STAGE 1 (IRON DEPLETED)	STAGE 2 (IRON DEFICIENT ERYTHROPOIESIS)	STAGE 3 (IRON DEFICIENCY ANEMIA)
Serum Ferritin (μg/L)	> 12	< 12	< 12	< 12
Marrow iron	2–3$^+$	0–1$^+$	0	0
TIBC (μg/dL)	300–360	360	390	410
Serum iron (μg/dL)	65–165	115	< 60	< 40
Transferrin saturation (%)	20–50	30	< 15	< 10
Free erythrocyte protoporphyrin (μg/dL)	< 50	< 50	100	200
Marrow sideroblasts (%)	40–60	40–60	< 10	< 10
Hemoglobin	Normal	Normal	Normal	↓↓↓
MCV	Normal	Normal	Normal	↓↓↓
RBC morphology	Normal	Normal	Normal	Microcytic hypochromic

(Stage 1 column bracketed "Early"; Stage 2 column bracketed "Intermediate"; Stage 3 column bracketed "Late")

Adapted from Hillman RS, Finch CA: Red Cell Manual, 5th ed, p 60. Philadelphia, FA Davis, 1985, with permission.

duce an increased demand for or loss of iron, *deficiency* eventually will occur that may finally be manifest as iron deficiency anemia.[73] The individual may not exhibit signs or symptoms of iron deficiency until the appearance of frank anemia. The sequential changes in development of iron deficiency are shown in Table 13-3.

Clinical Presentation

The presentation of iron deficiency anemia is similar to that of any other form of anemia. The usual range of symptoms, such as fatigue, breathlessness, and dizziness, brought greater than 60% of patients with iron deficiency to medical attention in one study.[9] These symptoms are related to reduced oxygen delivery to the tissues and so are typical of any anemia, regardless of cause. After the appearance of frank anemia, anemia progresses from mild to moderate, and even to severe, before the patient seeks treatment. This is because of the gradual onset that permits compensatory mechanisms to minimize the symptoms until the anemia is severe (Chap. 10).[75]

Because chronic blood loss is a significant cause of iron deficiency, some patients present with signs and symptoms related to their primary disease.[9] For example, a man may complain of epigastric pain related to ulcers or a woman may note menorrhagia. Iron deficiency may be detected when patients come to medical attention for such causes.

Another important clinical finding is the frequency with which patients report pica. Pica is a persistent, compulsive desire to eat a single food or nonfood item such as starch or something crunchy such as ice, clay, plaster, or crunchy foods. Pica appears to cease when iron intake increases.[22]

Physical Findings

A variety of epithelial changes are common in iron deficiency anemia, particularly disturbances related to the gastrointestinal system such as angular stomatitis (cracks in the corners of the mouth), glossitis (soreness of the tongue), and gastritis.[9] In some cases the gastritis progresses to gastric atrophy and results in achlorhydria. Another interesting epithelial change sometimes encountered is koilonychia, a flattening and spooning of the nails (Fig. 13-2).

This appears to be much more common in adults although it does occur in some iron-deficient infants.[46] Splenomegaly is rare,[9] and neurologic changes such as those seen in vitamin B_{12} deficiency are not found in iron deficiency anemia.

Laboratory Findings and Correlations with Disease

Hematology

The CBC reflects a decreased Hb and hematocrit in the late stages of iron deficiency (see Table 13-3). The Hb may be markedly decreased (8 g/dL or lower) before the patient complains of anemia-related symptoms.[93] Severe iron deficiency anemia is characterized by a reduced MCV, MCH, and MCHC. In one study of 115 patients all RBC indices were decreased: the average MCV was 75 fL (with a range of 59–80 fL); MCH was 21 pg (range 15–26 pg); and MCHC was 28 g/dL (range 22–31 g/dL).[5] On the blood film erythrocytes appear microcytic and hypochromic (Fig. 13-3). In severe iron deficiency only the outer rims of the cells are visible. A moderate anisocytosis with some cells in the normal size range may be seen and may be reflected in an elevated RDW. The increasing RDW may be an indicator of impending or overt iron deficiency, although this remains to be confirmed.[68] A variety of abnormal erythrocyte shapes are also observed on the blood film, including elongated cells, tailed elliptical cells, and tiny microcytes.[93]

Platelet counts may be low, normal, or high. Often, however, the platelet count is increased to about twice the reference range.[78] In such cases the etiology of the anemia may be related to chronic hemorrhage.[26] Increased platelet counts may occur in infants.[36] Leukocyte and reticulocyte counts usually are within the reference range and are therefore not particularly diagnostic.[70] The reticulocyte production index (RPI) gradually falls below 2.0 as iron deficiency progresses, because the bone marrow cannot compensate for the anemia without sufficient iron stores.

Bone Marrow

Study of the marrow is rarely necessary to make the diagnosis. When it is performed, the sample is stained for

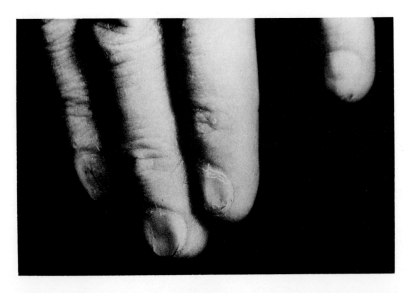

FIG. 13-2.   Koilonychia, the flattened, spooned nails seen in some cases of chronic iron deficiency. (From Hoffbrand AV, Pettit JE: Essential Haematology, 2nd ed, Oxford, England: Blackwell Scientific Publications Ltd, p 33. 1984, with permission.)

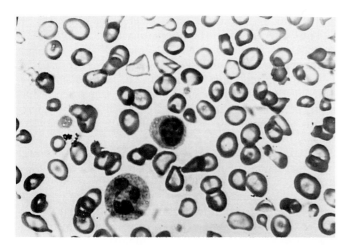

FIG. 13-3.   Microcytic, hypochromic erythrocytes in iron deficiency anemia. Note marked anisocytosis and poikilocytosis. (Courtesy of Dr. Paul I Liu.)

Prussian blue reactivity to estimate iron stores (Chap. 29). Iron stores are severely decreased in the first stage of iron deficiency development (see Table 13-3). This simply confirms the deficit of stored iron indicated by the decreased serum ferritin. Also notable are the marrow sideroblasts (iron-containing nucleated red blood cells), which are decreased in the second stage of anemia development.

Chemistry

Chemical analysis of iron status is important to identify the various stages of iron deficiency. Of particular importance is the serum ferritin level and FEP,[27,67] although, as noted earlier, there is disagreement on whether the serum ferritin or FEP measurement is the first to indicate the early stages of iron depletion. In any case both measurements are commonly used in the diagnosis of iron deficiency today because serum ferritin levels decrease and FEP levels increase in the early to intermediate stages (see Table 13-3), much before red cell morphology or Hb levels show any sign of abnormality.[44]

Other useful tests of iron status are serum iron, TIBC, and percent transferrin saturation. All of these measures become abnormal at around the same time as the FEP, although one report states that FEP does not increase until 2 to 3 weeks after the decrease in percent transferrin saturation.[31] As iron loss progresses, transferrin saturation and serum iron decrease, whereas the TIBC increases because of the lack of iron available for transport.

Ferritin is an acute-phase protein and will therefore be elevated during an inflammatory response. When iron deficiency and inflammation are concurrent, ferritin may be elevated, masking the iron deficiency.[63] Therefore, if inflammation is present when iron deficiency is suspected, other measures of iron status must be considered before the diagnosis can be made.

Serum erythropoietin levels are expected to be elevated in iron deficiency.[72] However, the erythropoietic mechanism is unable to respond without sufficient iron stores.

Differential Diagnosis

Several anemias fall into the category of those with microcytic, hypochromic erythrocytes. Table 13-1 indicates

TABLE 13-4. Recommended Laboratory Tests to Assist in Diagnosis of Iron Deficiency	
Required most frequently	CBC (with RBC morphology)
	Serum ferritin or FEP
	Reticulocyte count 7–12 days after start of iron therapy
Required occasionally	Serum iron
	TIBC
	Percent transferrin saturation
Required rarely	WBC differential

how these anemias may be distinguished. Appropriate diagnosis is important, because the treatments for these anemias differ significantly. Discussion of anemia of chronic disorders, sideroblastic anemia, and lead poisoning follows in this chapter. Thalassemia is discussed in Chapter 15. Table 13-4 provides a list of tests recommended to assist in the diagnosis of iron deficiency.

Effects of Treatment on Laboratory Results

Iron deficiency anemia is treated by giving iron supplements, controlling bleeding, or both as appropriate. Iron therapy should produce an increase in the reticulocyte count and RPI (> 3) within a few days, reaching a maximum at 7 to 12 days. Hemoglobin values increase until the patient's normal level is achieved, usually within 2 months. A dimorphic population of red cells becomes evident as new iron-normal erythrocytes increase in number while the iron-deficient erythrocytes disappear. Red cell histograms also document this replacement of iron-deficient red cells by normal cells. Patients should continue iron therapy after Hb levels normalize to reestablish adequate iron stores, which are reflected in normalization of the laboratory indicators of iron status.

If iron therapy does not produce the expected results, it must be discontinued and the diagnosis reevaluated. Continued iron therapy in the absence of iron deficiency can produce iron overload and delay appropriate therapy.

ANEMIA OF CHRONIC DISORDERS

Populations Affected

Anemia of chronic disorders is found in association with infectious, inflammatory, or malignant diseases of more than 1 or 2 months' duration.[15] This mild to moderate anemia is common, second only to iron deficiency as a cause of anemia, and in hospital populations, it may be the most common form. Some of the primary disorders producing this form of anemia are listed in Table 13-5.

Pathophysiology

Several mechanisms may be involved in the pathogenesis of this anemia. The first mechanism proposed is decreased iron release from storage in macrophages. This may be related to activated macrophages or monocytes that release a substance, interleukin-1, also identified as leukocyte endogenous mediator.[57] One effect of this compound is stimulation of synthesis of the acute-phase reactant apoferritin (the substance with which iron binds to form ferritin) within macrophages. If apoferritin levels are increased, iron

TABLE 13-5. Causes of Anemia of Chronic Disorders

CHRONIC INFLAMMATORY DISEASES
Infectious[16]
   Tuberculosis[34]
   Pulmonary infections, pneumonia
   Pelvic inflammatory disease
   Chronic fungal disease
   Subacute bacterial endocarditis
   Osteomyelitis
   Meningitis
Noninfectious
   Rheumatoid arthritis[76,82]
   Thermal injury[2]
   Systemic lupus erythematosus[29]
   Myocardial infarction[39]
MALIGNANT DISEASES[33,42,43]
Carcinoma
Hodgkin disease
Lymphosarcoma
Leukemia

attaching to the apoferritin might be effectively trapped within the macrophages,[50,54] reducing the amount of iron circulating to marrow sideroblasts. This is reflected in low serum iron and a reduced number of marrow sideroblasts (see Table 13-1) in the presence of adequate to increased storage iron.

The second proposed pathophysiologic mechanism is shortened erythrocyte survival.[13] Evidence suggests that the early demise of erythrocytes in chronic disease is attributable to some extracorpuscular factor, and a number of possible causes have been proposed.[14] One suggestion is that nonspecific stimulation of macrophages causes them to increase their activity, one consequence being increased erythrocyte destruction.

A third possible mechanism producing anemia of chronic disorders is impaired marrow response to the shortened red cell life span. The marrow should be able to increase its production and release of erythrocytes to compensate for the early destruction. However, in some individuals with anemia of chronic disorders, erythropoietin levels are not increased as would be expected from the anemia.

A review of studies relating to the pathogenesis of anemia of chronic disorders is available to those who wish to pursue the topic further.[57]

Clinical Presentation and Physical Findings

By definition the individual with anemia of chronic disorders has some primary infection, inflammation, or malignancy, and the presenting symptoms and physical findings usually are those of the primary disorder. These are, of course, quite varied and beyond the scope of this text. Occasionally the primary complaints will be related to the patient's anemia. This is more likely to occur if the patient has some existing condition that would reduce oxygen delivery to the tissues, such as severe pulmonary disease. In this circumstance the mild anemia would produce symptoms.[92]

Laboratory Findings and Correlations with Disease

Hematology

The anemia is mild to moderate, with the Hb perhaps 1 to 2 g/dL below the patient's normal baseline. For some patients this is within the normal reference range for the patient's age and sex. The hematocrit is usually mildly decreased or in the low reference range.[15] The anemia is normochromic, normocytic, although hypochromia with an accompanying decrease in MCHC is frequently observed. Microcytosis is not as common, but when it does occur, it is not usually as marked as in iron deficiency anemia.[14] A moderate degree of anisocytosis may occur, but poikilocytosis is minimal.[93]

The reticulocyte count typically is normal, although slight increases may occur.[92] However, the RPI may be less than 2.0, reflecting the hypoproliferative nature of this anemia. The leukocyte count, differential, and platelet count are of little diagnostic significance, although the leukocyte count may be of value in the diagnosis of the primary disorder associated with the anemia.

Bone Marrow

Marrow samples stained with Prussian blue confirm the patient's iron status. Stored iron is identifiable in macrophages and may, in fact, be increased as predicted by increased serum ferritin levels. Sideroblasts are few in number, which might be predicted from the low levels of circulating iron.[5] The bone marrow does not show the erythroid hyperplasia expected as a compensatory mechanism in anemia[92]; thus, the categorization of anemia of chronic disorders as a hypoproliferative anemia (Chap. 10).

Chemistry

Iron studies are particularly useful. Serum iron levels are low, similar to those found in iron deficiency anemia. The TIBC is low in chronic disorders, whereas it is elevated in iron deficiency. The combination of low iron and low TIBC in some cases produces a reduced transferrin saturation. Serum ferritin levels are elevated, in contrast to the low levels in iron deficiency, making this laboratory test a reliable differentiating means for these two disorders.[62] The increased ferritin levels reflect the normal to increased storage iron found in chronic disorders (see Table 13-1). Free erythrocyte protoporphyrin is also elevated.

Erythropoietin levels have been reported by some to be either decreased[28,29] or normal[28] in anemia of chronic disorders. In the latter case some unidentified abnormality is suppressing the marrow response to the hormone.

No specific tests can be recommended to diagnose anemia of chronic disorders because it is secondary to some disease process. That primary disease is the main focus of diagnostic and treatment protocols in anemia of chronic disease.

Effects of Treatment on Laboratory Results

Treatment is directed at the primary disease. Iron therapy is avoided because the patient has adequate tissue iron stores, and exogenous iron could cause overload unless there is an accompanying iron deficiency anemia.[15]

SIDEROBLASTIC ANEMIAS

The sideroblastic anemias are a diverse group identified by the common feature of abnormal iron kinetics. This results in excess accumulation of iron, which is deposited in the mitochondria of normoblasts. These iron deposits are identified using Prussian blue stain, and the resulting abnormal cells are identified as *ringed sideroblasts*. Sideroblasts are iron-containing normoblasts found in normal bone marrows.

There are three types of sideroblasts, sometimes referred to as Types I, II, and III, with Type III being the pathologic ringed sideroblast.[86] The iron in the Type I sideroblast is in the form of ferritin aggregates, and as many as four aggregates can be identified in approximately 50% of the normoblasts in a normal healthy individual. In some situations when iron is not used effectively for red cell production, the number of ferritin aggregates increases to more than six per cell, creating the Type II sideroblast.[41] In both instances this ferritin iron is randomly distributed in the cytoplasm and stains weakly with Prussian blue. The Type III pathologic ringed sideroblast of sideroblastic anemia shows larger granules situated in a ring or collar around the nucleus of the normoblast (see Plate 33). The iron has been identified as being in iron-laden mitochondria. For a diagnosis of sideroblastic anemia, at least 15% of the normoblasts must be Type III ringed sideroblasts.[7]

Although the various types of sideroblastic anemia have the common feature of ringed sideroblasts in the bone marrow, they appear to have differing etiologies. Sideroblastic anemias typically are classified as hereditary or acquired. Acquired sideroblastic anemias are further classified as idiopathic (refractory) or secondary to drugs and toxins (Table 13-6).

Hereditary Type

Genetics

The rare inherited form of sideroblastic anemia has been reported to occur in at least two forms. The most frequent is an X-linked recessive trait found predominantly in males of affected kindreds, although abnormal red cell morphology is observed in female carriers.[48,55] A few cases may arise from an autosomal recessive trait.[12]

Pathophysiology

Most patients with hereditary sideroblastic anemia have decreased δ-aminolevulinic acid synthase (ALA-S) activity.[55] The first enzyme in the porphyrin and heme synthesis pathway (see Fig. 13-1) is ALA-S, which is a mitochondrial enzyme that requires pyridoxal-5'-phosphate, a metabolically active form of vitamin B_6, as a coenzyme. There

are several possible causes of the decreased ALA-S activity. The enzyme may have a reduced affinity for the pyridoxal cofactor.[55] Another possibility is that the ALA-S apoenzyme is unusually sensitive to a degrading mitochondrial protease.[4] In both of these situations patients apparently respond to pyridoxine therapy. In the first, high doses of pyridoxine compensate for the low affinity. In the second, pyridoxine appears to protect the enzyme from protease degradation. Some cases do not respond to pyridoxine therapy and thus apparently have some as yet unidentified enzymatic malfunction.

Clinical Presentation and Physical Findings

Hereditary sideroblastic anemia is apparent in some affected individuals during infancy. However, most subjects are not identified until early adulthood[48] and a few only after 60 years of age.[64]

Patients typically display signs and symptoms of anemia. Patients may also have manifestations of iron overload, including mild to moderate splenomegaly and hepatomegaly, although liver function remains near normal. Diabetes related to iron deposits in pancreatic cells occurs in as many as one third of the patients. Late in the disease, cardiac arrhythmias may occur secondary to accumulating iron deposits in myocardial cells.[93]

Laboratory Findings and Correlations with Disease

HEMATOLOGY. The anemia is severe with an average Hb of 6.0 g/dL. Red cell morphology reveals a microcytic, hypochromic picture with anisocytosis, poikilocytosis, and target cells. Basophilic stippling is also observed. A dimorphic population of erythrocytes is common in sideroblastic anemias, including microcytic, hypochromic cells and normocytic, normochromic cells (Fig. 13-4).[48] The leukocyte and platelet counts usually are normal.[93]

BONE MARROW. Examination of the marrow is remarkable because of erythroid hyperplasia with excessive iron stored in macrophages. As many as 40% of the normoblasts are of the pathologic ringed sideroblast type (see Plate 33) with rings in the polychromatophilic or orthochromic

TABLE 13-6. Classification and Causes of Sideroblastic Anemia

HEREDITARY (rare)
ALA synthase deficiency
Other enzymatic deficiencies (?)
ACQUIRED
Primary (idiopathic)
Acute myeloid leukemia
Myelodysplastic syndromes
Myeloma
Secondary
Alcoholism
Lead poisoning
Chloramphenicol
Drugs used in treatment of tuberculosis
Isoniazid
Cycloserine
Pyrazinamide

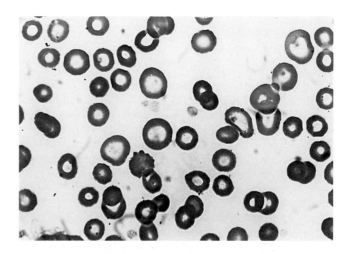

FIG. 13-4. Dimorphic erythrocyte population. Two distinct groups of cells, one group being microcytic and the other normocytic, is a common feature of sideroblastic anemias. (Courtesy of Dr. Paul I Liu.)

stage of normoblast maturation.[38] Megaloblastic changes are sometimes observed (Chap. 12).[48]

CHEMISTRY. Iron studies reflect the iron loading in these patients who are unable to use it effectively (see Table 13-1). Ferritin levels are high, consistent with the large amounts of stored iron. In addition, serum iron is high, as is transferrin saturation, indicating that iron is being delivered effectively to the developing erythrocytes in the bone marrow. The TIBC generally is normal. As discussed under Pathophysiology, however, the iron is not utilized in Hb synthesis and so it piles up in the mitochondria, creating the ringed sideroblasts.

Because the enzymatic defect of hereditary sideroblastic anemia actually affects the production of the porphyrin ring structure, FEP levels may be low or normal. In some circumstances the dimorphic cell population is also dimorphic with respect to FEP; the FEP level is normal in normal cells and low in the microcytic, hypochromic cells.[58]

Effects of Treatment on Laboratory Results and Prognosis

Pyridoxine typically is the treatment of choice. In some patients a remarkable response is observed with reticulocytosis and increasing Hb levels, while serum iron levels decline and FEP levels normalize. Unfortunately, more often than not, pyridoxine therapy produces a less than optimal response, with only slight improvement in the Hb level, and in some instances, pyridoxine produces no improvement.[48,58] In individuals whose bone marrow demonstrates megaloblastic changes, folic acid is added to the treatment regimen.

Some consideration may also be given to removal of the excess accumulated iron. Although this measure may not improve the patient's hematologic picture, the risk of problems related to iron overload (hemochromatosis) is reduced.[48]

The prognosis is variable and is to some degree dependent on the patient's response to pyridoxine therapy. Some live comfortably for many years.[48] Those who do not respond usually succumb to problems related to iron overload, such as cardiac arrhythmias, liver disease, or complications of diabetes.[93]

Idiopathic Type

Populations Affected

The idiopathic form of sideroblastic anemia (the primary classification of this anemia), which most frequently occurs in individuals older than 50 years, is referred to by a variety of names, the most popular being refractory anemia with ringed sideroblasts (RARS) and idiopathic acquired sideroblastic anemia (IASA).[86] This anemia is uncommon but not rare and affects both sexes about equally.[92]

Pathophysiology

Although the mechanism producing IASA is not clear, decreased activity of ALA-S has been found consistently in a number of patients.[3,55,74] The enzymatic defect appears similar to that described in individuals with hereditary sideroblastic anemia, namely, either an increased rate of degradation of ALA-S[4] or an abnormally high requirement for the cofactor pyridoxal-5′-phosphate to maintain active

ALA-S.[55] In a few individuals with IASA, low levels of heme synthase (ferrochelatase) have been documented.[10,74] These are not consistent findings, however. The finding of reduced levels of heme synthase would explain the observation of elevated FEP in IASA, because it is heme synthase that catalyzes the addition of ferrous iron to protoporphyrin to form heme (see Fig. 13-1). The cause of the increased FEP remains a mystery in most cases.

In approximately half the cases of IASA, chromosomal changes have been identified.[74] None of these changes is specific for IASA, as the same changes are found in other myelodysplastic disorders. Leukemic transformation, common in the myelodysplastic disorders, occurs in as many as 25% of individuals with IASA.[17,60]

Clinical Presentation and Physical Findings

Because IASA is insidious in its onset in older adults, the disease frequently is found in patients on routine examination or in patients whose complaints are not related to anemia. Some patients have the usual symptoms related to anemia. Physical findings include mild enlargement of the spleen or liver or both in about 40% of patients.[92,93]

Laboratory Findings and Correlations with Disease

HEMATOLOGY. Idiopathic acquired sideroblastic anemia is usually a moderate anemia with Hb in the range of 7 to 10 g/dL. The mean hematocrit has been reported as 0.27 L/L.[93] The anemia is normocytic or slightly macrocytic, and some cells are hypochromic. Dimorphism is evident in these patients, as in the hereditary form of the disease (see Fig. 13-4) although the population of hypochromic cells may be small. Anisocytosis may be marked, as may poikilocytosis, with the presence of some fragments, target cells, and heavily stippled, hypochromic cells.

Leukocyte and platelet counts usually are normal, although they may be slightly decreased. Leukocyte alkaline phosphatase scores have been reported to be below the normal range in about half the patients with IASA.[92,93]

BONE MARROW. Examination of the marrow reveals significant erythroid hyperplasia with a myeloid–erythroid (M:E) ratio approaching 1:1, whereas the reference value for normal adults is approximately 3:1 or 4:1. The bone marrow may resemble the erythroleukemic marrow. The two may be distinguished by the fact that the positive periodic acid Schiff (PAS) staining characteristics of erythroblasts in erythroleukemia are minimal in IASA.[93] There is an increase in the number of ringed sideroblasts among the basophilic normoblasts, which distinguishes hereditary and secondary sideroblastic anemia from primary IASA. Iron stains also show increased amounts of stored iron in macrophages and as many as 95% of the normoblasts as ringed sideroblasts.[38] If folic acid deficiency is present, megaloblastic changes also can be observed in the marrow.

CHEMISTRY. Iron studies (see Table 13-1) show very high transferrin saturation levels, exceeding 90% in some patients.[56] Ferritin levels are also elevated as a result of the equilibrium of high levels of stored iron with circulating ferritin. Similarly, FEP levels are elevated. Serum iron usually is increased.

Although the liver is involved in the disease in that there are excessive iron stores, liver dysfunction is slight, and bilirubin levels are only modestly affected.[93]

Differential Diagnosis

Table 13-7 lists tests recommended to assist in the diagnosis of sideroblastic anemia, whether inherited or acquired.

Effects of Treatment on Laboratory Results and Prognosis

In a number of patients with IASA no treatment is required because the anemia typically is nonprogressive and usually is not incapacitating. A therapeutic trial of pyridoxine is usually given, however, and at least partially relieves the anemia in some patients. As in the hereditary form of the disease, however, pyridoxine produces extremely variable results. In the patient with significant cardiovascular symptoms related to the anemia, packed red cells may be given, but this adds to the patient's iron overload.

Bone marrow findings may be a useful prognostic indicator. It appears that in patients with more than 30% ringed sideroblasts and apparently normal granulopoiesis and megakaryocytopoiesis, a benign course and a long life can be predicted. In contrast, if there are fewer than 30% ringed sideroblasts in combination with dysplastic granulopoiesis and megakaryocytopoiesis, a poor prognosis is likely, with possible progression to leukemia and a survival time of 1 to 2 years.[41]

Secondary Type

Populations Affected

Secondary sideroblastic anemia follows exposure to certain drugs and toxins. Among the drugs known to produce sideroblastic anemia are chloramphenicol,[35] ethanol,[45] and those used in the treatment of tuberculosis[55,88] and neoplastic disease.[23] Lead toxicity produces a unique form of sideroblastic anemia discussed later in this chapter.

Pathophysiology

The mechanisms for production of secondary sideroblastic anemias all apparently affect heme synthesis. Some variation in the mechanisms occurs, although most drugs and toxins appear to interfere with the activity of either ALA-S or heme synthase or both (see Fig. 13-1). Isoniazid, cycloserine, and pyrazinamide (all drugs used in the treatment of tuberculosis) reportedly inhibit reactions requiring pyridoxal-5'-phosphate as a coenzyme,[47] apparently by interfering with the conversion of vitamin B_6 to its active coenzyme form. This, in turn, reduces ALA-S activity and

could produce sideroblastic anemia similar in appearance to the hereditary form. Chloramphenicol, another antimicrobial drug, appears to inhibit mitochondrial protein synthesis in general, producing decreases in available ALA-S[77] and heme synthase,[66] as well as in other mitochondrial enzymes.[32]

Acute ethanol ingestion reduces the activity of several enzymes in the heme synthesis pathway (see Fig. 13-1), including porphobilinogen synthase (PBG synthase),[49] uroporphyrinogen decarboxylase, coproporphyrinogen oxidase, and heme synthase.[69] The effects of ethanol on heme synthesis produce sideroblastic anemia in about 30% of hospitalized alcoholics.[45]

Clinical Presentation and Physical Findings

Because this group of anemias is related to the treatment of various inflammatory, infectious, and neoplastic diseases or to ethanol ingestion, the presenting symptoms and physical findings are generally those related to the primary problem. The patients may exhibit signs and symptoms of anemia, however.

Laboratory Findings and Correlations with Disease

HEMATOLOGY.   The anemia is moderate to severe, with Hb ranging from 6 to 10 g/dL in alcoholics.[45] The peripheral film characteristics are similar to those in other sideroblastic anemias. The MCV is normal or slightly increased in the alcoholic; the MCHC is normal or slightly reduced.[30] The red cell population is dimorphic.[45]

BONE MARROW.   The definitive feature of secondary sideroblastic anemias, as with the other sideroblastic anemias, is the characteristic finding of up to 65% ringed sideroblasts in the bone marrow. In the alcoholic patient the bone marrow may also show megaloblastic changes and vacuolization of the erythrocyte precursors.[45,61]

CHEMISTRY.   Nutritional folic acid deficiency is well documented in alcoholics and is responsible for the megaloblastic changes that accompany the sideroblastic changes in these patients. Storage iron in the marrow is increased. Iron studies reflect the elevated iron levels in the patient (see Table 13-1). Transferrin saturation is increased, averaging about 65%.[30]

Effects of Treatment on Laboratory Results and Prognosis

Removal of the offending agent is the principal means of treatment.[88] The administration of pyridoxine and folic acid along with good nutrition aids in reversal of the disorder. In cases where drug therapy needs to be continued, supplementary pyridoxine may be helpful, but complete remission will not occur until the offending drug is removed.[37]

LEAD INTOXICATION

Populations Affected

Lead intoxication occurs in both children and adults. Children may receive excessive exposure to lead secondary to ingestion of lead-containing paint, such as when the child eats chips from flaking lead paint or chews articles so

TABLE 13-7. Recommended Laboratory Tests to Assist in Diagnosis of Sideroblastic Anemia

Required most frequently	CBC
	RBC morphology
	Serum ferritin or FEP
	Bone marrow; Prussian blue stain
Required occasionally	Serum iron
	TIBC
	Percent transferrin saturation
Required rarely	WBC differential

painted. It also is associated with use of improperly glazed pottery for cooking or eating.[51]

Pathophysiology

Elevated lead levels produce several injuries that reduce the circulating red cell mass. One effect is to inhibit activity of at least three enzymes in the heme synthesis pathway.[10] The first and most sensitive of these is PBG synthase, which converts δ-ALA to porphobilinogen (see Fig. 13-1). Another enzyme profoundly affected by lead is heme synthase (see Fig. 13-1). As a consequence of the effects on these two enzymes, δ-ALA levels are increased, and porphobilinogen levels are normal.[18] This conformation distinguishes lead toxicity from acute intermittent porphyria, in which both δ-ALA and PBG are elevated.[93] Similarly, coproporphyrinogen oxidase (see Fig. 13-1) appears to be inhibited by lead.[18]

Lead also appears to injure the red cell membrane, possibly by inhibiting ATPase, thereby interfering with cation exchange.[92] Synthesis of α and β globin chains seems to be defective in lead poisoning.[90]

Clinical Presentation and Physical Findings

In a study of 50 cases of lead poisoning[24] the most common symptoms were abdominal pain, constipation, vomiting, pain other than abdominal, and muscle weakness. Neurologic and psychological symptoms were found less frequently. Other than hematologic signs of the disease, the most frequently observed sign of lead toxicity is the so-called lead line, a linear blue–black deposit of lead sulfide in the gums near the teeth.[6] Dental caries, abdominal tenderness, and motor disturbances were also reported in 30% to 60% of the patients.[24]

Laboratory Findings and Correlations with Disease

HEMATOLOGY. The anemia typically is mild to moderate, with Hb ranging from 8 to 13 g/dL. The red cells usually demonstrate mild to moderate hypochromia and microcytosis, with the MCHC averaging 31% and the MCV averaging 79 fL.[93] Coarse or fine basophilic stippling is present in the erythrocytes in many cases but is not a uniform finding. Stippling may disappear when samples are collected in EDTA.[91] The reticulocyte count is slightly increased. The leukocyte count may be normal or slightly elevated.[24] Platelets apparently are normal.

BONE MARROW. Marrow aspirates show erythroid hyperplasia. Ringed sideroblasts may be observed, particularly in the marrows of children with severe anemia. Iron levels tend to be normal to slightly increased in adults and decreased in children.[92]

CHEMISTRY. Free erythrocyte protoporphyrin is increased in erythrocytes to a much greater extent than in iron deficiency (see Table 13-1). Urinary ALA is elevated, and PBG is normal. Urinary coproporphyrins are increased.[19] In contrast to other iron metabolism disorders the measurements indicating iron storage, including serum ferritin, marrow iron, and sideroblasts, are normal in lead intoxi-

cation. Transferrin saturation is elevated, and TIBC is normal (see Table 13-1).

According to the US Public Health Service,[87] acceptable lead levels in children are 15 to 40 μg/dL of whole blood. Treatment as a medical emergency is indicated when that level exceeds 80 μg/dL. Urinary excretion of greater than 1 μg of lead per milligram of EDTA administered as a trial establishes the diagnosis of lead intoxication.

Effects of Treatment on Laboratory Results and Prognosis

Administration of EDTA to chelate lead is the recommended treatment. There is a risk of encephalopathy secondary to the lead chelate,[18] but if small amounts of EDTA are given, this complication is less likely to occur.[1] Urinary excretion of lead is rapid in EDTA treatment, and the Hb level should return to normal in a few weeks.[8]

CHAPTER SUMMARY

Many patients suffer from anemias secondary to abnormalities of iron metabolism caused either by iron deficiency or by inability to utilize body iron stores appropriately.

The most common form of anemia is iron deficiency anemia, which results from increased physiologic need for iron, a nutritional deficiency of iron, or loss of iron stores through bleeding. Iron studies in iron deficiency anemia demonstrate depleted iron stores (see Table 13-1).

Anemia of chronic disorders is a common mild to moderate anemia accompanying infections, inflammation, and neoplastic disease. Iron appears to be trapped in macrophages where old erythrocytes are catabolized. Therefore, iron is not made available for reutilization in normoblasts. The effective result is iron deficiency in the presence of adequate iron stores (see Table 13-1). The anemia is corrected when the primary disease is resolved.

Sideroblastic anemias are a diverse group of uncommon anemias. The cause may be genetic, idiopathic, drugs, or toxins. Apparently, porphyrin synthesis is reduced in these patients so that they are unable to complete adequate Hb synthesis. Iron is available and ready for incorporation into forming Hb, but enzymes of the Hb synthetic pathway, particularly δ-aminolevulinic acid synthase (ALA-S) fail. The common feature of the sideroblastic anemias is the appearance of ringed sideroblasts in bone marrow aspirates stained for iron. A dimorphic erythrocyte population is frequently observed. Pyridoxine (vitamin B_6), a coenzyme of ALA-S, is sometimes useful in therapy.

Lead intoxication follows exposure to or ingestion of excessive amounts of lead. Lead inhibits several enzymes in the Hb synthetic pathway and thereby produces a picture similar to that of sideroblastic anemia. Although a mild to moderate anemia is present in these patients, gastrointestinal and neuromuscular signs and symptoms also are significant. Confirmation of elevated lead levels in whole blood is important to the diagnosis. Treatment involves removal of the offending agent and, in cases of acute lead intoxication, chelation therapy with EDTA.

CASE STUDY 13-1

A 24-year-old black female college student presented with the chief complaint of being tired all the time. She reported that she lived in a dormitory without kitchen facilities and that she did not care for the cafeteria food. Her physical examination was unremarkable. She did not report unusually heavy menstrual bleeding. Her CBC was reported as follows: WBC 7.8×10^9/L; RBC 4.71×10^{12}/L; Hb 10.3 g/dL; HCT 0.33 L/L; platelets 384×10^9/L; MCV 70 fL; MCH 21.9 pg; and MCHC 31.2 g/dL. The RBC morphology was abnormal, with moderate hypochromia and marked anisocytosis with many small RBCs. Iron studies (with reference ranges in parentheses) revealed serum iron 14 μg/dL (42–135 μg/dL); TIBC 375 μg/dL (250–450 μg/dL); percent transferrin saturation 4% (20%–55%); and serum ferritin 0 (30–250 μg/L).

1. From the patient's age, sex, and history, what types of anemia might be expected?
2. How do the CBC and red cell morphology influence the differential diagnosis?
3. Do the chemistry findings confirm the suspected diagnosis? Explain.
4. How would this patient be expected to respond to a 10-day trial of ferrous sulfate?
5. Could a sound diagnosis have been made on the basis of the ferritin level and CBC alone?
6. Is a bone marrow study necessary in this case?

REFERENCES

1. Albahary C: Lead and hemopoiesis. Am J Med 52:367, 1972
2. Andes WA, Rogers PW, Beason JW et al: The erythropoietin response to the anemia of thermal injury. J Lab Clin Med 88:584, 1976
3. Aoki Y: Multiple enzymatic defects in mitochrondria in hematological cells of patients with primary sideroblastic anemia. J Clin Invest 66:43, 1980.
4. Aoki Y, Muranaka S, Nakabayashi K et al: δ-Amino-levulinic acid synthetase in erythroblasts of patients with pyridoxine-responsive anemia: Hypercatabolism caused by the increased susceptibility to the controlling protease. J Clin Invest 64:1196, 1979
5. Bainton DF, Finch CA: The diagnosis of iron deficiency anemia. Am J Med 37:62, 1964
6. Belknap EL: Differential diagnosis of lead poisoning. JAMA 139:818, 1949
7. Bennett JM, Catovsky D, Daniel MT et al: The French–American–British (FAB) co-operative group: Proposals for the classification of myelodysplastic syndromes. Br J Haematol 51:189, 1982
8. Berk PD, Tschudy DP, Shepley LA et al: Hematologic and biochemical studies in a case of lead poisoning. Am J Med 48:137, 1970
9. Beveridge BR, Bannerman RM, Evanson JM et al: Hypochromic anemia: A retrospective study and follow-up of 378 in-patients. Q J Med 34:145, 1965
10. Bottomley SS: Porphyrin and iron metabolism in sideroblastic anemia. Semin Hematol 14:169, 1977
11. Bowie EJW, Tauxe WN, Sjoberg WE et al: Daily variation in the concentration of iron in serum. Am J Clin Pathol 40:491, 1963
12. Buchanan GR, Bottomley SS, Nitschke R: Bone marrow delta-aminolevulinate synthetase deficiency in a female with congenital sideroblastic anemia. Blood 55:109, 1980
13. Bush JA, Ashenbrucker H, Cartwright GE et al: The anemia of infection. XX: The kinetics of iron metabolism in the anemia associated with chronic infection. J Clin Invest 35:89, 1956
14. Cartwright GE: The anemia of chronic disorders. Semin Hematol 3:351, 1966
15. Cartwright GE, Lee GR: The anaemia of chronic disorders. Br J Haematol 21:147, 1971
16. Cartwright GE, Wintrobe MM: The anemia of infection. XVII: A review. Adv Intern Med 5:165, 1952
17. Cheng DS, Kushner JP, Wintrobe MM: Idiopathic refractory sideroblastic anemia: Incidence and risk factors for leukemic transformation. Cancer 44:724, 1979
18. Chisolm JJ: Disturbances in the biosynthesis of heme in lead intoxication. J Pediatr 64:174, 1964
19. Chisolm JJ: Screening techniques for undue lead exposure in children: Biological and practical considerations. J Pediatr 79:719, 1971
20. Committee on Iron Deficiency, AMA Council on Foods and Nutrition: Iron deficiency in the United States. JAMA 203:407, 1968
21. Cook JD: Clinical evaluation of iron deficiency. Semin Hematol 19:6, 1982
22. Crosby WH: Pica. JAMA 235:2765, 1976
23. Dacie JV, Mollin DL: Siderocytes, sideroblasts and sideroblastic anaemia (suppl 445). Acta Med Scand 179:237, 1966
24. Dagg JH, Goldberg A, Lochhead A et al: The relationship of lead poisoning to acute intermittent porphyria. Q J Med 34:163, 1965
25. Dallman PR, Yip R, Johnson C: Prevalence and causes of anemia in the United States, 1976 to 1980. Am J Clin Nutr 39:437, 1984
26. Dincol K, Askoy M: On the platelet levels in chronic iron deficiency anemia. Acta Haematol (Basal) 41:135, 1969
27. Dine MS, Oski FA: What is the best test for iron deficiency? Pediatrics 72:909, 1983
28. Douglas SW, Adamson JW: The anemia of chronic disorders: Studies of marrow regulation and iron metabolism. Blood 45:55, 1975
29. Dubois EL, Tuffanelli DL: Clinical manifestations of systemic lupus erythematosus. JAMA 190:104, 1964
30. Eichner ER, Hillman RS: The evolution of anemia in alcoholic patients. Am J Med 50:218, 1971
31. Finch CA, Cook JD: Iron deficiency. Am J Clin Nutr 39:471, 1984
32. Firkin FC: Mitochondrial lesions in reversible erythropoietic depression due to chloramphenicol. J Clin Invest 51:2085, 1972
33. Freidell GH: Anaemia in cancer. Lancet 1:356, 1965
34. Glasser RM, Walker RI, Herion JC: The significance of hematologic abnormalities in patients with tuberculosis. Arch Intern Med 125:691, 1970
35. Goodman JR, Hall SG: Accumulation of iron in mitochondria of erythroblasts. Br J Haematol 13:335, 1967
36. Gross S, Keefer V, Newman AJ: The platelets in iron-deficiency anemia. I: Response to oral and parenteral iron. Pediatrics 34:315, 1964
37. Haden HT: Pyridoxine-responsive sideroblastic anemia due to antituberculosis drugs. Arch Intern Med 120:602, 1967
38. Hall R, Losowsky MS: The distribution of erythroblast iron in sideroblastic anaemias. Br J Haematol 12:334, 1966
39. Handjani AM, Banihashemi A, Rafiee R et al: Serum iron in acute myocardial infarction. Blut 23:363, 1971
40. Hartmann RC, Jenkins DE, McKee LC et al: Paroxysmal nocturnal hemoglobinuria: Clinical and laboratory studies relating to iron metabolism and therapy with androgen and iron. Medicine 45:331, 1966
41. Hast R: Sideroblasts in myelodysplasia: Their nature and clinical significance. Scand J Haematol 36 (suppl 45):53, 1986
42. Haurani FI, Burke W, Martinez EJ: Defective reutilization of iron in the anemia of inflammation. J Lab Clin Med 65:560, 1965
43. Haurani FI, Young K, Tocantins LM: Reutilization of iron in anemia complicating malignant neoplasms. Blood 22:73, 1963
44. Hillman RS, Finch CA: Red Cell Manual, 5th ed. Philadelphia, FA Davis, 1985
45. Hines JD, Cowan DH: Studies on the pathogenesis of alcohol-induced sideroblastic bone-marrow abnormalities. N Engl J Med 283:441, 1970
46. Hogan GR, Jones B: The relationship of koilonychia and iron deficiency in infants. J Pediatr 77:1054, 1970
47. Holtz P, Palm D: Pharmacological aspects of vitamin B_6. Pharmacol Rev 16:113, 1964
48. Horrigan DL, Harris JW: Pyridoxine-responsive anemia: Analysis of 62 cases. Adv Intern Med 12:103, 1964
49. International Union of Biochemistry Nomenclature Commit-

tee: Enzyme Nomenclature 1984. Orlando, Academic Press, 1984

50. Klasing KC: Effect of inflammatory agents and interleukin 1 on iron and zinc metabolism. Am J Physiol 247:R901, 1984

51. Klein M, Namer R, Harpur E et al: Earthenware containers as a source of fatal lead poisoning. N Engl J Med 283:669, 1970

52. Koenig HM, Lightsey AL, Schanberger JE: The micromeasurement of free erythrocyte protoporphyrin as a means of differentiating alpha thalassemia trait from iron deficiency anemia. J Pediatr 86:539, 1975

53. Koller ME, Romslo I, Finne PH et al: The diagnosis of iron deficiency by erythrocyte protoporphyrin and serum ferritin analyses. Acta Paediatr Scand 67:361, 1978

54. Konijn AM, Hershko C: Ferritin synthesis in inflammation. 1: Pathogenesis of impaired iron release. Br J Haematol 37:7, 1977

55. Konopka L, Hoffbrand AV: Haem synthesis in sideroblastic anaemia. Br J Haematol 42:73, 1979

56. Kushner JP, Lee GR, Wintrobe MM et al: Idiopathic refractory sideroblastic anemia. Medicine 50:139, 1971

57. Lee GR: The anemia of chronic disease. Semin Hematol 20:61, 1983

58. Lee GR, MacDiarmid WD, Cartwright GE et al: Hereditary X-linked, sideroachrestic anaemia: The isolation of two erythrocyte populations differing in Xgᵃ blood type and porphyrin content. Blood 32:59, 1968

59. Lennartsson J, Bengtsson C, Hallberg L et al: Characteristics of anaemic women: The population study of women of Goteborg 1968–1969. Scand J Haematol 22:17, 1979

60. Lewy RI, Kansu E, Gabuzda T: Leukemia in patients with acquired idiopathic sideroblastic anemia: An evaluation of prognostic indicators. Am J Hematol 6:323, 1979

61. Lindenbaum J, Lieber CS: Hematologic effects of alcohol in man in the absence of nutritional deficiency. N Engl J Med 281:333, 1969

62. Lipschitz DA, Cook JD, Finch CA: A clinical evaluation of serum ferritin as an index of iron stores. N Engl J Med 290:1213, 1974

63. Lorier MA, Herron JL, Carrell RW: Detecting iron deficiency by serum tests. Clin Chem 31:337, 1985

64. Losowsky MS, Hall R: Hereditary sideroblastic anaemia. Br J Haematol 11:70, 1965

65. Lynch SR, Dassenko SA, Morck TA et al: Soy protein products and heme iron absorption in humans. Am J Clin Nutr 41:13, 1985

66. Manyan DR, Arimura GK, Yunis AA: Chloramphenicol-induced erythroid suppression and bone marrow ferrochelatase activity in dogs. J Lab Clin Med 79:137, 1972

67. Marsh WL, Nelson DP, Koenig HM: Free erythrocyte protoporphyrin (FEP). I: Normal values for adults and evaluation of the hematofluorometer. II: The FEP test is clinically useful in classifying microcytic RBC disorders in adults. Am J Clin Pathol 79:655, 1983

68. McClure S, Custer E, Bessman JD: Improved detection of early iron deficiency in nonanemic subjects. JAMA 253:1021, 1985

69. McColl KEL, Thompson GG, Moore MR et al: Acute ethanol ingestion and haem biosynthesis in healthy subjects. Eur J Clin Invest 10:107, 1980

70. Miale JB: Laboratory Medicine Hematology, 6th ed. St Louis, CV Mosby, 1982

71. Milman M, Cohn J: Serum iron, serum transferrin and transferrin saturation in healthy children without iron deficiency. Eur J Pediatr 143:96, 1984

72. Movassaghi N, Shore NA, Hammond D: Serum and urinary levels of erythropoietin in iron deficiency anemia. Proc Soc Exp Biol Med 126:615, 1967

73. National Center for Health Statistics: Diet and Iron Status, A Study of Relationships, United States, 1971–74. Vital and Health Statistics, series 11, Data from the National Health Survey, No. 229. Hyattsville, MD, National Center for Health Statistics, DHHS publication no. (PHS) 83-1679, 1982.

74. Pasanen AVO, Vuopio P, Borgstrom GH et al: Haem biosynthesis in refractory sideroblastic anaemia associated with the preleukaemic syndrome. Scand J Haematol 27:35, 1981

75. Reynolds RD, Lewis JP: Blood-loss anemias and the iron-deficient states. In Koepke JA (ed): Laboratory Hematology, p 11. New York, Churchill Livingstone, 1984

76. Roberts FD, Hagedorn AB, Slocumb CH et al: Evaluation of the anemia of rheumatoid arthritis. Blood 21:470, 1963

77. Rosenberg A, Marcus O: Effect of chloramphenicol on reticulocyte δ-aminolaevulinic acid synthetase in rabbits. Br J Haematol 26:79, 1974

78. Schloesser LL, Kipp MA, Wenzel FJ: Thrombocytosis in iron-deficiency anemia. J Lab Clin Med 66:107, 1965

79. Schulman I: Iron requirements in infancy. JAMA 175:118, 1961

80. Simon TL, Hunt WC, Garry PJ: Iron supplementation for menstruating female blood donors. Transfusion 24:469, 1984

81. Stockman JA, Weiner LS, Simon GE et al: The measurement of free erythrocyte porphyrin (FEP) as a simple means of distinguishing iron deficiency from beta-thalessemia trait in subjects with microcytosis. J Lab Clin Med 85:113, 1975

82. Strandberg O: Anemia in rheumatoid arthritis. Acta Med Scand (suppl) 454:1, 1966

83. Thomas WJ, Koenig HM, Lightsey AL et al: Free erythrocyte porphyrin: Hemoglobin ratios, serum ferritin, and transferrin saturation levels during treatment of infants with iron-deficiency anemia. Blood 49:455, 1977

84. Tietz NW: Textbook of Clinical Chemistry, 3rd ed. Philadelphia, WB Saunders, 1986

85. Tietz NW: Fundamentals of Clinical Chemistry, 3rd ed. Philadelphia, WB Saunders, 1986

86. Travis WD, Pierre RV: Preleukemia/dysmyelopoietic syndrome. Lab Med 16:147, 1985

87. US Public Health Service: Medical aspects of childhood lead poisoning: The Surgeon General's policy statement. Pediatr 48:464, 1971

88. Verwilghen R, Reybrouck G, Callens L et al: Antituberculous drugs and sideroblastic anaemia. Br J Haematol 11:92, 1965

89. Ward HP, Kurnick JE, Pisarczyk MJ: Serum level of erythropoietin in anemias associated with chronic infection, malignancy and primary hematopoietic disease. J Clin Invest 50:332, 1971

90. White JM, Harvey DR: Defective synthesis of α and-β globin chains in lead poisoning. Nature 236:71, 1972

91. White JM, Selhi HS: Lead and the red cell. Br J Haematol 30:133, 1975

92. Williams WJ, Beutler E, Erslev AJ et al: Hematology, 3rd ed. New York, McGraw-Hill, 1983

93. Wintrobe MM et al: Clinical Hematology, 8th ed. Philadelphia, Lea & Febiger, 1981

94. World Health Organization: Nutritional Anaemias. World Health Organization Technical Report Series No. 503. Geneva, World Health Organization, 1972

14

Anemia of Abnormal Globin Development— Hemoglobinopathies

Carolyn J. Pearce
Patricia Dow

TABLE 14–1. Basic Hemoglobinopathy Terms

TERM	DEFINITION	EXAMPLE
Hemoglobin variant	The abnormal hemoglobin caused by a globin chain structural abnormality	Hb S
Hemoglobinopathy	The condition diagnosed when the presence of a variant is confirmed in the blood by laboratory tests	Sickle cell disease (Hb SS) Sickle cell trait (Hb AS)
Qualitative globin chain abnormality	An abnormality in the *amino acid sequence* of the globin chain, not in the amount of globin produced	Substitution for one or more amino acids in globin chain with other amino acids
Structural globin chain abnormality	Abnormalities in globin chain composition that produce hemoglobin variants	Deletion of amino acids from globin chain Addition of extra amino acids to globin chain

Hemoglobinopathies are conditions caused by qualitative structural abnormalities of the globin polypeptide chains that result from alteration of the deoxyribonucleic acid (DNA) genetic code for those chains. The disorders may or may not cause clinical or laboratory abnormalities. Understanding hemoglobinopathies depends on understanding the basic structure of the hemoglobin (Hb) molecule (Chap. 7).

These abnormalities cause the production of abnormal hemoglobins known as *hemoglobin variants*. Table 14-1 explains the basic terminology of hemoglobinopathies. Hereditary abnormalities of the beta (β) globin chain are the most common causes of hemoglobinopathies. For example Hb S, the most common variant, is caused by a β-chain abnormality. Abnormalities of the alpha (α), gamma (γ), and delta (δ) chains are much less frequent but do occur. When hemoglobin variants are produced the patient is said to have a *hemoglobinopathy*. Thalassemias (Chap. 15), in contrast, are conditions caused by a *quantitative* abnormality

in globin chain production (*i.e.*, reduced or no production). Hemoglobinopathies and thalassemias are found worldwide. Figure 14-1 shows the overall geographic distribution of the more common hemoglobinopathies and thalassemias.

GENETICS OF ABNORMAL GLOBIN CHAIN PRODUCTION

Inheritance of hemoglobin variants follows Mendelian patterns (Fig. 14-2). A person who has two hemoglobin variants (*e.g.*, Hb SC) is said to be doubly heterozygous, having inherited a different abnormal variant from each parent. Another category of double heterozygosity is the combination of an abnormal globin chain and thalassemia.

By convention, genotypes for hemoglobin inheritance always indicate the hemoglobin of greater concentration first. For example, when Hb S is inherited from one parent and Hb A from the other, Hb A is present in higher concentration, so the genotype is written Hb AS.

NOMENCLATURE

Hemoglobin variants have both a common name and a scientific designation. The common names generally refer to the associated morphology (*e.g.*, Hb S for sickle cells, Hb C for intracellular crystals) or to the city, district, province, or hospital where they were discovered (*e.g.*, Gun Hill, Constant Spring). The M hemoglobins have been so designated because they are associated with the presence of methemoglobinemia.

The scientific designation denotes (1) the affected polypeptide chain, (2) the sequential amino acid number(s) affected, (3) the helix number involved, and (4) the nature of the abnormality (amino acid substitution, deletion, addition, or globin chain fusion). Table 14-2 lists the scientific designations of major β-chain variants.

The primary hemoglobin structure consists of amino acids in a specified sequence, 1 to 141 for α chains and 1 to 146 for β chains. The secondary hemoglobin structure is divided into eight rigid helical segments (A through H) that contain groups of amino acids (see Fig. 7-3). There are also seven nonhelical segments (*e.g.*, NA, AB, CD) that provide flexibility and allow physical bending of the globin chain (see Fig. 7-3). Thus, the scientific designation of Hb S

TABLE 14–2. Common Names and Scientific Designations of the Well-Known Hemoglobin Variants

MOLECULAR ABNORMALITY	HEMOGLOBIN COMMON NAME	AFFECTED CHAIN	AMINO ACID NUMBERS AFFECTED	HELICAL NUMBERS AFFECTED	β-CHAIN SUBSTITUTION	SCIENTIFIC DESIGNATION
Amino acid substitution	S	β	6	A3	Glu→Val	$\beta^{6(A3)Glu \rightarrow Val}$
	C	β	6	A3	Glu→Lys	$\beta^{6(A3)Glu \rightarrow Lys}$
	D-Los Angeles D-Punjab	β	121	GH4	Glu→Gln	$\beta^{121(GH4)Glu \rightarrow Gln}$
	E	β	26	B8	Glu→Lys	$\beta^{26(B8)Glu \rightarrow Lys}$
	O-Arab	β	121	GH4	Glu→Lys	$\beta^{121(GH4)Glu \rightarrow Lys}$
Amino acid deletion	Gun Hill	β	91–95	F7-FG2	NA	$\beta^{91-95 \ (F7-FG2) \ Leu \ His \ Cys \ Asp \ Lys \rightarrow 0}$
Amino acid elongation	Constant Spring	α	NA	NA	NA	$\alpha^{+31c \ (142 \ Gln)}$
Globin chain fusion	Lepore-Baltimore	$\delta\beta$	NA	NA	NA	$\delta^{(1-50)}\beta^{(86-146)}$

Key: Glu, glutamic acid; His, histidine; Leu, leucine; Lys, lysine; Pro, Proline; Thr, threonine; Val, valine; NA, not applicable.

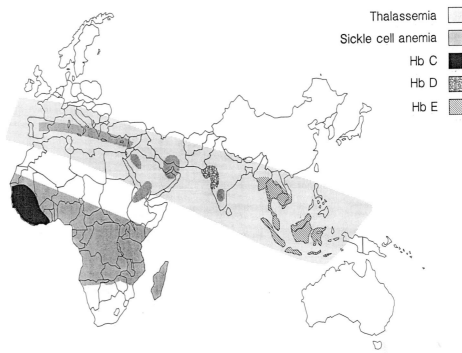

Thalassemia ☐
Sickle cell anemia ☐
Hb C ■
Hb D ▦
Hb E ▨

FIG. 14-1. The geographic distribution of the more common structural hemoglobin abnormalities and the thalassemias. (From Hoffbrand AV, Pettit JE: Essential Haematology, 2nd ed. London, Blackwell Scientific Publications, 1984, with permission.)

FIG. 14-2. Examples of Mendelian inheritance patterns of hemoglobinopathies: (1) All offspring of a normal parent (genotype AA) and one who has sickle cell anemia (genotype SS) have sickle cell trait (genotype AS). (2) Offspring of one normal parent and one with the sickle trait have a 50% chance of inheriting a normal hemoglobin genotype and a 50% chance of inheriting the sickle trait. (3) Offspring of two parents with sickle trait have a 25% chance of inheriting a normal hemoglobin genotype, a 50% chance of inheriting the sickle trait, and a 25% chance of inheriting sickle cell anemia. (4) Offspring of one parent who has sickle cell anemia and one who carries the sickle trait have a 50% chance of inheriting the trait and a 50% chance of having the disease. (5) All offspring of two parents with sickle cell anemia have sickle cell anemia.

	S	S
A	AS	AS
A	AS	AS

(1)

	A	S
A	AA	AS
A	AA	AS

(2)

	A	S
A	AA	AS
S	AS	SS

(3)

	S	S
A	AS	AS
S	SS	SS

(4)

	S	S
S	SS	SS
S	SS	SS

(5)

is $\beta^{6(A3)Glu \rightarrow Val}$. This is interpreted as a β chain variant affecting the sixth sequential amino acid position, which is the third position in the A helical segment. The variant is caused by a substitution in that position of valine (Val) for the normal glutamic acid (Glu).

CLASSIFICATION OF HEMOGLOBINOPATHIES

The hemoglobinopathies may be classified according to molecular or functional abnormalities.

Classification by Molecular Abnormality

From a molecular or structural standpoint, hemoglobin variants may result from a single amino acid substitution (the most common form of hemoglobinopathy) in the α or β chain, multiple amino acid substitutions, amino acid deletions, globin polypeptide chain elongation, or globin chain fusion. Table 14-3 lists the total number of known variants in each category of molecular abnormality and classifies them according to which chain is affected.

Classification by Functional Abnormality

Some hemoglobin variants cause a number of abnormal conditions (Table 14-4), whereas others produce no detectable clinical disability.

Aggregation

Hemoglobins that aggregate and have reduced solubility are capable of polymerizing or crystallizing (Hbs S and C, respectively) within the red cell. This causes distortion of cell shape, decreased "deformability," and consequent susceptibility to hemolysis.

TABLE 14–3. Molecular Abnormalities That Cause Hemoglobin Variants

ABNORMALITY	NUMBERS OF VARIANTS					EXAMPLES
	TOTAL	α CHAIN	β CHAIN	γ CHAIN	δ CHAIN	
Single amino acid substitution	294	93	175	16	10	S, C, D, E
Two amino acid substitutions	4	1	3	—	—	C-Harlem
Deletion	11	—	11	—	—	Gun Hill
Fusions*	7	—	7	6	1	Lepore
Elongated chains	8	6	2	—	—	Constant Spring
TOTALS*	324	100	198	22	11	

* The total of 324 molecular abnormalities is seven less than the actual sum of the totals of the last four columns because the fusion hemoglobins are listed in two columns since they involve two globin chains but represent a single hemoglobin variant.
(From Wintrobe MM: The abnormal hemoglobins: General principles. In Wintrobe MM et al: Clinical Hematology, 8th ed, p 804. Philadelphia, Lea & Febiger, 1981, with permission.)

Unstable Hemoglobins

Unstable hemoglobins are characterized by reduced solubility and a tendency to precipitate, forming intracellular inclusion bodies known as Heinz bodies that are rigid and incapable of traversing the splenic microcirculation. Affected red cells lose membrane and eventually are trapped and destroyed in the spleen. These hemoglobins are also sensitive to heat (i.e., 50°C) in vitro. Hbs Köln and Gun Hill are examples of unstable hemoglobins. Unstable hemoglobins may or may not have altered oxygen affinity; others may cause methemoglobinemia.

Methemoglobins

This abnormality is associated with five variants of Hb M, all of which cause iron to remain permanently in the oxidized (ferric) form referred to as methemoglobin. Because methemoglobin cannot bind oxygen, cyanosis results.

Oxygen Affinity

Increased oxygen affinity is associated with some variants (e.g., Hb Gun Hill). When release of oxygen to the tissue from hemoglobin is decreased, decreased oxygen tension in the tissues results in increased production of erythropoietin and erythrocytes (erythrocytosis). Some of these variants also are unstable.

Hemoglobins with decreased oxygen affinity also occur (e.g., Hb Kansas) and some are unstable. Since these hemoglobins release more oxygen per gram of hemoglobin, slight anemia may occur. Some variants do not cause detectable symptoms or signs. Others may cause cyanosis due to decreased oxygen saturation.

See Table 14–5 for a summary of molecular abnormalities associated with each group of functional abnormalities.

GENERAL LABORATORY FINDINGS

Laboratory findings vary from no detectable abnormalities to striking alterations, depending on which hemoglobin variant is involved. Patients who are homozygous for the more common β-chain variants (Hbs S, C, D-Los Angeles, and E) may demonstrate anemia. Target cells often are found on the peripheral blood film. Heinz bodies are characteristic of the unstable hemoglobins.

MOST USEFUL LABORATORY TESTS FOR DIAGNOSING HEMOGLOBINOPATHIES

The most significant laboratory tests for diagnosis of the hemoglobinopathies are outlined in Table 14–6. Two of the most useful tests include (1) hemoglobin electrophoresis, for variant identification by cellulose acetate at alkaline pH and by citrate agar at acid pH, and (2) the dithionite tube test for sickling hemoglobins (also known as the solubility test).

The alkali denaturation test for fetal hemoglobin (Hb F) quantitation is useful to help identify conditions in which Hb F is characteristically elevated, such as sickle cell anemia (Hb SS) and Hb S–thalassemia conditions, and to differentiate hemoglobinopathies from thalassemias.

Globin chain electrophoresis at acid or alkaline pH is a more specialized test performed when a high degree of specificity is needed that is not possible with routine electrophoresis.

Hb A_2 quantitation (Chap. 15) may be performed to rule out the possibility of thalassemia or the doubly heterozygous Hb S–thalassemia conditions. Hb A_2 is usually normal in Hb SS and AS, but increased in Hb S-thalassemia and other thalassemic syndromes.

Tests for unstable hemoglobins can also be diagnostic.

TABLE 14–4. Functional Abnormalities of the Hemoglobinopathies

FUNCTIONAL ABNORMALITY	CLINICAL CONDITION	EXAMPLE
None	None	Hb G-Philadelphia
Aggregation with reduced solubility	Hemolytic anemia; painful crisis (homozygous state)	Hb S
Instability with reduced solubility	Hemolytic anemia (heterozygous state)	Hb Köln Hb Gun Hill
Methemoglobinemia	Cyanosis	Hb M
Increased oxygen affinity	Erythrocytosis	Hb Chesapeake
Decreased oxygen affinity	Cyanosis or no clinical condition	Hb Kansas

(Modified from Wintrobe MM: The abnormal hemoglobins: General principles. In Wintrobe MM (ed): Clinical Hematology, 8th ed, p 815. Philadelphia, Lea & Febiger, 1981, with permission.)

TABLE 14–5. Functional Abnormalities of Hemoglobin Variants

	NUMBERS OF VARIANTS			
ABNORMALITY	SINGLE AMINO ACID SUBSTITUTIONS α CHAIN	β CHAIN	AMINO ACID DELETIONS	ELONGATED GLOBIN CHAINS
None or unknown	65	71	1	6
Aggregation	0	4		
Unstable	9	32	2	1
Methemoglobin	2	3		
Increased oxygen affinity	10	29	3	1
Decreased and oxygen affinity	3	10		
Unstable and increased oxygen affinity	3	18	4	
Unstable decreased oxygen affinity	1	8	1	
TOTAL	93	175	11	8

(From Wintrobe MM: The abnormal hemoglobins: General principles. In Wintrobe MM et al: Clinical Hematology, 8th ed, p 815. Philadelphia, Lea & Febiger, 1981, with permission.)

Dithionite Tube Test for Hemoglobin S[33,42,55,58]

The dithionite tube test is a screening test for the detection of sickling hemoglobin (*e.g.,* Hb S). It gives rapid results, is inexpensive, and has a high degree of accuracy, although it is not specific for Hb S. Several prepackaged kits are available.

DIOTHIONATE TUBE TEST
Principle

Red cells are lysed by saponin, allowing hemoglobin to escape. Sodium dithionite binds and removes oxygen from the test environment. Hb S polymerizes in the resulting deoxygenated state and forms a precipitate in a high-molarity phosphate buffer solution. The precipitate consists of tactoids, which are liquid crystals. The tactoids refract, deflect light, and make the solution turbid.

Specimen Requirements

Whole blood collected in ethylenediaminetetraacetic acid (EDTA), heparin, or sodium citrate is recommended (store at 4°C until testing). Do not store more than 3 weeks. Some procedures call for whole blood; others require packed erythrocytes. The cells should be separated just before the test is performed.

Reagents

Kits are available with prepackaged supplies and reagents. The National Committee for Clinical Laboratory Standards (NCCLS) sickle solubility procedure[58] provides instructions for laboratory reagent preparation.

Quality Control[58]

A positive and a negative control should be run with each set of tests. The positive control specimen should contain approximately 30% to 45% Hb S and have a hemoglobin value of 12 ± 2 g/dL. The negative control should have normal adult percentages of Hb A and A$_2$ and no Hb S.

Procedure

Manufacturer's instructions should be followed closely. The following procedure is an example of one that requires packed red cells.

1. Label three 12 × 75 mm test tubes: *Patient, Neg. control, Pos. control.*
2. Pipet 2 mL working solution at room temperature into each tube. Add 10 μL packed erythrocytes. Mix and wait 5 minutes.
3. Observe specimen for turbidity by holding tube 2.5 cm in front of newsprint or a reader card with thin black lines, or by placing the tube in a special reading rack designed for this test.

TABLE 14–6. Recommended Laboratory Tests for Diagnosis of Hemoglobinopathies

TESTS	COMMENTS
MOST FREQUENTLY REQUIRED	
Complete blood count RBC morphology evaluation Sickle cell solubility test Hemoglobin electrophoresis, cellulose acetate (pH 8.4–8.6)	
Hb electrophoresis, citrate agar (pH 6.0–6.2)	To distinguish/identify some abnormal Hbs detected on cellulose acetate electrophoresis
Supravital stain for Heinz bodies	To screen for unstable Hb; not a specific test since it also indicates G6PD and related deficiencies
Hb F quantitation	Alkali denaturation to quantitate Hb F in 2–40% range
Hb A$_2$ quantitation	Column chromatography (see Chap. 15)
OCCASIONALLY REQUIRED	
Heat denaturation test	To screen for unstable Hb
Isopropanol precipitation test	To screen for unstable Hb
Globin chain electrophoresis, acid or alkaline pH	To differentiate Hb S, D, G, and Q or Hb A$_2$, C, E, and O-Arab
RARELY REQUIRED	
P$_{50}$ quantitation	To screen for abnormal oxygen affinity
2,3-DPG quantitation	

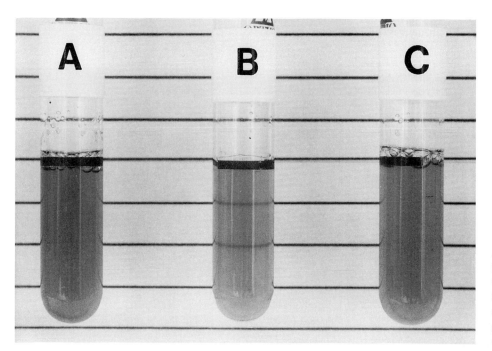

FIG. 14-3. Dithionite solubility test. Tube A is the positive control, tube B is the negative control, and tube C is the patient's blood. The patient's sample is positive for sickling hemoglobin because the heavy lines on the card behind the tube cannot be seen.

Interpretation of Results

Figure 14-3 shows the results of a positive control (A), negative control (B), and a positive patient sample (C). Turbidity indicates the presence of sickling hemoglobin regardless of the genotype (*e.g.*, SS, AS, S–thalassemia). If the solution is clear and lines are visible through it, the result is considered negative.

This test is not specific for Hb S. It is positive in the presence of other abnormal hemoglobins, such as Hb Barts and Hb I, and some unstable hemoglobins, such as Hb Sabine. Hb C-Harlem,[5,6] Hb C-Ziguinchor,[32] and Hb S-Travis[52] also cause a positive result. These last three hemoglobins have the same amino acid substitution abnormality as Hb S, but each also has an additional unique β-chain substitution.

The tube solubility test is used only for screening purposes. Normally, it should be performed after electrophoresis (at alkaline *p*H) to determine whether a hemoglobin band that travels in the Hb S or Hb C position is a sickling hemoglobin. The test may be performed as a quick screening procedure prior to electrophoresis in a laboratory where only a few electrophoresis requests are received each week; however, specimens should not be stored for more than 10 days before hemolysate preparation for electrophoresis.

Comments and Sources of Error

A positive solubility test must always be confirmed by electrophoresis at alkaline *p*H, and sometimes at acid *p*H.

Blood from infants younger than 6 months of age should not be tested by this method because production of the abnormal β chain that causes Hb S may not yet be working at full capacity.

If whole blood is used, false positive or false negative results may occur (Table 14-7).

If the patient's hemoglobin value is less than 7 g/dL and whole blood is used, double the amount of whole blood to avoid a false negative result.

Using 10 × 75 mm test tubes may cause a false negative result as the smaller tube diameter may allow the reader to see the black lines even if the solution is turbid.

A false negative result may occur if the patient has had a recent transfusion or if reagents are outdated.

All solutions must be at room temperature prior to use for testing. Reagents are usually stored in the refrigerator.

SPECIMEN COLLECTION FOR ELECTROPHORESIS PROCEDURES[13,57]
Specimen Requirements[57]

Venous blood may be collected in EDTA, heparin, sodium citrate, acid-citrate-dextrose (ACD), or citrate-phosphate-dextrose (CPD). Whole blood should be stored at 4°C for no longer than 10 days before the hemolysate is made.

HEMOLYSATE PREPARATION USING WATER AND ORGANIC SOLVENT
Procedure

1. Centrifuge whole blood at a relative centrifugal force (RCF) of 1500 to 2000 × g for 10 minutes to separate cells and plasma.
2. Remove plasma with a disposable pipet.
3. Wash cells three times with 0.85% NaCl solution (normal saline) and remove final wash solution.
4. Lyse cells by adding six volumes of distilled water to washed cells and a half volume (half the volume of washed cells) of toluene, chloroform, or carbon tetrachloride. One of the

TABLE 14–7. Sources of Physiologic and Technical Errors in the Sickle Solubility Test

FALSE POSITIVE RESULTS	FALSE NEGATIVE RESULTS
Erythrocytosis	Anemia (Hb <7 g/dL)★
Hyperglobulinemia★	Patient was recently transfused with normal blood
Extreme leukocytosis★	
Hyperlipidemia★	Holding tube too close to card when reading results
More blood added to reagent than called for by test procedure	Testing blood from infant younger than 6 months
Deteriorated reagent	Deteriorated reagent
	Use of 10 × 75-mm test tubes

★ May be avoided by using packed erythrocytes instead of whole blood and following appropriate methods for use of packed erythrocytes in this test.

latter two solvents is preferred if only 1 mL red cells or less is available, since the hemolysate appears as the top layer after centrifugation with these solvents but at the bottom with toluene. (Caution: These organic solvents are toxic when inhaled and should be handled under a fume hood.)

5. Shake vigorously by hand or by vortex mixer until bright red uniform mixture appears (approximately 5 minutes).
6. Centrifuge 25 minutes at approximately 1500 to 2000 × g. (The calculation for converting relative centrifugal force to revolutions per minute is provided in Appendix B).
7. If toluene is used, remove top toluene and cell stroma layers with a suction apparatus. If carbon tetrachloride or chloroform is used, clear hemolysate solution will be at the top.
8. Filter hemolysate through a layer of Whatman No. 1 filter paper.
9. Hemolysate may be stoppered and stored at 3 to 5°C after addition of 2 or 3 drops of 3% KCN per 5 mL hemolysate to convert methemoglobin to cyanmethemoglobin (methemoglobin could interfere with test interpretation).

Comments and Sources of Error

The organic solvents used in this procedure may produce denaturation and precipitation of Hb Barts, H, and other unstable hemoglobins. Only water should be used to lyse red cells if unstable hemoglobins are suspected, and the solution should be centrifuged at 2000 × g for 30 minutes to remove stroma. If turbidity remains, filter through two layers of Whatman No. 1 filter paper.

HEMOLYSATE PREPARATION USING HEMOLYSATE REAGENT
Procedure

This method is faster, easier (e.g., for large-scale screening), and useful when only a small sample can be obtained, as from an infant, but it is not very reproducible and not adequate for tests requiring larger amounts of hemolysate or stroma-free hemolysate. Either saponin or EDTA hemolyzing reagent may be used.

For saponin hemolysate, dissolve 0.1 g saponin (pure, certified grade) in 100 mL distilled water. Mix. Transfer to storage bottle and add 40 mg KCN. Mix and store at 25°C (room temperature).

To make EDTA hemolysate, dissolve 0.25 g EDTA (tetrasodium salt) plus 5 mg KCN in 80 mL distilled water. Adjust volume to 100 mL with distilled water. Mix and store at 25°C.

Prepare hemolysate by adding 1 volume washed red cells (2 drops) to 3 volumes hemolysate reagent (5 drops) and shaking vigorously for about 10 seconds. The Centers for Disease Control (CDC)[13] recommends 3 drops hemolysate reagent for every 50 μL washed red cells. Add 1 drop 3% KCN. NCCLS[57] states that blood taken by skin puncture may be drawn directly into one of the above reagents to prepare a hemolysate for electrophoresis.

Cellulose Acetate Hemoglobin Electrophoresis[7,13,34,57,70]

Cellulose acetate electrophoresis is a relatively simple method for detection and preliminary identification of both normal and abnormal hemoglobins, particularly Hbs A, F, S, and C. It provides for sharp band resolution in a short time. Abnormal hemoglobins found on cellulose acetate require confirmation by other methods (e.g., sickle solubility test, citrate agar electrophoresis). When either Hb F or A₂ appears to be elevated, it must be quantitated by other methods.

CELLULOSE ACETATE METHOD
Principle

A small quantity of red cell hemolysate is placed on the cellulose acetate membrane between the center and the cathode (negative pole) of an electrophoretic chamber. An electrical field is created in the chamber through the use of a power supply and generation of current through a buffer at alkaline pH. Hemoglobin molecules have a net negative charge at alkaline pH and migrate on the membrane toward the anode (positive pole). Owing to variations in the amino acid content of different hemoglobins, the net charge of each hemoglobin type varies, and this determines each hemoglobin's rate of mobility in the electrical field.

Specimen Requirements

Whole blood collected in EDTA, heparin, ACD, CPD, or sodium citrate is acceptable. Specimens may be stored at 4°C until the hemolysate is made, but no longer than 10 days.

Reagents

Buffer

Tris-EDTA-boric acid (TEB) buffer, pH 8.4–8.6 (may be purchased): Tris (hydroxymethyl) aminomethane, 10.2 g; EDTA, 0.6 g; boric acid, 3.2 g; distilled water, to 1 L. Store at 4°C and check pH before each use.

Stain

Ponceau S stain (may be purchased): Ponceau S powder, 0.5 g; trichloroacetic acid, 5.0 g; distilled water, to 100 mL. Store at room temperature; stable indefinitely.

Counterstain

This stain is required only when differentiation of heme from nonheme proteins is required and to detect minor bands. o-Tolidine dihydrochloride solution: o-tolidine dihydrochloride (handle with gloves), 1.0 g; glacial acetic acid, 25 mL; distilled water, to 100 mL. Store at room temperature in dark bottle. For counterstain, use 5 mL o-tolidine dihydrochloride solution. Add 3% hydrogen peroxide (stored in refrigerator), 3 mL; 1% sodium nitroferricyanide in distilled water, 5 mL; 3% acetic acid, 10 mL. These reagents are mixed only on the day of the test.

Solution for Destaining

Five-percent glacial acetic acid in distilled water (store at room temperature; stable indefinitely).

Solution for Dehydration

Absolute methanol (95% to 100%).

Clearing Reagent

Glacial acetic acid, 100 mL; absolute methanol, 400 mL; polyethylene glycol 400 (Carbowax, PEG 400), 25 mL (optional).

Quality Control

An Hb A₁FSC control as well as a normal A₁A₂ patient sample should be run with each set of patient samples on every plate. The patterns of unknown samples should be compared to the known samples run on each individual plate, since variations in current, buffer lots, or application may cause variations in migration rate with each run. Results should be rechecked occasionally using duplicate samples.

Procedure

The following procedure is a general one. If a specific system is used, the manufacturer's instructions should be followed.

1. Pour 100 mL TEB buffer into each of two outer compartments of an electrophoresis chamber. Add ice to the inner compartments if high amperage is anticipated.

2. Soak a paper wick in each outer compartment, then drape a wick over each of the inner ridges. Cover chamber.

3. Label cellulose acetate plate on corner of glossy side to indicate sequence of patient samples and to identify different sets of patients.

4. Place plates in rack with cellulose acetate sides all facing forward. Lower rack very slowly (over approximately 10 seconds) into container of buffer. Allow to soak for the amount of time specified by the manufacturer.

5. Clean sample well plate with distilled water and dry wells with cotton-tipped swabs. Prepare an additional plate and load with distilled water for rinsing.

6. Load up to 6 sample hemolysates and the two controls into clean, dry plate wells using a 5-μL microdispenser.

7. Prime sample applicator by depressing several times into sample wells then depressing once on a blotter. Place applicator back over sample wells. If procedure will be delayed more than 2 minutes, remove applicator and cover samples with a glass slide to prevent evaporation.

8. Remove a cellulose acetate plate from the buffer. Blot between two blotters quickly and evenly to remove excess moisture.

9. Place plate, cellulose acetate side up, in aligning base (labeled corner at bottom left).

10. Quickly depress applicator button three times to load samples on delivery tips.

11. Rapidly set applicator in aligning base with sample No. 1 on left side. Quickly and firmly push button down and hold for 5 seconds, to allow sample application on cellulose acetate plate. The jolt of delivery tips contacting cellulose acetate quickly and firmly causes tips to empty properly.

12. Immediately place plate, cellulose acetate down, in chamber, making sure wicks make good contact with cellulose acetate. Samples should be closer to the cathode to allow for migration to the anode (positive pole). Place a weight (*e.g.*, glass slide, coin) on top of the plate to ensure good contact.

13. Apply voltage according to manufacturer's instructions. From 250 to 400 V will be required for a period of time that depends on the type and size of cellulose acetate used. Immediately turn off power, remove plate, and begin staining.

14. General Staining, Destaining, Dehydration, and Clearing Procedure

    Stain in Ponceau S for at least 3 minutes. Drain on paper towels for 5 to 10 seconds.

    Destain in three to four successive 2-minute washes of 5% glacial acetic acid or until plate background is white. Drain on paper towels for 5 seconds between each wash.

    Fix plate in two successive 3- to 5-minute washes of absolute methanol. Drain for 5 seconds between washes.

    Move plate to clearing solution for 5 minutes.

    Air dry vertically for 1 to 2 minutes.

    Dry in incubator oven at 56°C for 3 to 6 minutes, acetate side up, on a blotter pad. Do not overdry.

15. Scan plate with densitometer to semiquantitate separated hemoglobin bands. (*Note:* Carbonic anhydrase released from red cells will also stain as a narrow band close to the application point.)

16. Label plate and place in a protective cover for permanent storage.

17. Counterstaining option.

If after the above procedure is followed a hemoglobin variant appears to be migrating in a position nearer the cathode than carbonic anhydrase, a second cellulose acetate plate should be run using a double or triple application of the specimen and a control. This plate should be stained with Ponceau S and then with a counterstain (described under reagents) for a few minutes until desired color appears; it is then rinsed with 5% acetic acid. The counterstain stains hemoglobin fractions purple, while nonheme protein remains pink or red. Specimen results must be compared to the control specimen. Commonly, counterstaining is used to differentiate Hb G_2 from carbonic anhydrase. Hb G_2, an α-chain variant, appears as a bluish purple band that migrates only a short distance (between application point and carbonic anhydrase). Other α-chain variants may migrate in a similar position.

Interpretation of Results

Interpretation of results may be based on known migration patterns of various hemoglobins (Fig. 14-4) and by comparison with controls. Hemoglobin percentages may be calculated manually or by computer, based on densitometry results.

Reference Ranges

Hb A_1, 97%; Hb A_2, 2% to 3.5%; Hb F, at birth 60% to 90%, < 1% after age 1 year. Each laboratory should determine its own reference ranges.

Comments and Sources of Error[57]

Definitive diagnosis of abnormal hemoglobins cannot be made on the basis of electrophoresis performed at a single pH. Citrate agar electrophoresis at acid pH provides another method to confirm the presence of certain variants. The sickle solubility test is always performed as a confirmatory measure when a hemoglobin band migrates in the S position on cellulose acetate.

Errors may result from use of unacceptable reagents, equipment, or samples, including buffers of incorrect pH or ionic strength or ones that are contaminated or cloudy; sample wells, applicator tips, blotters, or cellulose acetate plates contaminated with dirt, blood, or other proteins; and hemolysates that are old or discolored, contain red cell stroma, or are bacterially contaminated, all of which may cause poor separation, artifacts, or smearing of hemoglobin bands.

Technical errors include (1) improper loading of plates into buffer, which can cause trapped air or peeling; improper sample application, or improper blotting that leaves plates excessively wet or dry; (2) lack of contact between buffer and cellulose acetate; (3) excessive heat during electrophoresis (this can be controlled by placing ice in the center compartments [not the buffer] or by reducing voltage); (4) application points that are too close to the anode; (5) any delay in sample application, applying current to plate, or staining after electrophoresis; and (6) failure to remove leukocytes from specimen with increased leukocyte count may lead to migration of a band that is much faster than any known Hb variant. This band is thought to be leukocyte-derived myeloperoxidase.

In blood of poorly controlled diabetic patients, a band of glycosylated hemoglobin may appear slightly toward the anode from Hb A.

Citrate Agar Hemoglobin Electrophoresis[13,39,51,56]

Citrate agar electrophoresis routinely is performed at acid pH as a compliment to cellulose acetate electrophoresis, which is performed at alkaline pH. It differentiates some hemoglobin variants that migrate together on cellulose acetate. For example, it is used to differentiate Hb S from D and G, all of which migrate similarly on cellulose acetate. Citrate agar is also used to differentiate Hb C from C-Harlem, E, and O-Arab which also migrate together on cellulose acetate (see Fig. 14-4).

This procedure is useful for detecting small amounts of either Hb A or F in the presence of large amounts of the

Hemoglobin Electrophoresis

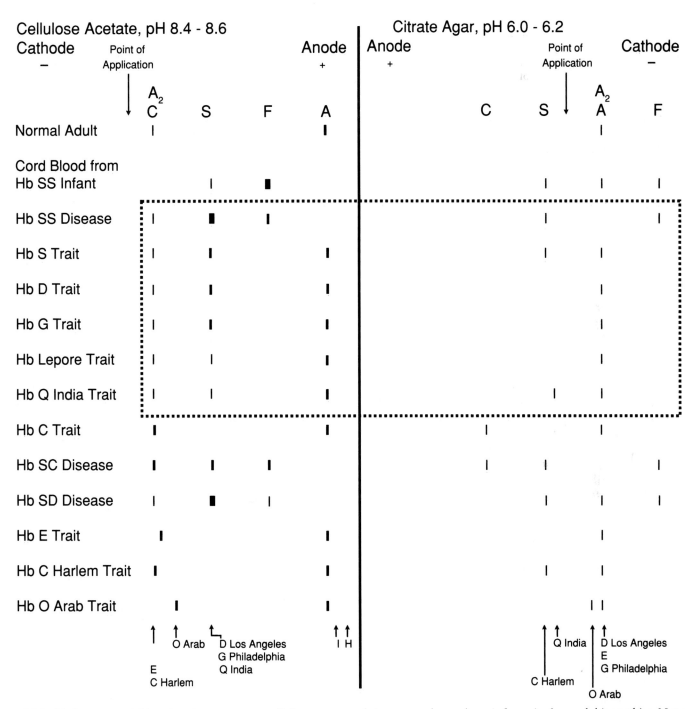

FIG. 14-4.   Hemoglobin migration patterns on cellulose acetate and citrate agar electrophoresis for major hemoglobinopathies. Note points of sample application and locations of anodes and cathodes for each method. Box around patterns in cellulose acetate electrophoresis indicates hemoglobins that are indistinguishable from Hb S at alkaline pH but distinguishable on citrate agar at acid pH. Hb I and Hb H (migration patterns not shown) both migrate faster than all other hemoglobins depicted on cellulose acetate.

other and in revealing small amounts of adult Hbs A and S present at birth in cord blood.

CITRATE AGAR METHOD
Principle

Hemoglobins are separated based on the interactions among hemoglobin variants, agar, and citrate buffer ions in addition to the altered electrical charge of the various hemoglobins at acid

pH. Hemoglobin variants are identified by their migration toward the anode and cathode and comparing the migration to that of known control samples. The test is strictly qualitative: the percentage of each hemoglobin present cannot be determined accurately using this method.

Specimen Requirements

Specimen requirements are similar to those stated earlier for cellulose acetate electrophoresis. NCCLS[56] recommends that specimen hemoglobin levels be checked and, if necessary, diluted with distilled water to about 0.5 to 1.0 g/dL for adult samples or 4g/dL for umbilical cord blood.

Equipment

Equipment is the same as that used for cellulose acetate electrophoresis, except that citrate agar plates (stored at 4° to 6°C) are used instead of cellulose acetate, and sponge wicks may be used instead of paper. Citrate agar plates may be made in the laboratory[56] or purchased commercially. No densitometer is used in this procedure.

Reagents

Stock Citrate Buffer (0.5 mol/L)

To 147 g sodium citrate and 4.3 g citric acid, add distilled water to 1000 mL.

Citric Acid

To 30 g citric acid, add distilled water to 100 mL.

Working Citrate Buffer (0.05 mol/L; pH 6.0 to 6.2)

Dilute 100 mL stock buffer to a total volume of 1000 mL with distilled water. Adjust pH to 6.0 to 6.2 by adding drops of citric acid (30 g/100 mL). Store at 4°C for up to 3 months.

Quality Control

Each new lot of agar plates should be tested to ensure good separation of known control samples. If Hb O-Arab is suspected, a Hb O-Arab control should be run if one is available. Strict adherence to expiration dates is required. Plates made in house are usually acceptable for 1 month when stored at 4°C. An Hb A₁FSC control should be run on each plate with patient samples.

Procedure

The following is a general procedure provided for information. Each manufacturer of citrate agar systems provides specific instructions that should be followed.

1. Allow citrate agar plate to come to room temperature. Put an identifying mark on back of plate to indicate position of sample No. 1.
2. Pour 100 mL working buffer into each outer section of chamber. Soak a wick in each section and drape wicks over shoulders of each compartment if wicks are required by system used.
3. Mix diluted hemolysate and control to ensure homogeneous samples. Adjust hemoglobin concentration for adult samples to about 0.5 to 1.0 g/dL and cord blood to about 4 g/dL.
4. Load sample application plate as described for cellulose acetate procedure. Use immediately or cover with slide.
5. Remove spring from applicator to allow sample tips to sit on agar surface.
6. Clean hemolysate applicator as described for cellulose acetate procedure. Prime applicator according to manufacturer's instructions.
7. Press applicator tips into sample wells three or four times.
8. Apply samples lightly (with sample No. 1 closest to identifying mark) to agar, approximately 3 cm from anode end of plate or in center. Do not break agar surface.
9. Let plate stand for several minutes to allow hemolysate to be completely absorbed into agar.
10. Place plate, agar side down, over bridges in chamber and ensure good contact with wicks if they are used. Place lid over chamber.
11. Follow manufacturer's instructions for voltage and time. If lid becomes warm to touch, place a cool pack on the lid or surround chambers with ice. Alternatively, perform electrophoresis in a cold room.
12. Prepare stain only on the day of its use and discard after use. During electrophoresis, mix 10 mL o-tolidine dihydrochloride (or o-dianisidine) stock stain with 5 mL 3% hydrogen peroxide. Avoid contact with skin.
13. Put citrate agar plate in staining dish and puddle stain over plate. Stain a few minutes until desired intensity is achieved.
14. Rinse for 10 minutes in distilled water. Water stops the staining reaction.
15. Allow to air dry or dry in oven at 100°C for 2 to 3 hours. Interpret hemoglobin bands according to controls.
16. Cover and seal for storage. Plates are stable for 3 months. A method for permanent storage is available.[35]

Interpretation of Results

Figure 14-4 shows the migration pattern of normal hemoglobins and some common variants on citrate agar at acid pH.

Comments and Sources of Error

Cellulose acetate and citrate agar electrophoresis together confirm the presence of Hb S, C, O, and several others. Other hemoglobins (e.g., Hb D-Los Angeles and Hb G-Philadelphia) cannot be defined solely by these two methods. Globin chain separation may be required.

Using the citrate agar method, hemoglobin mobilities are more affected by concentration and state of the hemoglobin, small changes in buffer composition, electrical conditions, and other factors than in other methods. Use of controls is therefore imperative.

Many of the same technical errors that may occur in performing cellulose acetate electrophoresis also apply to citrate agar.

Agar-impregnated cellulose acetate is an alternative to the medium described above.[56,72]

Alkali Denaturation Test for Fetal Hemoglobin[3,41,59,77]

Fetal hemoglobin (Hb F) is increased in a number of conditions (Table 14-8). The alkali denaturation test provides accurate and precise quantitation of the percentage of Hb F in blood, particularly when it appears to be elevated. It is the method recommended by NCCLS for quantitation of Hb F in the range of 2% to 40%.[59] Radioimmunoassay is more accurate when Hb F concentration is less than 2%, and column chromatography is more accurate when it is greater than 40%.[59] Quantitation of Hb F by densitometry of cellulose acetate electrophoretograms is *not* satisfactory.

TABLE 14–8. Conditions Commonly Associated with Increased Levels of Hb F

CONDITION	COMMENTS
Infancy	Newborns have 60 to 90% Hb F
Hemoglobinopathies	Particularly Hb SS
Unstable hemoglobins	
Doubly heterozygous conditions	SC, SD, Hb S–Thalassemia, Hb C–Thalassemia
Thalassemia	See Chapter 15
Hereditary persistence of fetal hemoglobin	See Chapter 15
Aplastic anemia	Some cases
Leukemia	Some cases
Pregnancy	Some cases

ALKALI DENATURATION METHOD

Principle

Hb F resists the denaturation exhibited by other hemoglobins at alkaline pH. After a specified period, denaturation is stopped by addition of saturated ammonium sulfate, which lowers the pH and precipitates any denatured hemoglobin. The test solution is filtered, leaving Hb F in solution that can be quantitated spectrophotometrically as a percentage of total hemoglobin.

Specimen Requirements

Whole blood collected in EDTA is recommended.

Reagents

1. Cyanmethemoglobin (Drabkin's) reagent, available commercially (Chap. 9).
2. Sodium hydroxide reagent (1.25 mol/L), available commercially.
3. Saturated ammonium sulfate (4.06 mol/L at 20°C). To 550 g ammonium sulfate add distilled water to approximately 1 L. Mix. Store in glass bottle at 20° to 25°C. Solution is stable up to 3 months. Undissolved crystals should always be present at bottom of bottle.

Quality Control

A specimen known to be normal and one with confirmed elevation of Hb F should be run with each batch of specimens tested. An elevated Hb F control may be prepared by mixing umbilical cord blood and normal adult blood of the same ABO group. It is not clear how long Hb F preparations are stable.

Procedure

The following recommended NCCLS procedure[59] should be performed at room temperature.

1. Prepare hemolysate as described earlier, using water and toluene (p. 190).
2. Determine hemolysate Hb concentration using standard cyanmethemoglobin methods (Chap. 9). Acceptable concentration is 8 to 12 g/dL.
3. Based on the Hb concentration of the hemolysate, calculate the amount of hemolysate to be added to 10 mL of cyanmethemoglobin reagent to make an approximately 5 g/L solution. If hemolysate Hb concentration is 8.0 g/dL, add 0.6 mL hemolysate to reagent. For each additional Hb g/dL, decrease the amount of hemolysate added by 0.05 mL. For example, for hemolysate Hb of 12.0 g/dL, add 0.4 mL hemolysate to 10 mL reagent.
4. Pipet 3.0 mL diluted hemolysate into each of three 17 × 100 mm tubes, two labeled Test and one labeled Total.
5. At 15- or 30-second intervals timed with a stopwatch, add 0.2 mL of sodium hydroxide reagent to each tube labeled Test. Mix well with vortex mixer.
6. Add 0.2 mL water to tube labeled Total.
7. Exactly 2 minutes after adding sodium hydroxide, add 2.0 mL saturated ammonium sulfate reagent to each tube (both tubes labeled Test and tube labeled Total).
8. After 5 minutes, filter contents of all three tubes through two layers of Whatman No. 42 (or No. 1) 7-cm filter paper folded into 5-cm short-stemmed funnels. Collect filtrates into clean, properly labeled tubes. Filtrates must be absolutely clear.
9. Prepare a blanking solution by mixing 3.0 mL cyanmethemoglobin reagent with 0.2 mL sodium hydroxide reagent and 2.0 mL ammonium sulfate reagent. Filter through two layers of filter paper as described for patient samples. Blank spectrophotometer at 540 nm.
10. Pipet 1 mL filtrate labeled Total into 4 mL distilled water; label Diluted Total.
11. Measure absorbance (A) at 540 nm of the two test filtrates and of the diluted total.

12. Calculate fraction of Hb F as a percentage:

$$Hb\ F(\%) = \frac{A_{Test}}{A_{Diluted\ Total} \times 5} \times 100$$

(A = absorbance; 5 is the additional dilution factor).

Reference Range

After 1 year of age, the reference range is < 1%.[3] Each laboratory should determine its own population reference range.

Comments

Difference between duplicate tests for each specimen must not exceed 0.5% Hb F for values less than 5%; 1% Hb F for values 5% to 15%; or 2% Hb F for values greater than 15%.[59]

Other acceptable methods exist for use with small samples, such as that described by Singer and coworkers[75] or NCCLS.[59]

Sources of Error

Possible sources of error in this procedure are poor technique (e.g., of pipeting and mixing); allowing more or less than 2 minutes reaction time; spectrophotometric errors (Chap. 9); filtrate turbidity; using outdated reagents or incorrect reagent concentrations; and using poor-quality filter paper.

GLOBIN CHAIN ELECTROPHORESIS[13,38,71,76]

Approximately 400 hemoglobin variants have been identified at present, so there are many that migrate together on both routine cellulose acetate and citrate agar electrophoresis. Globin chain electrophoresis provides another method that can be used to differentiate the variants. In this procedure, 2-mercaptoethanol is added to the hemolysate to separate globin chains from heme while urea is added to separate the α- and non-α chains. Subsequently, the sample containing free globin chains is electrophoresed on cellulose acetate at either alkaline or acid pH. Heme migrates toward the anode (positive pole) while globin chains migrate at varying speeds toward the cathode.

Since globin chain electrophoresis is not performed in most routine hematology laboratories, it will not be described here.

SYSTEMATIC LABORATORY DIAGNOSIS OF HEMOGLOBINOPATHIES

Figure 14-5 provides a basic systematic flow chart for laboratory testing of the hemoglobinopathies. The chart begins with electrophoresis on cellulose acetate and the test sequence thereafter is based on the preliminary results on cellulose acetate. This chart is also useful in selecting appropriate test procedures for differentiating thalassemia from hemoglobinopathies.

VARIANTS CAUSED BY β-CHAIN SUBSTITUTIONS

The β globin chain amino acid substitutions are the most common cause of hemoglobinopathies (see Table 14-5). The best known are single substitutions and include Hb S, C, D-Los Angeles, and E. Each affects millions of people worldwide.

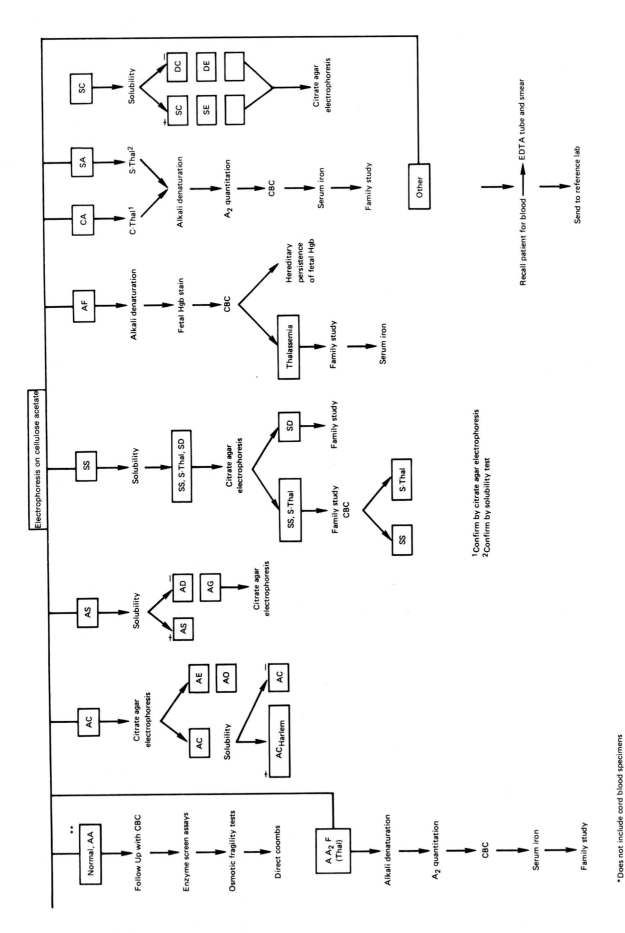

FIG. 14-5. Flow chart for laboratory diagnosis of hemoglobinopathies. (From Gillen LAF: Hemoglobins, myoglobin, and porphyrin. In Bishop ML, Duben–Von Laufen JL, Fody EP (eds): Clinical Chemistry–Principles, Procedures, Correlations. Philadelphia, JB Lippincott, 1985, with permission.)

Sickle Cell Anemia

Demographics and Genetics

Sickle cell disease is a worldwide disorder inherited as an autosomal codominant gene. Heterozygous inheritance of the sickle gene (AS) is frequently referred to as sickle cell trait, whereas the homozygous state (SS) is known as sickle cell anemia. The place of origin of the gene is probably Africa, where 20% to 40% of the population are heterozygous (see Fig. 14-1).[79] In the United States, 0.1% to 0.2% of the black population have sickle cell anemia, and approximately 8% are heterozygous.[53,69]

Hb S results from a point mutation for the sixth amino acid in the β chain in which one nucleotide base is substituted for another (GAG becomes GUG). As a result, valine is substituted for glutamic acid (see Table 14-2). Otherwise, Hb S is structurally the same as Hb A. Researchers have proposed that the Hb S gene mutation has provided resistance, but not immunity, from the malarial parasite *Plasmodium falciparum,* which is transmitted by mosquitoes.[2] When a red cell containing *P. falciparum* undergoes the sickling process, the parasite dies.[30] Geographic areas where *P. falciparum* is found coincide closely with areas where large numbers of persons carry the Hb S gene.[37] The molecular events resulting from the Hb S mutation include production of intramolecular hydrophobic bonds, which are responsible for the insoluble characteristics of Hb S. The amino acid substitution causes a loss of negatively charged ions on the molecule. Thus Hb S migrates slower than Hb A toward the positive pole in electrophoresis at alkaline *p*H (see Fig. 14-4).

Pathophysiology

When oxygenated, Hb S is fully soluble. Sickling occurs when oxygen decreases at the tissue level. When oxygen is released from the molecule, a conformational change occurs, which results in polymerization of hemoglobin molecules leading to the formation of tactoids or crystals, which cause the cells to become rigid (Fig. 14-6). Sickle cells impede blood flow to tissues and organs, resulting in tissue death, organ infarction, and pain.

Hemolysis is common. Sickled red cells are prematurely destroyed by the phagocytic system (extravascular hemolysis), especially the spleen, and by their inability to traverse the microcirculation (intravascular hemolysis). The bone marrow responds by increasing erythropoiesis. As a result, the marrow spaces widen and the bone cortex thins. Extramedullary hematopoiesis may be observed in severe cases.

Symptoms

Among sickle cell anemia patients aged 10 through 20 years, growth and sexual maturation generally lag behind that of normal adolescents. Symptoms can be severe. Every organ in the body is affected, and symptoms include pain of many types. Chronic hemolysis causes fatigue, weakness, pallor, and other symptoms of anemia. Many symptoms are associated with sickle cell crises.

Sickle Cell Crises

Painful sickle cell crises occur in patients of all ages. Any situation that produces excessive deoxygenation of the red cells may cause a crisis (*e.g.,* infection, dehydration, violent exercise, obstetric delivery, and high altitude [flying in unpressurized aircraft]). Low-grade fever is often found in association with crises.

Vasoocclusive crises occur when rigid sickle cells increase blood viscosity. Sickle cells are associated with development of microthrombi, vascular occlusions, and microinfarctions in the joints and extremities as well as in major organs, which can cause organ failure.

Infectious crises are a primary cause of death in sickle cell anemia.[82] *Streptococcus pneumoniae* is the major infectious agent among children. This may be partially attributed to abnormal splenic function.[74] Susceptibility to infection is also caused by depression of immune function.[31]

The first sites affected by decreased blood flow are frequently the small bones of the hands and feet at age 6 to 9 months. The condition is referred to as *hand-foot syndrome* or dactylitis. Affected patients experience painful swelling of the backs of the hands and feet. This swelling may be the first sign of sickle cell anemia. Infarctions of the small bones may cause fingers to grow to varying lengths. During puberty, affected sites include the femurs and humeri. The abnormally thin bone cortex is especially vulnerable to wearing and fracture.

In *bone, joint, and other crises,* pain may occur in the joints of arms and legs where sickle cells accumulate, in shafts of bones as sickle cells occlude the bone marrow sinusoids, and in the lungs, which are the site of frequent infarcts in adults due to sickle cell accumulation. Pulmonary infarcts can lead to severe chest or abdominal pain.

Splenic sequestration crises occur when sickle cells become trapped in the splenic microcirculation. The spleen enlarges as more cells are trapped, leading to hypovolemia (decreased blood volume), which may cause shock and even death. This usually occurs in children before age 6 years.

Aplastic crises are thought to be caused by infection and fever. They result in a temporary (usually 5 to 10 days) but significant reduction in erythrocyte count, hemoglobin, hematocrit, reticulocyte count, and bone marrow normoblasts. Leukocytes and platelets may or may not be affected.

Organs Affected by Sickle Cell Anemia

LIVER. Sickle cell sequestration in the liver sinusoids may cause hepatomegaly and liver malfunction in children

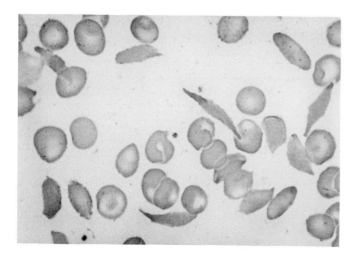

FIG. 14-6. Peripheral blood film from patient with Hb SS, sickle cell anemia.

and adults. It can also result in jaundice and hyperbilirubinemia.

HEART.   Iron deposition in the heart, mostly attributable to the frequent transfusions patients require, may lead to heart failure. Cardiomegaly may appear in early childhood.

SPLEEN.   Splenomegaly and abnormal splenic function may begin in early infancy (after 6 months of age). Later in childhood, splenic infarction and fibrosis occur due to sickle occlusion. Eventually, the spleen shrivels and becomes nonfunctional. In contrast, patients with Hb S–thalassemia or Hb SC disease usually exhibit splenomegaly.

SKIN.   An ulcer or scar on the leg, particularly the ankle, is common. It usually appears during adolescence.

KIDNEYS.   Infarcts may also occur in the kidneys, resulting in hematuria and failure of urine concentration.

LUNGS.   Infarctions in the lung tissue can occur due to infections and sickle cell occlusion.

Charache and colleagues[15] have published a valuable reference on management and therapy of sickle cell crises and organ involvement in sickle cell anemia.

Laboratory Findings

PERIPHERAL BLOOD.   Anemia is usually severe (Hb is 5 to 9 g/dL) and of the normocytic, normochromic type. It appears at about 6 to 9 months of age when Hb S is first produced. Anisocytosis is common and the most important poikilocyte is the sickle cell (see Fig. 14–6). Sickle cells must always be investigated and reported to the physician, even if they are seen only in an occasional microscopic field. Target cells usually are abundant. Ovalocytes and fragments (schistocytes) may also be seen. The red cell distribution width (RDW) is increased.

Cells that have transformed several times back and forth between the normal and sickle state generally become irreversibly sickled and appear as dense elliptocytes with areas where the hemoglobin has shrunk away from the cell membrane. Other findings include polychromasia, nucleated red cells (1 to 100 per 100 leukocytes), reticulocytosis (8.1% to 16.5%), and basophilic stippling. Howell-Jolly and Pappenheimer bodies indicate a nonfunctional spleen (autosplenectomy).

Leukocytosis (10 to 30 × 10^9/L) is common. The differential cell count reveals an increase in neutrophil percentage. If infection is present, a left shift may occur, causing immature leukocytes to appear in the peripheral blood. Thrombocytosis is also common (mean 440 × 10^9/L).[29] This is due to the fibrotic spleen, which cannot pool one third of the peripheral blood platelets as a normal spleen does. The megathrombocyte number is increased, especially during marrow infarcts.[17] During vasoocclusive crisis, total platelet and megathrombocyte numbers may decrease.[29]

SPECIAL HEMATOLOGIC TESTS.   All patients with Hb S in their genotype (*e.g.,* Hb SS, AS, S–thalassemia, SC, SD) should have a positive sickle solubility screening test (see Fig. 14–3).

Hemoglobin electrophoresis is performed to confirm the presence of Hb S. Quantitative hemoglobin electrophoresis results for Hb SS disease are shown in Table 14–9 in comparison to results found in other hemoglobinopathies. Quantitation of Hb S by densitometry reveals 80% to 90% Hb S. Hemoglobin F may be increased. It is usually no more than 10%, but occasionally it is as high as 20%. Hb A₂ is usually normal. If Hb A₂ or Hb F is increased, the possibility of a thalassemic condition interacting with Hb S should be investigated. Hb F should be quantitated by alkali denaturation and Hb A₂ by ion exchange microchromatography (Chap. 15).

Hemoglobins D-Los Angeles (also called D-Punjab), G-Philadelphia, and Q-India all migrate in the same position as Hb S on cellulose acetate (pH 8.4; see Fig. 14–4). Citrate agar electrophoresis (pH 6.0) helps separate Hb S from these other hemoglobins.

Diagnosis of sickle cell anemia in a fetus may be made as early as the second trimester of pregnancy by electrophoresis of blood from the placenta, but specimen collection can jeopardize fetal life.

Osmotic fragility is decreased, owing to the target and sickle cells whose large surface-to-volume ratio allows in-

TABLE 14–9. Results of Cellulose Acetate Electrophoresis (pH 8.6) for Major Hemoglobinopathies

HEMOGLOBINOPATHY	A (%)	F (%)	S (%)	C (%)	D (%)	E (%)	DEGREE OF CLINICAL ABNORMALITY†
Hb CC		1–7		>90			Mild
Hb AC	50–60	<2		40–50			None
Hb SC		1–7	50	50			Moderate to severe
Hb SS		1–10	80–90				Severe
Hb AS	55–70	<2	30–45				None or mild
Hb DD		<2			95		None
Hb AD	50–65	<2			35–50		None
Hb EE		1–5				95	Mild
Hb AE	60–80					20–40	None

* These are general figures to allow for comparison of major differences in the percentages of hemoglobin in the various disorders. Patients diagnosed with one of these conditions may have percentages slightly different from those shown. The numbers do not add up to 100 in some cases because these are approximations.
† Indicates whether patients experience any clinical signs or symptoms of illness.

creased water uptake before hemolysis. The erythrocyte sedimentation rate is low (*i.e.,* in the normal range) in spite of the anemia because sickle cells do not form rouleaux (rouleaux normally encourages erythrocyte sedimentation). The half-life of red cells containing Hb S is approximately 10 to 20 days (using ^{51}Cr), owing to their early hemolysis.

Bone marrow biopsy reveals erythroid hyperplasia. The myeloid:erythroid (M:E) cell ratio is approximately 1:1 (normal, 3:1).

CHEMISTRY. The generally increased values of lactate dehydrogenase, indirect (unconjugated) bilirubin, and urobilinogen, and the decreased serum haptoglobin level all reflect the hemolytic component of sickle cell disease.

Effects of Treatment on Laboratory Results

The primary goal of treatment is prevention of crises by avoiding situations that precipitate them. If a crisis does occur, the patient is hydrated, pain is alleviated with analgesics such as aspirin, and infection is treated with appropriate antibiotics. Patients are kept warm, because exposure to cold may precipitate a crisis. Excessive sweating must be prevented, since dehydration precipitates a crisis. Response to treatment may be crudely indicated on the blood film by a decrease in the number of sickle cells. Transfusions may be required when physical signs and symptoms warrant, although patients usually tolerate a hemoglobin value as low as 6.5 g/dL.[14]

Patients whose quality of life is poor may need repeated packed cell transfusions to maintain the Hb S level below 30%. After a cerebrovascular accident, transfusions must be continued for several years to prevent another stroke.[14] For surgical preparation, transfusions are required to raise the Hb A level to more than 50% with a hematocrit of 0.30 to 0.35 L/L.[23]

Many substances have been tested as antisickling agents, but none has proven to be totally satisfactory and research in this area is ongoing.[1] Cyanate has been used successfully for treatment by *in vitro* exposure of erythrocytes to cyanate, after which they are reinfused into the patient. This treatment increases the hemoglobin level and red cell survival time without causing toxic side effects.[47] Urea also has been studied because it is believed to prevent or reverse gelation of sickle cells. However, its benefit has not been proved.[1]

Nitrogen mustard is too toxic to administer *in vivo*, however, it may be useful in the treatment of red cells *in vitro* for reinfusion to prevent sickling.[15,66] Clinical trials are needed to prove or disprove its benefits.

Additional substances currently under long-term investigation fall into the category of cell membrane modifiers. They include zinc,[63] procaine hydrochloride,[61] Cetiedil, and piracetam.[1] Further studies are needed to evaluate all these agents.

A recent report on treatment of children with sickle cell anemia states that no chemical compound has satisfactorily met the criteria of efficiency, safety, and dependability and that pain control must still be provided.[73]

Bone marrow transplantation may be an alternative for selected patients.[44] Owing to the difficulty of finding a matching marrow donor and the problems of graft-versus-host disease, with its significant rates of morbidity and mortality, this treatment is generally reserved for special cases when there are virtually no other treatment choices until these problems can be overcome.

Prognosis

In the past, sickle cell anemia caused a shortened life span. As a result of genetic counseling of partners who carry the sickle gene, prenatal diagnosis, and education in the prevention of crises and in proper nutrition, life expectancy and quality of life have been improved to the point where some patients live a relatively normal and relatively long life.

The finding of Howell-Jolly bodies or pits or vacuoles in red cells upon careful observation of the blood film may be an early indication of immunodeficiency.[65] Prophylactic penicillin and vaccines are helping to prevent infections and reduce deaths.

Training parents to palpate the abdomen to monitor spleen size allows early detection of acute splenic sequestration crises and prevention of death owing to hypovolemic shock.

Sickle Cell Trait

Definition and Demographics

Sickle cell trait is the heterozygous (AS) state of sickle cell disease. The nomenclature for Hb S in sickle cell trait is $\alpha_2\beta_1\beta_2^{6\ Glu\rightarrow Val}$. Because Hb A is present in higher percentages than Hb S, Hb A compensates for Hb S, and these patients usually have no symptoms. The disorder may go undetected, but patients may experience the painful crises described for Hb SS if they encounter situations that cause extreme tissue hypoxia such as those caused by severe respiratory infection or exposure to extreme cold.

Among American blacks, the incidence of sickle cell trait is approximately 8%.[53,69] In some African tribes, the incidence is much higher. It is found in the same geographic areas as sickle cell anemia.

Laboratory Findings

PERIPHERAL BLOOD. Anemia generally is not present. Red cell morphology usually is normal, with the possible exception of a few target cells and an occasional sickle cell.

SPECIAL HEMATOLOGIC TESTS. The sickle solubility test is positive. Results of hemoglobin electrophoresis for heterozygous patients are shown in Table 14-9. Cellulose acetate hemoglobin electrophoresis reveals the presence of approximately 30% to 45% Hb S, with normal amounts of Hb F. Hb A levels should always be higher than Hb S in sickle cell trait.

URINALYIS. On rare occasions, hematuria may be present. In occasional patients the kidneys may fail to concentrate urine, causing hyposthenuria.

Prognosis

Patients have a normal life span and quality of life. Treatment is rarely required.

Hb S–Thalassemia

Hb S–thalassemia is a doubly heterozygous condition in which the mutant genes for both Hb S and thalassemia are inherited by a single individual. Thalassemia (Chap. 15) is characterized by a quantitative reduction or total absence of a globin polypeptide chain, most often the α or β chain.

Hb S–thalassemia has several forms. Although Hb S–α thalassemia is fairly common, it is usually clinically insignificant. On the other hand, one form of Hb S–β thalassemia is associated with clinical features similar to, although not as severe as, those of sickle cell anemia. There are two types of β thalassemia, $\beta°$ and β^+. Homozygous $\beta°$ thalassemia and Hb S–$\beta°$ thalassemia both demonstrate no β chain production, and thus no Hb A. Clinically, these forms are more severe than Hb S–β^+ thalassemia and similar in severity to sickle cell anemia. β^+ thalassemia and Hb S–β^+ thalassemia both demonstrate a reduced β chain production and decreased Hb A. The Hb S–β^+ thalassemias are classified as type 1 (clinically severe and hematologically abnormal, although less so than Hb S–$\beta°$) and type 2 (causes only a mild anemia and patients are asymptomatic). Because of the decreased production of β chains, there is a concomitant decrease in production of Hb A, and hence the percentage of Hb S per red cell is greater than one would expect in heterozygous conditions.

Demographics

Hb S–β thalassemia is a common sickling disorder among American blacks (1 in 1667 births), second only to Hb SC disease.[53] It is also prevalent in people of Greek, Turkish, Indian, North African, and Romanian ancestry and is the most common sickle disease variant in Mediterranean populations.[83] Blacks most often have type 2 Hb S–β^+ thalassemia, whereas nonblacks most often have type 1. Hb S–$\beta°$ thalassemia may be seen in any of these groups.

Physical Findings

In Hb S–$\beta°$ thalassemia, many of the same findings and crises that occur in sickle cell anemia occur, although the disease is somewhat milder. The spleen characteristically remains large into adulthood, a characteristic that may differentiate this disorder from Hb SS disease. Table 14-10 lists the physical findings from the various forms of Hb S–β thalassemia and compares them to those of Hb SS and Hb AS.

Laboratory Findings

ROUTINE HEMATOLOGY.   In severe Hb S–$\beta°$ thalassemia the Hb ranges from 5 to 10 g/dL and the reticulocyte count, between 10% and 20%. Erythrocytes are microcytic and hypochromic with marked anisocytosis (reflected by a high RDW), and there are many target cells. Sickle cells are found on the peripheral blood film (Fig. 14-7). In Hb S–β^+ thalassemia type 1 the Hb ranges from 7 to 10 g/dL and sickle cells may be found. The reticulocyte count may be normal or slightly decreased. In Hb S–β^+ thalassemia type 2 there is little or no anemia and few red cell abnormalities. Decreases in mean corpuscular volume (MCV) and mean corpuscular hemoglobin (MCH) may be the only clues to an abnormality.

SPECIAL HEMATOLOGIC TESTS.   Results of the sickle solubility test are positive, and the amount of Hb A detected on electrophoresis is smaller than the amount of Hb S, owing to the failure of or decrease in β-chain production. Hb A$_2$ and F levels are characteristically elevated. Hb S–$\beta°$ thalassemia often shows no Hb A although it may be as high as 15%. Blood of patients with Hb S–β^+ type 1 usually has only up to 15% Hb A, whereas that of Hb S–β^+ type 2 patients has 20% to 30% Hb A. Table 14-10 shows the distinct differences and similarities among the sickle cell and sickle cell–thalassemia disorders.

Measurement of α and β globin chain synthesis in reticulocytes is a helpful diagnostic tool. Hb S–$\beta°$ and S–β^+ thalassemia have a β to α chain ratio of approximately 0.5:1, whereas sickle cell anemia and sickle trait have a ratio of 1:1, which is normal.[10]

TABLE 14–10. Differential Laboratory and Clinical Features of Hemoglobinopathies and Hb S-Thalassemias

	Hb SS	Hb S–$\beta°$ THALASSEMIA	Hb AS	Hb S–β^+ THALASSEMIA*	NORMAL ADULT
Anemia	+++	+++	−/+	+/+++	−
Anemia classification†	N/N	M/H	N/N	M/H	−
Hb S (%)‡	80–95	80–95	20–40	55–75	0
Hb A (%)‡	0	0	60–80	5–30	97
Hb F (%)‡	0.5–10	≤5–20§	<2	≤5–20§	<2
Hb A$_2$ (%)‡	2.0–3.5	>3.5	2.0–3.5	>3.5	2.0–3.5
Sickle solubility	+	+	+	+	−
Peripheral blood sickle cells	++	+	+/−	+/−	−
β/α chains	1/1	0.5/1	1/1	0.5/1	1/1
Splenomegaly	−	++	−/+	−/++	−
Painful crises	+++	+++	−/+	−/+++	−
Hematuria	+	+/−	rare	−/+	−
Hemolytic episodes	++	++	−/+	−/++	−

* Hb S–β^+ thalassemia actually comprises two groups, types 1 and 2 (see text).
† N/N, Normocytic, normochromic; M/H, Microcytic, hypochromic.
‡ Percentages are based on cellulose acetate electrophoresis (alkaline pH). The percentages given are general guidelines. In reality, the results associated with any given case may vary from these ranges.
§ Fetal hemoglobin levels of 20% are also seen with Hb S–hereditary persistence of fetal hemoglobin.

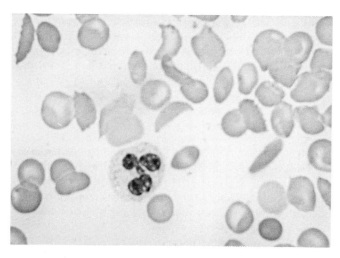

FIG. 14-7.   Peripheral blood film from patient with Hb S- and Hb S-thalassemia.

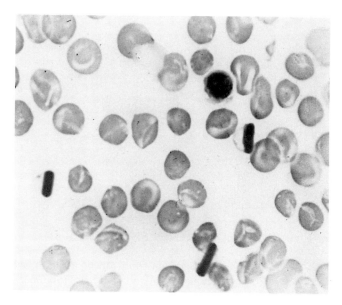

FIG. 14-8.   Peripheral blood film showing Hb C crystals and prominent target cells.

Effects of Treatment on Laboratory Results

Since treatment is mainly supportive, the hematologic laboratory findings generally do not change with treatment unless a transfusion of packed red cells is given, which would alter all erythrocyte values, including the indices. Transfusion also causes temporary dilutional effects and thus reduces the Hb S, Hb F, and Hb A_2 levels found on electrophoresis.

Prognosis

Patients with mild Hb S–β^+ type 2 live a normal life and require little medical attention. Because this condition is so variable, those with Hb S–β^+ type 1 and Hb S–β° may also live full lives with proper medical care. Other patients with Hb S–β thalassemia who have severe anemia and sickling crises require constant medical care. Bone marrow transplantation may constitute a therapeutic alternative.

Hb C Disease

The abnormal variant Hb C results from an amino acid substitution of lysine for glutamic acid at the sixth position of the β chain. This is technically written as $\beta^{6\ Glu\rightarrow Lys}$ Persons may be homozygous (Hb CC) or heterozygous (Hb AC) for this variant.

Hb CC tends to crystallize when dehydrated (hence the name crystal hemoglobin or Hb C). The cells most vulnerable to intracellular crystallization are older erythrocytes (approaching 120 days of age) because they tend to lose water as they age. Thus, older red cells containing Hb C are more rigid than normal cells. Fragmentation may occur in the microcirculation resulting in the production of microspherocytes. Hemoglobin C crystals are also produced in the microcirculation and are removed by the spleen. If the spleen is defective or nonfunctional, Hb C crystals are seen on the peripheral blood film (Fig. 14-8).

Demographics

Hemoglobin C is the second most common hemoglobin variant after Hb S. It is associated with the black race and is found mostly in Africa (see Fig. 14-1). Homozygous Hb

CC disease is estimated to affect 22 of every 100,000 American blacks.[53]

Clinical Findings

Persons with Hb CC disease commonly exhibit splenomegaly, which may cause abdominal pain. Hb CC, however, does not generally cause any other clinical abnormalities, and many patients have no symptoms even though they may have mild hemolytic anemia.

Laboratory Findings

PERIPHERAL BLOOD.   There is mild to moderate normocytic, normochromic anemia with numerous (40%–90%) target cells and a few spherocytes (see Fig. 14-8). Hexagonal or rod-shaped crystals may occasionally be observed on blood films, especially after splenectomy. These crystals are usually intracellular, elongated, and have parallel sides with both ends blunt. Hb CC crystals are significantly different from Hb SC crystals (see Figs. 8-31, 14-8, and 14-9). The Hb value ranges from 8 to 12 g/dL. The reticulocyte level is usually between 4% and 8%. Some patients do not experience anemia. The MCV and MCH are normal; MCHC is increased.

Red cell survival is decreased,[43] an effect attributed to early destruction by the spleen of red cells containing rigid Hb C crystals.

SPECIAL HEMATOLOGIC TESTS.   Hemoglobin electrophoresis results for Hb CC disease are shown in Table 14-9. Characteristically, most hemoglobin is Hb C; Hb F is increased in some instances and there is no Hb A. Hemoglobin C migrates with Hb A_2, E, and O-Arab on cellulose acetate (alkaline pH; see Fig. 14-4). It may be separated from all three by citrate agar (acid pH), because Hb C migrates farther toward the anode (positive pole) than the other variants in this medium (see Fig. 14-4). Column chromatography may also be used to separate and quantitate Hb C and Hb A_2 when both are present in one specimen.[40]

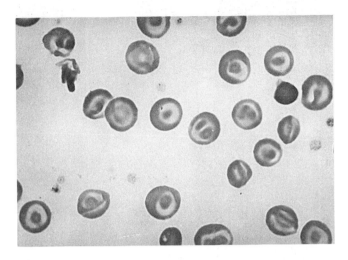

FIG. 14-9. Peripheral blood film from patient with Hb SC disease. Note SC crystal in upper left corner of field. Prominent target cells and characteristic "pocketbook" cells are also present.

Prognosis

Patients generally are asymptomatic and treatment is not required.

Hb C Trait (Hb AC)

Heterozygous Hb C (Hb AC) is found in about 3% of American blacks and is common in West Africans.[4] It produces no symptoms and no anemia. The red cells are slightly hypochromic, and approximately 40% are target cells. Results of hemoglobin electrophoresis are shown in Table 14-9 and Figure 14-4. The percentage of Hb A is higher than that of Hb C. The presence of microspherocytes along with a smaller percentage of Hb C suggests the possible presence of Hb C–α thalassemia.

Hb SC Disease

The incidence of Hb SC in American blacks is less than 1%, but it is one of the most common variants in Africa.[53] Persons who have Hb SC disease are said to be doubly heterozygous, because they inherited two hemoglobin variants. Hb SC disease differs from Hb SS disease in that clinical symptoms are milder (although similar) and complications are fewer.

Clinical Findings

Significant symptoms first occur during the teenage years, including anemia and joint, abdominal, and skeletal pain due to sickle cell vasoocclusion. Splenomegaly occurs in childhood and continues into adulthood, in contrast to the pattern in sickle cell anemia. In some cases, aseptic necrosis of the femoral heads can cause lameness. Diseases of the retina may result from blood viscosity that is higher than in sickle cell anemia. The concentration of sickle cells is higher in Hb SC than in sickle cell anemia since the hematocrit is higher in Hb SC than Hb SS disease. The resulting high blood viscosity can cause death.

Laboratory Findings

PERIPHERAL BLOOD. Anemia may or may not be present. When present, it is usually mild and classified as normocytic and normochromic. Target cells generally are present (see Fig. 14-9). In addition, folded, so-called pocketbook cells characteristic of Hb SC, an occasional spherocyte, and rare sickle cells may be found (see Fig. 14-9). Hb SC crystals, which have fingerlike projections ("Washington monument" projections) and usually protrude outside the cell membrane, can be found with careful searching (see Figs. 14-9 and 8-31).

SPECIAL HEMATOLOGIC TESTS. Results of the sickle solubility test are positive. Hemoglobin electrophoresis on cellulose acetate at alkaline pH reveals equal amounts of Hb S and Hb C (see Table 14-9). Hb F ranges from normal to 7%, and no Hb A is produced since no β chains are produced.[60]

Treatment and Prognosis

Therapy for Hb SC disease is similar to that for Hb S disease when crises occur. During childbirth, patients receive sodium bicarbonate to avoid acidosis. After childbirth, the mother may receive magnesium sulfate to prevent the formation of thrombi. Other patients may receive heparin for the same reason.[48]

The life span of the patient with Hb SC is normal. One of the most critical periods is pregnancy owing to the high blood viscosity and possibility of sickle crises. All patients are encouraged to have their retinas examined regularly for lesions, which can be detected early, before major damage or vision loss occurs.

Hb D

There are at least 16 β-chain variants and 6 α-chain variants classified as Hb D that migrate in the same position as Hb S but do not cause sickling.[82] Both homozygous (Hb DD) and heterozygous (Hb AD) conditions have been reported. Hb D may also be found in combination with Hb S or thalassemia. Many variants are named for the place where they were discovered, such as Hb D-Los Angeles (also known as Hb D-Punjab) in which glycine (Gln) is substituted for glutamic acid (Glu) in the 121st position of the β chain ($\alpha_2\beta_2^{121\ Glu\rightarrow Gln}$).

Demographics

Hemoglobin D-Punjab is found principally in Pakistan and northwest India (see Fig. 14-1). The frequency in India is estimated to be 3%.[48] Hb D-Los Angeles is probably the most common Hb D variant in the United States. It is found among black Americans and in Caucasians world wide. In general, Hb D is rare.

Clinical Findings

No clinical abnormalities are associated with the heterozygous state. Homozygous Hb D often is associated with splenomegaly, but patients are otherwise clinically normal.

Laboratory Findings

PERIPHERAL BLOOD. Homozygous Hb D disease usually is associated with mild hemolytic anemia and concomitant decreases in red cell parameters. Results of the sickle solubility test are negative. Indices are normal, but numerous flat target cells are seen on the blood film. The heterozygous state is not associated with hematologic abnormalities.

SPECIAL HEMATOLOGIC TESTS.   Cellulose acetate electrophoresis (alkaline pH) reveals 95% Hb D, which migrates in the same position as Hb S, and normal Hb A_2 and F in the homozygous state. There is less than 50% Hb D in the heterozygous state (the remainder being Hb A, A_2, and F; see Table 14-9). On citrate agar electrophoresis (acid pH), Hb D migrates toward the cathode in the same position as Hb A and A_2 while Hb S migrates toward the anode (see Fig. 14-4). Results of the solubility test are negative.

Hb SD

Hb SD is a doubly heterozygous condition. It has been reported for at least 9 of the 16 Hb D β-chain variants.[50] Only Hb SD-Los Angeles produces a clinical abnormality, a condition similar to mild sickle cell anemia.

Citrate agar electrophoresis is the definitive test for separation and verification of hemoglobins S and D. Results of the sickle solubility test are positive, but the citrate agar electrophoresis results separate Hb SS from SD (see Fig. 14-4).

Hb E

Hb E is a β-chain variant in which lysine is substituted for glutamic acid in the 26th position ($\alpha_2\beta_2^{26 \; Glu \rightarrow Lys}$). Both homozygous (Hb EE) and heterozygous (Hb AE) states exist.

Demographics

Hemoglobin E is the third most common hemoglobin variant in the world, affecting an estimated 30 million people.[26,28] It occurs with the greatest frequency in Southeast Asia (see Fig. 14-1), and has also been reported in American blacks.[48] Hb E frequently occurs in combination with β thalassemia causing a condition clinically similar to β thalassemia major.

Clinical Findings

Neither Hb EE nor Hb AE is associated with clinical abnormalities, except possibly splenomegaly associated with the homozygous state.

Laboratory Findings

PERIPHERAL BLOOD.   Laboratory findings for Hb E disorders are similar to those described for Hb D disorders. Hb EE disease causes mild microcytic, normochromic hemolytic anemia. Red cell survival time is slightly decreased. The hemoglobin is unstable. There are usually many target cells on the peripheral blood film.

Heterozygous Hb E may display an elevated red cell count and target cells. Red cell survival is normal, and patients are not anemic.

SPECIAL HEMATOLOGIC TESTS.   Hemoglobins E, C, O-Arab, and A_2 migrate closely on cellulose acetate (alkaline pH), although Hb E migrates slightly faster than C and A_2 (see Fig. 14-4). Typically, in homozygous persons, Hb E represents 92% to 98% of the hemoglobin and the amount of Hb F is normal or slightly increased (see Table 14-9). Hb E may be differentiated from Hb C and O-Arab on citrate agar electophoresis at acid pH as Hb E migrates with Hb A on this medium (see Fig. 14-4). Hemoglobins that migrate with Hb A_2 on cellulose acetate at alkaline pH must always be suspected when the Hb A_2 value estimated by densitometry is greater than 10%. Hb A_2 rarely exceeds 10% even when it is elevated in thalassemias.

In the heterozygous state (Hb AE), the concentration of Hb E is usually around 20% to 40%. This is high enough to indicate that there is a variant in the Hb A_2 position but lower than the 40% to 50% found more frequently in the heterozygous Hb C state (Hb AC). This may be related to the fact that because Hb E is unstable, a certain amount may be lost during specimen processing for electrophoresis.

Hb O-Arab

Hb O-Arab is a β-chain variant caused by the same type of substitution as in Hb C: glutamic acid is replaced by lysine—but the substitution point is the 121st amino acid instead of the sixth ($\alpha_2\beta_2^{121 \; Glu \rightarrow Lys}$).

Hb O-Arab is rare. It is found in Israel, Bulgaria, Egypt, Rumania, Jamaica, Kenya and in 0.4% of black Americans. Persons with Hb O-Arab are normal clinically, except for some homozygous persons who have splenomegaly. Heterozygotes are asymptomatic. If Hb O-Arab is inherited in conjunction with Hb S, a severe clinical condition results that is similar to that seen with Hb SS.

Laboratory Findings

Homozygotes demonstrate a mild hemolytic anemia with many target cells. Since Hb O-Arab migrates with Hbs A_2, C, and E on cellulose acetate, citrate agar electrophoresis is required for the differential diagnosis because only Hb O-Arab moves just slightly away from the point of application toward the cathode on this medium (see Fig. 14-4).

MULTIPLE AMINO ACID SUBSTITUTIONS

Hb C-Harlem

Hemoglobin C-Harlem (also known as Hb C-Georgetown) is a β-chain variant caused by two amino acid substitutions. One occurs at the sixth amino acid and is identical to the Hb S substitution. The other occurs at the 73rd position, where aspartic acid is replaced by asparagine ($\alpha_2\beta_2^{6 \; Glu \rightarrow Val; \; 73 \; Asp \rightarrow Asn}$). Hb C-Harlem, Hb C-Ziguinchor, and Hb S-Travis are among the few hemoglobins that cause a positive sickle solubility test owing to the same substitution as for Hb S (in addition to another in the β chain).

Hb C-Harlem is rare and occurs in both homozygous and heterozygous states. Double heterozygosity for Hbs S and C-Harlem is also possible.

Clinical Findings

The clinical picture for homozygotic persons is unclear, since few have been identified.[6] Heterozygotes are asymptomatic. Patients with Hb SC-Harlem have a clinical picture similar to that of Hb SC disease.

Laboratory Findings

Results of the sickle solubility test are positive in the presence of Hb C-Harlem in any genetic state. On cellulose acetate (alkaline pH), there is a band in the Hb C position. On citrate agar, Hb C-Harlem migrates with Hb S (see Fig. 14-4).

α-CHAIN SUBSTITUTIONS

Hb G-Philadelphia

Hb G-Philadelphia is the only α-chain variant of significance in the United States. It results from the replacement of asparagine by lysine in the 68th position of the α-chain ($\alpha_2^{68 \ \text{Asn} \rightarrow \text{Lys}} \beta_2$). It is found among West Africans and is the third most common variant among American blacks after Hbs S and C.[69]

The homozygous form of this disorder is not compatible with life, since the condition prevents production of normal α chains necessary for production of oxygen-carrying hemoglobin. Heterozygotes are asymptomatic.

Laboratory Findings

Hb G-Philadelphia migrates on cellulose acetate (ranging from 25% to 40%) in the Hb S position (see Fig. 14-4), but results of the sickle solubility test are negative. Citrate agar provides further evidence that the variant is not Hb S because Hb G-Philadelphia migrates with Hb A. Globin chain electrophoresis is important for confirmation, because at alkaline pH, the abnormal α chain moves farther toward the cathode than most other hemoglobins. In addition, these patients have both normal and abnormal forms of Hbs A_2 and F. The abnormal variants result from the abnormal α chains produced. Typically, the abnormal Hb A_2, known as Hb G_2, migrates as a minor, faint band toward the cathode (i.e., backward from the point of application, in the opposite direction from all other hemoglobins on cellulose acetate [alkaline pH]). It is identified by using a counterstaining procedure.

OTHER VARIANTS

Hb I

The Hb I variant is rare. It affects either the α or β chain at various positions; usually lysine is replaced by glutamic acid. Hb I migrates between Hb Barts and Hb H, all of which migrate farther toward the anode than Hb A on cellulose acetate (alkaline pH) (see Fig. 14-4). Hb I and Hb H are best differentiated on cellulose acetate electrophoresis at pH 7.0, where Hb H migrates but Hb I does not.[68,71] Hb I, when present, constitutes approximately 25% of the total hemoglobin.

Hb Barts and H

These two variants are found in patients with α thalassemia who are producing fewer α chains than normal. Hb Barts

occurs in the newborn infant and consists of four γ chains. Hb H occurs in older children (after the γ- to β-chain switch) and consists of four normal β chains. Both variants migrate farther toward the anode than Hb A on cellulose acetate (alkaline pH) (see Fig. 14-4).

AMINO ACID DELETION

Hb Gun Hill

Hb Gun Hill has a deletion of five β-chain amino acids (β 91 to 95). The hemoglobin structure is altered so that no heme can bind to the β chain at the normal point of contact between heme and globin. This is caused by unequal crossing over between the β-chain genes and production of two chains of unequal length.[10] The result is an unstable hemoglobin, which produces mild hemolytic anemia. On cellulose acetate (alkaline pH) Hb Gun Hill migrates close to the Hb A_2 position. On citrate agar, it migrates with Hb A or between Hb A and Hb S.

ELONGATION OF THE POLYPEPTIDE CHAIN

Hb Constant Spring

Hb Constant Spring (Hb CS) has an elongated α chain because 31 amino acids are added to the end of the chain. This is caused by replacement of a terminator codon, which normally stops amino acid addition, with a codon for glutamine, which results in the addition of 31 amino acids before another terminator codon is reached. Since the α chain is affected, the clinical picture resembles α thalassemia.[10] Often, Hb CS is inherited in a double heterozygous condition (Hb H Constant Spring) (Chap. 15).

Hb CS is prevalent among Greeks and Chinese. Homozygotes have mild microcytic, hemolytic anemia and 3% to 5% Hb CS. On cellulose acetate (alkaline pH), Hb CS migrates slower than Hb A_2. To rule out the possibility of a nonheme protein migrating in this position, the cellulose acetate should be counterstained with o-tolidine or o-dianisidine. Hb CS stains purple; nonheme protein remains pink. Hb CS heterozygotes have little or no anemia, red cells are microcytic, and target cells may be observed.[19]

UNSTABLE HEMOGLOBIN DISEASE

Unstable hemoglobin disease (congenital Heinz body hemolytic anemia) is very rare, although over 70 unstable variants have been identified. The pattern of inheritance is autosomal dominant. Only heterozygotes exist; apparently homozygous fetuses do not survive. In addition to being unstable, some variants have other functional abnormalities, including methemoglobinemia or decreased or increased oxygen affinity or some combination thereof. Table 14-11 provides examples of unstable hemoglobins. Molecular abnormalities that result in hemoglobin instability are frequently those that disrupt contact between heme and globin, alter amino acids involved in the interface between α and β chains, or significantly change the shape or structure of the globin molecule. Regardless of the abnormality, the result is denaturation and precipitation of globin chains. Precipitation of globin in erythrocytes leads to formation of Heinz bodies, which cling to the membrane and are removed as the cells pass through the spleen. This predisposes the cells to hemolysis.

Clinical Findings

Severity of disease depends on the variant. Clinical findings may be severe, moderate, mild, or nonexistent. Severe forms become apparent in infancy, and patients with moderate forms may have splenomegaly and episodes of jaundice and hemolysis. Most variants cause either a mild disorder or no symptoms. They are frequently detected after a sudden hemolytic crisis caused by an oxidative insult to the red cells by infection or drugs. Hb Köln, the most commonly reported unstable hemoglobin,[81] causes only a mild disorder.

Laboratory Findings

PERIPHERAL BLOOD. The Hb ranges from less than 7 g/dL in the most severe forms to normal in some mild forms. Reticulocytosis is common, although it may or may not be adequate to compensate for the degree of red cell destruction. Usually, the MCHC is decreased, sometimes as low as 25 g/dL. This may be so because (1) unstable hemoglobin is partially heme deficient; (2) some hemoglobin is lost when Heinz bodies are removed by the spleen; or (3) the hemoglobin in Heinz bodies is not measured by standard hemoglobinometry.[81]

The blood film reveals anisopoikilocytosis with some hypochromic cells, polychromatophilia, and basophilic stippling. Fragments and spherocytes may be seen in severe disease. Bite cells (keratocytes [Chap. 8]) formed by splenic removal of Heinz bodies may also be seen.

Heinz bodies—a classic finding in this disorder—consist of denatured globin seen in red cells after supravital staining (Fig. 14-10A). They are not visible on Wright-stained blood films because they have the same charge as normal hemoglobin. Usually, Heinz bodies appear during hemolytic episodes or after splenectomy. One report asserts that the Heinz bodies of unstable hemoglobin disease are larger and are found in younger cells than those associated with glucose-6-phosphate dehydrogenase (G6PD) deficiency.[67]

HEMOGLOBIN ELECTROPHORESIS. Routine hemoglobin electrophoresis may or may not identify unstable hemoglobins. Some migrate with Hb A, some slower, and some faster. Hb Köln migrates slower than Hb A. On average unstable hemoglobins that affect the β chain represent 25% of the total hemoglobin while those that affect the α chain represent only about 12%.[81] Hb A_2 and Hb F may be increased in association with β-chain variants.

SPECIAL HEMATOLOGIC TESTS. The chromium-51 half-life (Chap. 16) of erythrocytes that contain unstable hemoglobin correlates with the severity of disease (2 days in severe disease, 6 to 16 days in moderate disease, and 9 to 23 days in mild disease; normal half-life is approximately 28 days).[45] Increased oxygen affinity has been observed in at least 24 variants and decreased affinity in at least twelve.[81] Results of the heat denaturation test are positive for almost all unstable hemoglobins, as are those of the isopropanol precipitation test, although the latter test is plagued with false positive results. The only way to confirm unstable hemoglobin is by peptide analysis, which is performed in only a few research centers. This study is not necessary if the patient can be managed without knowing the exact identity of the unstable hemoglobin.

Treatment and Prognosis

For patients with mild unstable hemoglobin disorders, the aim of treatment is prevention of hemolytic crises. In some cases of moderately severe disease, splenectomy may be considered to reduce hemolysis. Splenectomy is not helpful in severe cases, apparently because the liver also phagocytizes the severely damaged red cells.[46,78] Prognosis still is unclear, since unstable variants are rare.

TABLE 14–11. Examples of Unstable Hemoglobin Variants and Their Other Functional Abnormalities*

VARIANT	UNSTABLE	INCREASED OXYGEN AFFINITY	DECREASED OXYGEN AFFINITY	METHEMO-GLOBINEMIA	DEGREE OF HEMOLYTIC DISEASE
Bristol	x		x		Severe
Casper/ Southhampton	x	x			Severe
Genova	x	x			Moderately severe
Torino	x		x		Moderately severe
Constant Spring	x				Mild
Gun Hill	x	x			Mild
Köln	x	x			Mild
M-Saskatoon	x	x		x	Mild
Seattle	x		x		Mild
Tacoma	x				No clinical abnormalities

* A complete list of the many hemoglobin variants and their functional abnormalities is available in Reference 80.
(From Wintrobe MM: The abnormal hemoglobins: General principles. In Wintrobe MM et al: Clinical Hematology, 8th ed, p 806. Philadelphia, Lea & Febiger, 1981.)

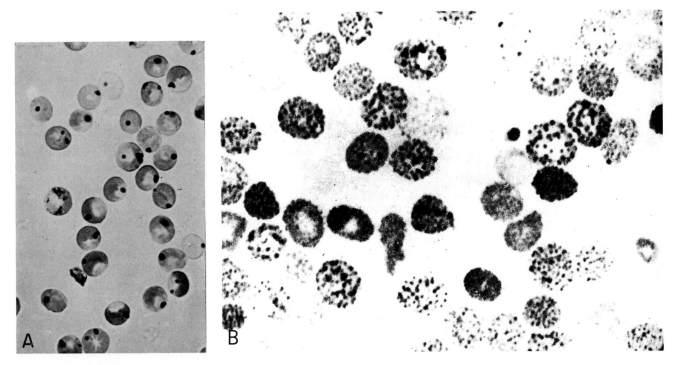

FIG. 14-10.   (**A**) Heinz bodies associated with unstable hemoglobin disease (crystal violet stain). (Reprinted by permission from Beutler E et al: Estimation of small percentages of hemoglobin. Nature 184:1877, copyright 1959 MacMillan Journals Limited.) (**B**) Hb H inclusion bodies from a patient with Hb H disease precipitated and stained with brilliant cresyl blue. (Reprinted by permission from Dittman WA et al: Hemoglobin H associated with an uncommon variant of thalassemia trait. Blood 15:975, 1960.)

MOST USEFUL LABORATORY TESTS FOR DIAGNOSING UNSTABLE HEMOGLOBINS

Many unstable hemoglobins are not detected by electrophoresis.[22] Tests specifically designed to detect unstable hemoglobins include the isopropanol precipitation test, the heat denaturation test, and the Heinz body staining technique.

ISOPROPANOL PRECIPITATION TEST[11]
Principle

Nonpolar solvents in a hemoglobin solution cause the internal bonding forces of the hemoglobin molecule to weaken and the molecule's stability to decrease. Thus, in a 17% isopropanol solution incubated at 37°C, stability of normal hemoglobin is borderline and it begins to precipitate after approximately 40 minutes. The presence of an unstable hemoglobin results in rapid precipitation, usually apparent within 5 minutes, and heavier flocculation after around 20 minutes' incubation.

Specimen

Use fresh anticoagulated whole blood (any anticoagulant is acceptable). Blood may be stored refrigerated up to 72 hours. Prepare hemolysate just prior to performing the test. Do not store hemolysate.

Special Reagents

Isopropanol-Tris Buffer

Add 12.11 g Tris (hydroxymethyl) aminomethane to 1-L volumetric flask; add 700 mL distilled water; add 170 mL 100% isopropyl alcohol, and mix. Adjust *p*H to 7.4 using concentrated hydrochloric acid. Add distilled water to make 1 L. This mixture is stable (tightly stoppered) in refrigerator for several weeks.

Quality Control

Run a normal blood sample as a negative control with the patient sample.

Hemolysate Preparation

Prepare hemolysate by water and organic solvent method described earlier in this chapter.

Procedure

1. Label two 10 × 75-mm tubes: one *Control,* one *Patient*.
2. Add 2 mL isopropanol-tris buffer to each tube and stopper. Place in 37°C water bath for 10 minutes.
3. Add 0.2 mL control hemolysate and 0.2 mL patient hemolysate to respective tubes.
4. Stopper tubes; invert gently a few times to mix; and place back in incubation.
5. Check tubes after 5, 20, and 45 minutes for precipitation or flocculation by gently tilting the tube horizontally and observing against a light source.

Interpretation of Results

Negative control should be clear at 5 and 20 minutes. Precipitation should appear at 45 minutes, otherwise buffer may be deteriorated. If patient sample shows precipitation within 5 to 20 minutes, unstable hemoglobin is indicated; report such results as positive.

Comments and Sources of Error[8]

If negative control does not precipitate at 45 minutes, prepare fresh buffer and repeat test.

When checking tubes, do not mix specimens. Precipitation can be broken up easily.

Incubation temperature must be maintained at 37°C.

Concentration of isopropanol (17%) in buffer is critical.

The pH of buffer solution is not critical but should be at least 7.2.

Addition of potassium cyanide to test system to oxidize all hemoglobin to methemoglobin has been recommended to reduce the possibility of a false positive result.[8]

Hb F levels greater than 4% may cause a false positive result.[8]

HEAT DENATURATION TEST[36,49,54]

Principle

Washed red cells are hemolyzed with water, a phosphate buffer is added, and the mixture is allowed to incubate at 50°C for 3 hours. Many unstable hemoglobins are heat sensitive and their partial denaturation causes the appearance of a flocculent precipitate within 1 hour of incubation, whereas normal blood shows little, if any, precipitate.

Specimen

Use fresh whole blood anticoagulated with EDTA or heparin. The normal control blood sample should be collected at the same time as the patient's blood.

Reagent

Phosphate Buffer, pH 7.4:

0.1 mol/L NaH_2PO_4 (13.8 g $NaH_2 PO_4 \cdot 2H_2O$ in 1 L distilled water); 0.1 mol/L Na_2HPO_4 (anhydrous) (14.2 g in 1 L distilled water). Add 19.2 mL 0.1 mol/L NaH_2PO_4 to 80.8 mL 0.1 mol/L Na_2HPO_4. Mix and let stand 10 minutes. Adjust pH if necessary.[1]

Quality Control

A normal blood sample serves as a negative control.

Procedure

1. Add 1 mL patient blood and 1 mL control blood to separate 16 × 100-mm tubes.
2. Wash cells four times with 0.85% saline. Discard each supernatant wash. Add 5 mL distilled water to each tube and mix to lyse erythrocytes.
3. Add 5.0 mL phosphate buffer and mix. Centrifuge tubes at 3000 rpm for 10 minutes.
4. Transfer upper 2 mL clear supernatant from each tube to clean, labeled tube. Incubate at 50°C for 60 minutes.
5. Record appearance of test and control solutions at 60 minutes.
6. Incubate for an additional 120 minutes and observe again.

Interpretation of Results

Normal control should show little if any precipitation. Positive results are indicated by copious flocculent precipitate after 60 minutes and even greater precipitation after 3 hours.

Comments and Sources of Error

If only a small amount of abnormal hemoglobin is present, or if it is relatively insensitive to heat, results may be negative.

Quantitative results may be obtained through calculation of the percent of unstable hemoglobin present in a sample based on the difference in absorbance of an unheated sample and a heated sample, divided by the absorbance of the unheated sample.[9,21]

HEINZ BODY STAINING TECHNIQUE[12,13,20,27,62]

Principle

Heinz bodies (see Fig. 14-10A) result from denaturation and precipitation of unstable hemoglobin. Denatured hemoglobin precipitates in erythrocytes, forming small inclusion bodies that adhere to the membrane. These inclusions are visible in vitro after supravital staining but not on Wright-stained films. Formation of Heinz bodies may be induced in normal red cells by treating them with highly oxidative substances, such as acetylphenylhydrazine, and incubating them for a long period.

Specimen Requirements

Whole blood anticoagulated with EDTA or heparin.

Reagents

Saline, normal, 0.85%

Sodium citrate ($Na_3C_6H_5O_7 \cdot 2H_2O$), 3 g/dL: Add 3.0 g sodium citrate to distilled water up to 100 mL.

Brilliant cresyl blue stain, 1 g/dL: Mix 0.5 g brilliant cresyl blue (water soluble) in 40.0 mL normal saline and add 10.0 mL 3 g/dL sodium citrate solution.

Quality Control

A negative control test should be run using a normal blood specimen drawn at the same time as the patient's specimen. A positive control test may be run if a specimen is available.

Procedure

1. Mark three 13 × 100-mm tubes: Patient, Negative control, Positive control.
2. Mix stain thoroughly before using and filter a small amount through Whatman No. 42 or 44 filter paper just prior to using it.
3. Mix whole blood and add 2 drops blood to 3 drops filtered stain in marked tubes and mix. Incubate at 37°C.
4. Make smears after 20 minutes, 1 hour, and 2 hours.
5. Cover tubes and let stand overnight at room temperature. Make smears at 24 hours.
6. Examine films from each time interval with oil immersion microscopy.

Interpretation of Results

Heinz bodies, which may be single or multiple in any given cell, appear refractile (see Fig. 14-10A). They may be round, oval, or serrated, and they stain pale blue with brilliant cresyl blue or deep purple with crystal violet. They vary from 1 to 4 μm and usually appear eccentrically, either near or attached to the cell periphery.

Normal, nonoxidized red cells should show no Heinz body formation, or at most, only rare Heinz bodies. Red cell populations that contain unstable hemoglobin from splenectomized persons contain significant numbers of Heinz bodies that become visible early in the incubation process. Red cells from patients who still have their spleen may have to be induced to form Heinz bodies by treating them with highly oxidative substances and long incubation.

Comments and Sources of Error

Heinz bodies may not circulate in patients with unstable hemoglobin unless the patient has been splenectomized.

Heinz bodies are not specific indicators of unstable hemoglobin; red cell enzyme deficiencies (e.g., G6PD) may also cause Heinz body formation if red cells are exposed to oxidant drugs.

TABLE 14–12. General Distinguishing Features of the Hb H and Heinz Body Inclusions Stained Supravitally with Brilliant Cresyl Blue*

FEATURE	HEINZ BODIES	Hb H INCLUSIONS
Staining characteristics	Pale blue	Greenish blue
Number per cell	1 or more	Multiple
Cell location	Eccentric	Cover the cell
Associated disorders	Unstable Hb	Hb H
	G6PD deficiency	

* In some cases, the two may be indistinguishable since this is only a screening test. Refer to Figures 14–10A and B for photomicrographic comparison of the two inclusions and to Figure 8-28 for comparison of these inclusions to stained reticulocytes.

Heinz bodies and Hb H inclusions (see Fig. 14-10B) are both stained with brilliant cresyl blue. Table 14-12 provides some clues to differentiating the two, although it is not always possible.

The isopropanol precipitation test or heat denaturation test should be run to confirm the results of a Heinz body screening test.

THE HEMOGLOBINS M

Five hemoglobin variants are designated as Hb M because they are associated with the presence of methemoglobin and congenital cyanosis. They include Hb M-Boston, Hb M-Iwate, Hb M-Saskatoon, Hb M-Hyde Park, and Hb M-Milwaukee. Either the α or β chain may be affected. Amino acid substitutions within the Hb M molecule prevent protection of iron from oxidation. Hence, Hb M contains iron in the ferric (Fe^{+++}) state (methemoglobin) and is incapable of carrying oxygen.

The pattern of inheritance is autosomal dominant. Hb M is found worldwide but is particularly prevalent in the Japanese. The homozygous state is not compatible with life. Heterozygotes, however, live a relatively normal life.

Clinical Findings

Patients have a lavendar blue (cyanotic) skin color that can be differentiated from the blue-gray color of cyanotic heart disease. In some cases, the fingers are clubbed at birth. Cyanosis is usually observed during the first day of life of babies with the α-chain variant, whereas infants with β-chain Hb M do not demonstrate cyanosis until after the second or third month of life (after the γ- to β-chain switch).

Laboratory Findings

The blood is characteristically brown. Some Hb M β-chain variants cause mild hemolytic anemia.[64] In addition, methemoglobin causes globin chain precipitation, so Heinz bodies may be seen in vitro. Hb M migrates slightly cathodal (i.e., slightly slower) to Hb A on cellulose acetate. Hb M accounts for 20% to 35% of the total hemoglobin in heterozygotes.[48] A pH of 7.1 is recommended for electrophoresis.[48] It is also recommended that all hemoglobin in the specimen be oxidized to methemoglobin by adding potassium cyanide before performing electrophoresis. Do-

ing so ensures that any migration differences observed are due to an amino acid substitution in the globin chains rather than to differences in the iron states.[48]

Spectrophotometric analysis of specimens is recommended for identification and quantitative analysis of Hb M.[48,84] Determining the absorption spectrum peaks of diluted hemolysates at various wavelengths and comparing them with the spectrum of normal blood allows for identification of Hb M variants.[24,25] Each variant has a unique absorption range.[48] Ultimately, Hb M must be confirmed by amino acid–chain studies, which usually are performed by reference laboratories.

Treatment and Prognosis

Treatment generally is not necessary. The condition must be diagnosed properly so that inappropriate treatment is avoided. For example, the presumptive diagnosis may be cyanotic heart disease (because of skin color) until laboratory tests reveal another condition.

HEMOGLOBINS WITH INCREASED OXYGEN AFFINITY

Certain alterations in the hemoglobin molecule result in decreased delivery of oxygen to the tissues (i.e., increased affinity between hemoglobin and oxygen). Many of these variants cause secondary erythrocytosis. Inheritance appears to be autosomal dominant and most patients are heterozygotes.

The first hemoglobin variant with increased affinity for oxygen was described in 1966[18] and named Hb Chesapeake. Presently, at least 60 such variants have been identified,[80] although all do not cause erythrocytosis. Hb Chesapeake is an α-chain variant in which arginine is replaced by leucine in the 92nd position.

Laboratory Findings

The Hb value usually ranges from normal to 20g/dL.[10] The leukocyte and platelet counts are usually normal. Some of these variants can be identified on either cellulose acetate or citrate agar electrophoresis, but a few cannot. The level of 2,3-DPG (diphosphoglycerate) should also be measured to rule out the possibility of abnormal oxygen affinity secondary to 2,3-DPG deficiency, which itself causes increased oxygen affinity when hemoglobin is normal. The steps required for identification of abnormal oxygen affinity hemoglobins are outlined elsewhere.[16]

The P_{50} is usually decreased in these patients (i.e., it takes less oxygen pressure than normal for hemoglobin to be half saturated with oxygen). This shifts the oxyhemoglobin dissociation curve to the left (Chap. 7).

Treatment and Prognosis

Most patients with high oxygen affinity hemoglobins live a normal life and require no treatment. Patient and family must be educated about the disorder to avoid unnecessary treatment of the erythrocytosis as a misdiagnosed myeloproliferative disorder or secondary erythrocytosis.

HEMOGLOBINS WITH DECREASED OXYGEN AFFINITY

Twenty-one hemoglobin variants have been identified that have decreased affinity for oxygen.[80] In some patients, the hemoglobin oxygen affinity is so low as to cause cyanosis. In others, decreased oxygen affinity causes increased release of oxygen to the tissues and resultant decreases in the number of red cells, and the patient appears anemic. The best known variant in this group is Hb Kansas, which is caused by a single amino acid substitution in the 102nd position of the β chain, where asparagine is replaced by threonine. The oxyhemoglobin dissociation curve is shifted significantly to the right and the P_{50} is greatly increased.

These variants may be stable or unstable. Stable variants usually cause cyanosis. Unstable variants frequently cause a mild hemolytic anemia. Cyanosis and normal arterial oxygen tension together are indicative of the presence of hemoglobin with decreased oxygen affinity. Most of these unusual hemoglobins may be detected by starch gel electrophoresis.[84]

CHAPTER SUMMARY

Hemoglobinopathies involve structured abnormalities in the α, β, δ, or γ chains, which may or may not cause clinical disorders. The abnormalities range from amino acid substitutions and deletions to chain elongation or fusion of two different chains.

Sickle cell anemia, caused by inheritance of two genes coding for Hb S, is the best known hemoglobinopathy. Hb S is an aggregating hemoglobin caused by an amino acid substitution in the β globin chain. Hb S has reduced solubility and is capable of polymerizing intracellularly, causing sickle cell formation. Sickle cell anemia is characterized in the laboratory by moderate to severe, normocytic, normochromic anemia, sickle cells on the blood film, a band migrating in the Hb S position on cellulose acetate, and a positive solubility test. It causes severe clinical abnormalities.

There are hundreds of variant hemoglobins, and a number of laboratory tests are necessary to identify them (see Table 14-6). Tests include cellulose acetate (alkaline pH), citrate agar (acid pH), and globin chain electrophoresis (alkaline and acid pH). The sickle solubility test is required to confirm any hemoglobin band migrating in the Hb S position on cellulose acetate. Special techniques for Hb A_2 and Hb F quantitation also may be useful in detecting patients who are doubly heterozygous and have both a hemoglobinopathy and thalassemia.

Unstable hemoglobins such as Hb Köln may also cause significant clinical abnormalities. Using the procedures described above as well as the Heinz body stain, isopropanol precipitation test, and heat denaturation test, the clinical laboratory may assist in confirming the presence of unstable hemoglobins.

Hemoglobin variants with an abnormal affinity for oxygen (increased or decreased) are identified by routine methods but may also require oxygen affinity studies, including quantitation of P_{50}.

CASE STUDY 14-1

A 12-year-old black boy was admitted to the hospital for the first time with fever, cough, and pain in the upper chest area. These symptoms had been present for 1 week. For years he had been troubled with recurring chronic ulcers in the lower tibial region (near the ankle). A 10-year-old brother had a similar illness, which was characterized by recurring attacks of fever and chronic ulceration of the legs. One sister had died 10 days earlier of unknown causes. The patient's father, mother, and four additional siblings were alive and well.

A blood count revealed the following data: WBC 22.0×10^9/L; RBC 1.4×10^{12}/L; Hb 4.0 g/dL. The differential cell count revealed 80% neutrophils, 17% lymphocytes, and 3% monocytes. On examination of erythrocyte morphology, a significant number of elongated red cells and many target cells were found, and the cells appeared normocytic and normochromic.

1. Based on the available data, what is the most probable diagnosis?
2. What screening test could be performed initially to support the diagnosis?
3. If the screening test is positive, what test should be performed next? What result is expected to confirm the diagnosis? Describe the appearance of the results.
4. What is the most likely cause of the elevated leukocyte count in patients with this diagnosis?

CASE STUDY 14-2

A 22-year-old black woman had developed a productive cough (a cough that brought forth sputum or mucus) 3 days prior to being admitted. The cough brought up yellow sputum that was not associated with chest pain, fever, or chills. On admission, the patient complained of pain in the shoulders, arms, and lower back.

Hematologic data included the following: WBC 9.0×10^9/L; RBC 3.78×10^{12}/L; Hb 11.0 g/dL; HCT 0.33 L/L; MCV 87 fL; MCH 29.1 pg; MCHC 33.6 g/dL. The differential cell count revealed: 79% neutrophils, 12% lymphocytes, 4% monocytes, 4% eosinophils, and 1% basophils. Platelet number appeared normal, and there was slight polychromasia. Abnormal erythrocyte morphology included an occasional unusual-looking, pointed crystal, pocketbook cells, target cells, and slight spherocytes.

Cellulose acetate electrophoresis indicated a moderately heavy band that migrated close to or in the Hb A_2 position and another moderately heavy band in the Hb S position when compared to the control.

1. What laboratory procedure would be recommended first in this situation to begin the diagnostic workup?
2. From the results obtained on cellulose acetate electrophoresis, name all the hemoglobins that possibly could be present.
3. What test should be used to confirm the diagnosis? How could the hemoglobins identified in question 2 be distinguished by the results of such a test?

CASE STUDY 14-3

A 21-year-old black man was seen for pain and stiffness in the right knee of 13 weeks' duration. He stated that at 2 years of age he had been found to have sickle cell anemia when he was hospitalized for swelling of his ankles and wrists. He was successfully treated with analgesics and blood transfusions. Since then, he had continued to have similar problems of varying severity.

Arthralgia (joint pain) was his main complaint for many years, but he had also suffered from back and chest pain and severe headaches. He had never experienced abdominal pain. Exertion, minor infection, and exposure to cold seemed to precipitate these symptoms. Other symptoms included shortness of breath and difficulty climbing stairs.

Family history revealed that four of seven siblings were dead. One was known definitely to have died from anemia; another was said to have "a touch of" sickle cell anemia. His mother was in good health, but nothing was known of his father.

A blood count revealed the following data: WBC 5.2×10^9/L; Hb 7.0 g/dL; HCT 0.22 L/L; MCV 84 fL; MCH 25 pg; MCHC 30 g/dL; platelets 440×10^9/L. Reticulocytes were 5.8%. Erythrocyte morphology review showed a rare sickle cell, moderate target cells, and moderate anisocytosis. Three nucleated red cells per 100 leukocytes were present, and the results of the differential cell count were normal.

Cellulose acetate electrophoresis revealed 21% Hb A and 70% Hb S along with Hb F and Hb A_2. Hb F quantitated by alkali denaturation was 4.9% and Hb A_2 quantitated by microchromatography was 4.1%.

1. Are hemoglobin abnormalities indicated by electrophoresis, alkali denaturation, or microchromatography results? Explain.
2. Which of the following hemoglobinopathies exhibit an increase in Hb F or A_2 values: sickle cell trait, sickle cell disease, sickle C (Hb SC) disease, Hb C disease, or Hb S–thalassemia?
3. Based on the rationale for your answer to question 2, what is the most likely diagnosis in this case?
4. Is the MCV generally consistent with the diagnosis given in answer to question 3?
5. If no Hb A had been found on cellulose acetate electrophoresis of this patient's specimen but Hb S, F, and A_2 were increased as in this patient's case, what would the most likely diagnosis be? Why?

REFERENCES

1. Aluoch JR: The treatment of sickle cell disease. A historical and chronological literature review of the therapies applied since 1910. Trop Geogr Med 36:Sl, 1984
2. Arends T, Bemski G, Nagel RL: Genetical, Functional and Physical Studies in Hemoglobins, pp 2, 8, 46, 175. Paris, S Karger, 1971
3. Betke K, Marti HR, Schlicht I: Estimation of small percentages of foetal haemoglobin. Nature 184:1877, 1959
4. Boggs DR: The frequency of heterozygosity for S and C hemoglobins in western Pennsylvania. Blood 44:699, 1974
5. Bookchin RM, Nagel RL, Ranney HM et al: Hemoglobin C Harlem: A sickling variant containing amino acid substitutions in two residues of the β-polypeptide chain. Biochem Biophys Res Commun 23:122, 1966
6. Bookchin RM, Davis RP, Ranney HM: Clinical features of hemoglobin C Harlem, a new sickling hemoglobin variant. Ann Intern Med 68:8, 1968
7. Briere RO, Galias T, Balsakis JG: Rapid qualitative and quantitative hemoglobin fractionation. Cellulose acetate electrophoresis. Am J Clin Pathol 44:695, 1965
8. Brosious EM, Morrison BY, Schmidt RM: Effects of hemoglobin F levels, KCN, and storage on the isopropanol precipitation test for unstable hemoglobins. Am J Clin Pathol 66:878, 1976
9. Brown BA: Hematology: Principles and Procedures, 4th ed, pp 148–152, 259. Philadelphia, Lea & Febiger, 1984
10. Bunn HF, Forget BG, Ranney HM: Human Hemoglobins, pp 31, 152–154, 166, 167, 178, 221, 225, 226, 268, 277, 279, 290. Philadelphia, WB Saunders, 1977
11. Carrell RW, Kay R: A simple method for the detection of unstable haemoglobins. Br J Haematol 23:615, 1972
12. Cartwright GE: Diagnostic Laboratory Hematology. New York, Grune & Stratton, 1963
13. Centers for Disease Control: Laboratory Methods for Detecting Hemoglobinopathies, p 129. Atlanta, Centers for Disease Control, 1984
14. Charache S, Lubin B, Reid CD (eds): Management and therapy of sickle cell disease, NIH Publication No. 85-2117. Bethesda, MD, National Institutes of Health, 1985
15. Charache S, Dreyer R, Zimmerman I et al: Evaluation of extracorporeal alkylation of red cells as a potential treatment for sickle cell anemia. Blood 47:481, 1976
16. Charache S: Haemoglobins with altered oxygen affinity. Clin Haematol 3:357, 1974
17. Charache S, Page DL: Infarction of bone marrow in the sickle cell disorders. Ann Intern Med 67:1195, 1967
18. Charache S, Weatherall DJ, Clegg JB: Polycythemia associated with a hemoglobinopathy. J Clin Invest 45:813, 1966
19. Dacie J: The Hemolytic Anemias, vol 1, pp 1–3. London, Churchill Livingstone, 1985
20. Dacie JV, Lewis SM: Practical Haematology, 6th ed. New York, Churchill Livingstone, 1984
21. Dacie JV, Lewis SM: Practical Haematology, 5th ed. New York, Churchill Livingstone, 1975
22. Dacie JV, Grimes AJ, Meisler A et al: Hereditary Heinz body anaemia. A report of studies on 5 patients with mild anaemia. Br J Haematol 10:388, 1964
23. Daniel SJ, Morris RC, Liu PI: Transfusion therapy in sickle cell disease. Ala Med 55:18, 1986
24. Drabkin DL: Spectroscopy, photometry and spectrophotometry, p 1039. In Glasser O (ed): Medical Physics, vol 2. Chicago, Year Book Medical Publishers, 1950
25. Dubowski KM: Measurement of hemoglobin derivatives. In Sunderman FW, Sunderman FW Jr (eds): Hemoglobin. Its Precursors and Metabolites, p 49. Philadelphia, JB Lippincott, 1964
26. Fairbanks VF, Gilchrist GS, Brimhall B et al: Hemoglobin E trait reexamined: A cause of microcytosis and erythrocytosis. Blood 53:109, 1979
27. Fertman MH, Fertman MB: Toxic anemia and Heinz bodies. Medicine 34:131, 1955
28. Flatz G: Hemoglobin E: Distribution and population dynamics. Humangenetik 3:189, 1967
29. Freedman ML, Karpatkin S: Elevated platelet count and megathrombocyte number in sickle cell anemia. Blood 46:579, 1975
30. Friedman MJ: Erythrocytic mechanism of sickle cell resistance to malaria. Proc Natl Acad Sci USA 75:1994, 1978
31. Gavrilis P, Rothenberg SP, Guy R: Correlation of low serum IgM levels with absence of functional splenic tissue in sickle cell disease syndromes. Am J Med 57:542, 1974
32. Goossens M, Garel MC, Auvinet J et al: Hemoglobin C-Ziguinchor α A2 β 62 (A3) glu•val β 58(E2) pro•arg: The second sickling variant with amino acid substitutions in 2 residues of the β polypeptide chain. FEBS Lett 58:149, 1975
33. Greenberg MS, Harvey HA, Morgan C: A simple and inexpensive screening test for sickle hemoglobin. N Engl J Med 286(21):1143, 1972
34. Helena Laboratories, Beaumont, TX. Hemoglobin Electrophoresis Procedure Using Cellulose Acetate Plate in Alkaline Buffer, 1985
35. Helena Laboratories, Beaumont, TX. Titan IV Citrate Hemoglobin Electrophoresis Procedure, 1983
36. Huehns ER: Disease due to abnormalities of hemoglobin structure. Ann Rev Med 21:157, 1970
37. Huehns ER, Shooter EM: Human haemoglobins. J Med Genet 22:48, 1965
38. Huisman THJ, Jonxis JHP: The Hemoglobinopathies: Techniques of Identification, p 201. New York, Marcel Dekker, 1977
39. Huisman THJ, Jonxis JHP: The hemoglobinopathies: Techniques of identification. Clin Biochem Anal 6:1, 1977
40. Huisman THJ: Chromatographic separation of hemoglobins A_2 and C. Clin Chim Acta 40:159, 1972
41. International Committee for Standardization in Haematology: Recommendations for fetal haemoglobin reference preparations and fetal haemoglobin determination by the alkali denaturation method. Br J Haematol 42:133, 1979
42. Itano HA: Solubilities of naturally occurring mixtures of human hemoglobin. Arch Biochem Biophys 47:148, 1953
43. Jensen WN, Schoefield RA, Agner R: Clinical and necropsy findings in hemoglobin C disease. Blood 12:74, 1957
44. Johnson FL: Bone marrow transplantation in the treatment of sickle cell anemia. Am J Pediatr Hematol Oncol 7:254, 1985
45. Jones RT, Koler RD, Duerst M et al: Hemoglobin Casper

G8β[106Leu•Pro]: Further evidence that hemoglobin mutations are not random. In Brewer GJ (ed): Hemoglobin and Red Cell Structure and Function, vol 28, p 79. New York, Plenum Press, 1972

46. Koler RD, Jones RT, Bigley RH et al: Hemoglobin Casper β[106(G8)Leu•Pro], a contemporary mutation. Am J Med 55:549, 1973

47. Langer EE, Stamatoyannopoulos G, Hlastala MP et al: Extracorporeal treatment with cyanate in sickle cell disease: Preliminary observations in four patients. J Lab Clin Med 87:462, 1976

48. Lehmann H, Huntsman RG: Man's Haemoglobins, 2nd ed, pp 164–172, 178–181, 269, 304–306, 310, 311, 404, 413–416. Philadelphia, JB Lippincott, 1974

49. Lehmann H, Huntsman RG: Man's Haemoglobins, p 293. Philadelphia, JB Lippincott, 1966

50. McCurdy PR: Hemoglobin S-G (S-D) syndrome. Am J Med 57:665, 1974

51. Milner PF, Gooden HM, General RT: Rapid citrate agar electrophoresis in routine screening for hemoglobinopathies using a simple hemolysate. Am J Clin Pathol 64:58, 1975

52. Moo-Penn WF, Schmidt RM, Jue DL et al: Hemoglobin S Travis: A sickling hemoglobin with two amino acid substitutions (β6[A3] glutamic acid•valine and β 142 [H20] alanine•valine). Eur J Biochem 77:561, 1977

53. Motulsky AG: Frequency of sickling disorders in US blacks. N Engl J Med 288:31, 1973

54. Motulsky AG, Stamatoyannopoulos G: Drugs, anesthesia, and abnormal hemoglobins. Ann NY Acad Sci 151:807, 1968

55. Nalbandian RM, Nichols BM, Camp FR et al: Dithionite tube test—A rapid, inexpensive technique for the detection of hemoglobin S and non-S sickling hemoglobin. Clin Chem 17:1028, 1971

56. National Committee for Clinical Laboratory Standards: Citrate agar electrophoresis for confirming the identification of variant hemoglobins: Tentative Guideline. NCCLS Publication H23-T. Villanova, PA, NCCLS, 1988

57. National Committee for Clinical Laboratory Standards: Detection of abnormal hemoglobin using cellulose acetate electrophoresis: Approved Standard. NCCLS Publication H-8A. Villanova, PA, NCCLS, 1986

58. National Committee for Clinical Laboratory Standards: Solubility test for confirming the presence of sickling hemoglobins: Approved Standard. NCCLS Publication H10-A. Villanova, PA, NCCLS, 1986

59. National Committee For Clinical Laboratory Standards: Quantitative measurement of fetal hemoglobin using the alkali denaturation method: Tentative Guideline. NCCLS Publication H13-T. Villanova, PA, NCCLS, 1988

60. Nelson DA, Davey FR: Erythrocytic disorders. In Henry JB (ed): Clinical Diagnosis and Management by Laboratory Methods, 17th ed, p 679, 685. Philadelphia, WB Saunders, 1984

61. Palek J, Liu A, Liu D et al: Effect of procaine HCl on ATP: Calcium-dependent alterations in red cell shape and deformability. Blood 50:155, 1977

62. Papayannopoulou T, Stamatoyannopoulos G: Stains for inclusion bodies. In Schmidt R et al (eds): The Detection of Hemoglobinopathies. Cleveland, CRC Press, 1974

63. Prasad AS, Ortega J, Brewer GJ et al: Trace elements in sickle cell disease. JAMA 235:2396, 1976

64. Pulsinelli PD, Perutz MF, Nagel RL: Structure of hemoglobin M-Boston, a variant with a five-coordinated ferric heme. Proc Natl Acad Sci USA 70:3870, 1973

65. Rodgers DW, Serjeant BE, Serjeant GR: Early rise in pitted red cell count as a guide to susceptibility to infection in childhood sickle cell anemia. Arch Dis Child 57:338, 1982

66. Roth EF Jr, Wenz B, Lee HB et al: Pathophysiological aspects of sickle cell vaso-occlusion. Prog Clin Biol Res 240:245, 1987

67. Schmid R, Brecher G, Clemens T: Familial hemolytic anemia with erythrocyte inclusion bodies and a defect in pigment metabolism. Blood 14:991, 1959

68. Schmidt RM, Brosious EM: Basic laboratory methods of hemoglobinopathy detection. DHEW Publication No. (CDC) 76-8266. Atlanta, Centers for Disease Control, 1975

69. Schneider RG, Hightower B, Hosty TS et al: Abnormal hemoglobins in a quarter million people. Blood 48:629, 1976

70. Schneider RG, Schmidt RM: Electrophoretic screening for abnormal hemoglobins. In Schmidt RM (ed): Abnormal Hemoglobins and Thalassemia—Diagnostic Aspects. New York, Academic Press, 1975

71. Schneider RG: Differentiation of electrophoretically similar hemoglobins—such as S, D, G, and P; or A₂, C, E, and O—by electrophoresis of the globin chains. Clin Chem 20:1111, 1974

72. Schneider RG, Hosty TS, Tomlin G et al: Identification of hemoglobins and hemoglobinopathies by electrophoresis on cellulose acetate plates impregnated with citrate agar. Clin Chem 20:74, 1974

73. Scott RB: Advances in the treatment of sickle cell disease in children. Am J Dis Child 139:1219, 1985

74. Seeler RA, Metzger W, Mufson MA: *Diplococcus pneumoniae* infections in children with sickle cell anemia. Am J Dis Child 123:8, 1972

75. Singer K, Chernoff AI, Singer L: Studies on abnormal hemoglobins. I. Their demonstration in sickle cell anemia and other hematologic disorders by means of alkali denaturation. Blood 6:413, 1951

76. Ueda S, Schneider RG: Rapid differentiation of polypeptide chains of hemoglobin by cellulose acetate electrophoresis of hemolysates. Blood 34:230, 1969

77. White JM: Fetal hemoglobin: Whole blood quantitation and intracellular distribution. In Schmidt RM et al (eds): The Detection of Hemoglobinopathies. Cleveland, CRC Press, 1974

78. White JM, Dacie JV: The unstable hemoglobins—molecular and clinical features. In Brown EB, Moore CV (eds): Progress in Hematology, vol 7, p 69. New York, Grune & Stratton, 1971

79. Williams WJ, Beutler E, Erslev AJ et al (eds): Hematology, 3rd ed, pp 509, 586, 593. New York, McGraw-Hill, 1983

80. Wintrobe MM: The abnormal hemoglobins: General principles. In Wintrobe MM et al: Clinical Hematology, 8th ed, p 816. Philadelphia, Lea & Febiger, 1981

81. Wintrobe MM: Unstable hemoglobin disease (congenital Heinz Body hemolytic anemia). In Wintrobe MM et al: Clinical Hematology, 8th ed, p 828. Philadelphia, Lea & Febiger, 1981

82. Wintrobe MM: Hemoglobinopathies S, C, D, E, and O and associated diseases. In Wintrobe MM et al: Clinical Hematology, 8th ed, pp 843, 858, 859. Philadelphia, Lea & Febiger, 1981

83. Wintrobe MM: The thalassemias and related disorders—quantitative disorders of hemoglobin synthesis. In Wintrobe MM et al: Clinical Hematology, 8th ed, p 888. Philadelphia, Lea & Febiger, 1981

84. Wintrobe MM: Methemoglobinemia and other disorders usually accompanied by cyanosis. In Wintrobe MM et al: Clinical Hematology, 8th ed, p 1016. Philadelphia, Lea & Febiger, 1981

Anemias of Abnormal Globin Development— Thalassemias

Carol N. LeCrone

The thalassemias are a diverse group of genetic disorders characterized by a primary, quantitative reduction in globin chain synthesis for hemoglobin (Hb). The thalassemias are probably the most common single-gene disorders in the world population.

Thalassemias involving reduced production of the alpha (α), beta (β), gamma (γ), and delta (δ) globin chains are discussed in this chapter. In addition, disorders caused by formation of structurally abnormal hemoglobins formed from normal globin chains or parts of normal chains will be described—to include Hb H (β_4), Hb Barts (γ_4), and Hb

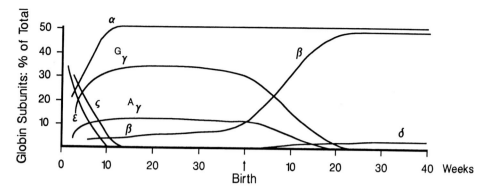

FIG. 15-1. Changes in globin subunits during human development from embryo to early infancy. (Adapted from Bunn HF, Forget BG: Hemoglobin: Molecular, Genetic and Clinical Aspects. Philadelphia, WB Saunders, 1986, with permission.)

Lepore. Since Hb Constant Spring presents with a thalassemic clinical picture, it is also discussed in this chapter.

HISTORY

Between 1925 and 1940, the clinical features of thalassemia were first described. Between 1940 and 1950, the genetic basis of the disorder was recognized. By 1960, it was obvious that the term *thalassemia* encompasses multiple genetic disorders. Since 1960, steady progress has been made in elucidating the structural nature of thalassemia; specific molecular defects have now been pinpointed.[62]

DEMOGRAPHICS

The thalassemias produce a massive public health problem in many countries but occur with particularly high frequency from the shores of the Mediterranean and Africa through the Middle East, the Indian subcontinent, Burma, and Southeast Asia (see Fig. 14-1).[54,60] This geographic distribution follows that of malaria, and recent studies show that *Plasmodium falciparum* survives less well in red cells from thalassemic subjects.[17] The thalassemias do occur sporadically in most racial groups.

GLOBIN SYNTHESIS DURING NORMAL HUMAN DEVELOPMENT

Human hemoglobin may contain any of seven different globin polypeptide chains—α, β, $^G\gamma$, $^A\gamma$, δ, ϵ, and ζ (Chap. 7). The changes in globin chain production during human development from the embryo to early infancy are shown in Figure 15-1. Table 7-2 summarizes the globin structure of human hemoglobins.

GENETICS

Structure of Chromosomes Associated with Thalassemia

Genetic information for the structure and production of a given globin chain is encoded in the nucleotide sequence of nuclear DNA. The DNA nucleotide sequence constitutes the gene or genetic locus on a chromosome. To understand the genetics of thalassemia, it is helpful to analyze the structure of chromosomes 11 and 16.

Figure 15-2 illustrates one of each pair of homologous chromosomes, thus depicting half of the full component of functional genes that direct specific globin chain synthesis. Note that the chromosome ends have been designated as 3' and 5'. On chromosome 11, one β and one δ gene, two γ genes, and a single ϵ gene are shown. Chromosome 16 has two α genes and one ζ gene. The genes designated with ψ are pseudogenes and are nonfunctional.[48,54] The two γ genes are denoted $^A\gamma$ and $^G\gamma$, indicating the two types of γ chains produced. $^A\gamma$ and $^G\gamma$ differ only in the 136th position, where the amino acid on $^A\gamma$ is *a*lanine and on $^G\gamma$ is *g*lycine. The genetic mechanism of globin chain production is discussed in Chapter 7.

Genetic Basis of Thalassemia

The inheritance of thalassemias follows Mendelian principles. Many thalassemic disorders result from known genetic abnormalities, but for some the exact defect is not understood.

The α and β thalassemias are the most common. The predominant cause of α thalassemia is gene deletion. Less frequently, α genes are present but one or more are nonfunctional.[20,42] In β thalassemia, the genetic abnormality usually is not associated with gene deletion; rather, the β genes are abnormal mostly because of point mutations in

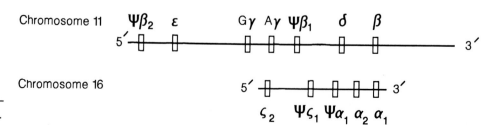

FIG. 15-2. Human globin gene arrangement on chromosomes 11 and 16.

the DNA code. Table 15-1 provides a summary of common genetic terms and definitions used to describe the thalassemias.

CLASSIFICATION OF THE THALASSEMIAS

The thalassemias are usually classified according to the particular globin chain whose synthesis is suppressed. The types are α, β, γ, δ, $\delta\beta$, and $\gamma\delta\beta$ thalassemia. It has also been determined that a hemoglobin variant known as Hb Lepore is actually a form of $\delta\beta$ thalassemia and that Hb Constant Spring is associated with α thalassemia. In addition, there is a less well defined group of hereditary disorders characterized by persistence of fetal hemoglobin (Hb F) production into adult life. Some of these conditions, which are collectively called hereditary persistence of fetal hemoglobin (HPFH), are now thought to represent extremely mild forms of thalassemia.

Many populations in which thalassemia is common also have a high prevalence of disorders that result from the inheritance of structural hemoglobin variants. Thus, it is not uncommon for a person who inherits one or more thalassemia genes to inherit and demonstrate a hemoglobinopathy as well (Chap. 14).[60]

GENERAL CONSIDERATIONS IN LABORATORY TESTING FOR THALASSEMIA

Table 15-2 lists the tests performed in the diagnostic work-up for thalassemia. Some generalizations may be made concerning laboratory characteristics of all thalassemias.

TABLE 15–2. Recommended Tests for Laboratory Diagnosis of Thalassemia

MOST FREQUENTLY REQUIRED
CBC (with red cell indices)
Red cell morphology evaluation
Serum ferritin
Hemoglobin electrophoresis, cellulose acetate
Hb F quantitation (alkali denaturation)
Hb A_2 quantitation (column chromatography)
Brilliant cresyl blue Hb H inclusion body test
Reticulocyte count
Reticulocyte production index
OCCASIONALLY REQUIRED
WBC differential
Serum iron
TIBC
Transferrin saturation (%)
Hemoglobin electrophoresis, citrate agar
NOT ROUTINELY REQUIRED
Bone marrow examination
DNA analysis
α/β Globin chain analysis

Hematology

In the thalassemia syndromes, erythrocyte indices generally indicate a microcytic and hypochromic anemia. The hemoglobin or hematocrit values vary with the type of thalassemia involved, and the reticulocyte production index (RPI) identifies the response of the bone marrow to anemia. The erythrocyte count is usually elevated relative to the degree of anemia. Erythrocyte abnormalities may include nucleated red blood cells, microcytosis, hypochromia, anisocytosis, poikilocytosis, polychromasia, basophilic stippling, and target cells. These abnormalities also vary with the type of thalassemia involved. Leukocytes and platelets usually are not affected.

TABLE 15–1. Summary of Genetic Terms and Definitions Used in the Thalassemias

TERMS TO DESCRIBE THALASSEMIAS	GENETIC REPRESENTATIONS	DEFINITION OF TERMS
Genes for globin production	Chromosome 11 Chromosome 16	$^G\gamma$, $^A\gamma$, β, δ, ϵ α, ζ
α Genes (genetic representation)	4 $\alpha\alpha/\alpha\alpha$	Normal number of α genes; two inherited from each parent
α-Gene deletions	$--/--$ $--/-\alpha$ $--/\alpha\alpha$ $-\alpha/-\alpha$ $-\alpha/\alpha\alpha$	(4-α gene deletion) (3-α gene deletion) (2-α gene deletion; both deletions inherited from one parent) (2-α gene deletion; one deletion inherited from each parent) (1-α gene deletion)
Nonfunctional α genes	$\alpha\alpha^T$	α Genes are present, but one or more may be nonfunctional
β Genes	2 β/β	Normal number of β genes; one inherited from each parent
Reduced β-chain production	β^+	+ Indicates decrease, but not total deficit, of β-chain production by that gene
No β-chain production	$\beta°$	° Indicates no β-chain production by that gene
δ and β gene deletions	$(\delta\beta)°$	Both δ and β globin genes deleted from chromosome 11
Hb Lepore designation	$(\delta\beta)$Lepore	Nonhomologous meiotic crossing over between δ and β globin genes on chromosome 11 (Fig. 15–4)

Special Hematologic Procedures

Bone marrow examination in thalassemia patients typically reveals hyperplastic red cell production, but it is seldom necessary for diagnosis. There may be specific diagnostic requirements necessitating the performance of α/β globin chain ratios or DNA analysis.

Hemoglobin electrophoresis on cellulose acetate at alkaline pH reveals variable results, depending on the type of thalassemia involved. Citrate agar electrophoresis at acid pH serves two major purposes. First, Hb F, which is often elevated in thalassemia, is effectively separated from Hb A. Second, hemoglobin variants may migrate differently in this medium, allowing them to be identified tentatively. The quantities of Hb A_2 and F and the presence of Hb H inclusions in erythrocytes can be diagnostic as well.

The acid elution slide test for Hb F is valuable to differentiate thalassemia from HPFH. In most thalassemias, Hb F occurs heterogeneously (*i.e.,* some cells contain Hb F and some do not) while there is a homogeneous distribution in pancellular HPFH.

Chemistry

Iron studies are often beneficial, particularly since thalassemia can mimic iron deficiency states (see Table 15-8). Differentiation of the two disorders is discussed later in this chapter. Among transfusion-dependent thalassemic patients, testing for iron overload is important, because overload can and does occur in thalassemia major and thalassemia intermedia. The possibility of iron overload is indicated by the persistence of serum iron levels in excess of 160 μg/dL and transferrin saturation greater than 60%.[21]

Testing in Early Infancy

Although most persons with thalassemia require no treatment, those who are transfusion dependent usually develop severe anemia during the first year of life.[62] Proper evaluation of infant hematologic values requires knowledge of the normal differences between infant and adult values. At birth, a normal infant's red cells are macrocytic, but the mean corpuscular volume (MCV) subsequently begins to

fall. At 10 months of age, the lower limit of the MCV reference range is 70 fL, which should not be confused with pathologic microcytosis. This gradually rises to adult levels (80–100 fL) by approximately age 12 years. Hb F is not diagnostic of β thalassemia in infants, since it is normally elevated in the first year of life.

Interference of Transfusion with Test Results

Knowledge of a patient's transfusion status is important for correct interpretation of electrophoresis results. Blood samples taken soon after transfusion contain both the patient's and transfused red cells. An abnormal hemoglobin fraction may be masked on hemoglobin electrophoresis as long as transfused cells are still circulating.

Effects of Concurrent Iron Deficiency on Test Results

Concurrent iron deficiency in thalassemia is known to lower the concentrations of Hb A_2 and Hb H[39,60] as well as serum iron and iron stores. This may mask the diagnosis of heterozygous β thalassemia and Hb H disease, respectively. Additionally, Hb H inclusions may be more difficult to detect in red cells. If a subject is iron deficient, iron stores should first be repleted; then diagnostic tests for thalassemia may be performed.

α THALASSEMIA

Nomenclature

The normal haploid genotype for α globin genes is designated $\alpha\alpha$. In α thalassemia, when gene deletion is involved two haplotypes are possible: one α-gene deletion, designated $(-\alpha)$ or two α-gene deletions $(--)$. A single α gene deletion is known as α thalassemia 2 or α^+ thalassemia,[60] whereas the double α-gene deletion is referred to as α thalassemia 1 or α° thalassemia.

Normally, a total of four α genes is inherited, two from each parent (see Fig. 15-2). These four genes produce α

TABLE 15–3. Genotypes of α Thalassemia

α-CHAIN GENES (CHROMOSOME 16)*	GENOTYPE	GENOTYPIC DESCRIPTION		DISORDER
██ ██	$--/--$	Homozygous α°thal	αthal 1/αthal 1	Barts hydrops fetalis
██ ██	$--/-\alpha$	Heterozygous α°thal/α^+thal	αthal 1/αthal 2	Hb H disease
██ ██cs	$--/\alpha^{cs}\alpha$	Heterozygous α°thal/Constant Spring	αthal 1/heterozygous Constant Spring	Hb H/Constant Spring disease
██ ██	$--/\alpha\alpha$	Heterozygous α°thal	αthal 1/normal	α thalassemia minor
██ ██	$-\alpha/-\alpha$	Homozygous α^+thal	αthal 2/αthal 2	α thalassemia minor
██ ██	$-\alpha/\alpha\alpha$	Heterozygous α^+thal	αthal 2/normal	Silent carrier (no disorder)
██ ██	$\alpha\alpha/\alpha\alpha$	Normal	Normal	None

* Four α globin chain genes (open rectangles) normally are present on the chromosome 16 pair. Gene deletions that cause α thalassemia are shown as black rectangles. (Modified from Fishleder AJ, Hoffman GC: A practical approach to the detection of hemoglobinopathies. Part I. The introduction and thalassemia syndromes. Lab Med 18:369, 1987, with permission.)

chains in a quantity equal to that of β chains, resulting in a β/α chain ratio of 1:1. Most forms of α thalassemia result from a decrease in the number of α chains produced because of a deletion in one, two, three, or all four α genes. Table 15-3 demonstrates the genetic structures of the various forms of α thalassemia, their associated genotypic descriptions, and resulting clinical disorders. Without α chains, excess γ and β chains accumulate and form the tetramers γ_4 (Hb Barts) and β_4 (Hb H). Severity of disease ranges from lethal when all four α genes are deleted to no clinical abnormality when one α gene is deleted.

In some populations there are structural hemoglobin variants such as Hb Constant Spring, which, because they contain α chains that are synthesized at a reduced rate, produce an α-thalassemia phenotype (see Table 15-3). Another type of α thalassemia involves a nondeletional form, which has a haplotype of $\alpha\alpha^T$. In this disorder, both α genes are present on chromosome 16, but defective synthesis of α chains results in an α thalassemia syndrome.[20,42]

Barts Hydrops Fetalis

Genetics, Demographics, and Pathophysiology

Barts hydrops fetalis is caused by the deletion of all four α globin genes ($--/--$), resulting in the production of Hb Barts (γ_4). Both parents of affected infants have heterozygous α° thalassemia ($--/\alpha\alpha$). Barts hydrops fetalis is observed almost exclusively in Southeast Asians, however, some infants in the Mediterranean island populations are also affected.[58,62] The disorder is lethal, and infants are usually stillborn or die within hours of birth. Survival into the third trimester of fetal life is attributed to the presence of Hb Portland ($\zeta_2\gamma_2$), which delivers oxygen to the tissues. Hb Barts, on the other hand, has a high affinity for oxygen and thus will not effectively release it to the tissues. Death results from hypoxia. Obstetric complications may lead to significant morbidity and mortality for the mothers of these infants.

Clinical Findings

Infants who are liveborn are underweight, edematous, demonstrate ascites (accumulation of serous fluid in the abdominal cavity), and have distended abdomens. There is usually marked hepatosplenomegaly.

Laboratory Findings and Correlations with Disease

Hemoglobin levels in cord blood vary from 4.0 to 10.0 g/dL, and the blood film shows red cells with gross thalassemic changes. These include marked variation in size and shape, hypochromia, variable reticulocytosis, and numerous nucleated red cell precursors.

Hemoglobin electrophoresis (alkaline pH) of cord blood hemolysates shows a fast-moving band made up of approximately 80% Hb Barts. In addition, there is about 20% of the embryonic Hb Portland and little or no Hb H, a band that moves even faster than Hb Barts (Fig. 15-3). There is no Hb A. This condition can also be diagnosed prenatally by performing DNA analysis on a chorionic biopsy specimen at about 8 to 10 weeks' gestation.[41]

Hb H Disease

Genetics, Demographics, and Pathophysiology

Hb H disease usually is caused by the deletion of three of the four α globin genes ($--/-\alpha$), but there are nondeletional forms ($\alpha\alpha^T/\alpha\alpha^T$ and $\alpha\alpha^T/--$). Family studies tend to show that one parent has heterozygous α° thalassemia and the other has heterozygous α^+ thalassemia (see Table 15-3). Hb H disease is widespread in Southeast Asia, parts of the Middle East, and in the Mediterranean island populations.[58,62] It can, however, occur sporadically in almost every ethnic group.

Lane	Hb	Origin	CA	CS	C Harlem / O Arab / E / C / A2	G / D / Lepore / S	F	A	Portland	Bart's	H
1	Bart's								‖	‖	(‖)^Δ
2	H		‖		‖			‖		(‖)*	‖
3	H/Constant Spring		‖	‖	‖			‖		(‖)*	‖
4	α Thal minor		‖		‖			‖			
5	α Thal (silent carrier)		‖		‖			‖			
6	AA2 (normal)		‖		‖			‖			

FIG. 15-3. Relative electrophoretic mobilities of hemoglobins on cellulose acetate, pH 8.4, of various α-thalassemia syndromes. (Lane 1) Barts hydrops fetalis cord blood (Δ, Hb H may or may not be present). Carbonic anhydrase (CA) and HbA$_2$ are not detectable at birth. (Lane 2) HbH disease (adult) (★, Hb Barts is present in ~10% of adult patients. (Lane 3) Hb H/Constant Spring (CS) (adult) (+, Hb Barts may or may not be present). (Lane 4) α-Thalassemia minor pattern in an adult is the same as that of a normal adult (Hb Barts = 2 to 10% at birth). (Lane 5) α-Thalassemia silent carrier (adult); the pattern is the same as in a normal adult (Hb Barts = 1 to 2% at birth). (Lane 6) Normal adult pattern.

This disorder results from the decreased synthesis of α chains and the resultant formation of the unstable hemoglobin Hb H (β_4). The concentration of Hb H is variable. Hb H tends to precipitate in older red cells, which are removed prematurely from the circulation by the spleen. The result is a lifelong, mild to moderate hemolytic anemia that is due to the instability of Hb H and the inability of the marrow to elicit an adequate compensation for the hemolysis. The severity of anemia depends on the degree of imbalance of the α/β chain ratio.

Clinical Findings

At birth, infants with Hb H disease appear well, but splenomegaly and anemia tend to develop by the end of the first year of life. Hepatomegaly occurs less often. The association of mental retardation and Hb H disease has been reported.[63]

Laboratory Findings and Correlations with Disease

In the adult steady state, Hb levels vary from 8.9 to 12.7 g/dL and the red cell indices are decreased.[54] There is a reticulocytosis of approximately 5%, but the reticulocyte production index (RPI) usually indicates an inadequate bone marrow response for the degree of anemia. This is a consistent finding in chronic anemia.

On the peripheral blood film, red cells are microcytic and hypochromic, with variation in size and shape. The electronically measured red cell distribution width (RDW) is increased in Hb H disease.[5] Almost all red cells have Hb H inclusions, which are visible microscopically when erythrocytes are incubated and supravitally stained with brilliant cresyl blue (BCB), a redox dye that causes the precipitation of Hb H in vitro. Cells containing Hb H resemble a golf ball because of the pitted inclusions. Individual inclusions appear similar to Heinz body inclusions, which are associated with precipitation of abnormally oxidized hemoglobin. Hb H inclusions (see Fig. 14-10B) generally occur in multiples and cover the cell surface, whereas Heinz bodies (see Fig. 14-10A) are usually eccentrically located and there are very few per cell.

Hemoglobin electrophoresis (alkaline pH) in affected neonates shows about 25% to 40% Hb Barts, but as β chains become available during the first few months of life, Hb Barts (γ_4) is gradually replaced by Hb H (β_4). Electrophoresis after this time shows Hbs H (which migrates faster than Hbs A and Barts), A, and A$_2$ (see Fig. 15-3). The Hb F level is normal. A small amount of Hb Barts is present in about 10% of adult patients.[54] One report states that Hb H levels can vary from 2% to 40%.[62] The range in 69 cases from Thailand was 2% to 24% (mean 9%).[36] The Hb A$_2$ levels are nearly always reduced.

Hb H may occasionally occur in certain acquired disorders such as erythroleukemia,[3] acute[40] or chronic granulocytic leukemia,[4] sideroblastic anemia,[67] and other myeloproliferative disorders.[56] In these cases, the Hb H level varies between 5% and 70% of the total hemoglobin.[60]

Treatment and Prognosis

Most patients with Hb H disease require no therapy; however, intercurrent infections should be treated promptly and oxidant drugs should be avoided. Patient development and life expectancy are usually normal.

Hb H—Constant Spring Disease

Genetics, Demographics, and Pathophysiology

A phenotype similar to Hb H disease may be caused by compound heterozygous inheritance of Hb Constant Spring (Hb CS) and $\alpha°$ thalassemia ($--/\alpha^{CS}\alpha$; see Table 15-3). Hb CS consists of two normal β chains, one normal α chain, and one abnormal α chain that has 172 amino acids as opposed to the normal 141 (i.e., 31 additional ones). This elongated α chain probably results from a mutation of the chain terminator codon. Therefore, inheritance of Hb CS causes a deficit in normal α chains, and when it is inherited along with a double α-gene deletion, it produces a disorder similar to Hb H disease.

Hb H/CS occurs frequently in Orientals and has been observed in Mediterranean populations. It represents up to 40% of all Hb H-like syndromes in Southeast Asians.[54]

Laboratory Findings and Correlations with Disease

The peripheral blood and blood film findings are very similar to those previously described for Hb H disease. Hemoglobin electrophoresis at alkaline pH reveals Hbs H, A, A$_2$, little or no Barts, and approximately 1.5% to 2.5% Hb CS. Hb CS migrates behind Hb A$_2$ (see Fig. 15-3), and because the percentage is small, it may be missed. Hemolysate should be applied heavily to the electrophoretic support medium when Hb CS is suspected.[16]

Treatment and Prognosis

Hemolysis may be more severe with Hb H/CS than in the typical three–α gene deletion Hb H disease. Treatment and prognosis are generally the same in both conditions.[54]

α Thalassemia Minor

Genetics, Demographics, and Pathophysiology

Alpha thalassemia minor (also known as α thalassemia trait) has two genotypic forms (see Table 15-3). One is termed heterozygous $\alpha°$ ($--/\alpha\alpha$) thalassemia and the other homozygous α^+ ($-\alpha/-\alpha$). The result in either form is a decrease in α-chain synthesis.

Both forms are common in Southeast Asians, Chinese, and Filipinos.[31] Homozygous α^+ thalassemia is common in American blacks (3.0%) and is also found among Mediterraneans. The heterozygous $\alpha°$ form is rare in blacks.[31] Neither condition produces clinical disease.

Laboratory Findings and Correlations with Disease

The hematologic findings are the same for both genotypes. Erythrocytes typically are microcytic and slightly hypochromic with decreased mean corpuscular volume (MCV) and mean corpuscular hemoglobin (MCH) levels; the mean corpuscular hemoglobin concentration (MCHC) is normal to slightly decreased. Target cells and other poikilocytes are common. Hematocrit and Hb levels are usually at the lower limit of the reference range. In some cases, there may be mild anemia. The erythrocyte count is usually above 5.5×10^{12} cells/L. The RDW is normal or only slightly increased.[27,57]

Newborns with α thalassemia studied in several racial groups exhibited 2% to 10% Hb Barts on hemoglobin electrophoresis (alkaline pH) of cord blood samples.[9,18,32,43,46,59,61,68] Therefore, Hb Barts concentrations greater than 2% may be helpful in diagnosing α thalassemia minor in newborns. Hb Barts disappears after the first few months of life; thereafter, the electrophoretic pattern is normal (see Fig. 15-3) even though Hb H is in fact present, but in concentrations too low for electrophoresis to detect. Hb H is detectable microscopically by induction of Hb H precipitation and staining with brilliant cresyl blue (BCB), as described earlier.

A modified BCB inclusion body test can be used to enhance the precipitation of Hb H, often causing the inclusions to be more visible.[25] A negative test result does not absolutely exclude either genotypic form of α thalassemia minor. A definitive diagnosis can be made by DNA analysis, but the test expense usually is not justified for this benign disorder. DNA analysis can be important, however, in determining specific genotypes for purposes of genetic counseling.

Differential Diagnosis

One study has shown that other disorders occurring with α thalassemia minor should be considered when the hematocrit is less than 0.31 L/L in women and children and less than 0.37 L/L in men.[31]

Microcytosis in the presence of normal Hb A_2 and Hb F levels is very suggestive of α thalassemia minor, particularly when other family members are similarly affected. Microcytosis with decreased iron stores, on the other hand, may indicate iron deficiency alone or thalassemia with coincident iron deficiency anemia.

The Silent Carrier

Genetics, Demographics, and Pathophysiology

The silent carrier form of α thalassemia, also known as heterozygous α^+ thalassemia, is associated with one α-gene

deletion ($-\alpha/\alpha\alpha$). This condition is common in Southeast Asians, Chinese, and Filipinos. Approximately 28% of American blacks have heterozygous α^+ thalassemia.[12] The silent carrier state is benign and is often discovered only during family studies.

Laboratory Findings and Correlations with Disease

The hematologic picture, including the blood count, is normal, or very minimally abnormal, with slightly decreased MCV and MCH values. Small percentages (1%–2%) of Hb Barts may be found in affected infants, but the electrophoresis pattern is normal in adults (see Fig. 15-3). Rare Hb H inclusions, occurring due to slight globin chain imbalance, may be found using the modified BCB inclusion body test.[25] Like α thalassemia minor, the silent carrier state cannot be ruled out on the basis of a negative BCB result. A definitive diagnosis can be made by DNA analysis. A summary of hematologic data on α thalassemia is presented in Table 15-4.

β THALASSEMIA

In β thalassemia, there is also unbalanced globin chain synthesis due to a lack of, or to the reduced production of, β chains. This causes an excess of α chains, which are very unstable. If the imbalance is relatively minor, unpaired α chains are simply removed by proteolysis during erythroid maturation; however, if the degradation process is overwhelmed by massive imbalance, excess free α chains precipitate, causing severe erythrocyte dysfunction. Many of the defective red cells are destroyed by bone marrow macrophages. The result is ineffective erythropoiesis and a massively enlarged erythron.

TABLE 15–4. Hematologic Features of α Thalassemia

DIAGNOSIS	GENOTYPE*	RED CELL MORPHOLOGY	HEMOGLOBIN ELECTROPHORESIS	MEAN GLOBIN CHAIN SYNTHESIS VALUES IN RETICULOCYTES (α/β RATIO)*	ANEMIA	LIFE EXPECTANCY
Hb Barts Hydrops Fetalis	$--/--$	$\downarrow$ MCV & MCH, $\uparrow$ NRBC	Hb Barts (80%)† Hb Portland	0:1	Severe	Fatal
Hb H Disease	$--/-\alpha$	$\downarrow$ MCV & MCH, $+++$ Hb H inclusions‡	Hb A Hb H (2-40%) $\pm$ Hb Barts $\downarrow$ Hb A_2	0.40:1	Moderate	Normal
α Thalassemia Minor						
Heterozygous α° or homozygous α^+ thalassemia	$--/\alpha\alpha$ $-\alpha/-\alpha$	$\downarrow$ MCV & MCH, $++$ Hb H inclusions‡	Normal	0.77:1	None or mild	Normal
Silent Carrier						
Heterozygous α^+ thalassemia	$-\alpha/\alpha\alpha$	Normal or sl $\downarrow$ MCV & MCH, $\pm$ Hb H inclusions‡	Normal	0.88:1	None	Normal

* Normal genotype is ($\alpha\alpha/\alpha\alpha$) and normal α/β ratio is 1:1.
† Cord blood sample
‡ Modified brilliant cresyl blue Hb H inclusion body test
Key: $\uparrow$, elevated; $\downarrow$, depressed; $+++$, marked; $++$, moderate; $\pm$, occasional or none.
(Modified from Todd D: Thalassemia. Pathology 16:5, 1984, with permission.)

TABLE 15–5. Classifications of β Thalassemias and Their Genotypes

CLASSIFICATION	GENOTYPE
Normal	β/β
THALASSEMIA MAJOR	
★Homozygous $\beta°$	$\beta°/\beta°$
Homozygous β^+ (Mediterranean form)	β^+/β^+
★Doubly heterozygous $\beta°/\beta^+$	$\beta°/\beta^+$
★Homozygous $(\delta\beta)$Lepore	$(\delta\beta)$Lepore$/(\delta\beta)$Lepore
THALASSEMIA INTERMEDIA	
★Homozygous $\beta°$	$\beta°/\beta°$
★Doubly heterozygous $\beta°/\beta^+$	$\beta°/\beta^+$
★Homozygous $(\delta\beta)$Lepore	$(\delta\beta)$Lepore$/(\delta\beta)$Lepore
Homozygous β^+ (black form)	β^+/β^+
Homozygous $(\delta\beta)°$	$(\delta\beta)°/(\delta\beta)°$
Doubly heterozygous $\beta°/(\delta\beta)°$	$\beta°/(\delta\beta)°$
Doubly heterozygous $\beta^+/(\delta\beta)°$	$\beta^+/(\delta\beta)°$
Doubly heterozygous $\beta°/(\delta\beta)$ Lepore	$\beta°/(\delta\beta)$Lepore
Doubly heterozygous $\beta^+/(\delta\beta)$ Lepore	$\beta^+/(\delta\beta)$Lepore
Doubly heterozygous $(\delta\beta)°/(\delta\beta)$ Lepore	$(\delta\beta)°/(\delta\beta)$Lepore
†Heterozygous $\beta°$	$\beta/\beta°$
Doubly heterozygous $\beta°/\beta^{sc}$	$\beta°/\beta^{sc}$
THALASSEMIA MINOR	
†Heterozygous $\beta°$ or β^+	$\beta/\beta°$ or β/β^+
Heterozygous $(\delta\beta)°$	$\beta/(\delta\beta)°$
Heterozygous $(\delta\beta)$ Lepore	$\beta/(\delta\beta)$Lepore
THALASSEMIA MINIMA	
Heterozygous β^{sc}	β/β^{sc}

Key: β, gene with normal β-chain production; β^+, gene with decreased β-chain production; $\beta°$, gene with no β-chain production; ★, some overlap between thalassemia intermedia and thalassemia major; †, overlap between intermedia and minor; sc, silent carrier.

There is a great deal of heterogeneity associated with β thalassemia. This most likely relates to the close proximity of the β, δ, and γ globin genes on chromosome 11. In the following discussion, β thalassemia will be the predomi-

nant term used; however, it is important to keep in mind that there may be abnormalities in all or part of the $\beta\delta\gamma$ globin complex.

Classification

Several classification schemes exist for the β thalassemias. There are many forms of β thalassemia, and they are most easily understood by grouping them into four clinical types, each of which includes many genotypes, some of which overlap between two groups (Table 15-5). The most debilitating clinical form is *thalassemia major*, in which there is typically severe anemia, often accompanied by iron overload. The second form is *thalassemia intermedia*, which is often associated with moderate anemia. Third is *thalassemia minor*, an asymptomatic form that may or may not produce mild anemia. Fourth is *thalassemia minima*, which causes no detectable clinical or routine laboratory abnormalities.

The β thalassemias occur most frequently in Europe, the Middle East, and North Africa (see Fig. 14-1). They are also common in China, India, and Central Africa.[13] A summary of the hematologic laboratory features and the severity of anemia differentiating the β thalassemias is presented in Table 15-6.

Thalassemia Major

There are four genotypes associated with β thalassemia major, three of which use the nomenclature $\beta°$ and β^+. $\beta°$ signifies no β globin chain production, and β^+ signifies decreased β globin chain production. The four genotypes include (1) $\beta°/\beta°$; (2) β^+/β^+ (Mediterranean form); (3) $\beta°/\beta^+$; and (4) $(\delta\beta)$Lepore$/(\delta\beta)$ Lepore (referred to as Hb Lepore). Table 15-5 summarizes the forms of thalassemia major.

Hb Lepore is composed of two normal α chains and two abnormal non-α chains formed by fusion of the N-terminal end of a δ chain and the C-terminal end of a β chain.[1] This

TABLE 15–6. Summary of Pertinent Hematologic Features of β Thalassemia

DIAGNOSIS	ERYTHROCYTE COUNT	ERYTHROCYTE MORPHOLOGY	HEMOGLOBIN ELECTROPHORESIS*	MEAN GLOBIN CHAIN SYNTHESIS VALUES IN RETICULOCYTES (β/α RATIO)	ANEMIA	LIFE EXPECTANCY (YR)
Thalassemia Major	↑	↓ MCV & MCH, ++ stippling, +++ NRBC, +++ targets	↑ Hb F, variable Hb A_2 ± Hb A†	0–0.3/1	Severe	20–30
Thalassemia Intermedia	↑	↓ MCV & MCH, + stippling, ± NRBC, ++ targets	N/↑ Hb F, variable Hb A_2 ± Hb A†	0–0.4/1	Moderate	Normal
Thalassemia Minor	↑	↓ MCV & MCH, + stippling, + targets	N/↑ Hb F, variable Hb A_2, variable Hb A	0.5/1	None to mild	Normal
Thalassemia Minima	Normal	Normal or slight ↓ MCV & MCH, ± stippling, ± targets	Normal	0.88/1	None	Normal

★ See Table 15–7
† Hb A is absent in genotypes containing only $\beta°$, $(\delta\beta)°$, or $(\delta\beta)$ Lepore genes (Modified from Todd D: Thalassemia. Pathology 16:5, 1984, with permission.)
Key: ↑, elevated; ↓, depressed; +++, marked; ++, moderate; +, slight; ±, occasional or none.

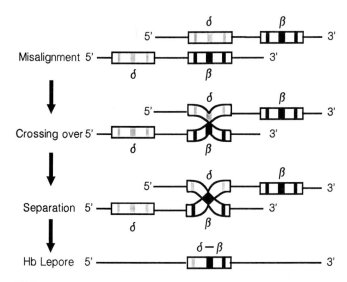

FIG. 15-4.   Illustration of the concept of nonhomologous meiotic crossing over in the genesis of Hb Lepore. (From Tietz NW [ed]: Textbook of Clinical Chemistry. Philadelphia, WB Saunders, 1986, with permission.)

abnormal hemoglobin is caused by nonhomologous meiotic crossing over between the δ and β globin gene loci (Fig. 15-4). The remaining portions of the δ and β genes form an anti-Lepore gene. The chromosome bearing the Lepore δβ fusion gene lacks intact δ and β genes. Three different Lepore hemoglobins have been described, including Baltimore, Boston, and Hollandia. Each differs in the point at which crossing over occurs. Hb Lepore-Boston is the most common Lepore hemoglobin seen. All Hbs Lepore are ineffectively synthesized, causing a β thalassemia syndrome.

Clinical Findings

Thalassemia major patients usually present with severe anemia within the first year of life. They tend to have a difficult clinical course. Bone marrow expansion resulting from excessive ineffective erythropoiesis causes marked skeletal deformities with frontal bossing (Fig. 15-5), cheek bone and jaw protrusions, distortions of ribs and vertebrae, and pathologic fractures of long bones. Often forward protrusion of the upper teeth and overbite lead to dental and orthodontic problems. Without adequate treatment, there is progressive hepatosplenomegaly, cardiomegaly, and other complications such as gallstones, chronic leg ulcers, and hypersplenism. Growth and sexual development are retarded, and intercurrent infections are common.[54]

Laboratory Findings and Correlations with Disease

PERIPHERAL BLOOD.   Without transfusion, Hb values range between 2.5 and 6.5 g/dL. There are numerous nucleated red cells on the peripheral blood film. Erythrocytes are microcytic and hypochromic and vary markedly in shape and size (Fig. 15-6). Target cells and basophilic stippling are typical. The RPI is generally less than 3.0. This is due to mild reticulocytosis, indicating ineffective erythropoiesis which does not adequately compensate for the se-

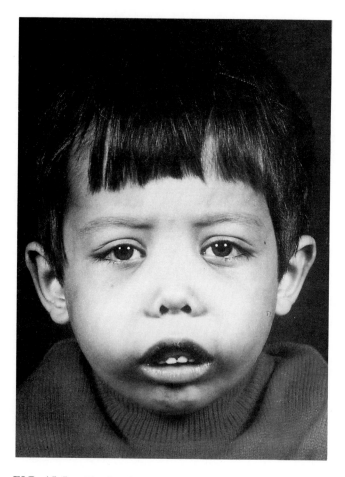

FIG. 15-5.   The facial appearance of a child with β-thalassemia major. The skull is bossed, with prominent frontal and parietal bones, and the maxilla is enlarged. (From Hoffbrand AV, Pettit JE: Essential Haematology, 2nd ed. London, Blackwell Scientific Publications, 1984, with permission.)

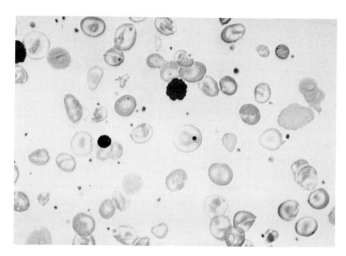

FIG. 15-6.   Peripheral blood film shows the morphologic appearance of red blood cells in homozygous β°-thalassemia (Cooley's anemia). There is marked variation in erythrocyte size and shape. Note microcytosis and hypochromia. Target cells and nucleated red cells are present. (From the American Society of Hematology Slide Bank, 2nd ed. Seattle, 1977, used with permission.)

verity of the anemia. Leukocytes characteristically are increased while the platelet count is generally normal.

BONE MARROW. The bone marrow is hypercellular, showing marked erythroid hyperplasia.

SPECIAL HEMATOLOGIC TESTS. The pretransfusion hemoglobin electrophoresis pattern (cellulose acetate, alkaline pH) in thalassemia major consists almost entirely of Hb F. Hb A_2 may be absent or the level may be reduced, normal, or slightly elevated (see Table 15-6). In homozygous $\beta°$ thalassemia ($\beta°/\beta°$) no β-chain synthesis occurs, so Hb A is absent. In the severe Mediterranean form (β^+/β^+) and in the $\beta°/\beta^+$ form of thalassemia major, Hb A may be detected once the switch from γ- to β-chain production takes place a few months after birth.

In homozygous Hb Lepore ([$\delta\beta$] Lepore/[$\delta\beta$] Lepore), approximately 10% to 20% of the hemoglobin on electrophoresis at alkaline pH is Hb Lepore, the remainder being Hb F (Table 15-7). Hb Lepore migrates to the same position as Hb S on electrophoresis at alkaline pH (Fig. 15-7). Hbs A and A_2 characteristically are absent since β and δ chains are not produced.

Hb Lepore produces a negative sickle solubility test result; however, this is not definitive for Hb Lepore. Citrate agar electrophoresis (acid pH) is required to definitively screen for Hb Lepore and, if present, to differentiate Hb Lepore from Hb S. Hb Lepore migrates to the Hb A position on this medium, while Hb S migrates in the opposite direction, toward the anode (see Fig. 15-7).

The acid elution technique for qualitative analysis of Hb F is helpful to differentiate the thalassemia major disorders, which all have increased Hb F, from HPFH. Thalassemia major reveals a heterogeneous distribution of Hb F in the red cells.[54] HPFH, in contrast, reveals a homogenous distribution, since all cells contain Hb F.

While not a particularly useful procedure, the osmotic fragility test is markedly decreased in thalassemia major. Some red cells do not even hemolyze in water owing to the large surface-to-volume ratio characteristic of target cells, which are common in thalassemia.

CHEMISTRY. The intramedullary hemolytic process associated with ineffective erythropoiesis results in a mild elevation of unconjugated bilirubin. Urine urobilinogen and fecal urobilin may also be increased. Serum ferritin and iron are elevated, and transferrin is often fully saturated owing to the iron overload problem in these disorders.

OTHER SPECIAL TESTS. The β thalassemia major syndromes can be diagnosed *in utero*. A new technique, DNA analysis of a chorionic biopsy specimen, has been carried out at 8 to 10 weeks' gestation. This will probably supplant amniocentesis sometime in the future, because the new procedure provides relatively large amounts of material for study and affords earlier diagnosis.[41]

EFFECTS OF TREATMENT ON LABORATORY RESULTS AND PROGNOSIS

In all cases of thalassemia major, the treatment and prognosis is generally the same. Without treatment, death usually occurs in the first or early second decade.[62] The mainstay of therapy is blood transfusion, which, however, necessitates the administration of an iron-chelating agent such as desferrioxamine to help forestall iron overload. Without the chelator, death occurs in the second or third decade of life, and this is due principally to myocardial damage. With iron chelation, life may be somewhat prolonged.

Other potential appoaches to treatment include the reactivation of γ globin gene expression, allogeneic bone marrow transplantation, and gene therapy.[38,52]

Thalassemia Intermedia

Thalassemia intermedia describes certain β thalassemias which are clinically milder than most thalassemia major syndromes but more severe than the thalassemia minor

TABLE 15–7. Hemoglobin Electrophoretic Results on Cellulose Acetate (Alkaline pH) in Various β Thalassemia Syndromes*

GENOTYPE	Hb A (%)	Hb A₂ (%)	Hb F (%)	Hb LEPORE (%)
THALASSEMIA MAJOR				
$\beta°/\beta°$	0	<2–6	90–98	
β^+/β^+ (Mediterranean form)	Present	<2–6	70–95	
$\beta°/\beta^+$	Present	<2–6	>75	
($\delta\beta$)Lepore/($\delta\beta$)Lepore	0	0	>75	10–20
THALASSEMIA INTERMEDIA				
β^+/β^+ (black form)	55–75	<2–6	20–40	
($\delta\beta$)°/($\delta\beta$)°	0	0	100	
($\delta\beta$)°/($\delta\beta$)Lepore	0	0	92	8
THALASSEMIA MINOR				
β^+/β or $\beta°/\beta$	>90	3.5–8	1–5	
($\delta\beta$)°/β	<90	<2–3	5–20	
($\delta\beta$)Lepore/β	Present	<2–2.6	1–3	5–15
THALASSEMIA MINIMA				
β^{SC}/β	95	2–3.2	<1	

* Normal hemoglobin concentrations are A, 95%; A_2, 2–3.2%; and F, <1%.
Key: β^+, reduced β-chain production; $\beta°$, no β-chain production; ($\delta\beta$)°, deletion of δ and β genes; ($\delta\beta$) Lepore, nonhomologous meiotic crossing over between δ and β globin genes on chromosome 11; SC, silent carrier.

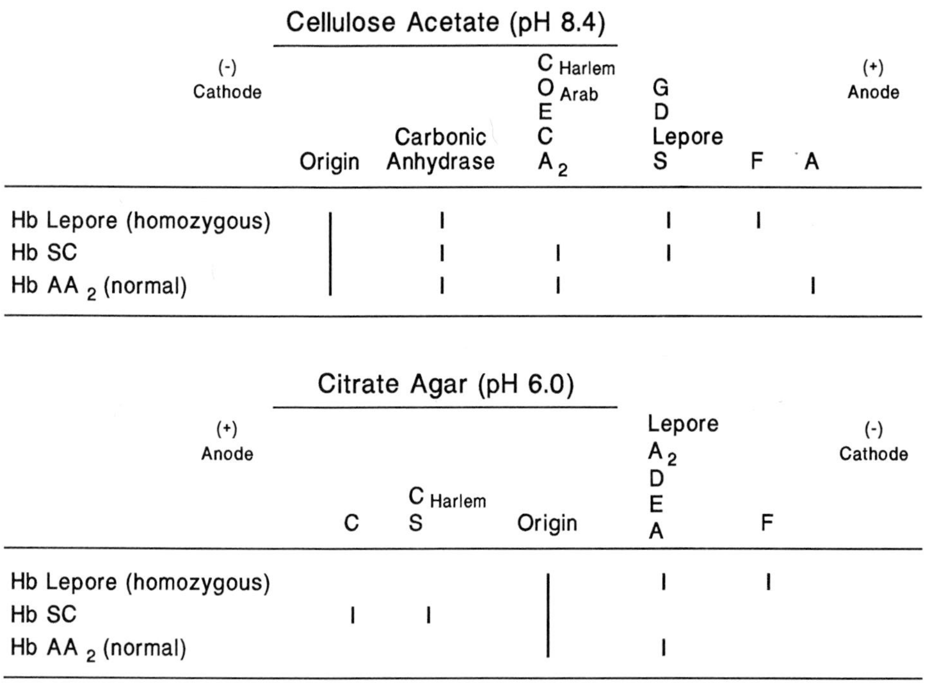

Cellulose Acetate (pH 8.4)

	Origin	Carbonic Anhydrase	C Harlem Arab / O / E / C / A_2	G / D / Lepore / S	F	A
	(-) Cathode					(+) Anode
Hb Lepore (homozygous)	|	I		I	I	
Hb SC	|	I	I	I		
Hb AA_2 (normal)	|	I	I			I

Citrate Agar (pH 6.0)

	C	C Harlem / S	Origin	Lepore / A_2 / D / E / A	F
	(+) Anode				(-) Cathode
Hb Lepore (homozygous)			|	I	I
Hb SC	I	I	|		
Hb AA_2 (normal)			|	I	

FIG. 15-7. Differentiation of hemoglobins Lepore and S using cellulose acetate electrophoresis, pH 8.4, and citrate agar electrophoresis, pH 6.0. Note that both hemoglobins migrate to the same position on cellulose acetate but are separated on citrate agar.

conditions. The genetic defects are variable, so there is some genotype overlap between thalassemia intermedia and thalassemia major and minor (see Table 15-5). The severity of the disorder ultimately differentiates the genotypes. Some of the more commonly encountered thalassemia intermedia conditions are described briefly below.

In thalassemia intermedia, it appears that the genes are less severely affected and that impairment of β chain synthesis is less than that usually seen in thalassemia major; alternatively, some other factor may compensate for the lack of β chains.

Homozygous β^+ Thalassemia (β^+/β^+) Mild Black Form

The β^+/β^+ form of thalassemia intermedia, also called the mild black form, is found among American and African blacks. There is less impairment of β-chain synthesis than in homozygous β^+ thalassemia of the Mediterranean type.[62] In the mild black variety, the β^+ gene produces β chains at approximately 50% of the normal rate, as compared to only about 10% for the β^+ gene in the thalassemia major Mediterranean form. The relative hemoglobin percentages associated with this disorder are shown in Table 15-7.

Homozygous $\delta\beta$ Thalassemia (($\delta\beta)°/(\delta\beta)°$)

Homozygous $\delta\beta$ thalassemia is caused by deletion of the δ and β structural genes on the chromosome 11 pair, which prevents the production of δ and β chains. $\delta\beta$ Thalassemia is milder than the thalassemia major syndromes because there is more efficient synthesis of γ chains. The γ chains bind with α chains to form Hb F, which constitutes 100% of the hemoglobin in these patients (see Table 15-7). Hbs A and A_2 cannot be synthesized since no δ or β chains are produced. The overall degree of α/non-α globin chain im-

balance is not as pronounced as in thalassemia major.[51] This disorder is found sporadically among American blacks, Arabs, Greeks, and Italians.

Doubly Heterozygous $\delta\beta$ Thalassemia Varieties

$\delta\beta$ Thalassemia may be found in conjunction with a variety of abnormal genes including $\beta°$, β^+, and Hb Lepore (see Table 15-5). Clinically, all of these present as thalassemia intermedia. In the $\delta\beta$ combinations with $\beta°$ and β^+ genes, Hb F is increased and Hbs A and A_2 are decreased or absent. In the case of $\delta\beta$ thalassemia and Hb Lepore, only Hbs F and Lepore are found on electrophoresis (see Table 15-7).

Clinical Findings

Growth and development of children with thalassemia intermedia is relatively normal. Clinical findings are similar to, but less severe than, those of thalassemia major; they include pallor, splenomegaly, and facial bone deformity. In adulthood, problems with iron overload may also be detected.

Laboratory Findings and Correlations with Disease

PERIPHERAL BLOOD. The peripheral blood picture is similar to that of thalassemia major, but the anemia is not as severe. Hemoglobin values range from 7 to 10 g/dL in untransfused patients. Generally these levels are sustained, and patients do not need to receive transfusions routinely. The erythrocytes are microcytic and hypochromic. Marked anisocytosis and poikilocytosis with target cells are common. Basophilic stippling and nucleated red blood cells are usually present on the peripheral blood film, although some patients may display neither.

BONE MARROW.   The marrow shows significant erythroid hyperplasia.

SPECIAL HEMATOLOGIC TESTS.   Hemoglobin electrophoresis at alkaline pH reveals a variety of patterns, depending on the genotype, and thus serves only as an initial screening procedure (see Table 15-7).

Effects of Treatment on Laboratory Results and Prognosis

Treatment for thalassemia intermedia is supportive rather than active, and most patients have a normal life span.

Thalassemia Minor

Thalassemia minor is generally an asymptomatic β thalassemia disorder in which there is little or no associated anemia, although peripheral blood erythrocyte morphology is significantly abnormal. There are three syndromes that are categorized as thalassemia minor (see Table 15-5), all of which are generally indistinguishable, clinically and hematologically, except for the heterozygous Hb Lepore state in which Hb Lepore is detected on electrophoresis.

Heterozygous β° (β°/β) or β^{+} (β^{+}/β) Thalassemia

This condition, also termed β thalassemia trait or high–Hb A_2 thalassemia, is caused by the combination of a normal β gene and either a β° or a β^{+} gene. Clinically, there seem to be no distinguishing features between the two genotypes. Differentiation can be accomplished by special DNA studies, if necessary. Hemoglobin electrophoresis may show an elevated Hb A_2 level (see Table 15-7).

Heterozygous $\delta\beta$ Thalassemia ($[\delta\beta]^{\circ}/\beta$)

In this disorder, the normal β gene produces normal β chains, whereas there is a deletion of the δ and β genes on the paired chromosome 11. Compensatory Hb F production occurs, with values ranging from 5% to 20%. Hb A_2 is normal or slightly decreased (see Table 15-7).

Heterozygous Hb Lepore ($[\delta\beta]$ Lepore/β)

In this disorder, one β globin gene is normal and Hb Lepore is produced from a second $\delta\beta$ fusion gene. Electrophoresis (alkaline pH) shows Hbs A, Lepore, F, and A_2. Hb Lepore is usually 5% to 15% of the total hemoglobin and Hb A_2 is either normal or slightly reduced. In most cases, Hb F is elevated (see Table 15-7).

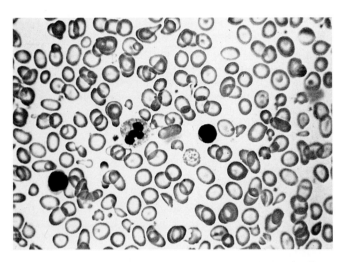

FIG. 15-8.   The morphologic appearance of red blood cells in heterozygous β-thalassemia (β-thalassemia trait) demonstrates microcytosis and varying degrees of hypochromia and poikilocytosis. Target cells and basophilic stippling are common findings. (From the American Society of Hematology Slide Bank, 2nd ed. Seattle, 1977, used with permission.)

Clinical Findings

Rarely are significant physical findings or symptoms caused by thalassemia minor, although in some cases of heterozygous β thalassemia, the hematocrit may be as low as 0.25 L/L during pregnancy.[62]

Laboratory Findings and Correlations with Disease

PERIPHERAL BLOOD.   Like thalassemia major and intermedia, heterozygous β thalassemia causes an increased erythrocyte count and often a marked decrease in MCV and MCH with a normal or slightly decreased MCHC. One study of 45 patients revealed a mean MCV of 65 fL, an MCH of 20.3 pg, and an MCHC of 31.2 g/dL.[44] Abnormalities in these parameters may be less dramatic in heterozygous $\delta\beta$ thalassemia.

Although patients are asymptomatic, the peripheral blood film, as in thalassemia major and intermedia, reveals striking morphology with microcytic, hypochromic red cells, anisopoikilocytosis, target cells, and basophilic stippling (Fig. 15-8). Unlike in thalassemia major and intermedia, nucleated red cells are not present on the peripheral film in thalassemia minor.

Anemia may be mild or absent. For thalassemia minor, studies have shown a mean Hb concentration for men of

TABLE 15–8. Laboratory Tests to Differentiate Iron Deficiency and Thalassemia Minor

	ERYTHROCYTE COUNT ($\times 10^{12}$ cells/L)	RDW	SERUM FERRITIN	SERUM IRON	TOTAL IRON-BINDING CAPACITY	TRANSFERRIN SATURATION (%)	ZnPP/H
Thalassemia minor	> 5.5	Normal or sl ↑	Normal or sl ↑	Normal	Normal	Normal	Normal
Iron deficiency	< 5.5	↑	↓	↓	↑	↓	↑

Key: sl, slight; ↑, elevated; ↓, depressed; ZnPP/H, zinc protoporphyrin/heme ratio.

12.9 g/dL[33,34,47] and for women, 10.9 g/dL.[34,47] The reticulocyte count may be slightly elevated if anemia is present.

In heterozygous β thalassemia, when the hematocrit value is less than 0.31 L/L in women and children and less than 0.37 L/L in men, other conditions in addition to thalassemia trait must be contributing to the anemia.[31]

BONE MARROW. The bone marrow shows slight erythroid hyperplasia.

SPECIAL HEMATOLOGIC TESTS. Relative electrophoretic percentages for the thalassemia minor syndromes are shown in Table 15-7. Characteristically an elevated Hb A$_2$ level is seen with heterozygous β° and β$^+$ thalassemia. Approximately half of these patients have a slightly elevated Hb F.[13] Special stains for erythrocyte inclusions are negative.

CHEMISTRY. It is important to perform chemical analysis to differentiate the microcytosis of β thalassemia minor from that of iron deficiency (Table 15-8). (See the section on Differentiation of Iron Deficiency and Thalassemia later in this chapter.)

Effects of Treatment on Laboratory Results and Prognosis

Usually no treatment is required in this condition, and affected people have a normal life span.

Thalassemia Minima (Silent β Thalassemia Trait)

Thalassemia minima describes a form of β thalassemia in which no clinical or laboratory abnormality is usually detected. The disorder is usually discovered accidentally or during family studies. The genotype, (β^{sc}/β), indicates the silent form (sc denotes silent carrier) of an abnormal β-globin gene. Results of electrophoresis are normal (see Table 15-7), the red cell morphology and count are within the reference range, and the MCV and MCH are within their reference ranges or slightly decreased. Globin chain synthesis studies reveal a slight decrease in β-globin production that results in a decreased β/α globin chain ratio.[60] Affected people have a normal life span. A summary of hematologic data in β thalassemia is presented in Table 15-6.

HEREDITARY PERSISTENCE OF FETAL HEMOGLOBIN

HPFH describes a heterogeneous group of inherited disorders characterized by increased levels of Hb F in adults in the absence of the usual clinical and hematologic features of thalassemia. HPFH is characterized by either deletion or inactivation of the β and δ structural gene complex. These disorders are sometimes classified in the thalassemia minor or minima scheme, depending on their clinical characteristics.

There is a compensatory persistence of γ-chain production into adult life, which prevents significant clinical abnormalities. There are two major categories of HPFH: (1) pancellular, in which all red cells contain increased levels

of Hb F as determined by the acid elution slide test, and (2) heterocellular, in which only a subpopulation of red cells contain increased Hb F.

Pancellular HPFH

The most common variety of pancellular HPFH in the United States is found in blacks and is associated with the synthesis of both ^{G}γ- and ^{A}γ-chain types of Hb F. The homozygous condition demonstrates 100% Hb F. In contrast to homozygous (δβ)° thalassemia, which also shows 100% Hb F, there is no anemia, but the red cells may be slightly microcytic and hypochromic. The blood picture in HPFH heterozygotes is characterized by the presence of 20% to 30% Hb F.[62] Hemoglobin levels, red cell indices, red cell morphology, and α/non-α globin chain synthesis ratios all are essentially normal.[10] There are other less common varieties of pancellular HPFH.

Heterocellular HPFH

Several types of heterocellular HPFH have been described, including British, Georgia, Swiss, Atlanta, and Seattle heterocellular HPFH.[60] While both ^{G}γ and ^{A}γ are usually present, their relative proportions vary. The total percentage of Hb F is only moderately increased in all types. For example, in the British type, Hb F ranges from 18% to 21% in homozygotes and 3.5% to 10% in heterozygotes.[65] There is no anemia, and the α/non-α globin chain synthesis ratios are balanced in both homozygotes and heterozygotes.

THALASSEMIA WITH HEMOGLOBIN VARIANTS

There are numerous well documented cases of the association of thalassemia with structural hemoglobin variants.[62] A common feature is the presence of microcytic, hypochromic red cells.[7] When the same type of globin chain is affected in subjects who are heterozygous for both thalassemia and a structural hemoglobin variant, the percentage of variant hemoglobin is usually greater than when it occurs in the simple heterozygous state. Sickle hemoglobin (Hb S), Hb C, and Hb E are all β-chain variants. When these hemoglobins coexist with β thalassemia, their concentration in red cells is higher than that of Hb A. On the other hand, when the affected globin chains are different—for example, when α thalassemia is inherited together with a β-chain variant—the β-chain variant is present in lower amounts than in the simple heterozygous state. In sickle cell–α thalassemia, for instance, the Hb S concentration is lower than that of Hb A.[54]

γδβ, γ, AND δ THALASSEMIAS

Inherited alterations of the γ and δ globin gene complex and combinations of γ, δ, and β thalassemia genes also produce a broad spectrum of disorders. However, these are not nearly as common as the α or β thalassemia syndromes.

γδβ Thalassemias

The γδβ thalassemias are rare and have not been found in the homozygous state. In newborn heterozygotes, the condition is usually associated with hemolytic anemia, microcytic, hypochromic red cells, and jaundice due to the defective synthesis of γ chains.[26] There is a remission of hemolytic anemia after a few months. Adult heterozygotes have hematologic changes similar to those of β thalassemia heterozygotes, except that the Hb A_2 and F levels are normal.[14,60]

γ Thalassemias

The γ thalassemias have been described only in isolated cases. It is usually identified by an abnormal ratio of $^Gγ$ to $^Aγ$ globin chains detected in cord blood screening surveys. Infants with total absence of $^Gγ$ globin chains, resulting from homozygosity of $^Gγ$ thalassemia, are clinically asymptomatic.[22] Homozygosity for γ thalassemia affecting both the $^Gγ$ and $^Aγ$ genes would be expected to be fatal *in utero*.

δ Thalassemias

The rare homozygous and heterozygous δ thalassemias present with an absence of, or diminished levels of Hb A_2, respectively.[15] Since Hb A_2 comprises only about 2.5% of the total normal adult hemoglobin, these thalassemias are clinically insignificant[54] and produce no clinical or hematologic abnormalities.

DIFFERENTIATION OF IRON DEFICIENCY ANEMIA AND THALASSEMIA

Presenting symptoms, physical findings, and the morphologic appearance of erythrocytes in the severe thalassemia disorders are generally so distinctive that there should be no confusion with iron deficiency. When microcytic indices are first detected, without such abnormal morphology or clinical findings, iron deficiency is often the first condition considered because it is more common. However, undiagnosed mild thalassemia minor should also be ruled out in these situations.

Laboratory tests for differentiation of iron deficiency and thalassemia are summarized in Table 15-8. The results of the erythrocyte count and RDW are distinctly different,[27,57] as are iron studies, including serum ferritin,[21,24,35] serum iron, total iron-binding capacity, and transferrin saturation.[53] Iron studies are discussed in Chapter 13.

The zinc protoporphyrin/heme (ZnPP/H) ratio is a measurement of iron status that is helpful for differentiating chronic iron deficiency[29] from thalassemia minor. This test is a measurement of the amount of ZnPP that is in excess of that used for hemoglobin synthesis. Excess ZnPP forms as a result of iron-deficiency states caused by various conditions. The ZnPP test may be used in place of the free erythrocyte protoporphyrin (FEP) test, which was developed prior to the discovery of ZnPP. In the FEP test, acid extraction causes the loss of zinc, leaving FEP in the test solution. Now, ZnPP may be measured directly with a hematofluorometer. This result may then be used to calculate the ZnPP/H ratio, which is elevated in iron deficiency but normal in thalassemia minor (see Table 15-8). The

ZnPP/H ratio increase in iron deficiency may be the first biochemical change that is readily measurable following a decline in iron status.[30]

Thalassemia minor may also have to be differentiated from disorders of iron metabolism (see Table 13-1).

MOST USEFUL LABORATORY TESTS FOR DIAGNOSING THALASSEMIA

Laboratory tests that are beneficial in diagnosing thalassemia are summarized in Table 15-2.

Hemoglobin Electrophoresis

Electrophoresis on cellulose acetate medium at alkaline pH is a useful screening procedure for separating hemoglobin variants (Chap. 14) which are interacting with thalassemia and the hemoglobins of the thalassemia syndromes such as Hbs H, Barts, Constant Spring, and Lepore (see Figs. 15-3 and 15-7). Electrophoresis at alkaline pH should not be the sole diagnostic test for thalassemia trait. The Hb A_2 elevation associated with β thalassemia trait may be suspected from careful inspection of the electrophoresis strip, but it must be confirmed quantitatively. The electrophoretic pattern in α thalassemia minor and silent α thalassemia is normal except in newborns.[55]

Citrate agar electrophoresis at acid pH is useful in differentiating some abnormal hemoglobins, which migrate together on cellulose acetate (*e.g.*, Hb Lepore and Hb S, see Fig. 15-7).

Quantitation of Hb F

There are numerous situations in which the quantitation of Hb F (see procedure in Chap. 14) is beneficial to further categorize certain thalassemia conditions. Significantly elevated Hb F levels are seen in homozygous $β^0$ and $β^+$ thalassemia (Mediterranean form), δβ thalassemia, Hb Lepore, and pancellular HPFH. Moderate or slight elevations in Hb F generally are seen in thalassemia minor conditions and the heterocellular forms of HPFH.

Quantitation of Hb A_2 by Microchromatography[37]

Very small amounts of Hb A_2 (up to about 3.5%) are found in normal adults. Elevated levels of this hemoglobin, usually 4.0% to 8.0%, generally indicate β thalassemia trait, but in some cases, homozygous β thalassemia may be indicated.

Hb A_2 may also be slightly elevated in association with Hb S trait or sickle cell anemia, unstable hemoglobin variants, and megaloblastic anemias.

Decreased Hb A_2 may be found in iron deficiency anemia, Hb H disease, δ and δβ thalassemia trait, many forms of HPFH, and Hb Lepore trait.

Hb A_2 BY MICROCHROMATOGRAPHY
Principle

In ion exchange chromatography, the interaction of charged groups on the anion exchange medium with charged groups on the hemoglobin molecules results in separation of different hemoglobin fractions. At a pH above 8.5, the majority of hemoglobins bind to the anion exchange support medium. At pH 8.3, Hb A_2 is eluted from the column. The remaining hemoglobins are eluted when a buffer of lower pH is passed through the anion exchange medium. The separated hemoglobins may be quantitated by spectrophotometry.

Specimen Requirements and Preparation

EDTA blood samples are required (may be stored at 4°C up to 10 days).

1. Centrifuge sample, remove plasma, and wash erythrocytes once in isotonic saline.
2. Centrifuge again and remove supernatant saline solution.
3. Lyse erythrocytes by adding 0.4 mL distilled water to 0.05 mL erythrocytes.
4. Vortex to mix.
5. Let stand 5 minutes at room temperature.

Quality Control

A normal and an elevated Hb A_2 control sample should be run with each set of samples. Duplicate testing is not required as long as the test system is in control. Such controls are commercially available, or they may be prepared.[23,49] Any specimen stored as a control should have tested negative for hepatitis and human immunodeficiency virus (HIV) antibody.

Reagents and Equipment

Columns may be prepared by the laboratory.[37] Microcolumns, available commercially, and already packed with anion exchanger in pH 8.5 buffer, are acceptable and much more convenient. Reagents include a stock buffer from which three additional buffers (pH 8.5, 8.3, and 7.0) are prepared, all of which may be prepared in house[37] or purchased commercially. A slurry, a suspension of anion exchanger in buffer, is also required if preparing columns in the laboratory, and may be prepared or purchased and poured into the columns on the day of analysis.

Procedure

This is a general procedure. If using commercially purchased equipment and reagents, follow package insert instructions.

1. Set up columns containing pH 8.5 buffer and anion exchange medium vertically in racks. Some procedures may require allowing columns to stand for a short period and drain.
2. Remove excess pH 8.5 buffer from top of column by aspiration using a Pasteur pipet, leaving a small residual layer of buffer (about 0.05 mL) to make the next step easier.
3. Using another Pasteur pipet, carefully apply 0.05 mL hemolysate to top of column, being careful not to disturb exchange medium. If hemolysate is dilute, use 0.1 mL. Allow hemolysate to soak into the top 5 mm of the column.
4. Fill reservoir with 6 mL pH 8.3 buffer. Collect approximately 6 mL effluent dripping from the bottom of the column into a 10-mL volumetric flask. This takes approximately 1 hour and represents fraction I. Final drops of effluent appear colorless. Dilute to volume with distilled water.
5. Add 6 mL pH 7.0 buffer to top of column. Collect this 6 mL effluent, which contains all remaining hemoglobin, in a 25-mL volumetric flask and designate as fraction II. Dilute to volume with distilled water. A small amount of red-brown color may remain at the top of the column. This is normal, but no red bands should remain in the ion exchange column.
6. Mix and measure absorbance of fractions I and II at 415 nm using pH 7.0 buffer as a blank.

Calculations

$$\text{Hb } A_2 \text{ (\% of total)} = \frac{\text{A fraction I}}{\text{A fraction I} + (2.5 \times (\text{A fraction II}))} \times 100\%$$

where A fraction I = Absorbance at 415 nm of Hb A_2 eluate after diluting to 10 mL volume
A fraction II = Absorbance at 415 nm of eluate (after diluting to 25 mL volume) containing all other hemoglobins after Hb A_2 has been eluted. (Multiplying by a factor of 2.5 corrects for the difference in dilution volumes between fractions I and II.)

Reference Range

Each laboratory must establish its own reference range. As a guideline, results for normal adults established by the CDC National Hemoglobinopathy Laboratory are 1.8% to 3.5%.[8]

Sources of Error

1. If reagents prepared by the laboratory are too acidic, the pH should not be adjusted with a base because this will cause salts to form and strip the hemoglobin from the column. In this situation, the reagent should be prepared again from scratch.
2. Inaccurate pH adjustment of anion exchange medium and buffers, and bubbles in the slurry will cause erroneous results.
3. Overloading columns with hemolysate sample may cause incomplete Hb A_2 separation.
4. Insufficient hemolysate sample may make visual collection of Hb A_2 fraction impossible.
5. Hbs A_2, C, E, and O (O-Arab) coelute using the microchromatography procedure, therefore, Hb A_2 cannot be quantitated in the presence of these hemoglobins. Any measured values for Hb A_2 of 10% or more should be assumed to indicate the presence of Hb C, E, or O.

Comments

1. Hemoglobin A_2 must be measured with considerable precision, because the diagnosis of β-thalassemia trait may hinge on the determination of an Hb A_2 value only 1% to 2% above the reference range.
2. When slow-moving hemoglobin fractions such as Hb S are present, this procedure must be modified slightly. Commercial kits are available for the quantitation of Hb A_2 when variants such as Hb S are present.[2,6]
3. Other methods may be used to measure Hb A_2, including elution from segments cut from cellulose acetate followed by spectrophotometry. Measurements are also possible using densitometric scanning of electrophoretic strips, but these methods may suffer from considerable imprecision.[19]

Brilliant Cresyl Blue Test for Hb H Inclusions[6,25]

In Hb H disease, α-thalassemia trait, and silent α thalassemia, the redox dye BCB can be used to induce precipitation of intrinsically unstable Hb H. Since inclusion-containing cells may be rare in the trait and in silent forms of α thalassemia, a modified procedure that enhances the development of Hb H inclusions is described.

BRILLIANT CRESYL BLUE STAIN FOR Hb H
Principle

Cells containing an unstable hemoglobin, such as Hb H, normally are removed promptly from the circulation by the reticuloendothelial system. When relatively young erythrocytes containing sufficient Hb H to form inclusions are released to the circulation, they are diluted in a population of cells with more nearly balanced globin chain synthesis and a normal life span.

When a blood sample is centrifuged to separate plasma and cells, the red cells taken from just below the buffy coat consist primarily of young, buoyant cells. These young cells are the most capable of forming the typical Hb H inclusions if α thalassemia is in fact present. Hb H inclusions, if present, are stained by BCB and may be viewed microscopically on blood films after staining.

Specimen Requirements

Fresh whole blood anticoagulated with EDTA.

Reagents

For 1% BCB solution combine sodium citrate, 0.4 g; normal saline, 100 mL; and BCB, 1.0 g. Filter before using. Solution must be stored in a dark bottle.

Quality Control

A significant number of reticulocytes should be visible on the patient specimen. If there are no reticulocytes, the specimen may not have been concentrated properly during preparation.

Procedure

1. Fill four microhematocrit tubes with blood and seal. Spin in microhematocrit centrifuge for 5 minutes. Score and break tubes approximately 3 mm above and 5 mm below the plasma-cell meniscus.
2. Expel contents of the four tube sections into a 12 × 75-mm test tube. Add 1 to 1½ drops of BCB stain to test tube and mix. Incubate at 37°C for 30 minutes.
3. Fill one microhematocrit tube with BCB-cell mixture. Balance this tube with an empty tube in microhematocrit centrifuge and spin for 5 minutes. Score and break tube approximately 4 mm below BCB-cell meniscus.
4. Expel cells and small amount of BCB solution onto microscope slide and mix. Remove buffy coat if it is expelled onto the slide.
5. Make a smear as for blood film. Let dry. Examine film under × 100 oil immersion lens for 20 minutes. This equates to looking at approximately 50,000 red cells. Count the number of cells with inclusions and report as number per 50,000 cells reviewed.

Interpretation of Results

Hemoglobin H inclusions, consisting of denatured β globin chains, typically appear as small, multiple, irregularly shaped greenish blue bodies with a pitted pattern similar to that of golf balls (see Fig. 14-10B). They usually are fairly uniformly distributed throughout the erythrocyte.

Almost all red cells contain inclusions in Hb H disease, whereas few to several cells may contain inclusions in α-thalassemia trait. Rare cells, perhaps as few as 1 in 50,000, may be positive in silent α thalassemia. Negative BCB results do not necessarily exclude the trait or silent forms of α thalassemia.

Comments and Sources of Error

1. Hb H inclusions must be distinguished from reticulocytes on the specimen film. Reticulocytes have a bluish purple, irregular, granular or filamentous pattern.
2. If conditions favor Heinz body formation (Chap. 14; see Fig. 14-10A), these red cell inclusions can be differentiated from Hb H inclusions by the fact that Heinz bodies are larger, fewer in number, and most often appear eccentrically along the membrane of the red cell.
3. Hb H is not entirely specific to α thalassemia, since rare

patients with erythroleukemia, granulocytic leukemia, or other myeloproliferative disorders have been described with this abnormality.

4. Gloves should be worn to perform this procedure.
5. Each BCB dye lot must be tested against red cells known to contain Hb H, since individual lots of dye vary in their ability to produce satisfactory preparations.

Acid Elution Slide Test for Hb F[8,28]

Frequently the intracellular distribution of Hb F is used to differentiate thalassemias with increased Hb F from pancellular HPFH. In thalassemia, there is nonuniform (heterogeneous) distribution of Hb F from cell to cell (i.e., some cells contain Hb F and some do not). In pancellular HPFH, all erythrocytes show nearly uniform (homogeneous) retention of Hb F.

It is important to recognize that a heterogeneous distribution of Hb F may also be found in sickle cell anemia and other hemoglobinopathies (Chap. 14), as well as in acquired aplastic anemia (Chap. 11), owing to the elevated Hb F concentration in these disorders.

ACID ELUTION OF Hb F
Principle

Blood films are prepared and fixed. All hemoglobins, with the exception of Hb F, are eluted from the red cell by citric acid-phosphate buffer at acid pH (3.3 to 3.5). Following the elution procedure, blood films are stained with Ehrlich acid hematoxylin and counterstained with erythrosin (eosin B; 0.1 w/v). Slides are then examined microscopically under high, dry magnification.

Specimen Requirements

Either EDTA-anticoagulated blood or blood obtained by microcollection may be used.

Quality Control

A known normal sample and a known sample of HPFH should be run with each set of slides. If a known HPFH sample cannot be obtained, an abnormal control is prepared by mixing 1 drop normal adult blood with 1 drop fresh cord blood, both of which must be ABO blood group compatible.

Procedure

1. Incubate citric acid–phosphate buffer in Coplin jar covered with Parafilm for 30 minutes at 37°C.
2. Dilute patient sample, normal, and abnormal control 1:1 with normal saline.
3. Make thin blood films using the patient, normal, and abnormal control specimens. Allow to air dry for 10 to 60 minutes.
4. Fix blood films in 80% (v/v) ethyl alcohol for 5 minutes. Rinse gently with distilled water.
5. Incubate slides in 37°C citric acid–phosphate buffer (step 1 above) for 6 minutes. Occasionally lift slides up and down to provide gentle agitation during incubation.
6. After 6 minutes, remove slides and rinse with distilled water. Stain in hematoxylin for 3 minutes. Rinse with distilled water. Counterstain with erythrosin for 3 minutes. Rinse with distilled water and air dry.
7. Examine under high, dry magnification using light microscopy.

Interpretation of Results

Cells containing Hb F will be stained bright pink to red, whereas normal adult cells that do not contain Hb F appear as "ghost cells" (only the outer cell membrane is visible).

Comments and Sources of Error

1. The elution time and pH of the citric acid–phosphate buffer must be carefully controlled.
2. High, dry magnification should be used to examine as much of the stained slide as possible. It is actually more difficult to focus on the acid-eluted and stained specimen using oil immersion microscopy, owing to the faint appearance of the ghost cells.
3. Kits are commercially available that measure the distribution of Hb F in red cells. Such kits may help to standardize the procedure, particularly in laboratories where this test is performed infrequently.
4. There are instances when the differentiation of HPFH and thalassemia may be difficult, even in laboratories with personnel experienced in looking at samples from patients with these disorders.

SPECIAL LABORATORY PROCEDURES FOR DIAGNOSING THALASSEMIA

Specialized testing, including globin chain synthesis and DNA analysis, may be performed to identify thalassemia and to elucidate specific genotypes when a conclusive diagnosis cannot be made by routine laboratory tests. On a case-by-case basis, the physician and laboratory personnel must decide whether the benefit of a complete diagnosis warrants the expense of further specialized testing.

Globin chain synthesis studies reveal the ratio of α to non-α globin chains. This is accomplished by incubating reticulocytes with a "radioactive" amino acid, usually leucine. The radioactive globin chains are then precipitated and separated by column chromatography. The fractions are counted for radioactivity, and the rate of synthesis for each chain is calculated to determine the production ratio of α to non-α chains.[8]

DNA analysis is also useful, both in the diagnosis of some thalassemias and in prenatal diagnosis. The procedure requires special equipment and reagents, as described elsewhere.[8] DNA analysis is usually required in special situations when a patient's genotype is necessary to make a diagnosis for proper treatment or for genetic counseling purposes.

CHAPTER SUMMARY

The thalassemias are a heterogeneous group of hereditary disorders found worldwide. They result from varied genetic mutations that lead to a quantitative reduction in globin chain synthesis. The α and β thalassemias are the most prevalent and result from a decrease in the synthesis of α or β globin chains.

The primary cause of α thalassemia is gene deletion; however, nondeletion types have been described. Infants with Barts hydrops fetalis (four α genes deleted) usually are stillborn and have severe hemolytic anemia. Hb H disease (three α genes deleted) causes mild to moderately severe hemolytic anemia. The two- and one-α gene deletions are essentially benign. Major hematologic features of the α thalassemias are summarized in Table 15-4.

The β thalassemias are classified as β° and β^+. In β° thalassemia, no β globin chains are produced by the mutant gene, whereas in β^+ thalassemia, some β globin chains are produced. Unlike α thalassemia, most β thalassemias are due not to gene deletion but to point mutations in the DNA genetic code. The β thalassemias, associated with various mutations in the β globin gene, may present as severe (thalassemia major), moderate (thalassemia intermedia), or benign (thalassema minor or minima) clinical syndromes.

Synthesis of other globin chains may also be impaired. For example, HPFH defines the persistence of Hb F synthesis throughout adult life without an associated thalassemia. Evidently, γ chain synthesis is able to compensate for the absence or decrease of β and δ globin production. In another group of related disorders, the $\delta\beta$ thalassemias, there is a decrease in or no β or δ globin synthesis but an increase in γ-chain synthesis. The increase in γ-chain synthesis is not as great as that in HPFH, and therefore a thalassemic phenotype results. Laboratory findings for some of the β thalassemias are summarized in Tables 15-6 and 15-7. Additionally, thalassemias and hemoglobinopathies may coexist (*e.g.*, Hb S/β° thalassemia).

Most thalassemias can be diagnosed by doing a few carefully selected laboratory procedures (see Table 15-2). Differentiation of thalassemia minor and iron deficiency through laboratory studies (see Table 15-8) is also important for appropriate patient therapy.

Treatment of symptomatic thalassemia generally consists of blood transfusion with the regular provision of chelating agents to help control iron overload. The vast majority of thalassemias are benign and do not require treatment.

CASE STUDY 15-1

A 22-year-old Italian man was hospitalized with a broken leg. He had always been in good general health, and this was his first hospitalization. Laboratory tests were ordered and the results (and corresponding reference ranges) were as follows: hematocrit 0.40 L/L (0.41–0.53); Hb 13.3 g/dL (13.5–17.5); RBC 6.35 × 10^{12}/L (4.7–6.1); MCV 63 fL (82–100); MCH 21 pg (27–33); MCHC 32 g/dL (31–35); WBC 7.4 × 10^9/L (4.0–10.0); serum iron 110 g/dL (65–165); TIBC 320 g/dL (300–360); percent transferrin saturation 34% (20–50); hemoglobin electrophoresis in cellulose acetate at alkaline pH, Hb A 92.2% (> 95%); Hb F 2.1% (< 1.0%): Hb A$_2$ 5.7% (1.8%–3.5%).

1. What diagnosis do these laboratory data suggest? Why?
2. What would be the expected red cell morphology on the Wright-stained peripheral blood film?
3. Does this diagnosed condition require treatment?
4. What is the life expectancy of this patient?
5. If the male in this case mated with a female who is heterozygous for β thalassemia (β°/β), what are the predicted chances that their offspring will be normal, homozygous, and heterozygous for thalassemia?

CASE STUDY 15-2

A 17-year-old Southeast Asian girl presented with a chronic, moderate, microcytic, hypochromic anemia. She had an enlarged spleen but was otherwise physically normal. Her reticulocyte count was increased to 5%. There was no anemia in her father's history, but her mother had a very mild, microcytic anemia with no associated clinical disabilities.

1. A complete blood count has already determined that the patient was moderately anemic. Since this probably is a hereditary disorder and the patient is Southeast Asian, what laboratory test might next be ordered?

2. Given the suspected diagnosis of an α-thalassemia syndrome, what is the probable genotype of this patient and why?

3. What are the most probable genotypes of the mother and father?

4. Considering the patient's suspected genotype, what results would be expected of the laboratory test recommended in answer No. 1?

REFERENCES

1. Baglioni C: The fusion of two peptide chains in hemoglobin Lepore and its interpretation as a genetic deletion. Proc Natl Acad Sci USA 48:1880, 1962

2. Baine RM, Brown HG: Evaluation of a commercial kit for microchromatographic quantitation of hemoglobin A_2 in the presence of hemoglobin S. Clin Chem 27:1244, 1981

3. Beaven GH, Coleman PN, White JC: Occurrence of haemoglobin H in leukaemia: A further case of erythroleukaemia. Acta Haematol 59:37, 1978

4. Beaven GH, Stevens BL, Dance N et al: Occurrence of haemoglobin H in leukaemia. Nature 199:1297, 1963

5. Bessman JD: New parameters on automated hematology instruments. Lab Med 14:488, 1983

6. Brown BA: Hematology: Principles and Procedures, 5th ed. Philadelphia, Lea & Febiger, 1988

7. Bunn HF, Forget BG: Hemoglobin: Molecular, Genetic and Clinical Aspects. Philadelphia, WB Saunders, 1986

8. Centers for Disease Control: Laboratory Methods for Detecting Hemoglobinopathies. Division of Host Factors, Center for Infectious Diseases, Centers for Disease Control, Atlanta, GA, 1984

9. Charache S, Conley CL, Doeblin TD et al: Thalassemia in black Americans. Ann NY Acad Sci 232:125, 1974

10. Conley CL, Weatherall DJ, Richardson SN et al: Hereditary persistence of fetal hemoglobin. A study of 79 affected persons in 15 Negro families in Baltimore. Blood 21:261, 1963

11. de Alarcon PA, Donovan ME, Forbes GB et al: Iron absorption in the thalassemia syndromes and its inhibition by tea. N Engl J Med 300:5, 1979

12. Dozy AM, Kan YW, Embury SH et al: α-Globin gene organisation in blacks precludes the severe form of α-thalassemia. Nature 280:605, 1979

13. Fairbanks VF: Hemoglobinopathies and Thalassemias. Laboratory Methods and Case Studies. New York, BC Decker, 1980

14. Fearon ER, Kazazian HH, Waber PG et al: The entire β-globin gene cluster is deleted in a form of $\gamma\delta\beta$-thalassemia. Blood 61:1269, 1983

15. Fessas P, Stamatoyannopoulos G: Absence of haemoglobin A_2 in an adult. Nature 195:1215, 1962

16. Fishleder AJ, Hoffman GC: A practical approach to the detection of hemoglobinopathies: Part I. The introduction and thalassemia syndromes. Lab Med 18:368, 1987

17. Friedman MJ: Oxidant damage mediates variant red cell resistance to malaria. Nature 280:245, 1979

18. Friedman SH, Atwater J, Gill FM et al: α-Thalassemia in Negro infants. Pediatr Res 8:955, 1974

19. Hamilton SR, Miller ME, Jessop M et al: Comparison of microchromatography and electrophoresis with elution of hemoglobin (Hb A_2) quantitation. Am J Clin Pathol 71:388, 1979

20. Higgs DR, Pressley L, Aldridge BE et al: Genetic and molecular diversity in nondeletion Hb H disease. Proc Natl Acad Sci USA 78:5833, 1981

21. Hillman RS, Finch CA: Red Cell Manual, 5th ed. Philadelphia, FA Davis, 1985

22. Huisman THJ, Reese MB, Gardiner MB et al: The occurrence of different levels of $^A\gamma$ chain and of the $^A\gamma$T variant of fetal hemoglobin in newborn babies from several countries. Am J Hematol 14:133, 1983

23. Huntsman RG, Carrell RW, White JM: Recommendations for selected methods for quantitative estimation of Hb A_2 and for Hb A_2 reference preparation. International Committee for Standardization in Haematology. Br J Haematol 38:573, 1978

24. Hussein HS, Hoffbrand AV, Leulicht M et al: Serum ferritin levels in β-thalassaemia trait. Br Med J Clin Res 2:920, 1976

25. Jones JA, Broszeit HK, LeCrone CN et al: An improved method for detection of red cell hemoglobin H inclusions. Am J Med Technol 47:94, 1981

26. Kan YW, Forget BG, Nathan DG: Gamma-beta–thalassemia: A cause of hemolytic disease of the newborn. N Engl J Med 286:129, 1972

27. Klee GG, Fairbanks VF, Pierre RV et al: Routine erythrocyte measurements in diagnosis of iron deficiency anemia and thalassemia minor. Am J Clin Pathol 66:870, 1976

28. Kleihauer E, Braun H, Betke K: Demonstration van fetalem Hamoglobin in den Erythrocyten eines Blutausstrichs. Klin Wochenschr 35:637, 1957

29. Labbe RF, Lamon JM: Porphyrins and disorders of porphyrin metabolism. In Tietz NW (ed): Fundamentals of Clinical Chemistry, 3rd ed. p 839, Philadelphia, WB Saunders, 1987

30. Labbe RF, Rettmer RL: Zinc protoporphyrin: A product of iron-deficient erythropoiesis. Semin Hematol 26:40, 1989

31. LeCrone CN, Detter JC: Screening for hemoglobinopathies and thalassemia. J Med Technol 2:389, 1985

32. Lopez CG, Lie-Injo LE: Alpha-thalassemia in newborns in West Malaysia. Hum Hered 21:185, 1971

33. Malamos B, Fessas P, Stamatoyannopoulos G: Types of thalassemia-trait carriers as revealed by a study of their incidence in Greece. Br J Haematol 8:5, 1962

34. Mazza U, Saglio G, Cappio FC et al: Clinical and haematological data in 254 cases of β-thalassemia trait in Italy. Br J Haematol 33:91, 1976

35. Mehta BC, Pandya BG: Iron status of β-thalassemia carriers. Am J Hematol 24:137, 1987

36. Na-Nakorn S, Wasi P, Suingdumrong A: Hemoglobin H disease in Thailand. Clinical and hematological studies in 138 cases. Isr J Med Sci 1:762, 1965

37. National Committee for Clinical Laboratory Standards: Standard for the Chromatographic (Microcolumn) Determination of Hemoglobin A_2, H9A, vol 8. Villanova, PA, NCCLS, 1989

38. Nienhuis AW, Anagnou NP, Ley TJ: Advances in thalassemia research. Blood 63:738, 1984

39. O'Brien RT: The effect of iron deficiency on the expression of hemoglobin H. Blood 41:853, 1973

40. Old J, Longley J, Wood WG et al: Molecular basis for acquired haemoglobin H disease. Nature 269:524, 1977

41. Orkin SH: Prenatal diagnosis of hemoglobin disorders by DNA analysis. Blood 63:249, 1984

42. Orkin SH, Old J, Lazarus H et al: The molecular basis of α-thalassemia: Frequent occurrence of dysfunctional α loci among non-Asians with Hb H disease. Cell 17:33, 1979

43. Pearson HA, McPhedran P, O'Brien RT et al: Comprehensive testing for thalassemia trait. Ann NY Acad Sci 232:135, 1974

44. Pearson HA, O'Brien RT, McIntosh S: Screening for thalassemia trait by electronic measurement of mean corpuscular volume. N Engl J Med 288:351, 1973

45. Pippard MJ, Callender ST, Warner GT et al: Iron absorption and loading in β-thalassaemia intermedia. Lancet 2:819, 1979

46. Pootrakul SN, Wasi P, Pornpatkul M et al: Incidence of α-thalassemia in Bangkok. J Med Assoc Thai 53:250, 1970

47. Pootrakul P, Wasi P, Na-Nakorn S: Haematological data in 312 cases of β-thalassaemia trait in Thailand. Br J Haematol 24:703, 1973

48. Pressley L, Higgs DR, Clegg JB et al: Gene deletions in α-thalassemia prove that the 5' ζ locus is functional. Proc Natl Acad Sci USA 77:3586, 1980

49. Schmidt RM, Brosious EM, Wright JM: Preparation and use of

a quality control hemolysate for microchromatographic determinations of Hb A$_2$. Am J Clin Pathol 67:215, 1977

50. Schroeder WA, Huisman THJ, Brown AK et al: Postnatal changes in the chemical heterogeneity of human fetal hemoglobin. Pediatr Res 5:493, 1971

51. Shchory M, Ramot B: Globin chain synthesis in the marrow and reticulocytes of β-thalassemia, hemoglobin H disease and βδ-thalassemia. Blood 40:105, 1972

52. Stamatoyannopoulos G, Nienhuis AW, Leder P et al: The Molecular Basis of Blood Diseases. Philadelphia, WB Saunders, 1987

53. Tietz NW (ed): Textbook of Clinical Chemistry. Philadelphia, WB Saunders, 1986

54. Todd D: Thalassemia. Pathology 16:5, 1984

55. University of Washington, Department of Laboratory Medicine: Handbook of Diagnostic Tests for Intrinsic Hemolytic Disorders and Thalassemia. Seattle, University of Washington, 1988

56. Veer A, Kosciolek BA, Bauman AW et al: Acquired hemoglobin H disease in idiopathic myelofibrosis. Am J Hematol 6:199, 1979

57. Walford DM, McPherson K, Deacon R: Discrimination between iron deficiency and heterozygous thalassaemia. Lancet 1:323, 1979

58. Wasi P, Na-Nakorn S, Pootrakul S: The α-thalassemias. Clin Haematol 3:383, 1974

59. Wasi P, Na-Nakorn S, Pootrakul S et al: Alpha- and beta-thalassemia in Thailand. Ann NY Acad Sci 165:60, 1969

60. Weatherall DJ (ed): The Thalassemias. Edinburgh, Churchill Livingstone, 1983

61. Weatherall DJ: Abnormal haemoglobins in the neonatal period and their relationship to thalassaemia. Br J Haematol 9:265, 1963

62. Weatherall DJ, Clegg JB: The Thalassaemia Syndromes, 3rd ed. Oxford, Blackwell Scientific Publications, 1981

63. Weatherall DJ, Higgs DR, Bunch C et al: Hemoglobin H disease and mental retardation. N Engl J Med 305:607, 1981

64. Winter WP (ed): CRC Hemoglobin Variants in Human Populations, vol 1. Boca Raton, FL, CRC Press, 1986

65. Wood WG, MacRae IA, Darbre PD et al: The British type of non-deletion HPFH: Characterization of developmental changes in vivo and erythroid growth in vitro. Br J Haematol 50:401, 1982

66. Wood WG, Weatherall DJ, Hart GH et al: Hematologic changes and hemoglobin analysis in β-thalassemia heterozygotes during the first year of life. Pediatr Res 16:286, 1982

67. Yoo D, Schechter GP, Amigable AN et al: Myeloproliferative syndrome with sideroblastic anemia and acquired hemoglobin H disease. Cancer 45:78, 1980

68. Zaizov R, Matoth Y: α-Thalassemia in Yemenite and Iraqi Jews. Isr J Med Sci 8:11, 1972

Introduction to Anemias of Increased Erythrocyte Destruction

Janice H. Parrish

Anemias may result from either decreased erythrocyte production or increased erythrocyte loss or destruction. When the rate of destruction exceeds the bone marrow's capacity to produce red cells, hemolytic anemia results. Since a normal bone marrow can increase its rate of production by as much as six to eight times normal, the red cell life span must be significantly shortened for anemia to develop. The term "hemolytic anemia" or "anemia of increased destruction" should be reserved for cases in which the rate of erythrocyte destruction is accelerated and the bone marrow is normal but is not capable of keeping up with the destruction.[12] The term implies increased erythrocyte destruction and production.

Some anemias result from a combination of decreased production and increased destruction. In megaloblastic anemias and thalassemias, decreased production is the major underlying problem. Because many of the developing red cells are very abnormal, there is even increased destruction of the cells before they leave the bone marrow (dyserythropoiesis or ineffective erythropoiesis). Other anemias, such as those associated with iron deficiency and chronic disease, may also have a somewhat shortened red cell life span. These anemias are said to have a hemolytic component, but because hemolysis is not the primary underlying cause, they should not be called hemolytic anemias.[41]

CLASSIFICATION

Hemolytic anemias may be classified according to several schemes (Table 16-1). Traditional classifications have included inherited and acquired disorders. Others have categorized hemolytic anemias according to the type of red cell defect—intrinsic or extrinsic. An intrinsic defect is one in which the patient's erythrocytes would not survive normally when transfused into a normal recipient (*i.e,* the erythrocytes themselves are defective). Transfused normal red cells have a normal life span in patients with an intrinsic red cell defect. An extrinsic defect is defined as one in which the life span of normal red cells would be shortened if they were transfused into the patient under investigation but the patient's red cells would survive normally if given to a normal recipient. Extrinsic defects result from abnormal environmental factors that damage normal red cells.

Most inherited hemolytic anemias are due to defects intrinsic to the erythrocyte (see Table 16-1). These defects may affect any part of the cell—the membrane (Chap. 17), metabolic systems (*i.e.,* enzyme deficiencies; Chap. 17), or hemoglobin molecule (*i.e.,* hemoglobinopathies; Chap. 14). Some inherited anemias are evident in infancy, while others do not become evident until adulthood.[27]

Most extrinsic hemolytic anemias are acquired (see Table 16-1). Red cells coated with antibodies or complement (Chap. 19), or damaged by some abnormal environmental factor (Chap. 18) or by liver or renal disease have a shortened life span, which may result in anemia. Prolonged sequestration of red cells in a hyperactive spleen (hypersplenism) can cause significant red cell destruction.

Abetalipoproteinemia and lecithin-cholesterol acyltransferase (LCAT) deficiency (Chap. 17) are examples of inherited disorders in which hemolysis is due to an extrinsic defect. These extremely rare disorders cause abnormalities in plasma lipids, which result in an erythrocyte membrane defect and subsequent hemolysis.

Another proposed method of classifying hemolytic anemias combines the mean corpuscular volume (MCV) with the red cell distribution width (RDW).[6] With this method, hemolytic anemias are placed in several categories; however, the utility of this system is still under investigation.

SITES OF ERYTHROCYTE HEMOLYSIS

Extravascular Sites

Most destruction of both normal and abnormal erythrocytes occurs in the organs of the reticuloendothelial system (RES), which include the spleen, lymph nodes, bone marrow, and liver. Most RES cells are fixed and free macrophages. The liver's RE cells are called Kupffer cells. There are also scavenger cells in the lungs called alveolar macrophages. The endothelial cells lining the sinuses in the liver, bone marrow, spleen, and lymph nodes are also considered part of the RES, as are circulating monocytes. Some hematologists now use the term *mononuclear phagocyte system* (MPS) for the RES, but the terms RES and MPS may be used interchangeably.[1] The term *extravascular hemolysis* is used to describe red cell destruction that occurs by phagocytosis of intact or fragmented red cells in the RES with release of hemoglobin into the macrophages.

In an immune reaction, cells in the circulation may become coated by immunoglobulin. Subsequently, the complement system cascade is initiated, which leads to generation of an intermediate complement component known as

TABLE 16–1. Classification of Hemolytic Anemias

INTRINSIC HEMOLYTIC ANEMIAS
Hereditary
Membrane defects
Hereditary spherocytosis
Hereditary elliptocytosis
Hereditary pyropoikilocytosis
Enzyme defects
G6PD deficiency
Pyruvate kinase deficiency
Glutathione reductase deficiency
Hemoglobinopathies
Hemoglobin SS, CC, SC, and S–β thalassemia
Acquired
Paroxysmal nocturnal hemoglobinuria
EXTRINSIC HEMOLYTIC ANEMIAS
Hereditary
LCAT deficiency
Abetalipoproteinemia
Acquired
Immune mediated
Mechanical, thermal, chemical damage
Infectious agents
Hypersplenism
Secondary to liver or renal disease
Secondary to hypertension

C3b (Chap. 19). Cells coated with immunoglobulin and complement may be destroyed by the liver Kupffer cell macrophages since they have receptors for the complement component C3b. Attachment of C3b to the red cell surface is generally associated with extravascular hemolysis in the liver.

Severely damaged cells that enter the circulation may also be destroyed by the Kupffer cell macrophages. Clearance of cells correlates with the extent of shape alteration. In one study, 50% to 80% of cells that were extreme forms of echinocytes and stomatocytes were cleared by the liver. Cells that were only mildly altered and retained their disc shape were cleared principally by the spleen.[11]

Because of the unique structure of the splenic circulation, most destruction of both abnormal and normal (120-day-old) red cells occurs in this organ. The spleen consists of two functional parts called the red and the white pulp (Fig. 16-1). The white pulp (lymph nodes) consists of a germinal center, where lymphocytes are produced, and the periarterial lymphatic sheath, which contains lymphocytes. Most phagocytic activity occurs in the red pulp. It contains a system of vascular channels called sinuses. The areas separating the sinuses, called splenic cords, contain a high concentration of macrophages. The marginal zone is a spongy network filled with blood cells that separates the red and white pulp.

Blood flows into the spleen through the splenic artery, which branches into multiple central arteries. Right angle vascular branches skim off a portion of the plasma, causing hemoconcentration in the central artery. A portion of the blood in a central artery empties directly into the sinuses, or very near them where the venous system collects the blood. The other portion empties into the cordal tissue of the red pulp or into the marginal zone separating the red and white pulp. Red cells that arrive in this cordal area must slowly make their way into the venous sinuses, passing through openings in the wall (only 3 μm in diameter) that separate

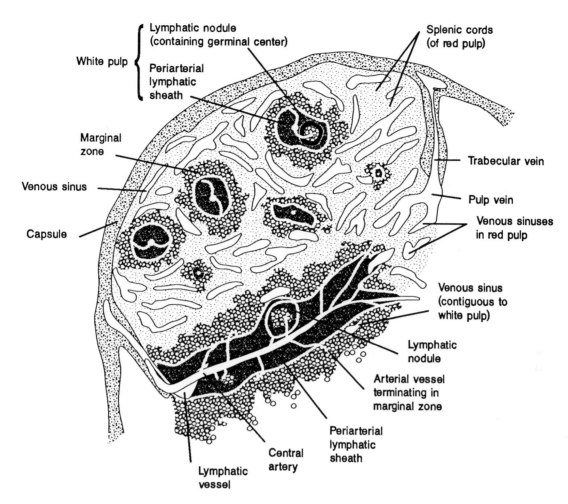

FIG. 16-1. Structure of the spleen. The white pulp consists of the periarterial lymphatic sheath and lymphatic nodules with germinal centers. The red pulp contains the splenic cords and sinuses. The marginal zone is interposed between white and red pulp. The central artery sends branches out into the marginal zone and then terminates in the red pulp. Blood from the splenic cords passes through a fenestrated wall into the sinuses and is then collected in the splenic veins. (Reprinted with permission of the publisher from Weiss L, Greep RO. Histology. Copyright 1977 by Elsevier Science Publishing Co, Inc, New York, NY.)

the cords from the sinuses.[2,16,31] Since the average red cell is 7μm in diameter, this slow, tortuous passage requires that red cells be easily deformable. It also brings them into prolonged contact with splenic macrophages and exposes them to conditions of low glucose concentration[25] and low pH,[33] which may lead to membrane damage. Blood leaves the spleen by way of the venous drainage system in the red pulp. Blood flows out through the trabecular vein into the portal circulation on its way to the liver.

Red cells that have lived their 120-day life span are termed *senescent*. As the erythrocyte ages, its ability to produce energy declines. Repeated passes through the spleen deplete the cells of glucose and decrease their surface area.[16] The spleen apparently recognizes subtle abnormalities in senescent cells and sequesters and destroys them. It also removes abnormal red cells that are not yet senescent. This process of removing senescent and abnormal red cells is termed *culling*.

Erythrocytes that contain inclusions (Chap. 8) are too rigid to pass easily through the spleen. Macrophages re-

move the inclusions along with a piece of the red cell membrane and a film of hemoglobin while leaving the red cell intact. This process is known as *pitting*. Patients without a spleen typically have a few circulating red cells that contain inclusions.

There are several conditions under which a red cell is unable to pass safely through the splenic circulation. Alterations in the membrane or increased volume can affect its flexibility. Pieces of membrane may be removed by macrophages, which recognize antibodies or complement attached to the red cell surface. Cells may also be rigid because of poor hemoglobin solubility. Difficulty in squeezing through the walls of the splenic sinuses can cause further damage. Eventually the cell is trapped and phagocytized.

If the spleen is enlarged, the splenic circulation is even more sluggish than normal. Cells with very mild abnormalities may lyse more readily than they would in a normal spleen. Increased splenic hemolysis causes further splenic enlargement.[23] Liver disease can cause both erythrocyte membrane abnormalities[10] and splenic congestion. As the abnormal red cells attempt to pass through the congested spleen, they are subject to damage, which eventually leads to hemolysis and more splenic enlargement.[24]

Intravascular Sites

When erythrocytes are severely damaged in the circulation they may be destroyed without phagocytic cell involvement. This *intravascular hemolysis* results in release of hemoglobin directly into the plasma. Intravascular hemolysis accounts for a small portion of normal erythrocyte destruction. It may be the predominant mode of hemolysis in extrinsic hemolytic anemias.

Intravascular hemolysis that is complement mediated involves more complement components than those associated with extravascular hemolysis, in which the final component leading to red cell destruction is generally C3b. When complement is further activated in intravascular hemolysis, a complex known as *C5b6789,* otherwise known as the *membrane attack unit* or *terminal complex,* is ultimately formed. This complex is so named because it is capable of penetrating the red cell surface, causing formation of a transmembrane pore. This damage may result in leakage of hemoglobin and other cellular components or osmotic swelling due to excessive permeability to water and electrolytes, both of which produce intravascular hemolysis. One example of this mechanism is found in hemolytic transfusion reactions due to major ABO incompatibility (Chap. 19).

There are several types of mechanical damage that can cause intravascular hemolysis (Chap. 18). In microangiopathic hemolytic anemias (MAHAs), which classically demonstrate red cell fragments on the blood film, red cells may be ruptured, for example, as they pass through diseased vessels or small vessels blocked by fibrin strands, a diseased cardiac valve, or a defective prosthetic valve. Malarial infestation, *Clostridium* septicemia, and severe kidney or liver disease may also cause intravascular hemolysis and anemia. Rare cases of intravascular hemolysis are caused by exposure to chemicals, physical trauma, and severe burns (Chap. 18).

ERYTHROCYTE CATABOLISM

Extravascular Hemolysis

When an erythrocyte is phagocytized in the extravascular system, the hemoglobin molecule is broken down into heme and globin in the phagocytic cell (Fig. 16-2). The globin chains are catabolized, and the amino acids are returned to the amino acid pool to be used again. Iron is released from heme, bound to the protein carrier molecule transferrin, and recycled. The enzyme heme oxidase opens the heme molecule to produce carbon monoxide and *biliverdin*. Biliverdin is immediately reduced to *bilirubin,* and released carbon monoxide is subsequently expired. Bilirubin is released from the macrophage into the plasma, where it binds to albumin and is carried to the liver. At this stage, it is termed *unconjugated (or indirect) bilirubin*. It is insoluble in water but highly soluble in fat. If the albumin-binding capacity is exceeded, unconjugated bilirubin is deposited in tissues that have a high lipid content.

Unconjugated bilirubin dissociates from albumin and passes across the hepatocyte membrane into the liver parenchymal cells. About 40% of this bilirubin flows back into the plasma, which accounts for the increase in unconjugated bilirubin in hemolytic anemias.[3] In the liver, bilirubin is conjugated with glucuronic acid by the enzyme glucuronyl transferase to form bilirubin diglucuronide. This form of bilirubin, called *conjugated (or direct) bilirubin,* is soluble in water but poorly soluble in lipids.

Conjugated bilirubin is excreted from the liver into the bile ducts by an active transport mechanism. The ducts direct the bile into the duodenum. In the terminal ileum and colon, the conjugated bilirubin is converted by bacterial enzymes into a group of pigments called *urobilinogens*. The majority of urobilinogen is excreted in the stool. Some urobilinogen is reabsorbed into the enterohepatic circulation, but most returns to the gastrointestinal tract. A small portion of urobilinogen is excreted into the urine.[28]

Intravascular Hemolysis

In intravascular hemolysis (or excessive extravascular hemolysis), free hemoglobin may be released directly into the plasma, where it typically exists in α-β dimers (Fig. 16-3). The free hemoglobin is bound to the plasma protein *haptoglobin*. The hemoglobin-haptoglobin complex is transported to the liver, where heme catabolism proceeds in the parenchymal cells along the extravascular pathway of degradation. Once haptoglobin releases hemoglobin in the liver, it is destroyed; it is not recycled.[9] Therefore, the haptoglobin level may be used as an indicator of the degree of hemolysis occurring *in vivo*.

The hemoglobin-haptoglobin complex is too large to pass the glomerulus; however, when the haptoglobin-binding capacity is exceeded, free hemoglobin may be detected in the plasma and filtered by the kidney into the urine. A certain amount of free hemoglobin is reabsorbed by the proximal tubules and degraded into bilirubin, but a portion of the iron is left in the renal epithelial cells as ferritin or hemosiderin.[36] Since renal epithelial cells are not capable of recycling iron, hemosiderinuria results within a few days as these cells are naturally sloughed into the urine. In severe hemolytic states, the maximum rate of reabsorption is exceeded and free hemoglobin passes into the urine, resulting in hemoglobinuria and methemoglobinuria.[34]

In the plasma, some free hemoglobin is taken up by the liver and some is oxidized to methemoglobin, from which the heme molecule and globin chains are readily extracted. Free heme is bound to the plasma protein *hemopexin*. Like haptoglobin, hemopexin is destroyed once it serves its function of delivering the heme molecule to the liver; however, hemopexin levels are not as indicative of hemolysis as haptoglobin levels. In severe hemolysis, when sufficient hemopexin is not available, the free heme is oxidized and bound to albumin to form *methemalbumin*. This complex remains in the plasma until more hemopexin is produced and made available by the liver. The heme from the heme-hemopexin complexes and hemoglobin-haptoglobin complexes is converted to bilirubin in the liver, conjugated with glucuronic acid, and excreted as urobilinogen through the gastrointestinal tract (see Fig. 16-3).[9,17]

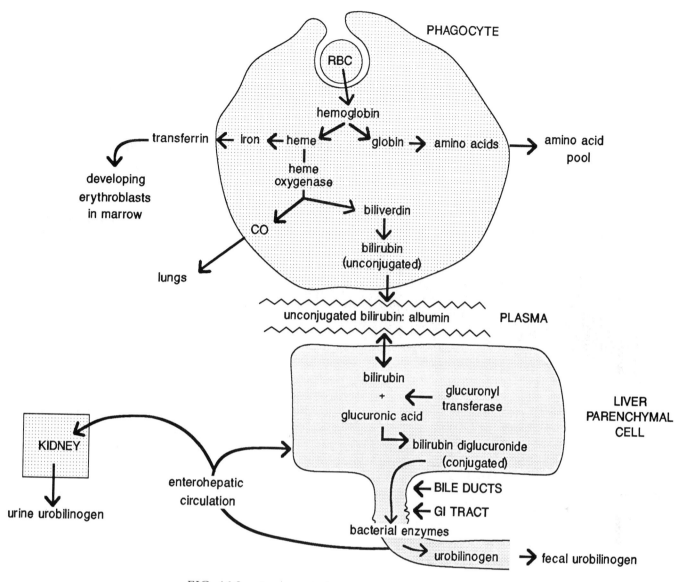

FIG. 16-2. A schematic diagram of extravascular hemolysis.

LABORATORY FINDINGS AND CORRELATIONS WITH DISEASE

In a patient with the usual complaints related to anemia, the presence of jaundice, splenomegaly, or occasionally dark urine suggests a hemolytic process. To establish hemolysis, laboratory data must show that both erythrocyte destruction and production are increased without evidence of blood loss. Table 16-2 summarizes the laboratory findings in hemolytic anemias. The results of tests marked in Table 16-2 for initial screening purposes are used in the decision to order more specific tests, which may be necessary to pinpoint the exact cause of the hemolysis and anemia. Table 16-3 summarizes the characteristics of important iron-containing compounds evaluated in the workup for hemolysis.

Hematology

The mean corpuscular volume (MCV) may help to limit the diagnostic possibilities. MCV varies, depending on the presence or absence of extreme reticulocytosis or red cell fragmentation. In hemolytic anemias, the degree of reticulocytosis and macrocytosis may correspond to the duration and degree of anemia. On the other hand, if the reticulocyte count is increased in response to acute hemorrhage or compensated hemolysis, the reticulocytes are only 5% to 8% larger than the mature erythrocytes, generally resulting in a normal MCV.[26] The decrease in hemoglobin, hematocrit, and red blood cell count reflect the degree of anemia. Increased leukocyte and platelet counts are typically associated with increased erythropoiesis but are more prominent in acute hemorrhage than in hemolysis. A decreased platelet count is a valuable clue to the recognition of microangiopathic hemolytic anemias such as disseminated intravascular coagulation (DIC).

Blood film evaluation may provide specific clues to the type of hemolytic anemia present. Polychromasia or polychromatophilic shift cells and nucleated red cells represent a response to increased levels of erythropoietin that is due to either blood loss or hemolysis. The finding of spherocytes, microspherocytes, target cells, sickle cells, echinocytes, el-

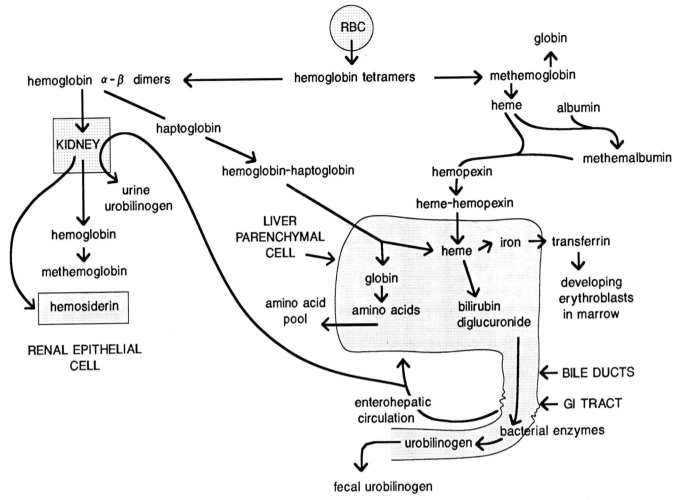

FIG. 16-3.   A schematic diagram of intravascular hemolysis. Note that the intermediate steps required for the conversion of heme to conjugated bilirubin are not repeated here (see Fig. 16-2).

liptocytes, schistocytes, ghost cells, agglutination, parasites, or other inclusions may reveal the underlying disorder that is leading to hemolysis. The presence of normal red cell morphology also helps exclude certain possibilities. Most hemolytic anemias have normal leukocyte morphology though occasionally, abnormalities such as erythrophagocytosis or the findings associated with septicemia may point to a specific problem. These findings allow for appropriate selection of special tests.

An increased reticulocyte count—and particularly an increased reticulocyte production index (RPI; Chap. 9)—support the suspicion that the anemia is due to increased loss or destruction of erythrocytes rather than to decreased production. An increased reticulocyte count and RPI may be seen in hemorrhage and following treatment for nutritional anemias, so these conditions must be excluded. A test for occult blood in the stool is performed easily and quickly and aids in confirming gastrointestinal blood loss as the cause of anemia and reticulocytosis.

In several conditions reticulocytopenia may confuse the picture. In some cases, reticulocytes completely mature in the bone àmarrow rather than in the peripheral blood, resulting in the paradox of a hyperplastic marrow

with a peripheral blood reticulocytopenia. Patients who experience an acute hemolytic episode may not show the expected reticulocytosis for 4 or 5 days. Abnormal reticulocytes, such as those produced in pyruvate kinase (PK) deficiency, may escape the bone marrow but be destroyed quickly in other areas of the RES. Consequently, the expected reticulocytosis may not always be observed in a PK-deficient patient with an intact spleen.[16] In any of these cases, the expected signs of increased production are absent while there is truly a hemolytic process present.

In the absence of blood loss, the RPI is a sensitive and specific indicator of hemolysis. If hemolysis is recent or chronic but mild, the RPI is expected to be two to four times the basal level. However, if hemolysis is chronic but moderate or severe, the RPI may be in the range of four to eight times the basal value.[27]

It should be recognized that the reticulocyte count remains elevated after hemolysis stops until the anemia is corrected, so reticulocyte counts should not be used to determine the need for therapy in hemolytic anemias, though they may be useful in determining the response to therapy in nutritional anemias.[5]

TABLE 16–2. Laboratory Findings in Hemolytic Anemias

SAMPLE	RESULTS	METHOD OF DETECTION
Plasma or serum	↑ Free hemoglobin	Visual/chemical
	↑ Methemoglobin	Visual/chemical
	↑ Methemalbumin	Visual/chemical
	↑ Unconjugated bilirubin★	Visual/chemical
	↓ Haptoglobin	Nephelometry
Urine	↑ Urobilinogen	Dipstick
	↑ Free hemoglobin	Dipstick/visual
	↑ Methemoglobin	Dipstick/visual
Urine sediment	+ Hemosiderin	Prussian blue stain
	+ Ferritin	Prussian blue stain
Bone marrow	Erythroid hyperplasia	Microscopic evaluation of Wright-stained concentrate
Whole blood	↓ RBC, Hb, HCT★	Automated counter
	↑ MCV (sometimes)★	Automated counter
	↑ Reticulocyte count★	Reticulocyte stain
Blood film	Polychromasia and morphology specific to underlying disease★	Microscopic evaluation of Wright-stained blood film
Feces	− Occult blood★	Chemical

★ Tests recommended for initial screening. Other tests may be performed, as indicated, based on results of initial screening tests. Key: ↑, elevated; ↓, depressed; +, positive result; −, negative result.

Bone Marrow Examination

Bone marrow examination should reveal erythroid hyperplasia with a myeloid-to-erythroid (M:E) ratio of approximately 0.5:1 instead of the usual 3:1 or 4:1. Cellularity is best judged on a biopsy section rather than an aspirate (Chap. 29).[40] However, if the clinical setting and laboratory data suggest a hemolytic anemia is present, bone marrow study usually is not required.[30]

Hemostasis

Disseminated intravascular coagulation (DIC) (Chap. 55) may be both the cause and result of certain hemolytic disorders. The coagulation pathway may be activated *in vivo* in cases of mechanical hemolysis because of the presence of substances in erythrocyte stroma that promote coagulation. Severe hemolytic transfusion reactions may occasionally be complicated by DIC, which results from interaction of the complement and coagulation systems.[7]

Prolongation of the prothrombin time (PT) and partial thromboplastin time (PTT) (Chap. 52), and decreased fibrinogen (Chap. 53) along with the presence of D-dimer (Chap. 54) are important coagulation laboratory findings in the diagnosis of hemolytic anemia owing to DIC. Tests for D-dimer are important because the presence of D-dimer is specifically diagnostic of coagulation *in vivo* by indicating only fibrin split products, whereas its predecessor, the fibrin split product test, indicates both fibrin and fibrinogen split products and so does not necessarily indicate actual coagulation *in vivo* (Chap. 54).

Chemistry

Much of the laboratory workup for hemolysis involves chemistry and urinalysis. Readers should refer to appropriate texts for details on the procedures discussed below.

Increased plasma *bilirubin* is one of the most sensitive indicators of hemolysis. There is usually a low level of unconjugated bilirubin (<1 mg/dL), which comes from the small amount of normal erythrocyte senescence and from the minute quantity of hemoglobin that is shed when the nucleus is extruded from developing erythrocytes. Total bilirubin levels reflect both the rate of erythrocyte destruction and liver function. Therefore, an increased total bilirubin can represent increased production from hemolysis, decreased hepatic clearance, or a combination of both. The unconjugated fraction is elevated in hemolysis. With normal liver function, chronic hemolysis cannot elevate the unconjugated bilirubin to more than 4 mg/dL.[5] In hypoproliferative anemias, the unconjugated bilirubin is usually less than 0.4 mg/dL; in ineffective erythropoiesis, it is usually greater than 0.7 mg/dL.[20]

Bilirubin concentration depends on total red cell mass. Other influences on bilirubin concentration include the patient's plasma volume, the concentration of albumin in the patient's plasma, and the presence of substances that can

TABLE 16–3. Important Iron-Containing and Related Compounds

COMPOUND	FUNCTION	LABORATORY ASSESSMENT	REFERENCE VALUES
Ferritin	Transmucosal transfer of absorbed iron, also reflects iron stores	Serum concentration	12–250 μg/L
Transferrin	Transport of iron to erythroid marrow	Serum concentration	220–400 mg/dL
Hemoglobin	O_2, CO_2 transport to and from tissues	Whole blood concentration as cyanmethemoglobin	14–16 g/dL
Methemoglobin	Iron oxidized to Fe^{+++}	Spectrophotometric analysis	0 g/dL or % of total hemoglobin
Myoglobin (muscle hemoglobin)	Involved in skeletal muscle function	Semiquantitative urine assay (performed in cases of suspected muscle necrosis)	Negative
Hemosiderin	Storage form of iron	Iron stain on marrow aspirate	1^+–2^+
Haptoglobin★	Carrier for free hemoglobin in plasma	Immunologic analysis, nephelometry	30–190 mg/dL

★ Haptoglobin itself is not composed of iron.

compete with bilirubin for binding with albumin.[5] Since a decrease in unconjugated plasma bilirubin concentration is the earliest indicator of a decreased rate of hemolysis, repeated determinations are useful indicators of the need for therapy (or lack thereof).[5]

Serum haptoglobin measurement is useful for identifying hemolytic disorders, especially now that simple and sensitive analytic techniques such as nephelometry are available. Levels below 25 mg/dL (reference range 30–190 mg/dL or 0.4–2.4 g/L) have been shown to be highly specific for identifying hemolytic disorders. Haptoglobin is usually absent when intravascular red cell destruction reaches two times the normal minimal rate.[8] Lowest values are found in cases of malfunctioning prosthetic cardiac valves, and consistently low values are associated with immune hemolytic anemias. Haptoglobin determination may be especially helpful for confirming the presence of hemolysis in cases where hemoglobinemia is undetectable.[32]

Because haptoglobin is an acute phase reactant, it may be increased in cases of inflammatory diseases such as systemic lupus erythematosus and rheumatoid arthritis, in neoplastic disease, and in infections. A patient with both a hemolytic anemia and one of these diseases may have a normal haptoglobin level. Therefore, failure to document a reduction in haptoglobin does not rule out hemolysis, although absence of haptoglobin does confirm hemolysis.[27,37]

Hemopexin is the plasma protein that carries free heme. It is expected to be decreased in hemolytic states, but this is not uniformly so. Hemopexin measurement is rarely necessary or useful in diagnosis;[42] nonetheless, hemopexin has been shown to be greatly decreased with severe hemolysis following cardiac surgery, in thalassemia major, and in some cases of Hb SS disease. It is minimally to moderately decreased in pernicious anemia, paroxysmal nocturnal hemoglobinuria, hereditary spherocytosis, and autoimmune hemolytic anemia. The degree of depletion is proportional to the concentration of free heme in the plasma and to the severity of hemolysis. Unlike haptoglobin, hemopexin is not an acute phase reactant, though it may be mildly increased in diabetes mellitus and infections.[35]

A *plasma hemoglobin* concentration of 10 to 40 mg/dL imparts a visible red tinge to the plasma. Measurement of plasma hemoglobin as oxyhemoglobin at 415 nm[19] is more accurate, although less sensitive, than the benzidine reaction.[18,39] The benzidine reaction is capable of detecting free hemoglobin when the level is less than 100 mg/dL. The cyanmethemoglobin reaction[22] is less sensitive but may be used to detect levels in excess of 100 mg/dL. When plasma hemoglobin has been oxidized to form methemoglobin, the heme readily dissociates and binds to albumin. Both methemoglobin and methemalbumin impart a brownish color to the plasma, which may mask hemoglobinemia.[13] Methemalbumin circulates for a long time and is useful for confirming that moderate to severe hemolysis occurred several days earlier.[9] Hemoglobinemia, methemoglobinemia, and methemalbuminemia are rare and usually occur only when there is significant intravascular hemolysis; their absence does not rule out hemolysis.[27]

Lactate dehydrogenase (LD) serum levels are often increased in hemolytic anemias though not as much as those in megaloblastic anemias. In hemolytic anemias, isoenzyme LD-2 predominates, in megaloblastic anemias, it is isoenzyme LD-1. Increased total LD is a rather nonspecific finding, since it occurs in myocardial infarction, liver disease, and ineffective erythropoiesis.[27] A normal LD level indicates almost certainly that hemolytic anemia can be ruled out.[38]

Urinalysis may reveal hemoglobinuria and methemoglobinuria when hemolysis is severe and haptoglobin-binding capacity is saturated.[34] The urine may be red or brown, depending on the oxidation state of heme. Free hemoglobin gives a positive urine dipstick (*e.g.,* Multistix) reaction. Microscopic urine examination is necessary to exclude the presence of intact red cells, which lyse in hypotonic urine and also cause a positive test result for hemoglobinuria.[20] *Hemosiderinuria,* the presence of hemosiderin (an insoluble form of storage iron) in the urine, is a valuable sign of current or recent intravascular hemolysis.[13] A Prussian blue stain of urine sediment reveals the presence of iron in renal epithelial cells that have been shed into the urine. Hemosiderinuria is especially useful to document mild intravascular hemolysis.[13] Iron remains in the urine sediment for several days after hemoglobinuria ends.[34]

Hemosiderinuria may also result from frequent red cell transfusions, but most patients who require repeated transfusions are already known to have a severe hemolytic anemia. Patients with hereditary hemochromatosis (an iron metabolism disorder characterized by abnormal iron deposition in the tissues causing a bronze skin pigmentation) may occasionally show increased urinary iron excretion, but this condition is readily distinguished from hemolytic anemia by other clinical and laboratory findings. Serum iron is normal in transfusion-induced hemochromatosis but increased in hereditary hemochromatosis.[13]

Increased *urine urobilinogen* reflects increased hemolysis, but urine urobilinogen levels are also affected by liver and kidney function[15] and by urine *p*H,[29] so it may not accurately reflect the degree of heme degradation. Because unconjugated bilirubin is insoluble in water, it is not present in the urine. Bilirubinuria would be seen in hemolytic anemia only if the patient also had liver disease and increased serum levels of conjugated bilirubin.

In the past, quantitation of fecal urobilinogen was used as an indicator of the rate of heme degradation. Today it is seldom used, because of various factors that are difficult to control and may cause inaccurate results.[15,28] Occult blood in feces should be negative in hemolytic anemias. A positive occult blood indicates gastrointestinal bleeding rather than hemolysis.

ERYTHROKINETICS

Red Cell Survival Studies

Determination of erythrocyte survival by erythrokinetic studies is rarely necessary to document hemolysis as the cause of an anemia. However, a brief explanation of the procedure is provided here because it may be useful in obscure cases where other laboratory findings are equivocal and in determining the exact site of erythrocyte destruction.[32]

The International Committee for Standardization in Haematology has published the reference method for red cell survival studies.[21] Approximately 10 mL of the patient's blood is anticoagulated with sterile ACD. A calculated amount of radioactive chromium (^{51}Cr) in the form of chromate ion (^{51}CrO$_4$$^{-2}$) diluted in normal sterile saline is added to the erythrocytes and incubated for 15 minutes, either at room temperature or in a 37°C water bath to allow red cell binding of ^{51}Cr. The cells are washed twice in sterile isotonic saline to remove unattached ^{51}Cr, are resuspended, and are administered intravenously to the patient.

An EDTA-anticoagulated blood sample is taken 10 minutes, 60 minutes, and 24 hours after the labeled cells are injected. Further samples are taken three times between days 2 and 7, and twice weekly until the blood radioactivity is minimal. A precisely measured volume of each sample is lysed, transferred to a counting tube, and gently mixed, and the radioactivity is counted on a well-type scintillation counter.

The radioactivity levels of all subsequent samples are compared on a percentage basis to the day 0, 100% sample (usually the 60-minute sample) to determine the percentage of radioactivity remaining in the circulating blood. These percentages are plotted on semilogarithmic paper against the number of days into the study to determine average red cell half-life, T$_{1/2}$, the number of days that have passed when 50% of the radioactive red cells have disappeared, while 50% remain in circulation (Fig. 16-4).

Since normal erythrocyte life span is approximately 120 days, the half-life would be expected to be 60 days, but the rate of elution of ^{51}Cr from erythrocytes is considered to be 1% per day, which causes a reduction in the expected half-life value. Additionally, because the patient sample is a random peripheral blood sample, the red cells vary in age from 0 to 120 days. Consequently, the reference range for erythrocyte half-life using this method is 25 to 32 days.

A half-life of 20 to 25 days suggests mild hemolysis, 15 to 20 days, moderate hemolysis, and less than 15 days, severe hemolysis (see Fig. 16-4). Measuring radioactivity over the spleen, liver, and heart may be useful in determining whether the spleen is a major source of erythrocyte destruction.[31] This test may be performed in conjunction with an erythrocyte production study, using radioactive iron to determine whether significant extramedullary erythropoiesis is occurring (Chap. 6).[4] Results of the two studies may aid in determining the major role of the spleen (*i.e.*, erythrocyte production or destruction) and whether splenectomy would have therapeutic value.

This test is logistically complex, requires a number of days to complete, requires that the patient be in a physiologic steady state (no change in the rate of hemolysis, no transfusions, no change in blood volume), exposes the patient to ionizing radioactivity, and is expensive. It is only available in specialized centers. In most cases, the hemoglobin concentration and RPI are sufficient to estimate the rate of hemolysis; measurement of erythrocyte life span would only confirm and quantify what is already evident from clinical findings and simpler laboratory determinations.[27,40]

Plasma Iron and Erythrocyte Iron Turnover

Measurements of plasma iron turnover and erythrocyte iron turnover use radiolabeled iron to evaluate total erythropoiesis and effective erythropoiesis, respectively. These tests have many of the same disadvantages as the ^{51}Cr red cell survival studies. Since the results correspond well to more readily available procedures (*e.g.*, the RPI and the bone marrow examination for hypercellularity), these more sophisticated tests are rarely indicated.[40]

CHAPTER SUMMARY

Hemolytic anemias occur when the erythrocyte's life span is shortened and the bone marrow's capacity to produce erythrocytes is exceeded by erythrocyte destruction. Hemolytic anemias may be inherited or acquired. Most inherited ones result from intrinsic erythrocyte defects. Acquired hemolytic anemias usually are due to extrinsic abnormalities that damage erythrocytes.

Most phagocytosis of both normal and abnormal erythrocytes occurs extravascularly in the spleen. Erythrocytes with extreme abnormalities may be destroyed in the liver or bone marrow. Abnormal erythrocyte destruction may also occur intravascularly.

Characteristic laboratory findings (see Table 16-2) include decreased hemoglobin and hematocrit values, decreased erythrocyte count, and an increased reticulocyte count and RPI. Polychromasia and specific morphologic findings on the blood film may indicate the underlying disease. Bone marrow examination is rarely required but usually shows erythroid hyperplasia. If ^{51}Cr erythrocyte survival studies are performed, a short-

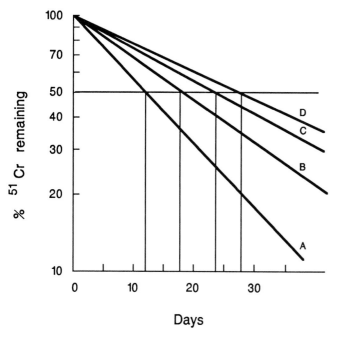

FIG. 16-4.   Chromium 51 erythrocyte survival study. The time required for half the radioactivity to disappear from the circulation is expressed as erythrocyte half-life (T$_{1/2}$). Normal T$_{1/2}$ is about 28 days when measured by ^{51}Cr survival methods. Decreasing T$_{1/2}$ corresponds to the severity of the hemolysis and increasingly shortened erythrocyte survival time. The four patient studies on this graph represent (A) severe hemolysis, (B) moderate hemolysis, (C) mild hemolysis, and (D) normal (no hemolysis). In this example, the respective half-lives were (A) 12 days, (B) 18 days, (C) 23 days, and (D) 27 days.

ened half-life is expected. Chemistry results include an increase in serum levels of unconjugated (indirect) bilirubin, free hemoglobin, methemoglobin, methemalbumin, and LDH. Haptoglobin and hemopexin levels are generally decreased. Urobilinogen, hemosiderin, hemoglobin, and methemoglobin may be detected in the urine. The physician uses preliminary laboratory data to confirm hemolysis and to aid in the selection of more specific tests and appropriate treatment.

CASE STUDY 16-1

An 8-year-old boy first presented with acute rheumatic fever and congestive heart failure and was treated with digitalis and penicillin. At age 14 years he underwent mitral valve replacement with a prosthetic valve and was treated with oral iron therapy because his hematocrit level was 0.29 L/L.

At age 24 he was admitted to the hospital with a 6-week history of coughing up blood, shortness of breath, and massive ankle-edema. He was a heavy smoker and consumed about a pint of alcohol daily. Physical examination revealed massive hepatomegaly and jaundice. The physician was unable to hear the expected clicking of the prosthetic valve. Echocardiography showed poor motion of the valve, suggesting the presence of an infection or clot, or both. Radiography showed massive lung hemorrhage.

Laboratory data were as follows: WBC 8.7×10^9/L; RBC 3.26×10^{12}/L; Hb 9.1 g/dL; HCT 0.29 L/L; MCV 88 fL; MCHC 32 g/dL; and platelets 70×10^9/L. Results of the differential cell count were 90% neutrophils, 1% bands, 6% lymphocytes, and 3% monocytes; neutrophils displayed moderate toxic granulation and marked vacuoles. Red cell morphology showed marked anisocytosis with macrocytes and microcytes; moderate poikilocytosis with target cells, schistocytes, echinocytes, and microspherocytes; moderate hypochromia and moderate polychromasia. Results of coagulation studies were prothrombin time, 19.4 seconds (reference range 10–14 seconds), partial thromboplastin time, >150 seconds (reference range 28–35 seconds).

There are several possible causes for this patient's anemia. Most patients with artificial valves have some hemolysis, but iron supplementation is usually sufficient to prevent anemia. Alcohol abuse and the increased erythropoiesis secondary to chronic hemolysis can lead to folate deficiency anemia. Liver disease may be associated with macrocytic anemia.

1. Are the red cell distribution width (RDW) and reticulocyte count expected to be normal, increased, or decreased in this case?
2. What red cell morphologic findings suggest that the anemia is due to hemolysis?
3. How is the clot or infection in the prosthetic mitral valve related to hemolysis?
4. What might the coagulation study results indicate? What other laboratory results in chemistry, urinalysis, and coagulation would support the preliminary diagnosis of hemolytic anemia?

REFERENCES

1. Beck WS: Reticuloendothelial (mononuclear phagocyte) system, lymphatic system, and spleen. In Beck WS (ed): Hematology, 4th ed. Cambridge, MA, The MIT Press, 1985
2. Bennington JL: Saunders Dictionary & Encyclopedia of Laboratory Medicine and Technology. Philadelphia, WB Saunders, 1984
3. Berk PD, Howe RB, Bloomer JR et al: Studies of bilirubin kinetics in normal adults. J Clin Invest 48:2176, 1969
4. Berlin NI: Erythrokinetics. In Williams WJ, Beutler E, Erslev AJ, Lichtman MA (eds): Hematology, 3rd ed. New York, McGraw-Hill, 1983
5. Berlin NI, Berk PD: Quantitative aspects of bilirubin metabolism for hematologists. Blood 57:983, 1981
6. Bessman JD, Gilmer PR, Gardner FH: Improved classification of anemias by MCV and RDW. Am J Clin Pathol 80:322, 1983
7. Brozovic M: Acquired disorders of blood coagulation. In Bloom AL, Thomas DP (eds): Haemostasis & Thrombosis. Edinburgh, Churchill Livingstone, 1981
8. Brus I, Lewis SM: The haptoglobin content of serum in haemolytic anaemia. Br J Haematol 5:348, 1959
9. Bunn HF: Erythrocyte destruction and hemoglobin catabolism. Semin Hematol 9:3, 1972
10. Cooper RA, Kimball DB, Durocher JR: Role of the spleen in membrane conditioning and hemolysis of spur cells in liver disease. N Engl J Med 290:1279, 1974
11. Cosgrove P, Sheetz M: Effect of cell shape on extravascular hemolysis. Blood 59:421, 1982
12. Crosby WH, Akeroyd JH: The limit of hemoglobin synthesis in hereditary hemolytic anemia. Am J Med 13:273, 1952
13. Crosby WH, Dameshek W: The significance of hemoglobinemia and associated hemosiderinuria, with particular reference to various types of hemolytic anemia. J Lab Clin Med 38:829, 1951
14. Dacie JV, Lewis SM: Practical Haematology, 4th ed. New York, Grune & Stratton, 1968
15. Elder G, Gray CH, Nicholson DC: Bile pigment fate in gastrointestinal tract. Semin Hematol 9:71, 1972
16. Erslev AJ, Gabuzda TG: Pathophysiology of Blood, 2nd ed. Philadelphia, WB Saunders, 1979
17. Gillen LAF: Hemoglobins, myoglobin, and porphyrins. In Bishop ML, Duben-Von Laufen JL, Fody EP (eds): Clinical Chemistry—Principles, Procedures, Correlations. Philadelphia, JB Lippincott, 1985
18. Hanks GE, Cassell M, Ray RN et al: Further modification of the benzidene method for measurement of hemoglobin in plasma. J Lab Clin Med 56:486, 1960
19. Harboe M: A method for determination of hemoglobin in plasma by near-ultraviolet spectrophotometry. Scand J Clin Lab Invest 11:66–70, 1959
20. Hillman RS, Finch CA: Red Cell Manual, 5th ed. Philadelphia, FA Davis, 1985
21. International Committee for Standardization in Haematology: Recommended method for radioisotope red cell survival studies. Br J Haematol 45:659, 1980
22. International Committee for Standardization in Haematology: Recommendations for haemoglobinometry in human blood. Br J Haematol 13(Suppl):68, 1967
23. Jacob HS, MacDonald RA, Jandl JH: Regulation of spleen growth and sequestering function. J Clin Invest 42:1476, 1963
24. Jandl JH: The anemia of liver disease: Observations on its mechanism. J Clin Invest 34:390, 1955
25. Jandl JH, Aster RH: Increased splenic pooling and the pathogenesis of hypersplenism. Am J Med Sci 253:383, 1967
26. Karnad A, Poskitt TR: The automated complete blood count: Use of the red blood cell volume distribution width and mean platelet volume in evaluating anemia and thrombocytopenia. Arch Intern Med 145:1270, 1985
27. Le Celle PL, Lichtman MA: Anemia with reticulocytosis: Hemolytic disorders. In Lichtman MA (ed): Hematology for Practioners. Boston, Little, Brown & Co, 1978
28. Lester R, Schumer W, Schmid R: Intestinal absorption of bile pigments. IV. Urobilinogen absorption in man. N Engl J Med 272:939, 1965
29. Levy M, Lester R, Levinsky N: Renal excretion of urobilinogen in dogs. J Clin Invest 47:2117, 1968
30. Lichtman MA: An approach to the diagnosis of reduced blood cell counts. In Lichtman MA (ed): Hematology for Practitioners. Boston, Little, Brown & Co, 1978
31. Macpherson AIS, Richmond J, Stuart AE: The Spleen. Springfield, Charles C Thomas, 1973
32. Marchand A, Galen RS, Van Lente F: The predictive value of serum haptoglobin in hemolytic disease. JAMA 243:1909, 1980

33. Murphy JR: The influence of *p*H and temperature on some physical properties of normal erythrocytes and erythrocytes from patients with hereditary spherocytosis. J Lab Clin Med 69:758, 1967

34. Pimstone N: Renal degradation of hemoglobin. Semin Hematol 9:31, 1972

35. Reich PR: Hematology: Physiopathologic Basis for Clinical Practice. Boston, Little, Brown & Co, 1978

36. Sears DA, Anderson PR, Foy AL et al: Urinary iron excretion and renal metabolism of hemoglobin in hemolytic diseases. Blood 28:708, 1966

37. Simmons A: Technical Hematology, 3rd ed. Philadelphia, JB Lippincott, 1980

38. Van Lente F, Marchand A, Galen RS: Diagnosis of hemolytic disease by electrophoresis of erythrocyte LDH isoenzymes on cellulose acetate or agarose. Clin Chem 27:1453, 1981

39. Vanzetti G, Valente D: A sensitive method for determination of hemoglobin in plasma. Clin Chim Acta 11:442, 1965

40. Wintrobe MM, Lee GR, Boggs DR et al (eds): Clinical Hematology, 8th ed. Philadelphia, Lea & Febiger, 1981

41. Yip R, Mohandas N, Clark M et al: Red cell membrane stiffness in iron deficiency. Blood 62:99, 1983

42. Zinkham W, Vangrov J, Dixon S et al: Observations on the rate and mechanism of hemolysis in individuals with hemoglobin Zurich: I. Concentrations of haptoglobin and hemopexin in the serum. Johns Hopkins Med J 144:37, 1979

There are three major categories of hereditary disorders causing anemias that are due to abnormal erythrocyte destruction. Of these, intrinsic erythrocyte membrane structural abnormalities and erythrocyte enzymopathies are the most common and best understood. Extrinsic plasma constituent abnormalities are a rare cause of hereditary hemolytic anemia.

HEREDITARY ERYTHROCYTE MEMBRANE ABNORMALITIES

The erythrocyte membrane skeleton is responsible for preserving red cell shape and integrity. The normal membrane is composed of equal amounts of lipid and protein (Chap. 6). Membrane abnormalities that result in hemolytic anemia often are due to alterations in structural proteins. The abnormalities may be caused by a deficiency of a particular structural protein or a defective skeletal protein structure. Membrane lipid content and cation transport abnormalities may also be involved. Erythrocyte destruction results from loss of membrane surface area, increased rigidity, fragmentation, or deformation. Red cells become trapped in the spleen and are prematurely destroyed. Disorders characterized as erythrocyte membrane abnormalities include hereditary spherocytosis, hereditary elliptocytosis, hereditary pyropoikilocytosis, and hereditary stomatocytosis.

Hereditary Spherocytosis

Definition
Hereditary spherocytosis (HS) is a hemolytic disorder characterized by numerous microspherocytic erythrocytes on the blood film.

Genetics and Demographics

Inheritance of HS is usually autosomal dominant, and therefore is manifest in heterozygotes. Several cases are often found in one family. In 25% of cases, neither parent is affected[30]; this may be the result of a spontaneous mutation, reduced penetrance of the dominant gene, or a recessive form of the disease.[29] HS is the most common hemolytic anemia in people of Northern European extraction (incidence 1 in 5,000).[29]

Pathophysiology

The basic abnormality in HS is a defect in red cell membrane protein composition. Three groups of proteins are important to red cell membrane structure.[38] The first, spectrin, forms dimers linked end-to-end to form tetramers (Fig. 17-1). Spectrin dimers are linked together by another protein known as actin. The spectrin–actin linkage is mediated by a third protein, protein 4.1. Two additional proteins are involved in attaching spectrin to the membrane lipid bilayer. Ankyrin binds to the spectrin fiber and attaches to an integral membrane protein, protein 3.

Two membrane protein defects may cause HS.[36] The first, defective binding of spectrin to protein 4.1,[48] is inherited as an autosomal dominant trait. The second abnormality, spectrin deficiency, is much less common, and its inheritance appears to be autosomal recessive.

Combination of the basic red cell defect and the splenic microcirculation leads to loss of membrane surface area and hemolysis. Two consequences of the defect relate to hemolysis. First, membrane permeability to sodium is increased.

To protect against osmotic lysis, the excess sodium is actively transported out of red cells; this transport requires abnormally high levels of adenosine triphosphate (ATP). Second, membrane lipid content is decreased. Despite these abnormalities, the cells' survival time is decreased only when the spleen is present. When red cells enter the spleen, circulation slows, glucose levels fall, and ATP generation declines. Accumulation of intracellular sodium results in osmotic swelling and increased membrane rigidity. In addition, lipids are readily lost from the membrane when red cells are deprived of energy.[25] Red cells with such an abnormal and rigid membrane are unable to negotiate the splenic microcirculation. Splenic entrapment and phagocytosis causes spherocyte formation, further splenic trapping, and eventually, destruction of erythrocytes (Fig. 17-2).

Clinical Presentation and Physical Findings

Three characteristic clinical features of HS are anemia, jaundice, and splenomegaly. The severity of the clinical course varies, typically being more severe in younger patients.[33] Patients usually present with HS before age 10 years, but mild cases may not be detected until adulthood. Increased metabolism of bile pigment (e.g., bilirubin and biliverdin) may cause pigment gallstones.

An uncommon but serious complication of HS, especially in children, is aplastic crisis in which peripheral blood pancytopenia develops due to lack of marrow cell production. The resulting anemia can be severe and life threatening. These self-limited crises are often precipitated by viral

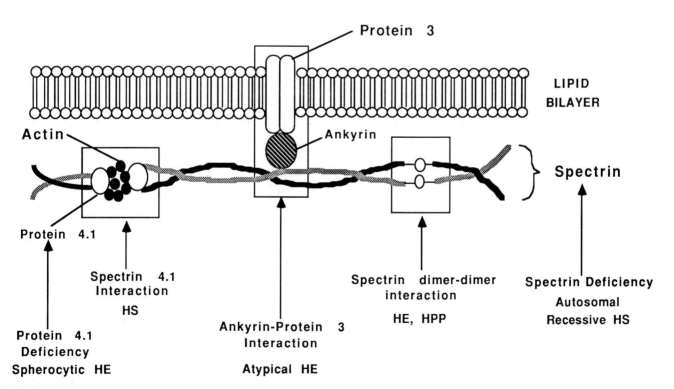

FIG. 17-1.   Diagram of the sites of erythrocyte skeletal defects in, from left to right, spherocytic hereditary elliptocytosis (HE); the most common form of hereditary spherocytosis (HS); atypical HE; the most common form of HE; hereditary pyropoikilocytosis (HPP); and the less common form of HS inherited as an autosomal recessive trait. Modified from Palek J, Lux SE: Red cell membrane skeletal defects in hereditary and acquired hemolytic anemias. Semin Hematol 20:189, 1983, and from Wolfe LC: A genetic defect in the binding of protein 4.1 to spectrin in a kindred with hereditary spherocytosis. N Engl J Med 307:1367, 1982, with permission.

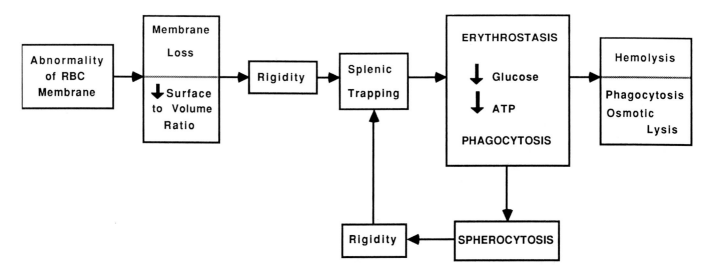

FIG. 17-2.   Pathophysiology of spherocyte formation and red cell destruction in hereditary spherocytosis.

infections. Leg ulceration is common and may be a patient's primary complaint.[41]

Skeletal abnormalities may be detected due to chronic bone marrow hyperplasia, which causes expansion of the medullary cavity. This may cause thickening of the facial bones. Some patients present with the same facial abnormality seen in thalassemia major (Chap. 15).

Laboratory Findings and Correlations with Disease

COMPLETE BLOOD COUNT (CBC).   Anemia is usually mild. Adults frequently have a hemoglobin (Hb) value above 10 g/dL, whereas infants and young children have lower levels (8–11 g/dL).[30] The mean corpuscular volume (MCV) is generally between 77 and 87 fL although it can be increased or markedly decreased.[47] The mean corpuscular hemoglobin concentration (MCHC) is increased in half to two thirds of patients.[25] Hereditary spherocytosis is distinguished as basically the only disease in which the MCHC is elevated above the reference range. Reticulocyte counts are usually between 5% and 20% but are more dramatically increased in some cases, particularly during recovery from aplastic crisis.[33,47]

The RDW generally is normal[2] but may be increased, depending on the degree of reticulocytosis. Aplastic crisis causes a marked decrease in Hb and a low reticulocyte count.

PERIPHERAL BLOOD FILM.   Numerous microspherocytes on the blood film (see Fig. 8-6) are characteristic. They appear small and dark and lack central pallor. Although anisocytosis may occur due to a mixture of microspherocytes and large polychromatophilic cells, there is little poikilocytosis other than the spherocytes.

BONE MARROW.   The bone marrow displays erythroid hyperplasia. An aplastic crisis causes marrow hypoplasia.

SPECIAL HEMATOLOGY TESTS.   The confirmatory test for HS is the osmotic fragility test. Red cells in HS have increased osmotic fragility (see procedure below). The di-

rect antiglobulin test is negative. Another special diagnostic procedure used occasionally is the autohemolysis test. The pattern of reaction is often indicative of HS. Autohemolysis is greatly increased in HS; however, this phenomenon does not occur if either glucose or ATP is added to the test system. Other disorders do not yield the same results. The autohemolysis test is discussed in a later section on Pyruvate Kinase Deficiency, where this test is more applicable to the diagnosis.

CHEMISTRY.   Other laboratory findings common to hemolytic processes support the diagnosis of HS. A slight to moderate rise in unconjugated (indirect) bilirubin, elevated fecal urobilinogen, and decreased haptoglobin levels may be observed. The intravascular hemolytic indicators of hemoglobinemia, hemoglobinuria, and hemosiderinuria do *not* appear in HS.

Most Useful Laboratory Tests for Diagnosing Hereditary Spherocytosis

The most useful diagnostic test for HS is the osmotic fragility test, but other tests (Table 17-1), including the incubated osmotic fragility and the direct antiglobulin test, may be helpful. Step-by-step procedures for these tests may

TABLE 17–1. Recommended Laboratory Tests to Assist in Diagnosis of Hereditary Spherocytosis

MOST FREQUENTLY REQUIRED
CBC with MCHC
Peripheral blood film examination
Osmotic fragility test
Reticulocyte count
OCCASIONALLY REQUIRED
Autohemolysis test
Direct antiglobulin test
Serum unconjugated (indirect) bilirubin
Serum haptoglobin
RARELY REQUIRED
Bone marrow examination

be found in the references provided and in some cases, in manufacturer's test kit enclosures.

OSMOTIC FRAGILITY TEST[16]

Principle

Osmotic fragility reflects the shape of erythrocytes. Because of the decreased surface area-to-volume ratio, spherocytes have a limited capacity to expand in hypotonic solutions and therefore lyse at higher concentrations of saline than normal biconcave red cells. This behavior is referred to as increased osmotic fragility. In contrast, cells that are hypochromic or flatter (*e.g.*, hypochromic cells in iron deficiency, target cells in thalassemia and sickle cell anemia, and sickle cells themselves) have decreased osmotic fragility (Fig. 17-3). They have a greater capacity to expand in hypotonic solution and lyse at lower concentrations of saline than normal cells.

Specimen Requirements

Fresh heparinized blood is preferred. Fifteen to twenty milliliters of defibrinated whole blood, prepared by placing whole blood into a flask with glass beads, also may be used. Anticoagulants containing oxalates are undesirable because they alter *pH*.

Reagents

The various saline concentrations may be prepared in the laboratory or purchased prepackaged. Saline concentrations already prepared by a manufacturer (*e.g.*, the osmotic fragility kit produced by Becton Dickinson, Rutherford, NJ) may be preferable for ease of use, time savings, and more reliable results.

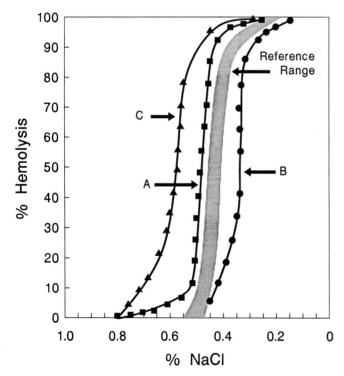

FIG. 17-3.   Results of erythrocyte osmotic fragility test under various conditions. Curve A shows the increased osmotic fragility of cells in hereditary spherocytosis. Curve B shows the decreased fragility of target cells in thalassemia. Curve C shows the markedly increased fragility in hereditary spherocytosis when the incubated osmotic fragility test is used. Compare each curve to the reference range.

General Procedure

The test is performed by suspending red cells in a series of saline (NaCl) solutions ranging from 0.85% to 0.1% and incubating for 30 minutes at room temperature. After each test suspension is centrifuged, the absorbance of each supernatant is measured at 540 nm. Using this absorbance, percent hemolysis is calculated (see below) by comparing each test solution to the 0.85% NaCl solution, in which no hemolysis is expected. More details on this procedure may be found in many laboratory procedure manuals.

Quality Control

A fresh normal specimen should always be run and plotted with the patient's specimen for comparison purposes and accurate test result interpretation.

Calculations

Calculation of percent hemolysis is based on absorbance of the supernatant of each NaCl concentration ($A_{x\%}$). The calculation is as follows:

$$\% \text{ Hemolysis} = \frac{A_{x\%} - A_{0.85\%}}{A_{0.0\%} - A_{0.85\%}} \times 100\%$$

For example, if the absorbance of the 0.20% NaCl supernatant is 0.77, the absorbance of the 0.00% (100% hemolysis) NaCl supernantant is 0.89, and that of the 0.85% NaCl is 0.05, the calculation of percent hemolysis for the 0.20% NaCl test suspension is

$$\% \text{ Hemolysis} = \frac{0.77 - 0.05}{0.89 - 0.05} \times 100\%$$
$$= 85.7\%$$

Percent hemolysis is plotted against NaCl concentration on linear graph paper (see Fig. 17-3). Note that the denominator should represent the largest amount of change in absorbance of all the test solutions because complete hemolysis is expected in 0.00% NaCl, which is essentially water. All other NaCl concentrations are compared to complete hemolysis to obtain their percent hemolysis. The 0.85% absorbance is subtracted from the numerator and denominator to correct for any incidental hemolysis that might result from specimen handling rather than true osmotic fragility. Normal erythrocytes should not lyse in 0.85% isotonic saline.

Reference Range

The reference range at 20°C is shown in Table 17-2. Hemolysis begins around 0.45% and generally is complete between 0.35% and 0.30% NaCl in clinically normal subjects.

TABLE 17–2. Reference Ranges for Osmotic Fragility at 20°C*

NaCl (%)	HEMOLYSIS (%)
0.00	100
0.10	100
0.20	100
0.30	97–100
0.35	90–97
0.40	50–90
0.45	0–45
0.50	0–5
0.55	0
0.60	0
0.65	0
0.70	0
0.85	0

* Hemolysis normally begins around 0.45% and generally is complete between 0.35% and 0.30% NaCl.

INCUBATED OSMOTIC FRAGILITY

In mild forms of HS, osmotic fragility may be normal. A test variation calls for measurement of the osmotic fragility following sterile incubation of the originally drawn whole blood specimen for 24 hours at 37°C, which enhances osmotic fragility if HS is present. Following 24-hour incubation, the test is repeated with new saline solutions using the same procedure as that for the unincubated osmotic fragility. Figure 17-3 demonstrates the increased fragility found in HS when the incubated method is used.

Comments and Sources of Error

It is important to obtain the blood sample with a minimum of stasis and trauma, and the test must be performed as soon as possible after the specimen is obtained. Saline solutions must be chemically pure, dilutions must be accurate, and the temperature and pH (7.4) must be kept constant.[26] In the incubated osmotic fragility test, the major source of error is bacterial contamination. To avoid this, flasks with beads used to collect defibrinated blood should be sterilized and plugged with sterile cotton before being used. While incubating blood, the flask should be plugged with sterile cotton.

If plasma color is abnormal (e.g., jaundiced or lipemic) it may be necessary to replace plasma with isotonic saline prior to testing, to avoid test interference. When a decreased hemoglobin level and poikilocytosis are both present in a specimen, these conditions may cause decreased osmotic fragility, most likely due to the decreased hemoglobin.

Occasionally the highest absorbance reading will occur in a test solution at or below 0.30% NaCl (it is normal to have 100% hemolysis in 0.30% NaCl). If this happens, use the highest absorbance reading obtained in place of the 0.00% reading in the denominator of the calculation.

Increased osmotic fragility is characteristic of HS but may also be seen in other acquired hemolytic anemias that typically have spherocytes (e.g., hemolytic disease of the newborn and autoimmune hemolytic anemia).[35] A greater increase in the incubated osmotic fragility is seen in HS than in other anemias.

Microcapillary[31] and automated[17] methods are also available for osmotic fragility testing.

DIRECT ANTIGLOBULIN TEST

Because the laboratory findings in HS are similar to those in immune hemolytic anemias, the direct antiglobulin test (DAT) is useful in the differential diagnosis. The DAT detects antibody on the red cell surface, so a negative result rules out immune-mediated hemolytic anemias and is expected in HS. The DAT procedure can be found in immunohematology textbooks.

Effects of Treatment on Laboratory Results

The usual treatment for HS is splenectomy, which removes the agent of red cell destruction and prevents complications such as aplastic crisis and gallbladder disease. Splenectomy should be delayed as long as possible because the spleen is important in the developing immune system, particularly in adolescence. Splenectomized patients have a normal life expectancy.

Following splenectomy, spherocytes persist on the peripheral blood film, and Howell-Jolly bodies are a prominent feature. Spiculated cells may also be present.[48] Reticulocyte counts decrease to normal levels, and if anemia was present, hemoglobin increases. Bilirubin levels decrease but may remain in the high normal range.[37] The osmotic fragility curve becomes more symmetric and less shifted than before splenectomy.[44]

Hereditary Elliptocytosis

Definition

Hereditary elliptocytosis (HE) is a heterogeneous group of disorders characterized by large numbers of elliptical erythrocytes on the blood film.

Genetics and Demographics

HE is only about one fifth as common as hereditary spherocytosis[20] and is found in all racial groups.[30] Inheritance is generally autosomal dominant. In some families the defect is linked to the genes for Rh blood factor.[1]

Pathophysiology

The factors that determine the elliptical shape of red cells are unknown. Since bone marrow normoblasts and circulating reticulocytes are normal in shape, red cells appear to assume the elliptical shape as the cells age. Studies indicate that the membrane structural defect involves spectrin or the proteins with which spectrin closely associates.[14] Three skeletal defects have been described (see Fig. 17-1).[36] The first is a deficiency of protein 4.1, which is necessary for association of spectrin and actin. This disorder is referred to as spherocytic HE. Other defects involve abnormal skeletal protein interaction, including spectrin dimer-dimer interaction and a defective ankyrin–protein 3 interaction, known as atypical HE.

What factors differentiate the hemolytic variety (found in 10% to 15% of patients with HE) from the asymptomatic condition remain unknown. Red cells in HE are known to utilize more ATP than normal cells and to demonstrate an increased rate of sodium efflux (a flowing out of the cell), a bipolar concentration of hemoglobin (as demonstrated by electron microscopy), and polarization of cholesterol in the membrane. Neither the biochemical nor the structural lesion of patients with HE correlates with the degree of hemolysis. The mechanism of hemolysis is known to involve membrane loss, decreased red cell "deformability," and shortened red cell survival due to splenic destruction.

Clinical Presentation and Physical Findings

Most affected people have no clinical manifestations. When present, hemolysis is usually mild and accompanied by anemia, jaundice, and splenomegaly.

Laboratory Findings and Correlations with Disease

COMPLETE BLOOD COUNT. The red cells in HE are normochromic and normocytic. Characteristically, the Hb value is greater than 12 g/dL and the reticulocyte count is less than 4%.[42]

PERIPHERAL BLOOD FILM. The peripheral blood film reveals greater than 25% elliptocytes and oval erythrocytes (see Fig. 8-14).[35,47] At least three types of HE have been described based on red cell morphology and clinical presentation: common HE, spherocytic HE, and stomatocytic HE.[29,36] Common HE, the most prevalent form, reveals typical HE red cell morphology. Hemolysis ranges from nonexistent to moderate. Spherocytic HE accounts for approximately 10% to 20% of cases, and the blood shows a significant number of rounded elliptocytes and spherocytes. Stomatocytic HE is rare.

BONE MARROW.   Bone marrow normoblasts are normal in shape. Erythroid hyperplasia correlates with the degree of compensation for hemolysis.

SPECIAL HEMATOLOGIC TESTS.   Osmotic fragility and the autohemolysis test usually are normal. In cases of spherocytic HE, values of these test results are increased.

CHEMISTRY.   Increased serum unconjugated bilirubin and fecal urobilinogen and decreased serum haptoglobin levels can be observed when hemolysis is present.

Effects of Treatment on Laboratory Results

In most cases no treatment is necessary. People with moderately severe hemolytic disease may benefit from splenectomy, which ameliorates anemia and restores a normal reticulocyte count, but elliptocytosis on the peripheral film persists. Other forms of poikilocytes may increase because they are not removed by the spleen.

Hereditary Pyropoikilocytosis

Definition and Genetics

Hereditary pyropoikilocytosis (HPP) is an extremely rare hemolytic disorder characterized by extreme anisocytosis and micropoikilocytosis with budding red cells, fragments, spherocytes, elliptocytes, and other bizarre-shaped cells.[29,36,49] Inheritance is autosomal recessive and the disorder characteristically occurs in black children.

Pathophysiology

The red cell membrane structural abnormality in HPP is related to a spectrin dimer-dimer association defect (see Fig. 17-1).[36] This defect is similar to that in some forms of HE, and evidence indicates a relationship between the two disorders. The extreme instability of the red cell membrane in HPP leads to both extreme morphologic abnormalities and thermal instability of the cells. As in HS, the mechanism of hemolysis appears to be related to membrane loss and rigidity. HPP red cells also are characterized by elevated calcium content with increased inflow and reduced outflow of calcium, but this abnormality appears to be secondary to the membrane structural defect.

Clinical Presentation and Physical Findings

HPP presents in infancy or early childhood with severe, often transfusion-dependent hemolytic anemia. In addition, jaundice, splenomegaly, and gallbladder disease may be present.

Laboratory Findings and Correlations with Disease
COMPLETE BLOOD COUNT.   The most striking feature is extreme microcytosis. The MCV often is between 25 and 55 fL.[46] Hemoglobin is decreased in proportion to the degree of hemolysis. Reticulocyte counts are elevated, but the reticulocyte production index depends on the ability of the patient's bone marrow to respond to anemia.

PERIPHERAL BLOOD FILM.   There is striking anisocytosis and poikilocytosis with microspherocytes, fragmented cells, elliptocytes, and other bizarre forms (Fig. 17-4). Polychromasia is also present.

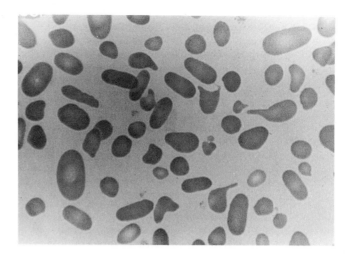

FIG. 17-4.   Blood film demonstrates hereditary pyropoikilocytosis. Note microspherocytes, fragments, elliptocytes, and bizarre forms. From McKenna RW, Hoffman GC, Horwitz CA, Ward PCJ: Laboratory approach to the diagnosis of hemolytic anemias. Workshop manual. Chicago, IL, American Society of Clinical Pathologists, 1984, with permission. Photomicrograph by Robert W. McKenna.

SPECIAL HEMATOLOGIC TESTS.   Suspected HPP red cells should be tested for thermal sensitivity. In contrast to normal cells, which fragment at temperatures above 49°C, red cells in HPP fragment at temperatures as low as 45° to 46°C. HPP is also characterized by an increased osmotic fragility, especially after incubation, and a markedly elevated autohemolysis test result.

Effects of Treatment on Laboratory Results

Hemolysis is reduced but not always corrected by splenectomy. Abnormal red cell morphology remains following splenectomy.[49]

Hereditary Stomatocytosis (Hydrocytosis) and Hereditary Xerocytosis

Definition

Hereditary stomatocytosis, also known as hydrocytosis, and hereditary xerocytosis are a heterogeneous group of red cell membrane disorders. They are characterized by mild to moderate hemolytic anemia, altered membrane permeability to cations, and most commonly, autosomal dominant inheritance.

Pathophysiology

Red cell water content is dependent on the cellular concentration of sodium and potassium cations. Red cells in hereditary stomatocytosis are characterized by increased permeability and flux (flow into and out of the cell) of both sodium and potassium, resulting in increased water content and swollen cells. There is a net increase in cellular sodium and a net decrease in potassium. The defect in sodium permeability is greater than that of potassium, causing a net *increase* in cellular cation concentration, which stimulates the entry of water into the cells to maintain osmotic equilibrium. These cells swell and take on the appearance of stomatocytes (from the Greek word *stoma,* mouth) on the peripheral blood film (*i.e.,* they have a mouth-like area of central pallor; see Fig. 8-10). Stomatocytes have an increased volume and a decreased surface-to-volume ratio, leading to decreased ability to deform and increased splenic destruction.

More commonly, however, the efflux (outflow) of potassium is greater than the influx (inflow) of sodium. In this condition, there is a net *decrease* in cellular cation concentration, which stimulates the movement of water out of the cells. The cells become dehydrated and are known as xerocytes (from the Greek word *xeros,* dry). Xerocytes have an increased surface-to-volume ratio, so the peripheral blood film reveals the presence of target cells[45] and cells with hemoglobin concentrated at one pole of the cell. The cells are not very deformable and are subject to reticuloendothelial destruction.

The structural basis for these membrane abnormalities is poorly understood. Increased membrane lipids, particularly phosphatidylcholine, have been reported in some cases.[45] Diminished phosphorylation of spectrin has also been implicated in hereditary stomatocytosis. Hemolysis is related to decreased red cell deformability and osmotic lysis in the spleen.[32]

Clinical Presentation and Physical Findings

The clinical features of hereditary stomatocytosis and xerocytosis are similar to those of other chronic hemolytic anemias. The degree of hemolytic anemia is usually mild but varies both within and between families.[35]

Laboratory Findings and Correlations with Disease
COMPLETE BLOOD COUNT.   Hemoglobin is rarely less than 8 to 10 g/dL. Reticulocytosis is usually moderate (10%–20%), but variations range from normal to as high as 45%. The MCV usually is increased in both conditions, and the MCHC is generally decreased in stomatocytosis and increased in xerocytosis.

PERIPHERAL BLOOD FILM.   In some cases of hereditary stomatocytosis, 10% to 50% of circulating red cells are stomatocytes. Target cells predominate in hereditary xerocytosis; some cells demonstrate the concentrated area of hemoglobin toward one pole of the cell.

SPECIAL HEMATOLOGIC TESTS.   Osmotic fragility is increased when stomatocytes persist, due to the decreased cellular surface-to-volume ratio. On the other hand, osmotic fragility is decreased when the target cells of xerocytosis, with their increased surface-to-volume ratio, predominate.[32] Autohemolysis (see procedure later in this chapter) is increased and may or may not be corrected by addition of glucose.[45]

CHEMISTRY.   Increased serum bilirubin and decreased serum haptoglobin reflect the degree of hemolysis. Confirmatory tests include abnormal red cell cation content and increased cation transport; these tests are performed by a special chemistry or reference laboratory.

Effects of Treatment on Laboratory Results
Splenectomy has proven beneficial in correcting hemolysis in patients with hereditary stomatocytosis. Those with hereditary xerocytosis generally do not benefit from splenectomy, presumably because xerocytes are being destroyed in areas other than the spleen.

HEREDITARY ERYTHROCYTE ENZYMOPATHIES

Normal erythrocyte metabolism in the Embden-Meyerhof (E-M) pathway and pentose phosphate pathway (PPP) is discussed in detail in Chapter 6. A number of hereditary enzymopathies cause abnormalities in these pathways.

Ninety percent of the energy in red cell metabolism is produced by anaerobic glycolysis through the E-M pathway, which produces ATP necessary for normal cell function and survival. Enzymopathies in this pathway are numerous and are referred to collectively as congenital nonspherocytic hemolytic anemias. Many lead to varying degrees of hemolytic anemia. The most common, pyruvate kinase (PK) deficiency, is discussed in detail. Other enzymopathies of this pathway are extremely rare.

The PPP is responsible for aerobic glycolysis, which generates 10% of the red cell's energy. This pathway generates reduced nicotinamide adenine dinucleotide phosphate (NADPH), which is linked to glutathione reduction, which in turn protects enzymes and hemoglobin from oxidation. Enzyme deficiencies of this pathway result in build-up of hydrogen peroxide, oxidative denaturation of hemoglobin, and hemolysis, usually as a result of oxidant stress. The most common enzymopathy of the PPP is glucose-6-phosphate dehydrogenase (G6PD) deficiency, which will also be discussed in detail.

Pyruvate Kinase Deficiency
Definition
Itself a rare disorder, pyruvate kinase is the most common enzyme deficiency of the E-M pathway. The disease results in mild to moderately severe hemolytic anemia.

Genetics and Demographics
Although most cases are found in people of northern European origin, PK deficiency occurs worldwide. It is inherited as an autosomal recessive trait. PK mutants are numerous, and most people with hemolytic anemia are doubly heterozygous for two mutant genes.[43] Heterozygous PK deficiency generally demonstrates about half the normal PK activity and is not associated with anemia or other hematologic changes.[40] Acquired PK deficiency occurs in some cases of dyserythropoietic syndromes.[34]

Pathophysiology
PK catalyzes the formation of pyruvate from phosphoenol-pyruvate (PEP) and is accompanied by the transformation of adenosine diphosphate (ADP) to ATP (Fig. 17-5). Thus, PK deficiency leads to a marked reduction in ATP production, which is necessary for maintenance of the

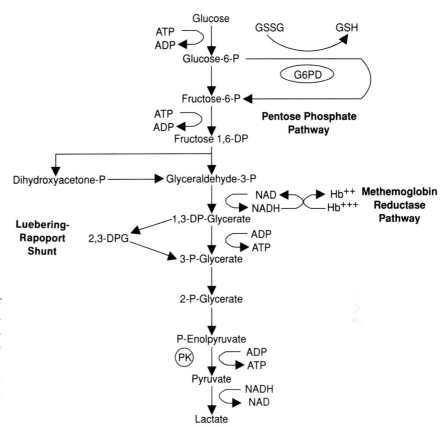

Embden-Meyerhof Pathway

FIG. 17-5. Anaerobic (Embden-Meyerhof [E-M] pathway) and aerobic (pentose phosphate pathway) glucose metabolism in erythrocytes. In E-M pathway note role of pyruvate kinase (PK) in production of ATP, pyruvate, and lactate. See Figure 6-7 for a more detailed diagram of these pathways. GSSG, oxidized glutathione; G-SH, reduced glutathione; Hb⁺, hemoglobin; Hb⁺⁺, methemoglobin.

membrane sodium-potassium pump. Potassium and water are lost from the cell, resulting in cell shrinkage, distortion of shape, and spiculation. Irreversible membrane injury resulting from potassium loss and an increase in membrane calcium causes decreased deformability and premature destruction in the spleen.

Reticulocytes in PK deficiency have an inordinate susceptibility to hemolysis. Reticulocytes derive their energy principally through mitochondrial oxidative phosphorylation rather than glycolysis. As mitochondria are lost during maturation, reticulocytes are very vulnerable to the effects of their glycolytic defect and are destroyed in the spleen.

Metabolic intermediates, such as 2,3-diphosphoglycerate (2,3-DPG) accumulate in PK deficiency as a result of the block in glycolysis. The cellular concentration of 2,3-DPG may exceed two to three times normal.[27] This increase is responsible for a shift to the right in the oxyhemoglobin dissociation curve, which causes red cells to release oxygen more readily to the tissues to compensate for anemia.

Clinical Features and Physical Findings

The clinical features of PK deficiency are highly variable. Some newborns require exchange transfusion; others have fully compensated hemolytic anemia and experience no symptoms. The disease is usually detected in infancy or early childhood, but occasionally it is not detected until adulthood. The signs and symptoms are those associated with chronic hemolysis, including anemia, splenomegaly, jaundice, and gallstones.

Laboratory Findings and Correlations with Disease

COMPLETE BLOOD COUNT. Hemoglobin ranges widely from 6 to 12 g/dL.[34] Red cells generally are normochromic and normocytic, although the MCV may be elevated when reticulocytosis is marked. Before splenectomy, reticulocyte counts range from 2.5% to 15%[47]; following splenectomy counts as high as 56% are not uncommon.[40] Leukocytes and platelets generally are normal.

PERIPHERAL BLOOD FILM. There are no prominent morphologic features. Polychromasia, poikilocytosis, and variable numbers of nucleated red cells may be found. Microspherocytes usually are not present.

CHEMISTRY. Serum unconjugated bilirubin is moderately elevated and haptoglobin levels are decreased. Erythrocyte glycolytic intermediates such as 2,3-DPG and PEP are increased, whereas ATP, lactate, and pyruvate, which require PK for production, are decreased.

SPECIAL HEMATOLOGIC TESTS. Results of the osmotic fragility test are normal, but the incubated fragility test may show variable degrees of abnormality. Autohemolysis is quite variable; some patients show mildly increased hemolysis that is partially prevented by glucose, and others have a greater increase that is not prevented by glucose. This test is discussed in detail below. Heinz bodies are not demonstrated, and the result of the direct antiglobulin test is negative.

Most Useful Laboratory Tests for Diagnosing Pyruvate Kinase Deficiency

Readers should refer to the references provided for detailed procedures for performing the tests outlined below.

FLUORESCENT SPOT TEST AND QUANTITATIVE PK ASSAY[3,4,9]

The PK fluorescent spot test is the recommended screening test for PK deficiency. An abnormal spot test result must be confirmed by the quantitative PK assay.

Principle

Both the qualitative and quantitative methods involve the same reaction. In the spot test, reaction mixture (containing phosphoenolpyruvate [P-enolpyruvate], NADH, and LD, which are incubated with the patient hemolysate) is added to filter paper and observed for fluorescence. PK is required to catalyze the conversion of P-enolpyruvate to pyruvate, followed by reduction of NADH to NAD by pyruvate, and finally, the formation of lactate, which requires the presence of lactate dehydrogenase (LD) (see Fig. 17-5). Loss of fluorescence of NADH under ultraviolet light indicates PK activity. PK-deficient erythrocytes fail to complete this reaction, and fluorescence persists for more than 60 minutes. In the quantitative assay, the change in absorbance of the reaction mixture is measured spectrophotometrically at 340 nm to quantify PK activity.

Specimen Requirements

Whole blood anticoagulated with EDTA, heparin, or acid-citrate-dextrose (ACD) solution is acceptable. Red cell hemolysates are prepared for analysis.

Reference Range

The reference range for quantitative PK activity is wide. It is reported in units (U) per gram of Hb, and is highly dependent on the method used. Most deficient people have 5% to 25% of the normal mean activity.[40] Heterozygous carriers have approximately half the normal activity.

Comments and Sources of Error

Leukocytes contain about 300 times as much PK as red cells and must be completely removed from the sample before the hemolysate is prepared. Also, a recent transfusion provides normal cells that may obscure PK deficiency until the donor cells are removed from circulation in 3 to 4 months.

AUTOHEMOLYSIS TEST[16]

The main value of this test is as a screen for PK deficiency and G6PD deficiency, each of which produces a different test result. A third result is obtained using cells from patients with hereditary spherocytosis (HS), but the osmotic fragility test should be the principal diagnostic tool used to investigate HS.

Principle

The autohemolysis test measures the spontaneous lysis of red cells incubated at 37°C for 48 hours. During this time, depletion of glucose and ATP results in membrane loss and spherocyte formation. Glucose or ATP added to the blood may protect against autohemolysis partially or completely.

Specimen Requirements

Sterile, defibrinated blood is the specimen of choice.

General Procedure

Defibrinated blood from the patient and a control are incubated alone and with glucose (or ATP) for 48 hours. After 48 hours a number of steps (which may be found in a laboratory procedure manual) are required before performing an absorbance reading on the serum of each specimen and calculating the percentage of hemolysis.

Quality Control

A normal specimen must be run in duplicate for comparison purposes and correct interpretation of results.

Reference Range

Normal red cells incubated under these conditions exhibit 0.2% to 2.0% hemolysis. With the addition of glucose, 0% to 0.9% hemolysis is seen, or with ATP, 0% to 0.8% is seen.

Comments and Sources of Error

Dacie[16] describes three patterns of autohemolysis.

Type I. Autohemolysis is slightly to moderately increased but is partially corrected by glucose. This is seen in G6PD deficiency, hereditary elliptocytosis, and unstable hemoglobin disease.

Type II. Autohemolysis is greatly increased and glucose has no effect, however, ATP corrects the hemolysis. This is associated with pyruvate kinase deficiency.

Hereditary Spherocytosis. Autohemolysis is greatly increased but can be corrected with either glucose or ATP. This pattern has also been found in triose phosphate isomerase deficiency.

The autohemolysis test is neither sensitive nor specific, so it is not used widely today. It may only be used to screen for PK and G6PD enzymopathies, since more specific enzyme assays are now available and are recommended for diagnosing these deficiencies.

Effects of Treatment on Laboratory Results

Treatment of PK deficiency involves transfusion therapy in severe cases of hemolytic anemia and exchange transfusions to prevent neonatal hyperbilirubinemia. Although it is not curative, splenectomy is indicated for patients who require regular blood transfusions. Following splenectomy, the hemoglobin value increases by 1 to 2 g/dL in most patients,[34] reticulocyte counts are markedly increased, and echinocytes are more prevalent on the peripheral blood film.[28]

Glucose-6-Phosphate Dehydrogenase Deficiency

Definition and History

G6PD deficiency is the most common red cell enzymopathy associated with hemolysis.[6] The disorder results from the inheritance of any one of a large number of abnormal genes that code for the G6PD enzyme. The course of the disorder varies from episodic hemolysis induced by drugs and other oxidant stresses to severe, chronic nonspherocytic hemolytic anemia. G6PD deficiency was discovered in the 1950s after it was observed that some black soldiers receiving the antimalarial drug primaquine developed hemolytic anemia.[18]

Genetics

G6PD deficiency is an X-linked inherited disease, so it is fully expressed in men with the genetic abnormality. In women it is fully expressed only in homozygotes. Because of X chromosome inactivation (Lyon hypothesis) in which one of the two X chromosomes of each cell is believed to be inactive, heterozygous women have two populations of erythrocytes. One population has normal enzyme activity (the genetically defective X chromosome was inactivated), and the other population is G6PD deficient (the normal X chromosome was inactivated).[39] Heterozygous women are clinically normal, although on the average their cellular G6PD concentration is about half the normal level.[33]

Genetic Variants and Demographics

G6PD deficiency is most common in West Africa, the Mediterranean, the Middle East, and Southeast Asia. Black people often have a mild deficiency (10%–60% of normal activity), Orientals have a more severe deficiency, and Mediterraneans the most severe.

There are over 150 genetic variants of the G6PD enzyme,[8] which generally are named for the geographic region in which they are prevalent (*e.g.*, G6PD Canton). Many G6PD variants can be classified according to enzyme activity, electrophoretic mobility, and clinical manifestations.[7,8] This chapter focuses on two well known variant groups in addition to a group of variants that produce similar laboratory findings.

The normal G6PD enzyme, designated as G6PD B, is found in all white people and most black people. Another variant, G6PD A, is prevalent among blacks and differs from G6PD B by a single amino acid substitution. The G6PD A and B enzymes have normal enzyme properties but differ in electrophoretic mobility due to the amino acid substitution. The variant G6PD A− (the minus sign indicates deficient enzyme activity) is the most common one associated with hemolysis. It is electrophoretically identical to G6PD A but has only 5% to 15% of the normal enzyme activity.[8] G6PD A− is found in 11% of American black men,[8] while about 25% of American black women are carriers.[11] Among Caucasians, the most common abnormal variant is G6PD Mediterranean, which affects 1 in 1000 people in Mediterranean regions.[20] The electrophoretic mobility of G6PD Mediterranean is identical to that of G6PD B, but its catalytic activity is often less than 1% of normal.[8] In addition, there is a large group of variants that express chronic hereditary nonspherocytic hemo-

lytic anemia. These variants are rare and occur sporadically among various ethnic groups.

Pathogenesis

Oxidative denaturation of hemoglobin is the major contributor to the hemolytic process in G6PD deficiency.[43] G6PD is necessary for converting glucose-6-phosphate (glucose-6-P) to 6-phosphogluconate and for the subsequent production of (6 PG) NADPH and reduced glutathione (GSH) (Figs. 17-5, 17-6). GSH protects enzymes and hemoglobin against oxidation by reducing hydrogen peroxide and free radicals. Hydrogen peroxide is generated in small amounts during normal red cell metabolism and in larger amounts when an oxidant drug interacts with oxyhemoglobin. Normal red cells exhibit sufficient G6PD activity to maintain adequate GSH levels. When G6PD is deficient, red cells cannot generate sufficient GSH to detoxify peroxide. Hemoglobin is then oxidized to methemoglobin (iron in the oxidized Fe^{+++} state). Heme is liberated from globin, and globin denatures, forming Heinz bodies. Heinz bodies attach to membrane sulfhydryl groups, inducing cell rigidity. At this point, red cells can no longer traverse the splenic microcirculation and lysis occurs.

Clinical Presentation and Physical Findings

The clinical features of G6PD deficiency vary, depending on the degree of oxidant stress, the race of the person, and the genetic variant involved. People who inherit the G6PD A− variant are not anemic, and hemolysis occurs more commonly with infections and only intermittently in association with exposure to oxidant drugs, diabetic acidosis, and the neonatal period. Numerous drugs and chemicals are known to induce hemolysis, including primaquine, phenylhydrazine (has been used to treat polycythemia vera), nitrofurantoin (an antibacterial used to treat urinary tract infections), nalidixic acid (an antimicrobial for gram-negative organisms), sulfanilimide (an antibacterial compound), methylene blue (used to treat methemoglobinemia), and naphthalene (formerly used as an antiseptic in diarrhea of typhoid fever).[5] The degree of hemolysis varies from asymptomatic to life-threatening episodes accompanied by abdominal pain, shock, and intravascular hemo-

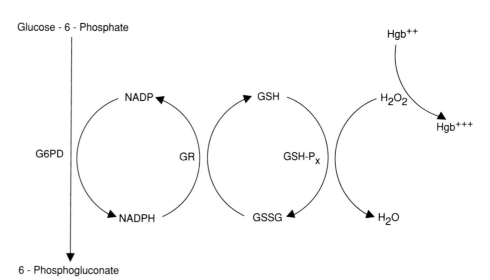

FIG. 17-6. Pentose phosphate pathway (hexose monophosphate shunt) where glucose-6-phosphate dehydrogenase (G6PD), nicotinamide-adenine dinucleotide phosphate (NADPH), and reduced glutathione (GSH) are necessary to detoxify hydrogen peroxide (H_2O_2) generated in erythrocytes and to keep hemoglobin in a reduced state (Hb^{++}). In G6PD deficiency, inadequate production of NADPH results in accumulation of oxidized glutathione (GSSG) and H_2O_2, oxidation of hemoglobin (Hb^{+++}), Heinz body formation, and hemolysis. (GR indicates glutathione reductase; GSH-Px, glutathione peroxidase).

lysis resulting in hemoglobinuria, jaundice, and pallor. Because G6PD activity declines more rapidly as cells age, hemolysis in G6PD-deficient black men is limited to older cells. Hemolysis usually subsides as the reticulocyte response increases, even if drug administration or infection persists, since reticulocytes have a nearly normal G6PD content.

In G6PD Mediterranean, G6PD levels are grossly deficient in red cells of *all ages*. Patients with this variant, like those with G6PD A−, commonly experience hemolysis that is initiated by infection. Hemolysis following oxidant stress in association with drugs is more common and more severe than that found in G6PD A−, and it is not self-limited. G6PD Mediterranean is occasionally associated with severe, potentially fatal hemolytic episodes following ingestion of fava beans (favism). Favism is not associated with G6PD A−. Patients with G6PD Mediterranean occasionally require transfusion when hemolysis is severe. G6PD Mediterranean is occasionally associated with hemolytic disease of the newborn.

Some of the rare types of G6PD deficiency are associated with chronic hereditary nonspherocytic hemolytic anemia. The deficiency of enzyme activity may be so great that chronic hemolysis occurs even without exposure to oxidants.

Laboratory Findings and Correlations with Disease
COMPLETE BLOOD COUNT.   In most cases Hb concentrations are decreased only following episodes of oxidant stress. Acute hemolysis is followed by a sudden decrease in Hb concentration of 3 to 4 g/dL below the reference range.[47] Anemia is normochromic and normocytic, and the reticulocyte count should begin to rise 4 to 5 days after the onset of hemolysis.

PERIPHERAL BLOOD FILM.   Even during hemolytic episodes, morphologic changes are neither striking nor specific. Polychromasia, poikilocytosis, and some spherocytes may be observed. "Bite" cells are often seen during acute hemolytic episodes (Fig. 17-7). The bites in these cells probably represent Heinz body craters. Bite cells are not diagnostic of G6PD deficiency and occur in acute oxidant hemolysis associated with unstable hemoglobins, in GSH deficiency, and in normal individuals following exposure to oxidizing agents.[27]

CHEMISTRY.   Signs of intravascular hemolysis include increased plasma hemoglobin and serum bilirubin levels, a decreased serum haptoglobin level, hemoglobinuria, hemosiderinuria, and increased urinary and fecal urobilinogen.

SPECIAL HEMATOLOGIC TESTS.   Heinz bodies, which represent denatured hemoglobin, cannot be seen by Romanowsky stains, but they may be observed through the use of a supravital staining procedure (Fig. 17-8) (Chap. 14). Patients with G6PD deficiency develop Heinz bodies in their red cells during hemolytic episodes.

In the past the autohemolysis test was used to screen for G6PD deficiency. G6PD-deficient cells show greater hemolysis than normal cells, and hemolysis is partially corrected by glucose or ATP. Increased autohemolysis is not

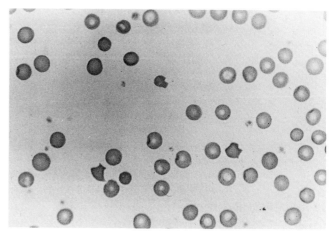

FIG. 17-7.   Bite cells in G6PD deficiency. From McKenna RW, Hoffman GC, Horwitz CA, Ward PCJ: Laboratory approach to the diagnosis of hemolytic anemias. Workshop Manual. Chicago, IL, American Society of Clinical Pathologists, 1984, with permission. Photomicrograph by Patrick CJ Ward.

specific for G6PD and has been replaced by more specific enzyme tests.[21]

Results of the direct antiglobulin test are negative, and it is often utilized to rule out immune-mediated hemolysis.

Most Useful Laboratory Tests for Diagnosing G6PD Deficiency
Table 17-3 lists tests that may assist in the diagnosis of G6PD deficiency. The discussion below covers three screening methods, describes a quantitative procedure for measuring G6PD enzyme activity, and summarizes the advantages and disadvantages of each. Readers should refer to references provided for exact test procedures.

G6PD FLUORESCENT SPOT TEST[3,4,9]
The G6PD fluorescent spot test is the recommended screening test for G6DP deficiency.

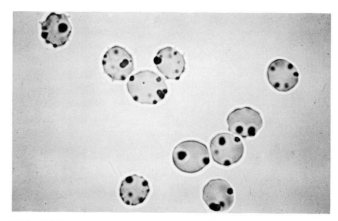

FIG. 17-8.   Heinz bodies in G6PD deficiency as visualized microscopically on a film made after red cells were supravitally stained. Note pitted golf ball appearance. From American Society of Hematology Slide Bank, 2nd ed. Seattle, ASH, 1977.)

TABLE 17–3. Recommended Laboratory Tests to Assist in Diagnosis of G6PD Deficiency

MOST FREQUENTLY REQUIRED
CBC
Peripheral blood film examination
Reticulocyte count
Erythrocyte enzyme screen
Heinz body stain
OCCASIONALLY REQUIRED
Serum unconjugated (indirect) bilirubin
Serum haptoglobin
Urine hemoglobin
Direct antiglobulin test
Erythrocyte enzyme assay
RARELY REQUIRED
Bone marrow examination
Autohemolysis test

Principle

The basic reaction involves the reduction of NADP to NADPH and the formation of 6PG (6-phosphogluconate) by G6PD in the presence of G6P (glucose-6-P). The reaction follows:

$$G6P + NADP \xrightarrow{G6PD} NADPH + 6PG$$
$$\text{(fluorescent)}$$

Blood is added to reagent, and after brief incubation, the mixture is placed on filter paper and observed for fluorescence of NADPH under fluorescent light. Blood with a normal G6PD level shows fluorescence; little or no fluorescence indicates a G6PD deficiency. Moderate fluorescence indicates a mild deficiency.

Specimen Requirements

Whole blood anticoagulated with EDTA, heparin, or ACD is required. Red cell hemolysates are prepared for analysis.

Quality Control

A normal control specimen should be run along with the patient's sample for comparison purposes, to ensure that the test system is working properly. Normal saline may be used to simulate a negative control. Fluorescence should not be observed in the negative control.

Interpretation of Results

Normal G6PD activity should cause strong fluorescence (similar to that from the normal control). A partial deficiency causes fluorescence only half as strong as that from the normal control. With severe deficiency, no fluorescence is observed (similar to the negative control).

Comments and Sources of Error

This test is highly specific, simple to perform, and inexpensive. In heterozygous women, the result may be normal. During acute hemolysis in patients with G6PD deficiency, the fluorescent spot test may be normal because of increased levels of G6PD in reticulocytes and younger red cells, which should be separated by removing the top portion of the erythrocyte population after centrifugation of the sample.[23] Otherwise, it is necessary to delay testing for 2 to 4 months or to utilize a more sensitive method. In addition, measurement of G6PD activity in red cells can be affected by the presence of leukocytes and platelets. Results are more accurate if the buffy coat is removed before testing.[19]

METHEMOGLOBIN REDUCTASE TEST[12,13]
Principle

This screening test indirectly detects NADPH generation by G6PD. In the test, methemoglobin is reduced to hemoglobin by transfer of a hydrogen ion from NADPH to methemoglobin with methylene blue as the facilitator. G6PD-deficient cells lack this ability.

Specimen Requirements

Fresh whole blood is required.

Comments and Sources of Error

This test is very sensitive and can detect G6PD deficiency even in the presence of hemolysis.[12] False positive results occur if blood is stored more than a few hours.[5] A modification of this procedure has been developed for detecting the percentage of affected cells in female heterozygotes.[22]

ASCORBATE CYANIDE TEST[24]
Principle

This test measures the ability of normal cells to detoxify hydrogen peroxide when incubated with ascorbate. Cyanide is used as a catalase inhibitor, since RBC catalase is an enzyme that also detoxifies hydrogen peroxide and would interfere with specific measurement of the glutathione peroxidase system. Red cells are oxidized by hydrogen peroxide generated by the interaction of ascorbate and oxyhemoglobin. In the absence of adequate G6PD activity, the reaction mixture develops a brown color due to methemoglobin formation.

Specimen Requirements

Heparin-, EDTA-, or ACD-anticoagulated blood is required.

General Procedure

Two milliliters whole blood is incubated with small amounts of ascorbate and cyanide solution at 37°C for 1 to 4 hours and observed hourly (after mixing the test specimen) for appearance of a brown color that indicates formation of methemoglobin. A normal control should be run along with the patient specimen. To ensure a valid test the control specimen should still be red when compared to the specimen from an abnormal patient, which turns brown. The brown color forms earlier in EDTA specimens than in heparinized or ACD specimens.

Interpretation of Results

Development of a brown color within 1 to 2 hours using an EDTA specimen or within 2 to 4 hours using a heparinized or ACD specimen indicates a G6PD deficiency. If the specimen remains red and looks the same as the normal control throughout the incubation period, G6PD activity is considered to be normal.

Comments and Sources of Error

This screening test is very sensitive and easy to perform. It will detect G6PD deficiency even in heterozygous women and in black men during hemolytic episodes (when G6PD is elevated because of reticulocytes), but it is nonspecific, and the result may be positive in pyruvate kinase deficiency, paroxysmal nocturnal hemoglobinuria, and in people who have unstable hemoglobins.[21]

QUANTITATIVE ASSAY FOR G6PD[4,9]
Principle

The assay is identical in principle to the fluorescent spot test, but this test is quantitative, because the exact change in absorbance is measured spectrophotometrically at 340 nm, which is converted to rate of NADPH generation. This correlates with a quantitative measurement of G6PD activity.

Reference Range

The reference range for G6PD activity is 8.34 ± 1.59 U/g hemoglobin.[9] Individuals with the G6PD A− variant show 10% to 60% normal enzyme activity, whereas those with

G6PD Mediterranean and chronic nonspherocytic hemolytic anemia have less than 10% of normal activity.[47]

Comments and Sources of Error

Results may be normal in heterozygotes and black men during hemolytic episodes. Attention must be paid to leukocyte and reticulocyte removal to prevent falsely elevated results. Normal donor cell G6PD activity in transfused blood may obscure G6PD deficiency. Tests for G6PD deficiency must, in these cases, be delayed 3 to 4 months to allow normal cells to clear from the circulation.

Effects of Treatment on Laboratory Results

There is no specific treatment for hemolysis due to G6PD deficiency. In most cases, it is sufficient to avoid exposure to potential sources of oxidant stress. This includes vigorous treatment of infection and withdrawal of offending medications. Following treatment, the hemoglobin level rises, the appearance of the peripheral blood film returns to normal, and Heinz bodies disappear. In variants that demonstrate chronic nonspherocytic hemolytic anemia, treatment such as exchange transfusion in newborns and transfusion during aplastic crisis may be necessary. Splenectomy generally is not helpful.

HEREDITARY PLASMA CONSTITUENT ABNORMALITIES

In this group of disorders, red cell survival is affected by abnormalities in lipid metabolism. The lipid composition of the red cell membrane depends on the lipid composition of plasma, so abnormalities in lipid metabolism (including abetalipoproteinemia and lecithin-cholesterol acyltransferase [LCAT] deficiency) may cause red cell membrane defects.

Abetalipoproteinemia

Definition and Genetics

Abetalipoproteinemia, also known as hereditary acanthocytosis, is a very rare but serious disorder caused by the absence of β lipoproteins in the serum. Inheritance is autosomal recessive. The disease is characterized by malabsorption of fat, retinitis pigmentosa (a degenerative condition of the retina), neurologic damage, and acanthocytosis of red cells.

Pathophysiology

The relationship between abnormal plasma lipid content and acanthocyte formation is not well understood. An increase in membrane rigidity appears to be the cause of a slightly increased rate of red cell destruction. Decreased deformability of the acanthocyte membrane results from an increase in sphingomyelin (a rigid layer) over lecithin (a more fluid layer).[15] Red cell membrane cholesterol is normal or only slightly increased, and phospholipid is normal or slightly decreased.

Clinical Features and Physical Findings

Hemolytic anemia is not a serious problem in abetalipoproteinemia, but complications due to nervous system and gastrointestinal disorders usually lead to early death.

Laboratory Findings and Correlations with Disease

COMPLETE BLOOD COUNT.   Anemia, when present, is mild, and red cell indices are normal. The reticulocyte percentage is normal or slightly increased.

PERIPHERAL BLOOD FILM.   Red cells are normochromic and normocytic. The most striking feature is the presence of large numbers of acanthocytes with irregular, pointed projections, some of which are long and spindly.

CHEMISTRY.   Serum lipids are markedly decreased. Plasma triglyceride levels are near zero, and plasma cholesterol is usually less than 50 mg/dL,[15] which is three to five times lower than the reference range.

SPECIAL HEMATOLOGIC TESTS.   Osmotic fragility is normal or slightly decreased and autohemolysis is increased.

Effects of Treatment on Laboratory Results

There is no definitive therapy for abetalipoproteinemia, and treatment of hemolysis usually is unnecessary.

Lecithin-Cholesterol Acyltransferase Deficiency

Familial LCAT deficiency is a rare inherited disorder characterized by mild normochromic, normocytic anemia. The disorder has been found only in Scandinavian families. Renal disease and corneal opacities are other features of the disease. Plasma LCAT deficiency leads to a reduction in plasma cholesterol esters and an increase in free cholesterol in the plasma. Prominent target cell formation results from increased red cell membrane cholesterol. Both hemolysis and decreased erythropoiesis have been implicated in the pathogenesis of anemia. The latter may be due to concurrent renal disease.[47]

CHAPTER SUMMARY

Hereditary hemolytic anemias involving red cell membrane and enzyme defects and plasma constituent abnormalities generally are characterized by normochromic, normocytic anemia, which is usually mild. Findings common to extravascular hemolytic processes (e.g., increased unconjugated serum bilirubin) are also seen.

In red cell membrane structural defects, hemolysis results from loss of membrane surface area, increased membrane rigidity, and premature destruction by the spleen. Hereditary spherocytosis (HS), the most common disorder of this group, is characterized by microspherocytes on the blood film and an increased osmotic fragility. An increased MCHC is a classic finding almost unique to HS.

Hereditary elliptocytosis (HE) is the second most common red cell membrane disorder, and anemia is present in only 10% to 15% of cases. The blood film characteristically reveals more than 25% elliptocytes. Hereditary pyropoikilocytosis (HPP) is a rare membrane disorder accompanied by severe anemia, extreme poikilocytosis and microcytosis, and red cell thermal sensitivity.

The membrane structural defect in hereditary stomatocytosis may involve altered membrane permeability to cations. In some cases, stomatocytes are present on the blood film, but more commonly, target cells are prevalent.

Enzyme deficiencies can occur in the red cell metabolic pathways. The most common are pyruvate kinase (PK) deficiency in the Embden-Meyerhof pathway and glucose-6-phosphate dehydrogenase (G6PD) deficiency in the pentose phosphate shunt.

PK deficiency may cause varying degrees of hemolysis. Persistence of test specimen fluorescence in the popular PK spot screening test indicates a PK deficiency. The autohemolysis test for PK is seldom used today because it lacks sensitivity. Quantitative PK assays provide a definitive diagnosis.

G6PD deficiency is an X-linked disorder that causes abnormal G6PD enzyme variants. The variant G6PD A−, which occurs principally in blacks, results in episodic hemolysis following oxidant stress. In G6PD Mediterranean, the most common variant in Caucasians, hemolysis tends to be more severe. Erythrocyte G6PD assays and the Heinz body stain are useful in diagnosing G6PD deficiency. Absence of fluorescence in the G6PD fluorescent spot screening test indicates a G6PD deficiency. The methemoglobin reductase test is another very sensitive G6PD screening assay. Performance of the ascorbate cyanide screening test is easy, but the test is not very specific for G6PD deficiency. The quantitative G6PD assay provides a definitive diagnosis.

Plasma constituent abnormalities such as abetalipoproteinemia and LCAT deficiency are rare disorders resulting from abnormalities in lipid metabolism. Acanthocytosis of red cells and decreased serum lipids are found in abetalipoproteinemia, and LCAT deficiency is characterized by prominent target cell formation.

CASE STUDY 17-1

A 13-year-old white boy was in apparent good health until he developed a severe case of influenza. He was seen by his family physician and complained of continued fatigue. Physical examination revealed pallor, mild jaundice, and splenomegaly. He had no previous history of anemia. Mild hyperbilirubinemia in the newborn period required phototherapy. The patient's brother was abnormally jaundiced at birth but was now in reasonable health. His mother had undergone splenectomy for a hematologic disorder. The complete blood count revealed: Hb 5.2 g/dL; HCT 0.19 L/L; RBC 1.8×10^{12}/L; MCV 78 fL; MCH 28.9 pg; and MCHC 37 g/dL. The reticulocyte count was 0.4%. The peripheral blood film revealed numerous microspherocytes and no polychromasia. The result of the direct antiglobulin test was negative and total bilirubin was 1.9 mg/dL.

1. What is the possible diagnosis and why?
2. What specific laboratory test would be recommended and what results are expected?
3. How do you explain the severe anemia and low reticulocyte count when the patient previously had been well?
4. What might family studies reveal?

CASE STUDY 17-2

A 6-year-old black boy was thought to be suffering from an acute hemolytic episode following a viral infection. The patient's older brother suffers from G6PD deficiency. The complete blood count revealed Hb 6.2 g/dL; HCT 0.19 L/L; RBC 2.2×10^{12}/L; MCV 86 fL; MCH 28.2 pg; and MCHC 33 g/dL. A Heinz body stain revealed Heinz bodies. The reticulocyte count was 22%. The ascorbate-cyanide test demonstrated early formation of a brown color while the control remained red. The result of the G6PD fluorescent spot test was positive for fluorescence, as was the normal control.

1. Identify and explain the discrepancy in the G6PD screening tests.
2. Identify the possible solution to the discrepancy.
3. Calculate the reticulocyte production index (RPI) (Chap 9). Does the indicated bone marrow response seem adequate?

REFERENCES

1. Bannerman RM, Renwick JH: The hereditary elliptocytoses: Clinical and linkage data. Ann Hum Genet (London) 26:23, 1962
2. Bessman JD, Gilmer PR, Gardner FH: Improved classification of anemias by MCV and RDW. Am J Clin Pathol 80:322, 1983
3. Beutler E: A series of new screening procedures for pyruvate kinase deficiency, glucose-6-phosphate dehydrogenase deficiency, and glutathione reductase deficiency. Blood 28:553, 1966
4. Beutler E: Red Cell Metabolism: A Manual of Biochemical Methods, 3rd ed. Orlando, Grune and Stratton, 1984
5. Beutler E: Hemolytic Anemia in Disorders of Red Cell Metabolism. New York, Plenum, 1978
6. Beutler E: Red cell enzyme defects as nondiseases and as diseases. Blood 54:1, 1979
7. Beutler E: Glucose-6-phosphate dehydrogenase deficiency. In Stanbury JB, Wyngaarden JB, Fredrickson DS et al (eds): The Metabolic Basis of Inherited Disease, 5th ed. New York, McGraw-Hill, 1982
8. Beutler E: Glucose-6-phosphate dehydrogenase deficiency. In Williams WJ, Beutler E, Erslev AJ et al (eds): Hematology, 4th ed. New York, McGraw-Hill, 1990
9. Beutler E, Blume KG, Kaplan JC et al: International Committee for Standardization in Haematology: Recommended methods for red-cell enzyme analysis. Br J Haematol 35:331, 1977
10. Beutler E, Blume KG, Kaplan JC et al: International Committee for Standardization in Haematology: Recommended screening test for glucose-6-phosphate dehydrogenase (G-6-PD) deficiency. Br J Haematol 43:465, 1979
11. Brewer GJ: Inherited erythrocyte metabolic and membrane disorders. Med Clin North Am 64:579, 1980
12. Brewer GJ, Tarlov AR, Alving AS: Methemoglobin reductase test: A new simple in vitro test for identifying primaquine-sensitivity. Bull WHO 22:633, 1960
13. Brewer GJ, Tarlov AR, Alving AS: The methemoglobin reduction test for primaquine type sensitivity of erythrocytes: A simplified procedure for detecting a specific hypersusceptibility to drug hemolysis. JAMA 180:386, 1962
14. Cooper RA: Hereditary elliptocytosis and related disorders. In Williams WJ, Beutler E, Erslev AJ et al (eds): Hematology, 3rd ed. New York, McGraw-Hill, 1983
15. Cooper RA, Jandl JH: Acanthocytosis. In Williams WJ, Beutler E, Erslev AJ et al (eds): Hematology, 3rd ed. New York, McGraw-Hill, 1983
16. Dacie JV, Lewis SM: Practical Haematology, 5th ed. New York, Grune & Stratton, 1975
17. Danon D: A rapid micromethod for recording red cell osmotic fragility by continuous decrease of salt concentration. J Clin Pathol 16:377, 1963
18. Dern RJ, Weinstein IM, LeRoy GV et al: The hemolytic effect of primaquine. J Lab Clin Med 43:303, 1954; 44:171, 1954
19. Echler G: Determination of glucose-6-phosphate dehydrogenase levels in red cell preparations. Am J Med Tech 49:259, 1983
20. Erslev AJ, Gabuzda TG: Pathophysiology of Blood, 3rd ed. Philadelphia, WB Saunders, 1985
21. Fairbanks VF, Fernandez MN: The identification of metabolic errors associated with hemolytic anemia. JAMA 208:316, 1969
22. Gall JC, Brewer GJ, Dern RJ: Studies of glucose-6-phosphate dehydrogenase activity of individual erythrocytes. The methemoglobin elution test for identification of females heterozygous for G6PD deficiency. Am J Hum Genet 17:359, 1965
23. Herz F, Kaplan E, Scheye ES: Diagnosis of the erythrocyte glucose-6-phosphate dehydrogenase deficiency in the Negro male despite hemolytic crisis. Blood 35:90, 1970
24. Jacob HS, Jandl JH: A simple visual screening test for glucose-6-phosphate dehydrogenase deficiency employing ascorbate and cyanide. N Engl J Med 274:1162, 1966

25. Jandl JH, Cooper RA: Hereditary spherocytosis. In Stanbury JB, Wyngaarden JB, Fredrickson DS (eds): The Metabolic Basis of Inherited Disease, 4th ed. New York, McGraw-Hill, 1978

26. Jandl JH, Cooper RA: Hereditary spherocytosis. In Williams WJ, Beutler E, Erslev AJ et al (eds): Hematology, 3rd ed. New York, McGraw-Hill, 1983

27. Keitt AS: Diagnostic strategy in a suspected red cell enzymopathy. Clin Hematol 10:3, 1981

28. Leblond PF, Lyonnais J, Delage J: Erythrocyte populations in pyruvate kinase deficiency anaemia following splenectomy. I. Cell morphology. Br J Haematol 39:55, 1978

29. Lux SE: Disorders of the red cell membrane skeleton: Hereditary spherocytosis and hereditary elliptocytosis. In Stanbury JB, Wyngaarden JB, Fredrickson DS et al (eds): The Metabolic Basis of Inherited Disease, 5th ed. New York, McGraw-Hill, 1982

30. Lux SE, Wolfe LC: Inherited disorders of the red cell membrane skeleton. Pediatr Clin North Am 27:463, 1980

31. McCormick JB: Microcapillary technic for red blood cell osmotic fragility. Am J Clin Pathol 46:392, 1966

32. Mentzer WC, Smith WB, Goldstone J et al: Hereditary stomatocytosis: Membrane and metabolism studies. Blood 46:659, 1975

33. Miale JB: Laboratory Medicine: Hematology, 6th ed. St Louis, CV Mosby, 1982

34. Miwa S: Pyruvate-kinase deficiency and other enzymopathies of the Embden-Meyerhof pathway. Clin Hematol 10:57, 1981

35. Nelson DA: Erythrocytic disorders. In Henry JB (ed): Clinical Diagnosis and Management by Laboratory Methods, 17th ed. Philadelphia, WB Saunders, 1984

36. Palek J, Lux SE: Red cell membrane skeletal defects in hereditary and acquired hemolytic anemias. Semin Hematol 20:189, 1983

37. Schilling RF: Hereditary spherocytosis: A study of splenectomized persons. Semin Hematol 13:169, 1976

38. Shohet SB, Lux SE: The erythrocyte membrane skeleton: Pathophysiology. Hospital Practice 19:89, 1984

39. Sullivan DW, Glader BE: Erythrocyte enzyme disorders in children. Pediatr Clin North Am 27:449, 1980

40. Tanaka KR, Paglia DE: Pyruvate kinase deficiency. Semin Hematol 8:367, 1971

41. Taylor ES: Chronic ulcer of the leg associated with congenital hemolytic jaundice. JAMA 112:1574, 1939

42. Torlontano G, Fontana L, DeLaurenzi A et al: Hereditary elliptocytosis. Haematological and metabolic findings. Acta Haematol 48:1, 1972

43. Valentine WN: Hemolytic anemia and inborn errors of metabolism. Blood 54:549, 1979

44. Weed RI, Bowdler AJ: Metabolic dependence of the critical hemolytic volume of human erythrocytes: Relationship to osmotic fragility and autohemolysis in hereditary spherocytosis and normal red cells. J Clin Invest 45:1137, 1966

46. Wiley JS, Gill FM: Red cell calcium leak in congenital hemolytic anemia with extreme microcytosis. Blood 47:197, 1976

45. Wiley JS, Ellory JC, Shuman MA et al: Characteristics of the membrane defect in the hereditary stomatocytosis syndrome. Blood 46:337, 1975

47. Wintrobe MM, Lee GR, Boggs DR et al: Clinical Hematology, 8th ed. Philadelphia, Lea & Febiger, 1981

48. Wolfe LC, John KM, Falcone JC et al: A genetic defect in the binding of protein 4.1 to spectrin in a kindred with hereditary spherocytosis. N Engl J Med 307:1367, 1982

49. Zarowsky HS, Mohandas N, Speaker CB et al: A congenital haemolytic anaemia with thermal sensitivity of the erythrocyte membrane. Br J Haematol 29:537, 1975

Acquired Nonimmune Anemia of Increased Destruction

Susan J. Leclair

The erythrocyte, despite its remarkable resilience, can be damaged and destroyed by various conditions that are neither inherited (Chap. 17) nor immune mediated (Chap. 19). This chapter deals with several situations in which such a hemolytic event can occur.

ACQUIRED EXTRACORPUSCULAR DEFECTS (FRAGMENTATION SYNDROMES)

Microangiopathic Hemolytic Anemia

Microangiopathic (*i.e.*, a disease of small blood vessels) hemolytic anemia (MAHA) can be a complication of one of several conditions in which there is a disturbance of the microvascular environment.[4] These primary states are many and varied. All the conditions discussed in this chapter appear to be associated with changes in the small vessels that are the result of (1) fibrin deposition, an activity that follows vessel injury and begins the repair process (Chap. 50); (2) severe systemic hypertension; or (3) vessel abnormalities. The conditions associated with MAHA included in this chapter are disseminated intravascular coagulation (DIC), thrombotic thrombocytopenic purpura (TTP), hemolytic uremic syndrome (HUS), abnormalities of blood vessel structure such as hemangioma, and abnormalities of blood vessels secondary to hypertension.

Pathophysiology

Erythrocytes undergo several different types of circulatory stress. Arterial blood pressure, cardiac output, *p*H, and variations in tonicity (tissue tension; in body fluid physiology, the effective osmotic pressure equivalent) are among the more prominent.[7] The shear force caused by the arterial blood pressure is sufficient to either fragment red cells that are caught by endothelial projections or have partially penetrated the endothelial cells of the vessel wall.[5] Abnormal deposition of fibrin, atheromas (a mass or plaque of degenerated, thickened arterial intima occurring in atherosclerosis), anatomic defects, and the like reduce the vessel lumen diameter, causing both a localized increase in blood pressure and an increased number of projections. The combination of this abnormal increase in the force of the moving cells and the smaller vessel cross-sectional area cause more pronounced injury and subsequent fragmentation of the red cells.[8] The physical findings in these cases are related to the primary disease, whereas signs and symptoms of fatigue, weakness, pallor, and dizziness are related to the degree of anemia.

Laboratory Findings and Correlations with Disease

PERIPHERAL BLOOD.   The peripheral blood picture varies, as it depends on the primary inciting event and the ability of the patient's bone marrow to compensate for hemolysis. As a result the anemia may range from nonexistent to severe, causing the erythrocyte count, hemoglobin (Hb), and hematocrit values to be slightly to severely decreased. Schistocytes (red cell fragments) are a characteristic finding, regardless of the hematocrit value. Generally, the number of schistocytes is an indication of the extent of hemolysis.

If hemolysis is active and the bone marrow competent, compensation results in a reticulocytosis, which is seen on the peripheral blood film as anisocytosis with a subpopulation of larger-than-normal cells and polychromasia. The reticulocyte count should be corrected for this by performing a reticulocyte production index (RPI) (Chap. 9). The RPI is usually greater than 3 in a hemolytic disorder if the bone marrow is capable of compensating for red cell destruction. If hemolysis is brisk and the marrow is attempting to compensate, nucleated red blood cells may be seen in the peripheral blood, although not to the extent that they can be found in some hereditary hemoglobinopathies. Occasional microspherocytes may also be observed.

Because of the variety of cell sizes that may be present, the red cell mean corpuscular volume (MCV) value should not be taken literally, for it represents the average of larger reticulocytes, smaller fragments and spherocytes, and normocytes, which yields an overall MCV in the low to normal range.[2] Bessman[3] and others have developed interpretations of the relationship of MCV, red cell distribution width (RDW) (Chap. 10), and the red cell histogram that have led to a more comprehensive analysis of the red cell populations found in these states. The RDW is reported to indicate the degree of actual cell size variability, which should be a more valuable laboratory parameter[3] than the MCV. If the RDW is more sensitive than the MCV in MAHA, the diagnosis and medical intervention might be made earlier. This remains to be confirmed.

Leukocyte counts vary with the primary disease state, although moderate leukocytosis is not uncommon. Thrombocytopenia may be found, since several disease states present with a consumption coagulopathy during which platelets and other coagulation factors are consumed at a faster rate than they can be replenished.

BONE MARROW.   Examinations of aspirates or biopsy specimens are not diagnostic and typically show normo-blastic (i.e., normal appearing nucleated erythrocytes) hyperplasia (abnormal increase in the number of cells in normal arrangement in the tissue), and occasionally hyperplasia of the megakaryocyte line. If the latter is present, the megakaryocytes appear to be somewhat immature.

COAGULATION.   Tests of the coagulation system must be performed to determine whether intravascular coagulation has initiated hemolysis.[36] Decreases in several components of the coagulation system, including factors I, II, V, and VIII (Chap. 50), are common if the coagulopathy is moderate to severe. If it is mild, performance of a test for fibrin D-d dimer (which reflects actual clotting and clot degradation in vivo) or other tests of the fibrinolytic system (which is responsible for normal clot breakdown [Chap. 54]) are useful for detection. The importance of evaluation of the coagulation system cannot be overemphasized, as it is essential for elucidating the patient's condition.

OTHER LABORATORY FINDINGS.   Other important findings in patient evaluation are increased plasma hemoglobin and decreased serum haptoglobin values. Urinary findings include occasional hemoglobinuria and hemosiderinuria.

Most Useful Laboratory Tests for Diagnosing Microangiopathic Hemolytic Anemia

Initially, a complete blood count and a differential leukocyte count are necessary to diagnose MAHA, including observation of erythrocyte morphology, specifically for the degree of schistocytosis. While frequent blood counts may be necessary to monitor hemolysis, generally, daily differential leukocyte counts are neither necessary nor helpful unless other complications arise. Bone marrow examination rarely, if ever, is necessary to make the diagnosis of MAHA.

Effects of Treatment on Laboratory Results

Since this condition is secondary to an underlying disorder, prognosis and treatment depend on what that disorder is; however, the hemolytic component of the syndrome may be adequately monitored in the following manner. If appropriate treatment for the underlying cause is effective, anemia should diminish gradually until the erythrocyte count, hemoglobin, and hematocrit values return to normal. The RDW should return to normal as the schistocyte and spherocyte populations decline and the erythrocytes become more uniform. The RPI should be performed periodically (not daily) to check for bone marrow compensation. RPI should remain greater than three as the red cell measurements return to normal if marrow compensation is adequate. Haptoglobin, plasma hemoglobin, and urinary hemoglobin levels are useful for diagnosis but not very useful in follow-up, because they are not particularly good indicators of the degree of hemolysis or marrow compensation.

Disseminated Intravascular Coagulation

When there is extensive damage to vessel endothelium or exposure to compounds that initiate clotting (e.g., thromboplastic substances that encourage coagulation or various proteolytic enzymes), DIC may follow.[33] As a direct result of fibrin deposition along and across the vessel lumen, erythrocytes can be fragmented or destroyed as they are pushed through the vessel by the action of blood pressure and rapidly flowing circulation (Fig. 18-1). DIC may occur at any age because it is strictly dependent on the primary disorders that can cause it, which are many. For further discussion of the pathophysiology of this condition, see Chapter 55.

Laboratory Findings and Correlations with Disease

PERIPHERAL BLOOD. Since DIC can be acute or chronic, the peripheral blood findings vary according to the degree of active hemolysis.[21] In acute DIC there is evidence of red cell destruction or signs of bone marrow compensation, as described in the general discussion of MAHA. Schistocytes are common but are a relatively insensitive indicator of DIC. Subtle alterations due to compensation are found in erythrocyte numbers, reticulocyte count, and erythrocyte morphology.[16] The presence of macroreticulocytes, microspherocytes, and unusually shaped or fragmented erythrocytes alters the MCV. The hemoglobin and hematocrit levels depend on the extent of blood loss, the amount of dehydration, and the duration of the coagulopathy.

Thrombocytopenia is an early and consistent finding that is due to platelet consumption by excessive coagulation. The leukocyte count varies depending on the marrow's ability to respond appropriately to the causative agent or event. Granulocytopenia may be a sign of the marrow's inability to compensate. Other abnormal findings in the leukocytes, particularly in cases associated with bacterial sepsis, might include toxic granulation, Döhle bodies, and an increase in the number of immature granulocytes (i.e., a shift to the left)[32] (Chap. 26).

BONE MARROW. Marrow examination is essentially nondiagnostic. Its value lies in ascertaining the state of the marrow's compensatory mechanism. In most patients with DIC, the marrow reflects normoblastic hyperplasia with occasional megakaryocytic hyperplasia. After prolonged episodes of DIC, the marrow may enter an "exhausted" stage and mimic an aplastic state in which it becomes hypocellular (Chap. 11).

COAGULATION AND FIBRINOLYSIS. These tests are required to correctly identify acute and chronic DIC. The reader is referred to Chapter 55 for a discussion of DIC and to other chapters on coagulation laboratory procedures in the Hemostasis section of this textbook.

CHEMISTRY. Chemical blood findings are important in chronic DIC because intravascular hemolysis is often at an indetectable level, at which compensation by the marrow is relatively easy. In these cases, chemical abnormalities are more diagnostic than hematologic parameters. Increased levels of serum lactate dehydrogenase (isoenzymes 1 [LD-1] or 3 [LD-3]) and decreased levels of haptoglobin are important findings in suspected chronic DIC and would be expected in acute DIC. Hemoglobinemia and hemoglobinuria occur during active periods of hemolysis.

SPECIAL TESTS. Red cell half-life (Chap. 16) in both acute and chronic DIC is decreased, indicating decreased red cell survival time, but this measurement is rarely necessary for diagnosis.

Effects of Treatment on Laboratory Results

Because DIC is the result of a primary disease state, treatment of the underlying cause must be initiated before any resolution is possible. If treatment is successful, abnormal laboratory findings should return to normal and schistocytes should disappear from the peripheral film.[31]

Thrombotic Thrombocytopenic Purpura

In contrast to DIC, which has no age preference, and to hemolytic uremic syndrome, which is more common in

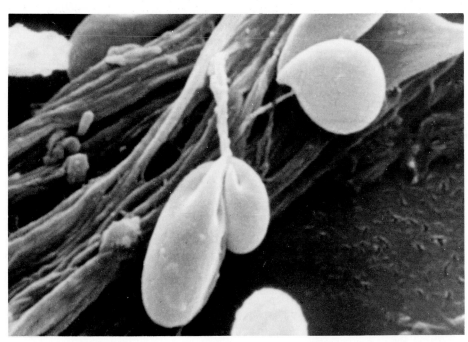

FIG. 18-1. Classic scanning electron micrograph of the so-called hanged red cell, which helped to clarify the pathogenesis of schistocyte formation in patients with inappropriate fibrin deposition (X 5200). Dense fibrin band in background formed from accumulations of finer strands, some of which are still evident. (From Bull BS, Kuhn IH: The production of schistocytes by fibrin strands. Blood 35:104, 1970, with permission.)

children, thrombotic thrombocytopenic purpura (TTP) is most often seen in young adults (peak incidence is in the third decade of life). Also known as Moschkovitz syndrome, TTP is characterized by fever, hemorrhagic signs such as petechiae, neurologic signs such as seizures (and coma in some cases), and renal disease.[23] Hemolytic anemia is a consistent finding. TTP shows striking pathology in the gray matter of the cerebral cortex and medulla of the brain secondary to vascular occlusions. These occlusions show extensive platelet aggregation, leading to excessive platelet consumption. Although many causes have been proposed, those cited most frequently are inappropriate immune response, decrease in prostaglandin formation, and stimulation by oral contraceptives.

Laboratory Findings and Correlations with Disease

Typically, the Hb value in TTP is below 10 g/dL. Initial values below 5 g/dL are not uncommon. Reticulocytosis is brisk, and normoblasts are present on the peripheral blood film. Large numbers of schistocytes are characteristic. Significant poikilocytosis includes bizarre and distorted forms. Thrombocytopenia is common; values can be as low as $10 \times 10^9/L$ (Fig. 18-2). While thrombocytopenia is common in both TTP and DIC, these disorders differ in the results of coagulation testing. Granulocytosis is common, and counts may exceed $20 \times 10^9/L$. Immature granulocytic forms may be present.

COAGULATION. In TTP results of tests of the coagulation system are usually within reference ranges, whereas they are abnormal in DIC.

BONE MARROW. As with DIC, a bone marrow examination is not necessary for diagnosis. Typically, however, the marrow shows normoblastic hyperplasia, and it may also demonstrate an increase in megakaryocytes.

CHEMISTRY. Intravascular hemolysis is the most likely cause of anemia in TTP, as plasma hemoglobin and unconjugated bilirubin levels are elevated, and the haptoglobin level is decreased.

Effects of Treatment on Laboratory Results

TTP is a serious, progressive, and rapidly fatal disease unless intervention with correct therapy occurs. Therapy includes the use of platelet inhibitors such as aspirin, dextran, and sulfinpyrazone; plasma exchange transfusion; high-dose corticosteroids; and splenectomy and heparin therapy if the concurrent presence of DIC has been confirmed. Most patients achieve a complete and long-lasting remission. With an effective therapeutic approach, some abnormal values begin to disappear within hours (*e.g.,* platelet counts increase and schistocytes disappear within 2 days).[24]

Hemolytic Uremic Syndrome

Hemolytic uremia, first described in 1955,[11] is a syndrome of infants and young children that involves acute intravascular hemolysis and renal failure. HUS has also been reported in women during normal pregnancy, and particularly in the postpartum period.[30] The syndrome involves hemolytic anemia of the microangiopathic type and variable amounts of platelet destruction. While the inciting event is not clearly defined, mild febrile illnesses, certain immunizations, and gastrointestinal disturbances have been implicated.[25] The onset of symptoms usually is acute. Typical signs and symptoms include increased blood pressure, vomiting, diarrhea, pallor, abdominal pain, and dark-colored urine. The syndrome often progresses to either oliguria or anuria. Hepatomegaly is common; splenomegaly is not. While there are some neurologic signs, such as drowsiness and convulsions, they are neither as frequent nor as severe as those seen in TTP. Purpuric (patches of purplish skin discoloration) and ecchymotic lesions (large black and blue marks in the skin) may be caused by either a low platelet count, ingestion of aspirin during the initial stages of the illness, or a combination of the two.

Laboratory Findings and Correlations with Disease

PERIPHERAL BLOOD. The Hb values of these patients are severely decreased, sometimes as low as 4 g/dL. The leukocyte count may be elevated with a predominance of neutrophils. Thrombocytopenia, when present, seems to be in proportion to the severity of the anemia. The peripheral blood film shows schistocytes, burr cells, and when compensation is occurring, moderate to marked polychromasia.

COAGULATION. Coagulation test results are usually within reference ranges.

CHEMISTRY. The hemolytic portion of HUS causes a marked elevation of plasma hemoglobin values. In many cases, this may be detected by examination of the plasma by the unaided eye. Haptoglobin is decreased and methemoglobin is present. Serum bilirubin values may be slightly elevated. Hemoglobinuria and hemosiderinuria also are present.

The uremic portion of HUS is demonstrated by other findings, such as extreme elevations of blood urea nitrogen (BUN) and serum creatinine.

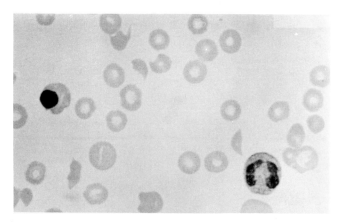

FIG. 18-2. Peripheral blood from a patient with thrombotic thrombocytopenic purpura shows helmet cells, schistocytes, spherocytes, immature forms (note nucleated erythrocyte), and severe depletion of platelet number. (From Kapff CT, Jandl JH: Blood: Atlas and Sourcebook of Hematology. Boston, Little, Brown, & Co, 1981, with permission.)

URINALYSIS. Protein (mostly albumin), erythrocytes, leukocytes, and casts are usually found during urinalysis.

Effects of Treatment on Laboratory Results

The increase in the recovery rate of children appears to be correlated with the increase in the treatment quality of the renal failure aspect of HUS. Current therapy includes conservative management of fluid, electrolytes, and blood gases together with a precise control of blood pressure.[6] Some more severely affected children may require peritoneal dialysis or hemodialysis. Laboratory values return toward normal after therapy has been established. Presently, therapy for the hemolytic component of the disease is somewhat controversial.

Abnormal Blood Vessel Structure

Hemangiomas (benign tumors of the blood vessels) may be associated with MAHA. They are found most often in the skin and liver. The proposed explanation for the hemolytic process is that local coagulation initiated by the presence of the abnormal vascular component causes the red cell fragmentation.

Malignant hypertension is a rapidly progressive form of high blood pressure associated with severe vascular damage.[19] This damage may cause a MAHA. Uremic changes in the form of peripheral blood burr cells may be noted (Fig. 18-3) in this condition.

A number of patients suffering from malignant disease have also been observed to have acute hemolytic episodes that are considered to be MAHA. In most of the cases studied, hemolysis appears to have been initiated by localized coagulation caused by the presence of abnormal endothelium or mucin production. Patients with carcinoma of the stomach, breast, or pancreas are more likely to have abnormal vessel construction than those with other forms of carcinoma. As with most MAHA, the erythrocyte fragmentation usually results from shearing of the cells as they are caught on fibrin strands produced in the coagulation process.

Laboratory Findings and Correlations with Disease

PERIPHERAL BLOOD. With hemangiomatous lesions, the hemolysis is chronic and mild, whereas with malignant hypertension the process is more acute. The Hb value may drop abruptly to an average of less than 10 g/dL. Thrombocytopenia is present. Evaluation of leukocytes and any immature red cells in the peripheral blood is difficult because it must take into account the possibility of an underlying disease process, which could be myelophthisis (replacement of the bone marrow) in the case of disseminated malignancy.

COAGULATION. Some patients have a consumptive coagulopathy, which is demonstrated by abnormal results of coagulation studies.

CHEMISTRY. Hemolysis is confirmed by the presence of elevated indirect (unconjugated) bilirubin levels, elevated LD-1 and LD-2 isoenzymes, and decreased haptoglobin levels.

Effects of Treatment on Laboratory Results

Standard treatment of hemangiomas involves irradiation of the tumor site or surgical removal if possible, either of which should end fragmentation. There is no standard therapy for MAHA in patients with carcinoma, and usually their prognosis is poor. In cases of hypertension, treatment with appropriate drug intervention should be sufficient to end erythrocyte fragmentation; however, treatment should include an appreciation of the possibility that antihypertensive agents such as aldomet (Chap. 19) can initiate autoimmune hemolytic anemia. In such cases, the drug being used should be discontinued immediately and a new mode of treatment should be sought.[26]

Mechanical Injury to Erythrocytes

Damage to the Heart and Aorta

Not uncommonly, patients who have aortic valvular disease such as aortic stenosis or a cardiovascular prosthesis develop a form of red cell fragmentation. Several mechanisms have been proposed for this hemolysis, including direct mechanical injury, abnormal turbulence, fibrin deposition, and autoimmune antibody formation.

LABORATORY FINDINGS AND CORRELATIONS WITH DISEASE. **Peripheral blood.** The peripheral blood in this anemia has no distinctive features. Patients have signs and symptoms that relate to the red cell damage. Normal erythropoietic response to the hemolysis may compensate for the anemia. If hemolysis is compensated, the peripheral blood numbers and picture may be normal, with macrocytic cells in association with a reticulocytosis in patients who usually have an MCV in the high normal range. If hemolysis is significant, the peripheral blood picture and other laboratory findings are identical to those of a microangiopathic hemolytic process (Fig. 18-4).

Chemistry. The rise in bilirubin value, especially the unconjugated fraction, parallels the severity of the hemolysis.

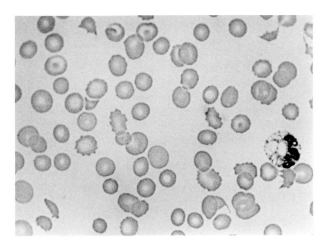

FIG. 18-3. The peripheral blood picture of a patient suffering from malignant hypertension shows both fragmentation and burr cells, indicating uremic changes. Note vacuolated, nearly destroyed appearance of granulocyte, which has almost no granules. (From Kapff CT, Jandl JH: Blood: Atlas and Sourcebook of Hematology. Boston, Little, Brown & Co, 1981, with permission.)

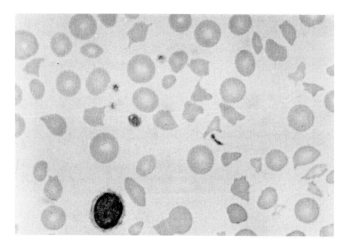

FIG. 18-4.   A typical representation of the mechanical injury that may be induced by prosthetic valves or great vessel abnormalities. (From Kapff CT, Jandl JH: Blood: Atlas and Sourcebook of Hematology. Boston, Little, Brown & Co, 1981, with permission.)

EFFECTS OF TREATMENT ON LABORATORY RESULTS.   If the hemolysis is severe enough to suggest the necessity for surgical intervention, replacement or repair of the anatomic lesion, whether valve, patch, or rupture, must be considered. Until that decision is made, bed rest and other palliative therapy is recommended. Only after the cause is corrected will hemolysis diminish.

Stress or March Hemoglobinuria

A rare form of hemolysis occurs in susceptible people (usually a young adult) who engage in extremely stressful exercise, typically involving forceful contact of some or all of the body with a hard surface. This transient hemolysis has been seen in soldiers after prolonged forced marches and in practitioners of karate and other vigorous exercise.

SYMPTOMS.   Since the hemolysis is transient and patient complaints are not severe, clinical evaluation often is not performed. Complaints include passage of dark urine after exercise and vague abdominal or lower back pains.

LABORATORY FINDINGS AND CORRELATIONS WITH DISEASE.   **Peripheral blood.** In this disease the peripheral blood may show polychromatophilia after recurrent episodes of hemolysis. Red cell measurements will decrease to a level consistent with the severity of the hemolysis.
   Chemistry. The plasma hemoglobin level may be elevated and serum haptoglobin decreased.

Miscellaneous Extracorpuscular Mechanisms of Injury

Infections and Infestations

Hemolysis can occur as a complication of exposure to a variety of infectious agents. Malaria, caused by any of the four species (*Plasmodium vivax, P. malariae, P. falciparum, P. ovale*), results in a hemolytic process initiated by the direct invasion of erythrocytes by the parasite. Anemia may be mild to severe and persists for some time after successful treatment of the infestation.[38] Infection with *Toxoplasma gondii,* occasionally contracted from domestic cats, has been associated with hemolytic events in children and adults.[22]
   Hemolytic episodes have also been associated with infections of various species of *Clostridium, Staphylococcus,* and *Streptococcus,* and many gram-negative bacilli. The mechanisms of these episodes are unclear, but they may be secondary to the activation of so-called T antigens on the red cell surface.

Exposure to Chemicals and Toxins

Hemolytic anemias also have been reported as complications of spider bites, bee stings, and snake venom. Again, the mechanisms are unclear.[34] A well known complication of hemodialysis has been the onset of a hemolytic event. Probable causes of this include oxidizing compounds in water supplies used for bacterial purification and additional contaminants in the water, such as nitrate or copper.[20]

Thermal Injury

Because mature erythrocytes are extremely fragile and sensitive to changes in osmotic pressure and mechanical injury, exposure to elevated temperatures caused by burns results in fragmentation and membrane loss. Thus, schistocytes and microspherocytes are found immediately on the peripheral blood film. Hemoglobinemia and hemoglobinuria are common the first day after a thermal injury. The morphologic damage seen in burn victims is self-limited and eventually resolves. The renal aspect of the hemolysis is of greater concern in the patient's prognosis. Hemolysis that occurs several days after the thermal event may be due to the infusion of fresh frozen plasma (to replenish lost plasma volume) that may contain hemolytic antibodies.[35]

ACQUIRED INTRACORPUSCULAR MECHANISMS OF INJURY

Paroxysmal Nocturnal Hemoglobinuria

Pathophysiology

Paroxysmal nocturnal hemoglobinuria (PNH) is a rare, acquired defect of insidious onset which arises in bone marrow stem cells. It occurs most often in the third to fifth decades of life, although it has been reported in childhood and old age. The cells arising from the affected stem cells show an abnormal sensitivity to complement in acidified plasma or a low ionic strength environment, which results in complement-mediated lysis. Because it affects the stem cells, all erythrocytes, granulocytes, and platelets arising from those cells possess the defect. In the erythrocyte line, cells appear to demonstrate three different types of sensitivity. PNH-I erythrocytes react normally in the presence of complement, whereas PNH-II cells are three to five times more sensitive. The cell population PNH-III reacts most strongly on average with 15 to 25 times more sensitivity. Patients generally appear to have a mixture of two of the cell subcategories, the combination of PNH-I and PNH-III being most common.[28]
   Patients with PNH have signs and symptoms associated with the chronic extravascular hemolysis and hemoglobinuria which occur chiefly at night, when blood pH falls.

Exercise, which also causes a slight reduction in blood pH, has been associated with hemolysis in these patients, but the association of acid pH with hemolysis still is unclear. While many different biochemical abnormalities have been demonstrated in the cells of patients with PNH, no one abnormality has been suggested as the major agent of hemolysis. Abnormalities have been indicated in the immune mechanism and structural protein or biochemistry of the erythrocyte membrane, among others. Recent evidence also points to defects in regulator proteins of C3 convertases, decay-accelerating factor (DAF), and the like.[17]

Clinical Signs and Symptoms

The clinical signs and symptoms are wide ranging, since the abnormal cell population varies. The hemolysis may be asymptomatic, or rarely, very severe. Typically, patients present with weakness, slight jaundice, abdominal pain of unknown origin, and splenomegaly. Hepatomegaly is unusual. Hemoglobinuria is not an obvious finding.[29]

Laboratory Findings and Correlations with Disease

PERIPHERAL BLOOD.   The hematologic findings are variable in severity and presentation. The Hb level may drop below 6 g/dL. Red cells can vary from macrocytic, normochromic to microcytic, hypochromic if there is increased urinary iron loss. Relative reticulocytosis does occur but it is usually inadequate for true compensation. Normoblasts may be found in the peripheral blood. Leukopenia is common, with neutropenia and relative lymphocytosis.[14] There is some speculation that neutropenia may be the result of a shift from the circulating to the marginating granulocyte pools (Chap. 23). Thrombocytopenia does occur, but the platelet life span appears to be normal.

BONE MARROW.   Marrow examination is not necessary for diagnosis. Most commonly, the marrow demonstrates normoblastic hyperplasia with some decrease in megakaryocyte number. One complication of PNH is the progression of the disease into aplastic anemia, in which case marrow examination is valuable for demonstrating the replacement of normally cellular areas with fat, which results in pancytopenia.

CHEMISTRY.   Some biochemical defects have been noted in the erythrocytes and granulocytes. Decreased leukocyte alkaline phosphatase (LAP) and acetylcholinesterase (AChE) have been found, although, according to the clonal theory, it is probable that there are two or more populations of leukocytes, one with normal enzyme content and one with decreased enzyme content.[10]

Most Useful Laboratory Tests for Diagnosing PNH

The diagnosis of PNH is based on two tests that amplify PNH erythrocytes' abnormal sensitivity to complement (i.e., the membrane-puncturing capability of activated complement). These tests include the so-called sugar water, or sucrose lysis screening test and the more specific Ham's acidified-serum test.

Because PNH erythrocytes are more sensitive to complement than their normal counterparts, they readily undergo hemolysis in these tests. The phenomenon occurs in the absence of any antibody.

SUGAR WATER SCREENING TEST[12]
Principle

Whole blood is incubated at 37°C in a low ionic strength sugar water solution, which promotes binding of complement components, particularly C3 (Chaps. 16 and 19) to the red cell surface. This environment strains the ability of erythrocytes to remain intact. Normal erythrocytes do not hemolyze under these conditions, but erythrocytes from patients with PNH, which are extremely sensitive to complement-mediated lysis, do hemolyze.

Specimen Requirements

Venous blood collected in citrate may be used (one part citrate to nine parts whole blood) or whole blood anticoagulated with oxalate (one part 0.1 mol/L sodium oxalate to nine parts whole blood). A defibrinated whole blood specimen (1–2 mL) is also acceptable. A normal specimen should be drawn in the same manner for use as a control.

Reagents

To make sucrose solution, add 9 to 10 g sucrose (commercial granulated sugar) to 100 mL distilled water. The pH should be approximately 7.4. Prepare fresh daily.

Quality Control

A fresh normal control sample should be tested as a negative control along with the patient sample.

Before the test is performed a small amount of the normal sample and the patient's sample should be centrifuged and the plasma checked for hemolysis due to traumatic venipuncture, which would cause a false positive test result. Hemolyzed specimens cannot be used for testing.

Procedure

1. Pipet 4.5 mL sucrose solution into each of two 13 × 100-mm test tubes; label one *Control,* one *Patient.*
2. Add 0.5 mL well mixed control blood and patient blood to respective tubes. Cover and invert both tubes gently to mix.
3. Place both tubes in a 37°C water bath for 30 minutes. (Room temperature incubation is acceptable also.) Centrifuge tubes to sediment red cells.
4. Observe supernatant for hemolysis.

Interpretation of Results

If patient's supernatant contains hemolysis, the result is positive and indicates the possibility of PNH as well as other hemolytic states. A normal control sample must yield a negative result, otherwise the test is invalid and should be repeated.

Comments and Sources of Error

1. If result is negative, no further testing is necessary because this test is quite sensitive for PNH.
2. The sugar water test is not very specific (i.e., a positive result does not necessarily indicate PNH). Therefore, if the result is positive, it must be confirmed by performing Ham's acidified-serum test.
3. Blood for this test should not be collected in heparin or EDTA; doing so causes erroneous results.
4. False negative results may be due to (A) lack of complement in the plasma or serum (it is therefore imperative to use fresh samples to ensure complement activity); (B) use of unbuffered sucrose solution (pH should be close to 7.4); and (C) recent massive transfusion of the patient with normal erythrocytes.
5. False positive results may be due to (A) traumatic venipuncture during which the specimen was hemolyzed; (B) a severely anemic specimen; and (C) a specimen from a patient with an immune hemolytic anemia, although hemolysis in this case is usually much less prominent than in PNH.

HAM'S ACIDIFIED SERUM TEST

Principle

Erythrocytes in PNH are abnormally sensitive to complement-mediated lysis in acidified serum. Several combinations of patient and normal serum and cells are mixed and some are acidified to maximize the hemolytic effect associated with PNH.

Specimen

Defibrinated whole blood from patient and a control sample are required. Both samples are centrifuged and serum and cells are separated. A small amount of normal serum must be heat-inactivated at 56°C for 30 minutes.

Procedure

1. Set up seven 12 × 75-mm tubes, as shown in Table 18-1. All serum is added in 0.5-mL quantities; all cells and 0.2N hydrochloric (HCl) acid are added in 0.05-mL quantities.
2. Mix and incubate for 60 minutes at 37°C.
3. Centrifuge and observe each supernatant for hemolysis.

Quality Control

Several quality control features are built into this test. Note on Table 18-1 that tubes 4 and 7 contain heat-inactivated serum and should therefore not demonstrate lysis, even with cells from PNH patients since complement is not available (except for patients with hereditary spherocytosis, see Comments). Tubes 5 and 6 should not show lysis because they contain normal serum and cells; the HCl in tube 6 should not cause lysis of normal cells. If any tubes expected not to exhibit hemolysis do show it, the test results are invalid and the test should be repeated, taking care to follow the procedure.

Interpretation

Table 18-1 demonstrates the lysis pattern in PNH when this procedure is followed. Note that tube 1 may have a trace of hemolysis or none. Hemolysis is often stronger with patient cells, HCl, and normal serum than with patient cells, patient serum, and HCl.

The lysis pattern for hereditary spherocytosis (HS) is also shown in Table 18-1. The differential result is in tube 4. Spherocytes will hemolyze in acidified serum without complement, thus if hemolysis occurs in tube 4, HS may be indicated; PNH cells do not hemolyze without complement, so the result in tube 4 will be negative in PNH.

Comments and Sources of Error

False negative results may occur if fresh serum is not used. Heat inactivation of serum must be complete (i.e., 56°C for 30 minutes), to prevent erroneous results.

In addition to PNH, results of the Ham's test may be positive in aplastic anemia, leukemia, and myeloproliferative disorders.[9] It is positive in 60% of cases[37] of the rare type II form of congenital dyserythropoietic anemia known as hereditary erythroblastic multinuclearity with positive acidified serum test (HEMPAS [Chap. 12]). Fortunately PNH and HEMPAS can be differentiated because in HEMPAS, lysis never occurs with the patient's own serum, only with normal serum. Also the result of the sugar water screening test is positive in PNH but negative in HEMPAS.

Differential Diagnosis

The diagnosis of PNH is difficult to make with any one procedure or symptom. Laboratory tests and symptoms must demonstrate idiopathic intravascular hemolysis with or without hemoglobinuria, pancytopenia with or without hypocellularity in the bone marrow, recurrent thrombotic episodes, and unexplained abdominal pain or headache in association with hemolytic episodes. A positive Ham's test result is also important to the diagnosis.

Effects of Treatment on Laboratory Results

There is no successful therapy for PNH, but bone marrow transplantation, hormone therapy, infusions of washed red cells, oral iron therapy, and anticoagulants have been used in various situations. Management should be conservative and given as needed. Treatment should be based on the degree and frequency of hemolytic episodes. As a result, laboratory values may retain many abnormalities throughout the course of the disease although, in some patients, over time, laboratory values have returned to normal. Prognosis is difficult to predict because some patients appear to achieve complete clinical remission; others remain in a chronic hemolytic state with increased possibility of thrombotic events; some progress into more malignant states; and still others enter an aplastic state that leads to

---

TABLE 18–1. Ham's Acidified Serum Test*

CONSTITUENTS	TEST TUBE NO.						
	1	2	3	4	5	6	7
Fresh normal serum	X	X			X	X	
Patient's fresh serum			X				
Heat-inactivated serum—Normal-ABO Compatible				X			X
Patient's erythrocytes	X	X	X	X			
Control erythrocytes					X	X	X
HCl, 0.2 N		X	X			X	X
	LYSIS PATTERNS						
Lysis pattern in PNH	−/TRACE	+++	+	−	−	−	−
Lysis pattern in hereditary spherocytosis	−	+	+	+	−	−	−
Normal specimen	−	−	−	−	−	−	−

* Mixtures of reagents, control, and patient specimen for the Ham's test. Expected pattern of hemolysis is indicated for PNH and for hereditary spherocytosis. No hemolysis is expected with a normal control specimen.
Key: X = add serum to tube in 0.5-mL quantities, add cells and 0.2 N HCl in 0.05-mL quantities; − = negative; + = slight hemolysis; +++ = marked hemolysis.

hemorrhage and infection, either of which may be fatal.[15,18,27]

ACQUIRED INTRACORPUSCULAR DEFECTS

Those anemias associated with such disease states as nutritional deficiencies (*e.g.*, iron [Chap. 13] and folate deficiencies [Chap. 12]); abnormalities in plasma constituents (*e.g.*, Waldenstrom's macroglobulinemia and multiple myeloma [Chap. 39]); severe liver disease; and certain acquired secondary enzymopathies have a hemolytic component which results from defective erythropoiesis and the abnormal environment to which the erythrocytes are exposed.

CHAPTER SUMMARY

The major causes of acquired extracorpuscular defects include various categories of microangiopathic hemolytic anemia (disseminated intravascular coagulation [DIC], thrombotic thrombocytopenic purpura [TTP], hemolytic uremic syndrome [HUS], and abnormal vessel construction, due, for example, to malignant hypertension and hemangioma), mechanical injury (from a valve prosthesis, aortic damage, or stress or forceful bodily contact with a hard surface), and miscellaneous other mechanisms of injury (heat, infections, toxins). Although hemolysis is important as a major complication, discovering it is less important than determining the initiating event. Proper therapy generally involves correction of the instigator rather than direct treatment of the hemolysis. In addition to the complete blood count, laboratory profiles of these patients should include studies of the coagulation system and renal or liver function testing as a way of discriminating among the various primary causes.

Paroxysmal nocturnal hemoglobinuria (PNH) is categorized as an acquired intracorpuscular injury. PNH cells are abnormally sensitive to complement. In an acid or low ionic strength environment, PNH cells bind complement, particularly the C3 component, and hemolyze through complement mediation. Differential laboratory diagnosis of PNH is best accomplished using the sugar water screening test and the more specific Ham's acidified serum test.

CASE STUDY 18-1

A 4-year-old boy complaining of fever, vomiting, and sore throat was seen in the pediatric outpatient clinic. He lived out of state and had been visiting his grandparents for the month. His grandmother gave no pertinent medical history except that he had experienced some kidney trouble in the past year and that his appetite was poor but had gotten worse in the last few days.

The child was pale, listless, and had a temperature of 39°C (normal, 37°C). His mucous membranes were pale. His throat was red and inflamed, with occasional white patches. Cervical lymph nodes were palpable. Small ecchymoses (blue–black hemorrhagic areas on the skin) were present on his thighs and upper arms. The child was unable to produce a urine specimen.

The CBC results were WBC 11.0 × 10⁹/L; RBC 3.41 × 10¹²/L; Hb 9.0 g/dL; HCT 0.30 L/L; MCV 88 fL; MCH 26.3 pg; MCHC 30.0 g/dL; and platelets 125 × 10⁹/L. The differential count revealed 64% neutrophils, 2% bands, 27% lymphocytes, 3% monocytes, and 4%

eosinophils. RBC morphology showed a dual population of cell size; some cells were normocytic and some microcytic with slight hypochromia. There was moderate poikilocytosis, with slight schistocytes and moderate burr cells.

1. In light of the child's presenting signs and symptoms and his available history, without considering the laboratory data, is it possible to make a clear diagnosis? What might the possibilities be?
2. Given the CBC and RBC morphology, is hemolytic uremic syndrome ruled out as a possible diagnosis?
3. What additional tests should be performed to confirm the diagnosis?
4. Assuming that the diagnosis is correct (see answer to question 2), what is the prognosis for this child?
5. A throat culture taken at the time of his presentation grew β-hemolytic *Streptococcus pyogenes*. Does this result have any relation to the child's present condition?
6. How could the variability in the red cell morphology be explained?

REFERENCES

1. Antman KH, Skarin AT, Mayer RJ et al: Microangiopathic hemolytic anemia and cancer: A review. Medicine 58:377, 1979
2. Bessman JD: Automated Blood Counts and Differentials. Baltimore, The Johns Hopkins University Press, 1986
3. Bessman JD, Gilmer PR, Gardner FH: Improved classification of anemia by MCV and RDW. Am J Clin Pathol 80:332, 1983
4. Brain MC, Dacie JV, Hourihane OB: Microangiopathic haemolytic anaemia: The possible role of vascular lesions in pathogenesis. Br J Haematol 8:358, 1962
5. Bull BS, Kuhn IH: The production of schistocytes by fibrin strands. Blood 35:104, 1970
6. Carvalho ACA: Bleeding in uremia—a clinical challenge. N Engl J Med 308:38, 1983
7. Cokelet GR: Rheology and hemodynamics. Ann Rev Physiol 42:331, 1980
8. Cokelet GR, Meiselman HJ, Brooks DE: Erythrocyte Mechanics and Blood Flow, vol 13. New York, Alan R Liss, 1980
9. Conrad ME, Barton JC: The aplastic anemia-paroxysmal nocturnal hemoglobinuria syndrome. Am J Hematol 7:61, 1979
10. Dockter ME, Morrison M: Paroxysmal nocturnal hemoglobinuria erythrocytes are of two distinct types: Positive or negative for acetylcholinesterase. Blood 67:540, 1986
11. Gasser WC, Gautier E, Spek A et al: Hämolytisch-urämische Syndrome: Bilaterale Nierenrindennekrosen bei akuten erworbenen hämolytischen Anämien. Schweiz Med Wochenschr 85:905, 1955
12. Hartmann RC, Jenkins DE Jr: The "sugar water" test for paroxysmal nocturnal hemoglobinuria. N Engl J Med 275:155, 1966
13. Hartmann RC, Jenkins DE Jr, Arnold AB: Diagnostic specificity of sucrose hemolysis test for paroxysmal nocturnal hemoglobinuria. Blood 35:462, 1970
14. Hurd WW, Miodovnik M, Stys SJ: Pregnancy associated with paroxysmal nocturnal hemoglobinuria. Am J Obstet Gynecol 60:742, 1982
15. Hirsch VJ, Neubach PA, Parker DM et al: Paroxysmal nocturnal hemoglobinuria: Termination in acute myelomonocytic leukemia and reappearance after leukemic remission. Arch Intern Med 141:525, 1981
16. Jacobson RJ, Jackson DP: Erythrocyte fragmentation in defibrination syndromes. Ann Intern Med 81:207, 1974
17. Kinoshita T, Medof ME, Silber R et al: Distribution of decay-

accelerating factor in the peripheral blood of normal individuals and patients with paroxysmal nocturnal hemoglobinuria. J Exp Med 162:75, 1985

18. Krause JR: Paroxysmal nocturnal hemoglobinuria and acute nonlymphocytic leukemia. Cancer 51:2078, 1983

19. Linton AL, Gavras H, Gleadle RI et al: Microangiopathic haemolytic anaemia and the pathogenesis of malignant hypertension. Lancet 1:1277, 1969

20. Lynn KL, Boots MA, Mitchell TR: Haemolytic anaemia caused by overheated dialysate. Br Med J 1:306, 1979

21. Merskey C: Defibrination syndromes or ...? Blood 41:599, 1973

22. Michelson AD, Lammi AT: Haemolytic anaemia associated with acquired toxoplasmosis. Aust Paediatr 20:333, 1984

23. Moschcowitz E: An acute febrile pleiochromic anemia with hyaline thrombosis of the terminal arterioles and capillaries: An undescribed disease. Arch Intern Med 36:89, 1925

24. Myers TJ, Wakem CJ, Ball ED et al: Thrombotic thrombocytopenic purpura: Combined treatment with plasmapheresis and antiplatelet agents. Ann Intern Med 92:149, 1980

25. O'Regan S, Robitaille P, Mongeau JG et al: The hemolytic uremic syndrome associated with ECHO 22 infection. Clin Pediatr 19:125, 1980

26. Physician's Desk Reference, 40th ed. Oradell, NJ, Medical Economics, 1986

27. Rosse WF: Paroxysmal nocturnal haemoglobinuria in aplastic anaemia. Clin Haematol 7:541, 1978

28. Rosse WF: Paroxysmal nocturnal hemoglobinuria—present status and future prospects. West J Med 132:219, 1980

29. Rosse WF, Parker CJ: Paroxysmal nocturnal haemoglobinuria. Clin Haematol 14:105, 1985

30. Segonds A, Louradour N, Suc JM et al: Postpartum hemolytic uremic syndrome: A study of three cases with a review of the literature. Clin Nephrol 12:229, 1979

31. Sharp AA: Diagnosis and management of disseminated intravascular coagulation. Br Med Bull 33:265, 1977

32. Siegal T, Seligsohn U, Aghai E et al: Clinical and laboratory aspects of disseminated intravascular coagulation (DIC): A study of 118 cases. Thromb Haemostas 39:122, 1978

33. Spero JA, Lewis JH, Hasiba U: Disseminated intravascular coagulation. Thromb Haemostas 43:28, 1980

34. Taylor EH, Denny WF: Hemolysis, renal failure and death, presumed secondary to bite of recluse spider. South Med J 59:1209, 1966

35. Topley E, Bull JP, Maycock WD et al: The relation of the isoagglutinins in pooled plasma to the haemolytic anaemia of burns. J Clin Pathol 16:79, 1963

36. Triplett DA (ed): Laboratory Evaluation of Coagulation. Chicago, ASCP Press, 1982

37. Verwilghen RL, Lewis SM, Dacie JV et al: HEMPAS: Congenital dyserythropoietic anemia (type II). Q J Med 42:257, 1973

38. Woodruff AW, Ansdell VE, Pettitt LE: Cause of anaemia in malaria. Lancet 1:1055, 1979

Acquired Immune Anemia of Increased Destruction

Sister Catherine Sherry

Immune hemolytic anemia is characterized by accelerated destruction or hemolysis of red cells by an antibody. The resultant anemia is due to the function, or in some cases malfunction, of the body's immune system. In the normal immune system, the presence of a foreign antigen results in the production of antibodies to that antigen as a self-defense mechanism. *Isoantibodies* (also called *alloantibodies*) develop when a person is exposed to antigens that are found in the same species but are not present on the exposed person's cells.

In some cases the normal process that prevents formation of antibodies to the host's own antigens is flawed, and the immune system produces antibodies called *autoantibodies,* which react with the host's own cell or tissue antigens.

A third type of antibody is induced in some persons by certain drugs. These antibodies may resemble autoantibodies, but they demonstrate several modes of formation and cell destruction.

The anemias caused by any of these mechanisms are all acquired (*i.e.,* they are never inherited). They are called acquired immune hemolytic anemias, and are classified as isoimmune, autoimmune, or drug induced (Table 19-1). In all of these hemolytic disorders, the bone marrow must increase red cell production to compensate for increased destruction, so an erythroblastic hyperplasia in the marrow may be expected in all cases of adequate response. Bone marrow examination usually is not required to diagnose an acquired immune hemolytic anemia, since the findings do not reveal the diagnosis unless the condition is a primary marrow disease, such as lymphoma or leukemia.

TABLE 19–1. Classification of Immune Hemolytic Anemias

ISOIMMUNE
   Hemolytic disease of the newborn (HDN)
   Hemolytic transfusion reaction
AUTOIMMUNE
   Warm-antibody
     Primary (idiopathic)
     Secondary
       Chronic lymphocytic leukemia (CLL)
       Lymphoma
       Systemic lupus erythematosus
       Viruses
       Iron deficiency anemia
   Cold-antibody
     Primary (idiopathic cold agglutinin syndrome)
     Secondary cold agglutinin syndrome
       Mycoplasma pneumoniae
       Infectious mononucleosis
       Lymphoproliferative disease
   Paroxysmal cold hemoglobinuria (PCH)
     Idiopathic
     Secondary
       Syphilis
       Viral disease
DRUG INDUCED
   Hapten (drug adsorption) mechanism
   Immune complex (innocent bystander) mechanism
   α-Methyldopa (autoimmune/unknown) mechanism

HEMOLYSIS IN ACQUIRED IMMUNE HEMOLYTIC ANEMIA

In the acquired immune hemolytic anemias, hemolysis may occur in the intravascular system or in the extravascular reticuloendothelial system, depending on the disorder. When hemolysis is caused by an immune mechanism, however, other components are involved in the process.

Role of Complement

The complement system plays an important role in acquired immune hemolytic anemias. It consists of serum proteins that interact to mediate certain effects of the inflammatory response. The complement system also interacts with the coagulation, fibrinolytic, and kinin systems (Chap. 50).

Two pathways of reactions are involved in the sequential activation of complement components, the classic pathway and the alternate pathway. The classic pathway is activated by immunoglobulin G (IgG) or IgM antibodies complexed with antigens. This pathway, the one associated with autoimmune hemolytic anemias, is defined in some detail in this chapter. The alternate complement pathway is activated by certain cells, particles, or microorganisms without the presence of antibody. Because the alternate pathway is a nonimmune mechanism of defense against these foreign elements,[24, 27] it is beyond the scope of this chapter.

Complement components are designated by Arabic numerals,[3] for example, C1 or C3 (Fig. 19–1). The C1 molecule is a unique component with three subunits designated as C1q, C1r, and C1s, all of which are stabilized by the presence of calcium in the molecule. The C1 component is also known as the recognition unit since it initiates the complement cascade by recognizing IgG or IgM antibodies on cell surfaces (see Fig. 19–1).

Activated components in the fluid phase (*i.e.*, not attached to a cell or particle surface) are designated by a bar over the component number (*e.g.*, C̄1). Activated components bound to cell surfaces do not have such an indicator. When a complement component is activated, complement fragments are produced. These are indicated by lower case letters as suffixes, for example, C2a and C2b are the fragments produced upon activation of C2 (see Fig. 19–1).

The role of complement in the extravascular and intravascular hemolytic processes is discussed in the following sections of the chapter. Figure 19–1 provides an overview of the classic complement pathway with comments on key features relating to the sequence of reactions.

Extravascular Hemolysis in Acquired Immune Hemolytic Anemia

In an immune reaction, cells in circulation may become coated by immunoglobulin. Subsequently, the complement system cascade is initiated, leading to generation of an intermediate component known as C3b. C3b is bound to the cell surface, and this attachment generally is associated with extravascular red cell destruction in the liver. Destruction of immunoglobulin and complement-coated cells by liver Kupffer cell macrophages may be attributed to Kupffer cell receptors for the complement component C3b.

C3b is generated through the initial reactions of the complement system (see Fig. 19–1) as a result of activation of two antibody-binding sites close to each other on the red cell surface. These two sites may be activated by attachment of a single IgM antibody or, less effectively, by two IgG antibodies. When activated, these sites fix complement, beginning with the C1q component. Generally speaking, activated C1 acts on C4, converting it to an active state. Activated C4 along with C1 converts C2 to an active form. Finally, the combination of activated C4 and C2, termed C4b2a (or C3 convertase), cleaves C3 into C3b and C3a. C3b remains attached to the red cell membrane. C3a, however, is released to the plasma, where it acts as an anaphylatoxin, which serves as a mediator of inflammation by inducing mast cell degranulation and histamine release. Ultimately, strong attachment of C3b to the red cell surface is responsible for liver Kupffer cell destruction of these red cells.

Complement System Control

A serum enzyme called C3b inactivator (see Fig. 19–1) readily cleaves C3b into C3c and C3d if membrane interaction or cell destruction does not occur rapidly. C3d, once bound to the red cell membrane, actually prevents cell destruction, because it does not bind to macrophage receptor sites, and it appears to prevent the further attachment of C3b to the membrane, thus preventing complement-mediated extra- or intravascular destruction.[2]

C4 inactivator and C1s inhibitor also serve to control and limit complement system activity. In addition, the C4b2a component is unstable, which provides another control mechanism.[24]

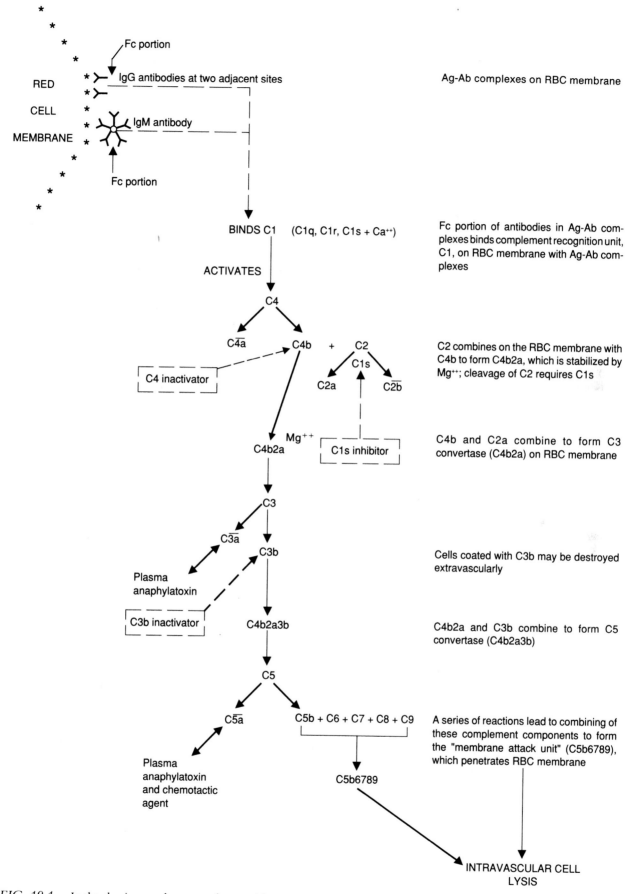

FIG. 19-1. In the classic complement pathway, either two IgG antibodies or one IgM antibody combines with antigens on the RBC membrane, forming antigen-antibody (Ag-Ab) complexes. The Fc portion of the antibodies may then bind the complement component Cl, thus activating the complement cascade.

Intravascular Hemolysis in Acquired Immune Hemolytic Anemia

Intravascular hemolysis that is complement mediated involves more complement components than those associated with extravascular hemolysis. The final component leading to extravascular red cell destruction is generally C3b. When the C3b component is further activated in intravascular hemolysis, a series of reactions leads to formation of C5b6789, otherwise known as the membrane attack unit, or terminal complex (see Fig. 19–1). This complex is so named because it is capable of penetrating the red cell surface by forming a transmembrane pore. This damage may result in leakage of hemoglobin and other cellular components or osmotic swelling due to excessive permeability to water and electrolytes, both of which result in intravascular hemolysis. One example of this mechanism of action is found in hemolytic transfusion reactions resulting from ABO incompatibility.

Complement System Control

This complement-mediated hemolytic process is limited by the same components as those associated with extravascular hemolysis. One further regulating component is the instability of the C4b2a3b enzyme complex,[24] also known as C5 convertase (see Fig. 19–1), which is needed for generation of the membrane attack unit.

ISOIMMUNE HEMOLYTIC ANEMIA

Isoantibodies (alloantibodies) are produced when one individual is exposed to antigens of another of the same species that are not already present on the first individual's cells. Isoantibodies do not react with the immunized person's antigens. Isoimmune hemolytic anemias are characterized by the presence of isoantibodies and are most commonly associated with either hemolytic disease of the newborn (HDN) or hemolytic transfusion reactions.

Hemolytic Disease of the Newborn

Definition

HDN is an anemia caused by destruction of the infant's red cells when a maternal antibody that is specific to an antigen on the infant's red cells crosses the placenta.

History

In 1940 Landsteiner and Wiener[17] discovered the Rh system of red cell antigens. It was thought that the Rh antigens might account for the observation of maternal antibodies in a case of erythroblastosis fetalis reported in 1939 by Levine and Stetson.[20] Landsteiner and Wiener discovered that the sera of rabbits and guinea pigs, immunized with Rhesus monkey red cells that carried the Rh antigen, agglutinated the red cells of most Caucasians tested. This newly described Rh antigen system did prove to provide the explanation for Levine's case of maternal-infant blood incompatibility.[18]

Pathophysiology

Transplacental passage of small amounts of fetal blood is relatively common, even during normal pregnancy. The mother's system may be stimulated to produce antibodies by the passage across the placenta of incompatible fetal red cells. The resulting antibody crosses back into the fetal circulation, and the fetus' red cells are destroyed. The most severe effects of such an event have been associated with Rh incompatibilities, although ABO incompatibilities can produce HDN with milder symptoms. Other blood groups, such as Kell, also have been implicated.[28]

Clinical Presentation and Common Symptoms

The affected infant is anemic and jaundiced with hepatosplenomegaly. The degree of jaundice parallels the severity of the anemia. Infants most adversely affected may develop bilirubin encephalopathy (brain damage), also known as kernicterus, central nervous system deficits, and mental retardation. Some infants may be stillborn.

Physical Findings

The infant's initially acceptable skin color becomes paler as the anemia increases, and then icteric as hemolysis continues. Edema and ascites may be observed. Lethargy and hypotonicity as well as hypoxia due to the severe anemia may occur in more severely affected infants.

Laboratory Findings and Correlations with Disease

CORD BLOOD HEMATOLOGY.   Cord blood shows a normal or decreased hemoglobin level (compared to infant reference ranges), reticulocytosis, and an increased number of nucleated red cells (hence the term erythroblastosis fetalis).[1] Red cell macrocytosis and polychromatophilia are prominent, due to the increased rate of erythropoiesis in response to antibody-mediated hemolysis.

CHEMISTRY.   The bilirubin levels in cord blood may be slightly to significantly elevated, depending on the severity of hemolysis. A progressively increasing level seen within 48 to 72 hours after birth represents the extent of hemolysis as well as the inability of the infant's immature liver enzyme system to conjugate and excrete bilirubin. Hyperbilirubinemia is due to unconjugated bilirubin.

IMMUNOHEMATOLOGY.   In HDN due to anti-Rh antibodies, the infant's red cells react positively in the direct antiglobulin test (DAT; previously called the Coombs test), which detects antibody-coated red cells. In ABO disease, negative or weakly reactive DAT results may be found. This may be due to the small number of A and B antigens on cord blood cells (when compared to adult cells), which limits the number of antibody molecules that are able to bind to the infant's red cells. This small number of antibodies may not be detectable by routine DAT methods. In such cases, the anti-A or anti-B antibodies from the mother that are coating the cells may be detected by techniques in which an eluate of the antibodies from the infant's cells is incubated with ABO-appropriate test cells.

Note that prenatal antibody detection tests on the mother's serum (indirect antiglobulin test) and amniotic fluid analysis for bilirubin may predict the onset of HDN in the infant.

Effects of Treatment on Laboratory Results—Prognosis

If the severity of the disease indicates, exchange transfusion is performed, which replaces the fetus' antibody-coated red cells with donor cells that do not carry the antigen that the mother's antibody is attacking. Afterward, results of the DAT soon become weak or negative, anemia is corrected, and a significant reduction in bilirubin level is observed. In less severe cases, phototherapy (exposure of the infant to fluorescent light) reduces bilirubin levels by oxidizing bilirubin to biliverdin and then to colorless non-bilirubin precursors. Phototherapy is quite effective.

More important, however, is prevention of HDN due to anti-Rh antibodies. This is accomplished by passive immunization of Rh-negative mothers (those who have not already developed anti-Rh antibodies during a previous pregnancy or from receiving a transfusion of incompatible Rh-positive blood) by administering anti-Rh antibodies in the form of commercially prepared Rh_o immunoglobulin, also known as Rh_o IgG. This treatment is administered to Rh-negative mothers immediately following amniocentesis, abortion, or delivery of an Rh-positive baby. Some of the baby's Rh-positive cells can enter the mother's circulation during delivery and stimulate an immune response that could adversely affect future fetuses unless Rh_o IgG is administered to prevent it. Properly administered, this program can and has reduced anti-Rh HDN significantly.

Babies born severely affected by anti-Rh antibodies have a 10% to 20% chance of surviving. Infants with mild to moderate disease who are promptly treated have excellent survival rates.[14]

Hemolytic Transfusion Reaction

Definition
A hemolytic transfusion reaction results from the transfusion of red cells bearing antigens that are foreign to the recipient's immune system. If antibodies to the antigens introduced by transfusion are already present in the plasma, there is an immediate transfusion reaction; otherwise, antibodies soon develop through a secondary immune response, causing a somewhat delayed reaction.

History
Recognition of hemolytic transfusion reactions followed the discovery of the ABO blood group system by Landsteiner in 1900 and the subsequent identification of other blood group systems, such as Rh and Kell.

Pathophysiology
Hemolysis of transfused cells may result from rapid intravascular destruction of the transfused cells (immediate hemolytic transfusion reaction) or from more gradual, less clinically serious extravascular destruction of antibody-sensitized red cells (delayed hemolytic transfusion reaction).

IMMEDIATE HEMOLYTIC TRANSFUSION REACTIONS. If the ABO system is involved, anti-A and anti-B antibodies of the IgM type cause immediate intravascular destruction of the transfused red cells mediated through the activation of two antibody-binding sites close to each other on the red cell surface. These activated sites fix complement, and activation of the complement cascade results in formation of the membrane attack unit, which causes hemoglobin to be released into the plasma.

DELAYED HEMOLYTIC TRANSFUSION REACTIONS. Sometimes the hemolytic process does not begin for 2 to 14 days. Such reactions are most often associated with IgG antibodies, which are less effective in activating antibody-binding sites and less potent than IgM. When the incompatibility involves recipient IgG antibodies, such as anti-Rh antibodies, which do not bind complement, or Duffy- or Kidd-system antibodies with sublytic complement activation properties (i.e., antibodies that activate complement to a small extent but not to the point of actual cell lysis by generation of the membrane attack unit), extravascular hemolysis may result. This is due either to sequestration of the C3b-sensitized, transfused red cells by the spleen or sequestration by the liver Kupffer cells. It should also be noted that red cells coated with IgG antibodies that do not bind complement (e.g., anti-Rh) are sequestered and destroyed in the extravascular system, primarily in the spleen. Destruction of IgG-coated cells may not be as severe as that associated with IgM- and complement-coated cells.

Clinical Presentation and Common Symptoms
Initial symptoms of transfusion reaction are facial flushing, anxiety, nausea, clammy skin, chest pain, and back and leg pain.

Physical Findings
Hypotension, fever, and increased respiratory and pulse rates may occur. In serious cases, renal failure and disseminated intravascular coagulation (DIC) may develop.

Laboratory Findings and Correlations with Disease
By examining the serum of a carefully drawn blood specimen, hemoglobinemia may be observed, particularly in severe cases involving the ABO system, in which immediate intravascular destruction of the transfused red cells occurs. Intravascular hemolysis can activate the coagulation system, which results in depletion of fibrinogen, factor VIII, and platelets. This is demonstrated by low levels of these factors in plasma and an increased partial thromboplastin time (PTT). The D-d dimer test may reveal intravascular coagulation. This test is specific for fibrin split products and thus indicates coagulation and fibrinolysis in vivo (Chap. 50). Hemoglobin and urobilinogen in the urine and subsequent hyperbilirubinemia may be observed.

The DAT demonstrates the sensitization or coating of the transfused cells with IgG antibodies such as anti-Rh_o. Anemia results from a transfusion reaction.

Effects of Treatment on Laboratory Results
The best treatment is prevention. ABO transfusion reactions are due to human error in blood typing or in clerical aspects of the transfusion. Treatment of an immediate transfusion reaction is usually focused on treating the hypotension and preventing renal failure by infusing a diuretic or a drug that increases renal blood flow. Reversal of abnormal laboratory test findings should occur as the patient's condition improves.

With delayed transfusion reactions, treatment is usually unnecessary. With time, the spherocytes seen on the blood film disappear as the damaged and hemolyzed cells are destroyed in the reticuloendothelial system.

Prognosis

If the amount of incompatible transfused blood is minimal or the antigen-antibody system involved has a weak reactivity, the prognosis is favorable with treatment.

AUTOIMMUNE HEMOLYTIC ANEMIA

The autoimmune hemolytic anemias (AIHA) include warm-antibody AIHA, cold-antibody AIHA (cold agglutinin syndrome), and paroxysmal cold hemoglobinuria (PCH) (Table 19-2).

In these disorders, the normal mechanism that prevents formation of antibodies to the host's own antigens is flawed, and the immune system produces antibodies called *autoantibodies* that react with the host's own cell or tissue antigens. Current evidence suggests that the production of this type of antibody occurs when T lymphocyte (T-cell) regulation of B lymphocytes (B cells) is impaired.[21]

Warm-Antibody Autoimmune Hemolytic Anemia

Definition

Warm-antibody AIHA occurs when the patient's own immune system produces anti-red cell antibodies that react most effectively in the laboratory at warm temperatures (37°C).[9]

History

Recent research based on newer and more accurate methods indicates that 30% of these anemias are primary whereas 70% are secondary to some other disorder.[11] The approximate incidence of the disorder is one in 80,000 persons. Approximately 75% of all AIHA is classified as warm-antibody type.[11]

Pathophysiology

These autoantibodies usually are IgG, although some may be IgM or IgA. They may or may not bind complement. The autoantibodies are called incomplete because they do not cause direct agglutination of red cells. By binding to red cell surfaces, they cause extravascular destruction of red cells, principally in the spleen (see Table 19-2). The warm-antibody type of hemolytic anemias are categorized as *primary* or idiopathic if the specific cause is unknown and *secondary* if the patient has another disease complicated by hemolytic anemia.[30]

Clinical Presentation and Common Symptoms

This disease is seen in both sexes but slightly more often in women. It may be acquired at any age, although the frequency of onset is higher after age 40 years. This is understandable, particularly in secondary warm-antibody AIHAs, which are associated with underlying diseases such as chronic lymphocytic leukemia, lymphoma, systemic lupus erythematosus (SLE), viral infections, and immune deficiency diseases. The course may be very mild, with gradually developing symptoms, or acute with fulminating symptoms.

Physical Findings

Progressive weakness, occasional acute fever, pain, hemoglobinuria, mild jaundice, splenomegaly, hepatomegaly, and lymphadenopathy are common.

Laboratory Findings and Correlations with Disease

Hemoglobin values vary with the severity of hemolysis. Red cells are often macrocytic, but there is marked anisocytosis. Spherocytes indicate the hemolytic process. Marked reticulocytosis is evident as the marrow tries to compensate for the hemolysis. With competent marrow, the reticulocyte production index (RPI) should be greater than three. Thrombocytopenia may also occur. The serum unconjugated bilirubin value is moderately increased. Hemoglobinemia and hemoglobinuria may be seen in severe cases.

The DAT is positive in the majority of cases, confirming the presence of IgG antibodies with or without complement on the red cells. The DAT test for IgG detection sometimes requires modifications, such as adding PVP

TABLE 19-2. Delineation of Common Antibodies and Other Key Features of the Acquired Autoimmune Hemolytic Anemias

	WARM ANTIBODY	COLD ANTIBODY	PAROXYSMAL COLD HEMOGLOBINURIA
Optimal reaction temperature	37°C	0–4°C	0–4°C (antibody binds to cell) 37°C (hemolysis takes place)
Thermal amplitude*	20–37°C	0–32°C	<15°C
Immunoglobulin type	Usually IgG (some IgM, IgA)	Usually IgM (some IgG)	IgG (Donath-Landsteiner autoantibody)
Antibody type	Incomplete†	Agglutinin	Hemolysin
Mechanism of antibody production	Immune response	Naturally occurring and immune response	Immune response
Complement (C′) activation	May bind C′	Binds C′	Binds C′
Protein structure	Polyclonal	Monoclonal or polyclonal	Polyclonal
Blood group specificity	Rh, Kell, others	Ii	Pp
Primary mechanism of cell destruction	Extravascular, principally splenic	Extravascular, principally hepatic	Principally intravascular
Severity of disease	Often severe	Often mild	Distinct episodes of severity
Treatment	Steroids, splenectomy, immunosuppressants	Avoid cold	Avoid cold
Transfusion requirements	Transfusions contraindicated	Rarely needed	Could be required

* Thermal amplitude refers to the temperature range in which antibody binds to the red cell surface.
† Incomplete antibodies do not cause direct agglutination of cells.

(polyvinylpyrrolidone) or Polybrene to increase sensitivity. The indirect antiglobulin test may also demonstrate autoantibody in the serum when there is active hemolysis. Warm autoantibodies usually have a specificity for Rh antigens, although other blood group specificities have been described.[7]

Effects of Treatment on Laboratory Results—Prognosis

For secondary warm-antibody AIHA, treating the underlying disease may reverse the hemolytic process. Transfusion as a treatment for severe anemia may be fraught with problems, from difficulty in accurate blood typing to finding a compatible blood unit in the presence of blood group-specific autoantibodies. Successful treatment with corticosteroids, which act to inhibit the clearance of IgG-sensitized red cells and suppress antibody synthesis, results in increased hemoglobin values. Intravenous immune globulins have sometimes been useful. Splenectomy for patients who do not respond to corticosteroids may result in hematologic improvement since the spleen is the major site of sequestration of IgG-sensitized cells.

Prognosis varies depending on the severity of the hemolytic episodes and the nature of the underlying disease in the secondary form.

Cold-Antibody Autoimmune Hemolytic Anemia (Cold Agglutinin Syndrome)

Definition

Humans normally have a small and harmless amount of cold autoantibody, including anti-I, anti-H, and anti-IH, but people who have cold agglutinin syndrome develop a pathologic form of anti-I antibody that leads to hemolysis.

Cold-antibody AIHA is caused by pathologic antibodies that react most effectively at cold temperatures (0°–10°C) *in vivo* and *in vitro*.

History

These cold-reacting antibodies were identified by Landsteiner[16] at the turn of the century and later were found to have a relationship to hemolytic anemia and Raynaud's phenomenon, a peripheral circulation abnormality. They are less common than warm antibodies. Wiener's discovery of the I antigen furthered the characterization of these autoantibodies.[39]

Pathophysiology

Pathologic cold autoantibodies usually are IgM antibodies against the I antigen (see Table 19-2). Because of their ability to bind and activate complement (e.g., C3b), destruction of red cells is primarily extravascular, in the liver, due to Kupffer cell C3b receptors. To a lesser extent, complement-mediated intravascular hemolysis may occur, as may hemolysis due to red cell shape changes caused by cold agglutinins.

Cold-antibody AIHA is categorized as primary (or idiopathic) cold agglutinin disease or as secondary cold agglutinin disease, in which infectious agents such as *Mycoplasma pneumoniae* or Epstein-Barr virus (the agent of infectious mononucleosis) or lymphoproliferative diseases constitute the major disorder.[26]

Clinical Presentation and Common Symptoms

Primary cold agglutinin disease is most common in elderly people, but secondary disease is seen in all ages, depending on the incidence of the underlying diseases. When the patient is exposed to cold, red cell agglutinates occur that obstruct the capillary circulation, causing numbness, pain, and blue or red skin discoloration. This circulatory abnormality is known as acrocyanosis or Raynaud's phenomenon. It usually involves exposed body parts, the tip of the nose, ear lobes, or fingers. Gangrene may develop in the extremities in severe cases.

Physical Findings

Acrocyanosis, anemia, and at times, mild jaundice are the result of hemolysis, and the principal findings in primary disease. In acute episodes, hemoglobinuria and renal failure may ensue. In secondary disease the underlying disease dictates the physical findings.

Laboratory Findings and Correlations with Disease

HEMATOLOGY.   Hemoglobin values decrease as hemolysis increases and may, in fact, vary seasonally with the temperature. Reticulocytes proliferate in relation to hemolysis. Leukocyte and platelet numbers generally are normal. Of importance is the effect of these cold agglutinins on laboratory procedures. Clumping of red cells while preparing blood films or when using an automated cell counter can result in erroneous values if it is not detected. Classically, the MCV for these samples is extremely elevated, and the MCH and MCHC appear entirely unrealistic. To overcome this problem, the blood sample should be warmed for at least 15 minutes at 37°C, and the equipment and reagents should be prewarmed if possible.

OTHER LABORATORY FINDINGS.   Bilirubin levels are mildly increased. Haptoglobin and complement levels may be decreased as hemolysis progresses. Mild hemoglobinemia may be observed.

A *cold agglutinin screening test* is helpful in diagnosis. It involves testing the ability of patient serum to agglutinate normal red cells suspended in saline after the mixture is first incubated at room temperature then in cold water at 20°C. If the patient's serum does agglutinate normal red cells at 20°C, the serum cold agglutinin must be titrated at 4°C and the thermal amplitude (the range of temperatures over which these antibodies attach to red cells) must be determined to provide information for the diagnosis. For patients experiencing hemolysis, the cold agglutinin titer at 4°C is usually over 1000, whereas that for healthy subjects generally is under 64. Pathologic anti-I antibodies have a broad thermal amplitude (0°–32°C), whereas healthy persons' values are less than 22°C. At 37°C, the agglutinating property of cold agglutinins is characteristically reversed. This is why blood samples from these patients require warming before being analyzed.

The astute technologist handling the blood sample at room temperature may provide the diagnosis by observing the clumping phenomenon seen from the outside of the tube along the tube walls.

Cold agglutinins show specificity for the I antigen of adult cells in most cases, or for the i antigen of fetal or cord red cells. The DAT usually is positive when a polyspecific antiglobulin serum is used that detects both complement and antibodies on the red cell surface. Complement is actually the only component being detected on the red cell, as demonstrated by a positive result with anti-C3–specific antiglobulin serum and a negative result with reagents lacking anti-C3.

Effects of Treatment on Laboratory Results—Prognosis

For patients with secondary cold agglutinin syndrome, keeping them warm and treating any underlying disease is the best therapy, since infectious disease and the related hemolytic process are ordinarily of limited duration. For persons who have the idiopathic syndrome, steroid therapy, immunosuppressive therapy, or alkylating agents such as chlorambucil may be effective in normalizing test results. Plasmapheresis to remove intravascular IgM antibodies may benefit acutely ill patients.

Transfusion to correct anemia is technically difficult, since blood typing and cross-matching results are affected by the presence of cold agglutinins. Cold blood should not be transfused, in order to avoid intravascular agglutination. The prognosis is variable, depending on the underlying disease.

Paroxysmal Cold Hemoglobinuria

Definition

PCH, an autoimmune disease similar to cold-antibody AIHA, is caused by binding of the Donath-Landsteiner autoantibody to the patient's red cells following exposure to cold, which results in intravascular hemolysis and gross hemoglobinuria.

History

PCH was one of the first hemolytic anemias to be described and correlated to cold exposure. A causative "autolysin" was suggested by Donath and Landsteiner in 1904.[10] The autoantibody responsible for PCH is still called Donath-Landsteiner (D-L) antibody and is demonstrated by the Donath-Landsteiner test. It has been suggested that genetic factors controlling immune responsiveness may dictate who develops this rare disease, which represents less than 1% of acquired AIHAs.[13]

Pathophysiology

The PCH autoantibody is an IgG antibody (as opposed to the IgM type found in cold-antibody AIHA), which is also a powerful hemolysin (see Table 19-2). Both idiopathic PCH[4] and PCH secondary to advanced syphilis and viral diseases, particularly among children with mumps, measles, chicken pox, infectious mononucleosis, or the flu, have been described.[8, 31] This antibody binds to red cells at temperatures below 15°C in the presence of complement and shows specificity for the Pp blood group system.[19] Hemolysis occurs on warming.

Clinical Presentation and Common Symptoms

After exposure to varying degrees and periods of cold, the patient may present with headache, vomiting, pain in the abdomen and extremities, severe chills and fever, and significant hemoglobinuria. Following the attack, patients often pass dark brown or black urine and complain of weakness. Patients are often free of symptoms between attacks, and the duration of symptoms during and after exposure is limited.

Physical Findings

Mild jaundice, splenomegaly, and hepatomegaly may be seen.

Laboratory Findings and Correlations with Disease

Hemoglobin values drop rapidly as hemoglobinuria is observed. Red cell morphology may include some spherocytes, fragmented red cells, and polychromasia. Leukopenia followed by leukocytosis occurs. The former is consistent with observed phagocytosis of red cells. Immature leukocytes may be found on the blood film.

Results of the Donath-Landsteiner test are positive. In this test, the patient's serum is incubated with normal group O, P–positive cells at 4°C, and then the mixture is warmed to 37°C, at which temperature complement is bound and hemolysis occurs if the D-L antibody is present.[22] A patient control and a normal control sample should be run to ensure valid results. The patient and normal control specimens are blood samples incubated for 60 minutes at 37°C. After centrifugation neither control should show hemolysis.

Urine contains hemoglobin and methemoglobin, as serum haptoglobin becomes saturated with hemoglobin from lysed cells. The DAT is positive at the time of attack if a complement-specific (i.e., nongamma globulin) antiserum is used and the test is performed at a cold temperature. Cells are coated by inactivated complement components. The serum bilirubin level may be mildly elevated after the attack.[33]

Effects of Treatment on Laboratory Results—Prognosis

In secondary PCH, successful treatment of the syphilis or infection most often relieves the symptoms. The short duration of viral diseases usually precludes specific therapy. In both instances, laboratory test values return to normal. In idiopathic primary disease, however, avoidance of cold is the preventive therapy of choice, and although results of the D-L test may continue to be positive, attacks and their associated abnormal laboratory test results are minimized by avoiding the cold.

DRUG-INDUCED IMMUNE HEMOLYTIC ANEMIA

In some people, certain drugs provoke abnormal antibody production that causes immune hemolytic anemia. These antibodies may resemble autoantibodies. Three principal modes of formation and cell destruction are involved: (1) the hapten or drug adsorption mechanism; (2) the immune complex or "innocent bystander" mechanism; and (3) the α-methyldopa or autoimmune (unknown) mechanism. These mechanisms are explained graphically in Figure 19-2 and summarized in Table 19-3.

Hapten (Drug Adsorption) Mechanism

Definition

When a hapten, a low-molecular weight substance (less than 5000) that rarely stimulates antibody production, is involved in drug-induced hemolytic anemia, a drug or one of its metabolites stimulates production of an antibody that complexes with the drug, which is already bound to the red cell membrane. The antibody-coated red cell then becomes susceptible to extravascular destruction.[23]

History
Increasing use of antibiotics such as penicillin in massive doses led to the development of this type of hemolytic anemia. This mechanism is also associated with some cephalosporins (e.g., cephalothin, a drug used to treat some bacterial infections and as a penicillin substitute).

Pathophysiology
Hapten groups are formed by the chemical reaction of a drug such as penicillin with serum proteins. These drug-protein groups adsorb nonspecifically to the red cell surface and induce production of an antibody specific for the drug. The antidrug (e.g., antipenicillin or anticephalothin) antibody then combines with the drug attached to the red cell (see Fig. 19-2). The antibody is usually IgG, warm reactive, and noncomplement binding. The IgG-coated red cells are then subject to extravascular destruction (see Table 19-3), mainly in the spleen.

Low levels of antipenicillin antibody have been found in normal persons, but about 3% of all patients who receive large doses of penicillin develop a positive DAT reaction. Of these, sensitization is more common following intramuscular penicillin therapy; only a small number who are receiving massive intravenous doses on a long-term basis develop overt hemolytic anemia.

Clinical Presentation
Patients with hapten-type drug-induced hemolysis develop this complication while under treatment for an underlying disease. If hemolysis ensues, the typical symptoms of anemia and hemolysis develop.

Laboratory Findings and Correlations with Disease
The most significant finding is the positive DAT. The patient's red cells react strongly with anti-IgG antiglobulin reagent. Eluates from these red cells fail to react with normal red cells but do react with drug-coated cells. Because normal people may have low levels of antipenicillin antibody, high titers must be demonstrated in order to implicate the drug.

An abrupt decrease in hemoglobin level followed by a gradual increase in reticulocyte count and RPI can be expected, along with an increased unconjugated bilirubin level. Thrombocytopenia and neutropenia have been reported, suggesting antibody-mediated suppression of development of penicillin-coated precursor cells.[25]

Effects of Treatment on Laboratory Results—Prognosis
Removal of the offending drug ordinarily reverses the hemolytic process, and the DAT result becomes negative over a period of a few days to weeks. If necessary, a drug that has previously induced hemolytic anemia can be given again if the patient is monitored carefully for the appearance of a secondary immune response.

Immune Complex (Innocent Bystander) Mechanism

Definition
The drugs in this mechanism cause complement-mediated intravascular hemolysis by nonimmune-mediated attachment of immunogenic complexes to the red cell surface. The red cell is an innocent bystander, because this complex is not binding specifically to a red cell antigen (see Fig. 19-2).

History
The innocent bystander type of hemolytic anemia was described in 1954 in a patient with schistosomiasis who was treated with the drug stibophen. Other drugs that may act in a similar manner are quinidine, quinine, sulfonamides, and phenacetin.[32]

Pathophysiology
Because drugs usually are small molecules, the drugs in this case first bind firmly to a plasma protein. This complex then reacts with antibody to the drug. In the second step of this mechanism, the drug-protein-antibody complex binds nonimmunologically on the red cell surface. The antibodies are either IgM or IgG and have the ability to bind complement, which results in intravascular hemolysis (see Table 19-3). Often complement may be found alone on the red cell surface, owing to dissociation of the drug-protein-antibody complex after complement fixation occurs (see Fig. 19-2).

TABLE 19–3. Summary of Mechanisms Causing Drug-Induced Immune Hemolytic Anemias

MECHANISM	DRUG TYPE	ANTIBODY TYPE	DAT* RESULT (POLYSPECIFIC)	HEMOLYSIS
Hapten (drug adsorption)	Penicillin (large doses), streptomycin, cephalothin	IgG	+	Extravascular, mainly splenic; develops slowly; severe in rare cases; stops with removal of drug
Innocent bystander (immune complex)	Stibophen (small doses), phenacetin	IgM or IgG	+	Intravascular, acute hemolysis; stops 1 to 2 days after removal of drug
α-Methyldopa (autoimmune/ unknown)	α-Methyldopa (dose-related), levodopa, mefenamic acid	IgG	+	May develop slowly in a few patients after 3 months or more of therapy; less than 1% of patients on methyldopa experience hemolysis; stops several days to a week after removal of drug

⋆ Direct antiglobulin test performed using polyspecific antiserum.

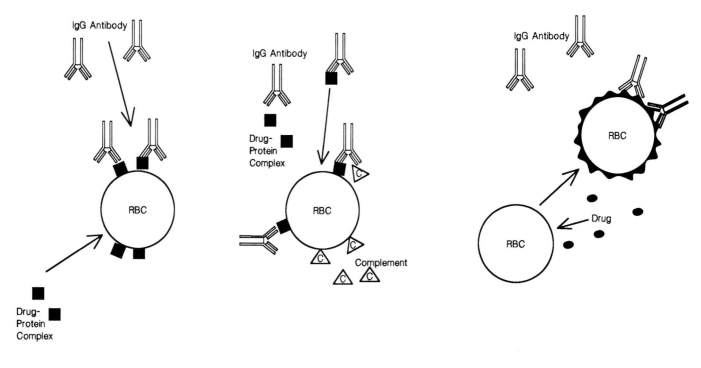

Hapten Type
Drug Adsorption Mechanism,
e.g., Penicillin

Innocent Bystander Type
Immune Complex Mechanism,
e.g., Phenacetin, Stibophen

Alpha-Methyldopa Type
Autoimmune/Unknown Mechanism,
e.g., Alpha-Methyldopa, Levodopa

FIG. 19-2.   The three mechanisms of drug-induced immune hemolytic anemia. In the *drug adsorption mechanism*, a drug-protein complex forms in the plasma and is adsorbed to the red cell membrane. This stimulates antidrug antibody production, and this antibody complexes to the drug on the red cell surface leading to hemolysis. In the *immune complex mechanism*, a drug-protein complex in the plasma stimulates antibody production and antibody binds to the drug-protein complex while it is still in the plasma. This complex binds nonimmunologically to "innocent" red cells. In the *α-methyldopa type*, production of autoantibody specific for Rh antigens on the red cell surface is induced by the drug circulating in the plasma. These antibodies bind to the cell surface, but the drug does not.

Clinical Presentation

The common symptoms of hemolysis occur when the drug is being administered. The acute onset of symptoms in the face of the underlying disease for which the drug was prescribed dictate the physical findings. Renal failure may ensue.

Laboratory Findings and Correlations with Disease

A decrease in hemoglobin occurs as intravascular hemolysis proceeds. Hemoglobinemia is apparent. Spherocytosis, leukopenia, and thrombocytopenia may be observed in some cases. The rapid hemolysis results in hemoglobinuria, and renal failure is a common finding. Elevated PTT and low factor VIII and fibrinogen levels reflect an intravascular coagulation process as well. Results of the DAT are positive when polyvalent or complement-specific reagents are used. Serum bilirubin rises as hemolysis progresses.

Effects of Treatment on Laboratory Results–Prognosis

Immediate removal of the offending drug may be the only therapy required. Steroids may be helpful when hemolysis is severe. Abnormal test results gradually become normal after the drug is removed, but the DAT may remain positive for up to 2 months, owing to the firm attachment of inactivated complement to red cells. Renal failure indicates a poor prognosis.

α-Methyldopa or Autoimmune (Unknown) Mechanism

Definition

In this AIHA, the drug induces the formation of antibody with specificity to a red cell antigen (rather than to the drug itself), which may result in hemolysis (see Fig. 19-2).

History

In 1966, the first reports were published of significant numbers of patients who had received α-methyldopa (Aldomet) for hypertension and developed a positive DAT result and in some cases, a hemolytic anemia.[6]

Pathophysiology

Hemolytic disease occurs in about 1% of patients who take α-methyldopa.[32] The autoantibody is produced only after several months of continuous therapy. It is directed not to the drug but to red cell antigens. The exact mechanism of this abnormal autoantibody production is unclear.

The antibody, an IgG, is similar in activity to those of the warm-antibody autoimmune type and has specificity for Rh antigens, presumably for some specific basic structural component of the Rh substance (see Table 19-3). The capacity of methyldopa to inhibit normal T-cell suppressor function has been suggested as the root of this aberration. This leads to abnormal, uncontrolled B-cell autoantibody production in some patients.[15]

Other drugs with similar modes of action are levodopa and mefenamic acid. In this disorder, the drug has no cross reaction with the red cell antigen that reacts with the antibody, but it appears to induce an immune process in which it does not participate.[13]

Clinical Presentation

The course of the disease is rather insidious; hemolysis may start from 18 weeks to 4 years after therapy begins.[32] Symptoms and physical findings are those associated with anemia.

Laboratory Findings and Correlations with Disease

Hematologic studies show decreased hemoglobin, a compensatory increase in reticulocytes, and moderate numbers of spherocytes. Bilirubin (total and unconjugated) levels are moderately elevated. Although the DAT is positive with anti-IgG sera in approximately 15% of patients who have been taking the drug for at least 3 months,[32] most show no evidence of overt hemolysis. The red cell antibodies are specific for Rh antigens.

Effects of Treatment on Laboratory Results—Prognosis

Removal of the drug methyldopa rapidly stops the hemolytic process. Corticosteroid therapy is sometimes useful, and transfusions may be necessary for severe cases. Results of the DAT are negative within a few months after the drug is discontinued. A number of patients so affected often have other autoantibodies (e.g., antinuclear antibody [ANA] or rheumatoid factor).[5]

CHAPTER SUMMARY

The combination of mild jaundice, fatigue, decreased hemoglobin, and a positive result on the direct antiglobulin test (DAT) may suggest an anemia of increased red cell destruction. The role of isoimmune antibodies (produced after exposure to foreign antigens from an individual of the same species) or autoimmune antibodies (abnormally produced against the host's own antigens) as causative agents should be considered. These antibodies are associated with acquired immune hemolytic anemia, which is classified in several categories (see Table 19-1).

Immune hemolysis is associated with both intravascular and extravascular hemolysis. The hemolytic process involves not only antibodies and antigens but also the complement system (see Fig. 19-1). Extravascular hemolysis is often associated with the formation of complement component C3b on the red cell surface, which is recognized by receptors in the reticuloendothelial system, thus leading to red cell destruction. Intravascular hemolysis is ultimately caused by the complement membrane attack unit, C5b6789, formed on the red cell surface, which penetrates the surface causing cell lysis.

Hemolysis due to isoimmune antibodies is more common than that due to autoimmune antibodies. It is seen in HDN, in which maternal IgG antibody crosses the placenta and attacks the infant's cells, which have the corresponding antigen. Although severe HDN due to Rh antibodies has decreased in incidence over the past 10 to 20 years owing to effective treatment with Rh_o IgG, HDN due to ABO or other blood group antibodies does occur.

Isoimmune hemolytic anemia due to transfusion reactions may be immediate or delayed for 2 to 14 days. Immediate transfusion reactions often occur with IgM anti-A and anti-B isoantibodies, which cause intravascular hemolysis when incompatible blood is transfused. Delayed transfusion reactions commonly occur with IgG antibodies that are less efficient in binding complement and usually cause extravascular sequestration of antibody and complement-coated red cells.

In the autoimmune hemolytic anemias, a disturbance of the normal immune system occurs in which antibodies to the host's own antigens are produced. The antibodies may be either warm reacting (37°C) or cold reacting (0°–10°C); the latter causes cold agglutinin disease (see Table 19-2).

Paroxysmal cold hemoglobinuria (PCH) is a rare autoimmune disorder caused by an autoantibody to the Pp blood group system. It may be idiopathic or secondary to viral disease.

Acquired immune hemolytic anemia may be caused by certain drugs that induce production of abnormal antibodies that destroy red cells. Three characteristic types of drug-induced immune hemolytic anemia exist (see Fig. 19-2): (1) drug adsorption or hapten type; (2) innocent bystander or immune complex type; and (3) α-methyldopa or autoimmune type.

CASE STUDY 19-1

On a cold February day, a 6-year-old boy was brought to the emergency room by his frantic mother because he had passed red urine and looked very pale. He was a normal, active boy, and in fact had played out in the snow the day before. He had had the "flu" for 1 week about 10 days before this episode. He had not received any medication except acetaminophen. On admission his CBC values were Hb 8.0 g/dL; HCT 0.22 L/L; RBC 3.0×10^{12}/L; platelets 350×10^9/L; WBC 12.2×10^9/L. The differential cell count was neutrophils 40%; bands 10%; lymphocytes 43%; monocytes 7%. The reticulocyte count was 0.9%.

1. Do the hemoglobin and hematocrit values match?
2. What is the most likely cause of the red urine?
3. What are the possible diagnoses?
4. What additional tests could help determine the diagnosis?
5. What treatment is indicated?

CASE STUDY 19-2

A patient blood sample was analyzed on routine admission using an automated cell counter. The results were WBC 7.1×10^9/L; RBC 3.2×10^{12}/L; Hb 13.5 g/dL; HCT 0.36 L/L; MCV 112.5 fL; MCH 42.2 pg; MCHC 37.5 g/dL.

1. Do the hemoglobin and hematocrit values match in this case? Is this to be expected given the red cell indices results?
2. Are all of the red cell indices above the usual reference range?
3. Do these abnormal results represent a laboratory error or a blood disorder? Why?
4. What can be done to verify accurate results for this patient?

REFERENCES

1. Allen FH, Diamond LK: Erythroblastosis Fetalis. Boston, Little, Brown & Co, 1957

2. Atkinson JA, Frank MM: Studies on the *in vivo* effects of antibody: Interaction of IgM antibody and complement in the immune clearance and destruction of erythrocytes in man. J Clin Invest 54:339, 1974

3. Austen KF, Becker EL, Biro CE et al: Nomenclature of complement. Bull WHO 39:935, 1968

4. Bird GW, Wingham J, Martin AJ et al: Idiopathic nonsyphilitic paroxysmal cold hemoglobinuria in children. J Clin Pathol 29:215, 1976

5. Breckenridge A, Dollery CT, Worlledge SM et al: Positive direct Coombs tests and antinuclear factor in patients treated with methyldopa. Lancet 2:1265, 1967

6. Carstairs KC, Breckenridge A, Dollery CT et al: Incidence of a positive direct Coombs test in patients on α-methyldopa. Lancet 2:133, 1966

7. Charles LT: Resolving incompatibilities in patients with warm reactive autoantibodies. J Med Technol 35:291, 1986

8. Colley EW: Paroxysmal cold haemoglobinuria after mumps. Br Med J 1:1552, 1964

9. Dacie JV: Autoimmune hemolytic anemia. Ann Intern Med 135:1293, 1975

10. Donath J, Landsteiner K: Uber paroxysmale Hämoglobinurie. Munch Med Wochenschr 51:1590, 1904

11. Issit PD: Applied Blood Group Serology, 3rd ed, p 514. Miami, Montgomery Scientific Publications, 1985

12. Issit PD: Applied Blood Group Serology, 3rd ed, p 540. Miami, Montgomery Scientific Publications, 1985

13. Issit PD: Applied Blood Group Serology, 3rd ed, p 548. Miami, Montgomery Scientific Publications, 1985

14. Kanto WP Jr, Marino B, Godwin AS et al: ABO hemolytic disease: A comparative study of clinical severity and delayed anemia. Pediatrics 62:365, 1978

15. Kirtland HH III, Mohler DN, Horwitz DA et al: Methyldopa inhibition of suppressor lymphocyte function. N Engl J Med 302:825, 1980

16. Landsteiner K, Levine P: On the cold agglutinins in human serum. J Immunol 12:441, 1926

17. Landsteiner K, Wiener AS: An agglutinable factor in human blood recognized by immune sera for Rhesus blood. Proc Soc Exp Med 43:220, 1940

18. Levine P, Katzin EM, Burnham L: Isoimmunization in pregnancy; its possible bearing on etiology of erythroblastosis foetalis. JAMA 116:825, 1941

19. Levine P, Celano MJ, Falkowski F: The specificity of the antibody in paroxysmal cold hemoglobinuria (PCH). Transfusion 3:278, 1963

20. Levine P, Stetson KE: An unusual case of intragroup agglutination. JAMA 113:126, 1939

21. Logue G, Rossi W: Immunologic mechanisms in autoimmune hemolytic disease. Semin Hematol 13:277, 1976

22. Mackenzie GM: Paroxysmal hemoglobinuria. A review. Medicine 8:159, 1929

23. Marchand A: Immune hemolytic anemia: Classification, manifestations, and mechanisms of destruction. Diag Med 5:51, 1982

24. Muller-Eberhard HJ: Complement. Ann Rev Biochem 44:697, 1975

25. Murphy MF, Riordan T, Minchinton RM et al: Demonstration of an immune-mediated mechanism of penicillin-induced neutropaenia and thrombocytopaenia. Br J Haematol 55:155, 1983

26. Pruzanski W, Schumak KW: Biologic activity of cold-reacting autoantibodies. N Engl J Med 297:538, 1977

27. Ruddy S, Gigli I, Austen KF: The complement system of man. N Engl J Med 287:489, 545, 592, 642, 1972

28. Weinstein L: Irregular antibodies causing HDN. Obstet Gynecol Surv 31:581, 1976

29. Wiener AS, Unger LJ, Cohen L et al: Type-specific cold autoantibodies as a cause of acquired hemolytic anemia and hemolytic transfusion reactions: Biologic test with bovine red cells. Ann Intern Med 44:221, 1956

30. Wintrobe MM et al: Autoimmune hemolytic anemia. In Wintrobe MM et al (eds): Clinical Hematology, 8th ed, p 926. Philadelphia, Lea & Febiger, 1981

31. Wishart MM, Davey MG: Infectious mononucleosis complicated by acute haemolytic anemia with a positive D-L reaction. J Clin Pathol 26:332, 1973

32. Worlledge SM: Immune drug induced hemolytic anemia. Semin Hematol 6:181, 1969

33. Worlledge SM, Rousso C: Studies on the serology of paroxysmal cold hemoglobinuria (PCH) with special reference to its relationships with the P blood group system. Vox Sang 10:293, 1965

20

Anemia

of

Blood

Loss

Linda C. Schumacher

An acute blood loss or hemorrhage, whether internal or external, can pose a serious threat to life if medical intervention is delayed. A minor loss (500 mL or less) generally is not serious and usually does not require laboratory analysis or transfusion unless bleeding continues, but in cases of extensive blood loss, the physician must assess the severity of hemorrhage through hematologic testing to help determine whether a transfusion is necessary. During this assessment, the patient's physical signs and symptoms must also be monitored closely by attending staff, because advanced complications, shock, and ultimately death may result from extensive blood loss. Together, hemorrhage and shock are a complex problem, which will be examined in this chapter along with the pathophysiology and laboratory findings associated with acute and chronic blood loss.

ACUTE BLOOD CELL LOSS

Pathophysiology

Many physiologic changes accompany acute blood loss. It is accepted generally that normal blood volume is 4.0 to 4.5 L for women and 5.0 to 5.5 L for men. Normal volume changes are kept under control by the interplay of various hormones, including antidiuretic hormone (ADH), aldosterone, and erythropoietin, and by an osmotic phenomenon known as plasma refill.[6] Changes in blood flow as a result of volume variations affect cerebral blood flow, leading to headaches and confusion. Changes in blood flow also affect renal blood flow, and cause decreased glomerular filtration and ultimately reduced urine formation. Other hormones, including catecholamines, cortisone, and growth hormone, can create a state of hyperglycemia when necessary. This provides glucose for energy during osmotic transfer of fluids from inside the blood cells into the extracellular space.[5] Unless the blood loss is extensive, the body's initial response is to maintain blood volume at all costs.

Blood loss affects both the hematopoietic and cardiovascular systems. The hematopoietic system is affected by blood volume depletion, as it must work at an accelerated pace to replace the lost blood cells, including erythrocytes needed immediately for delivery of oxygen to the tissues. The cardiovascular system is affected because of its sensitivity to volume shifts. With acute blood loss, cardiac arrest and death may occur. With minor bleeding, up to 20% of total blood volume may be lost, producing cardiovascular symptoms such as tachycardia and angina pectoris, but the symptoms disappear in 24 to 48 hours as fluid volume is totally replaced. Patients with such a minor loss may have an anemia for 2 to 3 months but are usually asymptomatic. In such patients, as well as those with severe blood loss, a shift to the right in the oxyhemoglobin dissociation curve (Chap. 7) causes oxygen to be more readily released from hemoglobin, thus partially compensating for the anemic state. The level of erythrocyte 2,3-diphosphoglycerate (2,3-DPG) also increases in blood loss situations, thus decreasing the hemoglobin's affinity for oxygen and making it more available to tissues.

Internally, blood flow is redistributed to the heart and brain away from skin, muscle, and kidneys. Epinephrine causes vasoconstriction, and heart rate and stroke volume increase as the body attempts to maintain adequate blood flow and pressure and tissue oxygenation. Further, vasoconstriction causes an auto-transfusion effect of about 500 mL in adults (i.e., vessel constriction temporarily reduces the circulatory volume that needs filling). Studies of the plasma refill phenomenon have indicated that 40 to 60 mL of extravascular fluid, containing electrolytes and protein, may flow into the circulation every minute during the first 6 to 10 hours after the blood loss. Refill is complete 30 to 40 hours later.[6]

Circulatory insufficiency and inadequate tissue perfusion are the hallmarks of shock. There are three types of shock that can occur in conjunction with blood loss—hypovolemic (hemorrhagic) shock, cardiogenic shock, and shock due to vasodilation. Hypovolemic shock follows severe blood loss (loss of more than 20% of total blood volume). Common causes of hypovolemic hemorrhagic shock include traumatic hemorrhage, gastrointestinal hemorrhage, operative hemorrhage, ruptured aortic aneurysm, obstetric complications, and massive hemoptysis. Cardiogenic shock is caused by inadequate or abnormal cardiac function (e.g., congenital heart disease or after acute myocardial infarction or blood loss). Shock due to vasodilation and hypotension occurs in a number of disorders including sepsis and anaphylaxis.

Clinical Presentation and Common Symptoms

Depending on the volume of blood lost, the patient may experience signs and symptoms of volume depletion as well as anemia. The degree of symptoms experienced depends to some extent on the patient's age. Elderly people are more likely to show symptoms of cardiac failure and anemia after losing a significant—or even a modest—amount of blood. In severe anemia of rapid onset, retinal hemorrhages may occasionally cause vision disturbances. Table 20-1 shows the progression of patient symptoms as the severity of blood loss increases. The signs and symptoms generally associated with any kind of shock include hypotension, weak and rapid pulse, shallow and rapid respiration, altered mental state, cold and pale skin, decreased urine output, and acidosis (decreased blood pH).

Laboratory Findings and Correlations with Disease

Hematology

During the first few hours after a blood loss episode, there is usually no change in hematocrit (HCT) or hemoglobin (Hb) values, owing to the initial compensatory vasoconstriction. Depending on the volume lost, the patient may experience signs and symptoms of volume depletion. After 3 to 4 hours, the HCT and Hb values may begin to decrease and the leukocyte count may rise because of an outpouring of neutrophils from the marginal pool (Chap. 23). The blood film may contain bands and metamyelocytes. Depending on the severity of the loss, nucleated red blood cells may also be seen.[9] It is not until 12 to 24 hours after the blood loss episode that the full extent of anemia becomes evident. Platelets may be increased, and after adequate fluid replacement, leukocyte counts of 30 × 10^9/L are common. After 3 to 5 days, the blood film may show slight macrocytosis with polychromasia, reflecting a 10% to 15% reticulocyte response resulting from bone marrow erythrocytic hyperplasia that may be expected to last 10 days or more, depending on the volume of blood lost.[4] The reticulocyte production index (RPI) should be greater than 3 after a number of days if the bone marrow is capable of adequate response to the blood loss.

Figure 20-1 demonstrates the initially slow decrease in the Hb level after a rapid loss of approximately 30% of the normal blood volume. The Hb value reaches its minimum level only after several days. Total blood volume returns to normal within approximately 7 days, whereas the Hb rises back to normal over a period of weeks. The graph also

TABLE 20–1. Signs and Symptoms Related to Degree of Blood Loss

BLOOD LOSS (%)	SIGNS AND SYMPTOMS
10	May be none at rest
	Lightheadedness
	Increased pulse on arising
20	Hypotension
	Exertional tachycardia
30	Decreased cardiac output
	Hypotension
	Rapid pulse
	Cold, clammy skin
40–50	Severe shock and death

Adapted from Reynolds RD, Lewis JP: Blood loss anemias and the iron deficient states. In Koepke JA (ed): Laboratory Hematology, vol 1. New York, Churchill Livingstone, 1984.

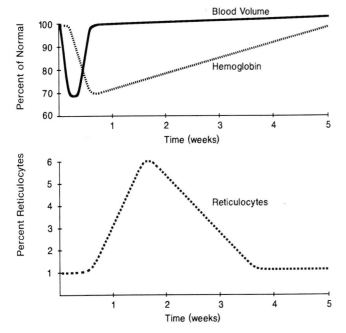

FIG. 20-1.   Relationship of blood volume to hematopoietic response in the event of acute blood loss.

represents the reticulocyte response associated with such a loss. Note that a maximal response generally is found within 1 to 2 weeks, and this tapers off over a period of weeks.

Chemistry

Serum ferritin is the best measure of the patient's iron storage status. It may be decreased if large amounts of iron are lost during the bleeding episode. Increased levels of plasma erythropoietin are found as erythropoietic activity is stimulated.

Effects of Treatment on Laboratory Results

In some cases it may be 20 to 60 hours before the full extent of the blood loss is known, so the immediate concern is to preserve fluid balance. Crystalloids and electrolyte solutions usually are administered as the initial treatment. Colloid solutions of plasma proteins or albumin are another option. All of these solutions may initially cause a relative decrease in hematocrit and thus, the appearance of more severe anemia. In the most severe cases, fresh whole blood may also be used, but a patient's normal compensatory mechanisms are preferred.[3] In these situations apparent anemia occurs as fluid enters the system and a dilutional effect ensues.[2]

Once bleeding is under control many patients receive oral iron therapy for a few months, to compensate for the iron loss.[10] If the bone marrow is capable of responding to the iron therapy, all red cell parameters should return to normal, over time, depending on the initial severity of the blood loss. Depending on the level of iron stores, Hb and HCT levels should begin to increase after about a week if iron is available. Platelet and leukocyte counts and the bone marrow status should also return to normal.

CHRONIC BLOOD CELL LOSS

Blood cell loss that continues for a long time is referred to as chronic. If chronic blood cell loss goes untreated, chronic iron deficiency (Chap. 13) may develop, with all the signs and symptoms of persistent anemia.

Pathophysiology

In contrast to the acute situation, chronic blood loss takes time to develop and produce symptoms. The normal menstrual whole blood loss of 35 to 80 mL per month reflects a loss of up to 40 mg iron per month. Since recycled iron from normal erythrocyte turnover and hemoglobin catabolism provides most of the 7 to 20 mg of iron required each day for normal bone marrow erythropoiesis, only 1 to 2 mg dietary ferrous iron normally is absorbed from the gastrointestinal tract each day. Significant monthly losses limit the amount of iron available for recycling and may result in chronic iron shortage.

Other chronic problems known to produce iron loss, particularly in men, include gastrointestinal bleeding. Occult carcinoma of the colon is a common cause of occult chronic blood loss; another is hookworm infestation. It is estimated that 20% of the world's population is infected with hookworm, which may cause a loss of up to 200 mL whole blood per day.[11]

Clinical Presentation and Common Symptoms

The symptoms are nonspecific and are the same as those of any anemia. With chronic blood loss, the symptoms of anemia may not appear until many months after the blood loss begins. Some patients may complain of an inability to concentrate, the result of decreased oxygenation of the tissues,[7] particularly those of the brain. Patients may also complain of tarry (tar-colored) stools, which are indicative of gastrointestinal bleeding. It takes only 60 mL of blood to cause a tarry stool, which may be one of the first symptoms of a gastrointestinal problem.

Laboratory Findings and Correlations with Disease

Since chronic blood loss leads to iron deficiency anemia, the peripheral blood film findings are the same as those described in Chapter 13. Briefly, the erythrocytes are microcytic and hypochromic; iron loss is moderate to severe.

With decreasing iron stores, the serum ferritin level is decreased while all red cell parameters remain normal in the early stages of iron loss. Total iron-binding capacity (TIBC), the capacity of transferrin to transport iron, is increased early in iron loss. Recently it was reported that a red cell distribution width (RDW) value of 15 or more identified 48 of 73 subjects who had reduced transferrin saturation (i.e., increased TIBC) due to iron deficiency.[7] Additional studies are necessary to determine the diagnostic significance of an increased RDW in these cases.

If chronic blood loss is allowed to continue and no treatment is instituted, the red cell count, Hb, and HCT values eventually decrease *after* the decrease in serum ferritin and increase in TIBC. If anemia is moderate to severe when the patient first presents, all iron and red cell parameters are abnormal. A positive result on a stool occult blood test is helpful in confirming gastrointestinal bleeding.

Effects of Treatment on Laboratory Results

Treatment with oral iron therapy should produce reticulocytosis within 7 to 10 days. It is imperative that the laboratory perform a reticulocyte count and RPI within 7 to 10 days to ensure that the patient is responding to the iron therapy. In some instances chronic blood loss is misdiagnosed as iron deficiency; the error is discovered when the patient fails to respond to oral iron therapy. When this happens, iron therapy is discontinued to avoid harmful iron overload.

Patients with a Hb value of less than 7 g/dL may require transfusions, depending on the body's ability to cope with a low Hb level. A unit of packed erythrocytes ordinarily raises the Hb concentration of an adult about 1 g/dL.[1] If bleeding continues and multiple transfusions are given, secondary platelet and coagulation complications may occur.

CHAPTER SUMMARY

The initial effects of acute and chronic blood loss may be somewhat dissimilar, but the long-term effects of iron depletion are the same. The concerns in acute loss are immediate maintenance of blood volume and control of bleeding. The resolution of chronic anemia is less critical but also important.

During the first few hours after blood loss, the HCT and Hb values generally remain steady, owing to initial compensatory vasoconstriction. After 3 to 4 hours, the values may drop and the leukocyte count may rise as immature granulocytes enter the peripheral blood secondary to an outpouring from the marginal pool. With severe blood loss, nucleated red blood cells are seen. After 12 to 24 hours the full extent of anemia is evident. Platelets may be increased, and after fluid replacements have stabilized, leukocyte counts of 30×10^9/L are common. The serum ferritin value may be decreased, reflecting iron loss. RPI should be greater than 3 after a number of days, if bone marrow response is adequate. Erythropoietin levels may be increased in order to stimulate erythropoiesis.

To preserve fluid balance, crystalloids and electrolyte solutions as well as plasma proteins or albumin can be given for initial treatment depending on the situation. These may at first cause a relative decrease in HCT and thus, the appearance of more severe anemia. Therapeutic iron is given if serum ferritin is decreased, and over time, all red cell parameters should return to normal if the bone marrow is functional.

Chronic blood cell loss occurs over time, most often because of excessive menstrual loss or gastrointestinal bleeding. The earliest diagnostic indicator is the serum ferritin value, which becomes abnormal before the other red cell parameters, including Hb, HCT, MCV, and MCHC.

Treatment of chronic blood loss requires treatment of the underlying disorder that is causing the loss. Usually patients are given therapeutic iron and their response is followed by reticulocyte count and RPI within 7 to 10 days to verify a response.

CASE STUDY 20-1

During his annual physical, a 40-year-old black man who was a hospital administrator had a complete blood count. The Hb value was 8.0 g/dL; MCV 70 fL; RDW 15.7; and peripheral blood red cells were described as microcytic and hypochromic.

1. What is the most common anemia to be expected with this blood picture?
2. What is the most likely cause of the anemia?
3. What simple laboratory procedure could be performed to help confirm the diagnosis?

REFERENCES

1. Baughan A, Hughes A, Patterson KG et al: Manual of Haematology. New York, Churchill Livingstone, 1985
2. Hall R, Malia RG: Medical Laboratory Hematology. Boston, Butterworths, 1984
3. Hillman RS: Acute blood loss anemia. In Williams WJ, Beutler E, Erslev AJ et al (eds): Hematology, 4th ed, p 700. New York, McGraw-Hill, 1990
4. Hoffbrand AV, Pettit JE: Essential Haematology, 2nd ed. Boston, Blackwell Scientific Publications, 1984
5. Kaufman CE, Papper S: Review of Pathophysiology. Boston, Little, Brown & Co, 1983
6. Kreis DJ Jr, Bane AE: Clinical Management of Shock. Baltimore, University Park Press, 1984
7. LaBounty LA: Iron metabolism and the identification of iron deficiency anemia. J Med Technol 3:81, 1986
8. Reynolds RD, Lewis JP: Blood loss anemias and the iron deficient states. In Koepke JA (ed): Laboratory Hematology, vol 1. New York, Churchill Livingstone, 1984
9. Schumacher HR, Garvin DF, Triplett DA: Introduction to Laboratory Hematology and Hematopathology. New York, Alan R Liss, 1984
10. Thompson RB, Proctor SJ: A Concise Textbook of Hematology. Baltimore, Urban and Schwarzenberg, 1984
11. Witts LF: Hypochromic Anaemia. Philadelphia, FA Davis, 1969

21

Systematic Laboratory

Evaluation

of Erythrocyte

Abnormalities

John A. Koepke

The preceding chapters in this section entitled Laboratory Evaluation of Erythrocyte Abnormalities include detailed discussions of the various types of anemia. With this knowledge in hand, this chapter seeks to put these chapters into perspective. It brings these discussions together for a global understanding of how to evaluate erythrocyte abnormalities from a laboratory standpoint when a disorder is first discovered but has not yet been diagnosed. Both physician and laboratory scientist should have a systematic (and hopefully similar) approach to laboratory evaluation of erythrocyte abnormalities, and they should work together for the patient's benefit.

The value of laboratory studies in the diagnosis of disease is probably best exemplified by the close relationship between hematologic examinations and clinical anemia. Indeed the identification of hematologic abnormalities frequently uses the laboratory characterization of the disorder as the name of the condition. Think, for example, of macrocytic or microcytic anemias, sickle cell anemia, pyruvate kinase deficiency, and many others.

Anemia may result from decreased synthesis of hemoglobin and erythrocytes, increased destruction of erythrocytes, or acute or chronic blood loss. As discussed in Chapter 10, the most useful classification, from a laboratorian's point of view, is based on the red cell measurements, particularly mean corpuscular volume (MCV) and mean corpuscular hemoglobin concentration (MCHC). Maxwell Wintrobe's pioneering work with the red cell indices was very important in the development of laboratory hematology and in guiding our approach to these problems.[9] These studies are reinforced by the evaluation of red cell morphology in the stained peripheral blood film.

THE PHYSICIAN'S ROLE IN THE DIAGNOSTIC PROCESS

The cause of anemia is identified by integrating clinical information with the results of laboratory studies. The patient's physician plays a key role in evaluating clinical information obtained from the medical history and physical examination, and incorporating erythrocyte measurements, including the reticulocyte count and reticulocyte production index (RPI), and sometimes serum iron or ferritin measurements, and bone marrow examination when necessary.

The exact diagnosis is not always obvious to the physician. More than likely the doctor will note that the patient is somewhat pale and in the subsequent history taking will seek to discover the possible cause of the anemia. Table 21-1 lists some clues in the patient's history that may suggest specific causes of anemia and in turn, indicate laboratory tests that may be useful in the diagnostic process.

Similarly, the physical examination may reveal significant clues to the cause of anemia. Table 21-2 lists some of these signs, which the physician will try to identify. Again, other definitive studies may be suggested.

Why does the physician order a blood count in the first place? What can be learned from it? In some cases if the count is to be used as a screening procedure, will the rapid report of a normal or abnormal count suffice? Or is the count being requested to monitor some aspect of the patient's condition? How do anemias affect the composition and morphology of the peripheral blood cells?

The definitive diagnosis of anemia depends, to a greater or lesser extent, on laboratory studies.[1,5,7,8,10] For many years blood films have been carefully examined in an effort to sort out the cause of anemia and of many other hematologic and systemic disorders. With the development of more and more sophisticated automated hematologic analyzers, which can, within a minute or two, provide an accurate and precise blood count, including the differential leukocyte count, there has been a tendency to downplay the importance of the blood film examination. It is helpful to use the instruments to make an initial sort of the specimens, separating normal from possibly abnormal cases. Flagging systems have been developed that can perform this function quite acceptably; when such systems are used properly, only flagged specimens require evaluation of the blood film. In the case of anemia, very useful information can be provided by the morphologic review of red cells on the blood film for clues, the search for concomitant abnormali-

TABLE 21–1. Patient History and the Cause of Anemia: Examples of Some Common Associations

HISTORY	ASSOCIATED ANEMIA
Chronic hepatic, renal, or other diseases (*e.g.,* cancer)	Anemia of chronic disease
Alcoholism	Folate deficiency
Vegetarian diet	Iron deficiency
Bleeding (gastrointestinal, menorrhagia, multiple pregnancies)	Iron deficiency
Exposure to toxic chemicals	Hypoplastic or aplastic anemia
Chronic drug ingestion	Megaloblastic, hypoplastic, or aplastic anemia

TABLE 21–2. Physical Signs and the Cause of Anemia: Examples of Some Common Associations

PHYSICAL SIGNS	ASSOCIATED ANEMIA
Jaundice (skin, sclerae)	Hemolytic anemia, anemia associated chronic liver disease
Leg ulcers (black patient)	Sickle cell anemia
Spooned nails	Iron-deficiency anemia
Dark line at base of teeth	Lead toxicity
Neurologic deficit	Megaloblastic (vitamin B_{12}) anemia
Lymph node enlargement	Anemia secondary to lymphoma, leukemia, or infection
Spleen enlargement	Hemolytic anemia, chronic liver disease, leukemia, lymphoma
Liver enlargement	Hemolytic anemia, metastatic carcinoma
Prominent forehead (frontal bossing)	Thalassemia, sickle cell anemia
Bone tenderness	Anemia secondary to myeloma or metastatic carcinoma
Bluish skin color	Methemoglobinemia
Oriental or Mediterranean ethnicity	Thalassemia syndromes

ties in the leukocyte or platelet population, or the finding of evidence such as red cell rouleaux or protein abnormalities.[6]

LABORATORY EVALUATION OF ANEMIA

Systematic Approach

About 25 years ago, William R. Best presented a systematic and logical way to use the laboratory efficiently. He developed a hemolytic anemia "tree" and a hemolysis "tree."[3] (Today the decision tree method is called an algorithm.) Figure 21-1 shows a more complete anemia algorithm, which serves as a tool for efficiently arriving at a possible diagnosis by obtaining key laboratory data in a step-by-step fashion. Each question is contingent on the answer to the preceding question, which is also a decision point in the physician's diagnostic thinking. This system, with its many branches, forms a logical approach to the diagnosis of the cause of anemia. The roots of the tree are the basic measurements (hemoglobin, hematocrit, and red cell count) that establish the presence or absence of anemia.

The Complete Blood Count

The basic hematologic study is the so-called complete blood count. This study, in all its many variations, includes some measurement of red cells, leukocytes, and platelets. In investigating anemia we may quantitate only the red cell population, or we may measure the oxygen-carrying capacity of the red cells by quantitating hemoglobin. The leukocyte count may be amplified with a differential leukocyte count, performed either with an instrument or by examining a Romanowsky-stained blood film. So the blood count may be performed in many different ways.

With the development of rapid, precise, and accurate hematology instruments, blood counts are now even more common. Any evaluation of cost versus benefit of care for the patient usually includes scrutiny of this test, since it is used so widely. But its popularity is well justified because

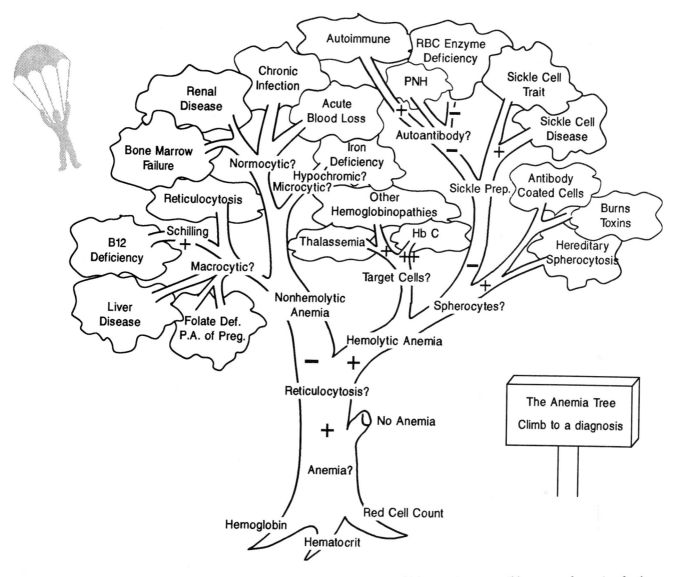

FIG. 21-1. Following the branches of the anemia tree leads the physician and laboratorian to possible causes of anemia of unknown origin. P. A. of Preg indicates pernicious anemia of pregnancy.

so many diseases produce identifiable, if at times nonspecific, changes in the blood count.

Because the blood count is, in reality, a *panel* of measurements or studies, it is conceivable that deleting some parts of the study (*e.g.*, the MCHC) will produce no significant loss of information. Conceivably it could be revamped to meet patient care needs better. It is quite evident that hematology instrumentation can be employed to examine patient specimens more efficiently. A basic premise for the most efficient use of currently available instrumentation is that if a carefully chosen set of quantitative and qualitative parameters are found to be within a prescribed set of limits, additional studies probably are not necessary and significant abnormalities are not likely to be found on a blood film. If such studies were not done, significant savings would be realized and technologists' efforts could be devoted to more useful work.[6] Recently, new parameters such as the red cell distribution width (RDW), a quantitative estimate of red cell anisocytosis, have been added to the battery of results

generated by hematology analyzers. This measurement has been proposed as an additional major factor in the classification of anemia.[2] If anemia is present, the next logical question is whether it represents a hemolytic or a nonhemolytic process. The reticulocyte count has served as a simple yet useful test for this step, counting the red cells most recently released from the bone marrow. If peripheral hemolysis is increased, increased numbers of reticulocytes will be found in the blood. Various estimates of reticulocyte production, particularly in the face of anemia, are being used, with good effect on the diagnostic and therapeutic process.

The Blood Film Evaluation

At this level of our "tree climbing," the time-honored blood film examination is employed in an effort to discover additional clues that may be helpful. Other laboratory tests (*e.g.*, the sickle hemoglobin screen) may be suggested at this level before the definitive diagnosis is achieved. Each chapter details the peripheral blood film changes associated with the various anemias that are discussed.

The Bone Marrow Examination

A final important hematologic test in the diagnosis of anemia is the bone marrow examination. In the most general sense, any patient with anemia is a candidate for a marrow study. The cause of an unexplained anemia may become evident following a careful study of the bone marrow, but there has been a significant decline in the number of marrow studies that are performed to investigate anemia. Formerly many anemic patients underwent marrow aspiration routinely as part of their diagnostic work-up, but it is evident that little additional information is provided by a bone marrow study, for example, in hemolytic anemia. Patients with possible iron-deficiency anemia may require an assessment of marrow iron stores; however, the development of peripheral blood assays for serum iron and ferritin allow more efficient estimation of iron stores without bone marrow aspiration or biopsy.

EPILOGUE

Viewers of Figure 21-1 may wonder just why the man is descending in a parachute, as shown in the corner of the picture. As I remember it, Dr. Best, at the end of a presentation, asked whether anyone in the audience had wondered why the parachutist was included. Then he said it certainly was possible for the parachutist to land on the proper branch (*i.e.*, the correct

diagnosis), but that his chances of hitting that exact branch were not very good. Consequently, he proposed that the use of the logical approach, climbing from the ground up, constitutes a more efficient way of arriving at the correct diagnosis.

REFERENCES

1. van Assendelft OW: Laboratory tests in the differential diagnosis of anemia. Labmedica 3:21, 1986
2. Bessman JD, Gilmer PR, Gardner FH: Improved classification of anemia by MCV and RDW. Am J Clin Pathol 80:332, 1983
3. Best WR: Differential diagnosis of hemolytic anemias. In Sunderman FW, Sunderman RW Jr (eds): Hemoglobin—Its Precursors and Metabolites, p 307. Philadelphia, JB Lippincott, 1964
4. Dacie JW, Lewis SM: Use of haematological techniques in clinical work. In Dacie JW, Lewis SM: Practical Haematology, 6th ed, p 132. Edinburgh, Churchill Livingstone, 1984
5. de Gruchy GC: General principles in the diagnosis and treatment of anaemia. In de Gruchy GC: Clinical Haematology, 4th ed, p 59. Oxford, Blackwell Scientific, 1978
6. Koepke JA, Dotson MA, Shifman MA et al: A flagging system for multichannel hematology analyzers. Blood Cells 11:113, 1985
7. Koepke JA, Koepke JF: Hematologic problems—Anemia. In Koepke JA, Koepke JF: Guide to Clinical Laboratory Diagnosis, 3rd ed, p 148. Norwalk, CT, Appleton and Lange, 1987
8. Wheby MS: Using a clinical laboratory in the diagnosis of anemia. Med Clin North Am 50:1689, 1966
9. Wintrobe MM: The erythrocyte in man. Medicine 9:195, 1930
10. Wintrobe MM: The diagnostic and therapeutic approach to hematologic problems. In Wintrobe MM et al: Clinical Hematology, 8th ed, p 3. Philadelphia, Lea & Febiger, 1981

PART *IV*
THE
LEUKOCYTES

22

Introduction

to

the

Leukocytes

Louann W. Lawrence

The terms *leukocyte* and *white blood cell* are used synonymously to refer to the colorless nucleated cells that circulate in peripheral blood and function as the body's main line of defense against foreign invaders such as bacteria, viruses, and other foreign antigens. In peripheral blood they are present in much smaller numbers than erythrocytes, and they are transported by way of the peripheral blood to areas where they enter the tissues and perform their functions. In this chapter five types of normal leukocytes found in the peripheral blood are introduced. Three different classification systems are reviewed. The formation and function of these important cells are outlined briefly. Specifics of each cell are presented in subsequent chapters. A system for the morphologic identification of these cells in conjunction with brief morphologic descriptions of each cell are included.

KINETICS

Our knowledge of leukocytes is not as extensive as that of erythrocytes. Leukocytes spend a relatively short time in the peripheral blood. The term *kinetics* refers to the dynamic forces that move cells into and out of different body compartments or tissues. Leukocytes are found in three different compartments in the body: bone marrow, peripheral blood, and tissues. When we examine and count leukocytes in a peripheral blood sample, we are looking at only a small fraction of the body's total leukocyte population. Blood vessels serve principally as a transport system to get the leukocytes to the tissues where most of their functions are carried out. The kinetics of each leukocyte are discussed in more detail in Chapters 23 and 24.

TABLE 22–1. Leukocyte Classification

GRANULOCYTES	NONGRANULOCYTES
Neutrophils	Monocytes
Eosinophils	Lymphocytes
Basophils	
POLYMORPHONUCLEAR	MONONUCLEAR
Neutrophils	Monocytes
Eosinophils	Lymphocytes
Basophils	
PHAGOCYTES	IMMUNOCYTES
Neutrophils	Lymphocytes
Eosinophils	
Basophils	
Monocytes	

CLASSIFICATION

Five principal types of leukocytes normally circulate in peripheral blood: neutrophils, eosinophils, basophils, monocytes, and lymphocytes. Several different criteria may be used to classify leukocytes (Table 22-1). According to granularity, leukocytes may be classified as granulocytes (neutrophils, eosinophils, basophils) and nongranulocytes (monocytes and lymphocytes). The granulocytes contain distinct granules in their cytoplasm, whereas the nongranulocytes lack prominent granules. This classification is not very satisfactory, because the so-called nongranulocytes do, in fact, contain granules (all monocytes contain small, indistinct granules and certain subtypes of lymphocytes contain large azure granules); however, their granules are not their primary identifying characteristic. Another morphologic classification is based on nuclear segmentation. Polymorphonuclear cells (neutrophils, eosinophils, basophils) contain a multilobed or segmented nucleus in their mature form, while mononuclear cells (monocytes and lymphocytes) contain a nucleus that may be variable in shape but is a single mass, not segmented. Again, this is not a very satisfactory classification, because the nuclei of immature polymorphonuclear cells are not segmented and because basophil nuclei do not necessarily segment. The third classification system, which is based on the *function* of the cells divides them into phagocytes and immunocytes. In this text the latter classification system is used. In Chapter 23, the phagocytic leukocytes (neutrophils, eosinophils, basophils, monocytes) will be discussed, and in Chapter 24 the immunologic leukocytes (lymphocytes).

FUNCTION

The primary function of leukocytes as a group is defense against any invader into the body that may be recognized as foreign. Each cell type has a specific function and behaves as a separate but related system. The phagocytes seek out foreign invaders to engulf and destroy them. The immunocytes are concerned with antibody production and other activities of the immune response to a foreign substance (antigen). These two functions are closely interrelated, and each depends on the other to operate with maximum efficiency. Cell functions are discussed in more detail in subsequent chapters.

FORMATION

Not all leukocytes are formed in the bone marrow as erythrocytes are, but it is the principal site of granulocyte production. Lymphocytes are normally formed in lymphoid tissues throughout the body as well as in the bone marrow. Leukocytes are believed by most investigators to be formed from a totipotent stem cell, which in turn gives rise to (1) partially committed lymphoid stem cells, capable of forming the immunocytes and (2) partially committed myeloid stem cells, capable of forming phagocytes as well as erythrocytes and platelets.

From the myeloid stem cell evolves another precursor cell, the colony-forming unit–neutrophil–monocyte or CFU-NM, which is the progenitor of both neutrophils and monocytes.[2] Neutrophils and monocytes are thus derived from the same cell. Even though they evolve into morphologically distinct cells, they both retain phagocytosis as their primary function. Research has indicated the possibility that an eosinophilic stem cell might also evolve from the partially committed myeloid stem cell. Colonies composed entirely of eosinophils have been observed to develop in cultures of progenitor cells from normal marrow.[6] Recent studies have indicated the possibility of a common circulating progenitor cell for eosinophils and basophils.[1] (See Chap. 5 for a more detailed discussion of hematopoiesis.)

MORPHOLOGY

The major routine method for studying the morphology of leukocytes is the stained peripheral blood film. The use of a Romanowsky type stain, such as Wright stain, allows for the classification of leukocytes by their various reactions to the different dyes in the stain. The granulocytes are named according to their staining reactions. Eosinophil granules stain bright orange-pink because they have an affinity for eosin, the acidic dye in the stain. Basophil granules stain dark purple-blue because they have an affinity for methylene blue, which is the basic dye in the stain. Neutrophil granules remain "neutral," showing minimal affinity for either the acidic or basic dye and appearing light pinkish purple or pink-tan. Thus, the pH of the staining system is very important for proper cell identification. Cell colors can vary slightly with each staining system. One should never attempt to identify leukocytes on a poorly or improperly stained film. The most competent morphologists can be fooled into making mistakes by an improper staining system. (See Chapter 3 for additional discussion of blood film staining.)

Table 22-2 contains a list of criteria for the identification of leukocytes. A competent morphologist keeps these criteria in mind and uses as many as possible when attempting to identify any leukocyte. The most valuable and reliable criterion, especially for deciding whether a cell is mature or immature, is the nuclear chromatin pattern. Several stages of chromatin maturity have been described. Euchromatin denotes immaturity and is characteristic of blast cells. It appears finely granular and is distributed uniformly, with very few if any tiny aggregates (Fig. 22-1). The amount of heterochromatin increases with maturity. It appears as coarse, granular areas forming medium-sized to large

TABLE 22–2. Criteria for Leukocyte Identification

1. Cell size
2. Nucleus-cytoplasm ratio
   a. High ratio: Nucleus occupies most of cell area with only a small rim of cytoplasm.
   b. Low ratio: Nucleus is small in relation to volume of cytoplasm.
3. Cytoplasm characteristics
   a. Color of background cytoplasm
   b. Presence or absence of granules
   c. Color and size of granules
4. Nuclear characteristics
   a. Shape
   b. Color
   c. Chromatin pattern
   d. Presence or absence of nucleoli

aggregates or clumps that are irregularly distributed. Parachromatin, the nonstaining or clear areas between the chromatin clumps, becomes more prominent as cells mature.[5]

The nuclear:cytoplasmic ratio may be used for mature cells, but it varies in dividing cells, depending on what point in the mitotic cycle the cell happens to be. Because color can vary with each staining system, it is the least reliable criterion for cell identification. Nuclear shape is also a relatively poor criterion, as it is highly susceptible to artifacts and can change considerably in disease states. It helps to compare already identified cells on the same slide with those that are more difficult to identify. One must also keep in mind that cell maturation is an ongoing process and that different stages of cell maturation evolve from one stage to the next rather than in a stepwise process, so that a specific cell may demonstrate characteristics of two maturation stages. A cell may lack one or more of the identification criteria for a particular stage; therefore, the competent morphologist uses as many features as possible to make the best decision.

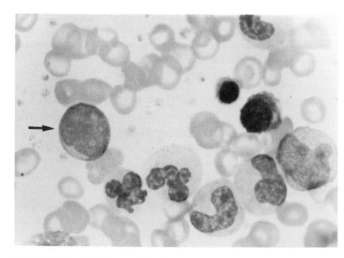

FIG. 22-1.   Differences in chromatin pattern. Compare the appearance of the chromatin pattern in the blast nucleus (*arrow*) to that in the surrounding, more differentiated cells. Note how the chromatin clumping increased between the neutrophil band forms and the segmented form. Note the denseness of the chromatin in the two red cell precursors.

A brief description of each cell as it appears under light microscopy on Romanowsky-stained films follows.[4] Detailed descriptions of each cell type are presented in subsequent chapters. The reference ranges listed below are for adults and should be considered as examples only.[3] Reference ranges must be established by each individual laboratory and may vary slightly.

Neutrophil, Segmented

See Plate 6.

Synonyms: Seg, polymorphonuclear neutrophil, poly, PMN
Diameter: 10 to 15 μm
Nucleus: Segmented into 2 to 5 lobes (some references regard 2–4 lobes as normal); lobes are connected by a threadlike filament that does not contain chromatin. Nuclear chromatin is dark purple and forms densely stained clumps separated by a network of lighter purple bands.
Cytoplasm: Stains light pink with numerous specific or secondary granules that are too small to be resolved individually with the light microscope and give the cytoplasm a grainy appearance. A few purple primary granules may remain.
Reference Range: Relative, 37% to 77%
           Absolute, 2.0 to 6.93 × 10⁹/L

Neutrophil, Band

See Plate 7.

Synonyms: Nonsegmented neutrophil, neutrophil staff or stab
Diameter: 10 to 15 μm
Nucleus: Elongated, curved, or sausage shaped with rounded ends and areas of dense clumping at each pole. The beginning of segmentation may be apparent, but the connecting band between lobes is wide enough to reveal two distinct margins surrounding nuclear material. Filaments are not present.
Cytoplasm: Identical to that of segmented neutrophil
Reference Range: Relative, 0% to 11%
           Absolute, 0 to 0.87 × 10⁹/L

Eosinophil

See Plate 8A.

Synonyms: Eo, acidophil
Diameter: 12 to 17 μm
Nucleus: Dark purple, chromatin pattern similar to neutrophil; usually band shaped or segmented into only two segments.
Cytoplasm: Filled with large, spherical, refractive granules of uniform size that stain bright orange-pink. The granules are usually evenly distributed but rarely overlie the nucleus.
Reference Range: Relative, 0% to 7%
           Absolute, 0 to 0.67 × 10⁹/L

Basophil

See Plate 9A.

Synonym: Baso
Diameter: 10 to 14 μm
Nucleus: Light purple staining, may be round, indented, band shaped, or lobulated. Usually difficult to see because of overlying granules. Chromatin pattern is smudged and indistinct.
Cytoplasm: Characterized by densely stained, dark violet to purple-black granules that are variable in size and unevenly distributed. Because the granules are water soluble, only vestiges of granules, sometimes contained within small vacuoles, may be found.
Reference Range: Relative, 0% to 1.6%
Absolute, 0 to 0.20 $\times$ 10^9/L

Monocyte

See Plates 10A and B.

Synonyms: Mono, mononuclear phagocyte
Diameter: 12 to 20 μm
Nucleus: Highly variable in shape; may be round, horseshoe shaped or lobulated, and usually shows some degree of folding or convolutions. Chromatin is light purple and arranged in loose strands or lacy pattern.
Cytoplasm: Abundant (*i.e.*, nuclear:cytoplasmic ratio is low). Dull, pale, faded, gray-blue, containing fine, indistinct granules giving it a ground-glass appearance. Cell outline may be irregular with occasional pseudopods, and occasional vacuoles may be seen.
Reference Range: Relative, 2% to 10%
Absolute, 0.03 to 0.90 $\times$ 10^9/L

Normal Lymphocyte

See Plates 20A and B.

Synonym: Lymph
Diameter: Small, 6 to 8 μm; medium to large, 8 to 12 μm
Nucleus: Deep purple, compact, densely packed clumps or blocks of chromatin with linear areas of parachromatin. Nucleoli may be visible. Shape may be round, oval, or indented.
Cytoplasm: Ranges from sparse in the smaller forms to abundant in the larger forms. Stains pale to bright sky blue. May contain a few prominent reddish (azurophilic) granules. May be indented by surrounding red cells.
Reference Range: Relative, 10% to 44%
Absolute, 0.6 to 3.44 $\times$ 10^9/L

Variant Lymphocyte

See Plates 24 through 26.

Synonyms: Reactive, atypical, stimulated lymphocytes
Diameter: Highly variable, 10 to 22 μm
Nucleus: May range from extremely dense to pale and immature-looking.
Cytoplasm: Usually abundant and ranges in staining intensity from deeply basophilic to pale blue.
Reference Range: Relative, 0% to 7.5%
Absolute, 0 to 0.66 $\times$ 10^9/L

REFERENCES

1. Denburg JA, Telizyn S, Messner H et al: Heterogeneity of human peripheral blood eosinophil-type colonies: Evidence for a common basophil-eosinophil progenitor. Blood 66:312, 1985
2. Golde DW, Groopman JE: Production, distribution and fate of monocytes and macrophages. In Williams WJ, Beutler E, Erslev AJ et al (eds): Hematology, 4th ed. New York, McGraw-Hill, 1990
3. Koepke JA, Dotson MA, Shifman MA: A critical evaluation of the manual/visual differential leukocyte counting method. Blood Cells, 11:173, 1986
4. National Committee for Clinical Laboratory Standards: Leukocyte Differential Counting—A Tentative Standard. NCCLS H20-T, vol 4, no 11. Villanova, PA, NCCLS, 1984
5. Shafer J: White Blood Cell Morphology Workshop Manual, ASMT Region III. Orlando, FL, 1975
6. Zucker-Franklin D, Grutsky G, L'Esperance P: Granulocyte colonies derived from lymphocyte fractions in normal human blood. Proc Natl Acad Sci USA 71:2711, 1974

23

The Phagocytic Leukocytes—

Morphology, Kinetics, and Function

Louann W. Lawrence

THE NEUTROPHIL

The neutrophil is the most common leukocyte in normal peripheral blood. In the mature form it is easily recognized on a Romanowsky-stained blood film by its distinctive segmented nucleus and pinkish purple or pink–tan granules in the cytoplasm. Six stages in the maturation of this cell have been defined—myeloblast, promyelocyte, myelocyte, metamyelocyte, band and segmented form. Collectively they are called the granulocytic or neutrophilic maturation series. It is important to be able to recognize the immature forms because they are seen in peripheral blood in many conditions. In addition, the ability to differentiate these cells in bone marrow specimens is a necessary skill in many medical center laboratories.

Morphology

In the past the three granulocyte types were usually approached as a group of cells differentiating from one identifiable blast cell (the myeloblast). Recent research has led us to believe that each cell may have its own precursor or blast cell. Although all blasts are recognizable by ordinary light microscopy, many are already committed to form a specific myeloid cell.[22] As more knowledge about the function of eosinophils and basophils is gained, it appears that the three granulocytes do not have as much in common as was once thought. Therefore, in this chapter eosinophils and basophils are discussed separately.

Myeloblast

The earliest recognizable form that can be identified by light microscopy as a cell that will mature into one of the myeloid cells is the myeloblast (Plate 11A). This cell has dark blue to blue cytoplasm that contains no visible granules. The nucleus is made up of a smooth, delicate, uniformly distributed chromatin pattern sometimes described as lacy. Myeloblasts usually have two or more distinct nucleoli, which disappear as the cell matures. The nucleus occupies most of the cell, leaving only a small rim of cytoplasm. This is referred to as a high nuclear-cytoplasmic ratio. The approximate cell diameter is 15 to 20 μm, depending on what stage in the mitotic cycle it is in. Cells become relatively larger just prior to mitotic division. Myeloblasts make up about 1% to 2% of the cells in normal bone marrow and normally are not seen in peripheral blood.

The French–American–British (FAB) Cooperative Group has introduced a modified definition of myeloblasts, which they believe may be more useful clinically in defining some hematologic disease states.[4] The cells are sometimes referred to as the European type I and type II myeloblasts. Type I is identical to the cell described in the previous paragraph, with *no granules* in the cytoplasm. Type II blasts have a few primary (azurophilic) granules in their cytoplasm. Their other characteristics are similar to those of the type I blasts, except that their nuclear-cytoplasmic ratio tends to be lower and the nucleus remains in a central position. They do not contain numerous cytoplasmic granules as does the promyelocyte, which is described in the next section (see Plate 11B and Chap. 34 for further descriptions and pictures of these two forms). Slight differences from one morphologist to another in identifying the various maturation stages are inevitable.

Monoblasts are presumed to exist but are not recognizable with ordinary light microscopy.[22] Most morphologists are very cautious in differentiating among types of blasts (myeloblasts, monoblasts, lymphoblasts) because light microscopy and Romanowsky stains result in such similar characteristics that it is difficult to distinguish among them. In leukemic diseases when blasts are seen in abundance in the peripheral blood and bone marrow, the use of cytochemical stains or immunologic cell markers helps to distinguish from which cell line the blasts arise. Cytochemical stains are special dyes used to stain a specific chemical constituent of a cell. The best rule when attempting to identify very immature cells on a peripheral blood film stained with Wright or a comparable type of stain is to call the cell a blast without attempting to distinguish its cell line. It is best to be aware of the limits of light microscopy and of the availability of more definitive methods of cell identification.

Promyelocyte

At the first appearance of cytoplasmic granules, the cell is placed in the promyelocyte stage, also called the progranulocyte. (The exception to this rule is the European type II blast described above.) It was once thought that promyelocytes could mature into any of the three granulocytes (neutrophil, eosinophil, or basophil), hence the term progranulocyte. It is now known that the cell is committed at a much earlier stage, perhaps during the stage that is recognizable as a blast, to becoming either an eosinophil, basophil, or neutrophil.

The promyelocyte is characterized by large, prominent, reddish purple granules in the cytoplasm called primary or azurophilic granules (see Plate 12). The background cytoplasm remains dark blue to blue, and the nucleus still appears fairly immature with a uniform, evenly distributed chromatin pattern. Nucleoli may or may not be visible. As the cell matures, the nucleus may be displaced off center and the nuclear-cytoplasmic ratio decreases. This cell is still rather large and may sometimes appear larger than the myeloblast, depending on its stage in the mitotic cycle. Promyelocytes make up 2% to 5% of cells in the bone marrow and normally are not found in the peripheral blood.

Synthesis of primary granules begins and ends during this stage. As the cell continues to divide, primary granules are diluted among daughter cells. These granules, which are rich in the enzyme peroxidase, are present in all stages including the mature segmented neutrophil, but they become less visible with Wright or a comparable stain. Evidence of this is the intense staining by peroxidase stains in the cytoplasm of mature neutrophils.

Myelocyte

Myelocytes begin to form a second set of granules referred to as secondary or specific granules. The primary granules become less visible as the secondary granules are being formed, thus cells in this stage may have varying amounts of each type of granule. Some investigators have proposed subdividing this stage into early and late, but it is not usually done because the distinction is not clinically relevant. Secondary granules are smaller and less easily resolved by most light microscopes and are the granules that eventually fill the cell and give it its characteristic pinkish tan color (see Plate 13A and B for two examples of myelocytes). The cytoplasm of the cell begins to lose cytoplasmic RNA (blue color), but a tinge of blue may remain, especially along the edges of the cell. As the pinkish specific granules begin to form in the Golgi region of the cell, a pink arc may be seen, which is sometimes called the "dawn of neutrophilia." The nucleus becomes more condensed and the chromatin pattern clumped; nucleoli usually are no longer visible. The nuclear:cytoplasmic ratio continues to decrease. The cell size ranges from 16 to 24 μm. Myelocytes are the last stage to undergo mitosis. Cells in subsequent stages continue to mature but do not divide. Neutrophilic myelocytes make up approximately 10% to 20% of marrow cells and normally are not seen in peripheral blood.

The secondary granules contain lysozyme, acid hydrolases, and a variety of other proteins but not peroxidase. The specific granule contents and their functions are discussed in the section on neutrophil biochemistry.

Metamyelocyte

The cell next matures into a metamyelocyte (also called a *juvenile*), and the shape of the nucleus becomes the chief identification criterion. Until this stage the nucleus has remained round or oval, but now it begins to flatten on one side and begins to constrict or indent (becoming kidney bean or peanut shaped) (see Plate 14). Nuclear chromatin condenses even more to become coarsely clumped. The cytoplasm has lost all traces of blue color (RNA) and appears uniformly pink with pinkish purple secondary granules evenly distributed, much as in the cytoplasm of the mature cell. Metamyelocytes make up approximately 15%

to 30% of marrow cells and normally are not found in the peripheral blood. To differentiate this stage from the next more mature stage (the band), the indentation of the nucleus must be less than half the width of the nucleus.

Band or Stab Cell

This is the last stage before the mature cell. Bands are normally present in a small percentage in peripheral blood. Probably the greatest source of variation and discrepancy in leukocyte morphology is identification of the band form. Because an increase in bands in peripheral blood can be clinically relevant, it is important to try to standardize criteria for band identification, at least within an institution. Extremes in band definitions range from "A cell is a band unless a filament is seen between segments" (normals range from 12%–18%) to "If it is indented over two thirds of the total width of the band at its widest point, it is no longer a band" (normals range from 0%–5%). In an attempt to standardize band definitions the College of American Pathologists Survey Committee makes the following recommendation: "Any mature cell of the granulocytic series which has a curved, band-shaped nucleus which has *not* developed a threadlike filament, shall be called a band. If any nuclear chromatin is seen in the bridge between the lobes, then the bridge is not a filament and the cell is a band." The committee also recommends, "Any cell in which the nucleus is so twisted that the entire outline of the nucleus is not visible, due to superimposition of one part of the nucleus upon the other parts, shall be classified as a poly (segmented neutrophil)."[10] By these criteria normal values range from 5% to 10%. Most clinical laboratories use these criteria but still may have discrepancies due to individual judgment and personal interpretation of each cell. Laboratories should develop quality control and training programs to keep band criteria standardized among their own personnel to aid physicians in identifying clinically relevant increases in band forms.

Segmented Neutrophil

This cell has several names, including segmented neutrophil, which is often shortened to "seg," and polymorphonuclear leukocyte, which is often shortened to "poly" or "PMN." It gets its name from the characteristic shape of the nucleus (Chap. 22). The normal relative reference range of mature segmented neutrophils in the peripheral blood is approximately 37% to 77% in adults (normal absolute value, 2.0–6.93 × 10^9/L).[25] Children normally have lower relative numbers of segmented neutrophils; however, since their total leukocyte counts tend to be higher than adults, the absolute values are very similar (3.0–4.0 × 10^9/L).[33]

Kinetics

Life Span and Pools

The life span of the neutrophil is approximately 9 or 10 days from myeloblast to death. The cell spends its life in three main areas of the body, passing from bone marrow to peripheral blood and into the tissues. The movement does not reverse: neutrophils do not go back into the blood after entering the tissues. In the bone marrow the cells can be pictured as in two separate pools: (1) mitotic and (2) maturation and storage (Fig. 23-1). The mitotic pool contains

myeloblasts, promyelocytes, and myelocytes. The maturation and storage pool contains metamyelocytes, bands, and segmented neutrophils. It has been estimated that the cells stay in the mitotic pool for 2 or 3 days and undergo four or five cell divisions. Cells spend 5 to 7 days in the maturation and storage pool, no longer undergoing division but progressively maturing. Under certain reactive or stressful conditions, maturation time may be shortened, divisions may be skipped, and release into the blood may occur prematurely.

Neutrophils move into the peripheral blood, where they remain only an average of 7 hours before passing into the tissues, where they perform their principal function and die a short time later. While in the blood they are continuously and rapidly exchanged between two intravascular pools, the circulating and marginal pools (Fig. 23-2). At any one time approximately half of blood neutrophils are not circulating freely but are adhering to vessel walls. These make up the marginal neutrophil pool (MNP). Shifts may occur during stress or exercise or after epinephrine is administered. Such movements from the MNP to the circulating neutrophil pool (CNP) cause transient leukocytosis. This may account for the elevated leukocyte count obtained from a fearful, crying child or an adult in a stressful situation. The value may be normal when it is checked under calmer conditions.[5]

If large numbers of granulocytes are removed experimentally by leukapheresis or by administration of a test dose of endotoxin, mature granulocytes are promptly released into the circulating blood from the marrow granulocyte reserve. This response is similar to the body's response to infection or trauma. In the first 1 or 2 hours the granulocyte count drops then rises by 3.0 to 5.0 × 10^9 mature cells per liter within about 4 to 5 hours. The initial drop is due to a shift of cells from the CNP to the MNP. The subsequent rise is due to a reversal of this shift as well as to cells being released from the marrow storage pool. The marrow pool is estimated to contain a 4- to 10-day supply of cells.[3] It is

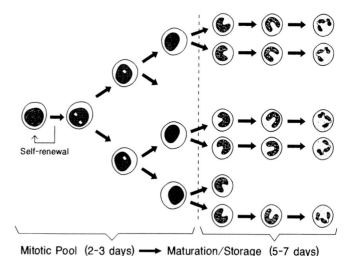

Mitotic Pool (2-3 days) ⟶ Maturation/Storage (5-7 days)

FIG. 23-1.   Bone marrow pools or compartments. Cells capable of division (stem cells, blasts, promyelocytes, and myelocytes) are in the mitotic pool. Nondividing cells (metamyelocytes, bands, and segmented forms) are in the maturation or storage pool.

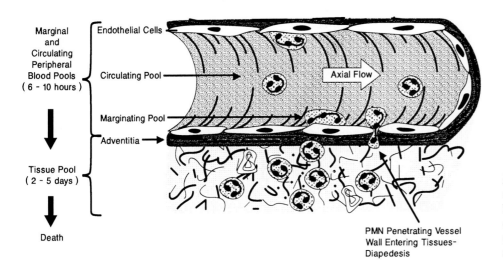

Marginal and Circulating Peripheral Blood Pools (6 - 10 hours)

Endothelial Cells

Circulating Pool

Axial Flow

Marginating Pool

Adventitia

Tissue Pool (2 - 5 days)

Death

PMN Penetrating Vessel Wall Entering Tissues- Diapedesis

FIG. 23-2. Neutrophil transit from marrow to tissues. The circulating blood has two neutrophil pools: those cells that are circulating (CNP) and those that are adhering to capillary endothelial cells (marginated or MNP).

not known whether granulocytes are released from the marrow on a first in–first out basis or randomly. The higher ratio of band to segmented cells in the marrow than in the peripheral blood tends to suggest selective release of segmented cells.[34]

Normally, neutrophils leave the blood and enter the tissues randomly with no relation to how long they have been circulating. They leave by the process of diapedesis, in which they squeeze between junctions in the endothelial cells of vessel walls (see Fig. 23-2). The production rate of neutrophils is an estimated 1.63×10^9 cells per kilogram body weight per day, which enter and leave the blood.[22] This production can increase dramatically in response to inflammatory stimuli.

Little is known about the cells after they move into the tissues. Their life span is thought to be short because they survive only 2 to 3 days in tissue cultures. If they are not utilized in an area of inflammation or infection they may leave the body by way of secretions in the bronchi or gastrointestinal tract, or in urine. They may die in the tissues, or may be destroyed by other phagocytic cells (monocytes or macrophages).

Regulatory Mechanism

Some humoral regulation of granulopoiesis is known to exist. Neutrophil numbers vary with time of day, exercise and diet. A two–part regulatory mechanism has been postulated—one factor to control differentiation of myeloid stem cells into granulocyte precursors and another to regulate marrow release into the blood.[7] Local control of stem cells by surrounding tissue in the bone marrow (hematopoietic microenvironment) may also play a part in granulocyte regulation. Current evidence suggests that differentiation of stem cells into granulocyte precursors is influenced by a group of humoral agents, referred to as colony-stimulating factors (CSF) or leukopoietin. Prominent sources of human CSF have been found to be blood monocytes and macrophages, activated T lymphocytes, endothelial cells, and fibroblasts. Not much is known about factors that influence release of CSF, but bacterial endotoxins and phagocytosis of bacteria are known to increase its release. There is strong evidence that CSF has a part in causing both proliferation and differentiation of granulocytic cells *in vivo*.[28] There is also thought to be a negative feedback mechanism of granulocyte production, which may work by inhibiting DNA synthesis in committed precursor cells.

Release of granulocytes from the bone marrow to the blood may be controlled by a substance called leukocytosis-inducing factor. In experimental studies, this substance appeared in the plasma after injection of bacterial endotoxins. When it was later reinfused, it caused an increased leukocyte number in peripheral blood and increased release of immature granulocytes from the marrow.[7]

Biochemistry

Energy Production

The priinicipal biochemical pathway to produce energy in the neutrophil is anaerobic glycolysis (Embden-Meyerhof pathway; Chap. 6). The hexose monophosphate shunt is also active in circulating leukocytes, but it accounts for less than 5% of the glucose consumed. Both pathways are stimulated to increase activity during phagocytosis. This is called a respiratory or metabolic burst and plays a role in the killing of microorganisms and detoxification of the cell.[29]

Granule Contents

The granules of neutrophils contain enzymes, most of which aid the cell in successfully killing bacteria. These enzymes are also sometimes useful in helping to identify immature cells of a specific cell line with the use of cytochemistry. The primary or azurophilic granules that first appear in the promyelocyte stage are membrane-bound lysosomes, which means that they contain acid hydrolases in inactive form that are used to digest phagocytosed bacteria intracellularly. Myeloperoxidase, lysozyme (muramidase), proteases, and bactericidal cationic proteins are among the many constituents of primary granules. Myeloperoxidase, together with hydrogen peroxide and a halide, aids in killing phagocytosed bacteria. Even though primary granules are not visible in the mature neutrophil, their contents are still present, as evidenced by the positive peroxidase staining of the mature neutrophil.

Lysozyme is capable of degrading glycopeptides and hydrolyzing carbohydrates that are constituents of the cell wall of some bacteria. There is evidence of its presence in both primary and secondary granules.[2] Monocytes contain larger quantities of lysozyme than neutrophils. The level of this enzyme in plasma or urine may be assayed to assess granulocytic and monocytic cell turnover or to distinguish among types of leukemia or monitor the clinical activity of the disease. Markedly increased lysozyme levels indicate involvement of the monocytic cell line, whereas moderately increased to normal levels are found when the granulocyte cell line is affected.[29]

Secondary granules contain lysozyme, lactoferrin, specific collagenases, and vitamin B_{12}-binding proteins, but no peroxidase. Lactoferrin is an iron-binding glycoprotein that competes with bacteria for iron, possibly inhibiting growth. It also may promote neutrophil adherence to endothelial cells.[16]

Alkaline phosphatase was originally thought to be a component of secondary neutrophilic granules. More recent studies have determined its location to be in a third set of granules, "tertiary granules." These granules have been described as a separate entity slightly less dense than the secondary (or specific) granules. They first appear during the late myelocyte stage, which corresponds with the appearance of alkaline phosphatase in the cell.[24,30] Although its function *in vivo* is not known for certain, the amount of enzyme activity tends to increase when cellular metabolism increases.

Function

Phagocytosis

The overall purpose of the neutrophil is to protect against infection. This function is quite separate from, but interrelated with, the protective function of the other leukocytes. The main mechanism used by the neutrophil is phagocytosis, which is the process of locating, ingesting, and killing bacteria and other foreign invaders. For discussion purposes this process is divided into five steps: motility, recognition, ingestion, degranulation, and killing (see Fig. 23-3).

MOTILITY. During locomotion, neutrophils acquire a distinct asymmetric shape that has been described as resembling a hand mirror. The "glass" of the mirror is formed by pseudopods and is called a lamellopod. It moves in a wavelike motion, or "ruffles," as it moves forward. The "handle" is a narrow tail of cytoplasm that seems to drag behind. The pseudopods that are formed during locomotion are filled with filament networks, which are polymers of actin, a muscle protein. Another muscle protein, myosin, also is present, and it catalyzes hydrolysis of adenosine triphosphate (ATP) to provide energy for the contraction of the

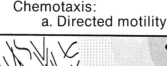

Chemotaxis:
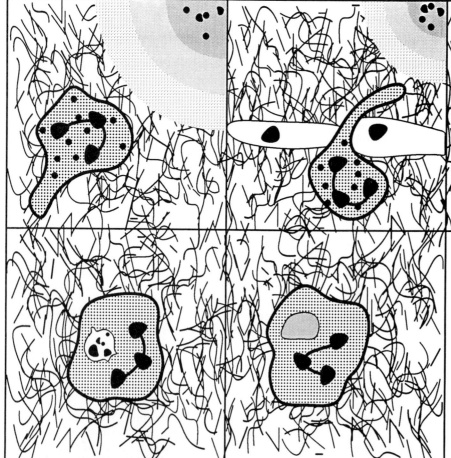

a. Directed motility   b. Diapedesis   c. Recognition and ingestion

d. Degranulation   e. Killing and digestion

FIG. 23-3. Phagocytosis is a function of neutrophils and monocytes. The act of phagocytosis includes directed motility, diapedesis, recognition and ingestion, degranulation, and killing and digestion.

actin fibers.[32] Neutrophils increase their glycolytic rate during locomotion and ingestion, in order to maintain a supply of ATP to sustain their motion and other activities.

The neutrophil normally moves in a zigzag motion referred to as *random* migration. In order to successfully attack invading microorganisms, the neutrophil is guided or drawn by a process called chemotaxis. In this process, chemical stimuli (chemotactic factors) are generated and released by interactions between tissues and microorganisms or other antigens. Chemotactic factors interact with the neutrophil through some type of reaction with membrane receptors, although little is known about the mechanism of action. Chemotactic factors form a gradient, and the neutrophil moves in the direction of the highest concentration of the chemical. Neutrophils tend to respond faster than monocytes to chemotactic stimuli. The end result is *directed* migration of the neutrophil toward the source of the stimulus.

One of the better known chemotactic factors is a low-molecular weight fragment, C5a, which is derived from the cleavage of proteins of the complement system. The C5a fragment is an anaphylatoxin that causes smooth muscle contraction and is also the most potent of the chemotactic factors.[32] Factors that are liberated from the bacteria themselves are also known to be chemotactic but are not well defined. One bacterial factor, endotoxin, is known to activate coagulation factor XII (Hageman factor), which initiates the coagulation and fibrinolytic systems. Fibrinopeptide B, plasminogen activator, and kallikrein are then generated from the activation of these systems and are known to be chemotactic factors. Other leukocytes, such as lymphocytes and monocytes, may liberate substances that are chemotactic for neutrophils. Other known chemotactic factors are metabolic products of arachidonic acid that are known to exist in inflammatory fluids and are produced by platelets.[31]

RECOGNITION.   Once the neutrophil has found its way to the site of invasion it must be able to recognize the offending organism or substance. Some bacteria resist recognition because of a capsule. Antibodies and complement substances that coat the organisms and aid the neutrophil in recognizing what to ingest are referred to as *opsonins,* from a Greek word meaning "to prepare for dining." Opsonins react with specific receptors on the neutrophil membrane, which in turn trigger the act of ingestion. Some bacteria can be recognized and ingested by neutrophils without any help, but other pathogens (*e.g., Streptococcus, Pneumococcus,* and *Meningococcus* organisms) are not ingested until they have been opsonized. The main opsonins are immunoglobulin G (IgG) antibodies and byproducts of the same complement-mediated reactions that produce chemotactic factors. Aided by IgM antibody a large fragment of the third component of complement, C3, binds to the surface of microorganisms and allows the neutrophil to recognize them. A glycoprotein found in plasma and the outer membrane of fibroblast and endothelial cells, called fibronectin, have also been shown to coat particles and enhance their ingestion by binding the particle to the phagocyte.[30,31]

INGESTION.   When a neutrophil comes into physical contact with a foreign particle, its lamellopod flows around the particle or microorganism and fuses together. This completely surrounds the particle in a phagosome. The neutrophil membrane also becomes sticky, to firmly adhere to the particle. If a neutrophil is moving randomly and happens to collide with an ingestible particle, it immediately forms a phagosome around the particle, even though no chemotactic factor is present.

DEGRANULATION.   Cytoplasmic granules within the neutrophil migrate to the phagosome and fuse with it. This fusion allows the contents of the granule to be released into the phagosome. Distintegration of the granule into the surrounding cytoplasm follows. This complex biochemical process requires increased energy from the neutrophil in the form of ATP, which is supplied by the metabolic burst described previously.

KILLING.   The neutrophil actively metabolizes oxygen to produce toxic substances for killing ingested foreign particles. The exact nature or location of the oxidizing agent is not known, but reduced pyridine nucleotide (NADPH) probably is the source of the reducing power. Two principal toxic metabolites produced are superoxide anion (O^-) and hydrogen peroxide (H_2O_2). Superoxide anion is the first reaction product of oxygen, and at acid pH is further reduced to hydrogen peroxide. As glycolysis increases during ingestion, lactic acid is generated, which effectively lowers the pH of the phagosome. The acid environment in the phagosome not only enhances the reduction of superoxide anion to hydrogen peroxide but is in itself bactericidal. Both superoxide and hydrogen peroxide permeate cell membranes and are highly toxic to bacteria (as well as to animal cells). The enzyme myeloperoxidase, which is found in the primary granules of the neutrophil, helps potentiate the killing action of hydrogen peroxide in the presence of ascorbic acid and halides. Lysozyme hydrolyzes the mucopeptide cell wall of a few species of bacteria.

Because the oxygen metabolites are toxic also to the host's cells, they are kept in check by several detoxification mechanisms. First, they are localized in the phagosomes and so, are sealed off from other parts of the cell. An enzyme, superoxide dismutase, rapidly converts any superoxide that escapes into the cell into hydrogen peroxide. Another enzyme, catalase, destroys hydrogen peroxide in the cytoplasm. Reduced glutathione and the hexose monophosphate shunt also act to detoxify hydrogen peroxide and to regenerate NADPH.

Disorders of Phagocytosis

A defect in any of the steps described above in the phagocytic process can result in a disease state. Patients with such defects suffer recurrent infections. An example of a defect in locomotion and ingestion is a disorder known as Chediak-Higashi syndrome. In this rare congenital disorder the inability of cells to respond to chemotactic gradients renders patients very susceptible to infections (Chap. 28).

Drugs such as corticosteroids, when taken in high doses and for protracted periods, can inhibit neutrophil migration, adhesiveness, and ability to ingest. Ethanol has also been shown to inhibit neutrophil locomotion and ingestion. Some systemic illnesses such as rheumatoid arthritis, uremia, multiple myeloma, systemic lupus erythematosus, and diabetes mellitus can impair neutrophil function, causing a decrease in chemotactic response or ingestion.[6]

Testing of Neutrophil Function

Measurement of the levels of serum immunoglobulins and complement will determine whether a functional disorder is related to production of opsonins and chemotactic factors that involve these two systems. Other tests of neutrophil function are usually performed *in vivo* and so, are difficult to standardize and reproduce, inconvenient, nonspecific, and usually done only in large medical facilities or research centers. These include the Boyden micropore filter technique to assay neutrophil migration in response to a chemotactic factor, and the Rebuck skin window procedure, which evaluates the speed, type, and number of phagocytes that respond to a skin abrasion.[31]

A third test that is performed to test neutrophil ability to kill certain organisms is the nitroblue tetrazolium (NBT) test (Chap. 30).

THE EOSINOPHIL

The eosinophil is classified as a phagocyte although its participation in phagocytosis is less pronounced than that of the neutrophil. It plays a major role in control of parasitic infections and in hypersensitivity reactions. Eosinophils are formed in the bone marrow and have recently been shown to have their own progenitor cell, which they may share with the basophil.[13] They undergo the same maturation stages as the neutrophil in the bone marrow and spend a short time in the blood in transit to the tissues where they perform their functions.

Morphology

The eosinophil can first be distinguished from the neutrophil at the promyelocyte stage. Eosinophilic promyelocytes, myelocytes, and metamyelocytes are difficult to distinguish because the size and numbers of granules tend to mask other morphologic features. Immature eosinophils have a few large blue granules, which are lost by attrition as the cell undergoes subsequent mitotic divisions. As the cell matures, specific granules form and take on a refractive, orange appearance. Because of the low percentage of these cells in the bone marrow and peripheral blood, they are not routinely differentiated into the several maturation stages; rather, they are merely divided into mature and immature forms. In pathologic conditions in which the percentage of eosinophils is greatly increased, it may be clinically relevant to identify the different stages (see Plate 8A and B). The mature eosinophil is described in Chapter 22.

Kinetics

The eosinophil goes through its maturation stages in the bone marrow, and cells are stored there several days before being released into the peripheral blood. The transit time is approximately 1 to 8 hours. They appear to survive longer in the tissues than neutrophils. Some studies have shown that eosinophils may reenter the circulation after being in the tissues, but most probably do not.[9] While in the tissues, they are found mostly in the skin or mucosal surfaces of the respiratory and gastrointestinal tracts. Of the body's total number of eosinophils, only approximately 1% are found in the blood. Death and elimination are similar to neutrophils.[1]

There is probably a humoral substance that regulates maturation of progenitor cells into eosinophils. Studies *in vitro* have shown a colony-stimulating factor (multi-CSF or interleukin 3) that possesses the ability to stimulate growth of a variety of colonies of cell types, including eosinophils.[28]

Biochemistry

The principal source of energy for eosinophils is glycolysis. They also experience a metabolic burst or increase in glycolysis prior to phagocytosis, just as is seen in neutrophils. All enzymes of the hexose monophosphate shunt are found in the eosinophil.

The outer, less dense matrix of eosinophil granules contains hydrolytic enzymes, one of which is peroxidase. The peroxidase in eosinophil granules is found in higher concentration and differs biochemically and antigenically from the peroxidase found in neutrophil granules. The inner core of the eosinophil granules contains basic protein rich in arginine and lysine, phospholipids, and possibly melanin. More than 50% of the protein is made up of major basic protein (MBP), an arginine-rich protein that may play a major role in the eosinophil's ability to damage parasitic invaders.[8]

When a large number of eosinophils disintegrate in secretions or exudates, Charcot-Leyden crystals may be seen. These hexagonal bipyramidal crystals have been found in nasal mucus of patients with allergic asthma, pleural fluid of patients with pulmonary eosinophilic infiltrates, and stool of patients with parasitic infections. Charcot-Leyden crystals were originally described as aggregates of the crystalloid core of eosinophil granules, but they have since been shown to be composed of lysophospholipase, which is localized in the plasma membrane of eosinophils.[20]

Function

Eosinophils function as phagocytes but appear to move more slowly and to have less intracellular killing ability than neutrophils. They respond to chemotactic factors such as bacterial products and complement components but appear to prefer factors secreted by mast cells and basophils (histamine) and antigen-antibody complexes. It has been proposed that eosinophils are drawn to the site of immediate hypersensitivity reactions by mast cell chemotactic factors and may contribute to the inactivation of mast cell products and local control of the reaction.[8]

Another important function of eosinophils is their ability to damage the larval stages of parasitic helminths. *Schistosoma mansoni* has been studied most extensively. Eosinophils attach to the parasite, which has been coated by antibodies, and extend long projections over the surface. They then degranulate and the contents of their granules break down the parasite. Degradation products of the parasite are then phagocytosed by a different population of eosinophils.

The entire process is antibody dependent and complement independent. Other leukocytes may assist in the phagocytosis part of the process.[19]

THE BASOPHIL

The basophil is the least common of the leukocytes and makes up 0.5% to 1.0% of total peripheral blood leukocytes and only 0.3% of nucleated blood cells in the marrow. Basophils are formed in the bone marrow, and their maturation stages parallel those of the neutrophil except that the nucleus does not always segment. Recent studies have shown evidence for a common circulating basophil-eosinophil progenitor cell[13] that is morphologically indistinguishable from the myeloblast.

Morphology

Because so few basophils are present in both peripheral blood and bone marrow, staging usually is not done, except to differentiate mature from immature basophils.

The mature basophil is described in Chapter 22. Basophil granules are water soluble and may disintegrate in the staining process, leaving a sparsely granulated cell.[18] The large size of the basophil granules helps in their differentiation from neutrophils with dark-staining (toxic) granules. The nucleus of the basophil is usually band shaped or bilobed with dense, irregular chromatin. In electron microscope studies basophil granules have been shown to have a substructure composed of dense particles embedded in a less dense matrix. A second population of smaller granules also is found, usually between the lobes of the nucleus. These are not observed with the light microscope.[14] Immature basophils have fewer granules, an immature-looking nucleus, and discernible basophilia in the cytoplasm (Plates 9A and B).

Relationship to Mast Cell

Mast cells are cells that resemble basophils and are normally distributed throughout the connective tissues, especially around blood and lymph vessels and peripheral nerves and rarely in the bone marrow. Mast cells are larger than basophils and usually have a small round nucleus and more abundant cytoplasm, which usually makes up about two thirds of the cell. Their granules stain darkly, like those of the basophil, but they are more numerous, more closely packed, and smaller. Usually the granules do not overlie or obscure the nucleus as they do in basophils (see Plate 17). Mast cells have a long life span and have been shown to proliferate in the tissues. Their cell of origin is unknown. In some—and perhaps all—species they develop from a hematopoietic progenitor cell.[17] Their relationship to basophils is still a matter of conjecture.

Kinetics

Basophils are thought to have a short life span, similar to that of the eosinophil. Exactly what happens to them after they enter the tissues is uncertain. The regulating mechanism for basophil production is unknown, but a T lymphocyte-produced basophilopoietin has been described in guinea pigs.[11] Recent studies have shown that mature basophils may be recruited from the circulation to sites of allergic reactions through lymphocyte-derived chemotactic signals. Increased numbers of basophil progenitor cells have been found in the circulation of atopic (i.e., allergic) persons. Basophil precursor cells may also be stimulated to differentiate into mature cells by a similar response. Basophil progenitor cells may arrive at allergen-stimulated tissue sites where they undergo differentiation. This process may also elicit further bone marrow release of basophil progenitors.[12]

Biochemistry and Function

The cytoplasmic granules of basophils and mast cells synthesize and store histamine and contain other mediators of the inflammatory response. Basophils are thought to be the repositories of virtually all of the histamine in normal human blood. Basophils have previously been reported to contain heparin, but some studies show they contain very little.[18] Basophil granules lack hydrolytic enzymes, although peroxidase activity is present. Aside from its granules, the cytoplasm of the basophil contains abundant deposits of glycogen, a small Golgi apparatus, a complex vesicular system, which is involved in degranulation, and only a few mitochondria, ribosomes, and strands of endoplasmic reticulum.[14]

Basophils have been reported to ingest sensitized erythrocytes and antigen-antibody complexes and to exert a sluggish motility. Their phagocytic capacity is substantially less than that of neutrophils or eosinophils. By far the more important function of basophils is their role in immediate hypersensitivity reactions. Basophils and mast cells have specific receptors for immunoglobulin E, which trigger degranulation when appropriate antigens are present. Clinical manifestations of this immediate hypersensitivity reaction may be some forms of bronchial asthma, urticaria, allergic rhinitis, and anaphylaxis to drugs, insect stings, and other antigens.[15]

Basophils also play a role in lymphocyte-mediated delayed hypersensitivity reactions. T lymphocytes stimulated by antigen or mitogen have been shown to generate substances that activate basophils to release histamine.[21] Basophils may account for 5% to 15% of infiltrating cells in allergic contact dermatitis and skin allograft rejection and an even smaller percentage of tuberculin and other classic delayed hypersensitivity reactions.[17]

THE MONOCYTE

The monocyte is sometimes classified with the lymphocyte because both are mononuclear cells and are morphologically similar. Functionally, however, monocytes more closely resemble the granulocyte, since phagocytosis is one of the monocyte's main functions. The monocyte also participates in cellular and humoral immunity in several other ways that will be discussed later in this chapter. The monocyte is often described as part of the mononuclear and phagocyte system, which includes macrophages found in tissues and body fluids. The term reticuloendothelial system was previously used to denote these same cells as well as various other tissue cells, but it is now considered inappropriate. The macrophage is the tissue cell counterpart of the blood monocyte. Both share phagocytosis as their major function, and kinetic studies indicate that the blood monocyte is the precursor of most, though perhaps not all, macrophages.[1]

Morphology

Promonocyte

The precursor cells of blood monocytes are monoblasts and promonocytes. Both precursor cells are very difficult to identify morphologically. Most morphologists agree that monoblasts are in the marrow but that they are probably indistinguishable from myeloblasts. Studies indicate that monocytes and neutrophils have a common precursor cell, but at which stage it becomes committed to form either cell line is not yet known.[26] Monoblasts have been identified in leukemic states, but these cells are products of a malignancy and do not necessarily resemble normal monoblasts. The earliest precursor cell to the monocyte that is recognizable by light microscopy is the promonocyte. Cytochemistry still may be required for positive identification. A promonocyte stained with a Romanowsky stain has the gray–blue cytoplasm characteristic of the mature monocyte and may have an indented or lobulated nucleus. The nuclear chromatin appears immature, with fine, evenly distributed chromatin. Nucleoli may or may not be visible. It is fairly large (12–18 μm) and has a high nuclear:cytoplasmic ratio (see Plate 15A and B).

Monocyte

Although the mature monocyte has a diameter similar to that of the neutrophil in a wet mount (12–15 μm), it often appears slightly larger than the other leukocytes on a peripheral blood film owing to its strong tendency to adhere and spread on glass surfaces. Monocytes are described in Chapter 22.

Differentiation of the Monocyte from Other Cells

Monocytes are most often confused with large lymphocytes, especially variant or atypical lymphocytes. The most reliable criterion to use to distinguish a monocyte is its nuclear chromatin pattern. It is loosely woven and linear. The lymphocyte has compact, clumpy nuclear chromatin. The monocyte nucleus also stains lighter than the lymphocyte nucleus, and the whole cell has a washed-out color rather than the deep purple nucleus and bright sky-blue cytoplasm of the lymphocyte. The nucleus of the monocyte may be round or lobulated, whereas lymphocyte nuclei usually are round or oval. Monocytes characteristically have much more abundant cytoplasm than lymphocytes and the nuclear:cytoplasmic ratio is lower. As many identification criteria as possible should be used, keeping in mind that the nuclear chromatin pattern is the most reliable.

Less frequently, monocytes may be confused with immature neutrophils, especially the band neutrophil if the monocyte has a band-shaped nucleus, which it frequently does. The best criterion in this case is still the nuclear chromatin pattern, although, with a good stain, the color of the cytoplasm should be very helpful. The band neutrophil cytoplasm should be pinkish with scattered distinct purple granules and the monocyte cytoplasm should be gray–blue with a ground-glass appearance. To differentiate monocytes from more immature neutrophils, which may have a bluish color to their cytoplasm and a round nucleus (such as the myelocyte), the nuclear chromatin pattern is the most reliable criterion. Immature granulocytes will have a more clumped chromatin pattern, which stains more darkly. Also, the immature granulocytes have more prominent cytoplasmic granules than monocytes do.

Kinetics

Life Span

Monocytes are formed in the bone marrow from the same progenitor cell that forms neutrophils. It is not known at which point in cellular maturation the cell becomes committed to be either a monocyte or a neutrophil. The first recognizable cell in the marrow is the promonocyte. The promonocyte is an actively dividing cell and undergoes at least three divisions as it matures to the monocyte, taking 30 to 48 hours. Monocytes lose their ability to divide and leave the marrow shortly after completing their last division, usually within 24 hours. There is no large marrow reserve pool for monocytes as there is for granulocytes—and probably no marginal pool once they reach the peripheral blood. Monocytes stay in the peripheral blood for about 70 hours and then move into the tissues, probably never to return to the blood. Previous studies suggesting a much shorter half-life in the blood and the existence of a substantial marginal monocyte pool have been disproved by more recent kinetic studies.[26,34] Once in the tissues, monocytes differentiate into macrophages and may remain in the tissue several months, possibly longer. Macrophage transformation in the peripheral blood usually denotes systemic infection (Chap. 26). Recent studies have shown other forms of tissue macrophages, such as osteoclasts, and dermal Langerhans cells, to have their origin in the bone marrow, suggesting development from blood monocytes.[23]

Regulatory Mechanism

Regulation of monocyte and neutrophil production is thought to be related to a group of hormones called colony-stimulating factor (CSF), which may act in a manner similar to erythropoietin on regulation of erythrocyte production. Although many tissues of the body produce CSF, cells of the monocyte-macrophage system are important sources, as are T lymphocytes, which are responding to mitogen or antigen.[27] Other substances released by macrophages, such as prostaglandins, are thought to inhibit monocyte production, thereby creating a balance. There is some evidence that under certain conditions some macrophages may be stimulated to proliferate in the tissues.[26]

Biochemistry

Energy Production

Monocytes depend on aerobic glycolysis for their energy and phagocytosis. They have only a small amount of stored glycogen, so they must depend on externally supplied substrates. Most macrophages depend on anaerobic glycolysis;

the exception is the alveolar macrophage, located in the lung, which relies heavily on aerobic glycolysis.

Granule Contents

Mature monocytes contain a variety of lysosomal enzymes, such as acid phosphatase, β-glucuronidase, lysozyme, lipase, peroxidase, and many others. Cytochemically, monocytes give a positive reaction for nonspecific esterases that are inhibited by sodium fluoride. These enzymes are helpful in the wide variety of monocyte functions. Monocytes are not as rich in peroxidase as the neutrophil, and the macrophage contains no peroxidase at all. Lysozyme is released continuously by monocytes and macrophages rather than during degranulation only, as in granulocytes. It functions mainly as a bacteriolytic enzyme, but it may have an enhancement effect on phagocytosis and a potential antineoplastic effect.

Receptors

Monocytes and macrophages have receptors for the Fc fraction of IgG and complement C3. Both have receptors for IgE.[26]

Function

Phagocytosis

The cells of the monocyte-macrophage system participate in phagocytosis in a manner similar, but not identical, to that described in the section on neutrophils. The neutrophil is generally thought to be the more efficient phagocyte, except when the particle to be engulfed is large in relation to the cell, in which case the monocyte is more efficient. Monocyte motility is slow compared to that of neutrophils. Studies using the Rebuck skin window show that neutrophils arrive at the scene of tissue damage first and monocytes tend to come along later to ingest cellular debris. Macrophages are influenced by a migration inhibition factor released by T lymphocytes which causes them to remain at the site of infection. Chemotactic factors that attract monocytes include antigen-antibody complexes, complement components, kallikrein, and factors released by activated T lymphocytes.

The killing potency of macrophages is greatly enhanced when the cells are "activated." Activation refers to the process of enhancing motility, metabolism, enzyme activity, and killing capacity. Activation may result from the cell coming in direct contact with microorganisms or their by-products, or from soluble substances, called lymphokines, released by sensitized T lymphocytes. Morphologically, activated macrophages are larger and have more granules; biochemically, metabolism of glucose increases by way of the hexose monophosphate shunt. Activated macrophages release greater amounts of enzymes, complement components, chemotactic factors for neutrophils, interferon, and pyrogen. They utilize the same oxygen metabolites (superoxide anion and hydrogen peroxide) as the neutrophil to kill foreign organisms. Microorganisms such as *Mycobacterium, Listeria, Salmonella, Brucella,* and certain fungi and protozoa that are known to parasitize macrophages and replicate within them may be inhibited or destroyed when the macrophages become activated. Macrophages have also been shown to eliminate viruses and virus-infected cells.[26]

Other Functions

In addition to phagocytosis, mononuclear phagocytes also play a role in cellular and humoral immunity in close association with T lymphocytes. Mononuclear cells phagocytize and process (degrade and chemically modify) antigens and present them to T lymphocytes. The T lymphocytes in turn respond by secreting lymphokines, which activate resting macrophages. After killing the microorganism, the activated macrophages liberate substances (prostaglandins) that suppress or turn off the T-cell reaction.

Macrophages release a soluble factor, interleukin 1 or lymphocyte activation factor, which stimulates T lymphocytes. This factor promotes replication of T lymphocytes that are responding to an antigen.[23] Mononuclear phagocytes also are known to secrete various substances that regulate the inflammatory response, numerous components of the complement system, and endogenous pyrogen that causes fever by its effect on the hypothalamus. They also produce interferon, which may participate in conferring protection against viral infections. Macrophages produce transcobalamin II, the primary transport factor for vitamin B_{12}. Monocytes and macrophages secrete substances such as plasminogen activator, plasmin inhibitor, platelet activation factor, and a tissue thromboplastin-like procoagulant, and thereby participate in the coagulation cascade and in fibrinolysis. The monocyte–macrophage system also secretes CSF, which promotes the proliferation of myeloid stem cells into the neutrophil and monocyte cell lines.

These cells phagocytize and remove old and degenerating cells, cellular debris, and particulate material such as activated clotting factors, denatured proteins, and antigen-antibody complexes. They secrete substances that stimulate the growth of fibroblasts and act in tissue repair at the site of inflammation. They utilize their Fc receptors to bind IgG-coated erythrocytes and phagocytize them as they traverse the spleen. They also play a role in hemoglobin degradation and iron transport by liberating iron from heme, storing the iron, and later transferring iron to transferrin for incorporation into developing erythrocytes. This latter process may be observed in the bone marrow as immature, developing erythrocytes surround a large macrophage. It is sometimes called the "nursing" or "suckling" phenomenon.

Finally, activated macrophages have been reported to kill several types of tumor cells in culture and in numerous animal studies. They may also perform a similar function *in vivo* but further studies are needed.

CHAPTER SUMMARY

The phagocytic leukocytes are significant as the body's main line of defense. By recognizing them morphologically on a stained blood film, their presence and concentration in the peripheral blood may be evaluated. It must be recognized, though, that this is a very incomplete picture because of the short time they spend in the vascular space. Recognizing the immature forms of these cells provides indicators of disease and marrow stress. The limitations of light microscopy when trying to identify immature cells must not be overlooked.

A discussion of the process of phagocytosis and its relationship to other functions of these cells has been presented. The interrelationship of all the cells and their functions is necessary for them to operate with maximum efficiency to keep the body free of foreign invaders.

REFERENCES

1. Ackerman SK, Douglas SD: Morphology of monocytes and macrophages. In Williams WJ, Beutler E, Erslev AJ et al (eds): Hematology, 3rd ed. New York, McGraw-Hill, 1983

2. Baggiolini M: The neutrophil. In Weismann G (ed): The Cell Biology of Inflammation. New York, Elsevier, 1980

3. Beck WS: Leukocytes I. Physiology. In Beck WS (ed): Hematology, 4th ed. Cambridge, MA, MIT Press, 1985

4. Bennett JM, Catovsky D, Daniel MT et al: Proposals for the classification of the myelodysplastic syndromes. Br J Haematol 51:189, 1982

5. Boggs DR, Winkelstein A: White Cell Manual, 4th ed. Philadelphia, FA Davis, 1983

6. Brayton RG, Stokes PE, Schwartz MS et al: Effect of alcohol and various diseases on leukocyte mobilization, phagocytosis and intracellular bacterial killing. N Engl J Med 282:123, 1970

7. Broxmeyer H, Van Zant G, Zucali JR et al: Mechanisms of leukocyte production and release XII. A comparative assay of the leukocytosis-inducing factor (LIF) and the colony-stimulating factor (CSF). Proc Soc Exp Biol 145:1262, 1974

8. Butterworth AE, David JR: Eosinophil function. N Engl J Med 304:154, 1981

9. Clark RAF, Kaplan AP: Eosinophil leukocytes: Structure and function. Clin Haematol 4:635, 1975

10. College of American Pathologists: Identification of Blood and Bone Marrow Cells, Quality Evaluation Program. Skokie, IL, CAP, 1972

11. Denburg JA, Davison M, Bienenstock J: Basophil production. J Clin Invest 65:390, 1980

12. Denburg JA, Telizyn S, Belda A et al: Increased numbers of circulating basophil progenitors in atopic patients. J Allerg Clin Immunol 76:466, 1985

13. Denburg JA, Telizyn S, Messner H et al: Heterogeneity of human peripheral blood eosinophil-type colonies: Evidence for a common basophil-eosinophil progenitor. Blood 66:312, 1985

14. Dvorak AM: Biology and morphology of basophilic leukocytes. In Bach MK (ed): Immediate Hypersensitivity: Modern Concepts and Developments. New York, Marcel Dekker, 1978

15. Dvorak AM, Dvorak HF: The basophil—Its morphology, biochemistry, motility, release reactions, recovery, and role in the inflammatory response of IgE mediated and cell-mediated origin. Arch Pathol Lab Med 103:551, 1979

16. Falloon J, Gallin JI: Neutrophil granules in health and disease. J Allerg Clin Immunol 77:653, 1986

17. Galli SJ, Dvorak AM, Dvorak HF: Morphology, biochemistry and function of basophils and mast cells. In Williams WJ, Beutler E, Erslev AJ et al (eds): Hematology, 4th ed. New York, McGraw-Hill, 1990

18. Galli SJ, Dvorak HF: Basophils and mast cells. Structure, function and role in hypersensitivity. In Gupta S, Good RA (eds): Cellular, Molecular, and Clinical Aspects of Allergic Disorders. New York, Plenum, 1979

19. Glauert AM, Butterworth AE, Sturrock RF et al: The mechanism of antibody-dependent, eosinophil-mediated damage to schistosomula of Schistosoma mansoni in vitro: A study by phase-contrast and electron microscopy. J Cell Sci 34:187, 1978

20. Gleich GJ, Loegering BS, Adolphson CR: Eosinophils and bronchial inflammation. Chest 87(Suppl):10S, 1985

21. Goetzl EJ, Foster DW, Payan DG: A basophil-activating factor from human T lymphocytes. Immunology 53:227, 1984

22. Golde DW: Production, distribution, and fate of neutrophils. In Williams WJ, Beutler E, Erslev AJ et al (eds): Hematology, 4th ed. New York, McGraw-Hill, 1990

23. Golde DW, Groopman JE: Production, distribution, and fate of monocytes and macrophages. In Williams WJ, Beutler E, Erslev AJ et al (eds): Hematology, 4th ed. New York, McGraw-Hill, 1990

24. Hayhoe FGJ, Quaglino D: Haematological Cytochemistry. New York, Churchill Livingstone, 1980

25. Koepke JA, Dotson MA, Shifman MA: A critical evaluation of the manual/visual differential counting method. Blood Cells 11:173, 1986

26. Lasser A: The mononuclear phagocyte system: A review. Hum Pathol 14:108, 1983

27. Schleimer RP, Fox CC, Naclerio RM et al: Role of human basophils and mast cells in the pathogenesis of allergic diseases. J Allerg Clin Immunol 76:369, 1985

28. Shadduck RK, Waheed A: The role of colony stimulating factor in the regulation of granulopoiesis. Blood Cells 10:163, 1984

29. Silber R, Moldow CF: Metabolism of neutrophils. In Williams WJ, Beutler E, Erslev AJ et al (eds): Hematology, 3rd ed. New York, McGraw-Hill, 1983

30. Smith GP, Peters TJ: Purification and properties of alkaline phosphatase from human polymorphonuclear leukocytes. Int J Biochem 17:209, 1985

31. Stossel TP: Leukocytes II. Phagocytosis and its disorders. In Beck WS (ed): Hematology, 4th ed. Cambridge, MA, MIT Press, 1985

32. Stossel TP, Boxer LA: Functions of neutrophils. In Williams WJ, Beutler E, Erslev AJ et al (eds): Hematology, 3rd ed. New York, McGraw-Hill, 1983

33. Van Assendelft OW: Reference values for the total differential leukocyte count. Blood Cells 11:79, 1985

34. Van Furth R, Raeburn JA, VanZweet TL: Characteristics of human mononuclear phagocytes, Blood 54:498, 1979

35. Wintrobe MM, Lee GR, Boggs DR et al: Clinical Hematology, 8th ed. Philadelphia, Lea & Febiger, 1981

36. Zucker-Franklin D: Eosinophils: Morphology, biochemistry, and function. In Williams WJ, Beutler E, Erslev AJ et al (eds): Hematology, 4th ed. New York, McGraw-Hill, 1990

24

Immune Leukocytes—

Maturation,

Kinetics,

and Function

F. Sue Allison

Lymphocytes play a major role in maintenance of health and in response to and recovery from disease. Variations in quality or quantity of lymphocytes provide diagnostic data and are indicators of the response to therapy. Accurate evaluation of lymphocytes depends on knowledge about their formation, migration, differentiation, and function. The surface markers and biochemical markers that are gained or lost and alterations in morphology that are demonstrated as these events occur assist in the laboratory evaluation of lymphocytes.

Microenvironment is as critical as genetic makeup to the development and function of lymphoid cells. The microenvironment of a cell includes its interaction with neighboring cells such as fibroblasts, dendritic cells, and endothelial cells.[14]

Three physiologic characteristics of lymphocytes that help distinguish them from other normal blood cells have been outlined by Müeller-Hermelink and are discussed below.[58]

Lymphocytes Are Not Obligate End Cells

An obligate end cell is a mature cell that is committed to perform a function and die. Granulopoiesis produces end cells (neutrophils) that vanish in the fulfillment of their function. Lymphopoiesis is different in that primary lymphoid organs provide a continuous supply of incompletely differentiated cells to peripheral lymphoid tissue. Subsequent to antigenic stimulation, lymphocytes either transform into effector (end) cells that perish in fulfilling their function or undergo blastic transformation to produce new lymphocytes to react with appropriate antigens.

Lymphocytes Are a Heterogeneous Group of Cells

Some lymphocyte precursors migrate to the thymus, where they become T cells, which are immunocompetent in cellular immunity. Other precursors develop into B cells, which will fulfill the function of humoral immunity (antibody production). Another group of lymphocytes is known as natural killer (NK) cells, which are capable of lysing a variety of target cells. The fraction of lymphoid cells that do not develop along either the T- or B-cell pathway is referred to as non-T, non-B cells. Differences in maturation, surface and biochemical markers, and responses to mitogenic stimulation exemplify the heterogeneity of these cells even though they may appear identical on examination with routine stains and light microscopy.

Lymphocytes Are Predestined to Migrate

Lymphocytes generally spend several hours to days in tissue and then migrate into the peripheral blood through efferent lymphatics and back to the lymphatic tissue by way of venules. Although other blood cells also migrate, they tend to go in one direction only (*i.e.*, they do not return to the blood). Both T and B cells are normal inhabitants of marrow and both freely migrate to and from body tissues.[76] The traffic of lymphocytes can be divided into two physiologic processes: the *migration* of dividing cells from marrow to thymus and to peripheral tissue that requires a long period of time; and the *recirculation* of small nondividing lymphocytes from blood into lymphoid tissue and back to blood, measured in hours.

LYMPHOPOIESIS

Sites of Formation

The lymphoid tissue consists of marrow, thymus, lymph nodes, spleen, tonsils, Peyer's patches, and numerous foci of subendothelial and subepithelial lymphocytes, monocytes and macrophages. These organs have been functionally divided into primary lymphoid organs (PLO) that supply the secondary lymphoid tissue (SLT) with partially differentiated lymphocytes. Lymphopoiesis in PLO is continuous and is not regulated by antigen. Secondary lymphoid tissue produces lymphocytes in response to antigen. Primary lymphoid production develops before the SLT during embryogenesis and occurs in the fetal liver followed by thymus and marrow.

Immunocompetent cells develop along defined pathways of lymphoid differentiation, which are determined, at least in part, by the microenvironment encountered by progenitor cells. The marrow supplies the thymus with prethymocytes or prothymocytes (pre-T cells) that require the thymic microenvironment to differentiate into T cells. The marrow also appears to be responsible in part for B-cell differentiation. While the origin of NK cells is controversial, there is evidence that NK cells are marrow dependent.[29,46,98] The developmental sites of non-T, non-B cells are unknown.

Bone Marrow Lymphopoiesis

The hierarchy of lymphoid cell development begins with the totipotent hematopoietic stem cells and has been the subject of several reviews.[9,27,66] Stem cells dwell primarily in the marrow and are capable of self-replication. Their progeny lose some totipotentiality with each cell division until they become committed to differentiate into a specific cell type. The *hematogone* has been described as an early precursor in the hierarchy of stem cell development.[92] Other authors have supported this view.[57,76,81,91] Hematogones are mononuclear cells that range in size from 10 to 20 μm and contain a large nucleus with strikingly homogeneous nuclear chromatin and no visible nucleoli.[51,57] The nucleus may be cleft. When cytoplasm is visible, it is medium to deep blue, extremely scant, and devoid of granules, inclusions, and vacuoles (see Plate 18).

The committed lymphopoietic stem cell or colony-forming unit–lymphocyte (CFU-L) produces functionally diverse cells (Fig. 24-1). Lymphopoiesis is monitored with antigenic markers and receptors on the cell surface and by cytochemical studies. The CFU-L is characterized by the presence of HLA-DR (Ia antigen in mice) and terminal deoxynucleotidyl transferase (TdT).[36]

Differentiation along the B-cell pathway may proceed in the marrow; however, the precursor cell usually migrates to a peripheral organ, frequently the spleen, where it acquires markers of a B cell.[78] The earliest recognizable B cell in humans (the pre-B cell) is a large, rapidly dividing cell with a convoluted nucleus, followed by a small pre-B cell that appears a few days later and divides slowly.[12] Large and small pre-B cells are present in the marrow throughout life. Small pre-B cells may be identified in blood from newborn infants, as well as in patients with aplastic anemia after marrow transplantation, and in lymph nodes after local antigenic stimulation (see Plate 19).

Pre-B cells retain the Ia-like antigen and a few test positive for TdT.[12] Stages of pre-B cell differentiation have been identified, but they are beyond the scope of this chapter except to indicate that an antigen known as the common acute lymphocytic leukemia antigen (CALLA) can be detected on normal pre-B cells and that intracytoplasmic heavy chains appear without accompanying light chains.

Immature (early) B cells, the next stage of differentiation, are characterized by the absence of the CALLA antigen and TdT, the first appearance of surface membrane immunoglobulin (sIg), intracytoplasmic heavy chains of IgM type, and the presence of B cell-specific antigens B4[61] and S-HCL2.[43]

Mature B cells are those that demonstrate sIg.[27,94] Shortly after the appearance of sIg molecules, light chains are synthesized, joined with heavy chains, and inserted into the plasma membrane. Light chain synthesis begins with an individual cell synthesizing either lambda (λ) or kappa (κ) chains, but not both. Receptors for the following are usually demonstrable on mature B cells: the Fc portion of IgG, IgM, IgA, and IgE isotypes, mouse erythrocytes (approximately 7% to 8% of peripheral blood lymphocytes), complement (C3b, C3d, C4b, C1q, C8, and C2 inhibitor), and Epstein-Barr virus (EBV).

Natural killer cells represent a morphologically homogeneous population of large granular lymphocytes (LGL), the majority of which are characterized by the presence of CD2, CD11b, CD16, and CD56 antigens and are nonadherent and nonphagocytic.[75,87] (CD stands for cluster designation. These were established by an international panel that clustered similar monoclonal antibodies into groups.) The most aggressive interleukin 2 (IL-2)-

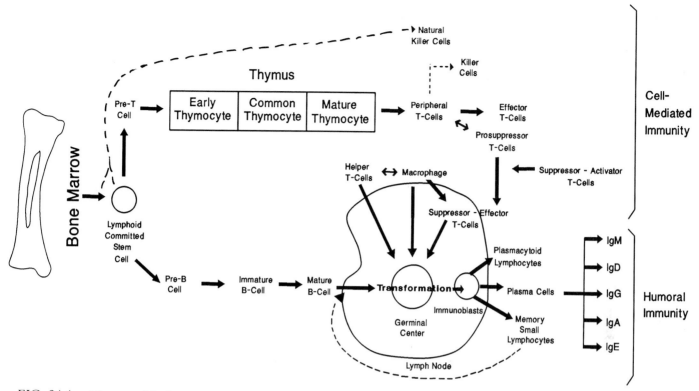

FIG. 24-1.   Diagram of the immune system. (Modified from Callihan TR, Holbert JM Jr, Berard CW: Neoplasms of terminal B-cell differentiation: The morphologic basis of functional diversity. In Sommers SC, Rosen PP (eds): Malignant Lymphomas, a Pathology Annual Monograph, p 172. Norwalk, CT, Appleton-Century-Crofts, 1983.)

dependent killer cells express NK cell-associated antigens CD16 and CD56 and lack markers characteristic of T cells.[49] An intact marrow microenvironment appears to be essential for differentiation into mature lytic NK cells.[28]

Marrow Lymphocyte Subpopulations

The distribution of lymphocyte subsets in normal marrow is summarized in Table 24-1.[10] In the aspirate, 7% of the cells were reported to be CALLA positive, indicating that many B cells were immature. Contamination by peripheral blood was assumed to account for the discrepancy between biopsy and aspirate data for T cells.

Thymus Lymphopoiesis

The prethymocyte (pre-T cell) originates from the CFU-L in marrow and migrates to the thymus to develop in the presence of thymic epithelial cells, macrophages, and thy-

TABLE 24–1. Distribution of Lymphocyte Subsets in Normal Marrow

CELL	SPECIMEN	
	BIOPSY (%)	ASPIRATE (%)
B	12	8
T	22–23	46–49
Non-T, non-B	55	30

(From Clark P, Normansell DE, Innes DJ, et al: Lymphocyte subsets in normal bone marrow. Blood 67:1600, 1986.)

mic factors.[73,94] There is evidence that the thymus, rather than genetic determinants, is responsible for differentiation of T cells.[55,79] Thymosin, a thymic hormone, appears to play a crucial role in the maturation of pre-T cells to T cells.

The thymus lies below the sternum and has a framework composed of epithelial cells. After infancy it slowly atrophies, essentially disappearing by adulthood. Internally, it is composed of a spongy network of endothelial cells organized into medulla (central region) and cortex (peripheral region) enclosed within a capsule (Fig. 24-2). The cortical region is distinguished by the presence of large lymphocytes that are dividing rapidly in the absence of antigen. Many of the cells remain in the thymus and die; others migrate to populate SLT; others undergo changes in surface antigens and become immunocompetent subpopulations of T lymphocytes as they migrate to the medulla. The majority of the latter group then migrate to SLT.

In humans pre-T cells are present in the thymus at about 8 weeks' gestation. These cells demonstrate TdT,[5] and possibly CALLA and Ia antigen.[19] They do not form rosettes with sheep erythrocytes (E) or demonstrate sIg.

Three discrete stages of intrathymic differentiation in humans have been outlined as early, common, and mature thymocytes, based on their reactivity with monoclonal antibodies (MAbs) (Table 24-2).[70] Less than 10% of thymocytes are classified as early and approximately 70% as common. Thymocytes lose surface marker characteristics of one stage and acquire others characteristic of another stage.[46,70,71] Mature peripheral blood T lymphocytes (stage IV), characterized by the loss of OKT10 reactivity, represent the final stage of maturation. The definitive marker for

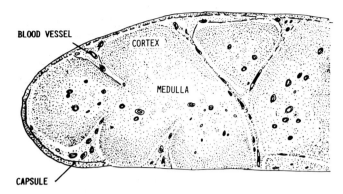

FIG. 24-2.   Diagram of thymus showing lobules composed of medullary and cortical tissue. (Modified from Burnet M: The thymus gland. Sci Am 207:53, 1962.)

T cells is the T cell antigen receptor (TCR). It is composed of two types, TCR-1 and TCR-2; the latter can be characterized into two separate populations, T-helper (CD4), and T-suppressor (CD8) cells.

Secondary Lymphoid Tissue Lymphopoiesis

The principal areas of dynamic lymphopoiesis in the spleen, lymph nodes, and Peyer's patches are the germinal centers in lymphoid follicles. Increased numbers of newly formed small lymphocytes are released by the spleen into the blood late in the course of an antibody response mediated by the spleen. This emphasizes that a portion of the recirculating pool is normally produced in the SLT as the result of continuous antigenic stimulation. B and T cells home to clearly defined areas, a process called *ecotaxis*.

Spleen

The spleen is composed of red pulp (primarily erythrocytes), white pulp (primarily leukocytes), and a marginal zone (Fig. 24-3). Major components of each include vessels, reticular cells, and free cells within a reticular meshwork.

T cells move from the marginal zone of the white pulp to the periarteriolar lymphoid sheaths (PALS) of the white pulp (T-dependent area). T cells then begin migrating from the spleen and are gone in 5 or 6 hours. B cells move from the marginal zone to the PALS to mix with T cells, then move to the upper part of the germinal centers of the white

pulp and return to the venous sinuses of the red pulp. This process requires approximately 24 hours.[21] These differences in migration patterns and times explain the predominance of B cells in the spleen.

Lymph Nodes

Lymph nodes have a capsule with a continuous endothelial lining. Afferent lymphatic vessels penetrate the capsule and transport lymph into the node to be filtered. The lymph exits through efferent lymphatics into the thoracic duct, which drains into the venous circulation. Within the capsule, lymph nodes are divided architecturally into the cortex and medulla (Fig. 24-4). The cortex contains primary and secondary follicles that are surrounded by a layer of lymphocytes referred to as the mantle zone. The medulla contains cordlike aggregates of lymphocytes as well as many plasma cells.

Two routes of lymphocyte entry into the lymph node are possible: (1) through afferent lymphatics and (2) from blood through the endothelial lining of postcapillary venules. The T cell journeys to the paracortex between the germinal centers and the medullary cords (see Fig. 24-4). These areas consist of dense accumulations of T cells scattered among interdigitating reticulum cells and epithelioid venules and are referred to as thymus-dependent zones. Interdigitating reticulum cells containing large amounts of Ia antigen are found only in T-dependent areas.[69] B cells congregate in the germinal centers,[21] move to the medulla, and exit the efferent lymphatics. Thus, germinal centers in the cortex of the lymph node and medullary cords in the deep portion of the lymph node constitute B cell-dependent zones.

Lymphoid follicles are organized to accomplish their primary function of antigen-induced, T cell-dependent, B cell proliferation and differentiation into plasma cells and memory cells. Germinal centers appear to be the site of the transformation of the B cell from a small to a large lymphocyte. Four morphologic types of cells exist in germinal centers: cells with cleaved nuclei, cells with round nuclei and prominent basophilic cytoplasm, macrophages, and dendritic reticulum cells. The transformed lymphocyte leaves the germinal center as an immunoblast and moves toward the medullary cords and continues its transformation into a plasma cell. Germinal centers contain predominantly B lymphocytes in transformation, while the medullary cords contain primarily immunoblasts, plasma-

TABLE 24–2. Stages of Intrathymic Differentiation

EARLY THYMOCYTE (STAGE I)	COMMON THYMOCYTE (STAGE II)	MATURE THYMOCYTE (STAGE III)	
		SUBSET 1	SUBSET 2
OKT9	CD1	CD2	CD2
OKT10	CD2	CD3	CD3
OKT11 (CD 2)	CD3 (OKT3, Leu 4)	CD4	CD5
TdT	CD4 (OKT4, Leu 3)	CD5 (OKT1, Leu 1)	CD8
OKT6, Leu 6 (CD 1)	CD7 (Leu 9)	CD7	OKT10
	OKT10	OKT10	

Key: OKT, Antibodies produced by Ortho Diagnostic Systems; Leu, antibodies produced by Becton Dickinson Monoclonal Center; CD, Cluster designation.
(Modified from Reinherz, Kung, Goldstein et al 1980, vol 77[70]; and Lanier, Allison, Phillips, 1986, vol 137.[45])

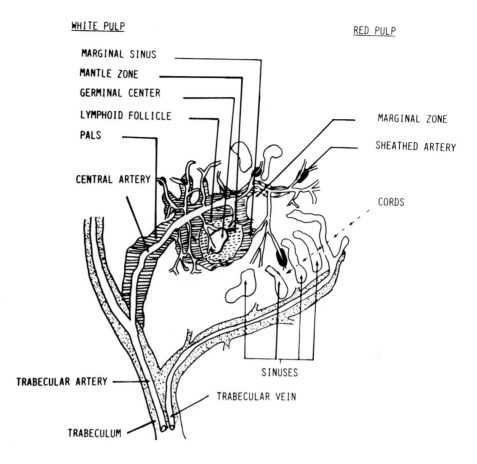

FIG. 24-3.   Diagram of spleen structure. White pulp contains periarteriolar lymphoid sheaths (PALS) and germinal centers with T cells concentrated close to the central arteriole and B cells in the follicle. Red pulp, separated from white pulp by the marginal zone, contains splenic cords and marginal sinuses. (Modified from Wintrobe MM, Lee GR, Boggs DR et al. Clinical hematology, p 260. Philadelphia, Lea & Febiger, 1981.)

cytoid lymphocytes, and plasma cells. Dense collars of predominantly B lymphocytes surround the germinal centers to compose the mantle zones.

The anatomy of lymph nodes is organized in such a way that lymph, loaded with antigen, enters a subcapsular sinus, where it comes in contact with many lymphocytes and macrophages. The subcapsular sinus communicates with cortical and subcortical sinuses that communicate with the medullary sinuses that empty into the efferent lymphatics.

The endothelium that lines these sinuses is discontinuous and enables efficient exchange of lymphocytes, macrophages, and antigen between lymphoid parenchyma and sinuses.

Lymphatic Aggregates

Dense accumulations of lymphocytes are found without a capsule in loose connective tissue throughout the gastrointestinal, respiratory, and urogenital tracts. Since much of

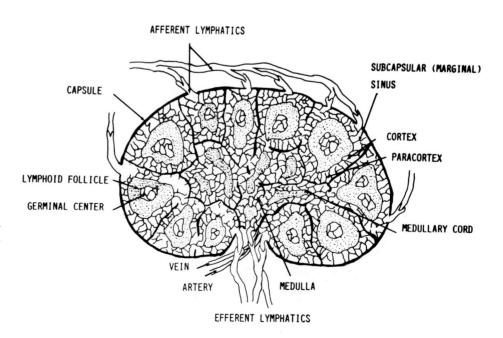

FIG. 24-4.   Diagram of the framework of a lymph node. T cells predominate in the paracortex, B cells in the germinal centers. (Modified from Wintrobe MM, Lee GR, Boggs DR et al. Clinical hematology, p 277. Philadelphia, Lea & Febiger, 1981.)

this lymphoid tissue is associated with mucosal surfaces, it is referred to as mucosa-associated lymphoid tissue (MALT).

LYMPHOKINETICS

Lymphokinetics is the process of lymphocyte multiplication, maturation, storage, and migration to tissues, including sites of infection or cell damage.

Mitosis and Multiplication

Radioisotopic labeling of lymphocytes provides information about cell division, kinetics, and life span of these cells.[12,94] The rate at which radioisotope-labeled cells appear in various tissues is used to measure their renewal and recirculation. The marrow has the fastest turnover of lymphocytes, the thymus, the next fastest turnover.

In humans, the rapidly dividing pre-B cell requires 30 to 36 hours to express B cell-specific antigens, Fc and C3 receptors, as well as sIg.[12,66] Pre-B cells represent approximately 0.6% of all nucleated cells in the marrow and approximately 6% of lymphoid cells.[12] In the peripheral blood, these are circulating lymphocytes that lack T- or B-cell surface markers.

Thymic lymphocytes appear at 8 weeks' gestation.[94] Precursor marrow cells (prothymocytes) migrate from the marrow to the thymus gland, where the microenvironment of thymic epithelial tissue and thymosin induce differentiation into T cells.

Life Span

Ottesen[64] reported two groups of lymphocytes with different life spans. One population (11%–22%), has a mean life span of 3 to 4 days; the other group (78%–89%) has a life span measured in months or even years. The short-lived B cell is the predominant cell in marrow.[76] The large volume of proliferative activity in marrow and thymus results in a high rate of lymphocyte death;[66] many short-lived cells never encounter an antigen.

Long-lived lymphocytes tend to predominate in peripheral tissues. The average life span of lymphocytes in the peripheral blood has been estimated at 4 years (±2.4 years); however, some may live up to 20 years.[8] Most small lymphocytes have been shown to be long lived and slowly replaced.

Migration of Lymphocytes

The process of migration involves the lymphocyte adhering to, traversing, and then detaching from endothelium.[67] Receptors on the surface of the different lymphocyte subpopulations appear to recognize determinants expressed by endothelial cells.[93] Once in the tissues, lymphocytes move among other cells, whether in lymph nodes, skin, spleen, lung, or intestinal mucosa. The time spent in blood or lymph is minimal compared to time spent moving through tissues. The small T cell takes 18 hours to recirculate and spends less than 1 hour in blood or lymph. Within the lymphoid tissue, rates and courses of movement differ according to cell type. For example, the following transit times have been obtained for lymphocytes migrating through the spleen: T cells, 5 to 6 hours; B cells, more than 24 hours; mesenteric and thoracic duct lymphoblasts, 4 to 5 hours; peripheral lymphoblasts, 8 to 10 hours.[67]

Migrating lymphocytes reenter the blood stream through the thoracic duct, migrate through endothelial cells of postcapillary venules, enter the lymph nodes through multiple afferent lymphatics, and leave by the efferent lymphatics.

When unimpeded the lymphocyte generally moves in a characteristic manner. The nucleus is displaced forward by an elongated "tail" (uropod) of cytoplasm. The uropod is the most adherent part of the cell, frequently becoming fastened to underlying support. Constraints by the physical environment may alter this typical hand-mirror appearance. Small lymphocytes in blood or nonstimulated lymphoid tissue are not very motile, whereas lymphoblasts are highly motile. Extrinsic agents influence lymphocyte locomotion.[67]

FUNCTION

The major function of the immune system is antigen recognition and the generation of an appropriate immune response. The interaction of T and B cells with each other and with other cell systems, such as endothelial and monocyte-macrophage systems, and factors such as type and amount of antigen, anatomic site of antigen entry, and complement, play crucial roles in the outcome of the immune response.

T cells perform regulatory and effector functions. Effector T cells are responsible for cell-mediated immunity, including defense against intracellular bacterial or fungal infections, cytolysis of virus-infected cells, allograph rejection, graft-versus-host reaction, and certain types of tumor immunity. Regulatory T cells induce or suppress proliferation and differentiation of effector T and B cells to moderate their functions.

B cells differentiate into plasma cells that secrete glycoprotein immunoglobulins (Igs) in response to stimulation by foreign antigens. This provides one mechanism of defense against pyogenic bacteria and some viruses.

NK cells appear to participate in many different immunologic functions. A major function is to recognize and lyse certain tumor cells and virus-infected cells without major histocompatibility (MHC) restriction. Previous sensitization or activation is not required for NK cell activity; however, this activity can be modulated by certain cytokines, including interferon (IFN-γ) and IL-2.[33] When exposed to IL-2, proliferation of NK cells occurs without requiring an antigen receptor.[90]

B Cells

The B cell system produces a variety of Igs that react with an infinite number of antigenic determinants. Synthesis of Igs by plasma cells is essential to the removal and degradation of many foreign substances. The binding of antigen by antibody begins a succession of events, including adherence of immune complex to receptors on leukocytes, complement activation, and neutralization of toxins and viruses.

The physical state of the antigen determines the type of cell interaction that is necessary to activate the resting B cell. For example, soluble antigens require modification by macrophages in addition to factors produced by T cells. Particulate antigens, such as bacteria, cells, and viruses, may be presented directly to lymphocytes or may require partial degradation by macrophages before presentation.

Lymphokines are biologically active substances produced by both B and T lymphocytes and macrophages. In certain situations, lymphokines may substitute for antigen. Several lymphokines produced by activated T cells directly regulate growth and maturation of B cells. These include B cell growth factors I and II, B-cell differentiation factor, IL-2, IFN-γ, and B-cell stimulatory factor-2.[6,30,40,48,52,56,63,64,68,80,83,96,99]

Resting B cells can be activated into the G_1 phase of the cell cycle by antigen or sIg cross-binding agents.[34,59] Once activated they are sensitive to lymphokines and progress to the S phase (DNA synthesis), although the steps involved are not clearly defined. In addition to T cell–derived growth factors for B cells, recent evidence indicates that normal stimulated B cells generate and respond to endogenous B-cell growth factor.[37,59]

Mitogens commonly used to evaluate lymphocyte function include pokeweed mitogen (PWM), lipopolysaccharide (LPS), *Staphylococcus aureus* Cowan I (SAC), and Epstein-Barr virus (EBV). Most B cells have receptors for EBV, the only known mitogen for man that is independent of accessory cells for its action and is the earliest B cell-specific surface marker identified so far for activated B cells infected with the virus.[86]

Various components of complement and prostaglandin E_2 (PGE$_2$) have been implicated in immunomodulatory roles. For example, C3 has been suggested as triggering the early stage of activation in the B cell and in generating memory B cells.[41] PGE$_2$ appears to play an important regulatory role in the magnitude of the B cell response *in vivo*.[85] The end result of B-cell activation is production of memory cells and plasma cells.

T Cells

The T-cell system consists of subsets with well defined effector functions (Table 24-3):

1. Helper T cells (T_H) induce other T cells and help B cells in the production of antibody.
2. Suppressor T cells (T_S) repress B- and T-cell responses.
3. Delayed hypersensitivity T lymphocytes (DHTL) respond to particulate and soluble antigens by producing chemotactic lymphokines (*e.g.*, macrophage chemotactic factors [MCF] and macrophage inhibitory factors [MIF]).

TABLE 24–3. T Cell Functional Characteristics

Helper T cells (T_H)
Suppressor T cells (T_S)
Delayed hypersensitivity T lymphocytes (DHTL)
Cytotoxic T lymphocytes (CTL)
Lymphokine production

---

4. Cytotoxic (or killer) T lymphocytes (CTL) destroy antigen-specific target cells on contact.

Helper and Suppressor T Cells

In response to antigen or mitogen stimulation the T-cell system orchestrates a complex and varied set of functions. Responses triggered by mitogens are like those that occur during activation by specific antigen. Phytohemagglutinin (PHA), concanavalin-A (con-A) and PWM are the best defined mitogens and have been used extensively to study T cells. While T_H cells are most responsive to PHA, T_S cells respond best to con-A; approximately equal numbers of B and T cells respond to PWM.[82]

T cells recognize antigen primarily when it is associated with membrane-bound products of the MHC complex. Allosensitized T_H cells recognize target cells bearing Ia-like antigens whereas T_S cells recognize HLA antigens.[53]

T-cell growth factor (TCGF/IL-2)[42] is defined as an inducible glycoprotein hormone synthesized and secreted by T cells following an encounter with antigen or lectin.[13] IL-2 is the essential signal for the proliferation and differentiation of activated T cells.[74] The production of IL-2 is dependent on IL-1, a monokine released by monocytes.[65] Thus, the induction of cytotoxic T cells involves IL-1 stimulating T cells to produce IL-2, which in turn stimulates other T cells to produce IFN-γ and to become cytotoxic.[17]

Although IFN-γ was characterized initially for its antiviral quality, other functions that have been attributed to it include inhibition of tumor cell growth, enhancement of NK cell and ADCC activities (see below), and alteration of cell membranes to increase antigen expression on B lymphoid, macrophage, and myeloid cell lines and activation of macrophages.[47] IFN-γ also drives the maturation of resting B cells to active immunoglobulin secretion.[80]

Ia-like antigen is expressed on approximately 40% of T_H cells, which proliferate in response to soluble antigen and produce lymphocyte mitogenic factor (LMF). Both Ia$^+$ and Ia$^-$ helper cells are required to synergistically help the B cell.[72] This is an example of an interaction between subsets of lymphocytes that demonstrates important inducer-suppressor populations.

Delayed Hypersensitivity T Lymphocytes

In response to appropriate antigen, DHTLs produce chemotactic lymphokines, which confine and activate macrophages (macrophage-inhibiting and -activating factor) and may recruit uncommitted lymphocytes. DHTL are involved in sequelae after microbial infections, such as the skin reaction used to test for exposure to *Mycobacterium tuberculosis* antigen. A second example of delayed hypersensitivity is allergic contact dermatitis produced by agents such as cosmetics or the plant allergens associated with poison ivy.

Cytotoxic T Lymphocytes

Both T_H and T_S subpopulations of lymphocytes contain CTL. Allosensitized T cells are directed at both classes of major histocompatibility complex antigens on target cells and have the ability to recycle to fulfill their function. For example, they can kill a target cell and then proceed to a second cell to continue their cytotoxic activity. Sheep erythrocyte receptors are easily demonstrated on CTL but difficult to demonstrate on killer (K) or NK cells.[18]

Natural Killer Cells

Other classes of human lymphoid cells are cytotoxic but lack clear markers for B or T cells (Table 24-4). These classes, each with large granular lymphocyte (LGL) morphology, and each with distinct activities, include NK cells, K cells, and lymphokine-activated killer (LAK) cells. LGLs reside primarily in the blood and spleen[2] and have the capacity to exert both natural killing and antibody-dependent killing.[7,22] LGLs represent a defined subset of mononuclear cells based on surface markers and mechanisms of cytotoxicity. They appear to be more efficient in the production of interferon, colony-stimulating factors, and IL-2 than other lymphocytes.[38] Differences among these cells are observed generally in the kinetics of activation, target cell specificity, stimulus responsible for activation, and the phenotype of the precursor.

Functions of NK cells have been summarized[75]: (1) recognition and lysis of certain tumor cells and virus-infected cells without MHC restriction; (2) resistance to certain bacterial, fungal, and parasitic agents; (3) immune regulation; (4) regulation of hematopoiesis; and (5) natural resistance to allogeneic grafts.

NK cells react spontaneously against a wide variety of syngeneic, allogeneic, and xenogeneic cells. Their activity is enhanced by interferon and is not restricted to malignant cells, since virus-infected cells, fetal cells, some subpopulations of thymus cells, marrow cells, and macrophages are also susceptible.[32] NK cells may fulfill an important function early in host defense before the antibody-dependent immune mechanisms have been mobilized.[97] The spleen and blood contain the majority of mature NK cells that exhibit maximum NK function.[1,2]

Killer Cells

There is a major difference in the cytotoxicity mechanism of K cells and CTLs. K cells do not react specifically with cell membrane antigens of their target cell, but effect binding and cytotoxicity by way of antibodies that are already bound to antigens in the cell membrane of target cells. This mechanism is referred to as antibody-dependent cell-mediated cytolysis (ADCC). The role that antibody plays in the specificity of K-cell killing also distinguishes them from NK cells. Abnormal K-cell activity has been demonstrated in virus infections, tumors, and autoimmune diseases.[58]

Lymphokine-Activated Killer Cells

LAK cells represent a subset of cytolytic cells that are activated directly by IL-2.[25] LAK cells do not express some NK surface antigens and thus are phenotypically different from NK cells.[24] Differences among these cells are observed generally in the kinetics of activation, target cell specificity, stimuli responsible for activation, and the phenotype of the precursor.

TABLE 24-4. Cytotoxic Non-B, Non-T Cells and Large Granular Lymphocytes

1.	Natural killer cells (NK)
2.	Killer cells (K)
3.	Lymphokine-activated killer cells (LAK)

Lymphokines

In addition to the lymphokines discussed previously and the specific and nonspecific helper and suppressor factors, activated B and T lymphocytes secrete a variety of other lymphokines. These lymphokines function principally to moderate effector cell number and function. Seven of these lymphokines will be discussed briefly.

Colony-stimulating factors (CSFs) are hematopoietic hormones secreted by monocytes, macrophages, and activated T cells that regulate proliferation and differentiation of granulocytes, macrophage precursors, and early and late erythroid precursors.[11,16,23,62]

Macrophage-inhibiting factor (MIF) is secreted by B and T cells, appears to share common structural elements with CSF, and inhibits normal monocytes and macrophages from migrating from capillary tubes. MIF has been shown to display potent colony-stimulating activity when assayed on human marrow cells.[39]

Lymphocyte migration inhibitory factor (LyMIF$_{35K}$) produced by B and T cells immobilizes lymphocytes at the site of inflammation.[50]

Lymphocyte chemoattractant factor (LCF) is a chemokinetic factor that increases migration of nonsensitized T cells.[50]

Histamine-producing cell-stimulating factor (HCSF) produced by activated T cells induces an increase in histamine produced by basophils or mast cells.[15]

T cell-activating factor is an antigen-independent lymphokine that activates CTL and NK cells to become cytolytic.[54]

Human lymphotoxin (HLT), which inhibits tumor cell growth, is produced primarily by T cells, although B cells produce it in certain circumstances.[95]

CHARACTERIZATION OF LYMPHOCYTES AND PLASMA CELLS

Romanowsky-Stained Films: Light Microscopy

Lymphocytes are divided arbitrarily by size into categories of small (diameter 7–10 μm) and large (diameter 11–25 μm). Small lymphocytes have a large nuclear:cytoplasmic ratio with relatively scanty cytoplasm. Large lymphocytes contain more abundant cytoplasm. The nucleus is round or oval (occasionally kidney shaped) and is composed predominantly of dense blocks of heterochromatin with central and peripheral areas of condensation. Areas of parachromatin are unstained or lightly stained and indistinct (see Plate 20). Lymphocytes are usually mononuclear; however, one or two binucleated lymphocytes per 10,000 may be observed.[4] The nucleolus may not be obvious when stained by ordinary techniques, especially in small lymphocytes. The scant amount of blue cytoplasm in a small lymphocyte is usually devoid of granules; however, medium-sized to larger cells with more cytoplasm may demonstrate azurophilic (red–violet) granules that are usually prominent (0.3–0.6 μm). The LGL as defined by some authors is difficult to distinguish from other lymphocytes containing granules[26,88,89] by light microscopy.

Transformed lymphocytes or variant lymphocytes are morphologically altered cells that reflect lymphocyte reaction to antigen. Their morphology is described in detail in Chapter 27.

Plasma cells are mononuclear cells of approximately 10 to 28 μm diameter with round or oval and smooth or irregular margins (see Plate 21). The eccentrically located nucleus is composed of blocks of heterochromatin resembling a tortoise shell.[4] Abundant nongranular cytoplasm usually appears deep blue owing to the presence of numerous ribosomes (RNA). The area immediately next to the nucleus containing the Golgi apparatus is unstained (perinuclear chromophobic area or area of Höf). The periphery of the cytoplasm appears to have a "layered look," which is explained by the presence of flattened parallel sacs of rough endoplasmic reticulum (RER). The cytoplasm may contain round, discrete globules that appear unstained, pale blue, or occasionally red. These globules contain immunoglobulin and are called Russell bodies. When they fill the cytoplasm, the cells may appear to contain a cluster of grapes and are referred to as morula, grape, or Mott cells (see Fig. 39-4).

Problems in Identification of Lymphocytes

Mononuclear cells with blue, nongranular cytoplasm frequently present difficulty in correct identification for novices. Generally, closer observation of nuclear chromatin structure or amount of cytoplasm, and comparing it with other cells on the same blood film are helpful.

Distinguishing Lymphocytes from Blast Cells
Common features of blast cells (particularly microblasts) and lymphocytes are similar size, a round purple nucleus which may contain nucleoli, and scant blue cytoplasm. The nuclear chromatin of the blast reveals delicate strands that have a stippled or sieve-like appearance (predominance of euchromatin) that stains evenly and lightly (pink-purple). In the lymphocyte, blocks of heterochromatin stain dark purple, with sharp demarcation of unstained or lightly stained parachromatin (compare Plates 20 and 11).

Distinguishing Lymphocytes from Monocytes
Large lymphocytes and monocytes may be confused unless the chromatin pattern is examined carefully. Whereas lymphocyte heterochromatin is in the form of blocks, the monocyte heterochromatin appears linear, lacy, stringy, or ropy and frequently with "brain-like" convolutions. The overall staining intensity of the monocyte nucleus is usually less than the lymphocyte. Nuclear shape may be of some help. The lymphocyte nucleus is round, ovoid, or kidney shaped, that of the monocyte is often folded or U shaped. Finally, the character of the cytoplasm may be of aid. Lymphocyte cytoplasm is clear blue whereas monocytes contain extremely small azure granules in a blue-gray cytoplasm that gives it an opaque or ground-glass appearance (compare Plates 10 and 20).

Distinguishing Lymphocytes from Rubricytes
Both lymphocytes and rubricytes may be of similar size and contain dense blocks of nuclear chromatin. The nuclear parachromatin of the lymphocyte tends to stain light purple with deep purple heterochromatin, giving the appearance of crushed velvet; parachromatin in the rubricyte appears

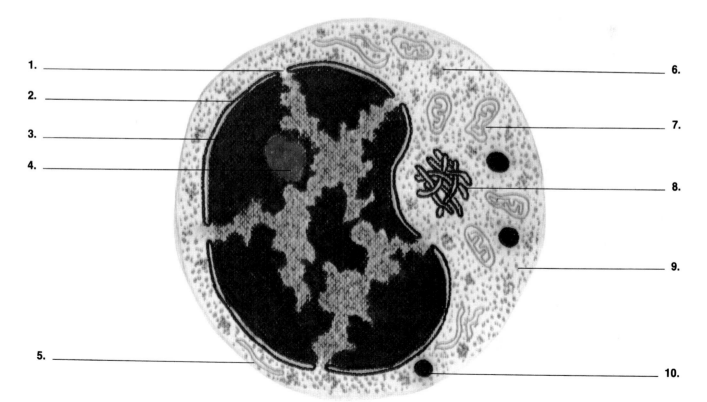

1. _____
2. _____
3. _____
4. _____
5. _____
6. _____
7. _____
8. _____
9. _____
10. _____

FIG. 24-5. A drawing of the electron microscopic appearance of a normal mature lymphocyte: (1) nuclear pore; (2) the nuclear envelope; (3) perinuclear chromatin; (4) nucleolus; (5) rough endoplasmic reticulum; (6) aggregate of glycogen; (7) mitochondrion; (8) Golgi complex; (9) polyribosome; (10) azurophilic granule (courtesy of Thomas F. Dutcher, MD).

TABLE 24–5. Summary of Cytochemical Features of Lymphocytes

CYTOCHEMICAL REACTION	T_H LYMPHOCYTES	T_S LYMPHOCYTES	T LYMPHOBLASTS	B LYMPHOBLASTS	B LYMPHOCYTES	NON-T NON-B LYMPHOBLASTS	PLASMA CELLS
Acid phosphatase	$1^+\star$	$1-2^+\dagger$	$2-3^+\star$	$0-1^+\dagger$	$0-1^+\dagger$	$0-1^+\dagger$	$3^+\star$
Alkaline phosphatase	0	0	0	$0-1^+$	0	0	0
α-Naphthyl acetate esterase	$2^+\star$	$0-1^+$	$0-1^+\star$	$0-1^+$	0	0	$0-2^+$
α-Naphthyl butyrate esterase	$1-2^+\star$	$0-1^+$	$0-1^+\star$	$0-1^+$	0	0	0
Fluoride-resistant esterase (acetate or butyrate)	$0-1^+\star$	$0-1^+$	$0-1^+\star$	$0-1^+$	0	0	0
Periodic acid–Schiff	$0-1^+$	$0-1^+$	$0-1^+$	$0-1^+$	$0-1^+$	$0-2^+$	$0-2^+$
Peroxidase	0	0	0	0	0	0	0
Sudan black B	0	0	0	0	0	0	0
Tartrate-resistant acid phosphatase	0	0	$0-1^+\star$	0	0	0	0

Key: ★, focal staining; †, diffuse staining.
Note: The intensity of reaction is graded on a scale from 0 to 4+: 0, no reaction; 4+, the strongest reaction.

more unstained, and the chromatin is in small dense spherical clumps, giving a checkerboard appearance. Generally, the cytoplasm of the lymphocyte tends to be clear blue, whereas the rubricyte may have a mingling of blue (RNA) and pink (hemoglobin), giving the overall color a "muddy" or gray appearance (Plate 3).

Electron Microscopy

Lymphocytes

Transmission electron microscopy of lymphocytes enables visualization of detailed nuclear structure and cytoplasmic organelles (Fig. 24-5). The nucleus has a double

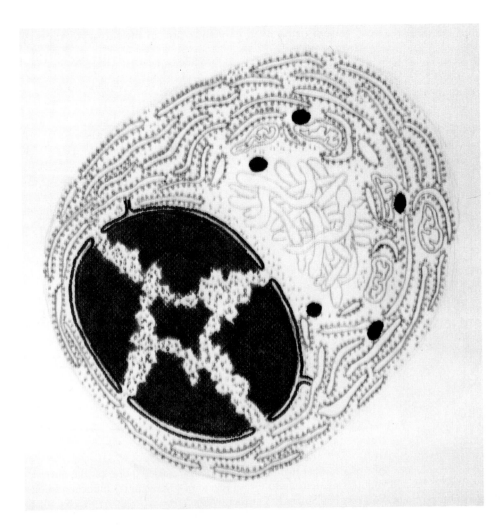

FIG. 24-6. Drawing of the electron microscopic appearance of a normal plasma cell (courtesy of Thomas F. Dutcher, MD).

TABLE 24–6. Recommended Cluster Designation (CD) Nomenclature

CLUSTER DESIGNATION	ANTIBODY	PRIMARY SUBPOPULATION
B CELL		
CD37	HD28, HH1, G28-1	B cell, (T, monocyte)
CD72	S-HCL2, J3-109, BV-40, BV-41	Pan-B cell; Pre-B cell
CD73	1E9.28.1, 7G2.2.11, AD2	B subset, T subset
CD74	LN2, BV-43, BV-45	B cell, monocyte
CDw75	LN1, HH2; EBV-141	Mature B cell, (T subset)
CD76	HD66, CR15-4	Mature B cell, (T subset)
CD77	38.13 (BLA), 424/4A11, 424/3D9	Resting B cell
CDw78	Anti-Ba, LO-pan B-a, 1588	B cell, (monocyte)
T CELL		
CD2R	T11.3, VITI3, D66	Activated T cells
CD27	VITI4, S152, OKT18A CLB-9F4	T subset
CD28	9.3, KOLT2	T subset
CD30	Ki-1, Ber-H2, HSR4	Activated T, B: Reed-Sternberg
CD38	HB7;T16	Reacts with lymphocyte progenitors, plasma cell
CD45RA	G1-15, F8-11-13, 73.5	T subset, B cell, granulocyte, monocyte
CD45RO	UCHL1	T subset, B cell, granulocyte, monocyte
CDw60	M-T32, M-T21, M-T41, UM4D4	T helper cell, cytotoxic T-effector cell
NK CELL		
CD16	BW209/2; HUNK2, 3G8 CLBFcGran1	NK cell, granulocyte, macrophage
CD56	Leu 19, NKH1, FP2-11.14, L185	NK cell, activated lymphocyte
CD57	Leu 7, L183, L186	NK cell, T, B subset

membrane containing nuclear pores. A large nucleolus is usually seen and frequently is surrounded by blocks of chromatin. The Golgi complex is small, and mitochondria are small and sparse. There is very little RER. Large granular lymphocytes contain cytoplasmic granules of different sizes located near the Golgi complex that are usually bound by unit membranes. Larger granules appear more electron dense than smaller ones.[26] Many vesicles are seen in the area immediately next to the Golgi apparatus.

Plasma Cells

The nucleus contains blocks of heterochromatin; the central block contains remnants of a nucleolus. Striking features of nuclear chromatin and cytoplasmic organelles are visible with transmission electron microscopy (Fig. 24-6). The cytoplasm is laden with RER, which surrounds the nucleus. The Golgi complex is large and pushes into the nucleus. Large, elongated mitochondria are present in the cytoplasm, usually around the Golgi complex. Sparse lysosomes may be observed.

Cytochemistry

Cytochemical reactivity routinely used to evaluate lymphocytes is summarized in Table 24-5. The various reac-tions are described in detail in the chapter devoted to cytochemistry (Chap. 30).

Cell Markers

Cell morphology in combination with cytochemical testing expedites making the diagnosis and prognosis of disease, but greater understanding relative to pathophysiology, treatment, and prevention of disease has been facilitated through the discovery of cell surface markers by the use of monoclonal antibodies (MAbs). The lymphocyte, with its unique subsets, has served as the prototype for these techniques.

A summary of the most frequently used monoclonal antibodies for lymphocytes, a brief description of the reactivity, and the recommended cluster designation (CD) nomenclature are included in Table 24-6.[3,20,31,35,43,44,60] The confusing array of names for various MAbs grew out of the practice of different manufacturers assigning different symbols for a simple MAb (e.g., Ortho, OKT series; Beckton-Dickinson, Leu series; Coulter, T series). The CD nomenclature represents an international effort to provide a simple, unambiguous, and adaptable system for classifying leukocyte differentiation antigens. A review of Table 24-6 will show how these correlate with one another.

CHAPTER SUMMARY

From their origin in marrow to differentiation in the thymus or secondary lymphoid tissue (SLT), lymphoid cells may become programmed for immediate action or may circulate "immortally" in anticipation of a summons to action. These characteristics make the lymphocyte a cell with remarkable capabilities. It differs from other defensive cells such as granulocytes in that it may have a life span of several years or may die *in situ* within hours or days without participating in the war on foreign agents.

Effective immunocompetence is dependent on the heterogeneity, quantitative balance, and interaction of subpopulations of lymphocytes with each other and with other cells in their microenvironment. The ability of lymphocytes to migrate from the marrow to thymus and SLT and for some cells to recirculate is dependent on the stickiness and motility of the cells. The microenvironment provided by endothelioid venules; receptors on endothelial cells, dendritic reticulum cells, interdigitating reticulum cells, monocytes, and macrophages; and the architecture of the primary and secondary lymphatic tissue play crucial roles in determining the fate of antigen.

Finally, it is essential for the clinical laboratorian to be able to morphologically identify resting small lymphocytes, large (granular or nongranular) lymphocytes, transformed lymphocytes, and plasma cells in blood and bone marrow. Identification of lymphoid cells through cytochemistry and cell markers is vitally important to evaluate and differentiate the numerous lymphocyte subpopulations.

REFERENCES

1. Abo T, Cooper MD, Balch CM: Characterization of HNK-1⁺ (Leu-7) human lymphocytes 1. Two distinct phenotypes of human NK cells with different cytotoxic capability. J Immunol 129:1752, 1982
2. Abo T, Miller CA, Gartland GL et al: Differentiation stages of

human natural killer cells in lymphoid tissues from fetal to adult life. J Exp Med 157:273, 1983

3. Bernard A, Boumsell L: The clusters of differentiation (CD) defined by the first international workshop on human leukocyte differentiation antigens. Hum Immunol 11: 1, 1984

4. Bessis M (Brecher G trans): Blood Smears Reinterpreted. Berlin, Springer International, 1977

5. Bollum FJ: Terminal deoxynucleotidyl transferase as a hematopoietic cell marker. Blood 54:1203, 1979

6. Boyd AW, Freedman AS, Anderson KC et al: Phenotypic changes occurring during *in vitro* activation of human splenic B lymphocytes. In Reinherz EL, Haynes BF, Nadler LM et al (eds): Leukocyte Typing II. Human B Lymphocytes p 429. New York, Springer-Verlag, 1986

7. Bradley TP, Bonavida B: Mechanism of cell mediated cytotoxicity at the single cell level. IV. Natural killing and antibody-dependent cellular cytotoxicity can be mediated by the same human effector cell as determined by the two-target conjugate assay. J Immunol 129: 2260, 1982

8. Buckton KE, Court Brown WM, Smith PG: Lymphocyte survival in men treated with x-rays for ankylosing spondylitis. Nature 214:470, 1967

9. Callihan TR, Holbert JM Jr, Berard CW: Neoplasms of terminal B-cell differentiation: The morphologic basis of functional diversity. In Sommers SC, Rosen PP (eds): Malignant Lymphomas, p 169. Norwalk, CT, Appleton-Century-Crofts, 1983

10. Clark P, Normansell DE, Innes DJ et al: Lymphocyte subsets in normal bone marrow. Blood 67:1600, 1986

11. Cline MJ, Golde DW: Cellular interactions in haematopoiesis. Nature 277:177, 1979

12. Cooper MD, Lawton AR: Pre-B cells: normal morphologic and biologic characteristics and abnormal development in certain immunodeficiencies and malignancies. In Pernis B, Vogel HJ (eds): P&S Biomedical Sciences Symposia, Cells of Immunoglobulin Synthesis, p 411. New York, Academic Press, 1979

13. Depper JM, Leonard WJ, Smith KA et al: Monoclonal anti-Tac blocks the action and membrane binding of human interleukin-2. In Oppenheim JJ, Cohen S (eds): Interleukins, Lymphokines, and Cytokines, p 19. New York, Academic Press, 1983

14. de Sousa M: Microenvironment to a lymphoid cell is nothing more than interaction with its neighbors. Adv Exp Med Biol 66:165, 1976

15. Dy M, Lebel B, Schneider E: Histamine-producing cell-stimulating factor (HCSF) and interleukin 3 (IL3): Evidence for two distinct molecular entities. J Immunol 136:208, 1986

16. Estrov Z, Roifman C, Wang Y-P et al: The regulatory role of interleukin 2–responsive T lymphocytes on early and mature erythroid progenitor proliferation. Blood 67:1607, 1986

17. Farrar WL, Johnson HM, Farrar JJ: Regulation of the production of immune interferon and cytotoxic T lymphocytes by interleukin 2. J Immunol 126:1120, 1981

18. Fast LD, Hansen JA, Newman W: Evidence for T cell nature and heterogeneity within natural killer (NK) and antibody-dependent cellular cytotoxicity (ADCC) effectors: A comparison with cytolytic T lymphocytes (CTL). J Immunol 127:448, 1981

19. Foon KA, Billing RJ, Terasaki PI et al: Immunologic classification of acute lymphoblastic leukemia: Implication for normal lymphoid differentiation. Blood 56:1120, 1980

20. Foon KA, Todd RF: Immunologic classification of leukemia and lymphoma. Blood 68:1, 1986

21. Ford WL: Lymphocyte migration and immune responses. Prog Allerg 19:1, 1975

22. Gastl G, Niederwieser D, Marth C et al: Human large granular lymphocytes and their relationship to natural killer cell activity in various disease states. Blood 64:288, 1984.

23. Greenberger JS, Krensky AM, Messner H et al: Production of colony-stimulating factor(s) for granulocyte—macrophage and multipotential (granulocyte/erythroid/megakaryocyte/macrophage) hematopoietic progenitor cells (CFU-GEMM) by clonal lines of human IL-2–dependent T lymphocytes. Exp Hematol 12:720, 1984

24. Grimm EA, Ramsey KM, Mazumder A et al: Lymphokine-activated killer cell phenomenon. II. Precursor phenotype is serologically distinct from peripheral T lymphocytes, memory cytotoxic thymus-derived lymphocytes and natural killer cells. J Exp Med 157:884, 1983

25. Grimm EA, Robb RJ, Roth JA et al: Lymphokine-activated killer cell phenomenon. III. Evidence that Il-2 is sufficient for direct activation of peripheral blood lymphocytes into lymphokine-activated killer cells. J Exp Med 158:1356, 1983

26. Grossi CE, Cadoni A, Zicca A et al: Large granular lymphocytes in human peripheral blood: Ultrastructural and cytochemical characterization of the granules. Blood 59: 277, 1982

27. Gupta S, Good RA: Markers of human lymphocyte subpopulations in primary immunodeficiency and lymphoproliferative disorders. Semin Hematol 17:1, 1980

28. Hackett J Jr, Tutt M, Lipscomb M et al: Origin and differentiation of natural killer cells. II. Functional and morphologic studies of purified NK.1 1+ cells. J Immunol 136:3124, 1986

29. Haller O, Wigzell H: Suppression of natural killer activity with radioactive strontium: Effector cells are marrow dependent. J Immunol 118:1503, 1977

30. Hirano T, Yasukawa K, Harada H et al: Complimentary DNA for a novel human interleukin (BSF-2) that induces B lymphocytes to produce immunoglobulin. Nature 324:73, 1986

31. Haynes BF: Summary of T cell studies performed during the second international workshop and conference on human leukocyte differentiation antigens. In Reinherz EL, Haynes BF, Nadler LM et al (eds): Leukocyte Typing II. Human T Lymphocytes, p 3. New York, Springer-Verlag, 1986

32. Herberman RB, Ortaldo JR: Natural killer cells: Their role in defenses against disease. Science 214:24, 1981

33. Hercend T, Schmidt RE: Characteristics and uses of natural killer cells. Immunol Today 9:291, 1988

34. Howard M, Nakanishi K, Paul WE: Soluble factors required for B cell proliferation and differentiation. In Oppenheim JJ, Cohen S (eds): Interleukins, Lymphokines and Cytokines, p 187. New York, Academic Press, 1983

35. International Union of Immunological Societies and World Health Organization Subcommittee: Nomenclature. J Immunol 135:659, 1985

36. Janossy G: Differentiation of human bone marrow cells and thymocytes. In Knapp W (ed): Leukemic Markers, p 45. London, Academic Press, 1981

37. Jurgensen CH, Ambrus JL, Fauci AS: Production of B-cell growth factor by normal human B cells. J Immunol 136:4542, 1986

38. Kasahara T, Djeu JY, Dougherty SF et al: Capacity of human large granular lymphocytes (LGL) to produce multiple lymphokines: Interleukin 2, interferon, and colony stimulating factor. J Immunol 131:2379, 1983

39. Kawaguchi T, Golde DW, Mednis A et al: T cell-derived migration-inhibitory factor and colony-stimulating factor share common structural elements. Blood 67:1619, 1986

40. Kehrl JH, Muraguchi A, Butler JL et al: Human B-cell activation, proliferation and differentiation. Immunol Rev 78:75, 1984

41. Klaus GGB, Humphrey JH: The generation of memory cells. I. The role of C3 in the generation of B memory cells. Immunology 33:31, 1977

42. Klein B, Rey A, Jourdan M et al: The role of interleukin 1 and interleukin 2 in human T-colony formation. Cell Immunol 77: 348, 1983

43. Knapp W, Reiber P, Dörkeu B et al: Towards a better definition of human leukocyte surface molecules. Immunol Today 10:253, 1989

44. Knowles RW: Immunochemical analysis of the T cell–specific antigens. In Reinherz EL, Haynes BF, Nadler LM et al (eds): Leukocyte Typing II. Human T Lymphocytes, p 259. New York, Springer-Verlag, 1986

45. Lanier LL, Allison JP, Phillips JN: Correlation of cell surface antigen expression on human thymocytes by multicolor flow cytometric analysis: Implications for differentiation. J Immunol 137:2501, 1986

46. Lanier LL, Phillips JH, Hackett J et al: Natural killer cells: Definition of a cell type rather than a function. J Immunol 137:2735, 1986

47. Lee SH, Aggarwal BB, Rinderknecht E et al: The synergistic antiproliferative effect of gamma interferon and human lymphotoxin. J Immunol 133:1083, 1984

48. Leibson JH, Gefter M, Zlotnik A et al: Role of gamma interferon in antibody-producing responses. Nature 309:799, 1984

49. Lotzova E, Savary CA: Generation of NK cell activity from human bone marrow. J Immunol 139:279, 1987

50. McFadden RG, Cruikshank WW, Center DM: Modulation of lymphocyte migration by human lymphokines. III. Characterization of a lymphocyte migration inhibitory factor (LyMIF$_{35K}$). Cell Immunol 85:154, 1984

51. McKenna RW, Bloomfield CD, Brunning RD: Nodular lymphoma: Bone marrow and blood manifestations. Cancer 36:428, 1975

52. Mayer LF, Thompson C, Fu SM et al: T-cell factors regulating B-cell activation and differentiation. Curr Top Microbiol Immunol 113:77, 1984

53. Meuer SC, Schlossman SF, Reinherz EL: Clonal analysis of human cytotoxic T lymphocytes: T4$^+$ and T8$^+$ effector T cells recognize products of different major histocompatibility complex regions. Proc Natl Acad Sci USA 79:4395, 1982

54. Milanese C, Siliciano RF, Schmidt RE et al: A lymphokine that activates the cytolytic program of both cytotoxic T lymphocyte and natural killer clones. J Exp Med 163:1583, 1986

55. Miller HC, Schmiege SK, Rule A: Thymosin-induced functional T cells from the bone marrow. Fed Proc 32:879A, 1973

56. Mond JJ, Thompson C, Finkelman FD et al: Affinity-purified interleukin 2 induces proliferation of large but not small B cells. Proc Natl Acad Sci USA 82:1518, 1985

57. Muehleck SD, McKenna RW, Gale PF et al: Terminal deoxynucleotidyl transferase (TdT)–positive cells in bone marrow in the absence of hematologic malignancy. Am J Clin Pathol 79:277, 1983

58. Müller-Hermelink HK, Lennert K: The cytologic, histologic and functional bases for a modern classification of lymphoma. In Lennert K (ed) (Frederick DD, Soehring M, trans): Malignant Lymphomas Other than Hodgkin's Disease, pp 3, 17. New York, Springer-Verlag, 1979

59. Muraguchi A, Nishimoto H, Kawamura N et al: B cell–derived BCGF functions as autocrine growth factor(s) in normal and transformed B lymphocytes. J Immunol 137:179, 1986

60. Nadler LM: B cell/leukemia panel workshop: Summary and comments. In Reinherz EL, Haynes BF, Nadler LM et al (eds): Leukocyte Typing II. Human B Lymphocytes, p 3. New York, Springer-Verlag, 1986

61. Nadler LM, Anderson KC, Marti G et al: B4, a human B lymphocyte–associated antigen expressed on normal, mitogen—activated, and malignant B lymphocytes. J Immunol 131:244, 1983

62. Nicola NA, Vadas M: Hemopoietic colony-stimulating factors. Immunol Today 5:76, 1984

63. Okada M, Sakaguchi N, Yoshimura N et al: B-cell growth factors and B-cell differentiation factor from human T hybridomas. J Exp Med 157:583, 1983

64. Ottesen J: On the age of human white cells in peripheral blood. Acta Physiol Scand 32:75, 1954

65. Palacios R: Mechanism of T-cell activation: Role and functional relationship of HLA-DR antigens and interleukins. Immunol Rev 63:73, 1982

66. Parks DE, Chisari FV: Production and distribution of lymphocytes and plasma cells. In Williams WJ, Beutler E, Erslev AJ et al (eds):Hematology, p 923. New York, McGraw-Hill, 1983

67. Parrott DMV, Wilkinson PC: Lymphocyte locomotion and migration. Prog Allerg 28:193, 1981

68. Paul WE: Nomenclature for B-cell stimulatory factors. Cell Immunol 84:461, 1984

69. Poppema S, Bhan AK, Reinherz EL et al: Distribution of T cell subsets in human lymph nodes. J Exp Med 153:30, 1981

70. Reinherz EL, Kung PC, Goldstein G et al: Discrete stages of human intrathymic differentiation: Analysis of normal thymocytes and leukemic lymphoblasts of T-cell lineage. Proc Natl Acad Sci USA 77:1588, 1980

71. Reinherz EL, Kung PC, Goldstein G et al: A monoclonal antibody reactive with the human cytotoxic/suppressor T-cell subset previously defined by a heteroantiserum termed TH$_2$. J Immunol 124:1301, 1980

72. Reinherz EL, Morimoto C, Penta AC et al: Subpopulations of the T4+ inducer T-cell subset in man: Evidence for an amplifier population preferentially expressing Ia antigen upon activation. J Immunol 126:67, 1981

73. Reinherz EL, Schlossman SF: Current concepts in immunology. Regulation of the immune response-inducer and suppressor T-lymphocyte subsets in human beings. N Engl J Med 303:370, 1980

74. Rey A, Klein B, Ilnicki C et al: The role of interleukin-2 in T-colony formation by human pre–T cells (pTCFC). Clin Exp Immunol 58:154, 1984

75. Ritz J, Schmidt RE, Michon J et al: Characterization of functional surface structures on human natural killer cells. Adv Immunol 42:181, 1988

76. Ropke C, Hougen HP, Everett NB: Long-lived T and B lymphocytes in the bone marrow and thoracic duct lymph of the mouse. Cell Immunol 15:82, 1975

77. Rosenthal N, Dreskin DH, Vural IL et al: The significance of hematogones in blood, bone marrow and lymph node aspiration in giant follicular lymphoblastoma. Acta Haematol 8:368, 1952

78. Ryser JH, Vassalli P: Mouse bone marrow lymphocytes and their differentiation. J Immunol 113:719, 1974

79. Scheid MP, Hoffmann MK, Komuro K et al: Differentiation of T cells induced by preparations from thymus and by nonthymic agents. J Exp Med 138:1027, 1973

80. Sidman CL, Marshall JD, Shultz LD et al: Gamma interferon is one of several direct B cell–maturing lymphokines. Nature 309:801, 1984

81. Smith CH: Blood Diseases of Infancy and Childhood, p 496. St Louis, CV Mosby, 1972

82. Stobo JD: Mitogens. Clin Immunobiol 4:55, 1980

83. Swain SL, Dutton RW: Production of a B cell growth-promoting activity (DL) BCGF, from a cloned T cell and its assay on the BCL 1 B cell tumor. J Exp Med 156(6):1821, 1982

84. Swain SL, Howard M, Kappler J et al: Evidence for two distinct classes of murine B cell growth factors with activities in different functional assays. J Exp Med 158(3):822, 1983

85. Thompson PA, Jelinek DF, Lipsky PE: Regulation of human B-cell proliferation by prostaglandin E2. J Immunol 133:2446, 1984

86. Thorley-Lawson DA, Mann KP: Early events in Epstein-Barr virus infection provide a model for B-cell activation. J Exp Med 162:45, 1985

87. Timonen T, Ortlando JB, Herberman RB: Characteristics of human large granular lymphocytes and relationship to natural killer and K cells. J Exp Med 153:569, 1981

88. Timonen T, Ranki A, Saksela E et al: Human natural cell-mediated cytotoxicity against fetal fibroblasts. III. Morphologi-

cal and functional characterization of the effector cells. Cell Immunol 48:121, 1979

89. Timonen T, Sakela E, Ranki A et al: Fractionation, morphological and functional characterization of effector cells responsible for human natural killer activity against cell-line targets. Cell Immunol 48:133, 1979

90. Trinchieri G, London L, Kobayashi M et al: Regulation of activation and proliferation of human natural killer cells. Adv Exp Med Biol 213:285, 1987

91. Vogel P, Bassen FA: Sternal marrow of children in normal and pathologic states. Am J Dis Child 57:245, 1939

92. Vogel P, Erf LA, Rosenthal N: Hematologic observations on bone marrow obtained by sternal puncture. Am J Clin Pathol 7:498, 1937

93. Vogler LB, Glick AD, Collins RD: B Cell neoplasms: Correlation of recent developments with the biology of normal B lymphocytes. In Stefanini M, Gorstein F, Fink L (eds): Progress in Clinical Pathology IX, pp 197. Orlando, Grune and Stratton, 1984

94. Vogler LB, Grossi CE, Cooper MD: Human lymphocyte subpopulations. In Brown EB, Moore, CV (eds): Progress in Hematology XI, p 1. New York, Grune and Stratton, 1979

95. Wintrobe MM, Lee GR, Boggs DR et al: Clinical Hematology. Philadelphia, Lea & Febiger, 1981

96. Wong GHW, Clark-Lewis I, McKimm-Breschkin JL et al: Interferon-gamma induces enhanced expression of Ia and H-2 antigens on B lymphoid, macrophage and myeloid cell lines. J Immunol 131:788, 1983

97. Yang J, Zucker-Franklin D: Modulation of natural killer (NK) cells by autologous neutrophils and monocytes. Cell Immunol 86:171, 1984

98. Yoda Y, Kawakami Z, Shibuya A et al: Characterization of natural killer cells cultured from human bone marrow cells. Exp Hematol 16:712, 1988

99. Zubler RH, Lowenthal JW, Erard F et al: Activated B cells express receptors for, and proliferate in response to pure interleukin 2. J Exp Med 160:1170, 1984

Laboratory

Evaluation

of

Leukocytes

Joan C. McNeely
Darlean Brown

This chapter emphasizes the procedures for manual counting and differentiation of leukocytes. Manual cell counts and differentiation were originally the only means of enumerating and classifying cellular elements in blood and body fluids. To a large extent the laboratory evaluation of leukocytes, erythrocytes, and platelets has now been automated (Chaps. 43 and 44). Leukocyte identification and classification is referred to in the laboratory as the *leukocyte differential* count.

If automated leukocyte evaluation is available, why must laboratory scientists learn manual techniques for evaluating them? There are several reasons.

For every automated method there should be a back-up method, and in some laboratories that method is the manual one. Results from automated methods may be evaluated by manual methods, although automated leukocyte and erythrocyte counts should be evaluated with a single-channel automated cell counter as a backup rather than a manual method.

Not all samples can be evaluated by automated methods for one reason or another. For example, when a leukocyte count is extremely low or high, it may be necessary to perform a manual count because of loss of instrument linearity (capability to count cells accurately) at the extreme ends of the spectrum. Other samples that may require manual cell counting include those with abnormal proteins, clumped platelets, or antibody elements in the plasma that interfere with an instrument's ability to count leukocytes.

Extremely abnormal leukocytes, such as those seen in leukemia, may not, in some cases, be accurately differentiated by automated methods, although today some methods are proving to be very accurate in identifying abnormal cells. For laboratories with automated leukocyte differential capabilities, the decision to perform manual differential counts on certain specimens is in the hands of each individual laboratory. The fact remains that there will be specimens that require a manual differential count for some time to come.

MANUAL LEUKOCYTE COUNTS

Manual cell counts are performed with the aid of an apparatus called a *hemocytometer* (Fig. 25-1). The areas of the hemocytometer generally used for counting leukocytes as well as erythrocytes and platelets (Chap. 59) are indicated in Figure 25-2. In practice erythrocytes no longer are counted manually on the hemocytometer because this is a very inaccurate method. Today, erythrocyte counts are performed on single-channel or multichannel instruments. The formulas presented for calculating total cellular elements in the procedures that follow may be applied to leukocytes, erythrocytes, and platelets. In today's automated laboratories manual counting is used principally for cells in abnormal specimens and in cerebrospinal fluid and other body fluids (Chap. 31).

MANUAL LEUKOCYTE COUNTS
Principle

A suitably diluted specimen is loaded onto a hemocytometer and the cellular elements are identified and counted microscopically and reported as number of cells per liter.

Specimen Requirements

Whole blood anticoagulated with EDTA is preferred, although heparin or ammonium potassium oxalate may be used. Specimens must not have any clots. Specimens diluted prior to receipt in the laboratory must be labeled with the name of the diluent and the ratio of specimen to diluent.

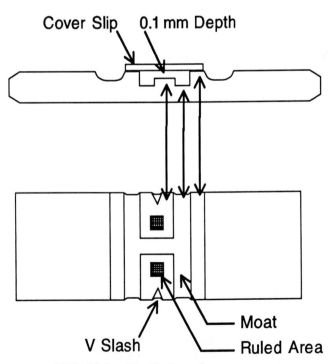

FIG. 25-1.   The Neubauer hemocytometer.

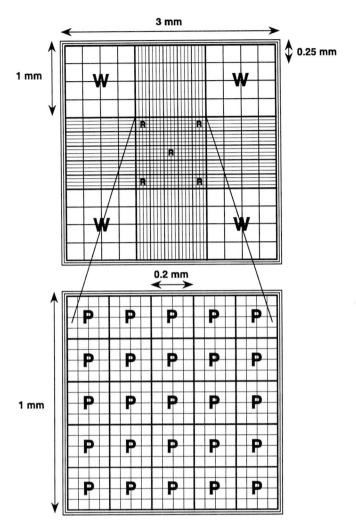

FIG. 25-2.   The ruled area of the Neubauer hemocytometer. There are nine large (1 mm) squares. Each of the four corner 1-mm squares is subdivided into 16 smaller squares and is marked **W** to indicate use for counting leukocytes. The center 1-mm square is subdivided into 25 smaller squares, each 0.04 mm². The squares marked **R** were used for counting erythrocytes when they were historically counted manually. The higher magnification of this center square (below) illustrates all 25 0.04-mm² squares marked **P** where platelets are counted.

Reagents and Equipment

Hemocytometer (Levy counting chamber with improved Neubauer ruling) (see Fig. 25-1). The two ruled areas on either side of the hemocytometer each have an area of 9 mm². These areas are divided into a counting grid that enables the microscopist to accurately count cellular elements (see Fig. 25-2). The depth of the chamber between coverslip and ruled area is 0.1 mm (see Fig. 25-1). Hemocytometers must meet the National Bureau of Standards (NBS) specifications, as indicated by the NBS initials on the chamber.

Cover slip, optically flat, designed for hemocytometers

Thoma diluting pipet or Unopette

Pipet suction apparatus (Clay Adams)

Diluents for leukocyte counting

Diluents for counting only leukocytes must be capable of lysing erythrocytes without destroying leukocytes. One of the following diluents may be used:

TABLE 25–1. Recommended Dilutions for Manual WBC Count Specimen Preparation Based on Anticipated WBC Count

ANTICIPATED WBC COUNT ($\times 10^9$/L)	RECOMMENDED DILUTION	TYPE OF THOMA PIPET
0.1–3.0	1:10	WBC
3.1–30.0	1:20	WBC
>30.0	1:100	RBC
≥100.0	1:200	RBC

Glacial Acetic Acid, 2% (v/v). Combine 2 mL acetic acid with distilled water to 100 mL in a volumetric flask. Always add acid slowly to water to assure good safety practice.

Hydrochloric Acid (HCl), 1% (v/v). Combine 1 mL concentrated HCl with distilled water to 100 mL in a volumetric flask.

Turk's Solution. Combine 3 mL glacial acetic acid, 1 mL aqueous gentian violet (1% w/v), and 96 mL distilled water. Turk's solution enhances leukocyte nuclear definition.

Diluents for platelet counting
Platelet-diluting fluids must preserve platelet integrity while inhibiting their aggregation (Chap. 59).

Diluents for CSF and other body fluids
See Chapter 31 for special handling of fluids. Cells in body fluids are counted without dilution in some cases.

General Procedure for Specimen Preparation

1. Place a dampened gauze square in bottom of Petri dish with two halves of a wooden stick placed on gauze to serve as a stand for the hemocytometer.
2. Place whole blood on rotator for at least 1 or 2 minutes or hand invert at least 60 times.[14] Complete but gentle inversion is required to mix blood but avoid hemolysis. Other body fluids must also be suitably mixed to ensure specimen homogeneity. Specimen samples for manual counts must be diluted immediately after the specimen is mixed.
3. Choose appropriate dilution for anticipated cell count (Table 25-1). Dilutions ranging from 1 part in 10 (1:10) to 1 part in 1000 (1:1000) may be made using Thoma pipets (Fig. 25-3). A 1:10 or 1:20 dilution is commonly made with the WBC pipet and a 1:100 or 1:200 dilution, with the RBC pipet.
4. Attach mechanical pipet suction device to WBC pipet.
5. To make a 1:20 dilution, draw a sample of whole blood specimen to exactly 0.5 mark (see Fig. 25-3) on pipet stem. If blood is drawn just slightly above this mark, use a nonabsorbent material to remove excess blood and ensure blood is at exactly 0.5 mark in pipet. If blood is drawn too far above

0.5 mark, the procedure should be repeated using a new pipet since excess blood causes an inaccurate dilution.

6. Tilt pipet so that stem is slightly above horizontal and wipe stem carefully with slightly dampened gauze, moving from pipet bulb toward tip. *Caution:* Do not allow capillary attraction to draw fluid from tip onto gauze. Gauze or any absorbent cloth tends to absorb the liquid portion of blood, causing an erroneous increase in cell counts.
7. Gently rotating pipet between forefinger and thumb, draw diluent steadily into pipet exactly to the 11 mark (see Fig. 25-3). This results in a 1:20 dilution of blood to diluent in the pipet bulb.
8. Immediately cover tip of pipet with middle finger and carefully remove suction device. Place thumb over open tip and vigorously rotate pipet back and forth, moving only the wrist, for 30 to 45 seconds. This ensures even dispersion of lysed erythrocytes (see Sources of Error). If a mechanical pipet shaker is available, shake pipet for approximately 3 minutes.
9. Repeat this procedure with a second pipet to obtain two dilutions of the same specimen.

Calculation of Dilution

When using a WBC pipet, divide value on stem to which blood sample is drawn by 10 to obtain sample dilution.

When using an RBC pipet, divide value on stem to which blood sample is drawn by 100 to obtain sample dilution. In each case the denominator (*i.e.*, 10 or 100) represents 1 unit less than the dilution mark above the bulb on the pipet (*e.g.*, for the WBC pipet, 11 − 1 = 10) (see Fig. 25-3). One part is subtracted to account for one part of diluent that remains in the pipet stem, which is not part of the mixture of sample and diluent in the pipet bulb.

For example, using a WBC pipet, if blood is drawn to the 0.5 mark and diluent to the 11 mark, the resulting dilution is 0.5:10 or 1:20. If blood is drawn to the 1 mark and diluent to the 11 mark, the dilution is 1:10. The same principle applies to calculating dilutions in the RBC pipet.

Sources of Error

Failure to mix blood specimen just prior to taking a sample for counting renders cell counts inaccurate.

Failure to immediately mix blood and diluent in Thoma pipet produces clumps of erythrocyte stroma, which entrap leukocytes and make accurate counting impossible.

Using diluent contaminated with blood causes erroneous results.

Bubbles in Thoma pipet cause an inaccurate dilution.

Drawing blood too far past the appropriate dilution mark and then drawing it out causes an inaccurate dilution because blood tends to stick to pipet walls.

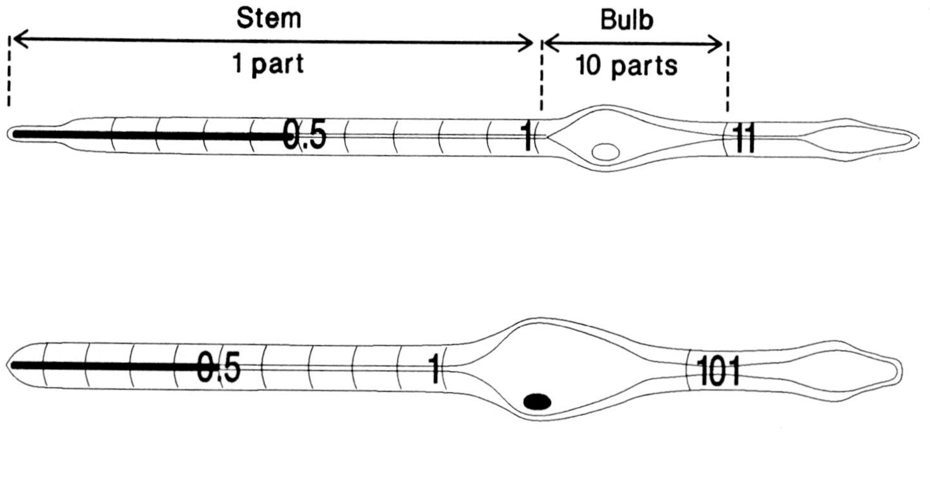

FIG. 25-3. Thoma pipets used to dilute specimens for cell counts. Upper pipet is used to make 1:10 or 1:20 dilutions. Lower pipet is used to make 1:100 or 1:200 dilutions for elevated leukocyte counts; this pipet was historically used for manual erythrocyte counts, which are no longer performed.

Unopette System for Manual Leukocyte Counts

The Unopette system (Becton Dickinson, Rutherford, NJ[5]) provides a series of reservoirs containing premeasured diluent and pipets that automatically measure the appropriate amount of sample required for diluting blood specimens in preparation for manual counting. Various reservoirs are available with appropriate diluting fluids for leukocyte, platelet, and eosinophil counts. Reservoirs are also available for performing dilutions to obtain a complete blood count from a skin puncture specimen or to measure erythrocyte osmotic fragility. The standard Unopette reservoir used for leukocyte counts contains 0.475 mL of a 3% aqueous solution of glacial acetic acid.

The technique for Unopette use is universal, no matter what laboratory procedure is to be performed. An over-

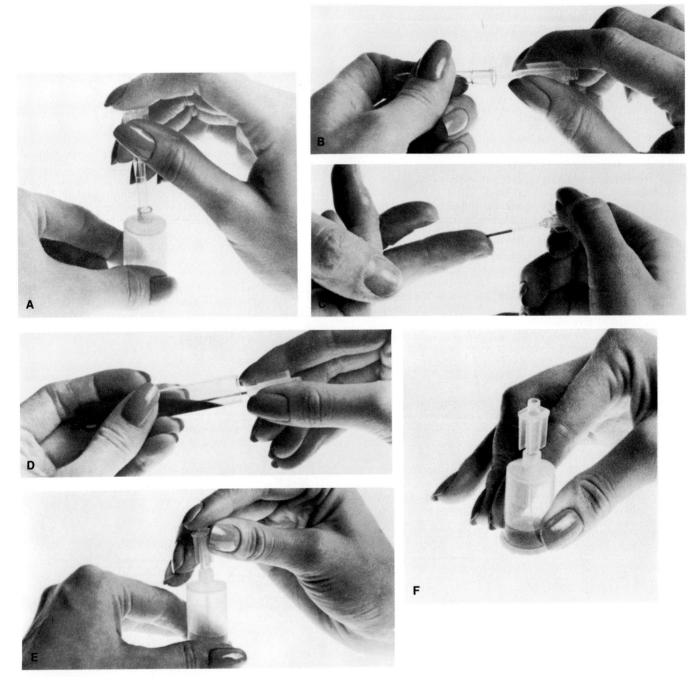

FIG. 25-4. Steps in the dilution of blood using the Unopette system. (**A**) Puncture diaphragm. (**B**) Remove shield from pipet assembly with a twist. (**C,D**) Draw sample into pipet from free-flowing skin puncture or tube. Remove excess blood on outside of pipet carefully with gauze. (**E**) Squeeze reservoir slightly to force out some air. Do not expel liquid. Cover opening of pipet overflow chamber with finger and seat pipet securely in reservoir neck. (**F**) Squeeze reservoir gently two or three times to rinse capillary bore, forcing diluent into, but not out of, overflow chamber.

view of the procedure is shown in Figure 25-4. Follow manufacturer's instructions carefully to ensure accurate results.

Preparing and Charging the Hemocytometer

Whether using a Thoma pipet or Unopette, the hemocytometer (Levy counting chamber with improved Neubauer ruling) is used to count the cells and must be scrupulously clean prior to use.

1. Just before using, always clean the hemocytometer and coverslip with distilled water followed by absolute methanol and dry thoroughly using only microscope lens paper to avoid leaving lint particles on cell counting grid area or coverslip. *Caution: Do not* use gauze for drying. It can scratch the grid surface. *Caution:* Carefully dry moat areas and do not allow fingers to touch any surface contacted by diluted specimen.
2. Place coverslip on hemocytometer so that it partially covers both V slashes (see Fig. 25-1).
3. Ensure that mixture in diluting pipet or Unopette is well mixed.
4. Charging from Thoma Diluting Pipet (follow instructions on package insert for charging from Unopette)
   a. Allow approximately one fourth of mixture in bulb to flow onto a waste cloth.
   b. Firmly place a *dry* finger over *dry* end of pipet to stop sample flow and place pipet tip on one of the hemocytometer V slashes at approximately a 30-degree angle. *Caution:* Do not disturb coverslip.
   c. Slowly release finger to allow mixture from bulb to flow evenly and completely under coverslip and over surface of ruled area. Be sure to fill area completely, but *do not* overfill or underfill.
   d. Use second dilution prepared in separate pipet to fill opposite side of hemocytometer and repeat loading procedure. Place hemocytometer in Petri dish and cover. Allow to stand for approximately 5 minutes to allow cells to settle.

Microscopic Cell-Counting Procedure

The cells included in the microscopic count of each square on the hemocytometer counting chamber are determined as illustrated in Figure 25-5. All cells touching any one of the triple lines at the top or left of the square being evaluated are counted. All cells touching any one of the triple lines at the bottom or to the right are excluded from the count. This convention is used to count any cellular element in any square of the hemocytometer. Standard areas of the counting chamber used for counting leukocytes (W), erythrocytes (R), and platelets (P) are illustrated in Figure 25-2. Though standard counting areas for these elements exist in modern laboratory practice, the actual areas counted vary

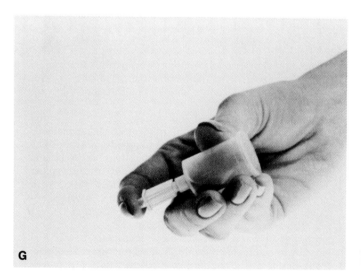

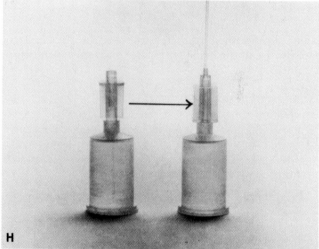

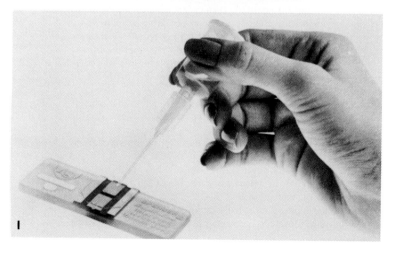

FIG. 25-4 (continued)
(**G**) Cover opening with finger and gently invert to mix. (**H**) Convert to dropper assembly. Mix well, invert, and expel first few drops of mixture on waste cloth. Maintain pressure on reservoir to avoid air bubbles. (**I**) Charge hemocytometer. (Courtesy Becton Dickinson Vacutainer Systems, Rutherford, NJ.)

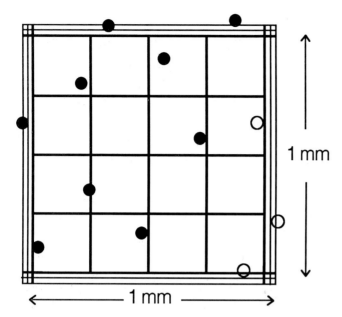

FIG. 25-5. Rules for microscopic counting of leukocytes on the Neubauer hemocytometer. One square millimeter is illustrated. Leukocytes are counted in eight of these 1-mm squares, four on each side of the hemocytometer. Leukocytes that touch the top or left triple boundary lines are counted; those that touch the bottom or right boundaries are not. (Solid circle, cells counted; open circle, cells not counted.)

widely. Professional laboratorians must be prepared to adapt the use of the hemocytometer to the specimen being examined.

MICROSCOPIC CELL COUNTING
Procedure

1. Rotate the low-power objective of the microscope into viewing position. *Caution:* This step is important to avoid damaging the hemocytometer and microscope objective lenses.
2. Carefully place hemocytometer on microscope stage. Move X/Y travel knobs so that center of one hemocytometer counting area is directly under objective.
3. To assist in focusing, move low-power objective as close as possible to hemocytometer, using coarse adjustment knob. *Do not force knob.*
4. While looking into oculars, turn coarse adjustment knob so that hemocytometer and low-power objective begin moving farther apart until grid lines come into focus. Leukocyte nuclei appear as slightly iridescent but not refractile objects. The cells should look like small dark or black dots. If necessary, adjust the light intensity or condenser to obtain an optimal field of view.
5. Using X/Y travel knob, move hemocytomer so that top left square of counting area is in center of field of view. This is where leukocyte count is begun.
6. Begin counting cells in upper left 1 × 1-mm square of ruled area.
7. For a standard leukocyte count, identify and count the cells over the four 1-mm² corners of each side of the hemocytometer (areas marked W in Fig. 25-2).
8. Calculate the number of leukocytes per liter for each side of the hemocytometer. Average the results and report this number.

Calculations

$$\text{Cells (x } 10^9/\text{L)} = \frac{\overset{\text{Total}}{\text{cells counted}} \times \overset{\text{Specimen}}{\text{dilution factor}}}{\text{mm}^2 \text{ counted} \times 0.1 \text{ mm}} \times 10^6$$

(*Note:* 0.1mm is the depth of fluid in chamber.) To calculate any dilution factor, set up this equation:

$$\frac{1}{\text{dilution}}$$

Example: 100 cells were counted on side A and 110 cells on side B in the four 1-mm² corners of the cell grid from a 1:20 dilution.

For this example, the dilution factor is then:

$$\frac{1}{1/20} = 20$$

$$\text{Side A} = \frac{100 \times 20}{4 \times 0.1} \times 10^6 = 5000 \times 10^6/\text{L} = 5.0 \times 10^9/\text{L}$$

$$\text{Side B} = \frac{110 \times 20}{4 \times 0.1} \times 10^6 = 5500 \times 10^6/\text{L} = 5.5 \times 10^9/\text{L}$$

$$\text{Average of} \atop \text{sides A and B} = \frac{(5.0 + 5.5)}{2} \times 10^9/\text{L} = 5.3 \times 10^9/\text{L} = \text{Final} \atop \text{WBC count}$$

In the past cell counts for blood and body fluids were reported in cells per cubic millimeter. It is now recommended that laboratories report these counts in SI units (Chap. 9), in which counts are reported as cells per liter (L), as in the formula above. By SI convention, cell counts are reported as illustrated in Table 25-2.

Quality Control

Quality control in manual counting is primarily a function of the technical expertise of the laboratorian. A quality control program for manual counts should monitor the following items:

Specimens must be checked individually for clots. Clotted specimens are unsuitable for counting any cellular element.

Diluting with either Thoma pipets or Unopettes must be done with scrupulous attention to technique. Only NBS Thoma pipets, which indicate on the stem the accuracy of pipet measurement (*i.e.,* ± 0.5%), should be used. Pipets with cracked or chipped tips should be discarded in a waste container designated for broken glass or sharp objects.

Only NBS hemocytometers should be used.

Levels of reservoir diluent in Unopettes should be checked visually to ensure that the volume appears correct. The reservoirs can be used only prior to their expiration date (check storage container for lot number and expiration date). Expired reservoirs are useful for practice.

Cells must be evenly distributed over the hemocytometer surface. For a standard leukocyte count within the reference

TABLE 25-2. Current SI Units Conversion from Former Reporting Units for Leukocytes (WBC), Erythrocytes (RBC), and Platelets (PLT)*

CELL TYPE	FORMER REPORTING UNITS	CURRENT REPORTING UNITS	FORMER EXAMPLE	CURRENT EXAMPLE
WBC	× 10³/mm³	× 10⁹/L	8.0 × 10³/mm³	8.0 × 10⁹/L
RBC	× 10⁶/mm³	× 10¹²/L	4.5 × 10⁶/mm³	4.5 × 10¹²/L
PLT	× 10³/mm³	× 10⁹/L	350 × 10³/mm³	350 × 10⁹/L

* The examples in the *Former* column are equivalent to those in the *Current* column.

range, there should be no more than a 15-cell difference between the highest and lowest total number of cells found among the eight 1-mm^2 corner squares counted.[6,19] For the standard erythrocyte count, the difference between the highest and lowest totals in the 10 0.04-mm^2 squares counted should be no more than 20. Counts that do not meet these standards should not be reported. Rather, the procedure should be repeated carefully using an acceptable, well mixed specimen.

Even with a skilled laboratorian and meticulous attention to detail, manual counting has a high percentage of error that cannot be avoided. This error is attributed to the small number of cells counted; the uncontrollable variation in cell distribution when the sample is loaded on the hemocytometer; the error in graduations of the pipet and hemocytometer; and various operator errors in the dilution process or loading process. For leukocyte counts, using a 1:20 dilution, the 95% confidence limits are approximately ±15%. For example, given a manual leukocyte count of 5.0×10^9/L performed using a 1:20 dilution, the 95% confidence limits for the count are approximately $5.0 \pm 0.8 \times 10^9$/L. For erythrocytes, the 95% confidence limits are generally ±20%. Given a hypothetical manual erythrocyte count of 5.0×10^{12}/L, the 95% confidence limits would be 4.0 to 6.0×10^{12}/L.

Leukocyte Reference Ranges

Each laboratory should determine its own population reference range (Chap. 46).

In 1952 the normal adult leukocyte reference range reported in one study was 4.5 to 11.0×10^9/L, based on manually counted samples.[2] Current published reference ranges are based on automated, electronically or optically counted samples.

Because leukocyte counts are age dependent, a single meaningful reference range cannot be established. Table 25-3 defines total leukocyte reference ranges as a function of age. These ranges were derived with automated cell counters. Other studies of absolute leukocyte reference ranges for adults have been published.[13,22] Many other factors cause variations in individual leukocyte counts, including time of day,[2,22] stress,[20] and exercise.[1] Black subjects consistently have lower reference ranges based on lower absolute neutrophil values.[7,15,31] (In one study of American blacks, a decreased neutrophil count was not evident.[13])

With more sophisticated automated instruments and greater care in selecting normal sample populations, the upper limit of the adult reference range may be lower than that based on manual counts.[25] With respect to lower limits, individual low values of 2.0×10^9/L in Caucasians and 1.5×10^9/L in blacks may be considered normal for certain individuals.

MANUAL DIFFERENTIAL CELL COUNTS

Performing differential cell counts is an art form. Skill is acquired only through practice based on a solid background of technical knowledge. Table 25-4 provides a summary of the steps required to perform a complete differential. These steps are discussed in detail below.

MANUAL DIFFERENTIAL CELL COUNTS
Principle

An appropriately prepared and stained blood film is systematically scanned microscopically to estimate leukocyte count, identify morphologic erythrocyte abnormalities, estimate platelet number, and classify leukocytes into group types.

Specimen Requirements

Whole unclotted blood is required for preparing the peripheral blood film. Fresh peripheral blood from a skin puncture is the specimen of choice for a manual differential count, but blood anticoagulated with an EDTA salt is used most often. EDTA is preferred since it prevents formation of artifacts and acceptably preserves blood for up to 3 hours. Use of an anticoagulant introduces certain morphologic changes in the leukocytes, which become increasingly exaggerated with storage time. Examples of these changes include vacuoles in the cytoplasm of granulocytes and karyorrhexis (nuclear disintegration). When final evaluations of blood films are made, the amount of time the cells were allowed to interact with EDTA before the films were prepared and stained should be taken into consideration.

Reagents and Equipment

The reagents and equipment for both manual and automated preparation and staining of peripheral blood films for manual differential counts are discussed in Chapter 3.

Microscope Preparation

Too often the microscope is taken for granted. Like other instruments, it requires daily performance checks. The Köehler

TABLE 25-3. Leukocyte Values in Man

AGE	TOTAL LEUKOCYTES ($\times 10^9$/L)	NEUTROPHILS			EOSINOPHILS	BASOPHILS	LYMPHOCYTES	MONOCYTES
		TOTAL	BAND	SEGMENTED				
12 hr	13.0–38.0	6.0–28.0	2.33★	13.2	0.02–0.95	0–0.5	2.0–11.0	0.40–3.6
		68%	10.2%	58%	2.0%	0.4%	31%	5.3%
1 wk	5.0–12.0	1.5–10.0	0.83	4.7	0.07–1.10	0–0.25	2.0–17.0	0.30–2.7
		45%	6.8%	39%	4.1%	0.4%	41%	4.8%
12 mo	6.0–17.5	1.5–8.5	0.35	3.2	0.05–0.70	0–0.2	4.0–10.5	0.05–1.1
		31%	3.1%	28%	2.6%	0.4%	61%	4.8%
6 yr	5.0–14.5	1.5–8.0	0–1.0	1.5–7.0	0–0.65	0–0.2	1.5–7.0	0.0–0.8
		51%	3.0%	48%	2.7%	0.6%	42%	4.7%
14 yr	4.5–13.0	1.8–8.0	0–1.0	1.8–7.0	0–0.50	0–0.2	1.2–5.8	0.0–0.8
		56%	3.0%	53%	2.5%	0.5%	37%	4.7%
21 yr	4.5–11.0	1.8–7.7	0–0.7	1.8–7.0	0–0.45	0–0.2	1.0–4.8	0.0–0.8
		59%	3.0%	56%	2.7%	0.5%	34%	4.0%

Values listed first for each age are absolute counts ($\times 10^9$/L); values listed second, as percentages, are relative counts.
★ Band count at 12 hours includes a small percentage of myelocytes.
(From Altman PL, Dittmer DS: Blood and Other Body Fluids, p 125. Bethesda, MD, Federation of American Societies for Experimental Biology, 1961, with permission.)

TABLE 25–4. Summary of Steps Required to Perform the Complete Differential Cell Count

Check Slide Identification
Perform Patient Specimen Orientation
Perform Low-Power (10×) Scan of the Blood Film
   Check Feather Edge for Fibrin Threads
   Examine Film Edges for Excessive Leukocytes
   Verify Acceptable Number of Leukocytes
   Verify Stain Quality
   Examine Erythrocyte Distribution Patterns and Shapes
Perform Oil Examination (100×) of the Blood Film
   Prepare Blood Film with Oil
   Estimate Platelet Count
   Estimate Leukocyte Count
   Perform Leukocyte Differential
      Classify 100 Leukocytes
      Report Results as Percentage of All Leukocytes
         Counted
      Keep Separate Count of NRBCs
      Note and Report Abnormal Leukocyte Morphology
      Grade Abnormal Erythrocyte Morphology
      Identify Miscellaneous Abnormal Cells

illumination procedure (Chap. 4) should be performed prior to each session with the microscope, particularly when performing differential counts, to ensure the best resolution and clarity in viewing hematopoietic cells.

Procedure

I. **Check slide identification.** Check blood film identification to ensure that film and automated count report identification match.

II. **Perform patient specimen orientation.** To become familiar with the patient specimen, carefully review the automated count report, noting the number of leukocytes and platelets, the number and size (MCV) of erythrocytes, and the hemoglobin concentration (MCHC) of erythrocytes. During the differential process, the above information is compared to the actual findings on the blood film. Any extreme discrepancy (e.g., a reference range platelet count on the automated report but only a rare platelet on the blood film) should be investigated immediately and resolved before the differential count is completed.

III. **Perform low-power scan to review blood film adequacy.**
  A. **Check feather edge (Fig. 25-6) for fibrin threads.** Fibrin threads may be present even in films made from specimens that do not contain gross clots. Fibrin threads tend to entrap larger leukocytes and are accompanied by platelet clumping. Neither a differential count nor a platelet estimate should be attempted on blood films that exhibit fibrin threads.
  B. **Examine film edges for excessive leukocytes.** The edges of even the best-prepared blood film have accumulations of granulocytes and monocytes, but in films that are spread too thin, most of the large cells are pushed to the film edges, leaving relatively more lymphocytes in the center. Blood film edges should contain less than 2 to 3 times more leukocytes than the number present in the body of the film.[21,30]
  C. **Verify acceptable number of leukocytes.** In a total leukocyte count of no less than 4.0×10^9/L, the acceptable working area should contain at least 300 leukocytes.[21] This may be quickly ascertained by someone experienced in scanning blood films.
  D. **Verify stain quality.** The stain should clearly distinguish between dark purple nuclear material and bright red–orange erythrocytes (Chap. 3).

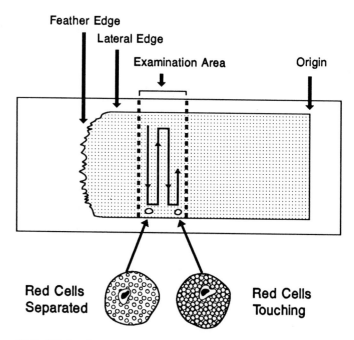

FIG. 25-6.   Illustration of a properly made push wedge peripheral blood film showing the battlement pattern for leukocyte differential procedure.

  E. **Examine erythrocyte distribution patterns and shapes.** Erythrocytes normally repel one another. In the examination area of a well prepared blood film, the erythrocytes should be distributed evenly and singly (or just slightly overlapping) in at least a lateral strip along the thinner end of the blood film. The cells should not be distorted. This strip should be the diameter of one low-power field. In the presence of abnormal serum globulins the erythrocytes may assume rouleaux formations (Chap. 8). In the presence of certain antibodies to RBC surface antigens (e.g., cold agglutinins), erythrocyte clumping or agglutination may be seen. The presence of either rouleaux or agglutination should be indicated on the differential report (Chap. 8).

  The presence of certain abnormal erythrocyte shapes can be readily detected under low-power scan (e.g., target cells, sickle cells, spherocytes). The many types of anisocytosis and poikilocytosis that should be indicated on the differential report are discussed in Chapter 8.

IV. **Perform oil-immersion examination of the blood film**
  A. **Prepare blood film with oil.** Evenly spread a thin layer of nondrying type B immersion oil over the blood film in the examination area toward the feather edge. Use oil sparingly and never substitute other types of lubricants for immersion oil, since substitutes may damage optical lenses.
  B. **Calculate ratio of electronic platelet count to platelets per oil-immersion field.** Before platelet estimates can be performed, the laboratory must calculate the ratio of the electronic platelet count to the number of platelets per oil-immersion (or high-power) field of view. This must be done once for every microscope brand in the laboratory used for platelet estimates owing to slight differences in the field of view of the various microscope brands. Once this ratio is calculated, it may be used to determine an estimation factor

for platelet estimates that may be used until there are major repairs or changes to the instrument used to obtain the electronic platelet counts or until a new microscope is used for the estimates. Any major changes of this nature warrant a close check of the current ratio, and possibly recalculation of the ratio, particularly when new equipment is introduced. The procedure for calculation of this ratio and estimation factor is as follows:

1. Perform electronic platelet counts on 30 consecutive fresh patient blood samples. Make sure the platelet count is in control.
2. Prepare and stain one peripheral blood film for each sample.
3. For each film, under oil immersion microscopy, find an area where 50% of the red cells are overlapping in doublets or triplets. Then count the number of platelets in 10 consecutive fields.
4. Divide the total number of platelets found by 10 to obtain the average number per single oil-immersion field.

5. Divide the electronic platelet count by the average number of platelets per oil field.
6. Add the numbers obtained in step 5 and divide by 30 (the number of observations in this analysis) to obtain the average ratio of the platelet count:platelets per oil-immersion field.
7. Round the number calculated in step 6 to the nearest whole number to obtain an estimation factor, the number of peripheral blood platelets represented by one platelet in an oil-immersion field.

Table 25-5 provides an example of this calculation. Each laboratory should perform this calculation using its own microscope and electronic equipment.

C. **Estimate platelet count.** Once the platelet estimation factor is calculated (step 7), the laboratory scientist may simply calculate the average number of platelets per oil-immersion field on all subsequent specimens and multiply this number by the estimation factor to obtain the platelet estimate. For example, in the hypothetical

---

TABLE 25–5. Calculation of the Platelet Count Estimation Factor★

SAMPLE NUMBER	ELECTRONIC PLATELET COUNT ($\times 10^9$/L)	AVERAGE NO. PLATELETS PER OIL IMMERSION FIELD (BASED ON 10 FIELDS)	ELECTRONIC PLATELET COUNT DIVIDED BY AVERAGE NO. PLATELETS PER OIL IMMERSION FIELD
1	252	17.1	14.737
2	301	24.1	12.490
3	282	18.6	15.161
4	60	4.0	15.000
5	257	16.8	15.298
6	388	26.1	14.866
7	290	18.9	15.344
8	246	15.9	15.472
9	450	29.1	15.464
10	56	4.1	13.659
11	10	0.8	12.500
12	312	19.3	16.166
13	252	16.2	15.556
14	90	5.8	15.517
15	136	8.6	15.814
16	298	21.0	14.190
17	362	22.9	15.808
18	95	5.8	16.379
19	280	18.3	15.301
20	157	12.0	13.083
21	240	15.5	15.484
22	200	12.8	15.625
23	15	1.5	10.000
24	281	18.9	14.868
25	195	13.5	14.444
26	198	13.1	15.115
27	71	4.4	16.136
28	262	18.1	14.475
29	328	21.3	15.399
30	188	12.9	14.574

$$\frac{443.925}{30} \quad \frac{SUM}{n} = 14.798 \approx 15.0$$

Therefore: 1 platelet per oil field $\approx 15.0 \times 10^9$/L

★ Due to slight differences in the field of view, this must be done for each microscope brand (e.g., Nikon, American Optical, Olympus) used in the laboratory, to obtain accurate peripheral film platelet estimates. This table presents sample platelet estimate data from a hospital laboratory showing platelet counts obtained from a Coulter Model S Plus IV and manual platelet counts obtained from peripheral blood films under oil immersion microscopy using the laboratory's own microscope brand. The ratio of platelet count to platelets per oil immersion field was calculated and the average of these ratios was taken to determine the actual number of peripheral blood platelets represented by one platelet on an oil immersion field.

laboratory represented in Table 25-5, if the average number of platelets found for any given sample on oil immersion fields is 17, the platelet estimate calculation would be:

$$17 \times 15 \times 10^9/L = 255 \times 10^9/L$$

The following guidelines are provided to facilitate platelet estimates:

1. The approximate reference range for platelets is 140 to $440 \times 10^9/L$.
2. There are approximately 10 to 40 red cells per platelet in normal peripheral blood. Thus, an oil-immersion field (1000 × magnification) containing 100 red cells should have three to 10 platelets, whereas a field with 200 red cells should have five to 20 platelets.
3. As with leukocyte estimates, platelet estimates in the presence of abnormal hematocrit values tend to be inaccurate.
4. Accurate estimates are possible only when there are no platelet clumps, or at most, rare clumps of two to three platelets. Larger or more numerous platelet clumps cause inaccurate estimates. If clumps are noted, the original blood specimen should be reexamined for clots. If clots are not found, platelet clumping in the presence of EDTA should be suspected and noted on the specimen report.
5. Platelet estimate reports and leukocyte differential count reports should also indicate the presence of large or morphologically abnormal platelets. Because of their size they may be counted by automated counting instruments as erythrocytes or even lymphocytes, and the result would be an inaccurate platelet total.
6. If different brands of microscopes are used in the same laboratory, they may have different field-of-view diameters, so a correction factor is required to calculate all counts performed on the microscope with the larger (or smaller) field of view to ensure consistency in reporting (Chap. 4). Otherwise, the estimation factor should be calculated for each microscope brand used in any given laboratory (see Table 25-5) and used appropriately for platelet estimates.

D. **Estimate leukocyte count.** Total leukocyte counts can be estimated roughly under either high-power scan (400 ×) or oil-immersion microscopy (1000 ×). The same procedure described in Table 25-5 for platelets can be applied to determining a calibration factor for leukocyte count estimates. Leukocyte count estimates should always be a part of the differential count, to verify the automated leukocyte count. Many laboratories report the estimated blood film leukocyte count only as low, normal, or high. In general, this is the best practice, since it is difficult to estimate the leukocyte count very accurately. Experience is the biggest factor in being able to perform leukocyte estimates accurately and consistently.

An accurate estimate depends on an acceptable anticoagulated specimen free from clots; a well prepared blood film; a well trained laboratory scientist; and development and use of a calibration factor appropriate for the microscope in use. A calibration factor must be determined for each microscope brand used in the laboratory. If there are any questions about the accuracy of an automated leukocyte count when it is compared to the estimate, the specimen identification should be rechecked, the automated count should be repeated, and

a new blood film should be prepared and evaluated. A manual count may also be performed if necessary.

Estimates should never be attempted without a knowledge of the hematocrit value of the specimen from which the film was made. As the hematocrit increases, the leukocyte estimate tends to be falsely decreased; as the hematocrit decreases, the leukocyte estimate tends to be falsely increased. Leukocytes should be evenly distributed over the examination area. Leukocyte clumping or the presence of endothelial or epithelial cells should be included in the comments of the differential count report.

E. **Perform differential leukocyte count.**
1. Classify 100 leukocytes. Leukocyte differentiation involves the counting and morphologic classification of 100 leukocytes reviewed while using a specific search pattern in the appropriate examination area of a blood film. The "battlement" track method is used to count leukocytes (see Fig. 25-6).[21] Each intact leukocyte must be classified, including distorted cells that can be clearly identified (e.g., fragile eosinophils). Skipping cells that are unfamiliar skews the results and is inaccurate and unacceptable practice. Chapters 23 and 24 present a detailed description of the appearance of mature and immature leukocytes.
2. Report results of the 100 cells classified as a percentage. These results are considered *relative* cell counts. For example, if 60 neutrophils were found among 100 leukocytes counted, this would be reported as 60% neutrophils. When manual differential counters are used, the technologist must verify that the sum of the percentages equals 100%.
3. Keep separate count of nucleated red blood cells (NRBCs). NRBCs are counted separately while classifying the 100 leukocytes. They should be reported as the number per 100 leukocytes counted. If more than 5 NRBCs are found per 100 leukocytes, the automated leukocyte count must be corrected, because NRBCs, being as large as small leukocytes, erroneously elevate the automated leukocyte count. The calculation for correction of the leukocyte count when NRBCs are present is discussed below in the section on Calculations.
4. Note and report abnormal leukocyte morphology. Leukocytes may appear abnormal or demonstrate inclusions, which must be noted on the differential count report. For example, toxic granulation in neutrophils is an indication of infection or chemical toxicity. Döhle bodies are an example of neutrophil inclusions which are associated with severe bacterial infections—and rarely, with platelet abnormalities. The many abnormal morphologic features that may occur are reviewed in Chapters 26 through 28.
5. Identify and grade abnormal erythrocyte morphology. Erythrocyte morphology is observed first under low-power scan for major abnormalities. It should be observed also during leukocyte differentiation, and finally, as a separate evaluation under oil immersion microscopy. Though abnormalities of erythrocyte shape and size may be observed under low power, erythrocyte inclusions such as malaria, basophilic stippling, Howell-Jolly bodies, and others can be visualized with certainty only by using oil-immersion microscopy (Chap. 8).
6. Identify and report in the differential comments any miscellaneous nonleukocyte abnormal cells, such as endothelial cells, basket cells, or NRBCs, that are

found during the differential. Such cells are not included in the 100-cell leukocyte differential count. Table 25-6 provides a description of well known miscellaneous cells and the normal and abnormal conditions under which they are found.

Quality Control for Differential Cell Counts

As for manual cell counts, quality control for differentials is basically a function of the expertise, alertness, and attention to detail of the laboratorian; however, when differentials are performed in an institution by a group of laboratorians, the following steps should be taken to ensure uniform reporting within the group:

Agree on the definition of all terms used (e.g., variant or atypical lymphocyte, Downey cell, Turk cell).

Establish 95% confidence limits within the group for differential performance and reporting (Table 25-7). This should be done on a cell-by-cell basis. Whenever available, a cell count from a properly calibrated automated instrument that counts large numbers of cells should be used as the true value. For example, if five technologists each perform a 100-cell differential on the same blood film, and the true number of peripheral blood lymphocytes according to the instrument count is 8%, then the reported value of each technologist, according to Table 25-7, should be between 3% and 16% lymphocytes.

This ensures that all personnel are reporting differential results within the 95% confidence limits. The automated three-part differential count, which includes granulocytes, lymphocytes, and monocytes, can be used as the mean or observed value "a" in Table 25-7, to establish confidence limits for manual differentials. Note in Table 25-7 that, as more cells are differentiated, the confidence interval range becomes tighter (i.e., the differential count becomes more accurate).

Regularly circulate unfamiliar slides among the group members and compare results with established confidence limits.

Establish a required level of accuracy that new laboratory personnel must achieve before being cleared to report differential count results.

Establish a list of abnormalities, which, if observed on the differential study, must be reviewed by the supervisor or clinical pathologist before results are reported (e.g., presence of blasts or any unclassified cells).

Calculations for Correction of Leukocyte Count in the Presence of Nucleated Erythrocytes

When more than five nucleated red blood cells are found during a 100-leukocyte differential count, correction of the

TABLE 25–6. Miscellaneous Cells That May Be Found During the Peripheral Blood Film Differential Count*

CELL TYPE	DESCRIPTION	NORMAL CONDITIONS UNDER WHICH CELLS ARE FOUND	ABNORMAL CONDITIONS UNDER WHICH CELLS ARE FOUND
Smudge cells	Nuclear remnants of lymphocytes; formed during blood film preparation. Appearance is similar to a thumbprint. Chromatin is structureless.	A few may be found normally	Disease characterized by abnormal proliferation of lymphocytes (e.g., chronic lymphocytic leukemia)
Basket cells	Nuclear remnants of granulocytic cells with netlike chromatin pattern; formed during blood film preparation.	A few may be found normally	Some leukemias
Necrotic cells	Granulocytic cells with pyknotic nuclei and an agranular cytoplasm	None	Prolonged exposure to EDTA; chemotherapy (rarely)
Phagocytic cells	Neutrophil that has engulfed foreign substance (e.g., bacteria, fungus)	None	Overwhelming septicemia, bacterial and fungal infections, erythrophagocytosis in which neutrophil engulfs RBC
Endothelial cells	These large cells (20–30 μm), which line the veins, often have a stretched, ovoid appearance. They have a single nucleus with dense chromatin and no nucleoli. Cytoplasm is abundant and appears translucent. Cells may appear in sheets. Usually found at feather edge; distinctive appearance when compared to blood cells.	Found occasionally in blood obtained by venipuncture	This cell is considered a contaminant of venipuncture. It must not be confused with clumps of malignant cells.
Megakaryocyte fragments	Medium to large, nude nuclei that stain dark purple.	Newborns	Aberrant platelet production, myelofibrosis, essential thrombocythemia
Nucleated red blood cells (NRBCs)	Varies according to cell maturity (see Chap. 6). Usually no attempt is made to classify the maturity of NRBCs; they are only counted, and the number per 100 WBC is reported.	Newborns	NRBCs may be found in many abnormal conditions (e.g., hemolysis, leukemia, myeloproliferative disorders, and others)

* These cells are not counted as part of the 100 leukocytes but should be mentioned in the comments when they are observed.

TABLE 25–7. Confidence Limits* for Percentages of Specific Cell Types Identified by Manual Differential Counts

a (OBSERVED PERCENTAGE OF SPECIFIC CELL TYPE)	n (TOTAL CELLS COUNTED IN DIFFERENTIAL)			
	100	200	500	1000
0	0 4	0 2	0 1	0 1
1	0 6	0 4	0 3	0 2
2	0 8	0 6	0 4	1 4
3	0 9	1 7	1 5	2 5
4	1 10	1 8	2 7	2 6
5	1 12	2 10	3 8	3 7
6	2 13	3 11	4 9	4 8
7	2 14	3 12	4 10	5 9
8	3 16	4 13	5 11	6 10
9	4 17	5 14	6 12	7 11
10	4 18	6 16	7 13	8 13
15	8 24	10 21	11 19	12 18
20	12 30	14 27	16 24	17 23
25	16 35	19 32	21 30	22 28
30	21 40	23 37	26 35	27 33
35	25 46	28 43	30 40	32 39
40	30 51	33 48	35 45	36 44
45	35 56	38 53	40 50	41 49
50	39 61	42 58	45 55	46 54

*Confidence coefficient, 95%.

Example: If 6% monocytes were identified in a 100-cell differential ($n = 100$), there is a confidence coefficient of 95% that the true value is between 2% and 13% and a 5% chance that it is not.

For a over 50, obtain confidence limits by reading limits for $100 - a$ in the table and subtracting them from 100.

Example: The 95% confidence limits for 75% neutrophils counted in a sample where 100 cells were counted ($n = 100$) are between 65% and 84%.

(From Rumke CL: Variability of results in differential counts on blood smears. Triangle, Sandoz Journal of Medical Science 4:156, 1960, Copyright Sandoz Ltd, Basle, Switzerland, with permission.)

automated leukocyte count is necessary. The correction calculation is as follows:

$$\frac{WBC \times 10^9/L \times 100}{NRBC\ per\ 100\ leukocytes + 100} = corrected\ WBC\ count$$

For example, given a WBC count of $24.0 \times 10^9/L$ and an NRBC count of 20/100 WBC,

$$\frac{24.0 \times 10^9/L \times 100}{20 + 100} = 20.0 \times 10^9/L,\ the\ corrected\ WBC\ count.$$

Calculation of Absolute and Relative Cell Counts

Performance of the routine leukocyte differential count yields results in terms of relative cell counts (*i.e.*, the percentage of total leukocytes represented by a specific cell type). Table 25-8 provides examples of how to convert relative cell counts to "indirect" absolute cell counts. The formula follows:

$$Indirect\ relative\ cell\ count \times \frac{Total\ WBC}{count} = \frac{Absolute}{cell\ count}$$

The percentage of each cell group observed on the differential is used in this formula to obtain the indirect absolute cell count for each cell type. The results should be compared to the established laboratory reference range. Table 25-3 pro-

vides a sample reference range chart for absolute leukocyte counts.

This calculation is referred to as the indirect absolute cell count because it is only an estimate of the actual number of cells per liter of any given cell type. The direct absolute cell count requires actually counting each cell type, either manually or by automated methods.

Absolute cell counts provide much more accurate assessments of the actual number of each cell type in the peripheral blood. As automated counting of specific cell types becomes more universal, absolute values are becoming the standard reporting format. Note in Table 25-8 two different specimens with the same "normal" differential count results. One has a leukocyte count of $8.0 \times 10^9/L$, which is within the adult reference range, and the other has a leukocyte count of $2.0 \times 10^9/L$, which is below the reference range. Calculation of the absolute neutrophil and lymphocyte counts reveals that, although the differential results appear normal for both, the specimen with the $2.0 \times 10^9/L$ leukocyte count indicates an absolute decrease in neutrophils and lymphocytes in the peripheral blood.

Leukocyte Differential Count Reference Ranges

Table 25-3 provides a relative mean leukocyte number for each normal leukocyte type for subjects ranging in age from newborn through adult. Ranges are shown for absolute counts. Table 25-9 provides a sample range for the leukocyte differential count in terms of relative numbers based on data from 507 healthy adults.[33] Each laboratory should develop its own reference range for the differential count. Relative cell counts should always be considered in terms of the total leukocyte count (*i.e.*, converted to an absolute count) for proper interpretation of the results, as discussed above.

Comments and Sources of Error

Although morphologic evaluation of a stained blood film is one of the most important hematologic procedures, the manual differentiation of leukocytes is an inaccurate and unreproducible method that is subject to errors that cannot be totally eliminated, including sampling errors, uncontrollable errors in cell distribution on the blood film, and human inconsistency in cell interpretation.

Certain cell types, particularly eosinophils and basophils, may be distributed in a nonrandom manner on a blood film. High percentages of these cell types, especially if found in a limited area of the film, should be rechecked before the numbers are reported.

Differential counts on leukocyte numbers in excess of $35.0 \times 10^9/L$ should be performed on 200 cells. As the leukocyte total rises, the total number of leukocytes counted should increase proportionally to ensure sampling from a sufficiently large portion of the examination area.

As leukocyte totals drop below $2.0 \times 10^9/L$, differential counts may be performed on fewer than 100 cells; however, when fewer cells are counted, the precision of the differential decreases tremendously (see Table 25-7), and counting fewer than 100 cells is acceptable only if it is absolutely unavoidable. If fewer than 100 cells are counted, the number of cells counted should be converted to 100% using the appropriate factor. For example, if only 25 cells are counted, each cell type identified should be multiplied by 4 to convert the 25 cell-differential to a 100-cell differential.

A note of the *actual* number of cells counted *must* be included in the differential report if more than 100 or fewer than 100 cells are counted; however, the differential should be converted to 100% for reporting purposes unless the laboratory manager directs otherwise.

For differentials on samples with a low leukocyte count, buffy coat preparations, in which leukocytes are concentrated before being spread on a glass slide, are sometimes used (Chap. 3). Buffy coat preparations have several drawbacks because the preparation method causes morphologic changes in the leukocytes and uneven distribution of cell types, and the procedure is somewhat time consuming.

Because of their life-threatening implications, certain blood film findings may have to be reported immediately to the attending physician: schistocytes, which may indicate a hemolytic condition; blast forms (if never or not recently reported in the patient); neutrophilic phagocytosis of microorganisms indicating the presence of systemic infection; sickle cells; and erythrocytic microorganisms, among others. Laboratory policies and procedures should clearly indicate which findings demand immediate reporting to the physician after confirmation by a supervisor or clinical pathologist.

ABSOLUTE EOSINOPHIL COUNTING PROCEDURE[26]

Occasionally, an absolute eosinophil count is still requested for diagnostic purposes because it may be more accurate and clinically meaningful to determine the absolute number of eosinophils in a volume of blood than to determine the relative number from the differential count. Decreased eosinophil numbers (eosinopenia) are associated with hyperadrenalism (Cushing's disease). Eosinophil numbers increase (eosinophilia) with allergic reactions, parasitic infestations, brucellosis, and certain leukemias.

Absolute eosinophil counts may be direct or indirect.

TABLE 25–9. Total Leukocyte Count and Relative Leukocyte Count Reference Ranges for Adults*

Total Leukocytes	$4.1–10.9 \times 10^9$/L
Neutrophils	47.0–79.5%
Lymphocytes	12.5–40.0
Monocytes	2.0–11.0
Eosinophils	0.0–7.5
Basophils	0.0–2.0

* Counts are based on analysis of blood from 507 healthy adults. Although not shown in this table, bands may also normally be seen in the peripheral blood (approximately 0.0 to 6.0%). These ranges will vary; therefore, each laboratory must determine its own reference ranges. Other chapters in this text list slightly different reference ranges for these cell types to emphasize the variance that normally exists in studies of different individuals from institution to institution. (From Zacharski LR, Elveback LR, Linman JW: Leukocyte counts in healthy adults. Am J Clin Pathol 56:148, 1971, with permission).

Calculation of the indirect count was discussed earlier and generally is used simply to verify the direct absolute count. The direct count procedure, to be discussed here, is similar to that of a manual leukocyte or erythrocyte count performed using a hemocytometer and microscope, but it is recommended that an automated method (*e.g.*, Technicon H-1, or a five-part differential instrument) be used, if at all possible, to obtain absolute eosinophil counts.

ABSOLUTE EOSINOPHIL COUNTS
Principle

Using a suitably diluted specimen and appropriate stain, eosinophils can be identified and counted microscopically, after specimen is loaded on a hemocytometer. Phloxine in the stain causes eosinophils to appear red under light microscopy. Red blood cells are lysed by propylene glycol in the diluting fluid. Heparin, if present in the diluting fluid, inhibits leukocyte clumping. Sodium carbonate enhances eosinophil granule staining. The count is reported in terms of cells per liter.

Specimen

Whole blood is anticoagulated with any dry anticoagulant, such as EDTA or heparin, which does not interfere with the action of the stain or diluent used to prepare the specimen. Skin puncture blood samples may also be used.

TABLE 25–8. Example of Conversion of Relative Cell Counts Obtained from Two Sample Leukocyte Differentials to Indirect Absolute Cell Counts*

	RELATIVE CELL COUNT (%)	×	TOTAL LEUKOCYTE COUNT ($\times 10^9$/L)	=	ABSOLUTE CELL COUNT ($\times 10^9$/L)	ADULT REFERENCE RANGE ($\times 10^9$/L)
PATIENT A SAMPLE: "NORMAL" DIFFERENTIAL WITH LEUKOCYTE COUNT IN REFERENCE RANGE						
Neutrophils	75%		8.0		6.0	1.8–7.7
Lymphocytes	18%		8.0		1.4	1.0–4.8
Monocytes	6%		8.0		0.5	0.0–0.8
Eosinophils	1%		8.0		0.1	0.0–0.45
PATIENT B SAMPLE: "NORMAL" DIFFERENTIAL WITH LEUKOCYTE COUNT BELOW REFERENCE RANGE						
Neutrophils	75%		2.0		1.5	1.8–7.7
Lymphocytes	18%		2.0		0.4	1.0–4.8
Monocytes	6%		2.0		0.1	0.0–0.8
Eosinophils	1%		2.0		0.02	0.0–0.45

* Both relative and absolute counts must be compared to laboratory reference ranges. Absolute counts provide a more accurate assessment of the types of leukocytes present in the peripheral blood as shown by comparison of the "normal" differential in a sample with a leukocyte count within the reference range to the exact same "normal" differential from a patient with a leukocyte count below the reference range. Note that comparison of the absolute values to the reference ranges shows that the neutrophils and lymphocytes are within the reference range for patient A but they are both below the reference range for patient B.

Reagents

A prepared kit is available that utilizes the Unopette system (Becton Dickinson, Rutherford, NJ)[5] for absolute eosinophil counts. The reservoir contains phloxine B solution in propylene glycol and distilled water. A 25-μL capillary pipet is used to aspirate the blood sample and make a 1:32 dilution in the reservoir. Alternatively, stains, including Pilot's solution or Randolph's stain, may be prepared by the laboratory as described elsewhere.[26]

Equipment

Thoma WBC diluting pipet (or eosinophil Unopette reservoir and 25-μL pipet).

A special hemocytometer with a larger counting volume than that of the Neubauer should be used for eosinophil counts. Either the Fuchs-Rosenthal or Speirs-Levy hemocytometer is acceptable.

Fuchs-Rosenthal hemocytometer (Fig. 25-7). This hemocytometer has two ruled areas each consisting of one 4 × 4-mm square. The hemocytometer's depth is 0.2 mm. Total volume in each ruled area is therefore (16 mm^2 × 0.2 mm) or 3.2 mm^3. Total volume that may be counted on the chamber is (2 × 3.2 mm^3) or 6.4 mm^3.

Speirs-Levy hemocytometer (Fig. 25-8). This hemocytometer has four counting areas, each consisting of ten 1 × 1-mm squares in two horizontal rows of five squares. Hemocytometer depth is 0.2 mm. Total volume of each counting area is (10 × 1 mm^2 × 0.2 mm) or 2.0 mm^3. Total volume that may be counted on the chamber is (4 × 2.0 mm^3) or 8 mm^3. Either two or all four counting areas may be counted during the procedure.

Quality Control

Quality control of eosinophil counts is similar to that for routine leukocyte counts. In addition, the manual absolute eosinophil count may be checked by performing a manual differential count and obtaining the automated total leukocyte count and calculating the indirect absolute eosinophil count (see Comments and Sources of Error).

Procedure

1. Make a 1:10 dilution by drawing well mixed blood to the 1.0 mark of WBC Thoma pipet and adding eosinophil stain

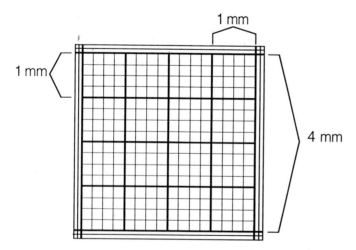

FIG. 25-7.   One ruled area of a Fuchs-Rosenthal hemocytometer. This special hemocytometer has two such counting areas, each with 16 1-mm^2 areas for increased accuracy of eosinophil and basophil counting. Chamber depth is 0.2 mm, so total volume is 6.4 mm^3 (0.2 mm × 16 mm^2 × 2 counting areas).

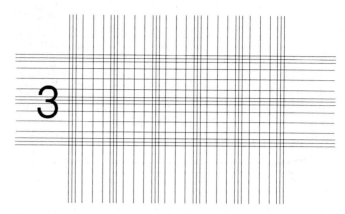

FIG. 25-8.   One counting area of a Speirs-Levy hemocytometer. This special hemocytometer has four such counting areas, each with ten 1-mm squares arranged in two horizontal rows of five. Eosinophils or basophils may be counted using this chamber. Chamber depth is 0.2 mm, so total volume is 8 mm^3 (0.2 mm × 10 mm^2 × 4 counting areas). An identification number engraved on the left side of each counting area and visible under the microscope facilitates orderly counting.

diluent to the 11 mark, using the exact procedure described for leukocyte counts. Alternatively, use a 25-μL pipet to aspirate the specimen and dilute in eosinophil Unopette reservoir to make a 1:32 dilution. If using Unopette method, follow manufacturer's instructions for further processing. If using Thoma pipet method, make a duplicate dilution. Mix both pipets for approximately 2 minutes.

2. Expel first four drops of mixture onto waste cloth and fill one side of counting chamber (if using Speirs-Levy chamber, fill both platforms of one side). Repeat the procedure using the other pipet for the opposite side of the chamber.

3. Place filled counting chamber into moist Petri dish. Allow 15 to 20 minutes for cells to settle, red cells to lyse, and eosinophils to stain.

4. Count eosinophils under low-power (10 ×) objective. Eosinophils stain reddish orange. Count the following areas, depending on which type hemocytometer is used. For Fuchs-Rosenthal hemocytometer, count entire ruled area on both sides of counting chamber. This yields the number of eosinophils in a total volume of 6.4 mm^3. For Speirs-Levy hemocytometer, count entire ruled area of two counting platforms on opposite sides of the hemocytometer. This yields the number of eosinophils in a volume of 4 mm^3. Alternatively, count all four platforms for a volume of 8 mm^3. For Neubauer hemocytometer, count entire ruled area on both sides of counting chamber. This gives a total volume counted of 1.8 mm^3.

Calculations of Absolute Direct Eosinophil Count

Eosinophils ($\times 10^9$/L) =

$$\frac{\text{Eosinophil count} \times \text{Dilution factor}}{\text{Volume counted (mm}^3)} \times 10^6$$

Below are examples of calculations using both types of hemocytometers. For each type, a sample calculation is given for the Unopette method and the Thoma WBC pipet method. Examples using Fuchs-Rosenthal hemocytometer:

Unopette $\dfrac{40 \times 32}{6.4} \times 10^6/L = 0.2 \times 10^9/L$

Thoma WBC Pipet $\dfrac{64 \times 10}{6.4} \times 10^6/\text{L} = 0.1 \times 10^9/\text{L}$

Examples using Speirs-Levy hemocytometer:

Unopette $\dfrac{50 \times 32}{4.0} \times 10^6/\text{L} = 0.4 \times 10^9/\text{L}$

Thoma WBC Pipet $\dfrac{70 \times 10}{4.0} \times 10^6/\text{L} = 0.2 \times 10^9/\text{L}$

Absolute Eosinophil Reference Range

The approximate reference range for adults is 0.0 to 0.45 × $10^9/\text{L}$ (0–450/mm^3). Table 25-3 presents sample ranges for various ages.[3] Each laboratory should determine its own reference range.

Comments and Sources of Error[6]

If a Thoma pipet and the Neubauer hemocytometer are used, there is an inherent error in the method of approximately 30%. Using a Thoma pipet and either the Speirs-Levy or Fuchs-Rosenthal chambers, the error is reduced to approximately 20%.[6]

Because the indirect absolute eosinophil calculation is not as accurate as that from the direct method, the results of the two calculations may not correlate very closely.

If oxalated blood is used, it must be diluted with the proper stain within 4 hours of being collected.

The Absolute Eosinophil Count and the Thorn Test

In the past, the Thorn Test was used to test adrenocortical function; however, it is rarely, if ever, used today. A short description is provided here for historical purposes only. The test involved a direct absolute eosinophil count. First, a specimen was drawn to calculate the fasting absolute eosinophil count. Next, the patient was given an injection of adrenocorticotropic horomone (ACTH). Four hours later, a second specimen was drawn for calculation of the absolute eosinophil count. With normal adrenocortical function, the second absolute count was expected to be at least 50% less than the fasting count. Fasting and 4-hour counts of approximately equal value indicated hypoadrenalism, in which the adrenal cortex is unable to respond to ACTH.

ABSOLUTE BASOPHIL COUNTING PROCEDURE[9]

Direct absolute basophil counts occasionally are requested for diagnostic purposes, as the indirect absolute count derived from the differential count is not very reliable, the differential reference range for basophils being 0% to 2%. This count may be used to confirm basophilia, an increase in the basophil count. It also may indicate basopenia, a decrease in the basophil count. Basophilia is associated with chronic myelogenous leukemia, polycythemia vera, myelofibrosis, myxedema, colitis, and sometimes chronic hemolytic anemia. Basopenia often occurs with allergic reactions. Refer to Cooper[9] for details on this seldom performed procedure, which calls for Cooper and Cruickshank stain and counting stained basophils on a Fuchs-Rosenthal or Speirs-Levy hemocytometer.

Absolute Basophil Reference Range

The approximate reference range for adults is 0.0 to 0.2 × $10^9/\text{L}$ (0–200/mm^3). Table 25-3 presents sample ranges for patients of various ages.[3] Each laboratory should determine its own reference range if possible.

Comments[9]

Counts may be completed in approximately 10 minutes with the method of Cooper; 30 to 60 minutes are required for methods described before that of Cooper. Blood dilution is stable, staining is fast, and counts may be performed up to 1 week after the mixture is prepared.

CONSIDERATIONS IN EVALUATING LEUKOCYTES FROM PEDIATRIC PATIENTS

Pediatric reference ranges for leukocytes and the morphologic appearance of children's leukocytes deserve special consideration because they are different from those of adults. A number of textbooks are available on the subject of normal and abnormal pediatric hematology.[18, 24]

The reference range of newborns' total leukocyte count is higher than for any other time of life (see Table 25-3). Although it declines significantly within 1 week, the high side of the reference range remains above that of adults into the teenage years.

One of the most striking features on the blood film of a newborn is the normal presence of nucleated red blood cells. There may be as many as 24 per 100 leukocytes differentiated, but normally they are seen only during the first few days of life.

Immature leukocytes are also typical on the newborn's blood film. Usually there is a shift to the left (Chap. 26), which reflects the finding of immature granulocytes, including metamyelocytes, myelocytes, and occasionally, a promyelocyte.[16] These immature cells generally disappear within the first few days of life.

Table 25-3 presents the leukocyte reference ranges in terms of absolute and relative numbers for various age groups. Note that 12 hours after birth, the absolute neutrophil and monocyte counts can be higher than at any other age. Within 2 weeks, however, the neutrophil count may drop to within normal adult ranges.[23] Monocytes are increased during the first year of life but are normal thereafter.[32] Eosinophil counts may be higher during the first year of life than at any other time, but also decline gradually with age.[10] No significance has been detected in the relationship of basophil counts and age.[32]

Note also that the absolute lymphocyte count at birth may be higher than that of adolescents and adults. Seven days after birth, the count may actually be higher than it was at birth, and this elevation may persist into the first year of life. The count begins to decline gradually with increasing age, although even teenagers may normally have a higher absolute lymphocyte count than adults.

Of particular interest in the pediatric differential count is evaluation of the lymphocytes, which can be baffling. There may be many variations in the appearance, size, and color of lymphocytes, which are caused by disease states in both adults and children. But in pediatric patients, the problem of identifying lymphocytes is compounded because the *normal* morphology of children's lymphocytes differs from that of adults' lymphocytes. Institutions where performance of pediatric differential counts is required should consult textbooks of pediatric hematology for guidance in establishing the criteria for differentiating between normal and abnormal lymphocytes.

LUPUS ERYTHEMATOSUS PREPARATION[11, 17]

The lupus erythematosus (LE) preparation is included here because it is a manual procedure that involves leukocytes and the diagnosis of systemic lupus erythematosus (SLE), an autoimmune disease, the exact cause of which is unclear. Patients' blood and body fluids contain so-called LE factor, a γ globulin that acts as an antibody to nuclear proteins. *In vitro,* this antibody can be induced to produce the classic LE cell.

The LE preparation was a very common procedure years ago, but during the last 10 to 15 years, its popularity has rapidly declined, owing in part to its replacement by the antinuclear antibody (ANA) test. ANA is one of five antibodies that make up the LE factor. (The methodology and significance of the ANA test is summarized later in this chapter.)

LUPUS ERYTHEMATOSUS PREPARATION
Principle

Blood is subjected to trauma by rotating anticoagulated blood with glass beads or by macerating a clotted sample through a sieve. Either action causes extrusion of nuclei from the leukocytes. Three factors must be present in the blood for the classic LE cell to form: (1) the LE factor; (2) extruded cell nuclei; and (3) phagocytic neutrophilic leukocytes. If the LE factor is present, it causes nuclear lysis, and this material invites phagocytosis by viable neutrophils, thus producing the LE cell.

Specimen Requirements

Five milliliters of whole blood anticoagulated with 0.5 mL dilute heparin is required for the procedure involving glass beads. A clotted specimen is required for the procedure involving maceration of a clot.

General Procedure

1. To prepare a clotted specimen, allow specimen to sit at room temperature for 2 hours. With a wooden stick, hold clot in tube and pour off serum. Place Petri dish under sieve. Place clot in sieve and macerate with a pestle.
2. To prepare heparinized specimen with glass beads, add five glass beads to sample tube of heparinized blood. Incubate for 30 minutes at room temperature. Place tube on rotator for 30 minutes. Incubate again for 1 hour at room temperature.
3. Transfer blood from Petri dish or heparinized tube to three or four Wintrobe ESR tubes using long-stemmed pipets. Centrifuge Wintrobe tubes for 10 to 20 minutes in balanced 13 × 100-mm test tubes at 2500 rpm to separate erythrocytes, buffy coat, and plasma (or serum).
4. Remove plasma (or serum) and discard carefully; do not touch buffy coat. Using a clean pipet, extract buffy coat and transfer one or two drops to each of several slides.
5. Place a second slide on top of each slide containing buffy coat and pull the two slides apart (Chap. 3) to make a smear. Allow smear to air dry, then stain either by manual or automated method using Wright stain. Examine smears under the 10 × or 40 × objective for the presence of the LE cell (see Plate 22).

Results

Results are reported as positive or negative. The LE cell is a neutrophil that contains a large spherical body in its cytoplasm. The inclusion is homogeneous and has no nuclear structure (see Plate 22). It stains pale purple.

The homogeneous mass may induce the formation of rosettes in which the mass is surrounded but not engulfed by neutrophils. These may be seen under low-power (10 ×) magnification. Rosettes do not indicate a positive test for LE.

Comments and Sources of Error

It is recommended that three slides be reviewed for 10 minutes each before the results of this test are reported. Either the 40 × or 10 × objective may be used, depending on the laboratorian's experience. Any suspected LE cell should be examined under oil immersion microscopy.

The presence of only a single LE cell does not constitute a positive result.

LE cells may be confused with tart cells. Tart cells are monocytes that have engulfed a mass, which may have a definite nuclear structure or may be pyknotic. Tart cells do not indicate a positive result for LE.

Table 25–10 summarizes common causes of positive, false positive, and false negative test results.

There are no advantages to the LE preparation procedure. It is time consuming to perform, and review of the smears can take from 10 to 30 minutes per patient, depending on cell recovery. If the preparation is suspicious (*i.e.,* if there are cells that look similar to an LE cell but are not definitive LE cells), the test is usually repeated for the next 2 days to afford several opportunities for the laboratory to demonstrate an LE cell and provide a conclusive report as to whether the test is positive or negative.

The test is positive only in about 80% of diagnosed cases of SLE. Once the patient starts taking corticosteroids, this percentage drops considerably, and the LE preparation cannot be used to monitor the status of the patient's remission.

The fact that the LE phenomenon cannot be produced consistently, especially in patients on therapy, and the incidence of false positives both have caused heightened interest in the ANA test for SLE. Although the ANA test is more sensitive, it is not specific for LE. An abnormal ANA result may indicate other disorders as well.

TABLE 25–10. Common Causes of Positive, False Positive, and False Negative Results in LE Cell Preparations

CAUSES OF POSITIVE OR FALSE POSITIVE RESULT	CAUSES OF FALSE NEGATIVE RESULT
Systemic lupus erythematosus	Adrenocorticosteroid therapy
Scleroderma	Leukopenia
Rheumatoid arthritis	
Hepatitis	
Drug therapy	
Hydralazine hydrochloride	
Anticonvulsant drugs (false positive)	
Drug sensitivities (false positive)	

ANTINUCLEAR ANTIBODY TEST[4,8,19,28,29]

The fluorescent ANA test is used in many laboratories to assist in the diagnosis of systemic rheumatic disease, including SLE. In most laboratories, the ANA test has replaced the LE preparation method, in which traumatized blood is used to demonstrate the LE phenomenon on a blood smear of concentrated buffy coat.

ANA is reported to occur in the 7S and 19S globulin components of the serum of some patients, including those with SLE, lupoid hepatitis, scleroderma, rheumatoid arthritis, and other disorders.[19]

Although a brief summary of the test will be presented here, a complete procedural description is beyond the scope of this text. The reader is referred to the references listed above.

QUALITATIVE INDIRECT FLUORESCENT ANTINUCLEAR ANTIBODY TEST
Principle

During incubation on a microscope slide, serum ANA reacts with various components of tissue cell nuclei, such as double-stranded DNA. By using a fluorescein-conjugated antihuman immunoglobulin, the ANA-nucleus antibody-antigen reaction may be detected with a fluorescence microscope as the fluorescent marker reacts with the bound ANA within the nucleus. Results are reported as positive or negative.

Comments and Sources of Error

This test is reported to be positive in most patients with SLE, but it is not specific for SLE, as it is also positive in most patients with lupoid hepatitis,[19] a large number of patients with scleroderma,[19] and approximately half of those with rheumatoid arthritis.[12, 19]

The staining pattern is variable. Fluorescence may cover the entire nucleus (most common in SLE), it may be concentrated at the periphery of the nucleus, it may be found only in discrete spots of the nucleus, or it may stain the nucleoli only. Staining patterns may indicate certain diagnoses more strongly than others.[8]

QUANTITATIVE INDIRECT FLUORESCENT ANTINUCLEAR ANTIBODY TEST[27]
Principle

Twofold serial dilutions of serum are prepared using positive and negative controls and patient specimens, and the indirect fluorescent ANA procedure is applied to each dilution. Using such dilutions, the highest dilution showing positivity provides a quantitative measure of the strength of the antibody and can assist in the diagnosis.

Interpretation of Results[27]

The slides are interpreted as positive or negative using fluorescence microscopy as described in the qualitative test comments above. Results are reported as the highest dilution of serum that gives a positive test (e.g., positive 1:20 dilution). Normal results are 1:10 to 1:20; the majority are 1:5 or below. SLE values are 1:20 to 1:40,960; the majority are 1:40 to 1:2560. Values in rheumatoid arthritis are 1:10 to 1:40,960, with the majority 1:10 to 1:320.

CHAPTER SUMMARY

Today the performance of manual leukocyte counts has been virtually replaced by automated counting techniques, but because instruments are not infallible, laboratory scientists are obligated to learn the art and science of manual leukocyte counting. In addition, manual leukocyte differential counts are increasingly being replaced by automation, but there will always be abnormal specimens that require manual review.

The Neubauer hemocytometer, Thoma pipet, and microscope are the key equipment used in leukocyte counting. Hemocytometers and Thoma pipets must meet NBS specifications. The proper specimen dilution must be selected, based on the approximate expected result (see Table 25-1). It is important to know the dimensions (length, width, depth) of the Neubauer chamber in order to correctly quantitate leukocytes (see Figs. 25-1 and 25-2). The formula for any cell count is as follows:

$$\text{Cells} \times 10^9/\text{L} = \frac{\text{Cells counted} \times \text{Dilution factor}}{\text{No. mm}^2 \text{ counted} \times \text{Depth}}$$

The dilution factor is calculated as 1 divided by the dilution. Leukocyte reference ranges, including the total count and absolute counts of each leukocyte type, depend on the patient's age (see Table 25-3).

The Unopette provides a convenient and acceptable alternative to using the Thoma pipet for preparing blood dilutions for leukocyte counts (see Fig. 25-4).

Table 25-4 provides a summary of the steps involved in performing a differential cell count. Leukocyte differentiation must be performed in a set pattern referred to as the "battlement" method (see Fig. 25-6). The differential count, during which procedure erythrocytes and platelets are evaluated as well, is reported in terms of the relative number or percentage of each leukocyte category on the peripheral film. This relative number can be converted to the absolute number of cells per liter of blood, which is a more valuable and accurate assessment of cell quantitites (see Table 25-8).

One method of ensuring quality control for the differential count is to set up a program for periodic comparison of laboratorians' results to one another, or preferably to automated results. Table 25-7 provides the 95% confidence limit ranges of expected results depending on the observed percentage of a specific cell type and the number of cells differentiated.

Manual eosinophil and basophil counts provide absolute cell count results that may be useful in certain diagnostic situations. The Fuchs-Rosenthal (see Fig. 25-7) or Speirs-Levy (see Fig. 25-8) hemocytometers should be used for these counts, because they allow for counting larger volumes than the Neubauer chamber.

In the past the LE preparation was performed routinely as part of the diagnostic work-up for SLE and other systemic rheumatic disorders. A positive LE preparation is reported upon finding the classic LE cell, a neutrophil that has engulfed a homogeneous mass (see Plate 22). Today the indirect fluorescent ANA test has replaced the LE preparation in most laboratories as a more accurate and reliable test.

EXERCISES

1. Two hundred fifty leukocytes were counted on a hemocytometer in the four WBC squares (each 1 mm^2) on side A and 265 were counted in the same areas on side B. A WBC pipet was used to dilute the patient's blood (0.5 part blood, and diluent drawn to the 11 mark). What is the final leukocyte count?

2. An automated leukocyte count was flagged as erroneous because it was above the linear range. After observing the peripheral blood

film, it was determined that there was an average of 70 leukocytes per oil-immersion field. The calculated calibration factor for the microscope in use was 1 WBC = 1.5×10^9/L peripheral blood leukocytes.

A. What is the approximate leukocyte count based on the peripheral blood findings and calibration factor?

B. What manual dilution should be made for counting on the hemocytometer? What type of pipet should be used?

C. Given this dilution and 170 cells counted in the four usual WBC (1 mm²) squares on side A and 184 counted in the same areas on side B, what is the final leukocyte count?

3. A differential count revealed 20 nucleated red blood cells per 100 leukocytes in a sample with 20.0×10^9/L leukocytes. Is a leukocyte count correction needed? If so, what is the corrected count?

4. Calculate leukocytes ($\times 10^9$/L) for the following values:

DILUTION OF BLOOD	NUMBER OF SQUARES	AREA OF EACH SQUARE	DEPTH OF CHAMBER	TOTAL CELLS COUNTED
A. 1:10	4	1 mm²	0.1 mm	194
B. 1:20	4	1 mm²	0.1 mm	383
C. 1:10	8	1 mm²	0.1 mm	273
D. 1:200	8	1 mm²	0.1 mm	207
E. 1:32	40	1 mm²	0.2 mm	50 (eosinophils)

5. On performing an eosinophil count using the Unopette system and a Fuchs-Rosenthal hemocytometer, 18 eosinophils were counted on side A and 22 on side B. What is the absolute eosinophil count?

6. A differential count showed 8 eosinophils in 100 leukocytes. Given a leukocyte count of 8.4×10^9/L, what is the indirect absolute number of eosinophils per liter? Show calculations. Is this result within the usual reference range?

CASE STUDY 25-1

During the monthly quality control check of laboratorians' differential performance accuracy and agreement, the following results were collected for a selected specimen for lymphocytes based on a manual 100-cell differential count. The same specimen was analyzed on an instrument that provides automated differentials based on examination of 10,000 leukocytes; this value is considered "truth."

Automated	Tech 1	Tech 2	Tech 3	Tech 4	Tech 5
10%	7%	14%	2%	17%	10%

1. Do all laboratorians' results fall within the 95% confidence interval for a 100-cell differential count, assuming that the automated result of 10% is the most reliable value? Explain.

REFERENCES

1. Ahlborg B, Ahlborg G: Exercise leukocytosis with and without beta-adrenergic blockade. Acta Med Scand 187:241, 1970

2. Albritton EC: Standard Values in Blood. Philadelphia, WB Saunders, 1952

3. Altman PL, Dittmer RS (eds): Blood and Other Body Fluids. Bethesda MD, Federation of American Societies for Experimental Biology, 1961

4. Barnett EV, Rothfield NF: The present status of antibody serology. Arthritis Rheum 12:543, 1969

5. Becton Dickinson and Company. Laboratory Procedures Using the Unopette Brand System, 8th ed. Becton Dickinson, Rutherford, NJ, 1977

6. Brown BA: Routine hematology procedures. In Brown BA: Hematology: Principles and Procedures, 4th ed, pp 33, 63. Philadelphia, Lea & Febiger, 1984

7. Caramihai E, Karayalcin G, Aballi AJ et al: Leukocyte count differences in healthy white and black children 1 to 5 years of age. J Pediatr 86:252, 1975

8. Clinical Sciences, Inc: Anafluor: An indirect fluorescent antibody (IFA) test system for detection and titration of antinuclear antibodies (package insert). Whippany, NJ, Clinical Sciences, Inc, 1986

9. Cooper JR, Cruickshank CN: Improved method for direct counting of basophil leukocytes. J Clin Pathol 19:402, 1966

10. Cunningham AS: Eosinophil counts—age and sex differences. J Pediatr 87:426, 1975

11. Dacie JV, Lewis SM: Practical Hematology, 5th ed. New York, Churchill Livingstone, 1975

12. Duke University Medical Center: Data on file. Contact Clinical Sciences, Inc, 30 Troy Road, Whippany, NJ 07981, 1986

13. England JM, Bain BJ: Total and differential leukocyte count. Br J Haematol 33:1, 1976; Br Med J 1:306, 1975

14. Fairbanks VF, Fahey JL, Beutler E: Clinical Disorders of Iron Metabolism, 2nd ed, p 178. NY, Grune & Stratton, 1971

15. Karayalcin G, Rosner F, Sawitsky A: Pseudo-neutropenia in Negroes. A normal phenomenon. NY State J Med 72:1815, 1972

16. Kato K: Leukocytes in infancy and childhood. A statistical analysis of 1,081 total and differential counts from birth to fifteen years. J Pediatr 7:7, 1935

17. Magath TB, Winkle V: Technic for demonstrating "L.E." (lupus erythematosus) cells in blood. Am J Clin Pathol 22:586, 1952

18. Mauer AM: Pediatric Hematology. New York, McGraw–Hill, 1969

19. Miale JB: Appendix—methods. In Miale JB: Laboratory Medicine Hematology, p 913. St Louis, CV Mosby Co, 1982

20. Milhorat AT, Small SM, Diethelm O: Leukocytosis during various emotional states. Arch Neurol Psychiatr 47:779, 1942

21. National Committee for Clinical Laboratory Standards: Leukocyte Differential Counting; Tentative Standard H20-T. Villanova, PA, NCCLS, 1984

22. Orfanakis NG, Ostlund RE, Bishop CR et al: Normal blood leukocyte concentration values. Am J Clin Pathol 53:647, 1970

23. Osgood EE, Baker RL, Brownlee IE et al: Total, differential and absolute leukocyte counts and sedimentation rates of healthy children four to seven years of age. Am J Dis Child 58:61, 1939

24. Oski FA, Naiman JL (ed): Hematologic Problems in the Newborn. Philadelphia, WB Saunders, 1982

25. Patrick CW, Keller RH: The New Morphology: Combining Traditional Cytomorphology with Automated Differential Information, Cytogenetics and Molecular Probes, Monoclonal Antibodies and Immunophenotyping, Laser Flow Cytometry and Cell Sorting. Workshop Manual, Annual Meeting, New Orleans, 1986. Washington DC, American Society for Medical Technology, 1986

26. Randolph TG: Differentiation and enumeration of eosinophils in the counting chamber with a glycol stain: A valuable technique in appraising ACTH dosage. J Lab Clin Med 34:1696, 1949

27. Ritchie RF: The clinical significance of titered antinuclear antibodies. Arthritis Rheum 10:544, 1967

28. Rothfield NF: Serologic tests in rheumatic disease. Postgrad Med 45:116, 1969

29. Shulman LE: Serologic abnormalities in systemic lupus erythematosus. J Chronic Dis 16:889, 1963

30. Stiene-Martin EA: Causes for poor leukocyte distribution in manual spreader-slide blood films. Am J Med Technol 46:624, 1980

31. van Assendelft OW et al: The differential distribution of leukocytes. In Koepke JA (ed): Differential Leukocyte Counting, p 11. Skokie, IL, College of American Pathologists, 1979

32. Wintrobe MM: Origin and development of the blood and blood forming tissues. In Wintrobe MM: Clinical Hematology, 8th ed, p 52. Philadelphia, Lea & Febiger, 1981

33. Zacharski LR, Elveback LR, Linman JW: Leukocyte counts in healthy adults. Am J Clin Pathol 56:148, 1971

PART V

LEUKOCYTE

ABNORMALITIES

(NONMALIGNANT)

Nonmalignant, Reactive Disorders of Phagocytes

E. Anne Stiene-Martin

Leukocytes function to protect the body against invasion by foreign organisms or antigens. In so doing they undergo visible changes (reactive or toxic changes) that are evaluated microscopically in the clinical laboratory. These changes are the most common leukocyte abnormality seen in the clinical hematology laboratory, and they are generally subdivided into quantitative variations (alterations in numbers) and qualitative variations (morphologic alterations). Such alterations must be distinguished from those seen in neoplastic leukocytes as well as those resulting from genetic abnormalities.

To discuss quantitative abnormalities in leukocytes, it is necessary to define reference ranges for total leukocytes as well as for each cell type. These may vary between laboratories because of differences in cell counting procedures, instrumentation, methods used to established reference values, and in patient populations. The lower level for total leukocytes in adults is usually somewhere between 3.0 and $4.0 \times 10^9/L$, and the high, between 10.0 and $11.0 \times 10^9/L$.[70] Pediatric values are significantly different. One source reports reference ranges for children to be 4.5 to 13.5 and for infants 6.0 to $17.5 \times 10^9/L$.[34] *Leukocytosis* (defined in adults as leukocyte counts greater than $11.0 \times 10^9/L$) may be caused by an increase in one or more of the cell types that normally circulate in peripheral blood or by the presence of abnormal cell types. Conversely, *leukopenia* is defined as a total leukocyte count of less than $3.0 \times 10^9/L$ and is due to a decrease in neutrophils (neutropenia or granulocytopenia), lymphocytes (lymphopenia), or all cell types (pancytopenia). Eosinophils, basophils, and monocytes are normally present in such low numbers that individual decreases do not produce leukopenia.

NEUTROPHILS

Quantitative Abnormalities

In determining whether an absolute increase or decrease in neutrophils exists, the age and ethnicity of the subject must be taken into account.[70] Children tend to have higher neutrophil counts than adults; blacks tend to have lower counts than caucasians.[61,70] When calculating the absolute value of circulating neutrophils (the product of the total leukocyte count and the percentage of neutrophils), all stages of neutrophil maturation, *excluding* blasts and progranulocytes, are included.

Neutrophilia

Neutrophilia may be defined as an absolute neutrophil count greater than 7.0 or 8.0 × 10^9/L.[34] Table 26-1 lists common reactive causes of neutrophilia and is subdivided into those involving pathology and those that are physiologic.

Three major causes for neutrophilia are infection, inflammation, and malignancy. Reactive neutrophilias may be either acute (transient) or chronic and frequently are accompanied by increased numbers of immature forms (neutrophilic left shift).

Bacterial infections, especially those caused by cocci, may produce striking neutrophilia. More moderate neutrophilic responses are characteristic of infections caused by bacilli such as *Escherichia coli*, certain fungal infections (actinomycosis), and viral infections (varicella, variola, rabies, herpes zoster). Neutrophilia is sometimes produced by spirochetes (*Leptospira ictohemorrhagiae*) and rickettsiae (typhus). Not all bacteria cause neutrophilia; some, in fact, suppress neutrophil production, resulting in a neutropenia to be described below.

The degree of neutrophilia produced by infections depends on virulence of the organism as well as the age and health (resistance) of the patient. Children tend to develop more profound neutrophilia than adults. Conversely, elderly persons, as well as those who have nutritional deficits or have received bone marrow replacement, may produce only moderate responses or none at all when challenged with the same infection.

Neutrophilia associated with inflammatory responses to tissue injury or destruction occur in a wide variety of situations (see Table 26-1). They include chronic serosal inflammation, such as that seen in rheumatoid arthritis, acute destruction represented by pancreatitis, colitis, myocardial infarction, severe hemolysis, surgical or traumatic wounds, thermal injury, and tissue destruction caused by a wide variety of chemicals (lead, mercury), drugs (digitalis, phenacetin), venoms (spiders, bees, wasps), and parasites (malaria, liver flukes).[75] The basic mechanism for neutrophilia in these cases is release of substances by dead or dying cells that act as chemotactic agents, marrow-releasing agents, or stimulators of marrow cell production.

Inflammatory responses may also occur in the presence of neoplasms, especially those that are growing fast or are producing substances that induce marrow output of neutrophils.[60] Metabolic disorders such as diabetes, renal dysfunction, or liver disease may produce circulating toxic substances (ketoacidosis, uremia, azotemia) and stimulate a neutrophilic response. Acute hemorrhage, especially when internal, stimulates neutrophilia,[23] presumably as a result of a combination of factors, including cell destruction and promotion of neutrophil release.

The mechanism by which adrenocorticosteroids cause neutrophilia is not clear, but it may be related to inhibition of neutrophil migration.[5] Lithium, a common antidepressant drug, has been the subject of recent investigation, because it appears to cause neutrophilia through direct stimulation of hematopoiesis.[7]

Physiologic neutrophilia is usually caused by a shift of marginated cells to the circulating pool, a condition sometimes referred to as pseudoneutrophilia. (See Chap. 23 for a discussion of marginal and circulating pools of leukocytes.) This neutrophilia is generally transient, lasting only a few hours, and is not characterized by any significant increase in immature forms. Such neutrophilias may be caused by physical stimuli (*e.g.*, exercise, excessive temperature changes, nausea and vomiting, pregnancy and labor) as well as by emotional stimuli (*e.g.*, rage, panic, stress).[49] Increased levels of epinephrine or norepinephrine may be the common factor in all these conditions.

Neutropenia

Neutropenia is the most common cause of leukopenia. It may be defined as a neutrophil count of less than 1.75 to 1.8 × 10^9/L. The term *agranulocytosis* is used to designate extreme neutropenia (<0.5 × 10^9/L). Profound neutropenia generally renders the patient vulnerable to infection; however, there is not always a consistent relationship between neutrophil count and the number of neutrophils delivered to the tissues, which may explain why some persons with neutropenia do not experience more infections.[76] Table 26-2 lists the major causes of neutropenia.

Decreased production of neutrophils may be inherited or acquired. Inherited forms are rare and include a variety of poorly understood syndromes. They include defective stem cell development (*e.g.*, reticular dysgenesis, cyclic neutropenia, infantile agranulocytosis, Fanconi's syn-

---

TABLE 26–1. Causes of Reactive Neutrophilia

PATHOLOGIC
 Infections (localized or generalized)
  Pyogenic bacteria
  Certain viruses
  Actinomyces fungi
  Some spirochetal and rickettsial organisms
 Inflammatory responses to tissue destruction
  Serosal
  Visceral
  Blood cell destruction
  Posttraumatic (surgical, accidental)
  Thermal injury
  Chemicals/drugs/venoms
  Parasitic invasions
 Other inflammatory responses
  Neoplastic growth
  Metabolic disorders
  Acute hemorrhage
 Drugs
  Corticosteroids
  Lithium
PHYSIOLOGIC
 Response to therapy
 Pseudoneutrophilia caused by physical or emotional stimuli

TABLE 26-2. Causes of Neutropenia

Decreased neutrophil production
  Inherited stem cell disorders
  Acquired stem cell disorders
    Chemical toxicity (*e.g.*, benzene)
    Marrow replacement
    Nutritional deficiencies
    Cytotoxic drugs
Increased neutrophil destruction
  Infections
    Overwhelming
    Certain bacteria
    Viral
  Immune reactions
    Isoimmune
    Autoimmune
    Drug-induced
  Sequestration
  Pseudoneutropenia
  Malignant myeloproliferative disorders

drome); genetic disorders of the immune system (*e.g.*, neutropenia with dysgammaglobulinemia); and disorders of cellular development or function that result secondarily in decreased circulating numbers (*e.g.*, Chediak-Higashi syndrome, lazy leukocyte syndrome) (Chap. 28).

Acquired forms of decreased neutrophil production are common. Destruction or injury to stem cell compartments generally results in hypoplastic or aplastic marrow with concomitant decreases in all cell types. Agents capable of causing moderate to severe marrow suppression include ionizing radiation, chemicals such as benzene, and a wide variety of cytotoxic drugs used in combating malignancy. Marrow replacement by tumor, fibrous tissue, or hematopoietic malignancy may result in pancytopenia. In some cases neutropenia may be a preleukemic manifestation.[39] Vitamin B_{12} or folate deficiency causes ineffective hematopoiesis that may lead to decreases in all cell types.

The second major category of neutropenic states includes those caused by increased neutrophil destruction due to infections, immune mechanisms or hypersensitivity states. Any infection that overwhelms the marrow's capacity to produce adequate numbers of neutrophils will result in neutrophils being consumed or recruited to the tissues faster than they are released by the marrow. This type of neutropenia is seen most frequently in debilitated patients who have little or no marrow reserves, elderly persons, and infants.

Typhoid, paratyphoid, and brucellosis are bacterial infections commonly associated with leukopenia and neutropenia. Rickettsial infections (Rocky Mountain spotted fever, scrub typhus, rickettsialpox) may or may not present with neutropenia.

Viral infections characterized by neutropenia include measles, yellow fever, infectious hepatitis, infectious mononucleosis and rubella.[53] The neutropenia of viral infections is often noted in the early stages of the disease.

Neonatal isoimmune neutropenia results from transplacental transfer of maternal IgG antibodies directed against fetal neutrophils.[37] Acquired autoimmune neutropenia has been described and is analogous to autoimmune hemolytic anemia or immune thrombocytopenic purpura, but not as common.[8] Antineutrophil antibodies have also been described in collagen vascular diseases (lupus

erythematosus, Felty's syndrome)[6] and following transfusion of blood products. Transient neutropenia during the first hour of hemodialysis is believed to be due to activation of the complement system and sequestration of neutrophils in the lungs.[15]

Drug hypersensitivity can result in severe neutropenia, referred to as agranulocytosis.[29] The list of drugs implicated in this disorder is extensive and growing. The first drug to be implicated, in the late 1920s, was amidopyrine. Since then, with the introduction of new drugs, isolated reports of agranulocytosis invariably followed. A recent report adds cephalosporin to the list.[52] Drug-induced agranulocytosis affects women more frequently than men (2.5:1) and is more often seen in middle age than in young adults. The underlying disorder may be a genetic defect that prevents proper metabolism of the drug. Removal of the offending drug generally results in prompt recovery.

A third mechanism of neutropenia is sequestration. Splenic enlargement, regardless of cause, may lead to neutropenia, which is usually relatively mild. Neutrophils may also be sequestered in pulmonary vasculature after chemotactic stimuli.[32]

Finally, patients may have a decreased number of circulating neutrophils because of shift from the circulating pool of neutrophils to the marginated pool. This may be referred to as *pseudoneutropenia* because the total blood granulocyte pool is not decreased. It may occur after injection of endotoxin, during hypersensitivity or viral infections, and after hypothermia.[64]

Qualitative Abnormalities

Morphologic alterations in neutrophils in response to stress, infection, or inflammation often are called *toxic changes*. These changes (Table 26-3) include the presence of increased numbers of immature forms (the so-called left shift) and morphologic evidence of maturation abnormalities, alterations in functional activity, or degenerative changes.

A neutrophilic left shift is defined as the presence of increased numbers of circulating nonsegmented or immature neutrophils. Release of marrow stores results in greater numbers of neutrophilic band forms and metamyelocytes. Continued marrow stimulus is accompanied by increased

TABLE 26-3. Toxic Neutrophil Morphology

Circulating immature forms
  Mild: Increased band and metamyelocyte forms
  Moderate: Circulating myelocytes and occasional promyelocytes
  Marked: Circulating blast forms
Morphologic abnormalities
  Cytoplasmic
    Toxic granules
    Döhle bodies
    Vacuolation
    Degranulation
    Pseudopods
    Swelling
  Nuclear
    Pyknotic and/or necrotic
    Hypersegmentation
    Nuclear projections
    Ring forms

marrow production of neutrophils and the presence of neutrophilic myelocytes in the circulation. Small numbers of promyelocytes and blast forms may be found in peripheral blood from individuals with severe or overwhelming infections. (See Chap. 23 for morphologic description of immature neutrophils.) The importance of recognizing and reporting the various stages of neutrophil development in peripheral blood is underscored by the fact that a change in the ratio of nonsegmented to segmented neutrophils appears to be one of the best indicators of the severity of infection.[13,46,47]

Morphologic evidence of neutrophil activation or degeneration can be subdivided into two categories of abnormalities: cytoplasmic and nuclear.

Cytoplasm

Cytoplasmic alterations in toxic neutrophils are those most frequently cited in the literature. They include toxic granulation, Döhle bodies, cytoplasmic vacuoles, degranulation, pseudopods, and swelling.

Toxic granules are believed to be altered primary granules.[41] Primary granules, although present in neutrophils under normal circumstances, are not prominent with ordinary Romanowsky stains. Neutrophil stimulation by foreign organisms or antigens may cause alterations in these granules, resulting in different staining characteristics.[43] Toxic granules are described as being larger than secondary granules (*i.e.*, resolvable with the light microscope) and dark blue-black in color after staining. Not all such granules are lysosomal. Some reports in the literature indicate that hemosiderin is present in some neutrophils with toxic granules[35] and may cause decreased neutrophil function.[72] Much has been written about the significance and prognostic value of quantitating toxic granulation. Generally it can be said that the greater the proportion of neutrophils affected, the graver the prognosis.[36] It is important to differentiate between true toxic granulation, artifactual granules caused by poor staining technique, and the abnormal metachromatic granules seen in some genetic disorders of mucopolysaccharide metabolism (Chap. 28). True toxic granules may be distinguished by their tendency to cluster within the cell and by the fact that not all neutrophils will be equally affected (Fig. 26-1). Dark granules caused by overstaining and Alder-Reilly bodies (Chap. 28) generally are distributed throughout the cell and all cells tend to be affected equally.

Döhle bodies (see Plate 23) are cytoplasmic inclusions consisting of ribosomal RNA arrayed in parallel rows.[4] They are found in segmented and band neutrophils. With Romanowsky stains they appear as pale blue, round or elongated bodies between 1 and 5 μm in diameter that are usually located in close apposition to cell membranes. It should be noted that the anticoagulant EDTA affects the staining characteristics of Döhle bodies so that they may be more gray than blue and may even disappear with time in EDTA. Döhle bodies are relatively nonspecific in that they are associated with a wide range of conditions, including pregnancy.[1] They are transient in that they are seen most often during the first 1 to 3 days after an insult (*e.g.*, infection, burn, surgery), after which they tend to disappear. What causes them to form is not known. They may reflect sudden storage pool release.

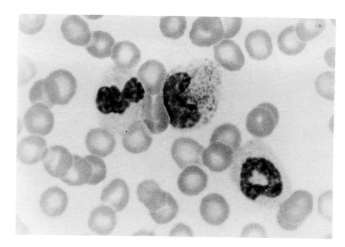

FIG. 26-1. Toxic granulation. Note that the center neutrophil contains toxic granules whereas the other two do not. This suggests that the granulation is not artifact. In addition, the neutrophil to the lower right contains a ringed nucleus.

It is important to differentiate between the transient Döhle body seen after infection or tissue damage and the larger spindle-shaped inclusion seen in May-Hegglin anomaly (Chap. 28). Transmission electron microscopy reveals structural differences,[11] however, most laboratories do not have access to electron microscopes. Light microscopic differentiation can usually be made based on size (May-Hegglin bodies often are greater than 5 μm in diameter), the cell types affected (May-Hegglin inclusions are found in all types of granulocytes), and the fact that May-Hegglin bodies are not transient.[11]

Cytoplasmic vacuolation is caused by phagocytosis, either of self (autophagocytosis) or of extracellular material. Autophagocytosis may be caused by drugs such as sulfonamides and chloroquine,[58] by prolonged storage of cells, and by degranulation on exposure to certain toxins or high doses of radiation.[30] Generally, autophagocytic vacuoles tend to be small in size (1–2 μm) and evenly distributed throughout the cytoplasm (Fig. 26-2). Phagocytic vacuolation due to ingestion is seen commonly in septic processes

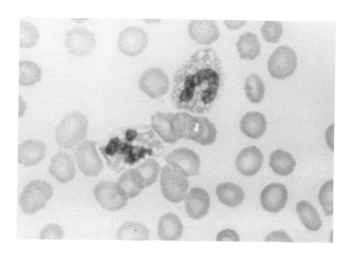

FIG. 26-2. Autophagocytic vacuoles. Note their small size and distribution throughout the cell.

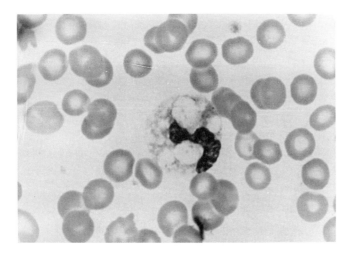

FIG. 26-3.   Phagocytic vacuoles. Compared to autophagocytic vacuoles, these are considerably larger and few in number.

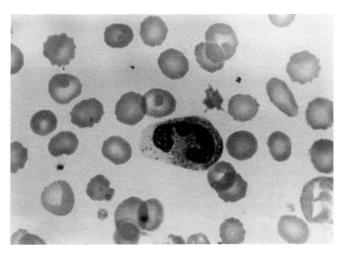

FIG. 26-4.   Granule-free cytoplasmic pseudopod. This may reflect either aberrant cell locomotion or prolonged delay in anticoagulant.

caused either by bacteria or fungi. Phagocytic vacuoles can be quite large (up to 7 or 8 μm), are not evenly distributed, and often are outlined by visible toxic granules (Fig. 26-3).

Numerous studies have correlated the presence of vacuolated neutrophils with bacteremia.[40,77] Vacuoles as well as toxic granulation are indicative of neutrophils with de-

creased bactericidal properties.[65] Consequently, assuming a fresh specimen, the presence of vacuolation in more than 10% of neutrophils can be very significant.[44]

True vacuolation must be distinguished from that due to excessive delay between blood collection and blood film preparation. Vacuolation due to delay tends to be auto-

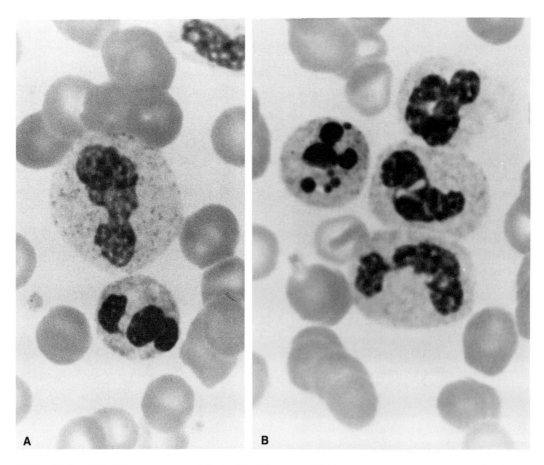

FIG. 26-5.   (A) The two neutrophils in this field are exhibiting anisocytosis or variation in size. In addition, the lower neutrophil contains a pyknotic nucleus. (B) Necrotic (dead) neutrophil on the left. Compare the nuclear structure of this cell to the three viable neutrophils to its right.

phagocytic (*i.e.*, small, evenly distributed vacuoles) and with neutral red the vacuoles are reported to stain yellow rather than red.[4]

Cytoplasmic degranulation is a normal function of neutrophils that have been activated or injured.[19] Primary granules are emptied into the phagosome, whereas secondary granules are secreted into the extracellular environment.[22] Degranulation often is accompanied by disruption of cellular membranes during the process of making the blood film.

Cytoplasmic pseudopods are rare alterations in toxic neutrophils. They are granule-free protrusions of cytoplasm that give the neutrophil an ameboid character (Fig. 26-4). They may be indicative of sluggish or depressed neutrophil locomotion known to be caused by a variety of bacterial and therapeutic agents.[20,21,74] They are seen most frequently in association with cytotoxic agents, whether therapeutic or released by other cells. Prolonged specimen storage in EDTA may cause artifactual pseudopods and must be distinguished from toxic cytoplasmic pseudopods.

Cytoplasmic swelling may be caused by actual osmotic swelling of the cytoplasm[55] or by increased glass adhesiveness of stimulated neutrophils. Regardless of cause, the result is perceptible variation in neutrophil size within a population, or neutrophilic anisocytosis (see Fig. 26-5A). A swollen or edematous neutrophil, sometimes referred to as a *macropolycyte,* must be distinguished from the large hypersegmented neutrophils resulting from vitamin B_{12} or folate deficiency.

Nucleus

Nuclear alterations in toxic neutrophils have received less attention in the literature. They include pyknosis, hypersegmentation, nuclear projections, and ring-shaped nuclei.

Pyknotic nuclei are shrunken and dense nuclei that apparently are dehydrated[58]; they may be in cells just about to die. They are seen most frequently in septic conditions. They should be distinguished from dead (necrotic) cells that are rarely seen in fresh specimens and whose nuclei are dense and broken into two or more rounded portions with no evidence of filamentous connections (compare Figs. 26-5A and 26-5B). Nuclear pyknosis also can result from poor staining or preparation techniques, but that can be detected, since most cells are equally affected. Unfortunately, there is some confusion in the literature because some authors also describe necrotic cells as being pyknotic.

Hypersegmented nuclei are commonly seen in long-term chronic infections. They may be either large or normal-sized. There may be more than one cause.[56] In some cases hypersegmented neutrophils may reflect borderline folate deficiency; in others, it may reflect a degenerative process.

Toxic nuclear projections are hairlike projections seen most frequently in band forms. The projections usually are only on the inner side of the band form, the side that faces the centriole (Fig. 26-6).[4] Toxic nuclear projections have been reported in patients with metastatic carcinoma or after irradiation.[18]

Ringed nuclei (see Fig. 26-1) are seen in both toxic states and malignant myeloproliferative states.[33,38] Small numbers of neutrophils with ringlike nuclei may be seen early in

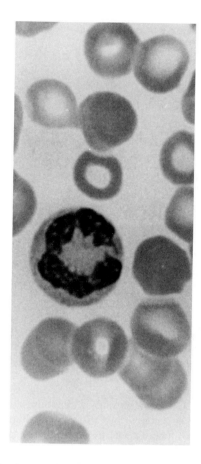

FIG. 26-6. Toxic nuclear projections. Note the hairlike projections on the inner side of the nucleus.

infections, when leukocytosis is prominent and band forms are increased to levels of 30% or more.

EOSINOPHILS

Quantitative Abnormalities

Eosinophilia

Eosinophilia (more than 0.7×10^9/L) may be inherited, malignant, or reactive. The eosinophilias seen in some hematopoietic malignancies are covered in Chapter 35. Hereditary eosinophilia has been reported in a few families as an autosomal-dominant trait.[54] The eosinophilia usually is benign, and the major concern is to differentiate inherited eosinophilia from reactive forms to be described below.

Reactive eosinophilia is most frequently associated with two categories of disorders (Table 26-4): parasitic invasion of tissue and hypersensitivity disorders. In addition, an eosinophilic response may be seen in collagen-vascular diseases, neoplastic disorders, and some immune deficiency states.[73]

Eosinophilia is associated with parasites that invade and cause tissue destruction, but it is not characteristic of protozoal infections. Eosinophils have unique capabilities for suppressing virtually all helminthic organisms (trematodes, nematodes, and cestodes). There is a significant positive correlation between eosinophil count and parasite

TABLE 26–4. Changes in Eosinophil Number

Eosinophilia
  Infestation by tissue-invading parasites
  Allergic reactions
    Respiratory (asthma, hay fever)
    Skin disorders (psoriasis, eczema)
  Hypersensitivity disorders
    Loeffler's syndrome
    Pulmonary infiltrates with eosinophilia (PIE)
    Tropical eosinophilia
  Malignancies of myeloid cells
  Certain infections (*e.g.,* scarlet fever)
  Miscellaneous disorders
    Familial
    Postirradiation
    Certain poisons
    Periarteritis nodosa
Eosinopenia
  Decreased production
  Acute bacterial infection
  ACTH administration

death.[16] Eosinophil attraction to parasites appears to be T lymphocyte-directed and antibody dependent.[9] Parasite killing is mediated through eosinophil degranulation,[42] release of crystalloid major basic protein and cationic proteins, and peroxidation.[25]

The role of the eosinophil in allergic reactions involves modulation of the inflammatory response resulting from basophil or mast cell degranulation. Immediate hypersensitivity reactions produce a wide variety of products that influence eosinophil traffic (Chap. 23). Activation of the immune system and basophil or mast cell degranulation may very well be the underlying mechanism for a wide variety of eosinophilia-producing conditions, including cutaneous disorders such as psoriasis and eczema; pulmonary disorders such as Loeffler's syndrome, pulmonary infiltrates with eosinophilia (PIE) and tropical eosinophilia; gastrointestinal disorders such as ulcerative colitis; certain types of tumors; and the mild eosinophilia that is associated with hemodialysis and irradiation.

The term *hypereosinophilic syndrome* is utilized to denote a condition in which there is persistent, extreme eosinophilia at levels above 1.5×10^9/L. The underlying cause may be parasitic, allergic, neoplastic (eosinophilic leukemia), or idiopathic (unknown). Persistent hypereosinophilia is cause for concern, since there tends to be eosinophil infiltration into all tissues with resulting tissue damage and organ dysfunction such as cardiomyopathy. Consequently, the hypereosinophilic syndrome is generally monitored carefully, and therapy to suppress eosinophils such as antihistamines, cytotoxic drugs, or leukapheresis may be instituted.

Eosinopenia

Eosinopenia is difficult to detect using routine differentials and total leukocyte count, since zero percent eosinophils is frequently considered to be within the normal range based on a 100-leukocyte differential count. If chamber counts are performed, eosinopenia may be defined as less than 0.05×10^9/L. It may result from production abnormalities similar to those listed previously for neutropenia. In addition, eosinopenia is a characteristic finding in most acute bacterial infections. Reappearance of eosinophils in the peripheral blood generally is a sign of recovery from the infection. The mechanism for the eosinopenia of acute infections is not known. It is not dependent on adrenal glucocorticosteroids and probably is not caused by mast cell degranulation. It may be a combination of factors, including sequestration, margination, and chemotaxis.[3]

Eosinopenia is also a well known outcome of ACTH administration if adrenal function is normal. Glucocorticoids, prostaglandins, and epinephrine will depress eosinophil levels.[78] The mechanism of these eosinopenias is felt to be a combination of increased margination and decreased marrow release.

Qualitative Abnormalities

Eosinophils exhibit some morphologic alterations that reflect activity. Circulating immature eosinophils (left shift) are extremely rare in reactive conditions, even in the face of markedly increased eosinophils. Morphologic evidence of stimulation and activity includes degranulation, vacuolation, and hypersegmentation.

Degranulation is probably the most prominent eosinophil alteration. The result is a cell with a few scattered eosinophil granules in pale blue to colorless cytoplasm (Fig. 26-7). The act of degranulation renders the cytoplasmic membrane somewhat vulnerable to the making of a blood film. Thus, eosinophilias frequently are characterized by increased numbers of broken or disrupted eosinophils on the blood film. Eosinophil degranulation should be reported only if the specimen is fresh, as eosinophils are prone to degranulate in stored blood. It should be noted that eosinophils with decreased granules may also be seen in malignant myeloproliferative disorders. These usually can be differentiated from reactive forms by the accompanying blood picture (*i.e.,* other evidence of malignancy).

Vacuolation of eosinophils is seen occasionally. The vacuoles tend to be quite small and their significance is unknown.

Hypersegmentation is the only relatively common nuclear alteration in reactive eosinophils. Since normal eosin-

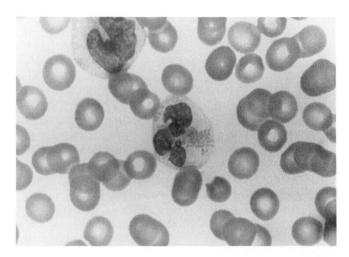

FIG. 26-7.   Reactive eosinophil exhibiting degranulation and three nuclear lobes (hypersegmentation).

ophils have only two nuclear lobes, eosinophil hypersegmentation is defined as three or more lobes or a mean greater than 2.5 lobes. The causes of eosinophilic hypersegmentation are probably similar to those described previously for neutrophils.

BASOPHILS

Quantitative Abnormalities

The normal number of circulating basophils is so low that reference values have been difficult to obtain, owing to the fact that 1000-cell differential counts would be necessary to calculate reliable absolute values.[24] Chamber counts using neutral red or Alcian blue are subject to relatively high coefficients of variation and so, are not totally satisfactory.[63] One reason for this may be that degranulation of basophils renders them unrecognizable in the chamber. The advent of flow cytometers that are capable of identifying basophils within populations of 10,000 leukocytes or more provides a means of defining the lower normal limits for basophils ($0.005-0.010 \times 10^9$/L); however, flow cytometers are not available in many clinical hematology laboratories. Consequently, the ability to detect basopenia remains beyond the capability of a large number of laboratories.

Basophilia

Basophilia may be defined as a basophil number greater than 0.3×10^9/L; it is present in many of the disorders that cause eosinophilia. This is not surprising in view of the evidence that eosinophils and basophils share a common stem cell.[17] Also, basophil activation, like that of eosinophils, appears to be controlled at least in part by T lymphocytes.[26]

Reactive basophilias are most frequently cited in association with immediate hypersensitivity reaction, long-term foreign antigen stimulation,[62] hypothyroidism, ulcerative colitis, and estrogen therapy.[67] There is a transient basophilia of unknown origin in newborn infants[50] and following exercise.[51] Striking basophilia is often seen in the myeloproliferative disorders (Chap. 35).

Basopenia

Basopenias have been described during acute infections, stress, hyperthyroidism, and increased levels of glucocorticoids.[67,75]

Qualitative Abnormalities

There is little or nothing in the literature about basophil morphology during reactive conditions. Immature forms do not circulate in reactive basophilia. Degranulation is the single morphologic alteration that may be detected. Degranulation may be seen after ingestion of a fatty meal[62] or as a consequence of antigen-related stimulation.[59] Evaluation of basophil degranulation presents some problems, as these granules are water soluble and may be lost during the staining of the blood film.

MONOCYTES

Quantitative Abnormalities

If reference ranges for monocytes are based on Romanowsky-stained morphology, the lower limits are between 0.03 and 0.09×10^9/L and upper limits are between 0.85 and 1.0×10^9/L. If, on the other hand, monocytes are identified using enzymatic[31] or surface markers, the upper limit of normal may be significantly higher (e.g., 1.8×10^9/L). It should be noted at this point that calculation of absolute values from a differential count should be based on at least a 200-cell differential count, because of the tendency of these cells to cluster along the edges of spreader-slide blood films.

Monocytosis

Monocytosis is defined here as numbers greater than 0.9×10^9/L. Owing to the fact that monocytes and neutrophils share a common stem cell, it is not surprising to note that many of the conditions listed above as causes of neutrophilia are also accompanied by absolute monocytosis. The increase in monocytes is usually inconspicuous in the presence of the more noticeable neutrophil response. For example, 6% monocytes in 25×10^9/L leukocytes represents an absolute monocytosis, which might be overlooked.

Monocytosis may be reactive or malignant. Inherited forms have not been described. The monocytosis seen in malignant myeloproliferative disorders is discussed in Chapters 33 through 35. Causes of reactive monocytosis are listed in Table 26-5.

Although a wide variety of acute bacterial infections have been reported to be accompanied by monocytosis, three in particular are cited most consistently: tuberculosis, subacute bacterial endocarditis (SBE), and syphilis.[12] Tuberculosis is thought to elicit increased monocytes because of their role in the cellular response to the bacillus (granuloma formation).[27] Monocytosis in such cases is believed to reflect active disease. Some of the monocytes in patients with SBE may mature in the peripheral blood, resulting in circulating histiocytes or macrophages. This is considered to be highly significant and is discussed below under qualitative changes. The spirochetes of syphilis cause widespread interstitial inflammation and invasion of lymphatic and vascular systems. In these patients monocytosis may be a response to inflammation or be related to the cells' role in the immune system.

TABLE 26–5. Causes of Monocytosis

Bacterial infection
    Tuberculosis
    Subacute bacterial endocarditis (SBE)
    Syphilis
Inflammatory responses
    Surgical trauma
    Tumors
    Collagen vascular disease
    Gastrointestinal disease
Recovery from neutropenia (relative)
Myeloproliferative disorders

Monocytosis may also be seen in inflammatory reactions to tissue destruction. These include such disparate conditions as surgical trauma,[28] tumors,[2] gastrointestinal disease,[45] and tetrachlorethane poisoning.[48]

There is little or no marrow storage of monocytes; therefore, they are released into the circulation before neutrophils are. Because of this, relative monocytosis frequently heralds recovery from agranulocytosis or marrow hypoplasia.

Monocytopenia

Monocytopenia (less than 0.03×10^9/L) may be seen following administration of glucocorticoids[66] or during overwhelming infections that also cause neutropenia. There are a few reports of inherited monocytopenia.[12]

Qualitative Abnormalities

A few morphologic expressions in monocytes may be considered to be reactive. These changes in appearance reflect basic monocyte responses to stimuli, including emergence of immature monocytes (Chap. 23) into the circulation (a type of monocytic left shift; Fig. 26-8)[32] and monocyte transformation into histiocytes, macrophages, or epithelioid cells.[69] Morphologic changes associated with transformation into histiocytes or macrophages include increases in cytoplasmic volume and spreading ability (cell diameters sometimes approach 50 μm), increased numbers of dense granules representing both primary and secondary lysosomes, and increased evidence of both phagocytic and pinocytic activity (cytoplasmic vacuolation, intracellular debris, and highly irregular cytoplasmic borders). In addition, the nuclear chromatin pattern may become reticular (netlike) and nucleoli, visible.[71] Nuclear shape varies from round to oval (Fig. 26-9).

The finding of histiocytes or macrophages in the peripheral blood of patients suffering from septic processes such as SBE has been described in the literature over several years. In this author's experience, these cells may make their appearance in the peripheral blood long before blood cultures

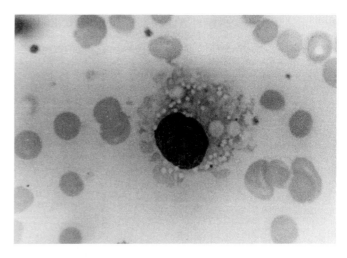

FIG. 26-9.   A circulating macrophage that was found in the feathered edge (tail) of a blood film taken from a patient who was septic.

are positive. Therefore, their identification is important. Generally speaking, they will most often be found in the edges of the blood film, owing to their large size.

A final monocyte alteration that might be considered a reactive change is an alteration in the nucleus to a long, thin, bandlike shape that frequently appears highly contorted (Fig. 26-10). Explanations for this finding are not found in the literature; however, they are seen frequently in the same preparations as hypersegmented neutrophils and may also reflect incipient folate deficiency.

SPECIFIC REACTIONS—DEFINITIONS

Two types of reactions should be defined and discussed, leukoerythroblastic reaction and leukemoid reaction.

Leukoerythroblastic reaction is defined as the presence on a blood film of both nucleated red cells and immature neutro-

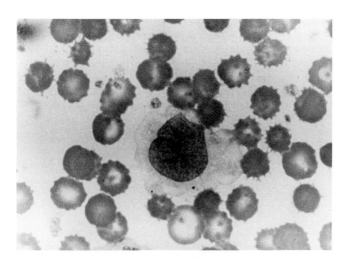

FIG. 26-8.   An immature-appearing monocyte reflecting a type of reactive monocytic "left shift."

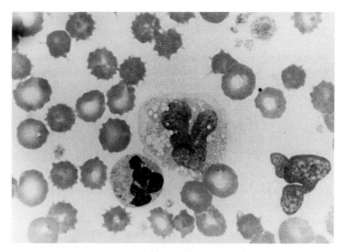

FIG. 26-10.   A toxic monocyte containing a highly contorted nucleus that may be reflecting incipient folate deficiency.

phils. Synonyms include leukoerythroblastic anemia and leukoerythroblastosis. The reaction may be mild or severe and may be present in a wide variety of conditions that have as a common feature stress or damage to marrow and evolution of extramedullary hematopoiesis.[14] The conditions most commonly associated with striking and sustained leukoerythroblastic reactions are those involving the presence of a space-occupying lesion in the marrow (myelophthisis) such as metastatic tumor, fibrosis, lymphoma, or leukemia. Mild and transitory leukoerythroblastic reactions may be a minor component of several conditions, including hemolytic anemia, severe infections, cardiac failure, uremia, and megaloblastic anemia.[14] Although it is a nonspecific reaction, leukoerythroblastosis provides important evidence of underlying disease or stress to the hematopoietic compartment.

Leukemoid reactions are reactive leukocytoses that resemble the blood findings seen in leukemia. Some investigators have defined a leukemoid reaction as one in which the total leukocyte count is greater than $50 \times 10^9/L$ or blast forms are found in the blood. It may be either myeloid or lymphoid.

Neutrophilic leukemoid reactions (NLR) most frequently present with excessively high leukocyte counts and a severe left shift, including occasional blast forms, and thus they resemble the blood picture of chronic myeloid leukemia (CML). They have been reported in patients with tuberculosis, metastatic tumor, and, in the experience of this author, they may accompany deep or occult abscesses. Differentiation between NLR and CML usually can be made on the basis of both morphology and cytochemistry. Morphologically, CML involves all granulocytes, so increased numbers of eosinophils, basophils with immature forms, or both is a hallmark of CML. NLR, on the other hand, generally involves only neutrophils, eosinophil and basophil numbers being normal or decreased. The neutrophil alkaline phosphatase value may be used to differentiate the two entities cytochemically. It tends to be increased in a neutrophilic reaction and decreased in CML. It suffices to say that the presence of circulating blast forms does not necessarily indicate leukemia and should be investigated further.

CHAPTER SUMMARY

The reaction of phagocytes to infection, stress, or trauma includes changes in numbers and in appearance. These alterations have been described for neutrophils, eosinophils, basophils, and monocytes. The importance of differentiating between true reactive morphology and artifact as well as distinguishing between reactive and malignant morphology has been stressed.

CASE STUDY 26-1

The patient, a 34-year-old white man complained of headache and drowsiness. History was negative except for severe sinusitis with accompanying fever 3 weeks prior to admission. The patient had no fever. Laboratory data include the following:

WBC	$106 \times 10^9/L$
RBC	$4.60 \times 10^{12}/L$
Hb	14.8 g/dL
HCT	0.45 L/L
MCV	98 fL
MCH	32 pg
MCHC	33 g/dL
PLT	$226 \times 10^9/L$

Diffential (300-cell) Count:

Blasts	2%
Promyelocytes	5%
Neutrophils*	
Myelocytes	7%
Metamyelocytes	14%
Bands	11%
Segs.	52%
Lymphocytes	6%
Monocytes	2%
Eosinophils	1%
Basophils	0%
NRBC/100 WBC	2

* Sixty percent of neutrophils contain toxic granulation; 5% of neutrophils contain Döhle bodies.

1. What is the evidence, pro and con, for a diagnosis of chronic myeloid leukemia?
2. Is the toxic granulation most likely true or artifactual? Why?
3. Is the monocyte number increased or normal?
4. The patient's neutrophil alkaline phosphatase value was 316 (normal, 65 to 165). What does this mean?

REFERENCES

1. Abernathy MR: Döhle bodies associated with uncomplicated pregnancy. Blood 27:380, 1966
2. Barrett ON Jr: Monocytosis in malignant disease. Ann Intern Med 73:991, 1970
3. Bass DA, Gonwa TA, Szejda P et al: Eosinopenia of acute infection: Production of eosinopenia by chemotactic factors of acute inflammation. J Clin Invest 65:1265, 1980
4. Bessis M: Living Blood Cells and Their Ultrastructure. Berlin, Springer-Verlag, 1973
5. Bishop CR, Rothstein CR, Ashenbrucker HE et al: Leukokinetic studies. XIII. A nonsteady state kinetic evaluation of the mechanism of cortisone-induced granulocytosis. J Clin Invest 50:1678, 1971
6. Bishop CR: The neutropenias of Felty's syndrome. Am J Hematol 2:203, 1977
7. Boggs DR, Jouce RA: The hematopoietic effects of lithium. Semin Hematol 20:129, 1983
8. Boxer LA, Greenberg MS, Boxer GJ et al: Autoimmune neutropenia. N Engl J Med 293:748, 1975
9. Butterworth AE: The eosinophil and its role in immunity to helminth infection. Curr Top Microbiol Immunol 77:127, 1977
10. Cassileth PA: Monocyte and macrophage disorders—self-limited proliferative responses. In Williams WJ, Beutler E, Erslev AJ et al (eds): Hematology, 3rd ed, p 861. New York, McGraw-Hill, 1983.
11. Cawley JC, Hayhoe FGS: The inclusions of the May-Hegglin anomaly and Döhle bodies of infection. Br J Haematol 22:491, 1972
12. Chilcote RR, Rierden WJ, Baehner RL: Neutropenia, recurrent bacterial infections and congenital deafness in patients with monocytopenia. Am J Dis Child 137:964, 1983
13. Christensen RD, Bradley PP, Rothstein G: The leukocyte left shift in clinical and experimental neonatal sepsis. J Pediatr 98:101, 1981

14. Clifford GO: The clinical significance of leukoerythroblastic anemia. Med Clin North Am 50:779, 1966

15. Craddock PR, Fehr J, Brigham KL et al: Complement and leukocyte-mediated pulmonary dysfunction in hemodialysis. N Engl J Med 296:769, 1977

16. David JR, Vadas MA, Butterworth AE et al: Enhanced helminthotoxic capacity of eosinophils from patients with eosinophilia. N Engl J Med 303:1147, 1980

17. Denburg JA, Telizyn S, Messner H et al: Heterogeneity of human peripheral blood eosinophil-type colonies: Evidence for a common basophil-eosinophil progenitor. Blood 66:312, 1985

18. Duplan JF, Bessis M, Breton-Gorious J: Les appendices nucleaires (caryoschizes) des granulocytes apres irradiation generale: etude au microscope electronique. Nouv Rev Fr Hematol 9:205, 1969

19. Falloon J, Gallen JI: Neutrophil granules in health and disease. J Allerg Clin Immunol 77:653, 1986

20. Ferrante A, Rowan-Kelly B, Scow WK et al: Depression of human polymorphonuclear leukocyte function by antimalarial drugs. Immunology 58:125, 1986

21. Forsgren A, Schmeling D: Effect of antibiotics on chemotaxis of human leukocytes. Antimicrob Agents Chemother 11:580, 1977

22. Gallen JI: Neutrophil specific granules: A fuse that ignites the inflammatory response. Clin Res 32:320, 1984

23. Gaylor MS, Chervenick PA, Boggs DR: Neutrophil kinetics after acute hemorrhage. Proc Soc Exp Biol Med 131:1332, 1969

24. Gilbert HS, Ornstein L: Basophil counting with a new staining method using Alcian blue. Blood 46:279, 1975

25. Gleich GJ, Loegering DA, Adolphson CR: Eosinophils and bronchial inflammation. Chest 87(Suppl):10S, 1985

26. Goetzl EJ, Foster DW, Payan DG: A basophil-activating factor from human T lymphocytes. Immunology 53:227, 1984

27. Groopman JE, Golde DW: The histiocytic disorders: A pathophysiologic analysis. Ann Intern Med 94:95, 1981

28. Grzelak I, Olszewski WL, Engeset A: Influence of operative trauma on circulating blood monocytes: Analysis using monoclonal antibodies. Eur Surg Res 16:105, 1984

29. Hartl W: Drug allergic agranulocytosis (Schultz's disease). Semin Hematol 2:313, 1965

30. Holley TR, vanEpps DE, Harvey RL et al: Effect of high doses of radiation on human neutrophil chemotaxis, phagocytosis and morphology. Am J Pathol 75:61, 1974

31. Horowitz DA, Allison AC, Ward P: Identification of human mononuclear leukocyte populations by esterase staining. Clin Exp Immunol 30:289, 1977

32. Issekutz AC, Ripley M: The effect of intravascular neutrophil chemotactic factors on blood neutrophil and platelet kinetics. Am J Hematol 21:157, 1986

33. Knecht H, Eichhorn P, Streuli RA: Granulocytes with ring-shaped nuclei in severe alcoholism. Acta Haematol 73:184, 1985

34. Koepke JA, Koepke JF: Guide to Clinical Laboratory Diagnosis, 3rd ed. Norwalk, CT, Appleton & Lange, 1987

35. Koszewski BJ, Vahabzadeh H, Willrodt S: Hemosiderin content of leukocytes in animals and man and its significance in the physiology of granulocytes. Am J Clin Pathol 48:474, 1967

36. Kugel MA, Rosenthal N: Pathological changes in polymorphonuclear leukocytes during progress of infection. Am J Med Sci 183:657, 1932

37. Lalezari P, Nussbaum G, Gelman S et al: Neonatal neutropenia due to maternal isoimmunization. Blood 15:236, 1960

38. Langenhuijsen MM: Neutrophils with ring-shaped nuclei in myeloproliferative disease. Br J Haematol 58:227, 1984

39. Lensink DB, Barton A, Appelbaum FR et al: Cyclic neutropenia as a premalignant manifestation of acute lymphoblastic leukemia. Am J Hematol 22:9, 1986

40. Lui CH, Lehan C, Speer ME et al: Early detection of bacteremia in an outpatient clinic. Pediatrics 75:827, 1985

41. McCall CE, Katayama I, Cotran RS et al: Lysosomal and ultrastructural changes in human "toxic" neutrophils during bacterial infection. J Exp Med 129:267, 1969

42. McLaren DJ: The role of eosinophils in tropical disease. Semin Hematol 19:100, 1982

43. Mackie PH, Mistry DK, Wozniak JT et al: Neutrophil cytochemistry in bacterial infection. J Clin Pathol 32:26, 1979

44. Malcolm ID, Flegel KM, Katz M: Vacuolation of the neutrophil in bacteremia. Arch Intern Med 139:675, 1979

45. Maldonado JE, Hanlon DG: Monocytosis: A current appraisal. Mayo Clin Proc 40:248, 1965

46. Manroe BL, Rosenfeld CR, Weinberg AG et al: The differential leukocyte count in the assessment and outcome of early onset neonatal group B streptococcal disease. J Pediatr 91:632, 1977

47. Marsh JC, Boggs DR, Cartwright GE et al: Neutrophil kinetics in acute infection. J Clin Invest 46:1943, 1967

48. Minot GR, Smith LW: The blood in tetrachlorethane poisoning. Arch Intern Med 28:687, 1921

49. Mishler JM, Sharp AH: Adrenalin: Further discussion of its role in the mobilization of neutrophils. Scand J Haematol 17:78, 1976

50. Mitchell RG: Circulating basophilic leukocyte counts in the newborn. Arch Dis Child 30:130, 1955

51. Morgan DJR, Moodley PI, Elliott EV et al: Histamine, neutrophil chemotactic factor and circulating basophil levels following exercise in asthmatic and control subjects. Clin Allerg 12 (Suppl):29, 1982

52. Murphy MF, Metcalfe P, Grint PCA et al: Cephalosporin-induced immune neutropenia. Br J Haematol 59:9, 1985

53. Nagaraju M, Weitzman S, Baumann G: Viral hepatitis and agranulocytosis. Am J Digest Dis 18:247, 1973

54. Naiman JL, Oski FA, Allen FH et al: Hereditary eosinophilia. Report of a family and review of the literature. Am J Hum Genet 16:195, 1964

55. O'Flaherty JT, Kreutzer DL, Ward PA: Neutrophil aggregation and swelling induced by chemotactic agents. J Immunol 119:232, 1977

56. Oria J, Yoneda S: Variation of the form and structure of the nucleus in various types of plurisegmented neutrophils. In Damashek W, Taylor FHL (eds): George R Minot Symposium in Hematology. New York, Grune & Stratton, 1949

57. Payne R: Leukocyte agglutinins in human sera. Correlations between blood transfusions and their development. Arch Intern Med 99:587, 1957

58. Ponder E, Ponder RV: The cytology of the polymorphonuclear leukocyte in toxic conditions. J Lab Clin Med 28:316, 1942

59. Pruzansky JJ, Ts'ao C, Krajewski DV et al: Quantification of ultrastructural variations in enriched blood basophils: Correlation of morphological changes and antigen-induced histamine release. Immunology 47:41, 1982

60. Robinson WA: Granulocytosis in neoplasia. Ann NY Acad Sci 230:212, 1974

61. Shaper AG, Lewis PP: Genetic neutropenia in people of African origin. Lancet 2:1021, 1971

62. Shelley WB, Jiuhlin L: Degranulation of the basophil in man induced by dietary lipemia. Am J Med Sci 242:221, 1961

63. Shelley WB, Parnes HM: The absolute basophil count. JAMA 192:108, 1965

64. Shenaq SA, Yawn DH, Saleem A et al: Effect of profound hypothermia on leukocytes and platelets. Ann Clin Lab Sci 16:130, 1986

65. Solberg CO, Hellum KB: Neutrophil granulocyte function in bacterial infections. Lancet 2:727, 1972

66. Thompson J, VanFurth R: The effect of glucocorticoids on the proliferation and kinetics of promonocytes and monocytes of the bone marrow. J Exp Med 137:10, 1973

67. Thonnard-Neumann E: The influence of hormones on the basophilic leukocytes. Acta Haematol 25:261, 1961

68. Thonnard-Neumann E: Studies of basophils; variations with age and sex. Acta Haematol 30:221, 1963

69. Tomkins E: The monocytes. Ann NY Acad Sci 59:832, 1955

70. van Assendelft OW: Reference values for the total and differential leukocyte count. Blood Cells 11:77, 1985

71. van Furth R, Raeburn JA, van Swet TL: Characteristics of human mononuclear phagocytes. Blood 54:485, 1979

72. Waterlot Y, Cantinieaux B, Hariga-Muller C et al: Impaired phagocytic activity of neutrophils in patients receiving haemodialysis: The critical role of iron overload. Br Med J 291:501, 1985

73. Weller PF, Goetzl EJ: The human eosinophil. Am J Pathol 100:793, 1980

74. Wilson ME: Effects of bacterial endotoxins on neutrophil function. Rev Inf Dis 7:404, 1985

75. Wintrobe MM, Lee GR, Boggs DR et al: Clinical Hematology, 8th ed. Philadelphia, Lea and Febiger, 1981

76. Wright DG, Meierovics AI, Foxley JM: Assessing the delivery of neutrophils to tissues in neutropenia. Blood 67:1023, 1986

77. Zieve PD, Haghsenass M, Krevans JR: Vacuolation of the neutrophil. Arch Intern Med 118:356, 1966

78. Zucker-Franklin D: Eosinopenia and eosinophilia. In Williams WJ et al (eds): Hematology, 4th ed. New York, McGraw Hill, 1990

Nonmalignant, Reactive Disorders of Lymphocytes

Virginia Haight

Nonmalignant disorders of lymphocytes are self-limited lymphoproliferative responses. Lymphocytic proliferation or the reactive lymphocyte morphology seen in these disorders is the result of normal lymphocyte response to antigen stimulation. Reactive lymphocytes are, and should be, found in normal blood, but in proportions greater than 20% they are considered significant and are found in a wide variety of conditions (Table 27-1).

The term *lymphocytosis* refers to an absolute increase in the number of circulating lymphocytes above the normal level of 4.0×10^9/L in adults; 9.0×10^9/L in infants and young children, and 7.9×10^9/L in older children.[14] Relative lymphocytosis refers to an increase in the percentage of circulating lymphocytes. A relative lymphocytosis does not necessarily reflect a true or absolute increase in lymphocytes.

TERMINOLOGY

Various terms have been used to describe the lymphocytes seen in nonmalignant reactive disorders—variant lymphocytes, reactive lymphocytes, atypical lymphocytes, virocytes, stress lymphocytes, Downey cells, transformed lymphocytes, transitional lymphocytes, and glandular fever cells, among others.

While *virocytes* is an adequate term to describe reactive lymphocytes in most patients who have a known viral infection, there are other causes of altered lymphocytes in which no virus is implicated. Because such lymphocytes are normal cells reacting to a stimulus, whether it be viral or other, the designation *reactive lymphocytes* has gained considerable popularity in several institutions. A less definitive but quite popular term is *atypical lymphocytes*. The National Committee for Clinical Laboratory Standards has proposed

TABLE 27–1. Causes of Lymphocytosis with and without Variant Morphology

Absolute lymphocytosis with variant lymphocytes
  Infectious mononucleosis
  Acute viral hepatitis
  Cytomegalovirus infections
Relative lymphocytosis with variant lymphocytes
  Toxoplasmosis
  Viral-related disorders
    Measles
    Mumps
    Chickenpox
    Rubella
    Viral pneumonia
  Immune disorders
    Drug reactions
    Serum sickness
    Idiopathic thrombocytopenia
    Autoimmune hemolytic anemia
  Nonviral infections
    Tuberculosis
    Syphilis
    Malaria
    Typhus
    Brucellosis
    Rickettsia
    Diphtheria
Absolute lymphocytosis with normal lymphocytes
  Acute infectious lymphocytosis
  Bordetella pertussis infection
Relative lymphocytosis with normal lymphocytes
  Neutropenia

variant lymphocytes as the term of choice. Table 27-1 lists the conditions in which variant (reactive) lymphocytes are found in peripheral blood.

HISTORY

Lymphocytes that show morphologic variation from normal small mature lymphocytes and yet are not leukemic cells have long been recognized in the peripheral blood of patients with a variety of clinical conditions. Türk first described these cells in 1907 in a patient whose disease had been diagnosed as acute leukemia but who later recovered. Türk described the cells as having an immature nucleus and basophilic cytoplasm similar to that of a plasma cell.[6] The benign nature of these cells was not recognized at that time. The first accurate description of them was published in 1923 by Downey and McKinlay in a paper entitled "Acute Lymphadenosis Compared with Acute Lymphatic Leukemia."[6] This paper described nine cases of *acute lymphadenosis* within a short period of time and suggested a common occurrence of the disease, which they categorized as a specific clinical entity. Study of the morphology of the lymphocytes showed atypical appearance to be a consistent finding. In all cases the morphology allowed correct diagnosis of a nonmalignant lymphocytosis, even though the clinical findings were similar to those of acute leukemia. In 1967 Wood and Frenkel addressed the important morphologic and biochemical characteristics of variant lymphocytes in various clinical entities.[21] Their studies of DNA synthesis utilizing thymidine-labeled lymphocytes showed that reactive lymphocytes actively synthesize DNA. It is now a well established fact that the variant or reactive

lymphocyte is a normal morphologic alteration reflecting a benign lymphoproliferative process. *Although the morphology is well documented, distinguishing benign from malignant disorders may be difficult, and often only clinical findings can establish the difference.*

MORPHOLOGY OF VARIANT OR REACTIVE LYMPHOCYTES

The most important feature of variant lymphocyte morphology is the recognition of its benign nature. The pertinent fact is that these lymphocytes are normal cells that have been altered as the result of a normal response to stimulus.

Downey and McKinlay, who provided the classic description of the reactive lymphocyte, found enough variation in its structure to classify variant (reactive) lymphocytes into three distinct types. In reactive lymphoproliferative disorders these cells are seen in the peripheral blood in either one or various combinations of the following three categories:

Type I

Also called plasmacytoid lymphocyte and Türk's irritation cell, type I cells are differentiated cells that are functionally immunocompetent and probably of B-cell origin.

Size: 9 to 20 μm diameter
Shape: Oval or round
Nucleus: Heavy strands or dense blocks of chromatin irregularly clumped with sharp, small, defined areas of parachromatin; nuclear shape may be indented or oval. Nuclear membrane is distinct.
Cytoplasm: Basophilia varies but usually the cytoplasm is moderately basophilic. It may be vacuolated, with darker areas of basophilia at the periphery. It may also have a foamy appearance and may contain azurophilic granules (see Plate 24).

Type II

Type II cells are sometimes referred to as the infectious mononucleosis (IM) cell because they are the predominant type in IM.

Size: 15 to 25 μm in diameter
Shape: Irregular or scalloped
Nucleus: The chromatin strands are coarse but not as condensed as those of type I. Rounded masses of chromatin are interspersed throughout. Nuclear shape is round or oval and is rarely lobulated. Nuclear banding frequently is seen in EDTA specimens. Nucleoli usually are not visible.
Cytoplasm: Abundant and often indented by surrounding structures. Nuclear:cytoplasmic ratio is 1:2 to 1:4. The cytoplasm has few vacuoles and usually is pale, except for basophilia at the periphery of the cytoplasm and radiating from the nucleus. This cell often has been described as resembling a fried egg or a flared skirt (see Plate 25).

Type III

Transformed lymphocytes or reticular lymphocytes are cells in an intermediate stage of transformation, the process through which the resting small lymphocyte undergoes blast transformation and ultimately becomes a fully immunocompetent T lymphocyte or plasma cell.

Size: 12 to 35 μm diameter
Shape: Round or irregular
Nucleus: Finely reticulated nuclear chromatin (immature). Chromatin strands are finely dispersed with loose, indistinct clumping and poorly defined parachromatin. Nucleoli are usually highly visible and elongated or irregular in shape.
Cytoplasm: Vacuolated with abundant basophilia and a clear perinuclear area (see Plate 26).

The size and shape of the nucleus contribute very little to the classification of the three types of variant lymphocytes, but chromatin structure (quantity and distribution) and parachromatin features are of paramount importance in distinguishing these cells from monocytes.

One major precaution should be noted here: Variant (reactive) lymphocytes are particularly vulnerable to effects of delay and anticoagulant (EDTA). Therefore, fresh specimens (*i.e.*, blood films made within 30 minutes of collection) are an absolute necessity. Prolonged exposure to EDTA can lead to bizarre morphology that mimics that seen in malignancy, such as clefted nuclei, mitotic forms, necrotic (dead) cells, and numerous broken cells.

Lymphocyte Transformation

The lymphocyte morphology described above reflects the cumulative events following antigenic stimulation in which the stimulated lymphocyte undergoes structural and biochemical changes, transforming the small lymphocyte to the blastlike cell, a process called blastogenesis (Fig. 27-1). Transformation can be produced *in vitro* by specific and nonspecific antigens. Several nonspecific antigens (mitogens) have been used to stimulate lymphocytes *in vitro*: phytohemagglutinin (PHA), pokeweed mitogen (PWM), streptolysin S *Staphylococcus* endotoxin (SLS), and antilymphocyte globulin (ALG). The most commonly used are PHA for T-cell stimulation and PWM for both T- and B-cell stimulation leading to mitosis. Cultures using PHA show nucleolar changes in 4 hours and RNA production within 8 hours; at the end of 72 hours most cells are transformed and in mitosis.

When lymphocyte transformation is studied with the transmission electron microscope, the nucleus becomes larger and clearer and the cytoplasm contains an enlarged Golgi apparatus, which increases rapidly and occupies a significant space in the cell's center. Ribosomes increase in number, and mitochondria increase in volume. The endoplasmic reticulum develops slightly if it is a T cell and considerably if it is a B cell. Azurophilic granules increase in number. Nucleoli become elongated and enlarged.

Scanning electron microscopy reveals a pronounced shape change from round to "hand mirror" shape—an indication of increased motility. A uropod (viscous posterior portion of the cytoplasm) becomes very prominent. The uropod region contains the Golgi complex, where proteins are accumulated.

Differentiation Between Reactive and Malignant Lymphocytes

Since both reactive and malignant lymphocytosis may exhibit immature-looking cells, to distinguish between the two entities requires skill and experience. The major morphologic differentiation lies in the heterogeneity of variant lymphocytes (polymorphism). This means that within a single specimen both large cells and small cells; basophilic cells and pale cells; cells with immature chromatin and cells with densely clumped chromatin are observed. Malignancies, on the other hand, usually are clonal, and all abnormal cells appear very similar to one another.

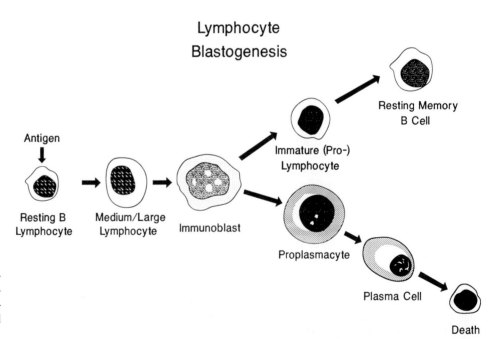

Lymphocyte Blastogenesis

FIG. 27-1. Diagram of morphologic changes associated with lymphocyte transformation in response to antigen stimulation. The B-cell line is used as an example.

ABSOLUTE LYMPHOCYTOSIS WITH VARIANT LYMPHOCYTE MORPHOLOGY

Infectious Mononucleosis

Definition

IM is a clinically acute contagious viral disease that affects primarily young adults and teenagers. It is not often seen before 10 years of age or after 40 years. When it does affect adults 40 years or older, it is generally more severe. The disease is self-limited and benign, but serious complications can occur which occasionally may be fatal. The disease is characterized by variant (reactive) lymphocytes in the peripheral blood and a heterophil antibody-positive serologic test.

History

As early as 1885, Filatov described idiopathic lymphadenopathy in children. Pfeiffer (1889) described what he considered to be a lymphatic reaction in children, and occasionally in adults, with nontender cervical glandular enlargement, absence of tonsillitis, abdominal pain, and enlargement of spleen and liver.[18] In 1920 Sprunt and Evans chose the term *infectious mononucleosis* to describe mononuclear leukocytosis following reaction to acute infections.[20] In 1923 Downey and McKinlay described the morphology of the reactive lymphocytes.[6] Serologic characterization was first described in 1932 by Paul and Bunnell and refined by Davidsohn and coworkers in 1955.[5] Thus a differential absorption test was developed and became widely accepted as a serologic test for the diagnosis of IM. Eventually, simple screening tests were devised. In 1964 Epstein, Achong, and Barr found that a herpeslike virus (Epstein-Barr virus, EBV) seen in lymphoblasts of patients with Burkitt's lymphoma was also seen in the lymphocytes of patients with infectious mononucleosis and that the sera from these patients contained large amounts of anti-EBV antibodies. The cause of IM remained obscure until 1968, when Henle found lymphocytes containing the EBV in the blood of a laboratory technician who had previously been negative for both heterophil and anti-EBV antibodies. Henle also showed a relationship between Burkitt's lymphoma and IM, which led to further studies that confirmed that EBV was the infective agent.[8,9,15]

Pathophysiology

Following the discovery that EBV was the agent of IM, many studies have been conducted to determine the pathophysiology. Studies have shown that asymptomatic infection with EBV occurs early in childhood, particularly in children whose socioeconomic environment is poor, and that by age 10 years, 60% to 90% of the population have been exposed to the virus.[12] Infection with the virus is often mild and asymptomatic in young children, and sera from these children is usually heterophil negative. By age 40 years most of the population have been exposed to and have acquired antibody to EBV antigen. Anti-EBV antibodies are believed to provide lifelong immunity for most persons. Adolescents who have not developed immunity (who are seronegative) are very susceptible to infection by EBV, and approximately 50% develop a clinically acute disease.

EBV selectively binds to specific receptors on B lymphocytes, enters at the histocompatibility locus, and takes over the genome of the cell, producing a virally altered cell surface. During the first week of the disease these B cells proliferate, producing infected clones of B cells. Immunoglobulin-secreting B cells also increase with the aid of T helper cells and in response to the infected B cells. Such a polyclonal B-cell response is reflected in hypergammaglobulinemia. The antibody response in turn activates T lymphocytes, inducing blastogenesis. Blastogenic T cell response is shown to increase with time, and during transformation, T lymphocytes acquire cytotoxic potential. The increased number of circulating reactive lymphocytes directly reflects this T-cell proliferation. During the second week of the disease, T-helper cell activity increases until finally T-suppressor cells become activated and shut down T-helper activity. In this way the interaction between T cells and infected B cells is controlled. The balance that is achieved between helper and suppressor cells invokes the immunoregulatory mechanism, returning the immune response to normal. Persons with immune disorders of impaired T cell function are not able to control proliferation of infected B cells; the result is long-lasting complications in which B cell lymphomas may develop. Occasionally, an antibody produced by EBV-infected B cells may be produced against platelet surface antigen or the i antigen on erythrocytes, producing either thrombocytopenia, autoimmune hemolytic anemia, or both. Following EBV infection, the virus may persist in the saliva and oropharynx as well as within a small proportion of B cells. This persistence of the virus in a latent form results in a persistence of antibody titers (immunoglobulin G [IgG]) against viral capsid, viral membrane, and EBV nuclear–associated antigen (EBNA).

Clinical Features

The incubation period of IM is about 11 days. Onset is usually accompanied by low-grade fever, which may then elevate to levels as high as 106°F. Fever, pharyngitis, and cervical lymphadenopathy are the presenting symptoms in more than 80% of cases. Occasionally the onset may be sudden, with shaking chills and high fever. Splenomegaly is found in about 50% of cases and hepatomegaly in approximately 10% of patients. A rash is present in 20% of cases. Occasionally, the patient may present at the prodromal stage, when the only manifestation is nonspecific malaise and fatigue and no hematologic or secondary changes are evident, making the diagnosis difficult. This prodromal stage may last 4 to 5 days, and the disease lasts for 1 to 3 weeks. Complications are rare, but when they occur they may be serious. Some of the complications are pneumonitis, meningoencephalitis, pericarditis, myocarditis, hepatitis, and laryngeal edema, all of which are related to lymphocytic infiltrates. Neurologic syndromes such as Bell's palsy and Guillain-Barré usually are reversible but can be fatal. Clinical complications include hemorrhage due to thrombocytopenia, airway obstruction due to enlargement of pharyngeal lymphoid tissue, and splenic rupture if splenomegaly is present. Spontaneous splenic rupture is rare. Out of 107 cases reported through 1978, only 18 were spontaneous.[19]

Laboratory Features

The major laboratory findings are in two areas, hematologic and serologic. The classic hematologic findings are absolute lymphocytosis ($>5 \times 10^9$/L), with more than 20% variant lymphocytes. In the first few days after infection, however, leukopenia may be present. Should a patient seek medical attention during these first few days, diagnosis could be difficult. The transient leukopenia is followed by a general increase in lymphocytes toward the end of the first week, which causes a rise in leukocytes to between 10 and 20×10^9/L. Children may present with leukocyte counts above 50×10^9/L. The peripheral blood contains a mixture of normal lymphocytes, variant lymphocytes, and an increased number of monocytes. Eosinophils also may be increased. The proportion of the various cell types changes as the disease progresses. All three types of variant lymphocytes (Downey cells) may be found, although type II predominates. Cells vary greatly in size and shape, in nuclear content (coarse to fine nuclear clumping), and in cytoplasmic features such as cytoplasmic vacuolation (foamy appearance) or smooth homogeneous cytoplasm. These lymphocytes usually appear 4 to 5 days after onset of the disease and persist for upward of 30 days. Since variant or reactive lymphocytes are found in a variety of other illnesses, the percentage may help to distinguish IM from other diseases. Forty percent or more is strongly suggestive of IM, and some investigators believe that serologic tests are unnecessary for diagnosis if atypia reaches 40% or more. Occasionally when clinical findings suggest IM, hematologic or serologic findings fail to confirm the diagnosis. In such instances cytomegalovirus (CMV) infection or toxoplasmosis should be suspected.

The classic serologic finding is the presence of the so-called heterophil antibody. When Paul and Bunnell discovered that sera of patients with infectious mononucleosis caused agglutination of sheep red cells, they called the antibody a heterophil antibody, meaning that it reacted with antigens that were not responsible for its production. Earlier, in 1911, Forssman had described a nonspecific antigen in the tissues of various animals, including the guinea pig. Antibodies to the Forssman antigen are present in sera of normal persons in low titers (<1:56). Infectious mononucleosis heterophil antibody *is not* absorbed or is absorbed only slightly by Forssman antigen and *is* absorbed by beef erythrocytes. Therefore, the presence of the heterophil antibody that is not absorbed by Forssman's antigen is the *sine qua non* (*i.e.*, diagnostic) of IM.

Two types of serologic tests for IM are available: the classic test described above and an antibody test specific for EBV. The classic test has been largely replaced by rapid tests (slide or tube) available from several manufacturers. The rapid tests use as the indicator cells fresh horse erythrocytes (which are more sensitive than sheep erythrocytes) and a suspension of guinea pig kidney and beef erythrocyte stroma for differential absorption. The specificity of these tests has been considered as reliable as the traditional differential absorption test, but they should be interpreted in conjunction with clinical and hematologic findings. Thus, if lymphocyte morphology resembles that in IM and results of the heterophil test are negative, then other viral diseases should be considered. Occasionally, the heterophil test is negative early in the course of the disease. If hematologic

and clinical findings support the diagnosis of IM, the serologic test should be repeated in a few days to 1 week.

For heterophil-negative or unusual cases, EBV-specific antibodies are assayed by immunofluorescence techniques. Immunofluorescent antibody tests are mandatory for diagnosis of infectious mononucleosis if other criteria have not been met. During the course of the disease, patients may develop a variety of EBV antibodies, which differ in reactivity and specificity. These include the heterophil group, which are IgM antibodies. Also included are IgG and IgM antibodies to viral capsid antigen (VCA), diffuse (D) component of early antigen (EA) complex, and IgG antibodies to EBNA (nuclear associated antigen). During acute infection and convalescence, antibodies are produced to various virus-specific and virus-determined antigens in a defined and predictable sequence. IgM antibodies arise during incubation and peak in 2 weeks then decline rapidly. IgA anti-VCA are seen in most patients and remain permanently. Failure to develop IgA antibodies appears to be associated with prolonged illness. Evidence that a patient is undergoing an episode of active IM is the presence of a high titer of IgG anti-VCA, the presence of IgM anti-VCA and anti-EA, and the absence of low-titer anti-EBNA.[7] Occasionally other antibodies are found in the sera of IM patients, including cold-reactive anti-i antibodies, and antinuclear antibodies.

If hepatitis is suspected as a complication, alkaline phosphatase, lactate dehydrogenase (LD), alanine aminotransferase (ALT), and aldolase values are elevated. Uric acid levels may be increased. Urine is usually normal, but occasionally there may be some proteinuria. If either hemolysis or impaired liver function is present, urobilinogen may be increased. Renal function usually is not impaired. Cerebrospinal fluid may contain lymphocytes up to 1×10^9/L, but protein and sugar values are normal.

Examination of bone marrow usually is not indicated, but occasionally it may be necessary to rule out leukemia. It is usually normal but may be hypercellular, with hyperplasia of the erythroid, myeloid, and megakaryocytic lines. Variant lymphocytes may be present but the overall number of lymphocytes usually is not increased.

Cytomegalovirus Infection

Definition and Clinical Features

CMV is a disease caused by cytomegalovirus that closely resembles IM. Clinical symptoms differ from those of IM inasmuch as patients do not have tonsilitis or enlarged lymph nodes. One of the most distinguishing features is that patients generally do not complain of a sore throat, usually the first and foremost manifestation of IM. Lethargy and cervical lymphadenopathy are unusual, and most CMV infections appear to be subclinical. Fever and splenomegaly are common in middle-aged adults. Lymphadenopathy usually is not a prominent finding. Hepatomegaly may be found in 50% of patients, as compared to only 10% in IM patients. Occasionally, a rash may be present. At onset of the illness, malaise, fever, and chills are common. Symptoms may persist for a longer period (3 weeks) than in IM. The incubation period is 35 to 40 days for adults and 20 to 25 days for children. CMV occurs commonly in adults, whereas IM is unusual after 35. Another distinguishing feature of CMV is that the heterophil antibody is negative although reactive lymphocytosis is present. Increased numbers of cases of CMV have been noted in homosexual men, and CMV has been implicated as a possible agent of Kaposi's sarcoma. CMV causes cytomegalic inclusion disease of newborns. CMV in newborns may cause hepatosplenomegaly, jaundice, cataracts, and mental retardation. It is thought that the disease is transmitted to the child perinatally from virus in cervical secretions, or possibly by blood transfusion.

Pathophysiology

The disease is caused by CMV, which was shown to be the cytotoxic agent when it was isolated from leukocytes of infected persons. It is a cell-associated herpes virus similar to EBV. The virus is found in urine, oral and cervical secretions, and semen, as well as in leukocytes. Since CMV resides in cervical secretions and semen, transmission in adults is primarily venereal. CMV was first recognized in 1962, when open heart surgery patients developed a severe febrile illness with skin rash, splenomegaly, and marked lymphocytosis that resembled IM. More than half of adults possess antibodies to CMV.

Laboratory Features

IgM and IgG antibodies to CMV antigen can be demonstrated. Complement-fixing antibody with a fourfold rise in the antibody titer is considered diagnostic. IgM antibody to CMV has also been found in patients with EBV mononucleosis. IgM cytolytic antibody to CMV-infected cells is seen in patients with primary CMV infection. Results of heterophil antibody tests are negative, and there is no increase in EBV titers. Lymphocytosis with variant or reactive lymphocytes similar to those seen in IM are always present. In contrast to infectious mononucleosis, T cells are not increased in CMV. The leukocyte count rarely exceeds $15 \times 10^9/L$; however, higher counts have been reported. A normochromic, normocytic anemia often occurs and results of the Coombs test may be positive. Platelet number may be decreased and may be low enough to produce petechiae. Occasionally, other laboratory abnormalities occur, including cold agglutinins, antinuclear antibodies, and cryoglobulins.

Post-transfusion syndrome is probably the best-known cause of CMV infection. It is acquired from transfusion of large amounts of fresh blood. CMV is found in the leukocytes of the transfused blood. Infection of the patient is due to direct transmission of CMV from donor blood or to activation of latent infection in the recipient. Symptoms appear 3 weeks to 3 months after transfusion. Seroconversion increases with the quantity of blood transfused (*i.e.,* 6%–10% with 1–5 units of blood and up to 40%–60% with 10–15 units of blood).

ABSOLUTE LYMPHOCYTOSIS WITH NORMAL LYMPHOCYTE MORPHOLOGY

Acute Infectious Lymphocytosis

Acute infectious lymphocytosis usually is found in children between the ages of 1 and 10 years, and occasionally up to 14 years of age. It is contagious, benign, and self-limited. The causative agent may be viral or nonviral; however, an enterovirus-coxsackie A subgroup has been isolated in stool specimens of 21% of patients and it may be responsible for the extreme lymphocytosis seen in this disease. The fact that the disease occurs in clusters and outbreaks is suggestive of a contagious agent. The incubation period appears to be between 12 and 20 days. The disease lasts from 3 to 5 weeks and may last as long as 2 months.

Clinical Features

Generally, patients with infectious lymphocytosis are asymptomatic. When symptoms accompany the disease, they usually are fever, upper respiratory infection, diarrhea, and abdominal pain. No organomegaly is noted.

Laboratory Findings

The one striking finding is an extreme leukocytosis that may exceed $100 \times 10^9/L$, although most patients exhibit leukocytes from 40 to $50 \times 10^9/L$. The leukocytosis is the result of marked T-lymphocyte proliferation. The morphology is that of small resting lymphocytes, uniform in size and structure with scanty cytoplasm. Variant or reactive morphology is conspicuously absent. Bone marrow examination reveals a slight increase in small lymphocytes. Serology is negative for the heterophil antibody.

Bordetella pertussis Infection

Bordetella pertussis is another infection in which 70% to 90% of leukocytes on the peripheral blood film are normal-looking lymphocytes. The increase in small lymphocytes may be due to redistribution from tissue pools to circulating pools caused by a lymphocyte-promoting factor (LPF). Studies in mice indicate that LPF attaches to lymphocytes and blocks their movement from blood to lymph nodes, thus increasing the number of circulating lymphocytes and decreasing lymphocytes in the lymph nodes. Leukocyte counts range from 15 to $50 \times 10^9/L$. The leukocytosis and lymphocytosis are more pronounced than in any other febrile illness except IM.

Lymphocytic Leukemoid Reaction

Any condition in which the lymphocytic leukocytosis is so marked that it gives the impression of possible leukemia qualifies as a lymphocytic leukemoid reaction. Infectious mononucleosis in children may present with leukocyte counts in excess of $50 \times 10^9/L$, which may lead to an impression of acute lymphocytic leukemia. Likewise, patients with infectious lymphocytosis may have a peripheral blood picture that is reminiscent of chronic lymphatic leukemia. Children who are critically ill with *Bordetella pertussis* infection may have a leukemoid response, with a leukocyte count above $50 \times 10^9/L$.

RELATIVE LYMPHOCYTOSIS WITH VARIANT LYMPHOCYTE MORPHOLOGY

Toxoplasmosis

A lymphadenopathic variety of *Toxoplasma* (*Toxoplasma gondii*) infection is similar in clinical presentation to IM, causing fever and enlarged lymph nodes. Hematologically, there is a relative but not absolute increase in reactive lymphocytes. The result of the heterophil antibody test is negative. Up to 10% of seronegative IM cases may be toxoplasmosis. The clinical symptoms ultimately help to differentiate between IM and toxoplasmosis. In IM, lymphatic involvement is often confined to posterior cervical lymph nodes, whereas there tends to be generalized involvement of lymphatic tissue in toxoplasmosis. Splenomegaly and sore throats are less common in toxoplasmosis. Laboratory features usually are benign, with normal hematologic parameters, the exception being a relative increase in lymphocytes and the presence of reactive lymphocytes. Rarely is absolute lymphocytosis seen. Morphology of the variant lymphocytes is variable; some may have scanty amounts of cytoplasm, making them resemble the lymphoblasts of acute leukemia. Cells of the IM type (type II) are not often seen. Current tests for confirmation are indirect fluorescent antibody and indirect hemagglutination techniques.

Miscellaneous Disorders

Lymphopenia and neutropenia develop soon after the onset of measles, mumps, chickenpox, hepatitis, and roseola, followed within a few days by a relative lymphocytosis. There is always a pleomorphic blood picture, and variant lymphocytes are a dominant finding. As recovery occurs and the blood picture normalizes, small lymphocytes increase and some of the large lymphocytes become plasmacytoid (type I). Immune responses, recent immunizations, hypersensitivity reactions, and autoimmune diseases all produce the same type of lymphoid reactions. The absolute number of lymphocytes does not increase, but an increase in mitotic forms and increased DNA synthesis are noted. Occasionally, immature lymphocytes (type III) may be seen. The immature appearance of these lymphoid cells may cause confusion with malignant lymphoproliferative disorders.

Ten percent of patients with thyrotoxicosis have neutropenia and relative lymphocytosis. The blood changes are probably due to a disturbance of adrenocortical function.

RELATIVE LYMPHOCYTOSIS WITH NORMAL LYMPHOCYTE MORPHOLOGY

Neutropenia

There is a wide variety of conditions in which the absolute number of neutrophils decreases, leaving relative lymphocytosis in which lymphocyte morphology is normal.

It should be noted that up to the age of 4 years, most normal children have greater numbers of circulating lymphocytes than granulocytes. Infants, especially those who are premature, may have circulating lymphoid cells with immature-looking chromatin and very scanty cytoplasm,

similar to those seen in acute lymphocytic leukemia. This probably reflects the seeding of peripheral lymphatic tissue by stem cells from bone marrow or thymus, an entirely normal phenomenon in this age group.

CHAPTER SUMMARY

This chapter has addressed abnormalities in lymphocyte number and morphology that are reactive in nature. Three major types of variant (reactive) lymphocyte morphology have been described in detail and those disorders that commonly result in reactive lymphocyte abnormalities have been discussed, with emphasis on infectious mononucleosis. The disorders have been classified according to whether they are characterized by absolute or relative increases in lymphocytes and whether reactive morphology is or is not present.

CASE STUDY 27-1

The patient is a 45-year-old woman with shaking chills and fever which began after she inhaled toxic fumes. Two days later she noticed a rash over her back and trunk. She was admitted to the hospital suffering from generalized body soreness, coughing, malaise, fever, and chills.

The patient was transfused with packed red cells and platelets on the second hospital day. The patient's condition began to stabilize on the fourth day. On the fifth day, the peripheral blood film showed 36% variant lymphocytes. The neutrophils no longer looked toxic, and there was no evidence of phagocytosis. Two weeks later, a marked reactive lymphocyte response was noted, which persisted for 2 weeks. The following laboratory results were obtained:

LABORATORY TESTS	ADMISSION	DAY 2	DAY 5
WBC (× 10⁹/L)	5.9		20.0
Hb (g/dL)	11.6	7.7	10.0
PLT (× 10⁹/L)	30	13	120.0
Neutrophils, seg (%)	24(toxic)		20
Neutrophils, band (%)	72		10
Lymphocytes (%)	2	(variant)	60
Monocytes (%)	2		10
Alkaline phosphatase (U/L)	494		
LD (U/L)	670		
AST (U/L)	196		
ALT (U/L)	132		
BUN (mg/dL)		40.0	
Monospot	Negative		
Fibrinogen (mg/dL)		100.0	

1. Judging from the clinical information and laboratory findings, what is the most likely cause of the thrombocytopenia and the left shift of the granulocytes?
2. Considering the patient's clinical history and treatment, what is the most likely cause of the reactive lymphocytosis? What laboratory tests are needed to confirm the diagnosis?

REFERENCES

1. Baumgartner J, Glauser MP, Burgo-Black AL et al: Severe cytomegalovirus infection in multiply transfused, splenectomized trauma patients. Lancet 2:63, 1982
2. Betts RF: Infectious mononucleosis syndromes. In Williams WJ, Beutler E, Erslev AJ et al (eds): Hematology, 4th ed, p 949. New York, McGraw-Hill, 1990
3. Bloedorn W, Houghton J: The occurrence of abnormal leukocytes in the blood in acute infections. Arch Intern Med 27:315, 1921
4. Cabot R: The lymphocytosis of infection. Am J Med Sci 145:335, 1911

5. Davidsohn I et al: The differential test for infectious mononucleosis. J Lab Clin Med 45:561, 1955

6. Downey H, McKinlay C: Acute lymphadenosis compared with acute lymphatic leukemia. Arch Intern Med 32:82, 1923

7. Fleisher G, Paradise J: Atypical lymphocytosis in children. Ann Emerg Med 10:424, 1981

8. Gerber P, Hamre D, Moy RA et al: Infectious mononucleosis: Complement-fixing antibodies to herpes-like virus associated with Burkitt lymphoma. Science 161:173, 1969

9. Henle G, Henle W, Diehl V: Relation of Burkitt's tumor-associated herpes-type virus to infectious mononucleosis. Proc Natl Acad Sci USA 59:94, 1968

10. Herz A: Die akute Leukamie. Leipzig, Franz Deuticke, 1911

11. Hewetson JF, Rocchi G, Henle W et al: Neutralizing antibodies to Epstein-Barr virus in healthy populations and patients with infectious mononucleosis. J Infect Dis 128:283, 1973

12. Klein E, Ernberg I, Masucci MG et al: T-cell response to B cells and Epstein-Barr virus antigens in infectious mononucleosis. Cancer Res 41:4210, 1981

13. Litwin J, Liebowitz S: Lymphocytes (virocytes) in virus diseases other than infectious mononucleosis. Acta Haematol 5:223, 1951

14. Miale J: Leukocytes. In Miale J: Laboratory Medicine Hematology, 6th ed, p 676. St. Louis, CV Mosby, 1982

15. Moses HL, Glade PR, Kasel JA et al: Infectious mononucleosis: Detection of herpes-like virus and reticular aggregates of small cytoplasmic particles in continuous lymphoid cell lines derived from peripheral blood. Proc Natl Acad Sci USA 60:489, 1968

16. Naegeli O: Blutkrankheiten und Blutdiagnostik. Berlin and Leipzig, Vereinigung wiss. Verleger W. de Gruyter & Co, 1919

17. Paul JR, Bunnell W: The presence of heterophile antibodies in infectious mononucleosis. Am J Med Sci 183:90, 1932

18. Pfeiffer E: Drusenfieber. Yahrb Kinderheilk 29:257, 1889

19. Rutkow I: Rupture of the spleen in infectious mononucleosis. Arch Surg 113:718, 1978

20. Sprunt T, Evans F: Mononuclear leucocytosis in reaction to acute infections. Johns Hopkins Hosp Bull 31:357, 1920

21. Wood T, Frenkel E: The atypical lymphocyte. Am J Med 42:923, 1967

Nonmalignant Hereditary Disorders of Leukocytes

Martha T. Thomas

INHERITED ABNORMALITIES OF GRANULOCYTE MORPHOLOGY

Nuclear Abnormalities

Morphologic abnormalities of the nucleus include hyposegmentation and hypersegmentation.

Pelger-Huët anomaly is hyposegmentation of the granulocyte nucleus with increased density and coarseness of chromatin. There are two forms of the anomaly: "true," which is inherited, and "pseudo," which is acquired. True Pelger-Huët anomaly is inherited as an autosomal dominant trait, and its distribution is worldwide. The cells appear to be both cytochemically and functionally normal.

Typically, in the heterozygous condition, the neutrophil nucleus either consists of two symmetric rounded lobes connected by a fine filament or fails to segment and thus resembles a peanut or dumbbell. The bilobed nuclei are commonly described as appearing like pince-nez spectacles (Fig. 28-1). Segmentation beyond two lobes is uncommon. In the rare homozygote, the nuclei remain round. Careful examination of the chromatin, which is coarse and densely clumped, indicates that these cells are fully mature.

The acquired or "pseudo" Pelger-Huët form is commonly associated with malignant myeloproliferative disorders, including preleukemia or myelodysplastic syndromes. It also has been reported in patients with infections or tumors that have metastasized to the bone. In the acquired form, a number of the cells contain round nuclei such as those seen in the homozygotic form of Pelger-Huët anomaly. In addition, the cytoplasm of cells in the acquired form frequently is hypogranular. The distinction between the two forms is based on morphologic evidence of diseases associated with the acquired form and on the family history.

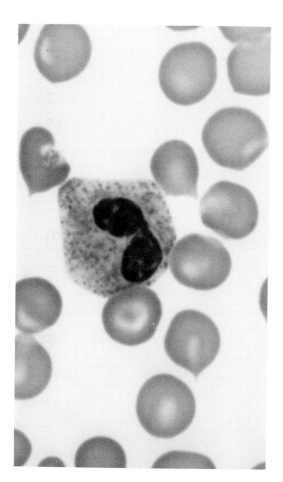

FIG. 28-1. Pelger Huët neutrophil showing typical nuclear shape (pince-nez or dumbbell) (original magnification × 1000).

It is of practical importance to recognize the Pelger-Huët anomaly so that it is not confused with a neutrophilic left shift. A differential on a patient with Pelger-Huët anomaly might be reported by the unwary as containing numerous myelocytes, metamyelocytes, and bands, when in actuality, all of the granulocytes are fully mature. These cells should be reported as mature neutrophils or placed in a separate category with a comment that they are Pelger-Huët cells. Careful observation of the nuclear shape and texture should facilitate the distinction.

Hereditary hypersegmentation of neutrophils is an autosomal dominant trait in which peripheral blood neutrophils are noticeably hypersegmented, with a mean of four lobes. Normally, segmented neutrophils seldom have more than five lobes, and a mean lobe count is usually slightly less than three. This condition, which is rare, is not associated with disease. It is important to be aware that hypersegmentation is not necessarily attributable to vitamin B_{12} or folic acid deficiency.

Cytoplasmic Abnormalities

May-Hegglin anomaly is a rare syndrome characterized by leukopenia, variable thrombocytopenia, giant platelets, and gray-blue spindle-shaped inclusions in the cytoplasm of the granulocytes and monocytes (see Plate 27). Inheritance

is autosomal and dominant. Most persons with this anomaly are in good health. However, approximately one-third of affected people develop hemorrhagic problems of variable severity.

The cytoplasmic inclusions resemble Döhle bodies but are larger and are present in cells other than neutrophils. Döhle bodies are granule-free areas of the cytoplasm containing parallel or laminar arrays of rough endoplasmic reticulum seen on electron microscopy. The inclusions of May-Hegglin anomaly are made up of dense fibrils thought to be messenger RNA.[10] The large platelets may be hypogranular. Platelet counts are most commonly in the 40 to 80 $\times 10^9$/L range. Bleeding times may be prolonged and clot retraction abnormal. The degree of abnormality seems to be proportional to the extent of thrombocytopenia. Platelet aggregation studies using ADP, collagen, and epinephrine are normal.

Alder-Reilly anomaly is inherited as an autosomal recessive trait and is characterized by the presence of abnormally large azurophilic granules resembling severe toxic granulation in the cytoplasm of granulocytes (Plate 28). Granules also may be seen in lymphocytes and monocytes. The inclusions do not appear to affect function. They are not seen consistently in the peripheral blood of patients exhibiting incomplete expression of the anomaly but can be found on careful examination of bone marrow macrophages. When the anomaly is completely expressed, all of the granulocytes, some of the lymphocytes, and even an occasional monocyte in both the bone marrow and the peripheral blood are affected. In addition, the granules of basophils and eosinophils are so bizarre that they can be differentiated from each other only by their peroxidase reaction, eosinophils being positive and basophils negative.[15] The abnormal neutrophil granules, in contrast to toxic granules, are not strongly positive for leukocyte alkaline phosphatase.

This anomaly may be seen in association with a group of storage diseases in which mucopolysaccharides accumulate in the cytoplasm of tissue and blood cells. These storage abnormalities will be discussed later in this chapter.

INHERITED ABNORMALITIES OF GRANULOCYTE FUNCTION

For proper function, phagocytes must be able to move randomly as well as directionally along a chemotactic gradient. Once they have arrived, they must be able to recognize and ingest the offending agent. Subsequently, they must be able to release their granule contents into the phagosome and undergo a respiratory burst to complete the destruction of the ingested antigen (Chap. 23). Defects in any of these abilities may result in disease. Job's syndrome and lazy leukocyte syndrome are examples of disease associated with defective motility of phagocytes.

Job's Syndrome

Job's syndrome is an uncommon condition in which the random movement of phagocytes is normal, but directional motility is impaired.[20] The mode of inheritance is unknown. The cells respond very slowly to chemotactic agents. As a result, bacteria have more time to multiply in the tissues before they are attacked. Like the biblical Job, the patients suffer from persistent boils and recurrent "cold" staphylococcal abscesses. (These abscesses are described as cold because the usual signs of inflammation [heat and redness] are absent.) The mechanism for the poor phagocyte response is unknown. However, because many of the patients described also have markedly increased levels of IgE,[20] it is possible that histamine released by the interaction between IgE and tissue mast cells is responsible for inhibition of phagocyte motility.

Lazy Leukocyte Syndrome

Lazy leukocyte syndrome is a rare condition in which, as its name suggests, both random and directed movement of the cells are defective.[14] The mode of inheritance is unknown. Bone marrow reserves of granulocytes are normal, but release of cells from the marrow to the peripheral blood is poor.[12] As a result, neutropenia is a consistent finding. The cells fail to respond to inflammatory stimuli but otherwise appear to have normal phagocytic and bactericidal activity. The clinical features include low-grade fever and recurrent infections involving the gums, mouth, and ears. Surprisingly, some patients have only mild clinical signs.

As is discussed in Chapter 23, normal neutrophils contain actin filaments that are closely associated with the cell's ability to form pseudopods and move. Ultrastructural and biochemical studies suggest that the cells in lazy leukocyte syndrome contain defective actin filaments.[2]

DEFECTIVE KILLING OF MICROORGANISMS

The inability to kill microorganisms may be secondary to a failure of granule release, as in the Chédiak-Higashi syndrome, or to inability to ingest the organism, as is seen in congenital deficiency of the complement component C3. In addition, defects in oxidative metabolism, as in chronic granulomatous disease of childhood, severe G6PD deficiency, and myeloperoxidase deficiency, will affect the bactericidal capacity of phagocytes.

Chédiak-Higashi Syndrome

Chédiak-Higashi syndrome is a genetic disorder first recognized because of the presence of giant cytoplasmic granules in the phagocytes and lymphocytes (Fig. 28-2). The syndrome affects at least six species: man, mink, cattle, mice, cats, and killer whales. It is inherited as an autosomal recessive trait and is manifested in all species in much the same way. It has been extensively studied because of the availability of animal models and because two animal models, cattle and mink, are of economic importance. The most striking feature is production of abnormally large cytoplasmic granules. Because all granule-producing cells are involved, the basic defect may well be in the Golgi complex, which is responsible for granule assembly. That is, the granules are believed to be normal in content but abnormally packaged.[16] Affected individuals display partial albinism, are more susceptible to a variety of common

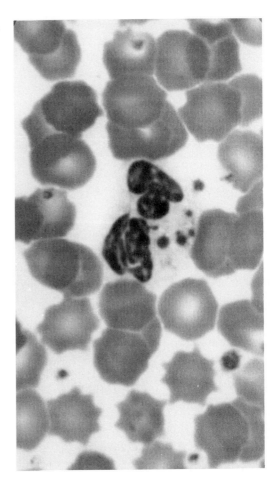

FIG. 28-2.   Chédiak-Higashi syndrome. Neutrophil exhibiting characteristic giant lysosomes. Source of this blood film was an Aleutian mink (original magnification × 1000).

infectious agents, and have hemorrhagic tendencies. In later or accelerated stages of the disease, hepatosplenomegaly, liver failure, lymphadenopathy with lymphomalike morphology, and neuropathy may develop. Death usually results from overwhelming infection.

Partial albinism is the result of a relative pigmentary dilution. Melanocytes are responsible for skin pigmentation. In Chédiak-Higashi syndrome, there is abnormal packaging of melanosomes into large melanin-containing structures, which, being fewer in number and more widely scattered, absorb less light. Thus, the skin, hair, and eyes of affected individuals appear lighter than normal. The patient often is described as having silvery hair and pale skin and suffers from photophobia.

Recurrent infections, most commonly with staphylococci and other gram-positive organisms, can be attributed to abnormal phagocyte function.[23] In addition to having abnormally large lysosomes, Chédiak-Higashi phagocytes do not move well in response to chemotactic stimuli (poor directional motility). Their plasma membranes appear to be in a constant state of abnormal movement (agitation)[18] and are more fluid than normal, possibly reflecting abnormal fatty acid content. Assembly of microtubules in the cytoplasm also appears to be disorderly.[8] Simultaneously, they show increased activity in the hexose monophosphate shunt and a more intense respiratory burst.[18] One might say they are in a constant state of low excitation that does not allow proper response to stimuli. In addition, there is defective granule release into phagosomes, with resultant poor bacterial killing. The abnormality also affects lymphocytes, which appear to lack natural killer activity.

The most striking laboratory feature is the presence of the large, abnormal cytoplasmic granules in granulocytes, monocytes, and occasionally, lymphocytes. The abnormal granules in phagocytes are peroxidase positive; those in lymphocytes are not. Routine coagulation studies are normal except for the bleeding time, which is prolonged. Platelet aggregation studies are abnormal regardless of the aggregating agent used because of the abnormal release of granule contents, with a decreased availability of ADP and serotonin. Anemia, leukopenia, and thombocytopenia frequently develop with time.

Congenital C3 Deficiency

Congenital C3 deficiency is rare and is inherited as an autosomal recessive trait. Heterozygous carriers have approximately half the normal C3 activity (adequate for disease resistance). Homozygotes suffer from repeated severe infections with encapsulated bacteria, which, because of the failure of opsonization by C3, are poorly recognized and inefficiently phagocytosed. (Chap. 23 discusses opsonins and their function.)

Chronic Granulomatous Disease

Chronic granulomatous disease (CGD) is a condition in which phagocytes ingest but cannot kill catalase-positive organisms because of the lack of an appropriate respiratory burst. (A respiratory burst occurs when phagocytes are activated by surface contact with agents such as opsonized bacteria or soluble agents such as C5a.) A drastic increase in oxygen uptake and generation of a series of oxygen metabolites that are deadly to biologic systems occurs. The metabolites produced include hydrogen peroxide, superoxide, hydroxyl radical, and singlet oxygen. The last named, which has the same molecular formula as atmospheric oxygen, has a distorted electron cloud around the two oxygen nuclei and is highly unstable. Its decay to the ground state is associated with the emission of light, a process called chemiluminescense.

There are two approaches to the evaluation of the respiratory burst. Chemiluminescense, which is the emission of low-level light pulses by stimulated cells, can be measured in luminometers.[22] Light pulses result from the oxidation of other molecules by the singlet oxygen produced in the burst. Normally, resting cells do not emit light, and activated cells do. In CGD, neither resting nor stimulated cells emit light. The respiratory burst can also be evaluated by nitroblue tetrazolium (NBT) reduction in the phagocyte. A yellow, water-soluble dye, NBT on reduction is converted to an insoluble blue formazan. Normal activated phagocytes reduce NBT with the peroxide they generate in the respiratory burst. Because burst activity is necessary for this reduction, patients with conditions in which the burst is lacking are unable to reduce NBT.

The clinical features of CGD are variable and may appear at any age. They include recurrent chronic pyogenic infections. Healing is often accompanied by granuloma formation (i.e., accumulations in the skin and other tissues of masses of macrophages and giant cells). Recurrent pneumonia is common and often is the cause of death.

There appear to be two modes of inheritance for CGD. In some families, the gene clearly is sex linked. In others, the condition appears to be transmitted as an autosomal recessive trait. The biochemical problem appears to be either a lack of the oxidase responsible for initial reduction of atmospheric oxygen to superoxide[9] or a failure of the membrane surface to stimulate a respiratory burst.[21] Catalase-positive organisms survive and multiply in the phagosome because they neutralize their own hydrogen peroxide. Catalase-negative organisms, which are unable to neutralize their peroxide, are destroyed in a normal fashion because they generate enough peroxide for the phagocyte's microbicidal system to function. From this standpoint, they might be considered "suicide" organisms.

Glucose-6-Phosphate Dehydrogenase Deficiency

Glucose-6-phosphate dehydrogenase deficiency, when severe, is similar to CGD. Absence of G6PD impairs the hexose monophosphate shunt, and phagocytes are unable to produce a respiratory burst, resulting in defective bactericidal activity. Screening tests for leukocyte G6PD are commercially available.

Myeloperoxidase Deficiency

Myeloperoxidase (MPO) deficiency is a relatively common disorder inherited in an autosomal recessive fashion. Its incidence has become apparent with the development of differential cell counters that use myeloperoxidase activity for cell identification.[13] It is a benign condition in which patients are rarely troubled by infections. In affected persons, MPO is either decreased or absent in neutrophils and monocytes but not in eosinophils. Apparently, by way of compensation, respiratory burst activity is increased. Without MPO, bacterial killing is slowed but complete. Laboratory testing for congenital MPO deficiency is of academic interest only.

INHERITED DISORDERS OF THE MONOCYTE–MACROPHAGE SYSTEM

Monocytes and macrophages are responsible for ingestion and disposal of foreign substances and unwanted metabolites. There are several mechanisms associated with macrophage overload, which results in macrophage storage disease. These mechanisms may be summarized as an enzyme lack, true overload that overwhelms the normal enzyme systems, and indigestibility of ingested particles. This section will cover those inherited storage diseases that are a result of the lack of single enzymes necessary for the degradation or catabolism of various lipids or carbohydrates, with brief consideration of true macrophage overload. The expression of each disease and the morphologic abnormalities observed vary with the particular product that is accumulating abnormally.

Mucopolysaccharidoses

Mucopolysaccharidoses are a group of closely related syndromes resulting from genetically determined deficiencies of specific enzymes involved in the degradation of mucopolysaccharides. They include Hurler (mucopolysaccharidosis I), Scheie (V), Hunter (II), Sanfilippo (III), Morquio or Morquio-Ullrich (IV), and Maroteaux-Lamy (VI) syndromes. In all but one form, the mode of inheritance is autosomal recessive; Hunter syndrome, the exception, is transmitted as a sex-linked recessive trait. Hurler and Hunter syndromes were given the name "gargoylism" because of the characteristic facial and skeletal abnormalities. The syndromes differ in severity and expression, depending on the extent of the enzyme deficiency and the particular tissues in which the abnormal product accumulates. The affected enzymes normally cleave terminal sugars from polysaccharide chains attached to a core protein. When there is a block in the removal of this terminal sugar, degradation of the rest of the polysaccharide is halted. These chains therefore accumulate within the lysosomes of cells in various tissues and organs, including leukocytes. Cells in affected tissues are swollen and have apparent ballooning and clearing of their cytoplasm. Electron microscopy shows the cleared areas to be full of minute vacuoles that contain mucopolysaccharides.[11] In peripheral blood and bone marrow, there is variable expression of the abnormalities consisting of metachromatic granules in leukocytes, as described under Alder-Reilly anomaly. It should be noted that these granules are sometimes referred to as "Alder-Reilly bodies" or as "Reilly bodies." Because they are metachromatic, they will stain purple with toluidine blue.

Lipidoses

Lipidoses are lipid storage diseases that are genetically determined and in which the macrophages of one or more tissues become overloaded with lipid. These diseases result from the lack of a functional enzyme required for breakdown of lipids that have been ingested by phagocytes. Expression of the disease depends on the particular enzyme that is depressed or missing. Transmission is autosomal recessive, and, except for Gaucher disease Type II, the highest incidence is seen in Ashkenazic (northern European) Jews, possibly reflecting an inbred population. Inherited lipidoses include Gaucher, Niemann-Pick, and Tay-Sachs disease. The last-named will not be discussed here, as there are no associated hematologic abnormalities.

Gaucher disease is the most common of the lipidoses. It is characterized by the lack of beta-glucosidase, with the resultant macrophage accumulation of glucocerebrosides in the spleen, liver, and bone marrow. Three types of Gaucher disease have been identified that differ in age of onset and severity.

Type I, the most common form, is called the "adult" form of the disease, although the symptoms usually begin in childhood or early adulthood. Accumulation of lipid-laden macrophages in the spleen causes pronounced splenomegaly. Liver macrophages interfere with the circulation of blood through the sinusoids, and liver function tends to deteriorate. The accumulation of Gaucher cells in the marrow causes bone lesions, and bone pain is probably the most

troublesome clinical problem from the patient's standpoint. The central nervous system is not affected. Some patients, depending on the age when the disease first appears, have normal life spans. Death may occur because of liver disease, bleeding, or sepsis.

Type II, the infantile or cerebral form of Gaucher disease, is much more severe because of central nervous system involvement. Neurologic deterioration progresses rapidly, and death usually occurs within the first few years of life.

Type III, the juvenile form of Gaucher disease, first becomes apparent in early childhood. The central nervous system is only occasionally involved. Hepatosplenomegaly and bone involvement develop rapidly, and the life expectancy is short.

Regardless of the type, leukopenia, thrombocytopenia, and various degrees of anemia are common and related to the extent of splenomegaly. The anemia is normochromic and normocytic. Masses of Gaucher cells may be found in the bone marrow, spleen, liver, and other affected tissues. The Gaucher cell is a large macrophage with a small, usually eccentrically placed, nucleus. Its cytoplasm is distended by glucocerebrosides, which give it a characteristic crinkled appearance like crumpled tissue paper (Fig. 28-3). These cells are strongly periodic acid-Schiff (PAS) positive. The measurement of beta-glucosidase in leukocytes is helpful in identifying homozygotes and heterozygotes and may be useful in genetic counseling. Characteriscally, serum acid phosphatase is markedly elevated in all forms of Gaucher disease and is helpful in comfirming the diagnosis.

Niemann-Pick disease is a disorder in which there is abnormal accumulation of sphingomyelin and cholesterol in mononuclear phagocytic cells and some parenchymal cells throughout the body because of a deficiency of sphingomyelinase. Five variants of the disease have been described, which probably differ on the basis of the particular isoenzyme involved and the severity of the deficiency. The most prevalent form develops in infancy and closely resembles the infantile form of Gaucher disease clinically. It is invariably fatal within the first few years of life.

In all forms of the disease, the bone marrow contains

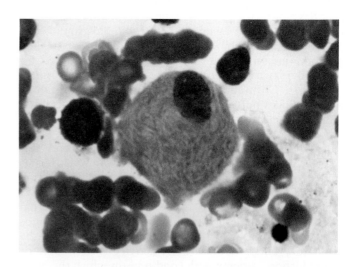

FIG. 28-3.   Gaucher cell. Note striations in cytoplasm of this abnormal macrophage (original magnification × 1000).

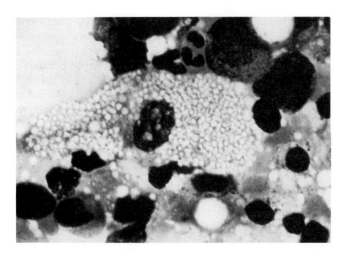

FIG. 28-4.   Niemann-Pick cell. Note lipid droplets in cytoplasm (original magnification × 1000).

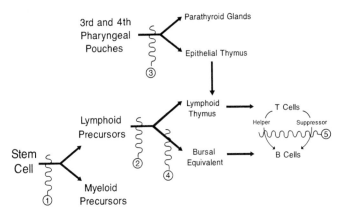

FIG. 28-5.   Ontogeny of immunocompetent cells. Points where development of these cells might be interrupted in pathologic conditions are indicated: (1) decrease in all cells—aplasia; (2) combined immunodeficiency; (3) defective T-cell production and cellular immunity; (4) defective B-cell production and antibody production; (5) defective communication between T and B cells or abnormal ratios of T to B cells.

numerous macrophages whose cytoplasm is swollen by numerous small, uniform lipid droplets. Such macrophages are often described as "foam" cells (Fig. 28-4). Peripheral blood monocytes and lymphocytes may also contain cytoplasmic vacuoles that appear by electron microscopy to be lipid. Their origin is not known.

Precise diagnosis and differentiation from similar lipidoses can be accomplished by identification of sphingomyelin in biopsies of tissues containing the affected cells or by establishing the deficiency of sphingomyelinase. Antenatal diagnosis can be made using fibroblasts cultured from amniotic fluid.

"Macrophage overload" may result in an increase in "foam" cells resembling those seen in the conditions described above. These cells may be seen in conditions associated with hyperlipidemia, such as diabetes mellitus and type I glycogen storage disease. "Pseudo"-Gaucher cells are commonly seen in chronic myelocytic leukemia, particularly after therapy. This is a situation where a normal enzyme system cannot process the enormous lipid burden presented by increased cell turnover.

Sea-blue Histiocytosis is a syndrome marked by hepatosplenomegaly, thombocytopenia, and accumulation in the spleen and bone marrow of histiocytes filled with lipid-rich granules that stain blue-green with polychrome stains such as Wright or Giemsa. Because the condition affects both sexes equally, inheritance is considered to be autosomal recessive. There is a high familial incidence. The nature of the stored lipid and the specific enzyme deficiency, if it indeed exists, has not yet been established. Indeed, there has been some disagreement about whether this is truly a specific syndrome, as sea-blue histiocytes have been described in a number of conditions, including chronic granulocytic leukemia and the adult form of Niemann-Pick disease.[4,5,19]

INHERITED DISORDERS OF IMMUNE LEUKOCYTES

Serious disease is associated with failure of lymphoid development in the bone marrow and thymus and with failure of the thymus itself to develop. Figure 28-5 summarizes the ontogeny of immunocompetent cells, the potential points of interruption, and the effects of interruption at each point. See Chapter 24 for a detailed discussion of lymphopoiesis. Immunologic deficiencies can be classified as B-cell deficiencies, T-cell deficiencies, and severe combined immunodeficiency disease.

B-Cell Deficiencies

Assessment of B-cell function is based both on the level of serum immunoglobulins and on the ability of the patient to produce immunoglobulins against antigens not normally encountered. A history of successful immunization against toxoids such as diphtheria or pertussis and normal levels of the expected anti-A and anti-B blood group antibodies are evidence of the previous development of a normal humoral response. The current humoral response can be evaluated by measuring the response to unusual antigens such as bacterial flagellin or keyhole limpet hemocyanin (KLH).[1] Circulating B cells can be enumerated by identification of Fc surface receptors or surface immunoglobulins. In addition, B cells can be concentrated and examined for their ability to respond to mitogens such as pokeweed mitogen or phytohemagglutinin (PHA). Infantile sex-linked agammaglobulinemia and common variable hypogammaglobulinemia are examples of true B-cell deficiency.

Infantile sex-linked (Bruton) agammaglobulinemia is transmitted by the mother to her male children. It becomes obvious when the infant is about 6 months of age and has essentially lost the protection of maternal IgG that crossed the placenta during intrauterine life. At this time, the child contracts a series of bacterial infections involving the usual childhood pathogens but fails to develop immunity against them. All classes of immunoglobulins are either absent or extremely low. Peripheral blood lymphocytes are normal in number; however, they tend to be exclusively T cells. It is clear that the T-cell system is functioning normally, as these children develop lasting immunity to most viral infections. Therapy includes the use of antibiotics and passive immunization with pooled human gamma globulin.

Common variable hypogammaglobulinemia is a far more common defect in which one or a combination of immunoglobulins is either missing entirely or is synthesized only in small quantities. Although the disease is produced by the inability of B cells to mature to functional plasma cells, the basic problem lies in the excessive production or activity of T suppressor cells.[1] Clinically, decreased resistance to infectious agents is seen only in those patients with impaired IgG production. Selective decreased production of IgA, both serum and secretory, is characterized by a malabsorption syndrome with noninfectious diarrhea and is closely associated with autoimmune diseases such as the collagen diseases and thyroiditis.

Patients with variable hypogammaglobulinemia cannot always be identified by quantitation of total gammaglobulins, as a decrease in one class may be masked by a selective increase in one or more of the others. It therefore is necessary to quantitate the immunoglobulin classes separately.

T-Cell Deficiencies

T-Cell deficiencies arise either from failure of development of the thymus or from a blockage of the stem cell destined to develop in the thymus.

There are a number of approaches to the laboratory evaluation of T-cell status. The first is study of hypersensitivity through skin testing with agents that induce a delayed hypersensitivity response in most normal adults. The lack of delayed hypersensitivity is known as "anergy." A history of normal recovery from viral infections supports the existence of normal cell-mediated immunity. Also, the numbers of circulating T cells can be measured using flow cytometry or sheep cell rosette techniques. Further information can be gained by studying the transformation of T cells in mixed lymphocyte culture, as this gives an indication of the functional capability of the T cells. Special enzyme studies for adenosine deaminase or nucleoside phosphorylase may also aid in the diagnosis: these are enzymes involved in purine metabolism and are present in healthy T cells. Nezelof's syndrome and DiGeorge's syndrome are classic examples of pure T-cell deficiency.

Nezelof's syndrome is an autosomal recessive disorder in which there is defective development of the lymphoid thymus. The block appears to be in or near the stem cell level and results in the inability to produce lymphocytes to populate the thymus. Because of the resulting failure of T-cell development, affected children are susceptible to repeated yeast, fungal, and viral infections.

DiGeorge's syndrome is almost indistinguishable from Nezelof's, the difference being that it is not of genetic origin. Its cause is unknown, but it may result from intrauterine infection.

Severe Combined Immunodeficiency Disease

Failure of both humoral and cell-mediated immunity is involved in severe combined immunodeficiency disease (SCID). Until recently, survival beyond infancy was rare in afflicted individuals. Many variants of this condition have been recognized, depending on the extent of T- or B-cell loss or both. A few of these will be described briefly.

Sex-linked agammaglobulinemia is a defect in the helper cellular immune mechanism leading to agammaglobulinemia. This disorder differs from Bruton agammaglobulinemia, in which only a B-cell defect exists. There is considerable variation from patient to patient in the immunoglobulin class that is deficient and in the extent of the loss. Life expectancy is short. The defect is seen only in boys and is a recessive characteristic.

Swiss-type agammaglobulinemia is inherited as an autosomal recessive and involves a loss of both B-cell and T-cell functions. Affected children are susceptible to a wide variety of severe infections and are unable to resist infection with even feeble pathogens, any one of which can contribute to early death. Little or no immunoglobulin is found in

TABLE 28-1. Hereditary *v* Acquired Morphologic Abnormalities

INHERITED FORM	ACQUIRED FORM	DISTINCTIONS	
Pelger-Huët (PH)	Neutrophilic left shift (NLS)	PH	Characteristic dumbbell shape; chromatin dense and clumped
		NLS	Chromatin in immature neutrophils is not dense; less clumping
	Pseudo-Pelger-Huët (PPH)	PPH	Presence of several round nuclei; hypogranularity and other evidence of malignancy
Hypersegmentation (HS)	B₁₂ or folate deficiency (B/F)	HS	Does not respond to therapy; is not transient
		B/F	Oval macrocytes
May-Hegglin (MH)	Döhle bodies (DB)	MH	Larger inclusions (>1 μm); present in all granulocytes and monocytes; accompanied by giant platelets
		DB	Smaller inclusions (1 μm or less) only in neutrophils
Alder-Reilly (AR)	Toxic granules (TG)	AR	All cells are affected; granules evenly dispersed in cells; granules not peroxidase positive
		TG	Granules clustered in neutrophils; not all cells affected; granules are strongly peroxidase positive
Chédiak-Higashi (CH)	Neutrophils with ingested organisms (IG)	CH	Patient history of lifelong infections; physical appearance (partial albinism); all cell types may have abnormal granules; granules are golden brown
		IG	Only phagocytes contain material; ingested organisms stain purple; other evidence of toxicity

the blood. The thymus is present in these children but lacks lymphoid elements.

Wiskott-Aldrich syndrome is a sex-linked recessive disorder characterized by repeated bacterial, viral, fungal, and protozoan infections. The basic problem appears to be failure to generate an adequate T-cell response. Total immunoglobulin levels may be normal in these patients; however, there is severe depression of IgM levels, with compensatory increases of IgA and IgG. Because the immunoglobulin decrease is limited to those cells that produce IgM, it is possible that the B-cell deficit is related to polysaccharide antigens[1] and to macrophages that process polysaccharide antigens for B cells. The T-cell defect is poorly understood. The thymus appears to be normal. Deficiency of T cells is seen only in peripheral lymphoid organs.

Ataxia telangiectasia is a rare condition in which there is ataxia (progressive loss of muscular coordination) associated with telangiectasia (dilatation of small blood vessels). It is transmitted as an autosomal recessive disease. About one-third of the patients exhibit peripheral blood lymphopenia, and almost all have an aplastic or hypoplastic thymus with a minimal T-cell population.[7] Skin test reactions to normal antigens of fungal origin are weak or absent. The IgG levels are normal or increased. Frequently, IgE levels are depressed. The virtual absence of IgA in 90% of patients is the cause of susceptibility to upper respiratory infections.[1]

CHAPTER SUMMARY

Genetically determined abnormalities of leukocytes may affect morphology, function, or both and may involve any cell line. All the abnormalities addressed in this chapter are relatively rare compared with reactive or malignant alterations. Because of this, there is always the concern that those disorders characterized by morphologic abnormalities might be mistaken for more common acquired morphologic abnormalities or vice versa. Table 28-1 lists those hereditary morphologic abnormalities that might be confused with acquired abnormalities and gives some possible distinctions.

CASE STUDY 28-1

A 5-year-old girl is admitted to the hospital for evaluation of recurrent infections, bleeding problems, and marked hepatosplenomegaly. She had been previously identified as having Chédiak-Higashi syndrome and displays subtle signs of partial albinism. Important laboratory findings are Hb 6.0 g/dL; platelets 81 × 10⁹/L; WBC 5.9 × 10⁹/L; reticulocytes 7%; differential is 30% neutrophils, 3% monocytes, 67% lymphocytes. Many cells contain abnormal granules pathognomonic for Chédiak-Higashi syndrome. Bone marrow aspirates and biopsy show widespread lymphohistiocytic infiltration characteristic of the accelerated (lymphomalike) phase of the syndrome. The abnormal blood chemistry findings are: total bilirubin 2.0 mg/dL; markedly elevated AST and ALT; prothrombin time 15 seconds (control 12 seconds); and markedly decreased IgG.

Her infection responds well to antibiotic therapy. Her anemia and thombocytopenia are treated with packed RBCs and platelets. Prednisone and vincristine are given to reduce the hepatosplenomegaly. However, these measures are of only transient help, and she requires repeated therapy periodically until her death a year later.

1. What is the most likely cause of the anemia and thrombocytopenia?
2. What factors contributed to her bleeding problem?
3. What laboratory results reflected progressive liver failure?

REFERENCES

1. Barrett JT: Textbook of Immunology, 4th ed, p 441. St Louis, CV Mosby, 1983
2. Boxer LA, Hedley-White ET, Stossel TP: Neutrophil actin dysfunction and abnormal neutrophil behavior. N Engl J Med 291:1093, 1974
3. Boyden S: The chemotactic effect of mixtures of antibody and antigen on polymorphonuclear leukocytes. J Exp Med 115:453, 1962
4. Dewhurst N, Besley GTN, Finlayson NDC et al: Sea blue histiocytosis in a patient with chronic non-neuropathic Niemann-Pick disease. J Clin Pathol 32:1121, 1979
5. Dosik H, Rosner F, Sawitsky A: Acquired lipidosis: Gaucher-like cells and "blue cells" in chronic granulocytic leukemia. Semin Hematol 9:309, 1972
6. Godwin HA, Ginsburg AD: May-Hegglin anomaly: A defect in megakaryocyte fragmentation? Br J Haematol 26:117, 1974
7. Gupta S, Good RA: Markers of human lymphocyte subpopulations in primary immunodeficiency and lymphoproliferative disorders. Semin Hematol 17:1, 1980
8. Haak RA, Ingraham LM, Baehner RL et al: Membrane fluidity in human and mouse Chédiak-Higashi leukocytes. J Clin Invest 64:138, 1979
9. Hohn DC, Lehrer RH: NADPH oxidase deficiency in X-linked chronic granulomatous disease. J Clin Invest 55:707, 1975
10. Jordan SW, Larsen WE: Ultrastructural studies of the May-Hegglin anomaly. Blood 25:921, 1965
11. Loeb H, Jonniaux G, Resibois A et al: Biochemical and ultrastructural studies in Hurler's syndrome. J Pediatr 73:860, 1968
12. Miller ME, Oski FA, Harris MB: Lazy leukocyte syndrome: A new disorder of neutrophil function. Lancet 1:665, 1971
13. Parry M, Root RK, Metcalf JA et al: Myeloperoxidase deficiency: Prevalence and clinical significance. Ann Intern Med 95:293, 1981
14. Patrone F, Dallegri F, Rebora A et al: Lazy leukocyte syndrome. Blut 39:265, 1979
15. Rampini VS, Adank W: Hamatologische Befunde bei Patienten mit Gargoylismus und heterozygoten Gerntrgern. Helv Pediatr Acta 19:101, 1964
16. Rausch PG, Pryzwansky KB, Spitznagel JK: Immunocytochemical identification of azurophilic and specific granule markers in the giant granules of Chédiak-Higashi neutrophils. N Engl J Med 298:693, 1978
17. Rebuck JW, Crowley JH: A method of studying leukocytic functions in vivo. Ann NY Acad Sci 59:757, 1955
18. Root RK, Rosenthal AS, Balestra DK: Abnormal bactericidal, metabolic and lysosomal functions of Chédiak-Higashi syndrome leukocytes. J Clin Invest 51:649, 1972
19. Sawitsky A, Rosner F, Chodsky S: The sea-blue histiocyte syndrome, a review: Genetic and biochemical studies. Semin Hematol 9:285, 1972
20. Schopfer K, Baerlocher K, Price P et al: Staphylococcal IgE antibodies, hyperimmunoglobulinemia E and *Staphylococcus aureus* infections. N Engl J Med 300:835, 1979
21. Seligmann BE, Gallin JI: Use of lipophilic probes of membrane potential to assess human neutrophil activation abnormality in chronic granulomatous disease. J Clin Invest 66:493, 1980.
22. Whitehead TP, Kricka LJ, Carter TJN et al: Analytical luminescence: Its potential in the clinical laboratory. Clin Chem 25:1531, 1979
23. Wolff SM, Dale DC, Clark RA et al: The Chédiak-Higashi syndrome: Studies of host defenses. Ann Intern Med 76:293, 1972

PART VI

SPECIAL

HEMATOLOGIC

EVALUATIONS

29

Preparation and Evaluation of Bone Marrow

Karen G. Lofsness
Ella M. Spanjers

The collection, processing, and examination of bone marrow is one of the more complex procedures in the clinical laboratory and one of the most difficult to perform properly. It is a technique that requires a great deal of skill and expertise, and it is not learned quickly. In order to obtain the maximum amount of information from the bone marrow sample, all steps must be executed carefully, from beginning to end.

The basic procedure described in this chapter is one that has been used effectively by our laboratory for many years.[21] It has been modified and updated as better equipment has become available and the demand for new diagnostic tests has multiplied. Figure 29-1 illustrates, in a flowchart format, our protocol for collecting, processing, and evaluating bone marrow samples. The portions of the procedure that are primarily the responsibility of the hematology laboratory are described in detail here.

Approximately 1800 bone marrow collections are performed by our laboratory each year. For almost all patients, the site of choice is the posterior iliac crest. Both a trephine biopsy and aspirated marrow are obtained in nearly all cases. The procedure used to collect these samples has been described thoroughly in a previous article.[5]

The authors realize there are probably as many methods of processing bone marrow specimens as there are laboratories collecting them. The procedure described in this chapter is recommended because it is flexible, there is a high yield of acceptable marrow samples, and almost every portion of the marrow obtained is utilized in some way. The various preparations complement each other and, when interpreted correctly, provide a great deal of information about the hematologic status of the patient.

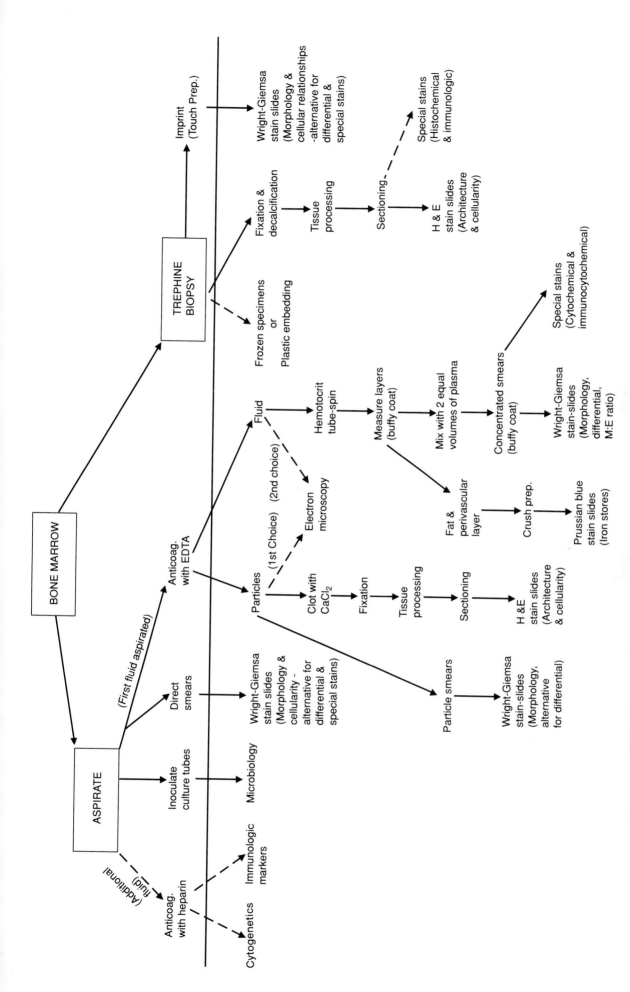

FIG. 29-1. Flowchart of protocol described in this chapter for collecting, processing, and evaluating bone marrow samples. Procedures above solid horizontal line take place at bedside; those below line are performed in laboratory. Solid arrows, routinely performed procedures; broken arrows, optional tests.

COLLECTION OF MARROW SPECIMENS

A medical technologist or medical laboratory assistant trained in preparing bone marrow specimens assists the person performing the bone marrow procedure. The assistant often has to act as a supportive influence, depending on the reaction of the patient to the procedure. Although a physician has usually described the test to the patient and obtained permission to perform it, the assistant may have to review the technique briefly. While assisting in the technical part of the bone marrow procedure and preparing the specimens, the assistant must be alert for any problems that might arise concerning the patient.

COLLECTION OF SPECIMENS
Necessary Supplies

Before the procedure is started, the assistant should clear a working area and have all supplies readily at hand. Disposable sterile bone marrow trays are commercially available, but additional supplies usually are necessary for obtaining the extra specimens that have become a part of the routine procedure in many hospitals and clinics. Trays designed by the laboratory can be set up and sterilized by the central supply area, and some of the supplies can be recleaned and reused. The following equipment is recommended for inclusion in this tray:

Aspiration needle (*e.g.*, University of Illinois sternal needle)

Trephine biopsy needle (*e.g.*, Jamshidi needle) (Note: Disposable needles are now recommended for all patients, and they cannot be sterilized with the tray. They may be distributed as a separate item with the tray.)

Two or more 30- to 35-mL syringes (glass or plastic) for aspiration

One small syringe (and accompanying needles) for local anesthetic

Sponges, forceps, medicine cups (for cleaning the area)

Towels for drapes

4 × 4-inch gauze squares

Lancet (for small incision)

Sterile gloves, solutions for cleaning the area, a local anesthetic, and tape for a pressure bandage can be obtained separately.

The supplies necessary for the bone marrow preparation at the bedside by the assistant can be carried in an inexpensive plastic carrying tray, approximately 9 to 14 inches long and 3 to 5 inches deep. This tray will easily hold the following necessary supplies:

Alcohol swabs

Lancets (for fingerstick)

Surgical blades (size 22)

2 × 2-inch gauze squares

Glass slides

Spreader device

Small battery-operated fan

Vials (17 × 80 mm) containing anticoagulant (EDTA) or commercially prepared EDTA tubes

Vials of freshly prepared Zenker fixative

Marking pencil

Additional supplies that can be carried in the tray or obtained as necessary include extra 30- to 35-mL syringes, extra aspiration and biopsy needles, heparin, saline, and various microbiologic culture tubes.

Blood Films

Whenever possible, fingerstick blood films should be prepared before the bone marrow is obtained, because stress to the patient can alter peripheral counts. A spreader device, such as that illustrated in Figure 29-2, should be used for all films. Twelve

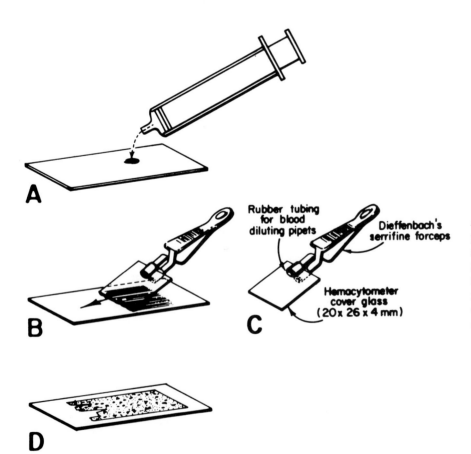

FIG. 29-2. Spreading technique used to prepare peripheral blood films and for direct and buffy coat preparations of marrow. Spreader device (*C*) consists of hemocytometer coverglass held by clamp forceps (Dieffenbach's serrefine) with rubber tubing on ends to lessen coverglass breakage. Small drop of blood or marrow is expressed onto clean glass slide (*A*). Marrow is quickly spread (*B*) and dried immediately. This technique produces thin uniform film slightly narrower than the slide (*D*). (From Brynes RK, McKenna RW, Sundberg RD: Bone marrow aspiration and trephine biopsy: An approach to a thorough study. Am J Clin Pathol 70:753–759, 1978, with permission.)

to fifteen blood films are made to ensure sufficient material for special stains as well as Wright-Giemsa staining. Ideally, anticoagulated blood is avoided for studying morphology because of the resulting changes in cell structure. Exceptions may be made in cases where a fingerstick could be harmful to the patient.

All films should be dried as quickly as possible to avoid drying artifact. A small fan may be used to dry films prepared at the bedside. This will enable the assistant to continue more quickly with the other steps of the procedure. For safety reasons, "waving" the slides dry is no longer recommended.

An alternative method for preparing films of blood and bone marrow is the coverslip technique. It provides even cellular distribution but requires more training to produce acceptable specimens. Coverslips are difficult to handle and process for both routine and special staining. Descriptions of the coverslip technique can be found in several references,[10,12,23] and it is described in Chapter 3.

Trephine Biopsy

The trephine (or core) biopsy should be obtained before the aspiration to avoid any disruption of marrow architecture at the site.[5] The trephine specimen is placed on gauze (which helps absorb excess blood), and immediately imprinted by touching the slide to the specimen. This avoids damaging the specimen with forceps and lessens the possibility of contamination. Several imprints from the same specimen should be made on at least two slides.

Bilateral trephine biopsies are frequently performed (on both the left and right posterior iliac crests), and more than one biopsy may be obtained from the same side. Each specimen should be imprinted separately and the slides labeled so that imprints from the same bone can be identified. This is important for counting purposes, special stains, and estimating cellularity. Occasionally, imprints are the only material available for morphologic and cytochemical study.

After imprinting, the biopsies are put into vials of Zenker working solution, which is prepared fresh daily. The biopsies from the right side should be fixed and processed separately from those from the left side, although all specimens from the same side can be processed together.

Aspiration

The aspiration of bone marrow follows immediately after the biopsy and usually is done on only one side. A 30- to 35-mL syringe is used to aspirate 1 to 3 mL of marrow. After the aspiration, the syringe should be kept horizontal with back pressure to avoid accidentally expressing the specimen until it is transferred to the vial described in the next paragraph. Speed in working with the aspirate is important, because the presence of megakaryocytes and the release of thromboplastin from tissue damage result in a shortened clotting time.

The aspirate is immediately transferred to a 2-dram (~10 mL) glass vial containing powdered disodium EDTA (1 mg/mL of marrow) and mixed gently. The surface should be such that megakaryocytes and platelets do not adhere to it. The amount of EDTA can be estimated after an initial weighing to visualize 1 mg. The amount used can vary somewhat without causing significant morphologic changes or clotting of the specimen. Preparing two vials, one for less than 1 mL of bone marrow and one for up to 3 mL, will help prevent problems. Commercially prepared dry disodium EDTA tubes can be used, but the smaller diameter of these tubes makes it more difficult to transfer the marrow. The larger vial surface area also provides faster and more thorough mixing with the anticoagulant and results in less clotting of the bone marrow specimen. Because the trephine biopsy is performed first, disruption of the area may initiate coagulation and cause clotting of the aspirate, even with speed and correct technique.

Direct Films

The small amount of marrow remaining in the syringe is sufficient for making direct films at the bedside. A drop of the marrow is expressed onto each of five or six slides and then distributed with a spreader device (see Fig. 29-2). If one large drop can be expressed onto a slide, the spreader can be dipped into the drop and then spread across individual slides. If the amount of marrow aspirated is insufficient for an anticoagulated specimen, as many films as possible should be made from the marrow in the syringe. This will provide slides for special stains, as well as Wright-Giemsa staining.

Occasionally, when a "dry tap" (the inability to aspirate marrow into the syringe) occurs, a small amount of marrow may be present in the aspiration needle. This marrow can be obtained for direct films if the top opening of the needle is covered with the index finger while it is being removed from the patient and a stylet is pushed into the needle as it is held over a slide.

If fluid cannot be aspirated for an anticoagulated specimen or for direct films, small pieces of an unfixed trephine specimen (after imprinting) can be cut off with a surgical blade and the freshly cut surface imprinted on a slide. One or more of these cut pieces also can be crushed between two slides. The slides are pulled apart in a parallel position while applying gentle pressure. These preparations often provide representative material for morphologic interpretation when the trephine does not imprint well, along with providing extra material for special stains. This procedure is done in the laboratory, and the specimen should be taken there on a gauze square slightly moistened with saline.

Special Procedures

Trephine biopsies for special preparations such as frozen sections, plastic embedding, or electron microscopy are usually obtained by cutting off, with a surgical blade, a representative piece of the biopsy after it has been imprinted. The remaining portion of the specimen is immediately transferred to Zenker fixative at the bedside, and the special preparation is taken to the laboratory on saline-moistened gauze for processing according to the procedure(s) requested.

Electron microscopy preparations are most satisfactory when made from particles of marrow. However, the buffy coat is more often available, and a technique has been described for processing it from a portion of the marrow aspirated for morphologic study.[15] Trephine specimens processed for electron microscopy are acceptable but are more difficult to section.

Bone marrow aspirates for special laboratory procedures are obtained after the specimen for morphologic study, because subsequent aspirations usually are more diluted with sinusoidal blood. The specimens for cytogenetic or immunologic studies are aspirated into individual 30- to 35-mL syringes that have been heparinized at the bedside with 0.5 mL of heparin (1000 USP U/mL) per 3 mL of marrow and capped to prevent loss of the fluid. Specimens for culture are drawn in a separate sterile syringe and transferred under aseptic conditions to the appropriate culture tubes.

Safety Precautions

All blood and bone marrow specimens should be considered potentially infectious and are to be handled using universal blood and body fluid precautions.[6] Gloves should always be worn when collecting or handling blood or bone marrow samples. Persons collecting bone marrow may wish to use additional barrier precautions, which include wearing a gown and mask as well as the gloves.

If a disposable tray has not been used, the entire marrow tray should be sterilized before being cleaned for reuse. Disposable trephine and aspiration needles are recommended for all patients. Any nondisposable laboratory supplies that have been exposed to blood or bone marrow during collection or processing of the specimen should be soaked for at least 1 hour in a solution of 1% sodium hypochlorite (bleach) or another recommended disinfectant before cleaning.

The further processing of blood and bone marrow specimens in the hematology laboratory should also be carried out using universal blood and body substance precautions. Gloves must be worn, and working behind a clear protective shield is recommended. Although a small fan may be used to dry films prepared in an individual patient's room, blood or bone marrow films prepared in the open laboratory area should not be dried with electric fans or by waving the slides in the air. In the laboratory, satisfactory drying of films can be accomplished by using a fan in a vented hood.

PROCESSING OF SPECIMENS

Aspirate

The bone marrow aspirate is a suspension of blood, fat, and solid units or particles of developing hematopoietic cells. The aspirate should be processed in the laboratory as soon as possible, preferably within 1 hour. Artifact caused by time delay will vary with different specimens.

The aspirate is gently mixed and poured into a disposable Petri dish. The fluid marrow is removed from around the particles with a 9-inch disposable Pasteur pipet and is transferred to one or more disposable Wintrobe hematocrit tubes. During this procedure, the fluid should be kept mixed by agitation with the tip of the Pasteur pipet to prevent uneven cellular distribution if more than one tube is filled. At the same time, gently tipping the Petri dish back and forth will aid in mixing and help to flow the fluid away from the particles, because it is important to retain them for films and section material. Even though particles are not always obtained in sufficient numbers for sectioning, films should still be made from any particles present.

Particle preparations are made by gently squashing a particle between two slides and then pulling the slides apart in a parallel position. Several particle films should be prepared. After the excess fluid is removed from the remaining particles, they are aggregated and clotted together by gently adding drops of 0.015 M $CaCl_2$ around the outside of the aggregate to prevent dispersing the particles. When they can be collected as a clot with a dissecting needle, the particles are transferred to Zenker fixative. Occasionally, no solid clot is obtained, and the particles are then aspirated into a Pasteur pipet and expressed gently into the fixative.

The Wintrobe tube containing the fluid specimen of marrow is covered and centrifuged for 8 to 10 minutes at 850 g (approximately 2800 rpm) in a tabletop centrifuge with a horizontal head. Normally, four main layers are present after centrifugation (see Fig. 29-8A). Reading from top to bottom, the layers and their reference ranges[5] are:

	ILIAC	STERNUM
Fat and perivascular cells	1%–3%	1%–3%
Plasma	No reference range	
Buffy coat (myeloid and erythroid nucleated cells)	3%–5%	5%–8%
Erythrocytes	No reference range	

The plasma and erythrocyte layers have no expected range, because they can vary widely depending on the amount of marrow dilution with sinusoidal blood. The total amount of fluid aspirated can be estimated from the Wintrobe tubes, as they hold approximately 1 mL. If less than 1 mL but more than 0.3 mL of marrow is present in the tube, the layer percentages can be calculated quite accurately.

Particles present in the centrifuged marrow will be found in either the fat layer or the buffy coat layer, depending on whether fat is present in the specimen. Usually, the presence of particles will not alter the volume of the layers significantly. Particles may also appear as a separate layer directly below the fat and then can be recorded independently.

The fat and perivascular layer is distinct and can be measured easily. However, the buffy coat may show several layers, and care must be taken to include the entire layer of nucleated cells. Erythroblasts usually layer just above the erythrocytes, and their respective colors may differ only slightly.

With a clean Pasteur pipet, "crush" preparations are made from the fat and perivascular layer using the method described for particle preparations. This layer is rich in macrophages and is used to demonstrate storage iron in the marrow by staining for the Prussian blue reaction. The more perivascular material present, the greater the reliability of the storage iron estimation.

The excess plasma is removed, leaving a volume equal to two times the buffy coat layer. Using a clean pipet (to avoid contamination with fat), the remaining plasma and the buffy coat layer are transferred to a paraffin-lined 10 × 35-mm disposable tissue culture dish or watchglass to make the concentrated preparations. The fluid is gently and thoroughly mixed with a glass stirring rod or the cleaned end of a Wintrobe tube and remixed after every four to five slides to prevent uneven distribution of cells. To ensure sufficient material for special stains, 20 to 25 films are prepared using the spreader device shown in Figure 29-2. If the buffy coat layer is small and more than one Wintrobe tube is available from the same aspirate, the buffy coat layers can be combined to obtain more preparations.

Clotted Specimens

Bone marrow aspirates containing fibrinous material or small clots are processed using the previously described techniques, but an attempt is made to avoid this material in the fluid to be centrifuged. Some of the megakaryocytes may be lost, but the other cellular distribution remains fairly reliable. If particles are not available, the clots should be processed for sectioning.

Solidly clotted marrow specimens or those containing large clots can be processed to obtain preparations for morphologic study and special stains, although the cellular distribution is unreliable. The clot is mashed to obtain fluid for centrifuging and processing by using a flat surface or cutting through it repeatedly with a Pasteur pipet. Particles are sometimes released with this procedure, and they can be spread and processed as described previously. If no particles are available, pieces of the clot should be processed for sectioning. Clotting of the specimen should be noted in the final report.

Material for Sectioning

Trephine biopsies and particle aggregates are processed for sectioning either mechanically or by hand. The biopsies and particles are prepared similarly, with the exception that trephine specimens must first be decalcified.

The paraffin block is sectioned at 4 μm, and cut at least half way through the specimen or until only a small amount of tissue is retained in the block. Serial sections from various areas of the ribboned material are mounted on albumin-coated slides and labeled separately, so that any specified area can be remounted if special stains are indicated.

The paraffin ribbons should be stored for a time to ensure they are available until all special stain requests have been completed. Special studies are often done in retrospect, and sections stored for 6 months or longer can still be mounted satisfactorily.

STAINING OF SPECIMENS

Routine Staining

All films should be well dried before they are stained; drying fixes the cells and helps prevent poor staining. A Romanowsky stain containing both Wright and Giemsa stains is preferred, because Giemsa increases the staining intensity of the azurophilic granules. However, an excess of Giemsa stain can cause difficulty in distinguishing between the neutrophilic and monocytic series because of the amount and intensity of reddish granulation produced.

Slides from each type of bone marrow preparation are stained for morphologic study. If sufficient material is available, it is recommended that the following be stained with Wright-Giemsa stain:

Three blood films
Two direct marrow films
Four or five buffy coat preparations
One particle preparation
One trephine imprint (from each biopsy)

One buffy coat film of marrow is also stained for iron by the Dacie and Lewis method[7] to check for the presence of sideroblasts. The crush preparation of the fat and perivascular layer is stained for storage iron by a Prussian blue method; if this specimen is not available, the buffy coat smear should be examined for iron-containing macrophages.

Evaluation of Stain Quality

The quality of the Wright-Giemsa stain should be assessed microscopically under oil by noting both the color and the contrast of cellular structures. Examination of the granulation in leukocytes is particularly important. Even the smaller granules, such as those in the neutrophil precursors, monocytes, and platelets, should appear sharp and distinct.

If the stain is not dark enough or the contrast in colors is not well defined, the slide usually can be improved by restaining. If the quality is still not acceptable, the staining solutions may be old or contaminated. They should be checked before attempting to stain fresh material.

Precipitated stain interferes with evaluating cell morphology and is not acceptable. If precipitate is present, it can sometimes be dissolved by rinsing the slide quickly in absolute methanol and immediately washing with water.

Special Stains

If possible, unfixed slides from each type of preparation are retained for special stains. The various cytochemical and immunocytochemical stains require different fixation methods, and the reactions may be decreased or completely inhibited if the wrong fixative is used. For example, absolute methanol decreases or completely inhibits the myeloperoxidase reaction.

Some of the special staining reactions are preserved longer if the films are desiccated. Storing some of the preparations in a desiccator is recommended if the type of special stain needed is not immediately apparent.

The more commonly performed cytochemical stains for bone marrow films include periodic acid-Schiff (PAS), myeloperoxidase, Sudan black, chloroacetate esterase, non specific esterase, and tartrate-resistant acid phosphatase (TRAP). These staining procedures are described elsewhere in the text. Immunocytochemical stains, such as TdT (terminal deoxynucleotidyl transferase), are becoming more popular as better procedures are developed and their diagnostic value becomes more apparent.

Staining Sectioned Material

Prior to staining, sections are fixed to the slides by heating in an oven at 58° to 62°C for 30 to 40 minutes and cooling to room temperature. Routine hydration of the sections is then carried out, and Zenker-fixed tissue is treated with an iodine and sodium thiosulfate solution to remove residual mercury.

The hematoxylin and eosin (H&E) stain is performed routinely on all sectioned material. For optimum staining, the times will vary for trephine and particle sections and even between specimens. Trephine biopsies fixed in Zenker solution need a longer hematoxylin staining time than those fixed in Formalin or B-5 (a mercury fixative containing formaldehyde). Particle sections need less staining time than trephine specimens.

After staining with hematoxylin, individual sections should be examined microscopically to evaluate the intensity of the stain. Sections can be restained before continuing if they appear too light, or decolorized with a recommended acid solution if they appear too dark.

The sections are counterstained in an alcoholic eosin solution and after transfer to the first xylene solution are checked microscopically for color contrast. Excess eosin, which can mask cellular detail, is removed by reversing the staining steps back through the various stages of alcohol. If the eosin color appears too light, the procedure is reversed back to the eosin step, the sections restained, and then carried through the stages of alcohol to xylene.

The preparation stained with H&E should appear crisp, with prominent nuclear detail, reddish eosinophil granules, and pale pink megakaryocyte cytoplasm.

Iron stains of sections should be done routinely on the particle sections only, as trephine biopsies lose some stainable iron in the decalcification process and cannot be used for an accurate estimation of storage iron. The enzyme stains are unsatisfactory on decalcified tissue, but other special stains such as PAS, reticulin, acid-fast, fungal, and many immunohistochemical stains can be done as requested, usually in specified areas of the sectioned material.

NORMAL MARROW CELLS

In addition to the developing hematopoietic cells described elsewhere in this text, several other cell types are present in normal marrow. Although macrophages, mast cells, osteoblasts, and osteoclasts are not seen frequently, it is important to be able to identify them because they may be confused with other cells, both normal and pathologic. Color plates 63 and 64 also illustrate some of these cells.

Macrophages

The most mature cell in the mononuclear phagocyte system is the macrophage or histiocyte. Macrophages are the progeny of the blood monocytes and perform essential phagocytic and immunologic functions. They are widely dispersed throughout the tissues of the body, and their morphology differs somewhat with their location.

In the bone marrow, macrophages are relatively large cells, with a diameter as much as 30 μm or more. On film preparations (Fig. 29-3) they are spreading, irregularly shaped cells, and pseudopods are often seen. The nucleus is usually oval, indented, or elongated. The chromatin, which stains lilac to light reddish purple with Romanowsky stains, is spongy or reticular in pattern. One or more nucleoli are often visible. The abundant cytoplasm is usually light gray to blue, although it sometimes has a pinkish tinge. The azurophilic granules vary in both number and size. In addition to the granules, cytoplasmic vacuoles are often seen and may be prominent. Other evidence of phagocytosis, such as engulfed erythrocytes, leukocytes, platelets, microorganisms, pigments, or other debris, may be present.

Macrophages stain positively with nonspecific (alpha-naphthyl acetate or alpha-naphthyl butyrate) esterase. They show negative to weakly positive activity with myeloperoxidase and chloroacetate esterase. Prussian blue stains may be used to demonstrate the increased storage iron that accumulates in macrophages in such conditions as sideroblastic anemia, excessive blood transfusions, and the anemia of chronic disease.

Because they are larger cells, macrophages tend to be pulled to the sides and feather edges of film preparations and should be searched for there. In normal marrow, macrophages comprise less than 1% of the nucleated cells. Their numbers are increased in disorders characterized by rapid cellular turnover, such as the hemolytic anemias, idiopathic thrombocytopenic purpura, and solid tumors.[22] Morphologically abnormal macrophages are seen in storage disorders such as Gaucher disease, in which a specific enzyme deficiency causes the accumulation of partially degraded lipid material in the macrophages, resulting in the characteristic cells.[11,22]

Mast Cells

The origin of mast cells (or tissue basophils) is uncertain, but they are widely distributed in the body. Tissue mast cells participate in inflammatory and hypersensitivity reactions, during which they release their granule contents outside the cell, causing localized edema and inactivation of toxic agents.[4]

On Romanowsky-stained bone marrow films, mast cells are from 12 to 25 μm in diameter (Fig. 29-4). They are usually rounded or oval, although they occasionally appear elongated or spindle shaped. The nucleus is round or oval and centrally located. It stains a uniform medium purple, but its structure is usually obscured by the intense cytoplasmic granulation. The background cytoplasm is colorless to slightly pink, and it is packed with densely staining dark purple to blue-black uniform spherical granules. Mast cells often stain so darkly that they are not easily recognized, and they may be mistaken for artifacts or cellular debris.

Mast cell granules contain both histamine and heparin, and they stain metachromatically with toluidine blue. Mast cells also stain positively with chloroacetate esterase.

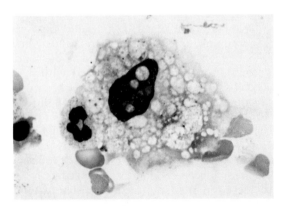

FIG. 29-3.   Macrophage. Abundant cytoplasm with prominent vacuoles, some of which overlie nucleus (original magnification × 1000).

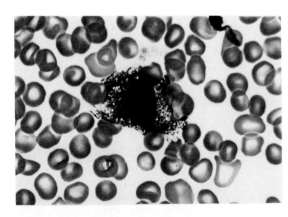

FIG. 29-4.   Mast cell. Nuclear structure obscured by dense, uniform granulation (original magnification × 1000).

Although mast cells superficially resemble basophils and may even share an ancestor, they are not the same cells. Mast cells are usually larger than basophils, and the granulation is more intense. In contrast to the irregular size and shape of basophil granules, the granules of mast cells are uniform and spherical. Mast cell granules are not water soluble.[22] The granules of both cell types contain histamine and heparin, and both stain metachromatically. However, mast cell and basophil granules differ ultrastructurally and in other chemical constituents.

Mast cells are rarely seen in normal bone marrow. They may be increased in refractory anemias, chronic renal failure, some lymphoproliferative disorders (*e.g.*, Waldenström macroglobulinemia), and systemic mastocytosis.[22]

Osteoblasts

Osteoblasts are specialized cells that synthesize new bone matrix. Although they are seen occasionally on films of aspirated bone marrow, osteoblasts are actually related to the marrow stromal network and are not part of the hematopoietic system.[22]

On film preparations, osteoblasts appear as oval, elongated cells approximately 30 μm in length (Fig. 29-5). The nucleus is round to oval, relatively small, and eccentrically located. It sometimes appears to be partially extruded from the cell, and the cytoplasm streams out behind the nucleus, giving the cell a "waterbug" or "comet" appearance. The chromatin is coarsely reticular, and one or more distinct nucleoli usually are seen. The basophilic cytoplasm is abundant, and the cytoplasmic border appears frayed or indistinct. There is often a rounded lighter-staining area (corresponding to the Golgi apparatus) within the cytoplasm at some distance from the nucleus. The texture of the cytoplasm is not smooth; it may have a grainy, fibrillar, or even slightly bubbly appearance. However, granules usually are not seen.

Morphologically, osteoblasts may be confused with plasma cells, as they both tend to have eccentric nuclei and basophilic cytoplasm. However, osteoblasts are larger than plasma cells, and the pale-staining area in the cytoplasm is separated from the nucleus. In plasma cells, this lighter area is perinuclear.

Osteoblasts often appear in clusters or aggregates and may be mistaken for tumor cells. They are seen occasionally in marrow films from infants and children but are rare in adult marrow except when active bone formation or repair is occurring, as in Paget disease, metastatic tumor, or at the site of a recent biopsy.[9]

Osteoclasts

Osteoclasts are large multinucleated cells that are involved in bone demineralization and resorption. It is likely that they are formed from the fusion of circulating monocytes and macrophages.[22]

The most distinctive characteristic of osteoclasts on a bone marrow film is their impressive size, which can reach 100 μm or greater (Fig. 29-6). These giant cells are irregularly shaped and have an indistinct ruffled cytoplasmic border. Osteoclasts contain a variable number of discrete nuclei, which are not connected to one another and may be scattered throughout the cell. The nuclei are round or oval and similar in size. They have a fine reticular chromatin pattern, and at least one prominent nucleolus usually is seen in each nucleus. The cytoplasm ranges from cloudy light blue to light pink. It is filled with azurophilic granules, which are irregular in both size and distribution within the cell. Larger purple–pink cytoplasmic inclusions are sometimes seen.

Because of their similar size and appearance, osteoclasts may be misidentified as megakaryocytes, and examination of the nuclear structure is the best way to distinguish them. In the osteoclast, each nucleus is separate; they are not attached to each other. Megakaryocyte nuclei are multilobulated; the segments are connected and may appear superimposed on one another (Fig. 29-7). Nucleoli, if visible in megakaryocytes, are small and inconspicuous. In addition, cytoplasmic granulation in megakaryocytes is much more uniform.

Like osteoblasts, osteoclasts are more common in the marrow of infants and children and are rarely seen in normal adult marrow. Osteoclasts are increased when bone remodeling or destruction is taking place, as in osteolytic bone disease. They may also be found associated with metastatic tumors[23] or at the site of recent marrow biopsy.[9]

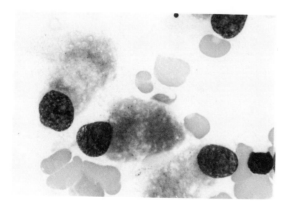

FIG. 29-5. Osteoblasts. Nucleus partially extruded, with cytoplasm streaming behind. Lighter cytoplasmic area separated from nucleus (original magnification × 1000).

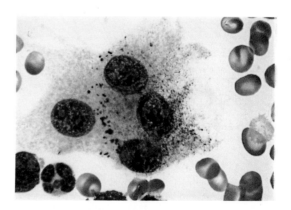

FIG. 29-6. Osteoclast. Separate nuclei, granular cytoplasm with larger inclusions (original magnification × 1000).

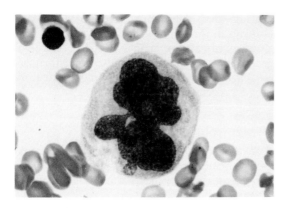

FIG. 29-7. Megakaryocyte. Multilobulated nucleus, uniform cytoplasmic granulation (original magnification × 1000).

EVALUATION OF MARROW PREPARATIONS

Prior to the microscopic examination of any bone marrow slides, the peripheral blood films obtained at the time of marrow collection should be evaluated. Erythrocyte, platelet, and leukocyte morphology are assessed, and except in cases of extreme leukopenia, a 300-cell differential (100 cells on each of three slides) is performed.

Cellularity and Composition of Sections

Because of the time involved in processing bone marrow sections, blood and marrow films will have been examined by the time the sections have been processed and stained. For continuity in interpreting bone marrow preparations,

the person examining the films from an individual case should also evaluate the architecture, cellularity, and morphology of the stained section material.

The ratio of marrow fat to hematopoietic elements is normally about 1:2 in adults. Iliac marrow may be slightly less cellular than sternal marrow. The amount of marrow fat generally increases with the age of the patient.[22] Less fat is seen on films than on sections because the aspirated marrow is somewhat diluted by sinusoidal blood. Although some biopsies show areas of variable cellularity, the overall cellularity of the specimen should be judged as normal, increased, or decreased. The relative cellularity of typical normocellular, hypercellular, and hypocellular marrows, comparing the buffy coat layer, the trephine sections, and the direct films of each, are shown as Figures 29-8 through 29-10.

Using low-power magnification, each section on each slide is evaluated for the following:
Cellularity
Cellular distribution (compare to film preparations)
Megakaryocytes
Abnormal aggregates or infiltrates (*e.g.*, tumor nodules or granulomata)
Fibrosis (confirm with reticulin stain)
Abnormal intracellular and extracellular material

Some findings may need further examination under oil magnification. Special stains of specific areas may subsequently be requested.

Low-Power Scan of Smears and Imprints

All bone marrow slides that have been Wright-Giemsa stained (direct, buffy coat, and particle preparations and trephine imprints) should first be examined under low

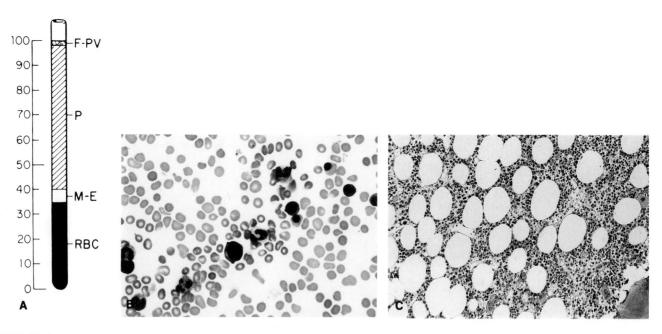

FIG. 29-8. Normocellular bone marrow (marrow transplant donor). Wintrobe tube (*A*) shows normal fat and perivascular layer (2%) and normal myeloid–erythroid (buffy coat) layer (5%). Direct film (*B*) at 400× original magnification and trephine biopsy section (*C*) at 100× original magnification are both normocellular. (Part *A* from Brynes RK, McKenna RW, Sundberg RD: Bone marrow aspiration and trephine biopsy: An approach to a thorough study. Am J Clin Pathol 70:753–759, 1978, with permission.)

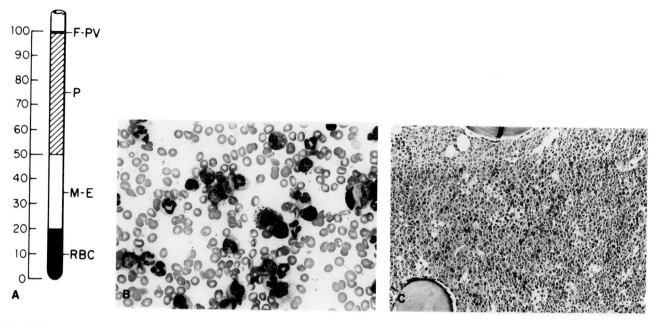

FIG. 29-9.   Hypercellular bone marrow (chronic myelogenous leukemia). Wintrobe tube (*A*) shows decreased fat and perivascular layer (trace) and markedly increased myeloid–erythroid (buffy coat) layer (30%). Direct film (*B*) at 400× and trephine biopsy section (*C*) at 100× are both markedly hypercellular. (Part *A* from Brynes RK, McKenna RW, Sundberg RD: Bone marrow aspiration and trephine biopsy: An approach to a thorough study. Am J Clin Pathol 70:753–759, 1978, with permission.)

power (×100 to ×200 total magnification). The entire slide is scanned for irregular cellular distribution and large or abnormal cells or aggregates. On film preparations, particular attention should be directed to the sides and feather edges, as larger cells and clusters of cells tend to accumulate there.

Although megakaryocyte numbers are best estimated from trephine sectioned material,[8] film preparations should also be examined, keeping in mind that any clotting will decrease the number of megakaryocytes. The feather edge of the concentrated or buffy coat preparation is the best area in which to evaluate megakaryocyte numbers and mor-

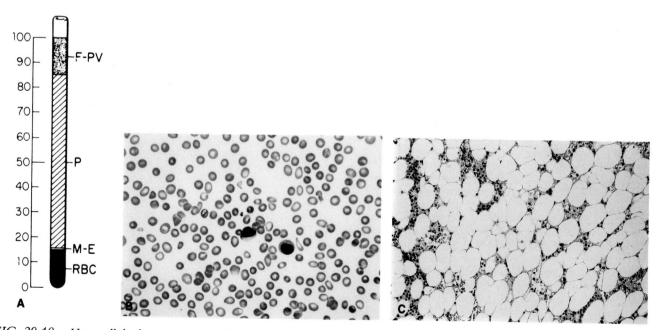

FIG. 29-10.   Hypocellular bone marrow (aplastic anemia). Wintrobe tube shows markedly increased fat and perivascular layer (15%) and decreased myeloid–erythroid (buffy coat) layer (trace). Direct film (*B*) at 400× and trephine biopsy section (*C*) at 100× are both markedly hypocellular. (Part *A* from Brynes RK, McKenna RW, Sundberg RD: Bone marrow aspiration and trephine biopsy: An approach to a thorough study. Am J Clin Pathol 70:753–759, 1978, with permission.)

phology. Normally, clumps of from two to six mega-karyocytes should be seen frequently along the feather edge, as well as scattered individually throughout the slide. In cases of peripheral blood thrombocytopenia, megakaryocyte numbers and maturation should be evaluated thoroughly.

Other large or unexpected cells that may be detected during the low-power scan include macrophages, mast cells, osteoblasts, and osteoclasts. Higher-power magnification should be used to confirm any unusual findings.

Tumor cells usually, but not always, occur in clumps or sheets in the marrow and sometimes will not be present on every preparation. When metastatic tumor is suspected, the entire set of stained slides (from both the trephine biopsy and the aspirate) must be examined completely before the marrow can be reported as being negative for tumor cells.

The last step in the low-power scan is the selection of the best slides and the optimal area for the differential count.

MARROW DIFFERENTIAL

After the low-power microscopic examination is completed, the marrow differential is performed. The concentrated (or buffy coat) specimen is preferable, as it is a relatively uniform preparation, most of the fat and particles having been removed by centrifugation. A large number of randomly distributed cells can be examined rapidly,[5] which is particularly advantageous with hypocellular marrows. However, the direct film, particle preparation, or touch imprint of the trephine biopsy also can be used for the differential count. These preparations have the advantage of being unaltered by anticoagulant.

MARROW DIFFERENTIAL
Procedure

A thin well-stained area of the slide in which the cells are evenly distributed and cellular damage is minimal should be selected and the differential performed using an oil immersion lens and ×1000 total magnification. Consecutive fields are examined, and all cells are identified. In addition to tallying the cell types, any morphologic abnormalities such as variations in cell size or structure, nuclear or cytoplasmic inclusions, mitotic figures, abnormal lobulation, or multinucleation should be recorded.

Unlike the peripheral blood differential, which includes only leukocytes in the total percentage, it is customary to include all nucleated hematopoietic cells in a bone marrow differential. However, because they are large cells and are not evenly distributed on the slide, megakaryocytes and macrophages are often reported as appearing increased, decreased, or normal in number rather than being included in the differential total.

It is recommended that at least 500, and preferably 1000 cells be counted for a marrow differential. This is best accomplished by counting 500 cells on each of two slides, which not only lessens the variability attributable to uneven cellular distribution, but also allows the examiner more opportunity to discover morphologic abnormalities. In cases of extremely hypocellular marrow or if only direct films can be obtained, fewer cells can be counted. However, the practice of routinely counting only 100 or 200 cells for marrow differentials should be discouraged, because the statistical variability is too great for this method to provide valid results.[17]

Reference Ranges

Although several "normal" marrow differential ranges can be found in the literature,[8,10,14,19,20,23] the variables involved in this procedure make it difficult to compare these studies or to adapt their data for use in one's own laboratory. The following factors can influence the determination of a reference range:
1. The number of subjects studied
2. Their age, sex, and state of health: were they randomly selected and truly "normal"?
3. The method used to collect and process the marrow
4. The amount of dilution with sinusoidal blood
5. The type of specimen used for counting: direct, concentrate, particle smear, or imprint
6. The counting procedure used
7. The number of cells counted
8. The criteria used for cell identification and classification
9. The number of observers and their expertise

Because of these variables, each laboratory should establish its own reference range if possible or at least compare a published range with known normals before adapting it.

The values used for adult bone marrow differentials on concentrated preparations in the authors' laboratory are shown (as an example) in Table 29-1. These ranges have been modified over the years and are considered guidelines rather than absolute limits between normal and abnormal. Our routine method of classifying and recording marrow differentials diverges somewhat from that in most published studies. Instead of subdividing cell lines into individual stages of maturity (i.e., neutrophil myelocyte, basophilic normoblast), we combine most cell lines and report them as a group (i.e., eosinophils and precursors). We have found this method to be advantageous for several reasons: it is faster; there is less variation in cell classification among individual observers; and the report is easier to interpret. When a significant increase or decrease in any specific stage of maturation is seen, it is always noted in the morphologic report. Type I and Type II myeloblasts and promyelocytes are tabulated separately because their percentages are important in the diagnosis and classification of the acute leukemias and the myelodysplastic syndromes according to the French-American-British (FAB) criteria.[1-3]

Pediatric bone marrow differential ranges are subject to the same variables listed previously. Most studies agree that the expected values in children differ somewhat from those of adults. In one study of normal infants, it was found that the number of marrow lymphocytes increases during the first month of life, and they remain the predominant leukocyte in the bone marrow at least through the 18th month. There is a corresponding decrease in both the granulocyte and the erythroblast populations.[16] Some of the small "lymphocytes" seen in the marrow of infants appear quite immature, with a fine, smooth chromatin pattern and relatively little cytoplasm.

TABLE 29–1. Guidelines for Adult Bone Marrow Differentials in Concentrated Smears, 1000-Cell Counts

CELL TYPE	RANGE (%)
Erythroblasts	18–24
Myeloblasts, Type I	0–1
Myeloblasts, Type II	0–2
Promyelocytes	1–4
Neutrophils and precursors	53–63
Monocytes	0–2
Eosinophils and precursors	1–3
Basophils and precursors	0–1
Lymphocytes	8–12
Plasma cells	0–2

These cells might well represent hematopoietic stem cells or progenitor cells.

Myeloid:Erythroid (M:E) Ratio

The relative proportions of the two principal bone marrow cell lines (myeloid and erythroid) can be expressed numerically as the M:E ratio. One method of determining this ratio compares the relative number of developing granulocytes (neutrophils, eosinophils, and basophils) with the relative number of erythrocyte precursors. For example, the M:E ratio for the following differential would be 60% myeloid to 15% erythroid, or 4:1:

50% neutrophils and precursors
8% eosinophils and precursors
2% basophils and precursors
20% lymphocytes
5% monocytes
15% erythroblasts

The expected marrow M:E ratio in adults ranges from 2:1 to 4:1. It may be somewhat higher in infants.[9,23]

Some authors exclude eosinophils and basophils and include only the neutrophils and their precursors in the myeloid component of the M:E ratio,[23] whereas others prefer a "WBC to Nuc RBC" ratio, including the lymphocytes, monocytes, and plasma cells with the granulocytes.[8] Which cell lines to include, and whether to express this ratio in reverse as an "E:M ratio," seems to be a matter of personal preference.

PREPARATION OF THE FINAL REPORT

The bone marrow report should describe all the significant findings, both positive and negative, in a concise and understandable format. The person preparing the final report should have examined all the different marrow preparations and reviewed the pertinent clinical information.

General information on the collection procedure, such as the anatomic site used, whether the biopsy was unilateral or bilateral, and whether any difficulty was encountered in obtaining marrow should be included. The approximate volume of marrow aspirated is recorded, along with the relative volumes (in percent) of the specific layers after centrifugation.

The differential report should state the preparation used for counting, the number of cells counted, and the relative percentages of each cell line, both normal and abnormal. Any irregularities in maturation or morphology are reported. The appearance of an abnormal or malignant population of cells, such as leukemic blasts, should be described in detail.

Megakaryocyte and macrophage numbers are reported as increased, decreased, or within normal limits. Any abnormal morphologic features in these cell lines should be described. If mast cells, osteoblasts, or osteoclasts are seen, their appearance is noted.

The results (both positive and negative) of all routine and special staining procedures are reported.

The cellularity of the marrow, as evaluated on the trephine sections, is reported as normocellular, hypercellular, or hypocellular. Any abnormalities of marrow architecture are described, and an estimate of megakaryocyte numbers from the sections is recorded.

The differential from the peripheral blood films taken at the time of marrow collection is included in the bone marrow report. Abnormalities of erythrocyte, platelet, and leukocyte morphology are described.

The report concludes with a summary of the significant findings, integrating data from all marrow and blood preparations examined. On followup marrow studies, comments comparing previous reports should be included. By interpreting these bone marrow findings in light of known clinical information and the results of other laboratory tests, the examiner arrives at a final impression (which may include or exclude a definite diagnosis). Confirmatory tests may be suggested or helpful references cited.

The final bone marrow report is the means by which the results of this complex study are communicated to the clinician. A variety of sample report forms for recording bone marrow studies have been published,[8,14,19,20] and computerized systems have been described.[13,24] It is the responsibility of each laboratory to consider the needs of the institution it serves and devise a bone marrow evaluation and reporting system that will provide the greatest benefit to clinicians and patients.

REFERENCES

1. Bennett JM, Catovsky D, Daniel MT et al: Proposals for the classification of the acute leukaemias. Br J Haematol 33:451, 1976
2. Bennett JM, Catovsky D, Daniel MT et al: Proposals for the classification of the myelodysplastic syndromes. Br J Haematol 51:189, 1982
3. Bennett JM, Catovsky D, Daniel MT et al: Proposed revised criteria for the classification of acute myeloid leukemia. Ann Intern Med 92:620, 1985
4. Bessis M: Blood Smears Reinterpreted. Berlin, Springer-Verlag, 1976
5. Brynes RK, McKenna RW, Sundberg RD: Bone marrow aspiration and trephine biopsy: An approach to a thorough study. Am J Clin Pathol 70:753, 1978
6. Centers for Disease Control: Recommendations for prevention of HIV transmission in health care settings. MMWR 36(suppl 2):1S, 1987
7. Dacie JV, Lewis SM: Practical Haematology, 4th ed. New York, Grune & Stratton, 1968
8. Diggs LW, Bell A: Bone marrow. In Schmidt RM (ed): CRC Handbook in Clinical Laboratory Science, vol 2, section 1. Boca Raton, CRC Press, 1980
9. Henry JB: Clinical Diagnosis and Management by Laboratory Methods, 17th ed. Philadelphia, WB Saunders, 1984
10. Kass L: Bone Marrow Interpretation. Philadelphia, JB Lippincott, 1979
11. Kitchens CS: Clinical observations of human bone marrow macrophages. Medicine 56:503, 1977
12. Koepke JA: Examination of the bone marrow. In Laboratory Hematology. New York, Churchill Livingstone, 1984
13. Martin PJ, Johnson-Taylor R: A simple questionnaire for use in computerizing bone marrow aspirate reports. Med Lab Sci 41:295, 1984
14. Miale JB: Laboratory Medicine, 6th ed. St. Louis, CV Mosby, 1982
15. Parkin JL, Brunning RD: Unusual configurations of endoplasmic reticulum in cells of acute promyelocytic leukemia. J Natl Cancer Inst 61:341, 1978
16. Rosse C, Kraemer MJ, Dillon TL et al: Bone marrow cell populations of normal infants: The predominance of lymphocytes. J Lab Clin Med 89:1225, 1977

17. Rumke CL: The statistically expected variability in differential leukocyte counting. In Koepke JA (ed): Differential Leukocyte Counting. Skokie, IL, College of American Pathologists, 1977

18. Rywlin AM: Histopathology of the Bone Marrow. Boston, Little, Brown, 1976

19. Schleicher EM: Bone Marrow Morphology and Mechanics of Biopsy. Springfield, IL, Charles C Thomas, 1973

20. Silver RT: Morphology of the Blood and Marrow in Clinical Practice. New York, Grune & Stratton, 1981

21. Sundberg RD: Aspiration biopsy of bone marrow. Bull U Minn Hosp 21:471, 1950

22. Trubowitz S, Davis S: The Human Bone Marrow: Anatomy, Physiology, and Pathophysiology. Boca Raton, CRC Press, 1982

23. Wintrobe MM, Lee GR, Boggs DR et al: Clinical Hematology, 8th ed. Philadelphia, Lea & Febiger, 1981

24. Youness E, Drewinko B: A computer-based reporting system for bone marrow evaluation. Am J Clin Pathol 69:333, 1978

30

Cytochemistry

Mary Ann Morris

ENZYMATIC TECHNIQUES
  Peroxidases
  Esterases
  Phosphatases

NONENZYMATIC TECHNIQUES
  Periodic Acid-Schiff Stain
  Sudan Black B
  Toluidine Blue
  Stain for Ferric Iron

IMMUNOCYTOCHEMICAL TECHNIQUES
  Enzyme Immunocytochemistry (Immunoperoxidase)
  Common Hematologic Uses

Morphologic classification of leukemia subtypes began in 1905 when Dr. John Auer[1] described a rod-shaped inclusion in the cytoplasm of "large lymphocytes" in a case of acute leukemia. Since that time laboratorians have striven to identify and classify the various cell types found in both acute and chronic leukemias. Initially, the only means available for subclassification was the appearance of cells (morphology) on Romanowsky-stained blood or bone marrow films under the light microscope. The reproducibility and validity of morphology at the light microscope level is questionable, as such examination is more of an art than a science and subject to the skill of the morphologist. Because advances in therapy have made accurate identification of cell types essential for clinical management, the use of cytochemical and immunocytochemical procedures has become commonplace in many laboratories.

Cytochemistry may be defined as the microscopic study and identification of chemical constituents within individual cells. The usefulness of cytochemistry includes identification of malignant cell types on the basis of cytoplasmic or nuclear chemistry; cellular constituents that are present in abnormal form or amount; lack of cellular constituents; and cells exhibiting functional abnormalities.

Rare variants of leukemia may be recognized with the aid of cytochemical stains. The use of specific staining techniques can establish the cell line involved in both acute eosinophilic and basophilic leukemias, as well as acute myelomonocytic leukemia with eosinophilia. Morphology is felt to be inadequate to establish the latter diagnosis, because the cells can be so abnormal that only a single granule, if any, is visible.

This chapter will describe methods and discuss recommendations of the International Committee for Standardization in Haematology (ICSH) where available,[22] as well

379

as interpretations and troubleshooting of methods. Cytochemical stains to be discussed are divided into three groups: enzymatic, nonenzymatic, and immunocytochemical.

In describing and discussing the methods, certain equipment and supplies are considered to be basic, being necessary regardless of the method being performed, and so will not be repeated for each procedure: Coplin jars, graduated cylinders, beakers, forceps, funnels, pipets, coverslips, filter paper, and neutralized mounting media.

Likewise, certain fixatives are common to several procedures. To conserve space, the makeup of the following two fixatives will be described only once:
Buffered formalin-acetone (pH 6.6)
 Dissolve in 30.0 mL H_2O
  Na_2HPO_4, 20 mg
  KH_2PO_4, 100 mg
 Add
  Acetone, 45 mL
  Formalin (40% formaldehyde), 25 mL
 Refrigerate when not in use. This is stable for as long as 1 month, depending on use.
Methanol-acetone fixative (pH 5.4)
 Mix
  Citric acid, 230 mg
  Distilled H_2O, 40 mL
  Acetone, 50 mL
  Methanol, 10 mL
 Adjust pH to 5.4 with concentrated NaOH
 Store in refrigerator (4°C).

ENZYMATIC TECHNIQUES

Peroxidases

Peroxidases are enzymes that catalyze the oxidation of substances by hydrogen peroxide.[7,8,23,30] The peroxidase reaction may be expressed as follows:

$$AH_2 + H_2O_2 \xrightarrow{\text{peroxidase}} A + 2H_2O$$

where A represents the oxidized substance or indicator (Fig. 30-1).

The peroxidase stain is used as a marker for primary neutrophilic granules. It is relevant for determining the presence or absence of a granulocytic component in an acute leukemia, and is routinely performed on all new acute

Diamino benzidine + H_2O_2 $\xrightarrow{\text{peroxidase}}$

+ $2H_2O$

Colored precipitate

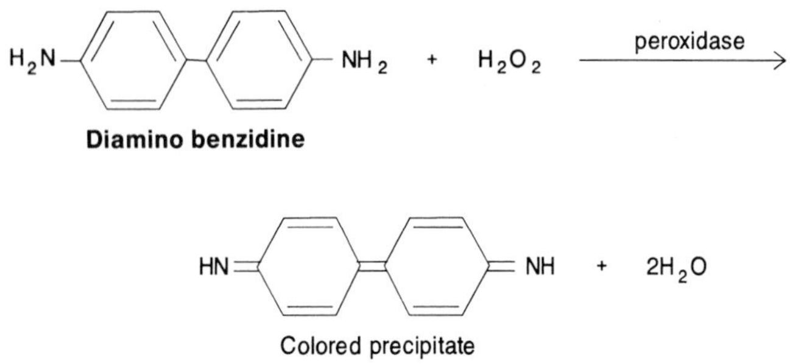

FIG. 30-1. Peroxidase reaction using diaminobenzidene as indicator. Oxidation results in formation of quinone rings (⬡), which are colored.

leukemias. Additionally, the peroxidase stain is recommended for the demonstration of Auer rods, because not all of these structures will be visible with Romanowsky stains.[8] A second peroxidase method that is particularly useful in identifying eosinophils and their precursors will also be described.

DIAMINOBENZIDINE METHOD
Reagents

Fixative: buffered formalin-acetone (pH 6.6)
Phosphate buffer, 0.07 M, pH 7.4 (refrigerate)
Phosphate buffer, 0.07 M, pH 6.64
Incubation mixture (prepare fresh for each batch)
 Phosphate buffer, 0.07 M, pH 7.4, 50.0 mL
 3,3-diaminobenzidine tetrahydrochloride, 37.5 mg
 3% hydrogen peroxide (H_2O_2), 0.15 mL
Giemsa stain, 10.0 mL

Procedure

Fix smears with cold buffered formalin-acetone for 30 seconds. Wash gently in cold water; fan dry.
Place slides in incubation mixture for 15 minutes at room temperature. Wash gently in running water.
Counterstain with Giemsa (10 mL stain/50 mL phosphate buffer, pH 6.64) for 40 minutes. Wash with water, air dry, and cover with coverslip.

Controls

A blood film from a normal donor will provide both positive (neutrophils) and negative (lymphocytes) controls. Such a control must be stained with the patient specimen.
Intraspecimen mature neutrophils or maturing neutrophil precursors and the pseudoperoxidase of red cells will also provide positive controls.

Interpretation

Peroxidase activity produces dark brown granules in the cytoplasm of granulocytes and monocytes.
Monocytes exhibit weak to moderate (scattered) activity compared with granulocytes, which generally are packed with positive granules.
Red blood cells stain diffusely brown because of pseudoperoxidase activity in Hb (Plate 29).

Remarks

The 3,3-diaminobenzidine (DAB) tetrahydrochloride may be a carcinogen and should be handled with caution in a hood using gloves and mask.

Troubleshooting

One should always begin with a careful evaluation of the control (normal neutrophils or maturing granulocytes). If there has been a technical error, such as failure to add hydrogen peroxide, negative staining will result. However, the red cells will still show staining of the pseudoperoxidase, which is not affected by the lack of hydrogen peroxide. The myeloperoxidase enzyme deteriorates during storage; therefore, specimens should be stained within 2 weeks of collection. Negative or weak staining will occur if storage is prolonged beyond this point.

Adequate fixation is critical, so reagents used for fixation should be chosen carefully. Peroxidases cannot withstand high concentrations of methanol. Likewise, fixation with formaldehyde will significantly decrease the peroxidase reaction.

ICSH Recommendation

The DAB reaction is thought to result in excellent localization and minimal diffusion of the reaction product. The panel felt that this was a simple method and is slightly better for the identification of Auer rods. The ICSH did not rule out other test methods such as 3-amino-9-ethyl carbazole and benzidine dihydrochloride, but rather thought that the choice should be based on availability of substrate, reagent carcinogenicity, and reviewer satisfaction with the reaction product.[22]

CYANIDE-RESISTANT PEROXIDASE STAIN

Eosinophilic leukemia is poorly understood. Morphologically, the blast cells may show little or no differentiation to the eosinophilic cell line. At times, one may see a single refractile granule or eosinophils with mixed abnormal granules (both eosinophilic and basophilic staining). The eosinophil peroxidase enzyme is different from that in other granulocytes because of the activity of the enzyme in the presence of sodium cyanide. Gabbas and Li[6] propose the utility of the cyanide-resistant peroxidase stain for the identification of the eosinophilic component of acute myeloid and acute myelomonocytic leukemias and also to aid in recognition of *de novo* acute eosinophilic leukemia.

Reagents

In addition to those already described for the DAB method, sodium cyanide (NaCN) and 1 N HCl will be required.

Procedure[13,29]

Fix and wash slides as described in the DAB method.
Incubation medium (filter the following):
    Phosphate buffer 0.07 M, *p*H 7.4, 50 mL
    3,3-diaminobenzidine, 37.5 mg
    3% hydrogen peroxide, 0.15 mL
Add 4.9 mg of NaCN to the incubation medium and titrate to *p*H 7.4 with 1 N HCL. Place slides in incubation medium for 5 minutes.
Rinse slides well in water.
Counterstain with Giemsa stain (10.0 mL of Giemsa/50.0 mL phosphate buffer, *p*H 6.64) for 40 minutes.
Wash with cold water and fan dry.
Apply a coverslip.

Controls

A normal blood buffy coat preparation to concentrate the number of eosinophils is recommended. Eosinophils should be strongly positive (brown), whereas neutrophils should be negative.

Troubleshooting

The troubleshooting of negative staining is similar to that for the peroxidase stain. If there is staining in the normal neutrophil, the observer should suspect that cyanide was not added to the incubation mixture.

Esterases

Esterases are enzymes that hydrolyze aliphatic and aromatic esters at acid or neutral *p*H (Fig. 30-2). At least nine esterase protein bands have been demonstrated by gel electrophoresis, and many are cell specific. Li and associates[12] demonstrated that isoenzymes 1, 2, 7, 8, and 9 are present in neutrophils. These isoenzymes can be stained with chloroacetate as the substrate and are commonly referred to as "specific" esterases. Isoenzymes 3, 4, 5, and 6 are present in monocytes as well as in certain other cell types and may be stained with either butyrate or acetate substrates. They are commonly termed "nonspecific."

In the following discussion, four esterase stains will be identified by their substrate specificity rather than as "specific" and "nonspecific" (Table 30-1). Use of the substrate component for stain identity is thought to be a more precise manner to communicate which stains were performed and

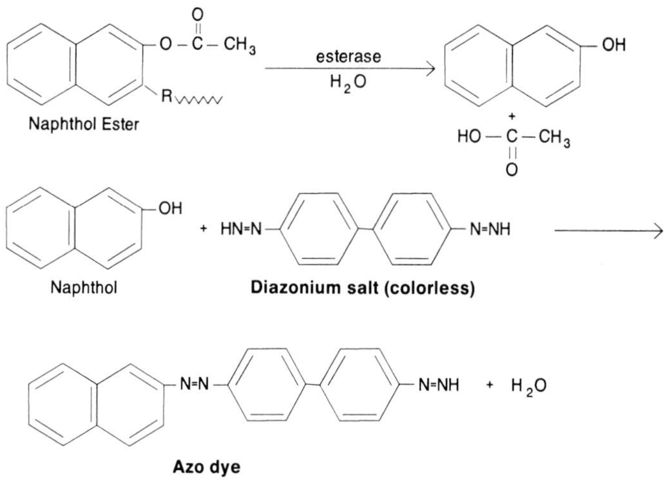

FIG. 30-2.   Esterase reaction using naphthol ester as substrate. Structure of R dictates type of ester (e.g., AS—D, AS—MX).

which cell type one is trying to demonstrate (Dr. C-Y Li, personal communication).

NAPHTHOL AS-D CHLOROACETATE ESTERASE

Naphthol AS-D chloroacetate esterase is a marker for mature and immature neutrophils and mast cells.[23,30] It is a stable enzyme that remains active after months of storage and can be demonstrated on paraffin-embedded sections. Because this enzyme may not be present in primitive myeloblasts, the stain is less sensitive than the peroxidase stain for the identification of primitive myeloid cells. The particular usefulness of the naphthol AS-D chloroacetate esterase stain is in demonstrating myeloid elements on paraffin-embedded sections such as of granulocytic sarcoma or the demonstration of mast cells in systemic mast cell disease.

Reagents

Fixative: buffered formalin-acetone (*p*H 6.6)
Sodium nitrite, 4%: dissolve 200.0 mg of sodium nitrite in 5.0 mL of distilled water. Store at 4° to 10°C. Stable for 1 week.
New fuchsin solution: dissolve 1.0 g of new fuchsin in 25.0 mL of warm 2 N hydrochloric acid. Filter when cool. Store at room temperature, away from direct sunlight. Stable for 2 months.
Hexazotized new fuchsin: mix equal volumes of new fuchsin and 4% sodium nitrite for 1 minute before use.
Naphthol AS-D chloroacetate solution: dissolve 10.0 mg of naphthol AS-D chloroacetate in 5.0 mL N,N-dimethylformamide. Store at 4° to 10°C. Stable 1 month.
Phosphate buffer, 0.07 M, *p*H 7.73
Mayer's hematoxylin

TABLE 30–1. Comparison of Esterase Substrates and Correlation with Isoenzymes and Cell Types

SUBSTRATE	ISOENZYME	POSITIVE CELLS
Naphthol AS-D chloroacetate esterase	1, 2, 7, 8, 9	Mast cells, neutrophils
Alpha-naphthyl acetate esterase	3, 4, 5, 6	Monocytes, megakaryocytes (strong), plasma cells, lymphocytes (focal)
Alpha-naphthyl butyrate esterase	2, 4	Monocytes, megakaryocytes (weak), lymphocytes (focal)

Procedure

Fix films with cold buffered formalin-acetone for 30 seconds. Wash with water.
Incubate films in the following medium (do not filter) at room temperature for 10 minutes:
    0.07 M phosphate buffer, pH 7.73, 38.0 mL
    Fresh hexazotized new fuchsin, 0.2 mL
    Naphthol AS-D chloroacetate solution, 2.0 mL
Wash with tap water.
Counterstain with Mayer's hematoxylin for 10 minutes.
Rinse in tap water, dry, apply coverslip, and examine.

Controls

Normal neutrophils are the positive control. A normal blood film is run simultaneously with the patient specimen.

Interpretation

Enzyme activity is seen as bright red granules in the cytoplasm of mast cells, neutrophils, and neutrophil precursors. Promyelocytes and many myeloblasts may also be positive. An occasional monocyte is weakly positive; eosinophils are negative.

ALPHA-NAPHTHYL ACETATE ESTERASE

Alpha-naphthyl acetate esterase (ANAE) staining identifies isoenzymes 3, 4, 5, and 6 and therefore can be used to demonstrate monocytes, megakaryocytes, plasma cells, and some lymphocytes.[12,30] The ANAE procedure yields a very strong reaction in monocytes and histiocytes and, with long incubation, a focal dotlike staining in certain lymphocytes. Lymphocytes that stain positively have been classified immunologically as T-helper lymphocytes.[10] This stain may have particular usefulness in chronic lymphocytic leukemia with T-helper phenotype. However, focal staining is weak or negative in the T-lymphoblasts of acute leukemia.

Reagents

Fixative: buffered formalin-acetone (pH 6.6)
Pararosanilin solution: dissolve 1.0 g of pararosanilin in 25.0 mL of warm 2 N HCl. This solution should be filtered when cool and kept at room temperature, away from direct sunlight. It is stable for 2 months.
Sodium nitrite, 4% (see chloroacetate method).
Hexazotized pararosanilin: mix equal volumes of pararosanilin solution and 4% sodium nitrite solution for 1 minute before use.
Alpha-naphthyl acetate solution: dissolve 100.0 mg of alpha-naphthyl acetate in 5.0 mL of ethylene glycol monomethyl ether. Refrigerate solution before use.
Phosphate buffer, 0.07 M, pH 6.64
Mayer's hematoxylin

Procedure

Fix films with cold buffered formalin-acetone for 30 seconds. Wash with water.
Mix and filter the following incubation medium and incubate films at room temperature for 2 hours:
    0.07 M phosphate buffer, pH 6.3, 38.0 mL
    Fresh hexazotized pararosanilin, 0.4 mL
    Alpha-naphthyl acetate solution, 2.0 mL
Rinse in water and counterstain with Mayer's hematoxylin for 10 minutes.
Rinse in running water for 10 minutes.
Fan dry and apply coverslip for examination.

Controls

Normal monocytes or histiocytes in bone marrow preparations or blood films act as positive controls.

Interpretation

Monocytes will stain red-brown. The pattern of staining for lymphocytes is dotlike. In reviewing the acetate stain for subclassification of acute monocytic leukemia, the observer must be aware that megakaryocytes and plasma cells will show significant staining.

Troubleshooting

Troubleshooting of all esterase stains will be discussed at the end of the section.

ALPHA-NAPHTHYL BUTYRATE ESTERASE

Alpha-naphthyl butyrate esterase (BE) is particularly useful in identifying monocytes, promonocytes, and monoblasts.[12] It stains isoenzymes 2 and 4. Although monocytes, megakaryocytes, and lymphocytes all may stain, morphology can usually identify mature nonmonocytic cellular elements. Butyrate esterase does not stain lymphoblasts, plasma cells, or megakaryoblasts. This stain is used to differentiate acute myelomonocytic, acute monocytic, and chronic myelomonocytic leukemias from other acute nonlymphocytic leukemias and dysmyelopoietic syndromes. It should be noted that Romanowsky stains can be particularly misleading in these diseases, especially with respect to distinguishing abnormal granulocyte precursors from abnormal monocyte precursors.

Reagents

Reagents for this procedure are similar to those described for the ANAE procedure except that the following substrate solution and phosphate buffer are substituted:
Alpha-naphthyl butyrate solution: dissolve 250.0 mg of alpha-naphthyl butyrate in 12.5 mL of ethylene glycol monomethyl ether. Refrigerate solution before use.
Phosphate buffer, 0.07 M, pH 6.64

Procedure

Fix films with cold buffered formalin-acetone for 30 seconds. Wash with water and fan dry.
Mix and filter the following incubation mixture and incubate the films for 45 minutes at room temperature.
    0.07 M phosphate buffer, pH 6.69, 38.0 mL
    Fresh hexazotized pararosanilin, 0.4 mL
    Alpha-naphthyl butyrate solution, 2.0 mL
Rinse in water and counterstain with Mayer's hematoxylin for 10 minutes.
Rinse in running water for 10 minutes.
Fan dry and apply coverslip for examination.

Controls

Normal monocytes in peripheral blood and histiocytes in bone marrow specimens may serve as positive controls.

Interpretation

Enzyme activity is noted as dark red precipitates in the cytoplasm of monocytes and histiocytes.

COMBINATION ALPHA-NAPHTHYL BUTYRATE-CHLOROACETATE ESTERASE

The advantage of a combination of alpha-naphthyl butyrate esterase and naphthol AS-D chloroacetate esterase on a single slide is the accurate review of the ratio of monocytic and neutrophilic components.[12] This stain allows the reviewer to distinguish the FAB subclasses M4, M5a, and M5b quickly from other subclasses of acute nonlymphocytic leukemia and chronic myelomonocytic leukemia from other subclasses of dysmyelopoietic disease (Plate 30).

Reagents

All reagents have been previously described.

Procedure

Fix films with cold buffered formalin-acetone for 30 seconds. Wash with water and fan dry.

Mix the BE incubation mixture described above. Incubate the films at room temperature for 30 minutes.

Rinse well in water.

Mix the CE incubation mixture described above, substituting 20 mg FastBlue BBN for the new fuchsin. Incubate the films at room temperature for 5 minutes.

Rinse well in water.

Counterstain with Mayer's hematoxylin for 10 minutes.

Rinse well in running water for 10 minutes.

Dry and apply coverslip for examination.

Controls

Normal monocytes and neutrophils in peripheral blood and histiocytes or developing neutrophils in bone marrow aspirates may serve as positive controls.

Interpretation

Enzyme activity is noted as dark red precipitate in the cytoplasm of monocytes and histiocytes. Blue granules appear in neutrophils and their precursors.

Troubleshooting

Troubleshooting for all esterase stains.

No staining reaction in monocytes or precursors

Check sodium nitrite. This solution must be made fresh and stored in the refrigerator no longer than 1 week.

Check for unforeseen dye lot changes. Different lots can have different dye strengths. Also, other components that accompany the specific dye within the reagent may inhibit the reaction.

Excess background staining

This problem usually occurs only with the combined esterase reaction using fast blue BB. One should be sure that washing has been complete.

No staining reaction in mature neutrophils with chloroacetate esterase (CE)

The reaction takes place in the first minute of preparation of the incubation medium. It is essential that this incubation mixture not be filtered nor made until immediately before it is used.

ICSH Recommendations

ICSH recommendations for all esterase stains.

Both alpha-naphthyl butyrate and alpha-naphthyl acetate are acceptable substrates for the identification of the monocytic series. The suggested pH for either test mode is 6.3, and pararosanilin is the suggested coupler, with good localization and minimal diffusion.[22] For T-lymphocyte identification, the ANAE reaction at pH 5.0 is recommended. Naphthol AS-D chloroacetate esterase is the accepted stain for the identification of mast cells and neutrophils. The advantage of the CE reaction over the peroxidase reaction is that CE does not stain the monocytic component. New fuchsin is the coupler of choice for CE because of its simplicity, chromogenicity, and stability.

Phosphatases

The acid phosphatase (AcP) enzymes are capable of hydrolyzing monophosphate esters at an acid pH. Li and coworkers[11,14] have demonstrated seven nonerythroid isoenzymes: 0, 1, 2, 3, 3b, 4, and 5 (Table 30-2).

Alkaline phosphatases (AkP) are a group of isoenzymes able to hydrolyze phosphate esters at an alkaline pH. In human hematopoietic tissues, alkaline phosphatase is present in neutrophils, osteoblasts, vascular endothelial cells, and sometimes, lymphocytes (Fig. 30-3).

TABLE 30-2. Isoenzymes of Acid Phosphatase

ISOENZYME	POSITIVE CELLS
0	Gaucher cells
1 and 4	Neutrophils and monocytes
3a	Lymphocytes and platelets
3b	Primitive cells and blasts
5	Hairy cells

ACID PHOSPHATASE

Acid phosphatase is present in all hematopoietic cells and is located in lysosomes.[14] Focal AcP staining has been noted in the blasts in 90% of acute T-lymphoblastic leukemias. This stain provides a simple test for identification of T-acute lymphocytic leukemia but should be evaluated with peroxidase and esterase reactions.

Reagents

Fixative: methanol–acetone mixture

Acetate buffer, 0.1 M, pH 5.2; refrigerate

Sodium acetate 3H$_2$O, 10.75 g

1 N acetic acid, 21.0 mL

Distilled water to 1000.0 mL

Substrate solution

Naphthol AS-BI phosphoric acid, 100.0 mg

N,N-dimethylformamide, 10.0 mL

This solution is stable at 4° to 10°C for 2 months.

Incubation mixture: 50.0 mL of acetate buffer, 0.5 mL of substrate, and 5.0 mg of fast garnet GBC salt.

Mayer's hematoxylin

Glycerin jelly

Procedure

Fix films with cold methanol–acetone mixture for 30 seconds.

Wash briefly with distilled water and air dry.

Place films in incubation mixture for 45 minutes.

Wash with water.

Counterstain with Mayer's hematoxylin for 5 to 20 minutes.

Wash with water, dry, and mount with glycerin jelly.

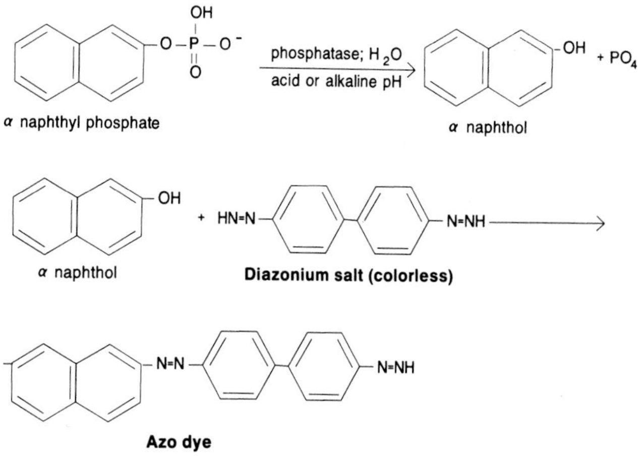

FIG. 30-3.   Acid or alkaline phosphatase reactions are essentially identical except for pH at which reaction is carried out. Note similarity to esterase reaction.

Controls

A film of normal peripheral blood will serve as a positive control, because all nucleated hematopoietic cells and the platelets contain some acid phosphatase.

Interpretation

Acid phosphatase activity is indicated as discrete purplish to dark red granules. The blasts of T-cell acute lymphoblastic leukemia usually show moderate activity confined to the Golgi area. The blasts of non-T-cell acute leukemia usually show negative or very weak activity throughout the entire cytoplasm.

ICSH Recommendations

Naphthol-AS-BI phosphate was selected as the substrate of choice. This substrate is highly chromogenic with distinct enzyme localization. Fast garnet GBC is the coupler of choice.

Troubleshooting

False-negative results may occur if the specimen has been stored for more than 2 weeks. Glycerin jelly is necessary as a mounting medium when using fast garnet GBC, as routine mounting media will leach the reaction product color within minutes.

TARTRATE-RESISTANT ACID PHOSPHATASE

In 1970, Li and colleagues[14] reported that the abnormal cells found in hairy cell leukemia (also known as leukemic reticuloendotheliosis) have a unique AcP in their cytoplasm. Using polyacrylamide gel electrophoresis, AcP isoenzyme band 5 was identified. This is the only isoenzyme that is resistant to L-(+)-tartaric acid (tartrate-resistant acid phosphatase; TRAP). This method is useful in leukopenic patients; as few as two cells with strong enzymatic activity are needed for the diagnosis of hairy cell leukemia.

Reagents

Reagents that differ from those of the previous method:
Substrate solution
    Acetate buffer, 0.1 M, pH 5.2, 100.0 mL
    Naphthol AS-BI phosphoric acid, 10.0 mg
    N,N-dimethylformamide, 0.5 mL
    This solution is stable at 4° to 10°C for 2 months
Incubation mixture
    Dissolve 1.0 mg of fast garnet GBC in 10.0 mL of substrate solution and 75.0 mg of L-(+)-tartaric acid. Adjust pH to 5.2. Filter before use and use immediately.

Procedure

Fix films with cold methanol–acetone mixture for 30 seconds.
Wash briefly with distilled water and air dry.
Incubate films for 1 hour in filtered incubation mixture.
Wash with water.
Counterstain with Mayer's hematoxylin for 5 to 20 minutes.
Wash with water, dry, and mount with glycerin jelly.

Controls

A patient specimen and normal blood film should be stained for acid phosphatase *without* the addition of L-(+)-tartaric acid. This acid phosphatase control is necessary to establish that normal enzyme activity is present in the specimen prior to tartrate inhibition. A normal blood film also should be run with the patient specimen in the tartrate-containing stain to confirm tartrate inhibition.

Interpretation

Acid phosphatase activity is indicated by discrete purplish to dark red granules in the cytoplasm of blood cells. The presence of tartrate in the incubation medium inhibits enzyme activity in

normal blood cells. The neoplastic cells of hairy cell leukemia are strongly positive. Histiocytes may have weak tartrate-resistant acid phosphatase activity. (Plate 31).

Troubleshooting

If staining is seen in normal neutrophils, tartaric acid was not added to the incubation mixture. Also, it is critical that the incubation mixture be used immediately after filtration. Falsely negative staining will occur if the specimen is more than 2 weeks old.

LEUKOCYTE ALKALINE PHOSPHATASE

Leukocyte alkaline phosphatase (LAP) is also known as neutrophil alkaline phosphatase or NAP, because neutrophils are the only leukocyte that normally contain various amounts of AkP.[20] Reactions are variable (Table 30-3). The main utility of this stain is in differentiating chronic granulocytic leukemia from leukemoid reactions or other myeloproliferative disorders. The reaction is depicted in Figure 30-3.

Reagents

Fixative
    Formalin, 40.0 mL
    Methanol, 360.0 mL
Store in freezer.
Tris buffer, 0.2 M, pH 9.1
    Trizma base, 48.44 g
    Distilled water, 200.0 mL
Adjust pH to 9.1 with 1N HCl
Substrate solution: dissolve 0.6 g of naphthol-AS-BI-phosphate in 10.0 mL N,N-dimethylformamide. Add 0.2 M Tris buffer to 2000.0 mL. Store in refrigerator.
Working solution: dissolve 50.0 mg of fast blue BBN in 50.0 mL of substrate solution (prepared just before use). Filter before use.
Nuclear fast red (see Sudan black B procedure)

Procedure

Immerse blood films in cold (4°–10°C) fixative for 30 seconds.
Wash well in either tap or distilled water.
Immerse fixed slides in working solution for 20 minutes at room temperature.
Wash well in tap water.

TABLE 30–3. Responses of Leukocyte Alkaline Phosphatases in Various Diseases

INCREASED
Polycythemia vera
Leukemoid reaction
Infections
Third trimester of pregnancy
Steroid therapy
Chronic granulocytic leukemia—blast crisis
Chronic neutrophilic leukemia
Chronic granulocytic leukemia with infections
NORMAL
Chronic granulocytic leukemia in remission
Secondary erythrocytosis
Chronic granulocytic leukemia with infections
DECREASED
Chronic granulocytic leukemia
Paroxysmal nocturnal hemoglobinuria
Sideroblastic anemia
Marked eosinophilia
Sickle cell anemia
Improper technique
Dysmyelopoietic disorders

Counterstain 20 minutes with nuclear fast red.
Wash in tap or distilled water.
Air dry.

Controls

Slides taken from pregnant women in their last trimester provide excellent positive controls, as their LAP score is above normal. One control is needed with each run of stains being done.

Scoring and Calculations

At least two patient slides are stained. Two observers, each using a different slide, should count 50 *segmented* neutrophils, scoring the staining reaction from 0 to 4[+] for each cell (0 = no granules; 1[+] = very few granules; 2[+] = moderate numbers of granules scattered throughout the cell; 3[+] = numerous granules that are starting to coalesce; 4[+] = cytoplasm packed with granules). Results are then compared; if the two 50 - cell counts are similar, they are combined for a total of 100 cells, and the score is calculated. In calculating the score, the number of cells seen in each particular grade is multiplied by that grade. The products are added together to arrive at the final score.

Interpretation

A normal LAP score at the Mayo Clinic is 40 to 100; however, every laboratory *MUST* establish its own normal values. This is especially important with this test because the scoring process is subjective.

Remarks

Segmented neutrophils, neutrophil bands, neutrophil metamyelocytes, as well as myelocytes may show AkP activity. Only segmented neutrophils are counted. Eosinophils do not stain and must be recognized by their nuclear structure and by the presence of refractile droplets (cytoplasmic granules) so they are not included in the count and mistakenly scored as 0.

Troubleshooting

Fixation time is important; if fixation is not adequate, the wash water hemolyzes the cells, resulting in streaked or even blank slides. It is most important that reagents and slides be kept at the required cold temperatures.

Because of the subjectiveness of the scoring procedure, the use of two individuals to perform the count is an invaluable quality control measure. If the two counts do not agree within approximately 10%, a third slide should be counted.

ICSH Recommendations

Recommendations were based on the usefulness of this test for the diagnosis of chronic granulocytic leukemia *v* other myeloproliferative diseases and leukemoid reactions.

Alpha-naphthyl phosphate is unsuitable as a substrate because of the decreased chromogenicity and water solubility. The substrate of choice is naphthol AS-BI phosphate, which yields a rapid result. Naphthol AS-MX phosphate was also thought to be suitable, although staining time is increased, and availability of this substrate is questionable.

NONENZYMATIC TECHNIQUES

PERIODIC ACID-SCHIFF STAIN

The Schiff reagent is a colorless solution capable of reacting with aldehyde groups in glycogen, mucoproteins, and other high-molecular-weight carbohydrates (Fig. 30-4). Glycogen is predominant in leukocytes. Positivity with periodic acid-Schiff (PAS) stain results in bright fuschia-pink staining. Staining intensity and the pattern of reaction vary with the cell type and maturity. The patterns of reaction are diffuse, granular (small or large), or a mixture.[23,27]

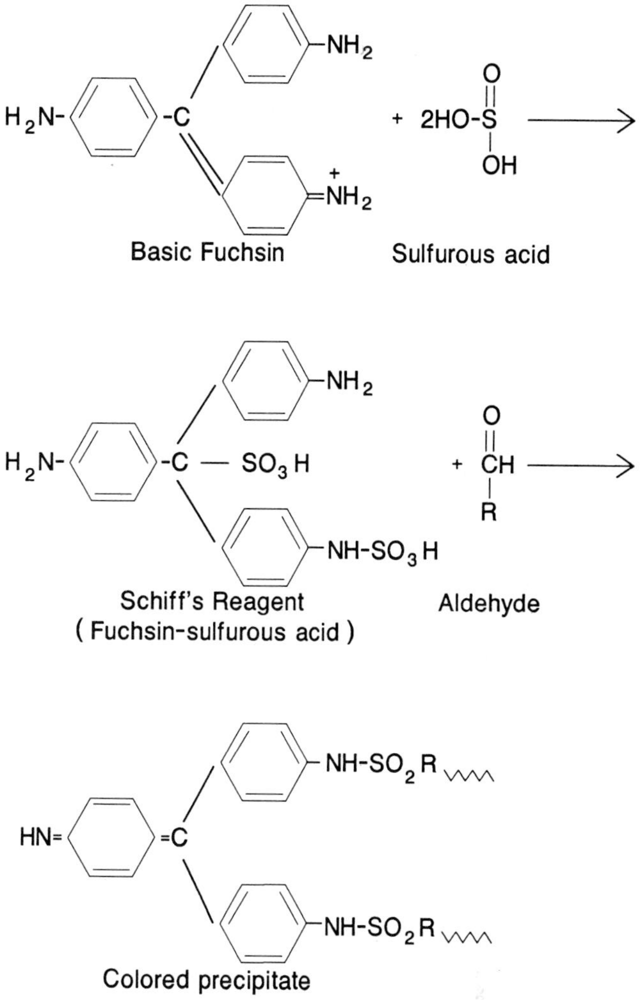

FIG. 30-4. Periodic acid-Schiff reaction. Treatment of basic fuchsin with sulfurous acid causes disappearance of quinone and hence a colorless solution (leukofuchsin). Treatment of cells with periodic acid exposes aldehyde groups in glycogen, which then react with leukofuchsin to restore a quinone and the color.

Reagents

Fixative: 10.0 mL of formalin and 90.0 mL of absolute methanol. Keep capped and refrigerated.

Periodic acid, 1%: 1.0 g periodic acid in 100.0 mL of distilled water. This reagent should be kept refrigerated when not in use and should be made fresh every 7 days.

Schiff's reagent: Commercially available. Keep refrigerated.
    Note: this reagent can be made by treating basic fuchsin with sulfuric acid and filtering through carbon; however, the technique is complex and time consuming, and therefore not cost effective. This reagent should be handled with care because, although it is colorless, it will stain hands and clothes a bright fuchsin pink. Schiff's reagent must be discarded if it turns pink or develops crystals.

Harris hematoxylin

Ammonia water (3–5 drops of concentrated NH_4OH in 50.0 mL of distilled H_2O).

Procedure

Fix films in formalin alcohol for 15 minutes.
Wash in running water for 15 minutes.
Incubate in 1% aqueous periodic acid for 20 minutes at room temperature.

Rinse three or four times in distilled water.
Incubate for 20 minutes in Schiff's reagent.
Wash in running water for 15 minutes.
Counterstain in Harris hematoxylin for 10 to 15 minutes.
Rinse quickly in dilute ammonia water.
Wash in distilled water.
Dry and apply coverslip for examination.

Controls

Intraspecimen mature neutrophils and platelets are positive, although there may be decreased positivity in some diseases. A separate control slide, normal blood or marrow film, should be run with the patient specimen.

Normal Findings

Neutrophils and their precursors are diffusely and finely granular. Positivity in neutrophils becomes more intense as the cell matures, with segmented neutrophils being strongly positive.

Basophils are positive, and eosinophil granules are negative.

Megakaryocytes are diffusely granular with large peripheral granules.

Monocytes are, at most, faintly positive with a few scattered small granules.

Lymphocytes are generally negative. Occasional lymphocytes (especially reactive forms) contain a few scattered small granules. Lymphoblasts are negative.

Erythrocyte precursors are negative.

Interpretation

At least a few neoplastic lymphoblasts will contain large ("chunky") granular PAS positivity in greater than 80% of acute lymphoblastic leukemia cases. Neoplastic myeloblasts may be positive in 10% of cases, but the positivity usually is finely granular or diffuse. The abnormal erythroblasts of erythroleukemia (M6) will contain granular positivity in the earlier forms (pronormoblasts and basophilic normoblasts). Diffuse positivity in later erythrocyte precursors (polychromatic and orthochromic) may be seen in M6 acute myelogenous leukemia and other conditions that stress red cell development such as megaloblastic anemia and thalassemia.

Troubleshooting

Should normal control neutrophils not stain intensely positive, the freshness of the periodic acid and of the Schiff reagent should be suspected. Annoying background staining may occur if the slides are not rinsed in running tap water for the specified amount of time.

SUDAN BLACK B

Sudan black B (SBB) is used for the demonstration of certain phospholipids and lipoproteins.[21,23] Its chemical structure is seen in Figure 30-5. The mechanism of action is uncertain in that it may be selective adsorption, a chemical reaction, or a combination. This stain is positive in granulocytes and monocytes–macrophages and negative in lymphocytes; therefore, the SBB reaction is similar to the myeloperoxidase reaction. An advantage of this reaction over the myeloperoxidase

stain is its stability to heat and storage. An SBB stain may be performed in retrospect on a specimen that is several months old. In addition, the SBB stain is believed to be slightly more sensitive to primitive myeloid cells than the myeloperoxidase stain. Another advantage is the fact that the reagents are not considered to be carcinogenic. The disadvantages of the SBB reaction when compared with the myeloperoxidase stain are the time necessary to perform the stain (1 to 2 hours) and its specificity. Because the SBB stain is a lipid stain, the user must be aware that there may be false-positive reactions in disorders characterized by cytoplasmic lipid vacuoles, such as Burkitt's lymphoma and occasionally, acute lymphocytic leukemia. A further disadvantage may be the increased background staining on bone marrow specimens secondary to the fatty nature of the bone marrow itself.

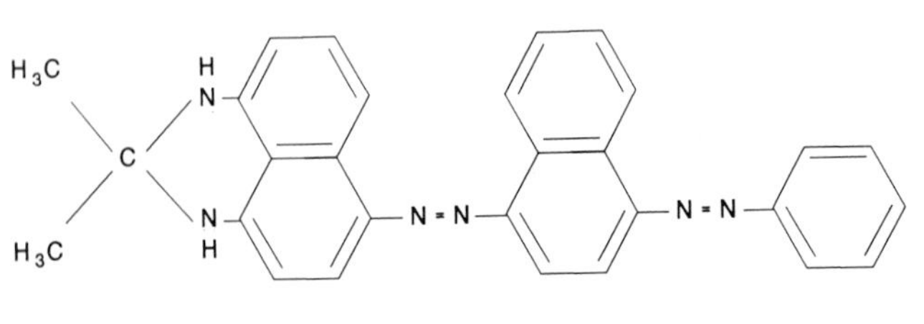

Reagents

Fixative: buffered formalin-acetone (pH 6.6)
Sudan black B: 0.3 g in 100.0 mL of absolute ethanol.
Phenol phosphate buffer
   Dissolve 16.0 g of crystalline phenol in 30.0 mL of absolute ethanol.
   Add phenol solution to 100.0 mL of distilled H_2O in which 0.3 g of hydrated disodium hydrogen phosphate ($Na_2HPO_4 \cdot 12 H_2O$) has been dissolved. The pH should be 7.0.
Working stain: add 40.0 mL of buffer to 60.0 mL of Sudan black B solution and filter by suction. Keeps 2 to 3 months, depending on usage. The pH of this stain should be neutral or only slightly alkaline (7.0–7.2).
Ethanol, 70%
Nuclear fast red counterstain
   Nuclear fast red, 0.1 g
   Aluminum sulfate, 5.0 g
   Distilled H_2O, 100.0 mL
   Dissolve aluminum sulfate in distilled water over warm water (indirect heat) until clear. Add nuclear fast red and continue heating until solution is clear.

Procedure

Fix air-dried films in cold buffered formalin-acetone fixative for 30 to 60 seconds.
Wash in running water for 1 minute.
Immerse in working stain for 1 hour.
Rinse in 70% ethanol for 2 minutes.
Wash in distilled water for 2 minutes.
Counterstain with nuclear fast red 10 to 15 minutes.
Wash, fan dry, and apply coverslip with glycerol mounting medium for examination.

Controls

A normal blood film (normal neutrophils) should be stained simultaneously with the patient specimen. Intraspecimen neutrophils also may be used as positive controls; however, neutrophils may be negative in certain myeloproliferative disorders. Lymphocytes should be negative.

Interpretation

Normally, myeloblasts are negative or contain a few sudanophilic granules in the area of the Golgi apparatus. Promyelocytes contain distinct granules throughout the cytoplasm. Neutrophil precursors contain increasingly numerous granules, with the segmented neutrophil being most intensely positive. Basophils may or may not be positive. Eosinophil granules are positive at their periphery with negative centers. Monocytes contain slight to moderate scattered positivity that may be obscured by the counterstain. Megakaryocytes are usually negative, as are platelets. Lymphoid cells and erythrocyte precursors generally are negative.

FIG. 30-5.   Sudan Black B (SBB) is a diazo dye because of presence of two azo groups (N=N) within structure.

Cells of acute monocytic leukemia (M5a and M5b) have a pattern of discrete positive granules. Cells in other nonlymphocytic leukemias contain groups of coarse granules, generally in the Golgi zone. Lymphoblasts (both normal and neoplastic) should be negative. Neutrophils and their precursors may have decreased sudanophilia in myeloproliferative disorders such as CML or the dysmyelopoietic syndromes.

Troubleshooting

Negative staining of normal neutrophils may occur if the *pH* of the staining solution departs from neutrality in either direction (acid or basic); consequently, it is advisable to check the *pH* of this solution at regular intervals. Because the material being stained with SBB is lipid, and because lipids tend to be soluble in acetone, false-negative results may occur if the specimen is left in the fixative for a long period. It should be noted that the original procedure used concentrated formalin vapors as a fixative for this very reason. The phenol present in the buffer acts as a mordant (intensifies the staining reaction), and false-negative reactions may occur if it is left out of the staining solution.

TOLUIDINE BLUE

Toluidine blue is a dye that can bind with acid mucopolysaccharides in blood cells to form metachromatic complexes.[23,30] Metachromasia is defined histochemically as a reaction product color that is significantly different from the color of the dye itself. For example, the granules of both basophils and mast cells are strongly metachromatic in that they stain reddish violet with toluidine blue. This stain is most useful in the recognition of mast cell disease and acute or chronic basophilic leukemias.

Reagents

Mota's fixative
  Lead subacetate, 0.5 g
  Reagent-grade methanol, 25.0 mL
  Distilled H_2O, 25.0 mL
  Glacial acetic acid, 0.25 mL
Toluidine blue, 0.1%
  Toluidine blue, 100.0 mg
  Absolute ethanol, 30.0 mL
  Distilled H_2O, 70.0 mL

Procedure

Fix films for 1 minute in Mota's fixative at room temperature.
Stain in 0.1% toluidine blue for 2 minutes.
Rinse quickly in tap water.
Dry and apply coverslip for examination.

Controls

Buffy coat preparations of normal peripheral blood (to concentrate normal basophils) are used as a positive control.

Interpretation

Nuclei will stain light blue. Metachromatic granules will appear reddish violet.

This stain is useful in identifying basophils and mast cells, especially neoplastic forms in which the number of granules may be significantly reduced. It is possible, however, for basophilic granules to be absent in neoplastic disorders of basophils. Consequently, a negative stain does not exclude the basophil neoplasms. A second use for this stain is the identification of the characteristic metachromatic granules in lymphocytes in disorders of mucopolysaccharide metabolism (*e.g.*, Reilly bodies).

Troubleshooting

Mota's fixative is used in this stain in order to make the metachromatic substance in the granules insoluble. Mucopolysaccharides are easily dissolved in an aqueous solution; therefore, proper fixation is critical. Negative staining may be artifactual if

the slides have been washed too vigorously or for too long a time.

STAIN FOR FERRIC IRON

Perls' reaction or a modification known as the Prussian blue reaction (Figure 30-6) is sensitive, technically simple, and widely used for the demonstration of ferric iron.[19] Intracellular ferric iron is demonstrable as storage iron in macrophages. One or two granules of intracellular iron may be found in a small percentage of normally developing red cell precursors (sideroblasts). Extracellular iron generally is considered to be artifactual unless it appears to be within fragments of iron-positive macrophage cytoplasm. Intramacrophage iron can be evaluated as bone marrow storage iron. Storage iron will be absent in iron deficiency anemia and increased in chronic diseases, frequent transfusion, and familial hemochromatosis. The presence of iron granules in otherwise mature, nonnucleated red cells (siderocytes) may be seen in iron overload or poor iron utilization syndromes.

Reagents

Fixative: absolute methyl alcohol
HCl, 2%: 8.0 mL of concentrated HCl in 400.0 mL of distilled H_2O
Potassium ferrocyanide, 2%
  40.0 g of potassium ferrocyanide
  2000.0 mL of distilled H_2O
Nuclear fast red (see Sudan black B stain)
Xylene and graded alcohols

Equipment

In addition to the basic equipment and supplies, a 37°C incubator is required.

Procedure

Bone marrow or peripheral blood films are fixed by flooding the slide with methyl alcohol for 1 minute, draining, and air drying. Paraffin sections are deparaffinized from xylene to 50% alcohol by standard procedures and rinsed in distilled water.
Place slide in Coplin jar containing one part 2% HCl to two parts 2% K ferrocyanide.
Place Coplin jar with slides and solution in 37°C incubator for 20 minutes.
Remove slides and wash with distilled H_2O.
Bone marrow or peripheral blood films are counterstained with nuclear fast red for 15 minutes, washed with distilled water, air dried, and covered with a coverslip for examination.
Paraffin sections are rinsed sequentially in 80% alcohol, 95% alcohol, absolute alcohol, absolute alcohol-xylene (50:50); covered with a coverslip, and examined.

Controls

Specimens from patients with increased iron are saved, and one slide is run as a positive control with each batch of iron stains. Positive staining is a blue to blue-green reaction with red nuclear staining. The concentrated bone marrow preparation yields the best preparation for examination of erythrocyte precursors.

$$4Fe^{+3} + 3K_4Fe(CN)_6 \xrightarrow{\text{HCl}} Fe_4[Fe(CN)_6]_3 + 12K^+$$

Potassium ferrocyanide   Ferric ferrocyanide

Blue–green precipitate

FIG. 30-6. Perls' or Prussian blue reaction.

Interpretation

Bone marrow iron storage is usually reported as absent, decreased, normal, or increased on the basis of a careful low-power review of marrow particles on fat and perivascular concentrates, bone marrow nucleated cell concentrates, or biopsy sections (Chap. 29). Interpretation of storage iron in biopsy sections should be tempered with the realization that the reaction is always decreased on paraffin sections secondary to leaching of the iron during the processing of the biopsy specimen. Negative staining should be reported with this caution. Each laboratory must establish its own criteria for the quantitation of storage iron.

The other principal use of the iron stain in hematology is the evaluation of red cell iron utilization. Impaired iron utilization causes accumulations of iron within the mitochondria that localize around the nucleus, forming a "ringed sideroblast." Recognition of ringed sideroblasts is necessary for the classification of dysmyelopoietic-preleukemic syndromes. Increased sideroblasts that are not ringed may be found in iron-overload syndromes (e.g., patients with a lifelong history of repeated blood transfusions). Iron granules in nonnucleated red cells (siderocytes) can be found in the peripheral blood in cases of iron overload and poor iron utilization, especially if the spleen is absent or not functional. Generally, the iron granules in siderocytes associated with ringed sideroblasts are larger and more distinct than those caused by simple iron overload.

Troubleshooting

The presence of excessive amounts of extracellular material that stains positive for iron can be caused by contaminated reagents, especially if tap water is used to rinse the slides (rust in water pipes). Negative staining in a positive control may be secondary to improper pH of the K ferrocyanide. The pH must be acid; therefore, if HCl is omitted from the staining reaction, false-negative results may occur.

IMMUNOCYTOCHEMICAL TECHNIQUES

Immunocytochemistry may be defined as the identification of the immunologic phenotype of a given cell population through the use of specific monoclonal or polyclonal antibodies against selected cell antigens. Various specimens may be used, including cell suspensions, paraffin or cryostat sections, smears, imprints, or cytospin preparations. A slide-based technique is advantageous because it allows for counting of designated cell populations and because a permanent slide can be filed for future review. During the last decade, antibodies have been produced against a large number of marker antigens, and many of these antibodies are commercially available. Immunocytochemistry is both practical and cost effective, as no expensive equipment is required. The specimen may be as much as 1 week old, which allows the reviewer to determine after collection which specific antibodies are appropriate. With these techniques, it is now possible to identify specific cell types or cell products that previously either were impossible to identify or required lengthy, expensive, and highly sophisticated procedures.

Application of these techniques in the hematology laboratory has been primarily for the identification of the cell types involved in acute or chronic leukemias. The ensuing discussion will review the cell types for which these techniques have been most helpful: lymphoid cells and megakaryoblasts.

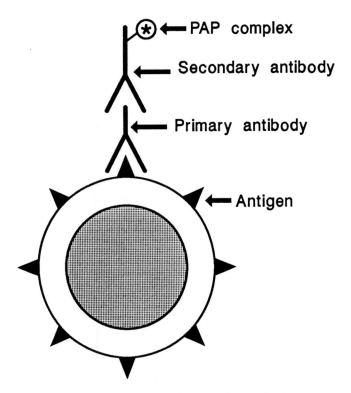

FIG. 30-7.   Diagram of peroxidase–antiperoxidase immunocytochemical staining method.

ENZYME IMMUNOCYTOCHEMISTRY (IMMUNOPEROXIDASE)

Enzyme immunocytochemistry uses an enzymatic reaction as an indicator and is applicable for the demonstration of surface, cytoplasmic, or nuclear substances.[15–17] The most common enzyme used is a plant enzyme: horseradish peroxidase. Peroxidase–antiperoxidase (PAP) staining has several advantages: it is easily obtainable and stable, endogenous peroxidase is easily blocked, a variety of chromogens are available to react with peroxidase to form a colored end product, and the test is inexpensive. Immunoalkaline phosphatase is another enzyme that can be used. Its advantage is the lack of cross-reactivity with the pseudoperoxidase of erythrocytes or granulocytes.

The PAP technique uses three reagents: a primary antibody that is specific for the antigen in question, a secondary antibody that will bind to the Fc portion of the primary antibody and carries the PAP complex as a tag, and the substrate used to make the peroxidase reaction visible (Fig. 30-7).

Method

Several kit methods are commercially available and will not be described here.

Controls

Controls are buffy coat preparations made from peripheral blood collected from healthy individuals. A separate control is run with each given antibody to monitor the performance of that antibody.

Interpretation

The reaction is seen as a color in the cytoplasm or nucleus of positively staining cells. Depending on the cell type being evaluated, positive cells may be counted or simply stated as being present. For example, when reviewing a peripheral blood film for an evaluation for chronic lymphocytic leukemia, positive cells usually are enumerated, and only lymphocytes (positive or negative) should be counted. On the other hand, if stains are requested on bone marrow, the reviewer may need only give an overall statement about the reaction within the cells in question.

Troubleshooting

Endogenous peroxidase has been a problem when dealing with peroxidase techniques and is found in neutrophils, monocytes, and eosinophils. Pseudoperoxidase is found in erythrocytes. Pretreatment with hydrogen peroxide or methanol and an acidic environment (pH 5.2 rather than 7.6) will minimize the degradation of peroxidase. The use of sodium azide with hydrogen peroxidase is an effective inhibitor of endogenous peroxidase without decreasing the intensity of the staining reaction. Sodium azide also eliminates the pseudoperoxidase of erythrocytes.

There is considerable lot-to-lot variability among monoclonal antibodies. Storage of the antibody is a critical factor in the use of the reagents. The manufacturer will state in the product literature what is the accepted temperature and time for storage. Products stored either too long or at incorrect temperatures will cause false-negative reactions. False-negative results also can occur if the specimens are more than 1 week old or if a procedural step is omitted.

The species from which the antibodies were derived (mouse, horse, rabbit, goat) are not always interchangeable. For example, rabbit-derived antimouse immunoglobulin should not be substituted for goat-derived antimouse immunoglobulin. If it is, negative staining may result because of slight differences in molecular structure that result in lack of binding.

Selection of the correct antibody is essential for the evaluation. For example, if one is evaluating an acute leukemia, the T-cell reagent should specifically identify early rather than mature T cells.

Errors also may occur during the enumeration of the positive cells. For example, in CLL, only positive lymphocytes versus negative lymphocytes should be counted. If the antibody reacts with more than the cell in question (e.g., HLA-DR reacts with lymphocytes, monocytes, and reactive T-lymphocytes), the observer must take care to count only the cell in question.

Remarks

The dilution factor for the primary antibody is dependent on the strength of the product in use. For most commercial products, a 1:25 dilution is adequate; however, the dilution may need to be adjusted.

Many monoclonal antibodies are available from different commercial sources. Confusion exists when reference is made to the commercial title rather than to the specific phenotype one is testing for. Generally, it is thought that one should use the specific cluster designation for descriptive purposes.

Common Hematologic Uses

Terminal Deoxynucleotidyl Transferase

Just as myeloperoxidase is used to identify primitive myeloid cells, terminal deoxynucleotidyl transferase (TdT) is considered a marker for primitive lymphoid cells (lymphoblasts). Until the relatively recent availability of anti-TdT antibodies, the only assay method was a biochemical one based on the fact that TdT catalyzes the polymerization of deoxynucleoside triphosphates by addition to the 3' hydroxyl ends without template instructions. Such assays are difficult to perform and thus are restricted to large reference laboratories and research settings. Additionally, the biochemical assay requires large quantities of cells and cannot evaluate heterogeneity among cells. The tagged antibody assay for TdT allows quick and specific identification of the enzyme in single cells. Polyclonal (antibovine) and monoclonal (antihuman) as well as purified serum antibodies are available, each resulting in slightly different reactions. The reagent of choice at this time is purified polyclonal antibovine TdT when using the slide-based technique. This product does not cross react with M_1 or M_0 myeloblasts and yields a clean reaction for the presence of lymphoblasts.

Megakaryocyte Precursors

The addition of M_7 (acute megakaryocytic leukemia) by the FAB Committee has pointed out the need for immunostaining to identify this subclass of acute leukemia because the early megakaryoblast is morphologically indistinguishable from the myeloblast. The marker of choice is one that identifies the IIb/IIIa glycoprotein complex (antigen) present on the cytoplasmic surface of platelets and megakaryocytes. Other markers that have been used to identify primitive megakaryoblasts immunochemically are platelet factor 4, factor VIII-related antigen, and platelet glycoprotein I.

Lymphocyte Subpopulations

It frequently is desirable to identify the phenotype of the neoplastic cell in lymphoid malignancies. This can be accomplished easily using immunocytochemical techniques and antibodies directed against the surface markers for the different lymphocyte subpopulations (B cells, T-helper cells, T-suppressor cells, etc).[18,28] Another group of diseases that necessitates the identification of lymphocyte subpopulations is the immune deficiency syndromes, both hereditary and acquired.

CHAPTER SUMMARY

Whether one is using cytochemical (Table 30-4) or immunocytochemical staining techniques, a systematic approach must be taken. Figure 30-8 is a suggested algorithm for the workup of acute leukemias. The myeloperoxidase is the first stain to be performed, regardless of the suspected cell type based on morphology. If the myeloperoxidase is positive, one would use the combined esterase stain to identify any monocytic component. If the myeloperoxidase is negative and one has ruled out a false-negative finding secondary to acquired myeloperoxidase deficiency, then the next major subtype is lymphoid (Table 30-5). To identify the lymphoid population, TdT is used. If there is a positive reaction with anti-TdT antibodies, further subtyping is performed using immunocytochemical techniques to identify the common acute lymphocytic leukemia antigen (CALLA), as well as specific T- and B-cell markers. Twu and coworkers[25] recently noted that the phenotype of the lymphocytic leukemias does not correlate with either the L_1 or the L_2 FAB subclassifications. Their initial data suggest that there is a difference in clinical course, presentation, prognosis, and karyotype based on the individual phenotype.

If the TdT stain also is negative, the uncommon phenotypes must be ruled out. These include basophilic, eosinophilic, megakaryocytic, and primitive myeloblasts. Rarely, the case remains undifferentiated.

The algorithm for chronic lymphocytic leukemia includes T_h-, B-, and T_s-cell subsets (Fig. 30-9). T-cell CLL is uncommon, but the recognition of the T subtype has clinical significance. Witzig and coworkers[28] have investigated the helper–

TABLE 30–4. Summary of Cytochemical Reactions

STAIN REACTION	CELL SPECIFICITY	CLINICAL APPLICATIONS
Peroxidase	Granulocytes, monocytes	Acute leukemia, M_1, M_2, M_3, M_4, dysmyelopoietic syndromes
Cyanide-resistant peroxidase	Eosinophils	Eosinophilic leukemia
Naphthol AS-D chloroacetate esterase	Neutrophils	Neutrophils, acute leukemia
Alpha-naphthyl acetate esterase	Monocytes, histiocytes, megakaryocytes, plasma cells	Acute leukemia, M_4, M_{5a}, M_{5b}, chronic myelomonocytic leukemia
Alpha-naphthyl butyrate esterase	Monocytes, histiocytes	Acute leukemia, M_4, M_{5a}, M_{5b}, chronic myelomonocytic leukemia
Combination alpha-naphthyl butyrate and naphthyl AS-D chloroacetate esterase	Neutrophils, monocytes	Acute leukemia, M_4, M_{5a}, M_{5b}, chronic myelomonocytic leukemia
Acid phosphatase	T lymphoblasts	Acute T-lymphocytic leukemia, T-cell lymphomas
Tartrate-resistant acid phosphatase	Hairy cells	Hairy cell leukemia
Leukocyte alkaline phosphatase	Neutrophils	Chronic granulocytic leukemia, leukemoid reactions
Periodic acid-Schiff	Abnormal blast cells	Acute leukemia, lymphocytes and erythrocytes (M_6)
Sudan black B	Granulocytes	Acute leukemia, M_1, M_2, M_3, M_4, M_{5a}, M_{5b}
Toluidine blue O	Basophils, mast cells	Acute basophilic leukemia, systemic mast cell disease
Iron stain	Iron	Iron stores, ringed sideroblasts, siderocytes

Modified from Sun T, Li CY, Yam LT: Atlas of Cytochemistry and Immunochemistry of Hematologic Neoplasms. Chicago, ASCP Press, 1985.

TABLE 30–5. Cytochemical Markers for Identification of Acute Lymphocytic Leukemia

LYMPHOBLAST TYPES	STAINS	SMEARS OR IMPRINTS
T cells	TdT, focal AcP, T antigens (Leu-1), E-rosette (Leu-5B, Leu-16, Leu-14)	TdT, focal AcP, T antigens (Leu-1)
B cells	SIg, CIg, B_1, B_4	SIg, CIg, B_1
Null cells	TdT, CALLA	TdT, CALLA

Abbreviations: AcP, acid phosphatase; CALLA, common acute lymphocytic leukemia antigen; CIg, cytoplasmic immunoglobulin; SIg, surface immunoglobulin; TdT, terminal deoxynucleotidyl transferase.
Note: the Leu series is produced by Becton-Dickinson Monoclonal Center, the B_1/B_4 series by Coulter Immunology.
Modified from Sun T, Li CY, Yam LT: Atlas of Cytochemistry and Immunochemistry of Hematologic Neoplasms. Chicago, ASCP Press, 1985.

TABLE 30–6. Markers and Tentative Subclassification of Chronic Lymphocytic Leukemias

MARKERS*	B CLL	B LSCL	T_h CLL	T_s CLL	T_m CLL
HLA-DR	+	+	−	−	−
B antigen	±	+	−	−	−
T antigen	−	−	+	+	+
Helper-T antigen	−	−	+	−	±
Suppressor-T antigen	−	−	−	+	+
Focal acid phosphatase	−	−	±	−	±
Morphology					
Nuclei	Round	Cleaved	Convoluted	Round	Convoluted
Azurophilic granules	−	−	−	+	−

Abbreviations: B LSCL, B-cell lymphosarcoma cell leukemia (leukemic phase of lymphoma); CLL, chronic lymphocytic leukemia; HLA-DR, Ia-like antigen; T_h CLL, T-cell CLL with helper/inducer T-cell characteristics; T_m CLL, T-cell CLL with mixed-cell characteristics, (i.e., both helper and suppressor T-cell characteristics); T_s CLL, T-cell CLL with suppressor/cytotoxic T-cell characteristics.
* These antigens are demonstrable by immunoperoxidase stain with monoclonal antibodies: for HLA-DR, OKI_{a1}; for B antigen, B_1 or B_2; for T antigen, Leu-4; for helper-T antigen, OKT_4; for suppressor-T antigen, OKT_8. The OK series is produced by Ortho Diagnostic Systems, the Leu series by Becton-Dickinson Monoclonal Center, and the B_1, B_2 series by Coulter Immunology.
Modified from Sun T, Li CY, Yam LT: Atlas of Cytochemistry and Immunochemistry of Hematologic Neoplasms. Chicago, ASCP Press, 1985.

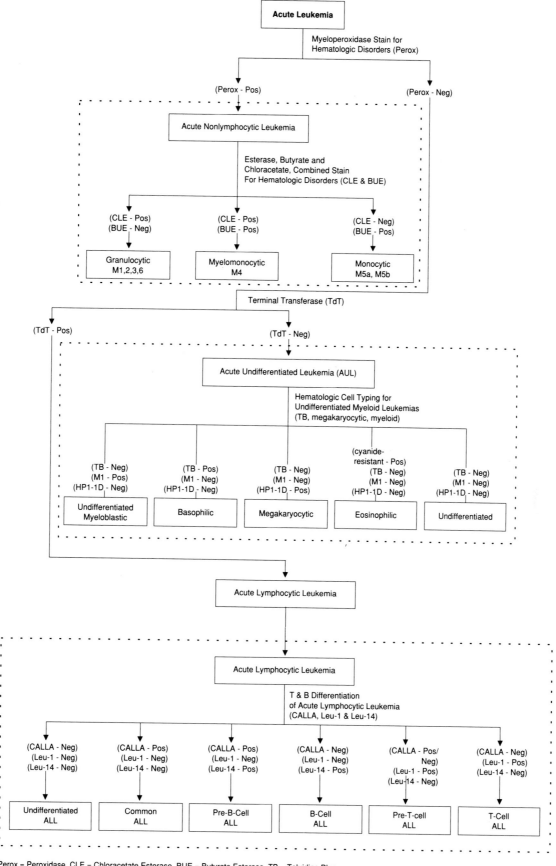

Perox = Peroxidase, CLE = Chloracetate Esterase, BUE = Butyrate Esterase, TB = Toluidine Blue,
cALLc = common Acute Lymphocytic Leukemia antigen

FIG. 30-8.   Algorithm for evaluation of acute leukemias. Inset: Further evaluation of acute undifferentiated leukemia.

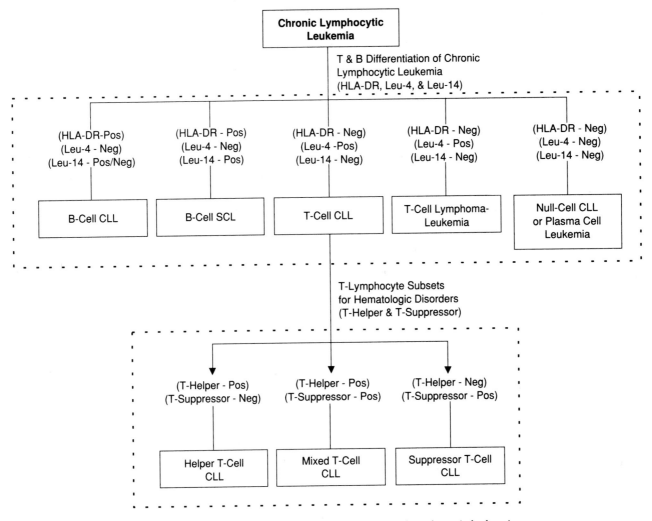

FIG. 30-9. Algorithm for evaluation of chronic lymphocytic leukemia.

inducer subtype and demonstrated that the T-helper CLL is associated with a worse prognosis than the B-cell CLL or T-suppressor CLL. T-suppressor lymphocytes are morphologically distinct, being large with abundant cytoplasm containing azurophilic granules. Patients with T-suppressor CLL may be asymptomatic, may not require chemotherapy, and generally have a long survival. A summary of tentative subclassifications is listed in Table 30-5.

In conclusion, morphology is an important component in the laboratory evaluation of leukemias. In a recent study by Browman and associates,[5] 63% concordance was achieved in intraobserver reviews using morphology based on Romanowsky-stained cells and the light microscope. When cytochemistry was applied, reproducibility improved to 89% and to 99% when phenotyping was included. Characterization of leukemic disease by morphology coupled with appropriate staining techniques and quality control of the methods yields results that will be most relevant clinically.

REFERENCES

1. Auer J: Some hitherto undescribed structures found in the large lymphocytes of a case of acute leukemia. Am J Med Sci 131:1002, 1906

2. Bennett JM, Catovsky D, Daniel MT et al: Proposals for the classification of the acute leukaemias. Br J Haematol 33:451, 1976

3. Bennett JM, Catovsky D, Daniel MT et al: Proposals for the classification of the myelodysplastic syndromes. Br J Haematol 50:189, 1982

4. Bloomfield CD, Brunning RD: FAB M7: Acute megakaryoblastic leukemia-beyond morphology. Ann Intern Med 103:450, 1985

5. Browman GP, Neame PB, Soamboonsrup P: The contribution of cytochemistry and immunophenotyping to the reproducibility of the FAB classification in acute leukemia. Blood 68:900, 1986

6. Gabbas AG, Li CY: Acute nonlymphocytic leukemia with eosinophilic differentiation. Am J Hematol 21:29, 1986

7. Graham T, Karnovsky ML: The early stages of absorption of injected horseradish peroxidase in the proximal tubules of mouse kidney: Ultrastructural cytochemistry by a new technique. J Histochem Cytochem 14:291, 1966

8. Harker JS, Laszlo J, Moore JO: The light microscopic demonstration of hydroperoxidase-positive Phi bodies and rods in leukocytes in acute myeloid leukemia. Histochemistry 58:241, 1978

9. Huang MJ, Li CY, Nichols WL et al: Acute leukemia with megakaryocytic differentiation: A study of 12 cases identified immunocytochemically. Blood 64:427, 1984

10. Knowles DM II, Halper JP, Machin GA et al: Acid alpha-

naphthyl acetate esterase activity in human neoplastic lymphoid cells: Usefulness as a T cell marker. Am J Pathol 96:257, 1979

11. Li CY, Ziesmer SC, Yam LT et al: Practical immunocytochemical identification of human blood cells. Am J Clin Pathol 81:204, 1984

12. Li CY, Yam KW, Yam LT: Esterases in human leukocytes. J Histochem Cytochem 21:1, 1973

13. Li CY, Yam LT, Crosby WH: Histochemical characterization of cellular and structural elements of the human spleen. J Histochem Cytochem 20:1049, 1972

14. Li CY, Yam LT, Yam KW: Acid phosphatase isoenzyme in human leukocytes in normal and pathologic conditions. J Histochem Cytochem 18:473, 1970

15. Li CY, Ziesmer SC, Yam LT et al: Practical immunocytochemical identification of human blood cells. Am J Clin Pathol 81:204, 1984

16. Nadji M, Morales AR: Immunoperoxidase: I. The technique and its pitfalls. Lab Med 14:767, 1983

17. Nadji M, Morales AR: Immunoperoxidase: II. Practical applications. Lab Med 15:33, 1984

18. Phyliky RL, Li CY, Yam LT: T cell chronic lymphocytic leukemia with morphologic characteristics of cytotoxic/suppressor phenotype. Mayo Clin Proc 58:709, 1983

19. Preece A: Gomori's iron reaction. In: A Manual for Histologic Technicians, 3rd ed, p 244. Boston, Little, Brown & Co., 1972

20. Rutenberg AM, Rosales CI, Bennett JM: An improved histochemical method for the demonstration of leukocyte alkaline phosphatase activity: Clinical application. J Lab Clin Med 65:698, 1965

21. Sheehan HL, Storey GW: An improved method of staining leukocyte granules with Sudan black B. J Pathol Bacteriol 59:336, 1947

22. Shibata A, Bennett JM, Castoldi GL et al: Recommended methods for cytological procedures in haematology. Clin Lab Haematol 7:55, 1985

23. Sun T, Li CY, Yam LT: Atlas of Cytochemistry and Immunochemistry of Hematologic Neoplasms. Chicago, ASCP Press, 1985

24. Travis WD, Li CY, Su WPD: Adult-onset urticaria pigmentosa and systemic mast cell disease. J Clin Pathol 84:710, 1985

25. Twu BH, Li CY, Smithson WA et al: Acute lymphocytic leukemia: Correlation of clinical features with immunocytochemical classification. Am J Hematol 25:13, 1987

26. Wick MR, Li CY, Pierre RV: Acute nonlymphocytic leukemia with basophilic differentiation. Blood 60:38, 1982

27. Wislocki GB, Rheingold JJ, Dempsey EW: The occurrence of the periodic acid-Schiff reaction in various normal cells of blood and connective tissue. Blood 4:562, 1949

28. Witzig TE, Phyliky RL, Li CY et al: T-cell chronic lymphocytic leukemia with a helper/inducer membrane phenotype: A distinct clinicopathologic subtype with a poor prognosis. Am J Hematol 21:139, 1986

29. Yam LT, Li CY, Necheles TF et al: Pseudoeosinophilia, eosinophilic carditis and eosinophilic leukemia. Am J Med 53:193, 1972

30. Yam LT, Li CY, Crosby W: Cytochemical identification of monocytes and granulocytes. Am J Clin Pathol 55:283, 1971

Laboratory Evaluation of Body Fluids

Carrie D. Brailas Ventura
Benjamin Drewinko

Examination of body fluids is an important function of the hematology laboratory. Understanding the origin of these fluids, their functions, and the proper procedures for accurate analysis is critical for every individual who assumes the responsibility of their examination.

BODY FLUID TYPES AND LOCATIONS

In general, three types of body fluids are examined in the laboratory: *cerebrospinal fluid* (CSF), *synovial fluid*, and *serous fluid*. The CSF is located in the space between the three meninges or membranes covering the brain and spinal cord and flows over the brain and spinal cord. Synovial fluid is located in joint cavities. Serous fluid is found in the body cavities that hold the abdominal organs, lungs, and heart, which are lined with a thin layer of connective tissue that forms a sac around the organs. The sac enclosing the abdominal organs is called the *peritoneum*; that enclosing the lungs is the *pleura*; and that enclosing the heart is the *pericardium*. Normally, there is a small amount of serous fluid within the sac surrounding each of these organs.

CEREBROSPINAL FLUID

Anatomy of the Central Nervous System

The body's central nervous system (CNS) consists of the brain and spinal cord. Bony structures, including the cranium and neural arches of the vertebrae, provide good

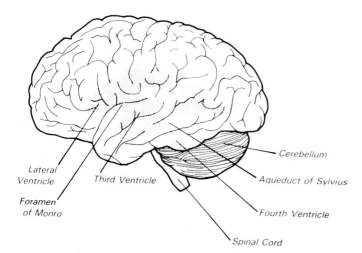

FIG. 31-1.   Inner ventricular system of CNS.

protection for the delicate CNS, and CSF provides a further cushion.

The CNS can be divided into an inner ventricular system and an outer subarachnoid system. The ventricular system (Fig. 31-1). consists of two lateral ventricles within the cerebral hemisphere, the third ventricle in the midline of the brain, the fourth ventricle between the brain stem and the cerebellum, and the central spinal canal, extending from the fourth ventricle down to the filum terminale of the spinal cord. The entire ventricular system is lined by a single layer of ciliated cuboidal cells called *ependymal cells*. The individual ventricles are connected to each other by several passages. The two foramina of Monro connect each lateral ventricle with the third ventricle, and the aqueduct of Sylvius connects the third and fourth ventricles.

The outer subarachnoid system covers the brain surface (Fig. 31-2). The meninges, which surround the brain and spinal cord, are composed of three membranes. The innermost is a delicate, closely applied pia mater. This is covered by the complex, weblike arachnoid membrane, which contains the surface cerebral blood vessels. The arachnoid membrane is in turn covered by the dura mater, a thick fibrous material containing several dural venous sinuses. The pia mater and arachnoid membrane collectively are called the *leptomeninges*. The thin area between them is the *subarachnoid space*.

Formation and Appearance of Cerebrospinal Fluid

In some areas, the capillaries of the pia mater form villi called the choroid plexuses that project into the ventricular system. Under normal conditions, CSF, which is a clear, colorless, modified ultrafiltrate of the blood, is formed by the choroid plexuses through ultrafiltration and secretion.[12]

The total CSF volume in adults is approximately 140 mL and is located in three areas: (1) 25 mL in the ventricular system; (2) 30 mL in the spinal subarachnoid space; and (3) 85 mL in the cerebral subarachnoid space. The total volumes are 10 to 60 mL in infants and 60 to 100 mL in children. There is a constant turnover of CSF, with approximately 500 mL being produced every 24 hours.[4]

Circulation, Absorption, and Function of Cerebrospinal Fluid

After production in the lateral ventricles, CSF passes through the foramen of Monro into the third ventricle and reaches the fourth ventricle through the aqueduct of Sylvius. It exits from the fourth ventricle through the foramina of Lushka and Magendie and enters the subarachnoid space, circulating downward along the spinal cord and upward over the cerebral hemispheres. It is then reabsorbed with the venous circulation through arachnoid villi in the dural sinuses and other specialized areas of the dura.

The CSF protects the brain from sudden changes in pressure and provides a site for metabolic exchange of nutrients and waste. The choroid plexus epithelium and the endothelium of all the capillaries in contact with the CSF anatomically form the blood–CSF barrier. This barrier regulates the passage of substances between the blood and CSF. The blood–CSF barrier and the cellular and chemical components of the CSF are altered in many disease states.

Lumbar Puncture and Laboratory Evaluation of Cerebrospinal Fluid

LUMBAR PUNCTURE
Indications

Lumbar puncture (spinal tap) is the most common method for obtaining CSF and is always performed under aseptic conditions. Another method of obtaining CSF involves a ventricular puncture performed by a neurosurgeon and the utilization of an Ommaya reservoir. This reservoir is placed under the scalp by a surgeon and stays in place for weeks to months to allow for

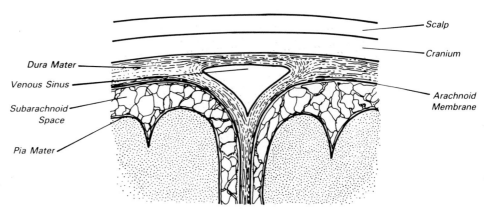

FIG. 31-2.   Outer subarachnoid system of CNS.

withdrawal of CSF specimens and for introduction of drugs for the treatment of CNS disease.

Examination of CSF is primarily a diagnostic tool used in confirming meningitis, encephalitis, brain abscess, CNS hemorrhage, leukemia and lymphoma, tumor, and demyelinating disease in which the myelin sheath of nerve tissue is destroyed or removed. The lumbar puncture can also be used therapeutically for the introduction of chemotherapy in patients with CNS leukemia and lymphoma, for the infusion of anesthetics and radiographic contrast media, and for the instillation of amphotericin B in fungal meningitis. Although the lumbar puncture is a simple procedure, problems and complications may occur. A thorough history and physical examination should be performed by a physician prior to the puncture. Funduscopic examination for papilledema (swelling of the optic nerve) must be included to rule out increased intracranial pressure: if there is increased pressure, extra care must be taken when removing CSF from the spinal canal; otherwise, the cerebellum may herniate into the foramen magnum, causing serious injury or even death. Lumbar puncture is contraindicated if septicemia or infection is present at the proposed puncture site, because meningitis can result from the spread of infection into the meninges.

Technique

The patient must lie on his or her side at the edge of a firm bed with the knees drawn up to hyperflex the spine. In adults, the puncture should be performed between the third and fourth vertebrae (L3–L4) or lower, whereas in children, L4 to L5 or lower is preferred to avoid spinal cord damage. A small-gauge needle should be inserted perpendicular to the plane of the back, with the forefingers of both of the operator's hands guiding it in. After it penetrates the skin, it is guided slightly upward (toward the patient's head) and pushed until a slight "give" indicates that the dura has been penetrated.[1]

The CSF pressure is the first measurement taken on passing the dura. Pressure is measured with a sterile graduated manometer affixed to the needle with a three-way stopcock that allows pressure to be measured and fluid to be withdrawn using a single needle. The normal pressure is 70 to 200 mm H_2O.[7] A low opening pressure indicates spinal block or leakage of CSF. High pressure may be secondary to meningeal inflammation, hemorrhage, cerebral edema, lesions, thrombosis of the venous sinuses, or congestive heart failure. The normal closing pressure is 40 to 100 mm H_2O.[7] If the initial pressure is not elevated and there is no significant fall in pressure when fluid is withdrawn, 10 to 20 mL of CSF can be removed without ill effects.

LABORATORY EVALUATION OF CEREBROSPINAL FLUID

The turbidity, color, and the cell count of CSF aid in the identification of infection, hemorrhage, malignant infiltration, and other diseases of the CNS.[2,3,11,12]

Specimen Requirements

As the fluid drips from the needle inserted in the patient, it is collected, using sterile technique, in three sterile tubes. Usually 1 to 4 mL is placed in each tube, and the tubes are numbered sequentially. Tube 1, containing the first fluid collected, should be used for chemistry and serology testing, tube 2 for microbiologic studies, and tube 3, with the last fluid obtained, for the cell count and differential. It is important to use tube 3 for hematologic studies because the last fluid collected will have the least peripheral blood contamination after a traumatic puncture. All tubes must be labeled with the patient's name and hospital number and the date. The accompanying requisition should include all information on the tube and the type of fluid, the tests requested, and the patient's diagnosis.

Delivery to and processing of the CSF by the laboratory should be immediate, because cell lysis can begin within 1 hour after collection. Refrigeration can help preserve the specimen for approximately 4 hours. The requisition should be stamped with the date and time of delivery to the laboratory.

MACROSCOPIC EXAMINATION
Principle
CSF turbidity is graded, and the color of the uncentrifuged sample (tube 3) is compared with the color of the supernatant fluid of the centrifuged sample (tube 1).

Procedure
1. Evaluate turbidity. Gently invert tube 3 and hold this uncentrifuged sample together with a tube of water against a newspaper. Grade turbidity 0 to 4^+: 0 = crystal clear fluid identical to water; 1^+ = slightly visible turbidity; 2^+ = turbidity present but newsprint can be read easily through tube; 3^+ = newsprint cannot be read easily; or 4^+ = newsprint cannot be read. The CSF may appear oily after injection of radiographic contrast medium. This finding should be reported.
2. Evaluate color. Gently invert tube 1 and record color of CSF. If color is present, centrifuge tube 1 for 5 minutes at 750 × g. Compare color of uncentrifuged tube 1 with that of supernatant fluid of the centrifuged tube. See Comments below for interpretation. Record color of CSF supernatant fluid of tube 1.

Reference Range
Normal CSF is clear and colorless. Any turbidity or color is abnormal.

Comments and Sources of Error
Failure to mix the specimen or using a clotted specimen causes erroneous results. Clotting occurs because of fibrinogen introduced in the traumatic tap. Turbidity is seen when the WBC count exceeds 200 × 10^6/L; the RBC count exceeds 400 × 10^6/L; or microorganisms are present.

Observation of the color of the supernatant fluid after centrifugation of tube 1 is vital. It is extremely important to differentiate a traumatic tap from pathologic CNS bleeding, which may be accomplished by following the procedure for color examination. Color in the supernatant fluid after centrifugation indicates a pathologic condition. The color may be pink, yellow, brown, or colorless. Pink indicates RBC lysis and Hb release; it can be seen 4 to 10 hours after a subarachnoid hemorrhage. Yellow or xanthochromic color indicates pathologic bleeding; it results from Hb breakdown to bilirubin in the subarachnoid space. Xanthochromia persists for 2 to 3 weeks after hemorrhage. It is also caused by a protein concentration greater than 2500 mg/L in the CSF or by liver disease. A brown color indicates the presence of methemoglobin formed after a subdural or intracerebral hematoma. Finally, if the supernatant fluid of tube 1 is colorless whereas the fluid in the tube was tinted before centrifugation, a traumatic tap has occurred.

MICROSCOPIC EXAMINATION: CELL COUNT
Principle
The RBCs and WBCs are counted manually using a hemocytometer with improved Neubauer ruling and a special thick coverslip.

Procedure
1. Use tube 3 for all counts unless it is not available, in which case use tube 1 (prior to centrifugation). Tube 2 must remain sterile for microbiologic testing.
2. Gently invert the tube and note the color and turbidity of the

specimen to determine which of the following counting procedures should be used.

3. If the CSF appears clear and colorless, charge well-mixed, undiluted specimen onto both sides of hemocytometer with a 100 μL pipet. If CSF appears turbid or tinted, dilute a small amount 1:1 with normal saline (0.9% NaCl) in a 12 × 75-mm test tube and plate on both sides of hemocytometer.

4. After 3 minutes, count the WBCs and RBCs in 1 μL of hemocytometer. This is nine large 1-mm^2 squares on one side and the center 1-mm^2 square of the opposite side.

5. Count each specimen in duplicate using both sides of hemocytometer and average the counts obtained from each side for the WBCs and RBCs. If sample has been diluted 1:1, multiply the results by two.

6. Record results as number of WBCs × 10^6/L and RBCs × 10^6/L or number/μL.

7. If the fluid contains too many RBCs to count on the hemocytometer, make a microdilution of the specimen and count RBCs using a single-channel electronic particle-counting instrument (Chap. 42). The WBCs may be counted manually after RBC lysis using a Unopette. Methods are described below.

Electronic RBC Count

a. Dilute 20 μL of CSF in a 10-mL 0.9% NaCl solution Unopette (1:500 dilution).

b. Expel the mixture into a particle-counting vial and perform the RBC count on this dilution using a single-channel electronic particle counter and standard procedure. Report the results directly from counter readout as RBCs × 10^6/L. If the count exceeds 10,000, it must be corrected for coincidence using manufacturer-provided charts.

Manual WBC Count

a. Dilute 20 μL of CSF fluid in a phase platelet Unopette (1:100 dilution). This causes RBC lysis. Plate on hemocytometer.

b. After 3 minutes, count WBCs (× 10^6/L) (as explained in steps 4 and 5 of microscopic examination procedure) and multiply by 100 to correct for dilution.

Reference Range

Table 31-1 presents CSF cell count reference ranges. Table 31-2 lists sample reference ranges for commonly ordered chemical, microbiologic, and serologic tests on CSF.[7,9,11]

Comments and Sources of Error

Failure to mix the specimen, counting microorganisms as cells, or using clotted samples cause erroneous results.

Other indications of a traumatic tap (besides clear supernatant fluid in tube 1 after centrifugation of a "tinted" CSF) to be distinguished from pathologic bleeding are a decrease in RBCs in the serial tubes (tube 1 having the most, tube 3 the

TABLE 31-2. Chemical Tests on CSF with Sample Reference Ranges and Commonly Requested Microbiologic and Serologic Tests

	REFERENCE RANGE	
TEST	SI UNITS	CONVENTIONAL UNITS
CHEMISTRY		
Albumin	70–360 mg/L	7–36 mg/dL
Calcium	1.05–1.35 mmol/L	2.1–2.7 mEq/L
Chloride	118–127 mmol/L	118–127 mEq/L
Glucose	2.75–4.40 mmol/L	50–80 mg/dL
Glutamine	0.41–1.10 mmol/L	6–16 mg/dL
5-HIAA	7.8–23.5 μmol/L	1.5–4.5 mg/dL
Immunoglobulins		
IgA	0–5 mg/L	0–0.5 mg/dL
IgG	10–40 mg/L	1–4 mg/dL
IgG/albumin	0.25–0.28	25–28%
IgG/total protein	0.05–0.12	5–12%
IgM	0–10 mg/L	0–1 mg/dL
Lactate dehydrogenase (LD)	0.1 of serum level	10% of serum level
Lactate	1.11–2.81 mmol/L	10–18 mg/dL
Lactic acid	1.1–2.2 mmol/L	10–20 mg/dL
Magnesium	1.2–1.6 mmol/L	2.4–3.1 mEq/L
Myelin basic protein	<4 mg/L	<4 ng/mL
Total protein	150–450 mg/L	15–45 mg/dL
pH	7.30–7.40	7.30–7.40
pCO_2	5.60–6.93 kPa	42–52 mm Hg
pO_2	5.33–5.87 kPa	40–44 mm Hg
Potassium	2.0–3.5 mmol/L	2.0–3.5 mEq/L
Protein electrophoresis Fraction		
Prealbumin	0.02–0.07	2–7%
Albumin	0.50–0.70	50–70%
Alpha-1 globulin	0.03–0.09	3–9%
Alpha-2 globulin	0.04–0.12	4–12%
Beta globulin	0.1–0.18	10–18%
Gamma globulin	0.03–0.09	3–9%
Sodium	144–154 mmol/L	144–154 mEq/L
Specific gravity	1.006–1.008	1.006–1.008
Urea	1.0–2.7 mmol/L	6–16 mg/dL
Uric acid	30–268 μmol/L	0.5–4.5 mg/dL
Zinc	0.31–0.92 μmol/L	2–6 μg/dL
MICROBIOLOGY		

Gram stain
Gram stain of sedimented CSF
Bacterial, fungal, viral cultures
Acid-fast stains (Ziehl-Neelsen or fluorescent rhodamine) and culture
India ink
Antibiotic sensitivities
Limulus amebocyte lysate test
Wet mount preparations, immunofluorescent methods, and electron microscopy for the identification of primary amebic meningioencephalitis

SEROLOGY
Countercurrent immunoelectrophoresis
Cryptococcal antigen
FTA (fluorescent treponemal antibody)
FTA-ABS (fluorescent treponemal antibody absorption test)
VDRL

least) or a clotted specimen. Crenation of the RBCs *cannot* be used as a distinguishing factor because it is seen in both traumatic taps and pathologic bleeding.

To determine if the CSF contains increased WBCs when large numbers of RBCs are present, compare the ratio of RBCs to WBCs in the patient's peripheral blood with that in the CSF. Normally, this ratio is 1000 RBCs to 1 or 2 WBCs.[11] If these two ratios are approximately the same, a traumatic puncture has occurred. A comment should be made on the report that the specimen is contaminated with peripheral blood. If the ratio is

TABLE 31-1. Reference Ranges for WBCs and RBCs in CSF

PATIENT AGE (YEARS)	WBC	
	SI UNITS (PER L)	CONVENTIONAL UNITS (PER μL)
<1	0–30 × 10^6	0–30
1–4	0–20 × 10^6	0–20
5–puberty	0–10 × 10^6	0–10
Adult	0–5 × 10^6	0–5
	RBC	
	SI UNITS (PER L)	CONVENTIONAL UNITS (PER μL)
All ages	0 × 10^6	0

lower in the CSF (*i.e.*, there are more than 1 or 2 WBCs per 1000 RBCs), the WBCs are actually present in the CSF and indicate a pathologic process in the CNS.

Methods of Concentration of Cells for Analysis and Differentiation

Differentiation of cells in the CSF provides important evidence of the nature and course of CNS diseases. A differential may be performed directly from the hemocytometer when a small amount of acidified crystal violet has been added to the CSF or by phase microscopy with unstained fluid. The one advantage of this method is that it requires no special equipment. Significant disadvantages include: (1) the inability to determine the exact cell type (only "mononuclear" and "polymorphonuclear" cells can be differentiated, and sometimes even these are difficult to identify; (2) only a few cells are available for classification; and (3) no permanent slide of the differential is retained.

Concentration of the cells prior to the differential count can provide more cells for greater precision in counting. Methods of cell concentration include centrifugation, sedimentation, membrane filtration, and cytocentrifugation.

In *centrifugation,* a 3- to 5-mL sample of CSF is centrifuged for 10 minutes. The supernatant fluid is removed, and a drop of 22% albumin is added to the sediment before the cells are spread on slides by the same technique used to make a peripheral blood film. Centrifugation is rapid and requires no special equipment. Also, the supernatant fluid can be used for other diagnostic tests. The disadvantages include variable and incomplete cell recovery and much cellular distortion and damage.

In the *sedimentation* method, 3 to 5 mL of CSF is placed in a plastic or glass cylinder. Cells settle by gravitational force onto a glass slide while the fluid is absorbed by surrounding filter paper (Fig. 31-3).[15] Excellent cell preservation results from this method. The disadvantages include the long sedimentation time (2 hours) and cell loss by absorbance into the filter paper.

In the *membrane filtration* technique, 3 to 5 mL of CSF is placed in a sterile syringe and forced through a small-pore filter. The wet filter is then removed, fixed, and stained. Preparation time is short, and excellent cell recovery results. Also, the noncellular portion of the fluid can be used for other diagnostic tests. The principal disadvantage is the inability to see fine cell structural characteristics.

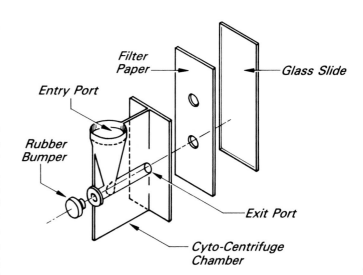

FIG. 31-4.   Cytocentrifuge technique for CSF concentration. Rubber bumper creates closed system between entry port where CSF is introduced and glass slide. This figure shows one of twelve chambers available in cytocentrifuge. The CSF and any cells contained therein leave chamber through exit port; excess fluid is absorbed by filter paper, and concentrated cells are deposited on glass slide. (Courtesy of Shandon, Inc., Publication No. CYTI, Pittsburgh, PA, December, 1976.)

In the *cytocentrifuge* method, 0.2 mL of CSF is centrifuged at low speed. The fluid passes through a tube, and the cells are deposited directly on a glass slide (Fig. 31-4).[16] Excess fluid is absorbed by filter paper. This method is rapid and simple. Good cell recovery results, with minimal distortion, from a small amount of sample.[3] Twelve slides can be spun simultaneously. The only disadvantage is the requirement for special equipment. When using the cytocentrifuge for cellular concentration, refer to Table 31-3 for quality control guidelines for the cell count and cellular recovery after cytocentrifugation.[2] Recount and respin if the cell count and recovery do not match.

Methods of Staining Cell Concentrates

Many staining methods are available for specimens concentrated on microscope slides. Wright or Wright-Giemsa stain are excellent for hematopoietic cells. Either stain is quick and easy and can be used after the slide has air dried.

The Papanicolaou stain is most useful in the diagnosis of nonhematopoietic tumors and is used primarily in cytopathology. This procedure is time consuming and requires immediate fixation, because the air-drying artifact can interfere with cellular morphology interpretation and diagnosis.

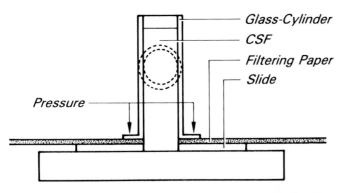

FIG. 31-3.   Chamber used in sedimentation technique for CSF concentration.

TABLE 31-3. Quality Control Guidelines for Cytocentrifuge Cell Recovery Based on Manual WBC Count

HEMOCYTOMETER WBC CELL COUNT ($\times 10^6$/L)	CYTOCENTRIFUGE CELL RECOVERY PER SLIDE
0	0–140
1–2	25–200
>3	>300

Many other stains can be performed on CSF concentrated preparations to achieve special diagnostic results, such as the Gram stain, peroxidase stain, periodic acid-Schiff (PAS) stain, esterase stain, and various stains for mycobacteria and fungus.

MORPHOLOGIC EVALUATION OF CELLS IN THE CEREBROSPINAL FLUID

Normal Cells

Many terms are used today to identify normal cells seen in CSF. The CSF normally contains lymphocytes and a few monocytes (Fig. 31-5).

Lymphocytes are the predominant cell in CSF, and they appear similar to those in the peripheral blood. A rare variant (reactive) lymphocyte may be seen in normal CSF (Fig. 31-6). These cells are reacting to various antigenic stimuli. Their nuclei may be eccentrically located and are round or indented with a chromatin pattern that ranges from dense to less dense. Nucleoli may be seen. The cytoplasm is intensely basophilic and may contain a few azurophilic granules. Lymphocytes function in the processes of humoral and cell-mediated immunity (Chap. 24).

Monocytes also are common in normal CSF. The ratio of lymphocytes to monocytes is approximately 70:30, although a higher percentage of monocytes is normal in newborns and young children. Monocytes have an irregularly shaped nucleus, which can be ovoid, kidney-shaped, or lobular (see Fig. 31-5). The chromatin is fine, and nucleoli may be seen. The cytoplasm is abundant and blue-gray and may contain vacuoles. Occasionally, fine pink granules are seen in the cytoplasm. Monocytes function as phagocytes, which remove cellular debris in the CNS during disease processes. Other terms used to describe monocytes are "reticulomonocytes," "histiocytes," "pia-arachnoid mesothelial cells," and "macrophages."

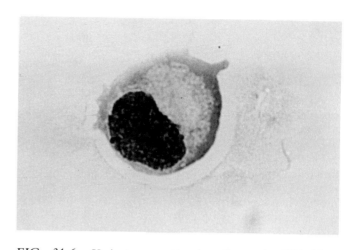

FIG. 31-6.   Variant or reactive lymphocyte in CSF. Note deeply basophilic cytoplasm and eccentric nuclear location. Absence of nuclear halo and presence of dense chromatin pattern identifies cell as lymphocyte rather than plasma cell. Slide made using cytocentrifuge (original magnification × 630; Wright stain).

Choroid plexus and ependymal cells line the CSF space and may be seen in normal and abnormal CSF. Choroid plexus cells are the most common (Fig. 31-7). These cuboid epithelial cells usually appear in groups without cell borders and contain small, round, condensed nuclei and abundant cytoplasm. They resemble the skin scrapings occasionally seen on a peripheral blood film. Ependymal cells are rare in CSF. They have small nuclei and an abundant amount of blue-gray cytoplasm, which is ciliated. The presence of either of these cells is of no diagnostic significance.

Nonmalignant Cells Secondary to Disease

Lymphocytes are diagnostically significant when the relative and absolute counts are increased. A large spectrum of lymphoid cells is seen in benign lymphocytosis of the CNS.

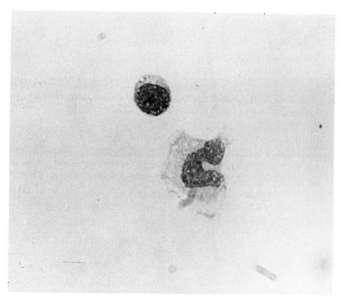

FIG. 31-5.   Normal cells in CSF. Upper cell is typical lymphocyte and lower cell, a monocyte. Slide made using cytocentrifuge (original magnification × 250; Wright stain).

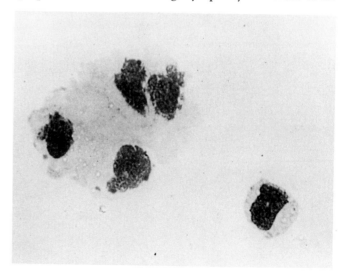

FIG. 31-7.   Choroid plexus cells in CSF. Note group formation. Single cell at right is a monocyte. Slide made using cytocentrifuge (original magnification × 250; Wright stain).

These small and large lymphocytes, plasmacytoid lymphocytes, transformed (atypical or variant) lymphocytes (see Fig. 31-6), and rare lymphoblasts can range from 6 to 20 μm in diameter. Table 31-4 details cell morphology and causes of pleocytosis (increased cells in the CSF). Plasma cells also may be found in CSF in certain disease conditions (see Table 31-4).

A pure monocytosis is uncommon in CSF. Increased monocytes and macrophages usually are accompanied by increased lymphocytes and plasma cells and may or may not be accompanied by increased neutrophils. A mixed presence of neutrophils, lymphocytes, plasma cells, and monocytes is seen in tubercular meningitis, chronic bacterial meningitis, fungal meningitis, leptospinal meningitis, and amebic encephalomyelitis and after the rupture of a brain abscess. Various numbers of lymphocytes, plasma cells, and monocytes are seen in viral meningioencephalitis, syphilis, and multiple sclerosis and after partial treatment of bacterial meningitis.

Macrophages with large amounts of cytoplasm and large vacuoles may be seen phagocytizing RBCs, WBCs, microorganisms, pigments, and lipids. Macrophages that contain RBCs are termed "erythrophages" and are seen a few hours after bleeding in the CNS. After 18 hours, these cells become siderophages or macrophages that contain iron as a result of RBC destruction.[10] These cells may remain in the CSF for months after bleeding.

Lipophages contain fat and can be seen in traumatic or liquefaction necrosis (tissue death followed by conversion to a fluid state), after cerebral infarcts, and after a myelogram. Macrophages may also be seen after intrathecal therapy (drugs introduced into the spinal canal), brain irritation, and pneumoencephalography (a procedure for examining the brain ventricles and subarachnoid spaces).

Neutrophils are not normal in CSF, but when present are morphologically the same as those in the peripheral blood. *In vitro*, they may degenerate rapidly and appear as shadows or smudges. Neutrophilia in the CSF is most significant in cases of bacterial meningitis, but neutrophils also are found in other disorders (see Table 31-4). A rare neutrophil should not be considered pathologic, as some concentration techniques, such as the cytocentrifuge, are sensitive enough to recover one neutrophil after microscopic peripheral blood contamination during lumbar puncture.

In the CSF, eosinophils are seldom seen, and basophils are rare and usually have no diagnostic significance. Erythrocytes also are not normal in the CSF. Cartilage and bone marrow cells and squamous epithelial cells from the skin are rarely seen and have no significance (see Table 31-4).

Cellular Picture in Nonmalignant Disease Processes

Bacterial meningitis causes increased WBC counts, ranging from 50 to 100,000 $\times$ 10^6/L, in the CSF. Neutrophils predominate, and intracellular and extracellular organisms may be seen. Later in the disease, after therapy, there is an increase in lymphocytes and plasma cells and in monocytes involved in phagocytosis. Common organisms causing bacterial meningitis are *Streptococcus pneumoniae*, *Neisseria meningitidis*, and *Hemophilus influenzae*.

Fungal meningitis is often first recognized when budding yeasts are seen during a manual CSF cell count. Such organisms can be seen more easily after concentration and Wright

TABLE 31-4. Nonmalignant Cells in CSF Secondary to Disease

	MORPHOLOGIC APPEARANCE	DISEASES CAUSING APPEARANCE IN CSF
Lymphocytes	Size and maturity vary; nuclei are round or indented and may contain nucleoli; cytoplasm ranges from scant to abundant and moderately to deeply basophilic	Antigen–antibody reaction, viral and fungal meningitis, tubercular meningitis, listeriosis, multiple sclerosis, and purulent encephalitis[11]
Plasma cells	Nuclei round or oval and eccentrically located; may be binucleated; chromatin very dense and may contain nucleoli; cytoplasm brightly basophilic and may contain prominent clear area	Herpes simplex meningioencephalitis and chronic diseases (*e.g.*, multiple sclerosis, tuberculosis, and syphilis)
Monocytes/macrophages	Monocytes appear same as in peripheral blood; macrophages may contain RBCs, iron, or fat	Pure monocytosis is unusual in CSF. Monocytes often found with neutrophils, lymphocytes, and/or plasma cells. Macrophages containing RBCs are seen a few hours after bleeding into CNS; these macrophages contain iron remnants 18 hours after CNS bleeding occurred. Macrophages containing fat are seen in traumatic or liquefaction necrosis, after cerebral infarcts, and after myelograms. Macrophages are also seen after intrathecal therapy, brain irritation, and pneumoencephalography
Neutrophils	Same as in peripheral blood	Bacterial meningitis, after hemorrhage or trauma to CNS, early stages of viral infection, tuberculous or fungal meningitis, and when CNS tumor is present
Eosinophils	Same as in peripheral blood	Parasitic infections, allergic disorders, and after myelograms
Basophils	Same as in peripheral blood	Rarely seen in chronic granulocytic leukemia involving the meninges
Erythrocytes	Same as in peripheral blood	After traumatic lumbar puncture, after CNS hemorrhage, and when malignancy is present
Bone marrow/cartilage/ squamous epithelial cells	Variable	Accidental puncture of vertebra and subsequent aspiration of cartilage or bone marrow during lumbar puncture. Epithelial cells result from skin contaminants

staining of the CSF, which causes the organisms to appear as small purple spheres separated by clear capsules. The organisms may appear intracellularly or extracellularly, sometimes in groups, and are smaller than lymphocytes (Fig. 31-8). In fungal meningitis, CSF cell counts range from normal to markedly increased. When they are increased, a mixed reaction of lymphocytes, plasma cells, monocytes, and neutrophils usually is present. Common causes of fungal meningitis are *Cryptococcus neoformans*, *Candida albicans*, and *Histoplasma capsulatum*.

Neurosyphilis causes an increase in the total leukocyte count, with lymphocytes and plasma cells predominating.

Tuberculous meningioencephalitis is indicated in its early stages by the occurrence of a mixed cell reaction, with an increase in CSF neutrophils, monocytes, lymphocytes, and plasma cells. Rarely, eosinophils also are increased. Later in the disease, there is an increase in lymphocytes, plasma cells, and monocytes.

Multiple sclerosis has no typical morphologic appearance. In some cases there is an increase in total CSF leukocyte count, plasma cells, and reactive lymphocytes.

Hemorrhage or stroke is immediately followed by an increase in CSF erythrocytes, neutrophils, and erythrophages. Later there is an increase in siderophages.

Malignant Cells

The CSF may contain malignant cells from three sources: primary brain tumors, metastatic tumors, and hematopoietic malignancies (leukemia, lymphoma, or plasma cell myeloma).

Solid-Tumor Cells

Solid-tumor cells are seen in CSF when the tumor reaches the subarachnoid space or the ventricular system. Whether these cells are recovered in processing also depends on the type of tumor, the site of the puncture, and the amount of specimen available for examination.

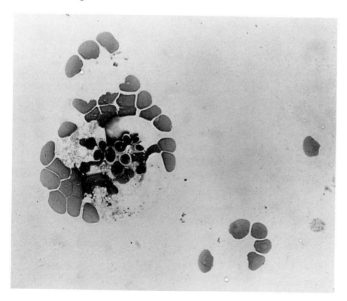

FIG. 31-8. Fungi (small dark spheres) in macrophage found in CSF. Slide made using cytocentrifuge (original magnification × 250; Wright stain).

In general, tumor cells are large and are often seen in clumps. The nuclei are large and contain prominent nucleoli and may be binucleated. The cytoplasm is basophilic and may contain cytoplasmic tags (Plate 36) seen as irregular blebs around the cell edge. Cells in mitosis are common. A single one of these characteristics is not sufficient to diagnose malignancy; one must weigh the overall cell picture before a decision is rendered.

Primary brain tumors include medulloblastoma, retinoblastoma, astrocytoma, ependymoma, meningioma, and pinealoma. Tumors that may be metastatic to the CNS include those of the lung, breast, and colon. Metastatic tumor cells have a greater tendency to exfoliate (slough off) and as a result are recovered more frequently than are cells from primary brain tumors.

Cells Associated with Hematopoietic Malignancies

Patients with CNS involvement by leukemia and lymphoma often present with symptoms of headache, nausea, and vomiting that may be misinterpreted as a result of drug toxicity or infection. The distinction can be made by finding leukemic or lymphoma cells in the CSF.

Patients usually do not present with CNS disease at the time of diagnosis. More often, malignant cells appear in the CSF after the disease has been established and after remission induced by chemotherapy. Leukemic and lymphoma cells may appear in the CSF during apparent remission.

Acute lymphocytic leukemia (ALL) is the most common leukemia to invade the CNS. Present therapy has extended the life span of these patients, so that more are relapsing in the CNS. Concentration devices for CSF have helped clinicians in their management of these patients, because they allow for earlier detection of CNS relapse. It is possible to see ALL cells in the CSF when the peripheral cell count is within the normal range and the patient has no neurologic symptoms. The blasts are similar to those in the bone marrow and peripheral blood. The nuclei are large and may contain nucleoli. The chromatin pattern ranges from fine to condensed. The cytoplasm is scant and basophilic and may contain tags (see Plate 37).

Acute nonlymphocytic leukemia (Chap. 34) less commonly invades the CNS. The blasts are larger than those seen in ALL. The nuclei have a fine chromatin pattern and prominent nucleoli. The cytoplasm is abundant, may contain a few granules and Auer rods, and may show tags. In acute progranulocytic leukemia, the malignant promyelocytes are large and similar to those seen in the peripheral blood (Chap. 34). Cytoplasmic tags may also be seen.

Leptomeningeal involvement may be found in patients with diffuse non-Hodgkin lymphoma. The most common types are lymphoblastic lymphoma, diffuse histiocytic lymphoma, and undifferentiated lymphoma. The malignant cells in the CSF resemble those seen in the lymph nodes, bone marrow, and other tissues. Much variation is found in these cells, including various amounts of basophilic cytoplasm and cytoplasmic tags. The nuclear shape ranges from round to irregular and may be notched or cleaved. The chromatin ranges from fine to condensed, and the nuclei may contain nucleoli (Plate 38).

Rarely, a population of plasma cells is recovered in cases of multiple myeloma involving the CNS. These malignant plasma cells have various amounts of intensely basophilic cytoplasm. A clear zone may appear adjacent to the nucleus, representing the Golgi apparatus. The nuclei are eccentric and may contain nucleoli.

Sources of Error in Cell Identification

Before interpreting leukemic, lymphoma, or plasma cells in the CSF, it should be verified that the CSF is not peripherally contaminated by a traumatic lumbar puncture, that bone marrow was not accidentally aspirated from the vertebra during the puncture, and that the invasion of immature cells is not the result of a completely different disease process.

Common sources of error in cell identification and interpretation are listed in Table 31-5.

OTHER BODY FLUIDS

Other body fluids examined in the laboratory are synovial (joint) fluid and serous fluid. Unlike CSF, synovial and serous fluids may accumulate abnormally in their respective body cavities. Such abnormal fluid is called an effusion.

Identification of Effusions as Transudates or Exudates

It is diagnostically helpful to divide effusions into the categories of transudates or exudates through laboratory analysis. *Transudates* result from filtration of blood serum across the physically intact vascular wall as the result of a systemic disease. *Exudates*, the active accumulation of fluid within body cavities in association with vascular wall damage, are caused by inflammation, malignancies, or infection. Several laboratory criteria, summarized in Table 31-6, are used to distinguish transudates from exudates.[14]

Synovial Fluid

Synovial fluid (SF), or joint fluid, is a clear, viscous liquid that provides lubrication and nourishment for the cartilage of joints. It is produced by dialysis of plasma across the synovial membrane, this fluid being combined with a hyaluronate-protein complex secreted by the synovial membrane.

COLLECTION

Aspiration of joint fluid, or arthrocentesis, is performed using aseptic precautions. The patient should be fasting if glucose testing is requested. A sterile disposable needle and sterile plastic syringe containing 25 units of heparin per mL of fluid to be withdrawn are used to collect the sample.[11] Because normal joints contain only 0.5 to 2.0 mL of SF, a dry tap is not uncommon unless an effusion is present. If sufficient sample is available for examination, it is collected in three tubes: 1 to 3 mL in a sterile tube for microbiologic examination; 1 to 5 mL in a heparin or liquid EDTA tube for cellular examination; and 1 mL in a plain tube for observation of clotting. These examinations are useful in detecting inflammatory and noninflammatory joint disease. Arthrocentesis also is performed to remove fluid and relieve symptoms. Medications may be injected at the end of the procedure.

TABLE 31-5. Common Sources of Error in CSF Cell Identification

PROBLEM	SOLUTION
1. Are abnormal WBCs seen in the CSF specimen actually present in the CNS or a result of peripheral contamination by a traumatic lumbar puncture?	Perform the cell count procedures and compare the RBC and WBC count in the CSF with the ratio in the peripheral blood. If the RBC:WBC ratio is lower in the CSF, the patient has a true increase in WBCs in the CNS
2. Are the clumps of cells malignant tumor cells or benign lining cells?	Benign Nucleus: small, round, with condensed chromatin Cytoplasm: abundant, lightly basophilic, with regularly defined cytoplasmic membranes Malignant Nucleus: large with prominent nucleoli; can be binucleated Cytoplasm: deeply basophilic; may demonstrate tags with an irregularly defined cytoplasmic membrane
3. Is the lymphoid proliferation malignant?	Usually a mixture of small, large, and variant (reactive) lymphocytes with a rare blast is seen in benign cases. Malignant cells are more monomorphic (similar in appearance)
4. Are the small, darkly staining purple spheres (with Wright stain) lymphocytes or fungi?	Small lymphocytes will contain a small amount of basophilic cytoplasm, whereas fungi will not. Perform India ink preparation to view the organisms or perform special stain to observe the capsule (such as PAS)
5. Are bacteria or a stain precipitate present?	Perform Gram stain to permit observation of bacteria if they are present
6. Have sufficient cells been recovered utilizing the cell concentration technique?	Scan working area of slide using low magnification (10× objective) to confirm location of all cells

---

TABLE 31-6. Effusion Differentiation into Transudates or Exudates

TEST	TRANSUDATE	EXUDATE
Color	Pale yellow	Yellow → red
Clarity	Clear	Cloudy
Total protein	<30 g/L	>30 g/L
Specific gravity	>1.015	<1.015
WBC	<300 × 10⁶/L	>1000 × 10⁶/L
Fibrinogen	Present (may cause clotting)	Not present

Causes	Systemic disease
	  Congestive heart failure
	  Cirrhosis
	  Hypoproteinemia
		Inflammation
		  Rheumatoid disease
		  Systemic Lupus
		    Erythematosus
		Malignancy
		  Metastatic
		    carcinoma
		  Lymphoma
		Infection
		  Tuberculosis
		  Bacterial or fungal
		    pneumonia
		  Bacterial or fungal
		    pericarditis

TABLE 31–7. Classification of Joint Diseases

I.	Noninflammatory	Osteoarthritis
		Osteochondritis dissecans
		Osteochondromatosis
		Traumatic arthritis
		Neuroarthropathy
II.	Inflammatory	Gout
		Pseudogout
		Reiter's disease
		Rheumatoid arthritis
		Systemic lupus erythematosus
III.	Septic	Bacterial infection, including tuberculosis
		Fungal infection
IV.	Hemorrhagic	Hemophilia
		Trauma
		Pigmented villonodular synovitis

From Glasser L: Reading the signs in synovia. Diagn Med 3(6): 35, 1980; with the permission of the Medical Economics Company.

CLASSIFICATION OF JOINT DISEASES

Joint diseases are classified in four categories, according to clinical and laboratory characteristics: noninflammatory, inflammatory, septic, and hemorrhagic disorders (Table 31-7). The laboratory features of each category are summarized in Table 31-8.[6]

GROSS EXAMINATION, VISCOSITY, AND MUCIN CLOT DETERMINATION

Immediate laboratory delivery of SF is important. Normal SF is clear and pale yellow and does not clot. Turbidity is indicative of leukocytosis, the presence of crystals, or cartilage debris. A few red cells usually are seen because of the trauma of aspiration, and the reference range is 0 to 2000 × 10⁶/L.[8] If bloody fluid is obtained, observation of the supernatant fluid after centrifugation can assist in differentiating a traumatic puncture (clear) from hemarthrosis or bleeding in the joint (color). Streaks of blood in the fluid indicate a traumatic puncture. Xanthochromia indicates previous bleeding in the joint, whereas red or brown is found if bleeding has been recent.

Viscosity is high in normal SF. It is measured by allowing SF to form a string by dropping it from a syringe into a beaker. If the string breaks before reaching 3 cm in length, viscosity is lower than normal. Low viscosity indicates joint inflammation.

The *mucin clot test* measures the concentration of hyaluronic acid in SF. To 0.5 mL of SF, about 2 mL of 2% acetic acid is added in a small beaker and allowed to stand for a few minutes. Normally, a firm clot will form, surrounded by a clear liquid. A weak clot or no clot formation indicates joint inflammation. Table 31-8 summarizes the results of this test and tests of viscosity for each of the four joint disease categories in comparison with reference ranges.

MICROSCOPIC EXAMINATION

The cell count on a normal SF may be performed on a standard hemocytometer. When counts are high, dilutions with normal saline should be made for counting on the hemocytometer or electronic counting equipment. Acetic acid cannot be used for WBC count dilutions, as a clot will form with the addition of acid. A viscous fluid may need to stand on the hemocytometer for 30 minutes to allow the cells to settle for counting. Reference ranges for the cell count and number of neutrophils per 100 WBCs are included in Table 31-8.[6]

The differential can be done by phase-contrast microscopy or by Wright stain of either unconcentrated SF or a concentrated specimen obtained by simple centrifugation, cytocentrifugation, or filtration. The differential usually is reported as the percentage of neutrophils. Normal SF contains less than 25% neutrophils and 75% normal lymphocytes and monocytes with no cartilage cells, cells with inclusions, or crystals.[9]

Neutrophils in SF are similar to those in the peripheral blood. An increased neutrophil percentage is seen in septic arthritis. In abnormal conditions, neutrophils may contain crystals or bacteria.

Macrophages may be seen in SF and resemble monocytes. They are large cells with abundant blue-gray cytoplasm that may contain crystals or hemosiderin after bleeding in the joint.

Synovial lining cells may be seen in SF and have no diagnostic significance. They have large amounts of basophilic cytoplasm and one or more round mature nuclei.

Ragocytes or RA cells are neutrophils containing small, dark gray inclusions. They are seen predominantly in rheumatoid arthritis but also in gout and septic arthritis. They may be identified using phase microscopy or immunofluorescent techniques. The inclusions consist of IgG, IgM, complement, and rheumatoid factor. Other cells seen in SF include mast cells, LE cells in patients with lupus erythematosus, and cartilage cells in patients with osteoarthritis. Malignant cells are rarely seen in SF. If malignancy is suspected, the specimen should be submitted for sectioned cytologic studies.

TABLE 31–8. Pathologic Classification of Joint Diseases Based on Laboratory Examination of Synovial Fluids

TEST	NORMAL	GROUP I (NONINFLAMMATORY)	GROUP II (INFLAMMATORY)	GROUP III (SEPTIC)	GROUP IV (HEMORRHAGIC)
Volume (mL)	<3.5	>3.5	>3.5	>3.5	>3.5
Color	Pale yellow	Yellow	Yellow–white	Yellow–green	Red–brown
Viscosity	High	High	Low	Low	Decreased
Mucin clot	Firm	Firm	Friable*	Friable	Friable
Leukocyte count (cells × 10⁶/L)	<180	200–2000	2000–100,000	10,000–>100,000	>5000
Neutrophils (%)	<25	<25	>50	>75	>25
Glucose (mg/dL)	Approx. same as blood glucose	Approx. same as blood glucose	>25 mg/dL lower than blood glucose	>25 mg/dL lower than blood glucose	Approx. same as blood glucose
Microbiologic culture	Negative	Negative	Negative	Often positive	Negative

* Friable = easily broken.
From Glasser L: Reading the signs in synovia. Diagn Med 3(6): 35, 1980; with the permission of the Medical Economics Company.

Wet preparation examination for crystals using polarized light should be performed on all SF, as their identification provides definitive diagnoses. Refer to textbooks on body fluids for a description of the many crystals that may be found in SF.[13]

Serous Fluid

Normally 1 to 10 mL of serous (serum-containing) fluid is found in the pleural, peritoneal, and pericardial cavities, where it reduces friction and facilitates movement between surfaces or membranes.[5] Formation occurs by plasma ultrafiltration. Other terms used to describe pleural fluid are *thoracentesis fluid*, *chest fluid*, or *empyema fluid*. Peritoneal fluid may also be called *abdominal fluid* or *ascitic fluid*. Pericardial fluid, which surrounds the heart, is also called *pericardiocentesis fluid*.

GROSS EXAMINATION

Serous fluid is aspirated for diagnosis, relief of symptoms, or instillation of drugs. Normal serous fluid is clear and pale yellow.

A fluid containing blood, also referred to as hemorrhagic, sanguineous (bloody), or serosanguineous (containing serum and blood), may indicate either a traumatic puncture or disease. Blood seen in a traumatic puncture usually is nonuniform in distribution and clears as the aspiration proceeds. Malignancy is the most common cause of a truly hemorrhagic fluid.

Chylous or pseudochylous specimens are milky white. Chylous specimens contain lipids and are caused by leakage from the lymphatic ducts secondary to trauma or malignancy. Pseudochylous fluids contain cholesterol crystals and cellular debris and are seen in tuberculosis and rheumatoid arthritis.

MICROSCOPIC EXAMINATION

Cell counts are routinely performed on serous fluids. Manual counts using the hemocytometer are preferred to electronic particle counts because debris or clots are often present that may falsely elevate the cell count or obstruct the instrument aperture. Hemorrhagic fluids may be diluted for RBC counts, and RBCs may be lysed with 3% acetic acid for the WBC count.

Serous fluid cells should be concentrated using cytocentrifugation, filtration, or sedimentation methods and stained for the differential. Wright stain is used in most hematology laboratories, whereas Papanicolaou stain is preferred in cytology laboratories. Differentials on serous fluids along with the total RBC and WBC counts are not always useful or diagnostic but can aid in classifying the effusion (see Table 31-6).

Lymphocytes are seen in most effusions and may be small, large, or reactive. They range from 9 to 15 μm in diameter and have round or indented nuclei. With Wright stain, they possess various amounts of basophilic cytoplasm, which may contain azurophilic granules. A lymphocytosis is seen in tuberculosis and carcinoma.

Plasma cells are similar to those found in CSF. They are seen in tuberculosis, malignancy, and rheumatoid arthritis and can accompany an increase in lymphocytes.

Monocytes appear similar to those in the peripheral blood, with irregularly shaped nuclei and abundant amounts of blue-gray cytoplasm, which may contain azurophilic granules. They are found in normal, reactive, and malignant fluids.

Macrophages can become extremely large, as much as 50 μm in diameter. The nuclei can be round or irregular in shape and usually have a lacy chromatin pattern. The cytoplasm is abundant and may contain whole RBCs and WBCs, cellular debris, iron, and microorganisms. Macrophages are commonly found in normal, reactive, and malignant fluids.

Neutrophils appear similar to those in the peripheral blood. However, they may also be hypersegmented or have an abnormal nucleus that is round and deeply stained. The cytoplasm may be vacuolated and exhibit a loss of granulation. Large numbers of neutrophils are seen in the early stage of inflammatory processes.

Serous fluids containing eosinophils are seen in many disease states. These cells, appearing similar to those in peripheral blood, are commonly seen in excess of 10% on the WBC differential of serous fluids in pneumothorax, infections, malignancy, infarction, chest trauma, and hypersensitivity syndromes.

Mature RBCs are present in most effusions. Increased num-

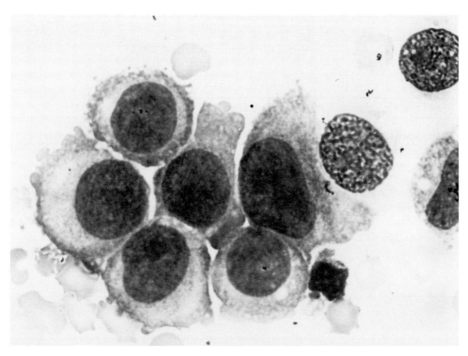

FIG. 31-9. Six mesothelial cells in pleural fluid. Note small lymphocyte (lower right). Slide made using cytocentrifuge (original magnification × 500; Wright stain).

bers are seen after a traumatic puncture or hemorrhage or during a malignant process. Nucleated RBCs may be seen after peripheral blood or bone marrow contamination and during a malignant process.

Mesothelial cells line the pleural, pericardial, and peritoneal cavities and usually make up at least 5% of the cellular elements on the serous fluid WBC differential. They range from 12 to 30 μm in diameter and can appear singly or in sheets. The abundant cytoplasm ranges from moderately blue to deep blue; it may have a light-staining hue near the nucleus, giving it a "fried egg" appearance (Fig. 31-9). Small cytoplasmic vacuoles may be present. The cells may contain one or several round nuclei, which are dark purple and stippled. Nucleoli are commonly found. Reactive mesothelial cells may contain large vacuoles and may exhibit phagocytosis. These cells are commonly confused with mononuclear phagocytes. They are also difficult to distinguish from malignant cells because they are large, possess basophilic cytoplasm, and are commonly found in sheets. However, the nuclei of malignant cells are larger and show more irregularity. Mesothelial cells are diagnostically insignificant and are found in most serous fluids. However, they are characteristically absent in tuberculous effusions.

Neoplastic disease is one of the most common causes of effusions. Malignant cells are commonly found in these fluids. Leukemia and lymphoma may invade body cavities, and the malignant cells in serous fluids of patients with these diseases resemble those seen in the peripheral blood, bone marrow, and lymph nodes. In these cases, the serous fluid or peripheral blood cell count is not always increased. Tumor cells are seen when the carcinoma has infiltrated the body cavity. The diagnosis of tumor involvement is usually made by the cytology laboratory.

Chemical and Microbiologic Determinations

Chemical tests commonly performed on synovial and serous fluids include glucose, total protein, lactate dehydrogenase (LD), amylase, and pH. Hyaluronic acid and uric acid also are measured on synovial fluid.

Common microbiology tests on both fluids include gram and acid-fast stains and aerobic, anaerobic, acid-fast, and fungal cultures.

Immunology tests may be ordered on synovial fluids, including rheumatoid factor, antinuclear antibody, complement, and immunoglobulin levels.

CHAPTER SUMMARY

Cerebrospinal fluid (CSF) flows over the brain and spinal cord, providing a protective cushion for the central nervous system (CNS). Examination of CSF provides important evidence concerning diseases affecting the CNS such as meningitis, brain abscess, and leukemia.

When performing an aseptic lumbar puncture to obtain a CSF sample, CSF pressure is measured first. Normally, it is around 70 to 200 mm H_2O. High pressure may indicate several disorders such as hemorrhage or malignancy. Low pressure indicates spinal block or CSF leakage. Three sterile tubes are used to collect CSF; usually only the third (last) tube is used for the cell count and differential, which should be performed within 1 hour of collection.

Normal CSF is clear and colorless. Turbidity, which is graded as 0 to 4^+, is caused by the presence of greater than 200×10^6/L WBCs or 400×10^6/L RBCs or by microorganisms. If color is present, the color of tube 1 before centrifugation is compared with the supernatant fluid of that tube

after centrifugation to distinguish between a traumatic tap, indicated by a colorless supernatant fluid, and a pathologic disorder, in which the supernatant fluid retains color. A pink color indicates erythrocyte Hb release; yellow (xanthochromic) may indicate pathologic bleeding, protein greater than 2500 mg/L, or liver disease; brown indicates methemoglobin.

The reference range for CSF cell counts differs with age (see Table 31-1). Table 31-2 lists sample reference ranges for other CSF laboratory tests.

Differentiation of cells in the CSF is best performed using a sample prepared by one of the cell concentration methods (*e.g.*, cytocentrifugation). Wright or Wright-Giemsa stain may be used to stain CSF cells. Lymphocytes and a few monocytes are normal in CSF (see Figs. 31-5 and 31-6).

Nonmalignant cells found in CSF secondary to disease (see Table 31-4) include lymphocytes, plasma cells, monocytes and macrophages, neutrophils, eosinophils, basophils, erythrocytes, and bone marrow, cartilage, and squamous epithelial cells.

Malignant cells in CSF include solid tumor cells and cells from hematologic malignancies including leukemia, lymphoma, and plasma cell myeloma. In general, tumor cells are large and are often seen in clumps. The nuclei are large with prominent nucleoli, and the cells may be binucleated. The cytoplasm is basophilic and may contain cytoplasmic tags (Plate 36).

Common sources of error in CSF cell identification and interpretation are included in Table 31-5.

Synovial (joint) fluid is examined to detect inflammatory and noninflammatory joint disease (see Tables 31-7 and 31-8). Normal joint fluid is clear and pale yellow. It does not clot and is highly viscous. Low viscosity indicates inflammation.

Serous (serum-containing) fluid is found in the pleural, peritoneal, and pericardial cavities, where it reduces friction and facilitates movement between surfaces. Normally, serous fluid is clear and pale yellow. Cell counts and differentials after specimen concentration are sometimes useful in diagnosis. Various cell types may be found in association with different disease states.

CASE STUDY 31-1

A 5-week-old girl was admitted to the hospital with bruising. A complete blood count revealed the following: WBC 283 × 10⁹/L; Hb 6.3 g/dL; HCT 0.19 L/L; and platelets 4 × 10⁹/L. The patient had 93 circulating blasts per 100 WBC in the peripheral blood. A bone marrow study was performed, and the diagnosis was acute lymphocytic leukemia, L1 type (Chap. 36). A lumbar puncture was performed, and the CSF cell count was WBC 2 × 10⁶/L and RBC 5180 × 10⁶/L. The CSF differential revealed blasts 80%, lymphocytes 14%, and monocytes 6%.

1. What is the reference range for CSF cell counts for a 5-week-old infant? Is the CSF cell count abnormal in this case?
2. Are the above data sufficient to determine if the blasts present in the CSF are a result of peripheral blood contamination or active CNS disease?
3. What calculations must be performed to identify or rule out peripheral blood contamination?
4. Does acute lymphocytic leukemia commonly invade the CNS?

CASE STUDY 31-2

A 31-year-old man was admitted to the hospital with a 4-week history of skin rash, pneumonia, and genital herpes. On admission he was found to have acquired immune deficiency syndrome (AIDS), *Pneumocystis carinii* pneumonia (PCP), and disseminated cryptococcus infection, with a positive lung biopsy and blood culture. A CSF cell count revealed no WBCs or RBCs.

1. Does the normal cell count rule out CNS infection?
2. Can a differential concentration technique such as the cytocentrifuge assist in the diagnosis?
3. Will the yeast organisms stain with Wright stain? What would stained organisms look like?
4. What other tests performed on the CSF can assist in the diagnosis of fungal meningitis?

REFERENCES

1. Cole M: Pitfalls in cerebrospinal fluid examination. Hosp Pract 4:47, 1969
2. Dalton W, Brailas CD: Cerebrospinal Fluid Morphology with Emphasis on Oncologic Specimens. American Society for Medical Technology Workshop Manual. Los Angeles, ASMT, 1983
3. Drewinko B, Sullivan MP, Martin T: Use of the cytocentrifuge in the diagnosis of meningeal leukemia. Cancer 31:1331, 1973
4. Fishman RA: Cerebrospinal fluid. In Boher AB, Boher LH (eds): Clinical Neurology. New York, Harper & Row, 1971
5. Glasser L: Evaluation: Serous fluids. Diagn Med 3(5):78, 1980
6. Glasser L: Reading the signs in synovia. Diagn Med 3(6):35, 1980
7. Glasser L: Tapping the wealth of information in CSF. Diagn Med 4(1):23, 1981
8. Hoeprich PD, Ward JR: The Fluids of the Parenteral Body Cavities. New York, Grune & Stratton, 1959
9. Kjeldsberg CR, Knight JA: Body Fluids: Laboratory Examination of Cerebrospinal, Synovial, and Serous Fluids: A Textbook Atlas. Chicago, American Society of Clinical Pathologists, 1982
10. Kölmel HW: Atlas of Cerebrospinal Fluid Cells, 2nd ed. New York, Springer-Verlag, 1977
11. Krieg AF: Cerebrospinal fluids and other body fluids. In Henry JB (ed): Clinical Diagnosis and Management by Laboratory Methods, 16th ed, vol 1, pp 635–645. Philadelphia, WB Saunders, 1979
12. Neely AE, Cheek KK: Cerebrospinal fluid. In Ross DL, Neely AE (eds): Textbook of Urinalysis and Body Fluids, pp 235–238. Norwalk, CT, Appleton-Century-Crofts, 1983
13. Neely AE, Cheek KK: Synovial fluid. In Ross DL, Neely AE (eds): Textbook of Urinalysis and Body Fluids. Norwalk, CT, Appleton-Century-Crofts, 1983
14. Neely AE, Cheek KK: Transudates and exudates. In Ross DL, Neely AE (eds): Textbook of Urinalysis and Body Fluids. Norwalk, CT, Appleton-Century-Crofts, 1983
15. Oehmichen M: Cerebrospinal Fluid Cytology: An Introduction and Atlas. Philadelphia, WB Saunders, 1976
16. Shandon, Inc., Publication No. CYTI, Pittsburgh, PA, December 1976

PART VII

MALIGNANT

MYELOPROLIFERATIVE

DISORDERS

Introduction

to the

Hematopoietic

Malignancies

E. Anne Stiene-Martin

Malignancy may be defined as the growth and proliferation of one or more clones of abnormal cells. Malignant blood cells do not respond to normal control or feedback mechanisms. In addition, they are believed to produce substances that inhibit the proliferation of normal cells. For a period of time, normal and malignant cells exist side by side in the bone marrow. Eventually, however, the malignant cells will fill the available space, and normal cells will be either inhibited or crowded to the point they cannot survive. These events are frequently manifested in the peripheral blood by decreases in red cells (anemia) and platelets (thrombocytopenia). The malignant cells may or may not circulate in the peripheral blood. If they do, the leukocyte count may be normal or increased; if they do not, there usually is a leukopenia. If not treated, the patient will succumb to infection secondary to the severe granulocytopenia or bleeding secondary to the lack of platelets.

The causes of malignant transformation in cells have not been completely elucidated. In at least some cases, these causes are known to include environmental agents, viruses, genetic susceptibility, or a combination thereof.

Sometimes, the fact that a cell or group of cells is malignant can be determined by their appearance (morphology). Table 32-1 lists various types of morphologic evidence of malignancy. Such evidence of abnormal growth, development, or proliferation is indicated by using the prefix "dys" before the term denoting growth and development (poiesis). For example, if one were to find giant, multinucleated red cell precursors, the term *dyserythropoiesis* might be used. Likewise, one might use the term *dysmegakaryocytopoiesis* if abnormally small or vacuolated megakaryocytes were seen.

Should abnormal cells be present in both the bone marrow and the peripheral blood, the term *leukemia* is used. If the abnormal cells are confined to the bone marrow and do not circulate, the term *aleukemic leukemia* is used. Another possibility is neoplastic growth of cells confined to lymphatic tissue (such as lymph nodes), resulting in solid lymphatic tumors. The term *lymphoma* is appropriate in these cases, the suffix "oma" meaning "tumor." Should the lymphoma spread to the bone marrow and peripheral blood, the term *leukemic lymphoma* is sometimes used.

Classification of the leukemias can be achieved in several ways. First, they can be classified according to the stem cell line involved (myeloid or lymphoid). The myeloid leukemias are those involving granulocytes, monocytes, erythrocytes, or megakaryocytes. Other terms that might be used to describe this group of malignancies are *myeloproliferative disorders* or *nonlymphocytic* leukemias. The latter term is used most frequently in reference to the acute nonlymphocytic leukemias (ANLLs) or acute myeloid leukemias (AMLs). Thus, "ANLL" and "AML" are used interchangeably. The lymphoid malignancies are those involving B cells or T cells and may either be leukemias or lymphomas.

Leukemias may also be classified into acute and chronic forms. These adjectives originally referred to the expected life span of the patient. That is, patients with acute leukemia had a life span measured in days or weeks, whereas patients with chronic leukemia might survive for 1 to 2 years. The advent of chemotherapy has drastically altered the life expectancy in these diseases, such that today, patients with "acute leukemia" may achieve a remission with therapy and live 5 to 15 years or longer. The terms *acute* and *chronic* have been retained, however, to denote the number of primitive (blast) cells in the peripheral blood or bone marrow. Leukemias are generally considered acute if greater than 30% blast forms are found in the peripheral blood or greater than 50% blasts are found in the bone marrow. Conversely, if a patient has less than 10% blasts in the peripheral blood, the leukemia is more likely to be con-

TABLE 32–1. Morphologic Evidence of Malignancy

NUCLEAR
  Shape abnormalities (clefting, contortions)
  Multinuclearity
  Megaloblastoid (nonresponsive to vitamin B_{12} or folate)
  Hyposegmentation (pseudo Pelger-Huët) or hypersegmentation
  Giant or prominent nucleoli
  Increased mitotic figures
CYTOPLASMIC
  Abnormal granules (*e.g.,* Auer rod)
  Mixed granulation (*e.g.,* basophil and eosinophil)
  Decreased granulation
  Increased fragility (cytoplasmic fragmentation)
OVERALL
  Abnormal size (gigantism or dwarfism)
  Tendency to cluster or clump
  Clonal morphology (all abnormal cells appear similar)

sidered chronic, depending on other findings. This leaves a gray area (10%–30% blasts), which is categorized as subacute, chronic, or chronic transforming into acute, depending on other hematologic findings and the clinical history.

As will be discussed in the following chapters, the acute leukemias have been further subdivided according to morphologic criteria by a group of representatives from France, America, and Britain (FAB classification). The acute myeloid or nonlymphocytic leukemias (AML or ANLL) have been subdivided into seven classifications (M1–M7),

whereas the acute lymphoblastic leukemias (ALL) have been subdivided into three classifications (L1–L3). These will be described in great detail in Chapter 34 (AML) and Chapter 36 (ALL).

The chronic leukemias have not been similarly subclassified as yet. The chronic myeloproliferative disorders include chronic granulocytic (myelocytic) leukemia (CML or CGL), polycythemia vera (PV), agnogenic myeloid metaplasia with myelofibrosis (AMM), and primary (essential) thrombocythemia (ET). These will be discussed in Chapter 35. The chronic lymphoproliferative leukemias include chronic lymphocytic leukemia (CLL), prolymphocytic leukemia (PLL), and hairy cell leukemia (HCL), which will be addressed in Chapter 37.

The solid tumors of lymphatic tissue (lymphomas) will be classified and discussed in Chapter 38, while Chapter 39 addresses a unique lymphoid malignancy that cannot be classified as either a leukemia or a lymphoma in the strictest sense: the plasma cell dyscrasias.

The concept of "preleukemia," in which there is morphologic evidence that leukemia might occur later, has fascinated investigators for several years. At present, the only definable syndromes that might be preleukemic are proliferative disorders of myeloid cells; lymphatic preleukemia is rare and poorly defined. The terms *myelodysplastic* or *dysmyelopoietic* syndromes are commonly used to refer to these disorders. These have also been subclassified by the FAB group and will be discussed in Chapter 33.

The

Dysmyelopoietic

Disorders

Robert V. Pierre

Chronic myeloproliferative disorders (CMPD) are conditions in which an abnormal pluripotential (stem) cell population arises in the bone marrow. This new line coexists in the marrow with the normal stem cell lines and has the potential to differentiate into mature end-stage cells. The new stem cell also has the potential to differentiate along a single cell line (clone) or along more than one cell line simultaneously. Examples are the production of predominantly granulocytes in chronic granulocytic leukemia, predominantly erythrocytes in polycythemia vera, and predominantly platelets in essential thrombocythemia. An example of the production of multiple cell lines is agnogenic myeloid metaplasia. These disorders are all clonal in nature.[12]

Although nearly all authors classify chronic granulocytic leukemia as a malignant process, the other chronic myeloproliferative disorders—polycythemia vera, idiopathic (essential) thrombocythemia, and agnogenic myeloid metaplasia—usually are not viewed as malignant until the later stages of the disorders, when they undergo transformation to acute leukemia. The reason for this conclusion is that in these disorders, cell maturation remains normal; there is little cellular dysplasia, and patients generally have long survival times.

A second group of clonal proliferative disorders of the myeloid cell lines is the dysmyelopoietic syndromes (DMPS). In these disorders, a new pluripotential stem cell line appears in the marrow. The process differs from the chronic myeloproliferative disorders in the absence of over-production and the presence of dysplasia of the myeloid cell lines. The DMPS are more often characterized by peripheral cytopenias secondary to either an absolute decrease in precursor cells in the marrow or ineffective cell production. There also is disagreement about whether these disorders are truly leukemic or instead represent qualitative stem cell abnormalities. All of these disorders have a great potential for transformation to an acute leukemic disorder. They have a clinical course that is shorter than that of the CMPD but usually longer than that of the acute leukemias.

The acute myeloid (nonlymphocytic) leukemias are also clonal proliferative disorders of the myeloid cell lines. They differ from the CMPD and DMPS in that they show little maturation and greater dysplasia and generally run a brief course.

This chapter will deal primarily with the second group of disorders, the dysmyelopoietic disorders.

HISTORY OF DISEASE DEFINITION

An article by Block, Jacobson, and Bethard in 1953 entitled "Preleukemic Acute Human Leukemia" was the first article describing the preleukemic disorders.[5] The first specific clinicopathologic entity described among this group of disorders was "refractory anemia with excess myeloblasts," by Dreyfus and associates in 1972.[11] In 1972, Zittoun, and coworkers described "chronic myelomonocytic leukemia."[38] Although these disorders have an increase in marrow blasts, the number of blasts are not sufficient to make a diagnosis of acute leukemia. In 1973, Saarni and Linman introduced the concept of a "preleukemic syndrome."[26] In this disorder, there must be dyspoiesis of at least two cell lines, and blasts must constitute less than 5% of the marrow cells. Other terms have been used by other authors for disorders that overlap in their features with the dysmyelopoietic syndromes (DMPS) and some forms of acute non-lymphocytic leukemia (ANLL). They include "refractory dysmyelopoietic anemia,"[25] "subacute myeloid leukemia,"[8] and "smoldering acute leukemia."[24]

The DMPS tend to be more frequent in males than females, similar to the male predominance that is found in overt ANLL.[35] These syndromes occur most frequently in patients 50 years or older,[23] but may be seen in any age group, including young children.

The causes of DMPS are not known, except that some cases may be secondary to X-ray therapy, chemotherapy with alkylating agents, or work or hobby exposure to toxic chemicals. Cases without a known history of such exposure are referred to as "primary DMPS."

The DMPS are being recognized with increasing frequency, although there is no known hereditary pattern or genetic role. Between 1967 and 1973, we saw 521 patients with suspected DMPS at the Mayo Clinic; in this same period, 426 patients with ANLL were seen.[23] This and subsequent experience has suggested to us that DMPS is more common than overt ANLL.

PATHOPHYSIOLOGY

The pathophysiology of DMPS can be explained by two simple hypotheses. The first is that DMPS represents the growth of an abnormal clone of cells in the marrow. Experimental work[6] has shown that leukemic cells can suppress the growth of normal cells, either by production of a humoral substance or perhaps by recruitment of T lymphocytes. If the DMPS clone has similar properties, suppression of the normal pluripotential stem cell line of the marrow can result in marrow hypoplasia and pancytopenia. If the suppression affects only the committed stem cell lines, selective marrow hypoplasia with isolated cytopenias in the peripheral blood may occur.

The second hypothesis is that the abnormal DMPS stem cell line has the ability to differentiate to mature end-stage cells that are abnormal in appearance and function.[2,30] Thus, the presence of dyserythropoiesis with ineffective erythropoiesis accounts for anemia with abnormal oval macrocytic red cells. The presence of neutropenia with abnormal mature forms such as pseudo–Pelger-Huët forms or degranulated neutrophils accounts for the frequent infections and fever. The suppression of megakaryocytopoiesis or dysplasia of megakaryocytes accounts for the thrombocytopenia and abnormal-appearing platelets, which frequently have abnormal function as well, resulting in bleeding manifestations.

CLINICAL PRESENTATION

The classic triad of symptoms in patients with DMPS is fatigue, fever, and bleeding. Many patients, particularly those with early stages of DMPS, are asymptomatic and are discovered on routine checkups or in the course of investigating other disorders. Physical examination is usually unremarkable, but pallor may be present secondary to anemia, fever may be present because of infection, and there may be petechiae or ecchymoses secondary to thrombocytopenia. The spleen may be slightly enlarged, but there is no lymphadenopathy.

PERIPHERAL BLOOD AND BONE MARROW ABNORMALITIES

Erythropoiesis

Erythropoiesis may show quantitative abnormalities that range from red cell aplasia to extreme erythroid hyperplasia. The hallmark of DMPS is dyserythropoiesis. The abnormal maturation is megaloblastoid in type. "Megaloblastoid" is used to signify the resemblance to the megaloblastic maturation typical of vitamin B_{12} deficiency. Megaloblastoid maturation is characterized by large precursors having an open chromatin pattern that is more coarse than that of megaloblastic maturation, and the chromatin may be attached to the nuclear membrane in large clumps. (Chap. 12 discusses the differences between megaloblastic and megaloblastoid morphology in more detail.) The nucleus may be irregular in shape, from simple indentation to complex cloverleaf forms. Multinuclearity may be present, and giant forms may be seen. There may be a left shift and an increase in the number of rubriblasts. In rare cases of pure red cell aplasia, only rubriblasts are seen.

Hemoglobinization of the cytoplasm of red cell precursors may be normal or impaired. Impaired hemoglobinization is associated with a hypochromic, microcytic, or dimorphic picture in the peripheral blood and increased stainable iron in the bone marrow with pathologic ringed sideroblasts. Pathologic ringed sideroblasts are those in which the iron granules consist of iron-laden mitochondria situated in a ring about the nucleus.

Granulopoiesis

Granulopoiesis may show quantitative changes ranging from decreased granulopoiesis to marked granulocytic hyperplasia. Dysgranulopoiesis is manifested by a left shift in granulocytic maturation with an increase in myeloblasts. There may be nuclear abnormalities such as hyposegmentation (Pelger-Huët forms) or hypersegmentation of neutrophils. The cells may also show dissociation of normal nuclear and cytoplasmic maturation, pseudonucleoli secondary to cytoplasmic intrusion into the nucleus, and nuclear blebs. Granule abnormalities are common; there may be hypogranulation of the neutrophils or coarse abnormal granules, the pseudo–Chédiak-Higashi abnormality. Rarely, eosinophils and basophils also show hypogranulation.

In some cases it is difficult to differentiate neutrophils from monocytes. There are atypical neutrophils with monocytoid features; this is particularly true in chronic myelomonocytic leukemia. There may also be cells that have the cytochemical features of both neutrophils and monocytes. This is not surprising, as the neutrophil and the monocyte are thought to be derived from a common precursor cell.

The French-American-British (FAB) group[4] has introduced a classification of DMPS in which they distinguish between Type I and Type II blasts. Type I blasts are myeloblasts with a centrally located nucleus, a fine nuclear chromatin pattern, and a prominent nucleolus. The cytoplasm contains no granules when stained with Romanowsky stain. Type II blasts are described as blasts with centrally located nuclei but slightly more mature nuclear chromatin pattern and a lower nuclear:cytoplasmic ratio. The cytoplasm contains large granules, one or many. This type of cell has also been referred to as an "abnormal progranulocyte (promyelocyte)." The combined total of Type I and Type II blasts is used to calculate the percentage of blasts. Tricot and coworkers[33] reported abnormal localization of immature precursors (ALIP pattern), which had prognostic significance for survival and progression to acute leukemia. In normal bone marrow, granulopoiesis is localized around the bone trabeculae, whereas erythropoiesis and megakaryocytopoiesis are located more centrally in the marrow space. In the ALIP pattern, clusters of blasts appear in the central marrow.

Megakaryocytopoiesis

Megakaryocytes may show quantitative abnormalities ranging from near absence to hyperplasia. Dysplasia of megakaryocytes is a common feature. The most frequent abnormality is a maturation arrest, with the majority of megakaryocytes being small to medium-size cells with a single or bilobed nucleus. The cytoplasm may show vacuolization and lack of granulation. In rare cases there are giant megakaryocytes with hypersegmentation of the nucleus (greater than the usual numbers of separate small individual nuclei). The peripheral blood platelets may be decreased, normal, or rarely, increased. They may be very large or hypogranular or have large fusion granules. Abnormalities of the dense tubular system or open canalicular system may give the platelets a Swiss cheese appearance.

SPECIFIC CLINICOPATHOLOGIC FORMS OF DYSMYELOPOIETIC SYNDROMES

The FAB group created a classification of the dysmyelopoietic syndromes or myelodysplastic syndromes. As in the acute leukemias, the FAB group did not describe these disorders but created diagnostic criteria for each of the entities.[4] The five entities follow:

1. Refractory anemia or refractory cytopenia (RA/RC)
2. Refractory anemia with ringed sideroblasts (RARS)
3. Refractory anemia with excess blasts (RAEB)
4. Chronic myelomonocytic leukemia (CMML)
5. Refractory anemia with excess blasts in transformation (RAEBIT)

Table 33-1 summarizes the principal criteria for these disorders.

Refractory Anemia

The principal feature of RA is dyserythropoiesis (Plate 39), which is manifested by megaloblastoid maturation of erythrocytic precursors and an anemia characterized by oval macrocytes. The patient may be mildly to severely anemic. The mean cell volume (MCV) and the red cell distribution width (RDW) usually are elevated. A dimorphic red cell picture may be observed. Dysplastic nucleated red cells, sideroblasts, and siderocytes may be found in the peripheral blood. The FAB group emphasizes that absolute reticulocytopenia is characteristic; however, in our experience, the relative reticulocyte percentage is often elevated, and prominent polychromatophilia may be seen on the blood film.

Dysgranulopoiesis is *not* a feature of RA. The total leukocyte count is normal or low; an elevated leukocyte count suggests an infection or other cause. The FAB group stipulates that less than 1% blasts be present in the peripheral blood and less than 5% in the bone marrow. Dyspoiesis of megakaryocytes is not a feature of RA; the peripheral platelet count is normal or slightly decreased.

The bone marrow cellularity is normal or increased. Erythrocytic hyperplasia is present with abnormal (megaloblastoid) maturation. The maturation abnormalities may be subtle and can easily be misidentified as normal or megaloblastic. No giant or bizzare multinucleated erythrocytic precursors are seen. A few patients have impaired hemoglobinization of erythrocytic precursors and a dimorphic peripheral red cell picture. Pathologic sideroblasts may be

TABLE 33–1. FAB Classification of Dysmyelopoietic Syndromes

	RA/RC	RARS	RAEB	CMML	RAEBIT
LEUKOCYTE COUNT	Norm to decr	Norm to decr	Norm to decr	Increased	Norm to decr
MONOCYTES					
MARROW	–	–	–	At least 20%	–
BLOOD	–	–	–	$>1 \times 10^9/L$	–
BLASTS IN PERIPH. BLOOD (%)	<1	<1	<5	<5	>5
BLASTS IN BONE MARROW (%)	<5	<5	5–20	5–20	20–30
DYSERYTHROPOIESIS	+++	++	+/–	+/–	+/–
DYSGRANULOPOIESIS	–	–	++	++	+/–
DYSMEGAKARYOCYTOPOIESIS	–	–	+/–	+/–	+/–
SIDEROCYTES/SIDEROBLASTS	+	+	+/–	–	+/–
RINGED SIDEROBLASTS	+/–	>15	+/–	–	+/–

seen in small numbers. Bone marrow iron is normal or increased. Type I and II blasts must account for less than 5% of all marrow cells. Bone marrow fibrosis is not a feature of RA.

Refractory Anemia with Ringed Sideroblasts (Idiopathic Acquired Sideroblastic Anemia)

The RARS disorder is similar to RA; however, the *sine qua non* is the presence of pathologic ringed sideroblasts (Plate 40) and impaired hemoglobinization of erythroid precursors with megaloblastoid maturation. Ringed sideroblasts must account for 15% or more of all nucleated marrow cells. Type I and Type II blasts must be less than 1% in the peripheral blood and less than 5% in the bone marrow. The peripheral blood picture is usually that of a dimorphic anemia with a combination of hypochromic microcytes and oval macrocytes. Sideroblasts and siderocytes may be present in the peripheral blood. The FAB group specifies that granulopoiesis and megakaryocytopoiesis should show minimal quantitative and qualitative changes.

Refractory Anemia with Excess Blasts

The RAEB disorder may display any of the erythroid changes of RA or RARS but must also have dysgranulopoiesis and peripheral cytopenias of two cell lines. The dysgranulopoiesis is more pronounced than in RA or RARS. Type I and Type II blasts must make up between 5% and 20% of all nucleated cells in the marrow. Up to 5% blasts may be observed in the peripheral blood film. There must be progression of granulocytic precursors to mature forms. Dysmegakaryocytopoiesis may be present with mononuclear or bilobed megakaryocytes and large, dysplastic platelets and thrombocytopenia in the peripheral blood.

Either RA or RARS may pass through progressive stages of the FAB classification before becoming leukemia. The FAB classification is a hierarchal classification in that the number of blasts takes precedence over other features. In cases of RA with marked erythrocytic hyperplasia and dysplasia, an increase in blasts to 5% or more causes the condition to be classified as RAEB; likewise, when blasts increase to 5% or more in RARS, the classification becomes RAEB in spite of prominent sideroblasts. Although RAEB is considered a DMPS, it has been found that when a child or young adult presents with a morphologic picture of RAEB, the disease will be rapidly progressive and should be classified as an M2 ANLL.

Chronic Myelomonocytic Leukemia

The CMML disorder has been included in the FAB classification as a DMPS. The term originally suggested by Zittoun and associates[37] has caused some confusion and may be an illogical usage. The FAB group does not believe that DMPS are early stages of leukemia or even necessarily preleukemic, yet the word "leukemia" is used in the name. The term *chronic myelomonocytic syndrome* might be more appropriate.

Although CMML may exhibit any of the dyspoietic features of erythropoiesis, granulopoiesis, and megakaryocytopoiesis described in RA, RARS, or RAEB, it has several distinctive features and, in fact, is more frequently confused with chronic myeloproliferative disorders than with acute leukemia or other forms of DMPS. The FAB criteria state that there must be between 0% and 20% blasts in the marrow and less than 5% blasts in the peripheral blood. The distinguishing feature is a prominent monocytic component in the bone marrow, at least 20% of the marrow cells, and more than 1×10^9 monocytes per liter of blood. The monocytes of the peripheral blood and the monocytic component of the marrow may be difficult to recognize because of the dysplasia of the neutrophils and monocytes. It is strongly recommended that a combined esterase stain[36] be used for both the peripheral blood and the bone marrow aspirate if CMML is suspected.

The FAB criteria may give a misleading impression that CMML is equivalent to RAEB with monocytosis, but CMML is quite different. Teereenhovi has pointed out (personal communication) that patients with typical RAEB may have transient episodes in which they have a peripheral blood monocytosis. The total leukocyte count in RA, RARS, and RAEB usually is normal or low; in CMML, it is most often elevated and may exceed $100 \times 10^9/L$. The marrow shows striking granulocytic hyperplasia with progression to mature forms. The mature neutrophils in CMML often show a striking hypogranular appearance. In our experience, there are many patients who are best classified as having CMML in whom the percentage of myeloblasts is lower than 5% in the bone marrow, and the process does not become blastic until it begins to transform to acute leukemia.

It is of interest that the FAB group did not recognize that CMML might exist in a transition stage between CMML and overt acute leukemia. We have seen patients with CMML with an increase of their marrow blasts to greater than 20% before supervention of ANLL. If such a patient were seen at this stage, the condition might be referred to as "CMML in transformation."

A syndrome occurs in infants or young children that resembles the CMML seen in adults, although it often has a more aggressive clinical course. This disorder characteristically has a deletion of chromosome 7 and may have other chromosomal abnormalities. This disorder has also been called Ph[1]-negative chronic granulocytic leukemia (CGL) or juvenile CGL.[6] A better name might be the "myelomonocytic syndrome of infants" or "monosomy 7 syndrome."[7]

A note should also be made at this point of a rare disorder described by Bearman and associates[3]: chronic monocytic leukemia. The original report described five cases, and review of the literature revealed an additional 28 cases. Although these patients have anemia, four of the five presented without peripheral blood monocytosis or bone marrow monocytic infiltrates. Peripheral blood monocytosis developed after splenectomy in four. Although this disorder may be confused with CMML after splenectomy, it should not be confused with DMPS at presentation because of the absence of peripheral blood or bone marrow changes.

Refractory Anemia with Excess Blasts in Transformation

Patients with RAEBIT may present with cytopenias and symptoms of brief duration, and their hematologic picture does not fit the definitions of RA, RARS, RAEB, or CMML or any of the FAB acute leukemia categories. The FAB criteria for RAEBIT are: (1) 5% or more blasts in the peripheral blood; (2) more than 20% but less than 30% blasts in the bone marrow (Plate 41); and (3) the presence or absence of Auer rods. The obvious diagnostic problem with RAEBIT is to differentiate it from M2 ANLL. The clinical course of RAEBIT is that of acute leukemia, particularly in young patients.[29]

DYSMYELOPOIETIC DISORDERS NOT INCLUDED IN THE FAB CLASSIFICATION

There are a variety of dysmyelopoietic syndromes not included in the FAB classification. Some have been well characterized, and others are less well defined (Table 33-2).

Refractory Cytopenia with Cellular or Hypercellular Marrow Not Meeting the Criteria for RA, RARS, RAEB, or CMML

The FAB group suggested the disorder not meeting the criteria for RA, RARS, RAEB, or CMML be included in a category of refractory cytopenia (RC). The majority of

TABLE 33–2. Dysmyelopoietic Disorders Not Included in FAB Classification

Refractory cytopenia not meeting criteria for RA, RARS, RAEB, or CMML
Secondary or therapy related
Postleukemic
Single cell line aplasias
Paroxysmal nocturnal hemoglobinuria
RARS with isodicentric X abnormality
Dysmegakaryocytopoiesis
  With the 5q⁻ chromosome abnormality
  Without the 5q⁻ chromosome abnormality
Acute myelodysplasia with myelofibrosis

cases of peripheral neutropenia or thrombocytopenia with hyperplasia of the corresponding precursors in the bone marrow and with maturation arrest are immune- or drug-related phenomena. In the author's experience such cases are rarely DMPS. In the past 19 years, we have observed two patients with a chronic idiopathic thrombocytopenic purpura picture, and another with a chronic immune neutropenia, that evolved into ANLL.

Secondary or Therapy-Related Syndromes

The secondary syndromes are an important group of DMPS. Studies have suggested that secondary or therapy-related ANLL is preceded by a preleukemic phase that may resemble the primary DMPS described above. Secondary DMPS usually follow the use of alkylator-type chemotherapy agents either alone or in combination with radiation therapy. Radiation alone produces a lower incidence of secondary DMPS and ANLL. The delay between therapy and the onset of DMPS is usually 2 to 3 years, but it may be as short as 2 months. Secondary DMPS often begins as a refractory macrocytic anemia or sideroblastic anemia. It differs from primary types in that it nearly always has pancytopenia and panmyelopathy with dysplasia in all marrow cell lines and frequently has a hypocellular marrow with an increase in fibrosis.

Postleukemic Syndromes

Foucar and coworkers described postleukemic DMPS.[14] They observed patients in whom DMPS had progressed to overt ANLL and, after therapy, reverted to their pretherapy DMPS status rather than to a normal marrow or persistence of ANLL. We likewise have observed patients who had attained a complete remission of their ANLL relapse as a DMPS rather than as a full-blown leukemia.

Single Cell Aplasias

Most cases of pure red cell aplasia represent immune disorders of marrow or injury by drugs such as chloramphenicol, but some cases represent DMPS. We followed seven cases of pure red cell aplasia over 18 years and observed one transformation to ANLL.

We have had one case of amegakaryocytic thrombocytopenic purpura that evolved to an ANLL. This disorder might be similar to a pure red cell aplasia in which a single cell line is initially affected.

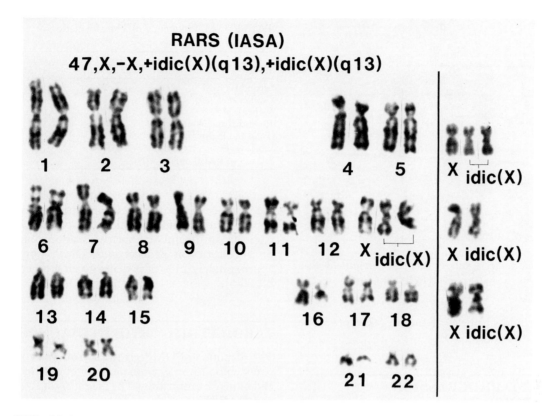

RARS (IASA)

47,X,-X,+idic(X)(q13),+idic(X)(q13)

FIG. 33-1.   GTG-banded 47,X,2idic(X)(q13) karyotype from patient with refractory anemia with ringed sideroblasts and 2idic(X)(q13) chromosome from three different metaphases (right).

Refractory Anemia with Ringed Sideroblasts and Isodicentric X Abnormality

We have observed a group of female patients with refractory sideroblastic anemia with an acquired isodicentric chromosomal abnormality (Fig. 33-1)[10] in whom the disorder rapidly transformed to ANLL. It is not known whether the breakpoints of this gene rearrangement are at or near the gene for the X-linked sideroblastic anemia.

Refractory Macrocytic Anemia with Megakaryocytic Abnormalities (5q⁻ Syndrome)

We believe that the 5q⁻ syndrome should be included among the DMPS, because in many cases, the condition goes on to ANLL.[34] The disorder is both a cytogenetic and a clinicopathologic entity. The patient must possess an isolated interstitial deletion of the long arm of chromosome 5 between bands q15 and q31. There is a striking female predominance in the disorder. The peripheral blood picture is that of a refractory oval macrocytic anemia with normal or increased platelets. The bone marrow is normocellular or hypercellular with megaloblastoid erythrocytic hyperplasia. The feature that distinguishes this disorder from refractory anemia is the numerous small or medium-size mononuclear or bilobed megakaryocytes, which frequently have vacuolated cytoplasm (Fig. 33-2). The type of megakaryocyte found in this disorder is not unique to the 5q⁻ syndrome. The combination of a refractory macrocytic anemia, the 5q⁻ chromosome, and atypical megakaryocytes is required for the diagnosis.

Dyspoietic Megakaryocytic Hyperplasia without 5q⁻ Chromosomal Abnormality or Marrow Fibrosis Abnormality

We have had several patients present with striking megakaryocytic hyperplasia and small mononuclear or bilobed megakaryocytes but no 5q⁻ chromosomal abnormality or marrow fibrosis. Slight dyspoiesis of both erythrocytes and granulocytes was observed (Fig. 33-3). In another variant of DMPS with megakaryocytic hyperplasia, the megakaryocytes are large and appear hypermature or hyperseg-

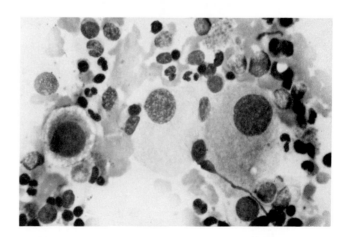

FIG. 33-2.   Bone marrow aspirate with three atypical "mononuclear" megakaryocytes from patient with 5q⁻ syndrome. One cell shows cytoplasmic vacuolization.

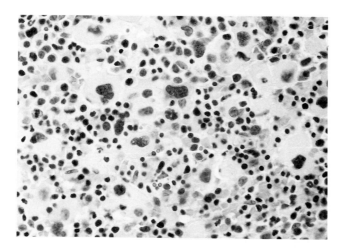

FIG. 33-3. Bone marrow biopsy section from patient with striking megakaryocytic hyperplasia (H&E stain).

mented. The individual nuclei of the megakaryocyte are separated and distinct (Fig. 33-4).

SURVIVAL AND PROGRESSION TO ACUTE LEUKEMIA

The median survival of patients with DMPS was approximately 2.5 years in a prospective study done at the Mayo Clinic.[23] Tricot and associates found a median survival of 18.5 months for patients with less than 5% marrow blasts and of only 7 months in patients with greater than 5% marrow blasts and noted that patients with the ALIP pattern have a shorter survival and more frequent transfor-

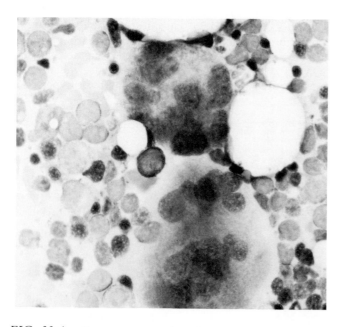

FIG. 33-4. Bone marrow aspirate from patient with a dysmyelopoietic syndrome characterized by megakaryocytic hyperplasia. Majority of magakaryocytes resembled large "hypersegmented" forms seen in this photomicrograph.

TABLE 33-3. Frequency of Transformation of DMPS to ANLL

SERIES	NUMBER OF PATIENTS	PERCENT WITH TRANSFORMATION
Second IWCL[28]	244	21
Coiffier et al[9]	193	32
Weber et al[35]	151	23
Rosenthal and Moloney[25]	117	24
Todd and Pierre[31]	326	22
Juneja et al★[18]	34	18

★ Cases of RAEB only.

mation to ANLL.[33] It is apparent that patients with DMPS die whether or not they develop acute leukemia, and they appear to die from complications of their anemia, neutropenia, or thrombocytopenia. Examination of a number of large series of patients with DMPS shows that only approximately 25% of patients go on to overt ANLL (Table 33-3).

LABORATORY TESTS IN DIAGNOSIS

The diagnosis of DMPS is made from the complete blood count, blood film examination, and bone marrow aspirate and biopsy examination. The diagnosis of RAEB, CMML, and RAEBIT can be made with great accuracy by these standard hematologic examinations and should present no problem to the experienced morphologist. Refractory anemia or refractory cytopenias pose a much more serious problem, because they are mimicked by a variety of disorders. In a prospective study of 325 patients with suspected DMPS followed for 16 years,[31] 31 patients had spontaneous resolution of their hematologic abnormalities and an additional 15 patients had their condition evolve into typical agnogenic myeloid metaplasia (AMM). Even in retrospect, these 46 (14% of the total) patients could not be distinguished from those whose condition eventually evolved into acute leukemia. All the patients whose condition resolved or transformed into AMM were initially said to have refractory anemia. No cases of RAEB, CMML, or RAEBIT were seen to resolve or transform into other chronic myeloproliferative disorders.

Because morphology alone is not adequate for identification of cases of suspected RA or RARS as DMPS, additional laboratory tests are mandatory. Serum vitamin B_{12} and folate levels should be measured in all cases, because early megaloblastic and megaloblastoid maturation can be indistinguishable. Serum iron and ferritin levels and iron stains on the bone marrow aspirate and biopsy should be performed. If pathologic sideroblasts are noted, they should be quantified by determining their percentage among all nucleated cells. A reticulin stain should be performed on the marrow to determine whether myelofibrosis is present. A peroxidase and a combined esterase stain should be done on both the peripheral blood and the bone marrow aspirate. The peroxidase stain is used to determine whether acquired peroxidase deficiency is present, and it may make Auer rods visible that are not seen on the Romanowsky stain. The combined esterase stain permits more accurate assessment of the percentage of monocytic cells in the peripheral blood and bone marrow.

The demonstration of a clonal chromosomal abnormality may be helpful in establishing the diagnosis of DMPS in problem cases of RA, RC, and RARS. The types of chromosomal changes observed in 40% to 60% of DMPS patients are similar to those observed in ANLL.[19] Secondary or therapy-related DMPS have the same chromosomal abnormalities as secondary ANLL. There is a higher frequency of chromosome abnormalities and abnormalities of chromosomes 5 and 7.[21] Cytogenetic studies are necessary to classify the 5q⁻ syndrome, the isodicentric X form of RARS, and the monosomy 7 syndrome of the infant and may be necessary to distinguish CMML from chronic granulocytic leukemia. In addition, the presence or absence of cytogenetic abnormalities gives prognostic information about both survival and likelihood of progression to acute leukemia.[19]

In atypical cases, particularly those that have pathologic ringed sideroblasts, muscle weakness, and neurologic abnormalities, toxic exposure to lead or arsenic should be ruled out by serum, urine, or tissue studies. We have seen a number of cases of lead or arsenic toxicity referred to us as suspected DMPS or subacute leukemia.

Progenitor cell assays or *in vitro* culture for stem cells, particularly for the CFU-GM, may be valuable for establishing the diagnosis of DMPS. However, these studies are mainly research tools and are not widely available for routine use.[16]

Flow cytometry analysis of bone marrow cells has been used to study DNA to determine the fractions of cells in the S and G_2 phases. Patients who have a higher fraction of cells in these phases have a more stable course.[22] These studies correlate with other types of labeling studies that show that reduction of proliferative activity correlates with a poor prognosis. Flow cytometry also has been used to measure DNA content and to identify aneuploidy.

FOLLOW UP OBSERVATIONS

For patients who appear to have a stable clinical course, follow up examinations are made at 6- to 12-month intervals. Repeat CBC and differential count results are sufficient. If any changes occur in the CBC or differential or in the patient's clinical status, a bone marrow examination should be done. Cytogenetic studies may show a change in the karyotype, with the development of a new abnormality or a change in the karyotype signifying clonal evolution. Evidence of a clonal change is suggestive of an imminent leukemic transformation.

TREATMENT

Treatment of patients with DMPS is dependent on two factors: (1) the clinical severity of the process and (2) the age of the patient.

Because patients with DMPS may have a long stable course, it is useful to observe the patient for some period. If the process is stable and the patient is asymptomatic, no therapy is recommended. If there are complications such as anemia, red cell transfusions may be required. Neutropenia and thrombocytopenia are of greater concern because long-term white cell or platelet transfusion therapy usually is not satisfactory.

One form of therapy being developed is based on the principle that leukemic and preleukemic cells can be induced to differentiate by "cell maturation agents." For example, human leukemic blasts can be induced to differentiate into mature neutrophils by exposure to drugs such as cytosine arabinoside, *cis*-retinoic acid,[17,30,32] or humoral factors that regulate granulopoiesis.[27] Trials of *cis*-retinoic acid and cytosine arabinoside in low dosage have induced complete remission in some patients and improvement in others, although the majority of patients do not show significant improvement.[13,15,20,30,32]

Age is an important factor in the selection of the therapeutic agents to be used. In young children or adults whose cytopenias are severe enough to warrant therapy, the disease should be treated as an acute leukemia. Aggressive antileukemic therapy has proved successful in young patients in inducing complete remissions with sustained survival, but unfortunately, only a small number of DMPS occur in young patients. Bone marrow transplantation has been done in a few patients and has proved successful in young patients.[1]

Understanding of the causes of acute leukemia and the nature of the intracellular changes that occur in the evolution of a preleukemic to leukemic process is still poor. With greater understanding, perhaps more effective therapy or prevention of this group of disorders will become possible.

CASE STUDY 33-1

The patient is a 77-year-old man who was admitted to the hospital for excision of a basal cell carcinoma in the nose. His admission CBC revealed a severe macrocytic anemia (Hb, 5.4 g/dL; MCV, 114 fL) and leukopenia (2.9×10^9/L), but platelets were normal. Blood film examination showed a shift-to-the-left with bands, metamyelocytes, and myelocytes present (a subsequent blood film revealed 1% blasts). The red cells were dimorphic with macrocytic, normochromic and macrocytic hypochromic cells exhibiting moderate poikilocytosis. Dacryocytes and oval macrocytes were frequent and occasional NRBCs were found. A bone marrow examination revealed 75% cellularity, decreased myeloid:erythroid ratio and erythroid hyperplasia. Erythroid precursors were megaloblastoid in appearance. Megakaryocytes were increased in number, and some had single round nuclei. Iron stain showed numerous (>25%) ringed sideroblasts.

1. What laboratory findings are compatible with the presence of a dysmyelopoietic disorder?
2. State the FAB DMPS classification most compatible with this patient's laboratory data and the two findings that are particularly characteristic of this subgroup.

Modified from Lotspeich-Steininger CA, McKenzie SB: Myelodysplastic syndromes: A review with case studies. J Med Technol 4:5, 1987, with permission.

REFERENCES

1. Appelbaum FR, Storb R, Ramberg RE et al: Allogeneic marrow transplantation in the treatment of preleukemia. Ann Intern Med 100:689, 1984
2. Baccarani M, Tura S: Differentiation of myeloid leukaemia cells: New probabilities for therapy. Br J Haematol 42:485, 1979
3. Bearman RM, Kjeldsberg CR, Pangalis GA et al: Chronic monocytic leukemia in adults. Cancer 48:2239, 1981
4. Bennett JM, Catovsky D, Daniel MT et al: Proposals for the

classification of the myelodysplastic syndromes. Br J Haematol 51:189, 1982

5. Block M, Jacobson LD, Bethard WF: Preleukemic acute human leukemia. JAMA 152:1018, 1953

6. Broxmeyer HE, Jacobsen N, Kurland J et al: *In vitro* suppression of normal granulocytic stem cells by inhibitory activity derived from human leukemic cells. J Natl Cancer Inst 60:485, 1978

7. Chessels JM, Sieff CA, Harvey BAN et al: Monosomy 7 in childhood: A preleukaemic state. Br J Haematol 49:129a, 1981

8. Cohen JR, Creger WP, Greenberg PL et al: Subacute myeloid leukemia: A clinical review. Am J Med 66:959, 1979

9. Coiffier B, Adeleine P, Viala JJ et al: Dysmyelopoietic syndromes: A search for prognostic factors in 193 patients. Cancer 52:83, 1983

10. Dewald GW, Pierre RV, Phyliky RL: Three patients with structurally abnormal X chromosomes, each with Xq13 breakpoints and a history of idiopathic acquired sideroblastic anemia. Blood 59:100, 1982

11. Dreyfus B, Rochant H, Sultan C et al: Les anémies réfractaires avec excès de myéloblastes dan la moelle. Presse Med 78:359, 1972

12. Fialkow PJ, Jacobson RJ, Singer JW et al: Philadelphia chromosome (Ph[1])-negative chronic myelogenous leukemia (CML): A clonal disease with origin in a multipotent stem cell. Blood 56:70, 1980

13. Flynn P, Miller W, Weisdorf D et al: Treatment of acute promyelocytic leukemia with retinoic acid: Correlation with cell culture studies. Blood 60 (suppl 1):155a, 1982

14. Foucar K, Vaughan WP, Armitage JO et al: Postleukemic dysmyelopoiesis. Am J Hematol 15:321, 1983

15. Gold E, Mertelsmann R, Moore MAS et al: Phase I trial of 13 cis retinoic acid in hematologic malignancies. Blood 58 (suppl 1):139a, 1981

16. Greenberg PL, Nichols WC, Schrier SL: Granulopoiesis in acute myeloid leukemia and preleukemia. N Engl J Med 284:1225, 1971

17. Housset M, Daniel MT, Degos L: Small doses of Ara-C in the treatment of acute myeloid leukaemia: Differentiation of myeloid leukaemic cell? Br J Haematol 51:125, 1982

18. Juneja SK, Imbert M, Joualt H et al: Haematological features of primary myelodysplastic syndromes (PMDS) at initial presentation: A study of 118 cases. J Clin Pathol 36:1129, 1983

19. Knapp RH, Dewald GW, Pierre RV: Cytogenetic studies in 174 consecutive patients with preleukemic or myelodysplastic syndrome. Mayo Clin Proc 60:507, 1985

20. Koeffler HP: Induction of differentiation of human acute myelogenous leukemia cells: Therapeutic implications. Blood 62:709, 1983

21. LeBeau MM, Albain KS, Larson RA et al: Clinical and cytogenetic correlations in 63 patients with therapy-related myelodysplastic syndromes and acute nonlymphocytic leukemia: Further evidence for characteristic abnormalities of chromosome nos. 5 and 7. J Clin Oncol 4:325, 1986

22. Montecucco C, Ricaardi A, Traversi E et al: Proliferative activity of bone marrow cells in primary dysmyelopoietic (preleukemic) syndromes. Cancer 51:1190, 1983

23. Pierre RV: Preleukemic states. Semin Hematol 11:73, 1974

24. Rheingold JJ, Kaufman R, Adelson E et al: Smoldering acute leukemia. N Engl J Med 268:812, 1963

25. Rosenthal DS, Moloney WC: Refractory dysmyelopoietic anemia and acute leukemia. Blood 63:314, 1984

26. Saarni MI, Linman JW: Preleukemia: The hematologic syndrome preceding acute leukemia. Am J Med 55:38, 1973

27. Sachs L: Regulatory proteins for growth and differentiation in normal and leukemic hematopoietic cells: Normal differentiation and uncoupling of controls in myeloid leukemia. In Ford RJ, Maizel AL (eds): Mediators in Cell Growth and Differentiation, p 341. New York, Raven Press, 1985

28. Second International Workshop on Chromosomes in Leukemia: Chromosomes in preleukemia. Cancer Genet Cytogenet 2:108, 1980

29. Scoazec J, Imbert M, Crofts M et al: Myelodysplastic syndrome or acute myeloid leukemia. Cancer 55:2390, 1985

30. Swanson GA, Picozzi VJ, Greenberg PL: Effects of retinoic acid and 1, 25 $(OH)_2$ vitamin D3 on hemopoiesis in normals and patients with myelodysplastic states. Blood 62 (suppl 1):155a, 1983

31. Todd WM, Pierre RV: Preleukaemia: A long term prospective study of 325 patients. Scand J Haematol 36 (suppl 45):114, 1986

32. Tricot G, DeBock R, Dekker AW et al: Low dose cytosine arabinoside (Ara C) in myelodysplastic syndromes. Br J Haematol 58:231, 1984

33. Tricot G, DeWolf-Peters C, Vlietinck R et al: Bone marrow histology in myelodysplastic syndromes: II. Prognostic value of abnormal localization of immature precursors in MDS. Br J Haematol 58:217, 1984

34. Van Den Berge H, Cassiman JJ, David G et al: Distinctive haematological disorder with deletion of long arm of no. 5 chromosome. Nature 251:437, 1974

35. Weber RFA, Geraedts JPM, Kerkhofs H et al: The preleukaemic syndrome. Acta Med Scand 207:391, 1980

36. Yam LT, Li CY, Crosby WH: Cytochemical identification of the granulocytes and monocytes. Am J Clin Pathol 55:283, 1971

37. Zittoun R, Berndou A, Bilski-Pasquier G et al: Les leucémies myélomonocytaires subaigues: Étude de 27 cas et revue de la litérature. Sem Hôp Paris 48:1943, 1972

Acute Myeloproliferative Leukemia (Acute Nonlymphocytic Leukemia)

Valerie J. Evans

DEFINITION

Acute nonlymphocytic leukemia (ANLL) is a general term applied to all acute leukemias involving cells other than lymphocytes. It is a progressive malignant disease of hematopoietic tissue and probably is a stem cell disorder. It is characterized by a predominance of immature marrow cells that have been blocked at an undifferentiated or partially differentiated stage of maturation with or without involvement of the peripheral blood. Normal myeloid elements are reduced in number, apparently as a result of crowding out by the leukemic cells, and eventually are replaced if the malignant proliferating clone remains unchecked. If untreated, ANLL has a rapidly fatal course, death usually being caused by the effects of the resultant pancytopenia, which are anemia, bleeding, and lack of resistance to infection. Acute nonlymphocytic leukemia is principally a disease of adulthood but may occur in all age groups. It has a slight predisposition for males.

ETIOLOGY

The cause of ANLL is not clear. It is likely a combination or interaction of several factors.[10]

Radiation

Evidence supporting the role of radiation exposure as a factor in the development of leukemia has come from three principal lines of study: (1) radiologists who were occupationally exposed prior to the establishment of safety standards and practices in clinical radiology; (2) patients treated by radiation for ankylosing spondylitis compared with others with the same disease who were not irradiated; and (3) survivors of the atomic blasts at Hiroshima and Nagasaki. Each of these groups has an increased incidence of leukemia.

Chemicals

Drugs and chemicals that cause bone marrow depression or aplasia are capable of producing leukemia and thus are referred to as *leukemogens*. Some of these chemicals are chloramphenicol, phenylbutazone, arsenic-containing compounds, sulfonamides, and some insecticides. Certain cytotoxic agents used in the treatment of neoplasms are likewise potentially leukemogenic. These include phenylalanine mustard and cyclophosphamide used to treat multiple myeloma; alkylating agents used to treat several types of cancer including Hodgkin disease, and immunosuppressants used to treat immunoinflammatory diseases. Benzene is the only chemical known unequivocally to produce cancer.

Genetics

Chromosomal aberrations, including aneuploidy and breakage, are demonstrated in a number of diseases associated with an increased incidence of ANLL. These diseases include Down syndrome (trisomy 21), Fanconi syndrome (excessive chromosomal breakage), Bloom syndrome (marked chromosomal breakage and rearrangement), and D-trisomy. Congenital leukemias are usually nonlymphocytic. Studies of cases of familial leukemia are also highly supportive of the genetic etiology of acute leukemia.

Viruses

There is no conclusive evidence that viruses are causative agents of human leukemia. However, type C RNA viruses are recognized as being the most common class of tumor viruses associated with animal leukemia and lymphoma. These viruses make use of an enzyme, reverse transcriptase (hence, the name retrovirus), which has been detected in human leukemic blood cells but not in normal cells. This enzyme facilitates the incorporation of viral genetic material into the host organism's genome. These retroviruses can carry genes responsible for the induction of cancer. Such genes, called *oncogenes,* are slightly altered versions of a normal one, which is referred to as a *proto-oncogene.* When retroviruses infect a human cell, they may pick up a proto-oncogene from the host cell. Somehow, the proto-oncogene is activated and becomes an oncogene after incorporation into the retrovirus genome. Normal cells subsequently infected with the oncogenic retrovirus are altered in some fundamental way to become cancer cells.[24]

CLASSIFICATION

Proper classification of the type of leukemia is necessary for clinicians to make educated treatment decisions and extend patient survival. Classification techniques use many cell features, among which are morphology, cytochemistry, and antigen analysis (immuno-chemistry).

Morphology alone is ineffective in identifying the lineage of all types of leukemia. For example, blast cell morphology, in which the cells are large with primitive nuclei, increased nucleoli, and basophilic cytoplasm, may be characteristic of lymphoblasts, myeloblasts, or monoblasts. Studies have demonstrated that many cases of acute leukemia have been improperly categorized by morphology alone and have had to be reclassified after cytochemical profiling. Additionally, batteries of special stains in many cases are negative, with no obvious maturation line or intermediate forms being present. These cases are referred to as *undifferentiated leukemias*.

In recent years, ultrastructural studies, and cytogenetic and immunologic techniques have been developed to help classify acute leukemia. The study of the ultrastructure of cells by electron microscopy makes it possible to identify specific organelles (*e.g.*, granules that cannot be seen with Romanowsky stains). Specific chromosomal abnormalities are associated with the different subgroups of ANLL and have a prognostic significance.[6] Many monoclonal antibodies have been developed that react with myeloid cells; these are used in an attempt to subclassify and to predict prognosis. However, immunotyping has not been as helpful in ANLL as it has in the lymphoid leukemias.

Morphologic Techniques

Categorization of the leukemias classically has been done by assessing the morphology of Romanowsky-stained specimens under light microscopy. This classification is based on the type of normal cell the malignant clone resembles and the stage of maturation of a given cell line. The presence of other abnormal cell types may provide clues to the cell line involved (*e.g.*, pseudo-Pelger-Huët cells would indicate that the affected cell line is granulocytic). The primary distinction to be made when classifying acute leukemias is whether the leukemia is lymphocytic or nonlymphocytic. Romanowsky staining of blasts in acute leukemia reveals certain morphologic characteristics that may be more definitive for one cell type than another. Some of the more important morphologic criteria used to identify blasts are the nuclear:cytoplasmic ratio, the shape of the nuclear outline, the number of nucleoli, and the degree of cytoplasmic maturation. The significance of one specific morphologic abnormality, the Auer rod, is considerable: it defines the leukemia as both acute and nonlymphocytic.

Cytochemical Techniques

Cytochemistry significantly enhances the classification of leukemia. The International Committee for Standardization in Haematology (ICSH) has recommended methods for these cytologic procedures.[23] Five enzymes have been standardized: peroxidase, alkaline phosphatase, acid phosphatase, nonspecific esterase, and chloroacetate esterase. Table 34-1 lists the cytochemical findings seen in the different categories of acute nonlymphocytic leukemia, and Chapter 30 describes the various cytochemical procedures.

TABLE 34–1. Cytochemical Findings in ANLL

| | SUDAN BLACK B AND PEROXIDASE | SPECIFIC ESTERASE (NAPHTHYL AS-D CHLOROACETATE) | NONSPECIFIC ESTERASE | | PAS |
			α-NAPHTHYL ACETATE	α-NAPHTHYL BUTYRATE	
Myelocytic M1, M2, or M3	Pos	Pos	Neg	Neg	–
Myelomonocytic M4	Pos	Pos	Pos	Pos	–
Monocytic M5	Neg or weak scattered positivity	Neg	Pos	Pos	Pos
Erythroleukemia M6	–	–	Pos	Neg	Pos
Megakaryocytic M7	–	–	Pos	Neg	Pos
Unclassified	Neg	Neg	Neg	Neg	–

–, generally not performed.

French-American-British System

In 1976, a group of French, American, and British investigators proposed a classification for the acute leukemias that would have as its basis Romanowsky-stained films of blood and bone marrow.[2] Known as the FAB classification system, its purpose was to provide a uniform method of subgrouping the different acute leukemias based on a standardized system of nomenclature and morphologic criteria. The criteria for subclassification are based on the morphology of the proliferating cells, principally nuclear morphology, as seen in bone marrow and peripheral blood. Cytochemical distinctions are made where appropriate. Table 34-2 lists some of the chief discriminating factors that may be used to subtype the ANLLs. Use of this standardized system has greatly facilitated the correlation of clinical and laboratory findings and responses to treatment between clinical investigators. It is of value principally in evaluating cases before cytotoxic drug treatment, which may alter morphology.

Specific morphologic criteria are based on two factors: the direction of cell line differentiation, and the degree of maturation of the proliferating cells. Seven subclassifications (Table 34-3) of the ANLLs are now recognized with M7, acute megakaryocytic leukemia, having been defined recently, almost 10 years after the original classification system was proposed.[1,4]

There is a great deal of morphologic heterogeneity and overlap between these subgroups. Counting bone marrow cells to determine the percentage of blasts is necessary, because the FAB classification is based on quantitative criteria, where the total number of blasts is compared with either the total of all nucleated cells or the total of nonerythroid cells in the bone marrow.

Basic to the morphologic criteria of this system is the definition of a blast, of which two types are recognized.[3] Type I blasts show no evidence of cytoplasmic differentiation (Fig. 34-1). Cytoplasmic granules are always absent, prominent nucleoli are observed, and the chromatin is stippled with no condensation. The nuclear:cytoplasmic (N:C) ratio of the smaller blasts tends to be higher than in larger ones. Type II blasts are similar to Type I but show some evidence of differentiation (Fig. 34-2). A few azurophilic granules may be observed in the cytoplasm. The nucleus

TABLE 34–2. Discriminating Factors in the Characterization of FAB Subgroups of ANLL

SUBGROUP	CLINICAL FEATURES	CYTOCHEMICAL POSITIVITY	CYTOGENETIC ABNORMALITIES	LABORATORY FINDINGS
M1	–	Sudan black B Peroxidase Naphthol AS-D chloroacetate esterase	–	
M2	–	Same as above	t(8q⁻; 21q⁺)	–
M3	DIC	Same as above	t(15; 17)	Prolonged PT and PTT values; low fibrinogen levels; positive fibrin split products test
M4	Tissue infiltrates; CNS involvement	Sudan black B Peroxidase Naphthol AS-D chloroacetate esterase α-Naphthyl butyrate and acetate esterase	Chromosome 16 (M4e)	Increased lysozyme
M5	Tissue infiltrates; CNS involvement	PAS α-Naphthyl acetate esterase α-Naphthyl butyrate esterase	t(9; 11) (M5a)	Increased lysozyme
M6	–	PAS α-Naphthyl acetate esterase α-Naphthyl acetate esterase	–	Significant peripheral normoblastosis
M7	Myelosclerosis	Acid phosphatase PAS	Chromosome 21	Platelet peroxidase

TABLE 34–3. Principal Morphologic Criteria in FAB Classification of ANLL

| SUBGROUP | CELL LINES | | NUCLEUS | CYTOPLASM |
	ORIGIN	CELL TYPES		
M1	Myelocytic	>30% myeloblasts (Type I and II blasts)	One or more nucleoli; fine stippled chromatin	Few azurophilic granules; Auer rods
M2	Myelocytic	>30% myeloblasts with >10% granulocytic component	One or more nucleoli; fine stippled chromatin	Various amounts; numerous azurophilic granules; Auer rods
M3	Myelocytic	Abnormal promyelocytes predominate	Reniform or bilobed shape	Heavy granulation; bundles of Auer rods (faggots)
M4	Myelocytic Monocytic	>30% blasts >20% granulocytic component >20% promonocytes and monocytes	—	—
M5a	Monocytic	Monoblasts predominate few promonocytes	Lacy chromatin with nucleoli	Basophilic; pseudopods; occasional granules
M5b	Monocytic	Blasts, promonocytes, and monocytes Promonocytes predominate in marrow Monocytes predominate in blood	Cerebriform shape with nucleoli	Grayish, ground-glass appearance; fine azurophilic granules
M6	Erythrocytic Myelocytic	>50% erythroid cells in all stages of maturation >30% myeloblasts	Multiple nuclear lobes Multiple nuclei Nuclear fragments Megaloblastic changes	Nuclear:cytoplasmic asynchrony; PAS positivity; gigantism; vacuolization
M7	Megakaryocytic	Megakaryoblasts predominate	Dense chromatin (lymphoid blasts) OR fine reticulated chromatin with nucleoli	Scant; blebs and vacuoles; platelet shedding

usually is centrally located, and the N:C ratio is lower. Cells are no longer classified as Type II blasts, but rather as promyelocytes, when the following morphologic changes occur: the nucleus becomes eccentric, a well-developed Golgi apparatus is apparant, chromatin has begun to condense, numerous cytoplasmic granules are present, and the N:C ratio diminishes.

M1: Acute Myeloblastic Leukemia Without Maturation
CLINICAL PRESENTATION. Acute myeloblastic leukemia (AML) without maturation is found in all age groups, with the highest incidence seen in adults. There is neither male nor female predominance. The onset may be sudden or insidious, taking months to years for symptoms to become apparent. Symptoms are related to the degree of

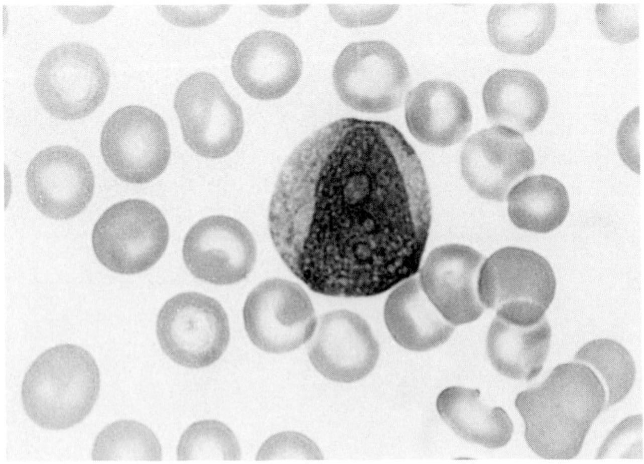

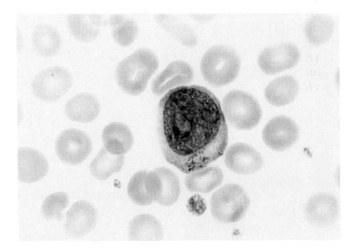

FIG. 34-1. Type I blast. Blood film from patient with M1 acute myelocytic leukemia without maturation. Note fine nuclear chromatin, prominent nucleoli, and absence of cytoplasmic granules (original magnification × 500; Wright stain).

FIG. 34-2. Type II blast. Blood film from patient with M1 acute myelocytic leukemia without maturation. Note fine nuclear chromatin, prominent nucleoli, and azurophilic granules in cytoplasm (original magnification × 500; Wright stain).

TABLE 34–4. Clinical Features of ANLL

	SIGNS AND SYMPTOMS	PATHOPHYSIOLOGY	SUPPORTIVE THERAPY
Anemia	Pallor Lethargy Dyspnea Fatigue Weakness	Bone marrow failure Dyserythropoiesis Decreased RBC survival	Red cell transfusion
Neutropenia	Fever Malaise Infection	Bone marrow failure Dysmyelopoiesis	Granulocyte transfusion Antibiotics Isolation techniques
Thrombocytopenia	Hemorrhage Bruising Purpura Epistaxis Gingival bleeding Menorrhagia	Bone marrow failure Coagulation defects Qualitative platelet abnormalities	Platelet transfusion

Organ infiltration	Bone tenderness
	Splenomegaly
	Hepatomegaly
	Lymphadenopathy
	Gum hypertrophy
	Skin infiltrates
	Ulceration of mucous
	  membranes
	Meningeal syndrome
	  Headache
	  Nausea
	  Vomiting
		Extramedullary
		  hematopoiesis
		Metastatic disease
			Radiotherapy

cytopenia that develops in the various cell lines and commonly include fever, malaise, fatigue, and petechiae (Table 34-4). Organomegaly is variable and may include enlargement of the liver, spleen, or lymph nodes; however, most individuals present with little or no organ involvement.

LABORATORY FINDINGS AND CORRELATIONS WITH DISEASE. Examination of the peripheral blood reveals that granulocytes, red cells, and platelets are reduced in number. The number of circulating blast cells is variable and usually is directly proportional to the total white count. In the early stages of AML, the white count may be normal or low, with few or no blasts in the peripheral blood, although blasts are increased in the bone marrow. The majority of cases present with leukocytosis secondary to high numbers of circulating blasts (Plate 42).

Nuclear:cytoplasmic maturational asynchrony is a common finding in the malignant cell populations. This may be

reflected morphologically (nucleus appears more immature than the cytoplasm) or functionally (*e.g.*, leukemic blasts exhibiting phagocytosis, which is a property of mature cells).

Characteristically, the bone marrow is hypercellular. Numerous morphologic abnormalities are found in all marrow cell lines, as observed by the presence of dysmyelopoietic neutrophil maturation, dyserythropoiesis, and morphologically abnormal megakaryocytes. Table 34-5 lists some of the more common changes.

The FAB categorization of M1 leukemia is based on evidence of granulocytic differentiation in the bone marrow. Blast cells may either be Type I or a combination of Types I and II. Some Type II blasts containing at least a few azurophilic granules, Auer rods, or both may be present. Further granulocytic maturation beyond the blast stage usually is seen in less than 10% of the cells.

The blast count is important, and the total of Type I and

TABLE 34–5. Morphologic Abnormalities Associated with ANLL

DYSMYELOPOIESIS	DYSERYTHROPOIESIS	DYSMEGAKARYOCYTOPOIESIS

Nuclear:cytoplasmic
  asynchrony
Leukemic hiatus
Nuclear abnormalities
Pseudo Pelger-Huët changes
Hypersegmentation
Unusual nuclear projections
Granule abnormalities
  Increased size and number
  Decreased number or absence
  Auer rods
Loss of cellular organelles
Irregular cytoplasmic basophilia
	Gigantism
	Multinuclearity
	Nuclear lobulation
	Nuclear fragments
	Pyknosis
	Megaloblastoid changes
	Cytoplasmic vacuoles
		Giant platelets (megathrombocytes)
		Hypernuclear and hyponuclear lobulation
		Micromegakaryocytes
		Granule abnormalities
		  Giant granules
		  Abnormal granules

II blasts must be at least 30% of the nucleated cells in the marrow. If the blast count is less than 30%, the case would be classified as a myelodysplastic syndrome rather than acute leukemia (Chap. 33).

Cytochemical demonstration of at least 3% Sudan black B- or peroxidase-positive blasts is essential to define the granulocytic nature of M1 acute leukemia. Auer rods will be positive in both reactions. The cytochemical profile for AML also includes positive chloracetate esterase staining and a negative acetate esterase reaction. It should be pointed out that the lack of positivity in normal myeloblasts and the presence of positivity in leukemic blasts is a reflection of the asynchrony between cytoplasmic and nuclear maturation characteristic of leukemic cells.

Laboratory studies for serum lysozyme and neutrophil alkaline phosphatase are generally nondiagnostic, demonstrating a wide range of results among cases. The results of CSF examination usually are negative because CNS involvement is almost never seen in AML.

M2: Acute Myeloblastic Leukemia with Maturation

CLINICAL PRESENTATION.   The presenting symptoms for the M2 form of AML are similar to those of the M1 type. These include manifestations of anemia, infection, and hemorrhagic tendency such as easy bruising, epistaxis, gingival bleeding, and petechiae. Organomegaly and extramedullary masses may also be present.

LABORATORY FINDINGS AND CORRELATIONS WITH DISEASE.   The peripheral blood findings commonly include a reduction in the number of normal blood cells and leukocytosis secondary to circulating blast cells (Plate 43). The bone marrow is hypercellular with the same morphologic abnormalities in all marrow cell lines that are described in M1. Some cases of M2 demonstrate a marked increase in basophils, eosinophils, or both. The M2 FAB subgroup is distinguished from M1 by the presence of granulocytic cells at or beyond the promyelocytic stage of maturation. In the bone marrow, Type I and Type II blasts account for more than 30% of the nucleated cells, with 10% or more additional granulocytic cells at various stages of maturation. Less than 20% of the cells are monocytes.

Leukemic alterations in morphology often are observed in peripheral blood, with the presence of pseudo-Pelger-Huët and hypogranular neutrophils being most common. Pseudo-Pelger-Huët changes are acquired from the leukemic cell line. The nuclei of these cells may appear rod shaped, dumbbell shaped, or round and nonsegmented. The chromatin may be abnormally condensed. It also is common to see mature neutrophils that appear to be devoid of cytoplasmic granules. Acquired myeloperoxidase deficiency can be demonstrated by cytochemical means. Even neutrophils that have granules may lack myeloperoxidase and may be identified incorrectly as monocytes.

Functional abnormalities may be acquired, with blocks at various stages of maturation. As a result, these cells may exhibit deficiencies in phagocytosis, microbial killing, random locomotion, or chemotaxis or in sequential combinations of these functions.

Cytochemically, M2 blast cells have the same profile as in M1 acute leukemia except that a larger percentage of the blast forms will be positive for peroxidase or Sudan black.

Serum lysozyme levels and neutrophil alkaline phosphatase also vary among cases of this type and do not contribute diagnostically.

Certain cytogenetic abnormalities have a relatively high incidence. A characteristic chromosomal translocation, t(8q$^-$;21q$^+$) has been reported in about 10% of cases. This abnormality is associated with low neutrophil alkaline phosphatase levels, a high incidence of cells containing Auer rods, and relatively long survival.

M3: Hypergranular Promyelocytic Leukemia

CLINICAL   PRESENTATION.   The M3 category of ANLL is found in all age groups similar to M1 and M2; however, it appears to have a greater predilection for males. The highest male:female ratios occur in the microgranular variant of M3. Clinical symptoms are similar to those of M1 and M2 acute leukemias except that these leukemias are frequently associated with disseminated intravascular coagulation (DIC), which is ascribed to the thromboplastinlike activity of the primary granules.

LABORATORY FINDINGS AND CORRELATIONS WITH DISEASE.   The majority of cells seen in M3 acute leukemia are abnormal promyelocytes, with heavy granulation filling the cytoplasm and sometimes overlying the nucleus. Indeed, the granules may be so abundant that they obscure the outlines of the nucleus. In contrast, M2 promyelocytes have less granulation, and granules do not obscure the nucleus. Bundles of Auer rods may be seen in the cytoplasm and are referred to as faggots. The nuclei are variable in size and shape, often being reniform or bilobed.

The cytochemical profile of M3 leukemia is similar to that of M1 and M2 except that in this case, most of the abnormal cells are intensely positive. Many of the hypergranular promyelocytes and the faggot-containing cells are disrupted easily during preparation of bone marrow films, resulting in granules and Auer rods lying free between and on top of cells. This film-making artifact must be distinguished from stain precipitate when interpreting cytochemical stain results (Plate 44).

M3m: Microgranular Promyelocytic Leukemia

A microgranular variant of acute promyelocytic leukemia is designated M3m.[11,22] Although clinically similar to M3 morphologically, it is dissimilar in that the cells appear devoid of granules. In fact, numerous granules are present in these promyelocytes but are below the normal resolution of the light microscope and therefore can be detected only by electron microscopy. For this reason, the term "microgranular" is preferable to "hypogranular." By morphology alone, these cases may appear to resemble a monocytic (M4 or M5) subtype. The blast cells are large, with a deeply notched or folded monocytoid nucleus. The cytoplasm is abundant and may appear to be finely dusted with granules that may lie over the folds of the nucleus. Few cells demonstrate prominent azurophilic granules. Auer rods may be observed. It is important to perform a cytochemical profile on these cases and to demonstrate absence of nonspecific esterase positivity so that these cells are properly distinguished from monocytes. Sudan black B, peroxidase, and chloracetate esterase staining should be intensely positive. Clinically, the prognostic outlook for the microgranular variant of M3 is the worst of this subgroup. The condition usually is heralded by initial high blast counts, unlike M3, which is more likely to present with leukopenia.

Cytogenetic studies have revealed a high incidence (almost 50%) of the chromosomal translocation t(15;17) associated with the M3 subgroup,[17] including the microgranular variant. The chromosomal changes in the acute myeloid leukemias are much less definitive than the Ph^1 chromosome found in chronic myelocytic leukemia (Chap. 35). The t(15;17) translocation is a poor prognostic sign. Other translocations have been observed, including t(9;22) and t(8;21).

M4: Acute Myelomonocytic Leukemia

CLINICAL PRESENTATION. Acute myelomonocytic leukemia is also known as Naegeli monocytic leukemia. Its clinical presentation is related to symptoms of progressive cytopenia, including fatigue, bleeding diathesis, fever, and organomegaly. Unlike the M1 to M3 types, this subgroup is associated with soft-tissue infiltrates, including gum hypertrophy and infiltration, rectal ulceration, and skin involvement. Meningeal symptoms also are common in M4 leukemia, with headache, nausea, vomiting, blurring of vision, and sometimes intracranial hemorrhage being manifested.

LABORATORY FINDINGS AND CORRELATIONS WITH DISEASE.   Most of the circulating cells in the peripheral blood are blasts and abnormal cells. Some of the highest white counts to occur in the ANLLs are seen in M4. Both granulocytic and monocytic differentiation is observed in the peripheral blood and bone marrow.

Several morphologic criteria are required for categorization as an M4. In the bone marrow, more than 30% of the nonerythroid cells must be blasts. The sum of myeloblasts, promyelocytes, and other maturing granulocytic forms is more than 30% but less than 80% of the nonerythroid cells. More than 20% of nonerythroid cells are of monocytic lineage in different stages of maturation. If the monocytic compartment exceeds 80% of the nonerythroid cells, the disease is classified as M5. More than 20% of peripheral blood white cells are monocytes or monocytic precursors (Plate 45).

Confirmation of the monocytic component of this subgroup requires cytochemistry. The profile includes positive reactions for Sudan black B or peroxidase and both specific and nonspecific esterase. Lysozyme, also known as muramidase, is a low molecular-weight enzyme found in neutrophils and monocytes. Monocytes contain larger amounts. Fifty percent of patients with M4 leukemia will excrete large amounts of lysozyme in their urine. Demonstration of serum or urine lysozyme is diagnostically important in M4 for the recognition of the monocytic component of these cells. Levels three times the upper limit of normal are considered significant.

A few cases of M4 leukemia are characterized by increased marrow eosinophils. Sometimes, these cells exhibit large basophilic granules mixed with the smaller eosinophilic granules. Nuclei may be single-lobed and unsegmented, similar to pseudo-Pelger-Huët changes. In contrast to normal eosinophils, these cells exhibit distinct chloroacetate esterase and PAS positivity. These leukemias are classified as M4e, which is associated with a deletion or inversion of the long arm of chromosome 16 and longer mean survival.

M5: Acute Monocytic Leukemia

CLINICAL PRESENTATION. Acute monocytic leukemia, also referred to as Schilling leukemia, is clinically similar to M4; however, the highest incidence of organ involvement is found in this subgroup. Extramedullary tissue masses and CNS involvement are characteristic. The etiology of these symptoms is related to the monocytic component. This leukemia is divided into two categories: M5a, poorly differentiated monocytic leukemia; and M5b, well differentiated monocytic leukemia. The M5b type differs from M5a clinically in that it is associated with a diffuse erythematous skin rash.

LABORATORY FINDINGS AND CORRELATIONS WITH DISEASE.   Morphologically, M5a is characterized in both blood and bone marrow by large blast cells with delicate, lacy chromatin (Plate 46A). One to three large, prominent vesicular nucleoli also are present. The cytoplasm of these cells is voluminous, and often, one or more pseudopods of basophilic cytoplasm are seen. Azurophilic granulation is rare. Some monocytes are found, along with a small percentage of promonocytes.

The M5b type is characterized by the presence of all stages of monocyte development: monoblasts, promonocytes, and monocytes (Plate 46B). The percentage of monocytes is usually higher in the peripheral blood than in the bone marrow, where the predominant cell is the promonocyte. Typical promonocytes have cerebriform nuclei with nucleoli. Their cytoplasm is less basophilic than that of monoblasts and has a grayish ground-glass appearance with fine azurophilic granules.

Normal bone marrow elements in both types of M5 leukemia are replaced by leukemic cells. Less than 10% of the nonerythroid cells are granulocytes, and greater than 80% are monoblasts, promonocytes, or monocytes. In M5a, more than 80% of the monocytic compartment is blasts, whereas in M5b, less than 80% of the monocytic cells are blasts. A few cells may contain Auer rods, but this finding is much less common than it is in other forms of ANLL. Cytochemically, these cells generally are negative for Sudan black B or peroxidase and specific esterase but are strongly positive for nonspecific esterase. Some cells may demonstrate weak scattered Sudan black B or peroxidase activity. The reactivity of these cells for nonspecific esterase will be inhibited by sodium fluoride.

Much as in M4, testing for serum and urine lysozyme reveals very high levels because of the monocytic component of this leukemia. Cytogenetic abnormalities are relatively nonspecific in M5 leukemia, with rearrangements involving chromosome 11, t(9;11) being the most common.

M6: Acute Erythroleukemia

CLINICAL PRESENTATION.   Erythroleukemia was first described by DiGuglielmo in 1917. The term erythroleukemia is used when there is a prominent percentage of both neoplastic myeloblasts and erythroblasts. Because of the overlapping morphologic characteristics, it is imperative to distinguish these cases from refractory anemia with excess blasts (RAEB), which is described in Chapter 33.

The clinical features of this subgroup are similar to those of the other categories of ANLL and may include fever, infection, purpura, and hemorrhage.

LABORATORY FINDINGS AND CORRELATIONS WITH DISEASE. Peripheral blood findings include a variable white count, pancytopenia, and most notably, numerous nucleated red blood cells (NRBCs). The presence of NRBCs in the circulation is accompanied by a wide variety of changes in red cell morphology, including anisocytosis, poikilocytosis, macrocytes, oval macrocytes, schistocytes, or mixed populations of hypochromic and normochromic red cells. None of these changes is specific in itself, but together, they are an indication of dyserythropoietic changes in the bone marrow.

The erythrocytic compartment of an M6 leukemia exceeds 50% of the nucleated cells in the bone marrow. The erythroid cells exhibit various degrees of bizarre morphology, including multiple lobulation of the nucleus with variation in lobe size, multiple nuclei, nuclear fragments, gigantism, vacuolization, and megaloblastoid features (Plates 47A and B). These findings are referred to as "dyserythropoietic changes." Additionally, greater than 30% of the nonerythroid cells in the bone marrow must be Type I or Type II blasts. These blasts may contain Auer rods. An M6 leukemia frequently progresses to M1, M2, or M4 leukemia.

The red cells in erythroleukemia are cytochemically unusual in that they often demonstrate PAS positivity. This positivity is the result of staining of glycogen and is localized in the cytoplasmic vacuoles of the erythroblasts. As the cells mature, they become richer in glycogen, and the pattern of positivity becomes diffuse rather than localized. Although this reaction is nondiagnostic, it is important to note that most other disorders with megaloblastoid maturation do not demonstrate this pattern of PAS positivity (*i.e.*, a change from granular to diffuse during maturation). The M6 erythroblasts also demonstrate positivity when stained for alpha-naphthyl acetate esterase.

M7: Acute Megakaryocytic Leukemia

Megakaryoblasts are nearly impossible to recognize by conventional light microscopy techniques. Early reports in the literature describing megakaryocytic leukemia were cases in which there was morphologically recognizable megakaryocytic differentiation. Because ultrastructural staining techniques and surface marker studies have only recently been developed for the recognition of this cell type, M7 was late in being described in the FAB classification system.

CLINICAL PRESENTATION. The symptoms are similar to those of the other subgroups, among which are fatigue, general malaise, fever, and bleeding tendencies.

LABORATORY FINDINGS AND CORRELATIONS WITH DISEASE. The blast cells of M7 were classified as undifferentiated by previous FAB criteria because of the cytochemical negativity for Sudan black B, peroxidase, and esterase. Blast cells in some cases are small and round with scanty cytoplasm and nuclear chromatin that is dense and heavy, giving the cells a lymphoid appearance. Megakaryocytes in other cases have an undifferentiated appearance, with nuclei that are round with finely reticulated chromatin and one to three prominent nucleoli. There may or may not be granules in the cytoplasm. There is marked heterogeneity in blast cell size, and some of the blasts can be two to three times the size of normal lymphocytes. Some blasts have cytoplasmic blebs or vacuolization (Plate 48B). According to the FAB criteria, some cells may appear as small differentiated megakaryocytes (micromegakaryocytes) with platelets shedding from the cytoplasm (Plate 48A). Others may be seen as naked nuclei with groups of platelets surrounding them. Abnormal giant platelets are a prominent finding in the peripheral blood, and platelet counts may be normal or increased. Examination of the bone marrow frequently reveals diffuse reticulin myelofibrosis with aggregates of megakaryocytes localized among sheets of blasts or fibroblasts.[12]

Previously, megakaryoblastic leukemia was largely underrecognized. Today, its identification is facilitated by cytochemical and immunologic techniques. Platelet peroxidase (PPO) is an enzyme synthesized early during megakaryocyte maturation.[5] Distinct from myeloperoxidase, PPO is recognized as a specific marker for cells of megakaryocytic origin. Ultrastructural staining for PPO reveals that this enzyme is localized in the nuclear envelope and endoplasmic reticulum but not in the Golgi apparatus or granules of megakaryocytes. This is unlike myeloperoxidase, which is found in the endoplasmic reticulum, Golgi apparatus, and granules of other cell types.

Cytochemical positivity for the alpha-naphthyl acetate esterase reaction with a negative reaction with alpha-naphthyl butyrate esterase is unique to megakaryoblasts.[14] Monocytes react positively with both esterase substrates. Acid phosphatase is another cytochemical marker for megakaryoblasts. Diffuse strong positivity is readily seen in the immature stages of this cell line. However, this pattern is common in other types of acute leukemia also. Cells from acute T-cell ALL demonstrate focal areas of paranuclear acid phosphatase activity; therefore, the acid phosphatase reaction cannot be used as a diagnostic marker for megakaryoblasts. Megakaryocytes are rich in glycogen and will stain intensely with PAS. This reactivity is principally confined to differentiated megakaryocytes, with megakaryoblasts being negative. The strongest PAS reactions will be observed in cells displaying cytoplasmic budding. The associated platelets also are brightly PAS positive. Finally, some megakaryoblasts may be identified on the basis of their surface glycoproteins IIa and IIIb using immunologic techniques. See Chapter 30 for further discussion.

ANLL Not Included in FAB Classification

Several types of ANLL are not included in the FAB classification scheme. These include: (1) the ANLLs characterized by primitive blast cells, which are unclassifiable morphologically and are negative for all cytochemical stains. These types are referred to as "undifferentiated leukemias" and are sometimes given the designation M0; (2) acute mast cell or acute basophilic leukemias which are rare disorders in which the cells can be confused with abnormal progranulocytes; (3) hypoplastic acute myeloid leukemia;[18] (4) mixed leukemias, which demonstrate a combination of lymphoid and myeloid characteristics; and (5) secondary leukemias that have evolved from myelodysplastic syndromes. These types may be atypical and difficult to fit into the FAB classification format.

TREATMENT

General Considerations

The ultimate goal in treating ANLL is to return the bone marrow to its normal state of health and function and to achieve disease-free survival for the patient. Certain factors play an important role in determining how successful therapy will be, specifically the age and pretreatment status. The younger the patient, and the less symptomatic he or she is before treatment, the greater the chance of a significant response. The presence of infection at the time of treatment can reduce the chance of achieving remission by as much as 50%. Although the specific subtype of ANLL is not a significant prognostic factor, both patients with M3 disease who have DIC and those with M5 disease with increased likelihood of extramedullary relapse have a somewhat poorer prognosis. Other negative prognostic indicators are an abnormal karyotype at diagnosis and a history of radiation or chemotherapy.

The principal treatment modalities for ANLL are chemotherapy to induce clinical remission, radiation therapy to control leukemic infiltrates, immunotherapy to bolster the patient's immune response to the leukemia, and bone marrow transplantation. A decision to treat is made when one or more of the following conditions occurs: (1) progressive neutropenia with peripheral neutrophil counts falling to 0.5 to 1.0×10^9/L; (2) progressive thrombocytopenia with platelet counts falling to less than 50×10^9/L; or (3) the leukemic population in the bone marrow accounting for 50% or more of the total cellularity. If hyperleukocytosis (WBC values exceeding 100×10^9/L) is present at the time of diagnosis, an assessment of the risk of leukostasis must be made. Leukostasis is a pathologic condition in which thin-walled blood vessels are dilated with leukemic cells. Headache, visual problems, and dyspnea are the symptoms. To prevent intracranial bleeding and to minimize pulmonary leukostasis, therapeutic leukapheresis can be used to lower the white cell count rapidly. Leukapheresis also will minimize the risk of renal failure secondary to hyperuricemia.

Chemotherapy

The different subtypes of ANLL are treated similarly with the exception of DIC in acute progranulocytic leukemia. Standard treatment programs for ANLL utilize a combination of drugs with different mechanisms of action and dose-limiting toxicities to achieve the highest remission rates. The two most commonly used cytotoxic agents are cytosine arabinoside (ara-C) and daunorubicin. When used together, they can produce at least a 65% remission rate.[15] Amsacrine (m-AMSA) is an effective single drug in patients with resistant AML. Table 34-6 lists the mechanisms of action and toxicities of the common chemotherapeutic drugs.

Administration of chemotherapy is intravenous, usually through right-atrial catheters (e.g., Hickman), which have been placed surgically for permanent venous access.[19] Provided no complications develop, such catheters remain in place until induction and consolidation therapy (see below) are completed. They facilitate not only the giving of chemotherapy, but also the administration of blood products, fluids, and antibiotics. They can also be used to collect daily blood samples, eliminating the need for repeated venipuncture.

The therapeutic strategy for treating ANLL includes three stages: induction of complete remission (CR), consolidation, and maintenance of remission. Complete remission is achieved when bone marrow cellularity returns to normal with less than 5% blasts present. Anything less than a CR is associated with shorter survival and no possibility of a cure. Approximately 20% of patients in whom complete remission is achieved after first treatment will not relapse.[7] Failure to achieve remission can reflect resistant leukemias or marrow hypoplasia so severe that it fails to regenerate. Patients may die from infection or hemorrhage secondary to the effects of chemotherapy prior to achieving a complete remission. If leukemic infiltrates persist in extramedullary sites, even though the bone marrow has returned to normal, complete remission is not achieved.

Shortly after remission is achieved, therapeutic doses of chemotherapy are given to prevent the recurrence of leukemia (consolidation). The same cytotoxic drugs used to achieve the complete remission usually are given during the consolidation phase. Intensification treatment using non-cross-resistant drugs may be given over a longer period after consolidation. Both of these periods of chemotherapy may be more properly called *post-remission therapy*.

Treatment of ANLL requires hospitalization both to

TABLE 34-6. Common Chemotherapeutic Agents Used in the Treatment of ANLL

DRUG	MODE OF ACTION	TOXIC EFFECT
Cytosine arabinoside (ara-C)	Pyrimidine antimetabolite; a cytosine analogue that inhibits DNA synthesis	Myelosuppression; gastrointestinal epithelial injury causing nausea, vomiting, diarrhea, and oral mucositis
Daunorubicin (DNR)	Anthracycline antibiotic; binds to DNA and interferes with mitosis and inhibits DNA and RNA synthesis	Myelosuppression; alopecia; cardiac toxicity; nausea and vomiting
Amsacrine (m-AMSA)	DNA interaction	Myelosuppression; cardiac toxicity

manage the potential toxic drug effects such as nausea and vomiting and primarily, because of the clinical effects of the profound induced myelosuppression. Post-therapeutic susceptibility to infection and bleeding necessitates reverse isolation techniques, intravenous antibiotics, and transfusion support until the marrow recovers. Post-treatment peripheral white counts usually fall to less than 0.5×10^9/L and may be as low as 0.1×10^9/L. Platelet values usually will be less than 20×10^9/L. Characteristically, the differential white count reflects the severe neutropenia and relative lymphocytosis. Residual blast cells may demonstrate morphologic changes attributable to chemotherapy that may make them difficult to recognize. The cytotoxic therapy used in ANLL produces striking megaloblastic changes because of drug interference with DNA synthesis.[9] Additionally, toxic granulation, increased nuclear projections, and hyposegmented nuclei may be seen in the neutrophils. Monocytes and lymphocytes demonstrate reactive changes, with lymphocytes appearing to have plasmacytoid features, and monocytes demonstrating increased cytoplasm, increased granules, and vacuolization. Red cell morphology is variable. Spherocytes reflect transfused blood. Polychromasia will increase as red cell production returns to normal in the marrow, and some oval macrocytes may be seen because of the megaloblastoid effect of the antimetabolite therapy. Ineffective erythropoiesis also is evident as coarse basophilic stippling.

Examination of the bone marrow after therapy reveals aplasia with a relative increase in plasma cells, lymphocytes, and histiocytes. As the marrow begins to regenerate a few weeks after therapy, an abundance of myeloblasts and promyelocytes is observed that may be confused with a return of leukemia. Red cells in all stages of development may be seen and frequently demonstrate megaloblastoid changes. Myeloid and megakaryocytic morphology is largely normal but may be characterized by megaloblastoid changes.

Treatment of Effects of Cytopenias

The clinical effects of the cytopenias that develop as a consequence of either the crowding out of normal blood cells in the marrow by the leukemic clone or by the reduction of normal numbers of granulocytes, red cells, or platelets as a consequence of chemotherapy, require proper management to prevent early death. Transfusions of packed red cells, platelet concentrates, or granulocytes commonly are given. Heparin may be effective in managing bleeding secondary to DIC, antibiotics may be given to attempt prevention of infection, and allopurinol may be necessary to prevent urate nephropathy.[16]

Radiotherapy

Meningeal leukemia occurs in a small percentage of patients with ANLL, particularly those having an M4 or M5 subgroup and presenting with a total white count greater than 100×10^9/L. Because systemic chemotherapy cannot cross the blood–brain barrier, radiation or intrathecal chemotherapy is given. Although meningeal leukemia is less frequently associated with ANLL than with ALL, it must be treated effectively to prolong patient survival. The presence of blast cells in the CSF is diagnostic. Treatment usually involves a combination of cranial radiation and intrathecal chemotherapy. Radiotherapy also is given when there is evidence of local tumor masses (chloromas) in other body sites.

Immunotherapy

Immunotherapy has been used in both attempts to increase the patient's own immunity to the leukemic cells specifically or to increase the patient's immunity nonspecifically to provide an antileukemic effect. Several agents have been used, including BCG (a bacterium formerly used to immunize against tuberculosis) and irradiated leukemic cells. Currently, the evidence for the efficacy of immunotherapy is inconclusive.[8]

Bone Marrow Transplantation

The mechanism by which marrow transplantation provides an effective defense against leukemia is not well understood. To prepare for transplantation, total-body irradiation of 1000 rads and intensive cyclophosphamide therapy are given to destroy any residual leukemic cells. Candidates for transplantation must be in good clinical condition and in the first clinical remission for the greatest chance of success. Age also is important, with higher survival rates in younger (<30 years) patients.

The most serious complication of bone marrow transplantation is graft versus host disease (GVHD), in which the T lymphocytes of the donor marrow destroy the lymphohemopoietic cells of the recipient. The better the human leukocyte antigen (HLA) match, the less the likelihood of significant GVHD. Autologous transplantation is an attractive alternative to allogeneic transplant for this reason. Bone marrow is harvested during remission and treated with various agents to purge it of residual leukemic cells. However, it is difficult to be assured that all leukemic stem cells have been removed or killed; thus, autologous transplantation carries a risk of inducing a leukemic relapse.

Peripheral blood stem cell transplantation may also be used to reestablish hematopoiesis. The donor material is prepared by cytopheresis. This technique may be used when marrow cannot be harvested easily or when attempting to reduce the contamination of stem cell harvest by tumor cells.

In allogeneic transplants, some form of immunosuppression is necessary to minimize the development of GVHD. Some of the more common immunosuppressive agents are methotrexate, a combination of methotrexate and prednisone, or cyclophosphamide and cyclosporin. Until hematopoietic regeneration occurs, transplant recipient patients must be clinically supported to manage the complications associated with panhypoplasia and immunosuppression.

Differentiation Treatment

One of the newest concepts in the treatment of ANLL is that of manipulating the maturation and differentiation of leukemic cells rather than killing them.[13,20,21] Leukemic cells are thought to be blocked at an early stage of development and unable to mature to fully functional end-cells.

Chemically inducing their maturation and differentiation may be an important new modality that might not carry with it the toxic effects of current therapeutic strategies. Differentiation treatments now being studied include retinoic acid, phorbol esters, and dimethylsulfoxide (DMSO). At this time, only retinoic acid can be used in humans.

Despite current advances, 25% of patients treated for ANLL will die from complications within the first 12 to 18 months. There is about a 60% long-term survival rate for AML patients who have undergone transplantation during the first clinical remission and approximately a 30% long-term survival rate for those patients who have achieved a second remission.

CHAPTER SUMMARY

Acute nonlymphocytic leukemia (ANLL) is a progressive malignant disease of hematopoietic tissue. Although the etiology of leukemia is unclear, it may be the outcome of the interaction of several factors, among which are radiation, chemicals, genetics, and viruses. This group of leukemias has been identified and subtyped on the basis of cell morphology as seen on Romanowsky-stained films of blood and bone marrow. New classification techniques such as cytogenetic, cytochemical, immunologic, and ultrastructural studies are now being employed to aid in diagnosis.

The French-American-British classification scheme is an important method of categorizing acute leukemia that has as its basis standardized nomenclature and morphologic criteria. This system has greatly facilitated the uniform reporting and identification of these leukemias among clinical investigators. Using FAB criteria, the acute nonlymphocytic leukemias can be divided into seven distinct subgroups. These subtypes generally have similar clinical manifestations related primarily to the degree to which the numbers of normal blood cell elements are reduced.

Different subtypes of ANLL are treated similarly. The principal treatment modalities are chemotherapy, radiation, immunotherapy, and bone marrow transplantation. Various prognostic factors such as age and pretreatment status are important in determining the rate of therapeutic success. Managing the clinical effects of the profound myelosuppression is necessary after chemotherapy. The prognostic outlook for patients with ANLL is improving.

CASE STUDY 34-1

The patient is a 59-year-old white woman admitted for evaluation of a painful, swollen right lower extremity and marked leukocytosis. Physical examination data included distended abdomen and splenomegaly 3 to 4 finger breadths below the left costal margin. The entire right lower extremity was markedly swollen with tense edema and the leg was warm and tender to palpitation. There was no lymphadenopathy. Admission laboratory data included: Hb 7.4 g/dL; HCT, 0.22 L/L; WBC, 5.0×10^9/L; Reticulocyte count, 0.1%; differential, segmented neutrophils, 6%, lymphocytes, 16%; monocytes, 13%; promonocytes, 25%; monoblasts, 40%. Red cells were hypochromic and microcytic. Platelet count was 19×10^9/L. Bone marrow aspiration and biopsy were obtained with some difficulty. Sheets of abnormal cells resembling large primitive monocytoid cells with abundant light blue cytoplasm filled the marrow. The nuclei were spongy in appearance, contained one to three large vesicular nucleoli, and were consistently irregular in shape. Erythroid and normal myeloid elements were greatly decreased. Serum lysozyme levels were markedly increased.

1. Based on the above description and laboratory results, into what FAB classification would this patient's leukemia most likely fall?
2. What cytochemical determination would most likely be positive in the abnormal cells within this patient's blood and bone marrow?
3. The patient was treated with a course of cytosine arabinoside and achieved a remission. A subsequent bone marrow revealed red cell precursors with megaloblastoid morphology. What is causing the red cell precursor morphology?

REFERENCES

1. Bennett JM, Catovsky D, Daniel MT et al: Criteria for the diagnosis of acute leukemia of megakaryocytic lineage (M7). Ann Intern Med 103:460, 1985
2. Bennett JM, Catovsky D, Daniel MT et al: Proposals for the classification of the acute leukaemias: French-American-British Cooperative Group. Br J Haematol 33:451, 1976
3. Bennett JM, Catovsky D, Daniel MT et al: Proposals for the classification of the myelodysplastic syndromes. Br J Haematol 51:189, 1982
4. Bennett JM, Catovsky D, Daniel MT et al: Proposed revised criteria for the classification of acute myeloid leukemia. Ann Intern Med 103:626, 1985
5. Breton-Gorius J, Reyes F, Duhamel G et al: Megakaryoblastic acute leukemia: Identification by the ultrastructural demonstration of platelet peroxidase. Blood 51:45, 1978
6. Cork A: Chromosomal abnormalities in leukemia. Am J Med Technol 49:703, 1983
7. Coltman CA, Freireich EJ, Savage RA et al: Long term survival of adults with acute leukemia (abstract). Proc Am Soc Clin Oncol 21:389, 1979
8. Foon KA, Smalley RV, Riggs CW et al: The role of immunotherapy in acute myelogenous leukemia. Arch Intern Med 143:1726, 1983
9. Foucar K, Vaughan WP, Armitage JO et al: Postleukemic dysmyelopoiesis. Am J Hematol 15:321, 1983
10. Fraumeni JF Jr, Miller RW: Epidemiology of human leukemia: Recent observations. J Natl Cancer Inst 38:593, 1967
11. Golomb HM, Rowley JD, Vardiman JW et al: "Microgranular" acute promyelocytic leukemia: A distinct clinical, ultrastructural, and cytogenetic entity. Blood 55:253, 1980
12. Huang MJ, Li CY, Nichols WL et al: Acute leukemia with megakaryocytic differentiation: A study of 12 cases identified immunocytochemically. Blood 64:427, 1984
13. Koeffler P: Induction of differentiation of human acute myelogenous leukemia cells: Therapeutic implications. Blood 62:709, 1983
14. Koike T: Megakaryoblastic leukemia: The characterization and identification of megakaryoblasts. Blood 64:683, 1984
15. Lewis JP, Meyers FJ, Tanaka L: Daunomycin administered by continuous intravenous infusion is effective in the treatment of acute non-lymphocytic leukaemia. Br J Haematol 61:261, 1985
16. Lokich JJ: Managing chemotherapy-induced bone marrow suppression in cancer. Hosp Practice 11(8):61, 1976
17. Misawa S, Lee E, Schiffer CA et al: Association of the translocation (15;17) with malignant proliferation of promyelocytes in acute leukemia and chronic myelogenous leukemia at blastic crisis. Blood 67:270, 1986
18. Needleman SW, Burns CP, Dick FR et al: Hypoplastic acute leukemia. Cancer 48:1410, 1981
19. Reed WP, Newman KA, de Jongh C et al: Prolonged venous access for chemotherapy by means of the Hickman catheter. Cancer 52:185, 1983
20. Ross DW: Leukemic cell maturation. Arch Pathol Lab Med 109:309, 1985

21. Sachs L: Growth, differentiation and the reversal of malignancy. Sci Am 254:40, 1986

22. Savage RA, Hoffman GC, Lucas FV: Morphology and cytochemistry of "microgranular" acute promyelocytic leukemia (FAB M3m). Am J Clin Pathol 75:548, 1981

23. Shibata A, Bennett JM, Castoldi GL et al: Recommended methods for cytological procedures in haematology. Clin Lab Haematol 7:55, 1985

24. Weinberg RA: A molecular basis of cancer. Sci Am 249:126, 1983

RECOMMENDED READING

Bloomfield CD (ed): Chronic and Acute Leukemias in Adults. Boston, Martinus Nijhoff, 1985

Goldman JM, Preisler HD (eds): Hematology 1: Leukemias. London, Butterworths, 1984

Thiel E, Thierfelder S (eds): Leukemia: Recent Developments in Diagnosis and Therapy. Berlin, Springer-Verlag, 1984

Wiernik PH, Canellos CP, Kyle RA, Schiffer CA (eds):Neoplastic Diseases of the Blood, vol 1. New York, Churchill Livingstone, 1985

Chronic Myeloproliferative Disorders

Irma T. Pereira

The myeloproliferative disorders (MPDs) were identified in 1951 by Dameshek[19] as a unified group of independent yet similar conditions that previously had been classified as separate entities. The disorders are polycythemia vera (PV), chronic myelogenous leukemia (CML), agnogenic myeloid metaplasia (AMM), and essential thrombocythemia (ET). Chronic neutrophilic leukemia, a rare disorder, has recently been added to the group. One could speculate that the MPDs are all the same disease, each with a slightly different manifestation. The MPDs could be compared to identical quintuplets: all have the same parent (hematopoietic stem cell) and they look alike, but each has its own individuality.

This chapter seeks to explain the integral and sometimes confusing relations of the MPDs as well as to point out the exceptions to these generalizations. Although classic descriptions will be presented, it must be remembered that the MPDs can vary dramatically; and coexistence with or transformation to other MPDs or even lymphoid diseases can take place at any time during their course.

The majority of MPD cases may be diagnosed readily from the peripheral blood film. However, additional procedures usually are necessary to confirm the diagnosis or determine the prognosis.

GENERAL CONSIDERATIONS

Chronic MPDs usually are found in patients in their fifth and sixth decades. The abnormal proliferation of cells associated with the MPDs is not attributable to a normal hematopoietic response such as granulocyte production and release as a response to infection. Rather, the MPDs are considered to be clonal abnormalities (*i.e.*, they begin in a single abnormal cell). The abnormality probably arises in a pluripotential stem cell, because in most cases, more than one line of myeloid cells is involved.

The best evidence of MPD clonality comes from studies of women who are heterozygous for the G6PD enzyme, producing both isoenzymes A and B.[30] The gene for G6PD is carried only on the X chromosome; thus, G6PD is a sex-linked trait (Chap. 17). The female genotype for the G6PD isoenzymes may be homozygous ($X^A X^A$ or $X^B X^B$) or heterozygous ($X^A X^B$). According to the Lyon hypothesis (Chap. 5), one X chromosome in each cell is inactivated, and all progeny of that cell retain that inactivation. Therefore, in G6PD-heterozygous women, although each cell makes only one isoenzyme, any tissue, including hematopoietic tissue, will produce a mixture—some cells will produce isoenzyme A and others, isoenzyme B. However, when a hematopoietic neoplastic disease is present in a G6PD-heterozygous woman, all of the patient's hematopoietic cells produce only one isoenzyme. Meanwhile, the cells of other tissues continue to be mixed, some producing isoenzyme A and others, isoenzyme B. This finding has led to the conclusion that all the neoplastic cells come from a single cell, and that the MPDs have a clonal origin.

Cells involved in the MPDs include mature and immature granulocytes, erythrocytes, and platelets. Common clinical features are splenomegaly; mild to marked leukocytosis, thrombocytosis, and/or erythrocytosis; and various degrees of marrow fibrosis that are considered by some investigators to be a secondary feature resulting from increased numbers of abnormal megakaryocytes and platelets.[14,46,56] See Table 35-1 for the pathogenicity of the chronic MPDs.

All of the MPDs have strong interrelations, as demonstrated by the frequent transformations between them (Fig.

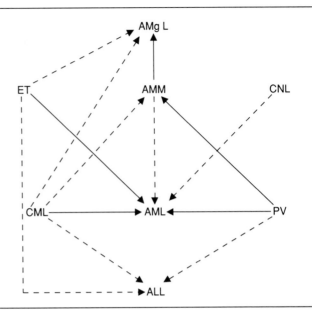

FIG. 35-1. Transitions in chronic myeloproliferative disorders. CML = chronic myelogenous leukemia; AMM = agnogenic myeloid metaplasia; ET = essential thrombocythemia; PV = polycythemia vera; CNL = chronic neutrophilic leukemia; AML = acute myelogenous leukemia; ALL = acute lymphoblastic leukemia; AMgL = acute megakaryocytic leukemia; solid arrow, frequent; dashed arrow, infrequent.

35-1). In addition, many MPDs terminate in acute myelogenous leukemia (AML) (blast transformation; Chap. 34). A small percentage of cases terminate in acute lymphoblastic leukemia (ALL) (Chap. 36).

POLYCYTHEMIA VERA

Polycythemia vera (*vera* is a Latin term meaning "true") is a chronic MPD characterized by panmyelosis (increase in all cellular bone marrow elements) and specifically by increased red cell mass (RCM) caused by a clonal stem cell

TABLE 35–1. Pathogenicity of Myeloproliferative Diseases

DISORDER	AGE (YEARS)	SEX	Ph[1] CHROMOSOME	MAIN CELL TYPE AFFECTED	SURVIVAL (YEARS)	MAIN CAUSE OF DEATH
CML	>30	M>F	+	Granulocytes	2–5	Blast transformation; hemorrhage; infection
PV	>50	M>F	−	Erythrocytes	~10–15	Thrombosis or hemorrhage; PPMM; blast transformation
AMM	>50	M=F	−	Fibroblasts	~5	Marrow failure; blast transformation; hemorrhage or thrombosis; heart, hepatic, or kidney failure; infection
ET	>50	M=F	−	Platelets	~1–5	Hemorrhage or thrombosis; blast transformation
CNL	?★	?★	−	Neutrophils	<4	Blast transformation; hemorrhage; infection

★ Not fully established; only 17 patients reported.

disorder. The condition also is known as "primary polycythemia." In polycythemia vera, erythrocyte counts are increased to greater than $5.9 \times 10^{12}/L$ in women and $6.6 \times 10^{12}/L$ in men. A true increase in the RCM and the plasma volume is characteristic. A mild granulocytic leukocytosis and a considerable thrombocytosis also occur frequently.

Other conditions may cause either a relative or an absolute (secondary) RCM increase and must be ruled out prior to diagnosing a condition as PV (Chap. 10). Relative polycythemia is associated with an elevated HCT secondary to decreased plasma volume rather than an increased RCM. Secondary polycythemia is an increase in RCM that is associated with some identifiable cause.

If the cause for an erythrocytosis cannot be found, a stem cell-related disorder is usually suspected[1] and may be tentatively diagnosed as PV (see Differential Diagnosis section).

Clinical Presentation

Symptoms

Patients commonly complain of various combinations of headaches, vertigo, ringing in the ears, blurred vision, itching eyes, upper gastrointestinal pain (sometimes secondary to peptic ulcers), a feeling of fullness after eating small amounts (probably because of splenomegaly), and red itchy skin (pruritus), especially after a hot bath. Thrombotic events, either venous or arterial, are common.[18]

Physical Findings

Most patients are between 50 and 60 years of age; however, the condition has been seen in all age groups. The mucous membranes and skin have a ruddy cyanotic (reddish purple) appearance. Hypertension occurs frequently. Hepatomegaly and, more often, splenomegaly, usually secondary to extramedullary hematopoiesis (cell formation outside the marrow), are common findings. Gout is also common because of the high uric acid levels caused by rapid cell turnover.[6]

Laboratory Findings

Peripheral Blood

The most obvious finding in the peripheral blood is an extremely high erythrocyte count, which may reach $10 \times 10^{12}/L$. This leads to increased Hb levels (males greater than 17.5 g/dL; females greater than 15.5 g/dL) and HCTs (males greater than 0.55 L/L; females greater than 0.47 L/L). The MCV and MCHC values are often low normal to slightly reduced because of the decreased or absent iron stores in the marrow as a result of chronic bleeding and phlebotomy and increased red blood cell production and turnover. An occasional normoblast (NRBC) may be found. The reticulocyte count generally is not significantly increased. The leukocyte alkaline phosphatase (LAP) score usually is increased.

Because panmyelosis is one of the distinguishing features of PV, the increase in RCM is only one element of this complex disorder. The patients also classically exhibit a granulocytic leukocytosis and thrombocytosis. Indeed, this is so often the case that the absence of an increase in these components should alert the physician to the likelihood of a condition other than PV.[71] Leukocyte counts can go as high

as 40 or $50 \times 10^9/L$. Granulocytic leukocytosis is most common, but occasionally, a slight left shift with a few metamyelocytes is seen. Basophil numbers frequently are elevated, and platelet counts can be as high as $2000 \times 10^9/L$. A moderate number of abnormal platelet forms may be present. Abnormal platelet aggregation and adhesiveness, as well as decreased levels of platelet factor 3 (PF3),[38] frequently are seen. It often is difficult to prepare a good peripheral blood film because of the increased blood viscosity. Even in the feather edge, the film appears crowded. To make a better film, equal parts of the blood specimen and normal saline may be mixed in a small test tube to reduce blood viscosity. There is no sign of marrow fibrosis in the peripheral blood early in the disease and usually little if any at the time of diagnosis.

Bone Marrow

The marrow is hypercellular with the fat spaces almost completely replaced by blood cells. Obvious features are increased megakaryocyte and normoblast numbers. Many megakaryocytes are large and abnormal in appearance. Basophils usually are increased, resulting in elevated levels of blood histamine, the probable cause of the itching that follows hot baths. Little, if any, fibrosis may be seen early in PV. However, marrow fibrosis tends to worsen as the disease progresses, possibly through the action of a number of factors, including megakaryocytic alpha granules releasing platelet-derived growth factor.[14,78,81] Iron is decreased or absent.[59,64]

Chemistry

Normal to elevated levels of serum B_{12}, increased B_{12} binding capacity, and decreased serum iron and ferritin levels are present. Serum erythropoietin levels are decreased or normal in spite of the high RCM.

Differential Diagnosis

In 1967, the Polycythemia Vera Study Group was organized. One of its main goals was to develop a set of diagnostic criteria for PV. Table 35-2 summarizes the criteria recommended by this group.[9]

Increased RCM may be caused by conditions unrelated to an MPD and may be categorized in one of two groups: secondary or relative. Both of these types of erythrocytosis are discussed in more detail in Chapter 10. A brief review is presented below.

In contrast to PV with its generally low erythropoietin levels, the *secondary polycythemias* show normal to increased erythropoietin production, which may be compensatory (appropriate) or inappropriate. Sensitive radioimmunoassays for the quantitation of erythropoietin are now available.[50] The *compensatory* erythrocytoses are associated with tissue hypoxia, which may result from living at high altitudes, cardiovascular or pulmonary disease, abnormal hemoglobins with an increased oxygen affinity (Chap. 14), and heavy smoking.[90] All of these disorders cause a decrease in the amount of oxygen delivered to the tissues, thereby stimulating erythropoietin production and the increased erythrocyte production that leads to secondary polycythemia. Secondary polycythemia with *inappropriate* increases in erythropoietin is associated with some kidney diseases[60,79] and with erythropoietin-producing renal tu-

TABLE 35–2. Polycythemia Vera Study Group Criteria for Diagnosis of Polycythemia Vera*

CATEGORY A	CATEGORY B
1. Increased red cell mass Male >36 mL/kg Female >32 mL/kg	1. Thrombocytosis Platelets >400×10⁹/L
2. Normal arterial O₂ saturation; >92%	2. Leukocytosis WBC >12×10⁹/L with no fever or infection
3. Splenomegaly	3. Increased leukocyte alkaline phosphatase score (>100) with no fever or infection
	4. Increased serum B₁₂ (>900 ng/mL or Increased unbound B₁₂ binding capacity (>2200 ng/mL)

* Diagnosis may be made if: (1) all characteristics in category A are present OR (2) category A characteristics 1 and 2 are present plus any two characteristics from category B. In addition, patients must have had the disease diagnosed no longer than 4 years and had no prior treatment except phlebotomy.
From Wasserman LR: The management of polycythemia vera. Br J Haematol 21:371, 1971, with permission.

mors, hepatocellular carcinoma,[68,82] ovarian tumors, uterine fibroids,[69] and cerebellar hemangioblastoma.[40] In these conditions the RCM is abnormally increased.

Relative polycythemia is not associated with a true increase in RCM. Rather, RCM, as measured by the microhematocrit, is elevated because the plasma volume has decreased for some reason. Causes of relative polycythemia include plasma loss (*e.g.*, from severe burns) and dehydration from vomiting, severe diarrhea, or lack of water.

The differential diagnosis of PV and secondary polycythemia is relatively simple from a clinical and laboratory viewpoint. Clinically, the spleen is rarely palpable in secondary polycythemia but is almost always palpable in PV. Thrombotic or hemorrhagic episodes are common in PV but rare in secondary polycythemia. From a laboratory viewpoint, the combination of a granulocytic leukocytosis, severe thrombocytosis, extreme erythrocytosis, and peripheral blood basophilia is so unusual that it almost always leads to the diagnosis of PV.

Testing for increased RCM is usually standard practice in suspected PV. It also is helpful in distinguishing relative and absolute erythrocytosis. The test involves collection of a blood sample from which the red cells are separated and labeled with a small dose of radioactive chromium(⁵¹Cr). After injection back into the patient, the labeled red cells are allowed to circulate for 15 minutes to allow them to disperse evenly in the circulation. At that point, a blood sample is removed and the amount of radioactivity in the erythrocyte portion determined. The lower the radioactivity measurement, the higher the blood volume. An RCM exceeding 36 mL/kg for males or 32 mL/kg for females is abnormally high and indicative of PV.[11] Plasma volume, which is normal or increased in PV, can be measured similarly using radioiodinated albumin. See Table 35-3 for other tests useful in the differential diagnosis of primary and secondary polycythemia.

Effects of Treatment on Laboratory Results

Patients may be treated with phlebotomy, radioactive phosphorus (³²P), myelosuppressive drugs, or a combination thereof. Continued phlebotomy tends to worsen the iron deficiency and may aggravate the thrombocytosis. Radiation is given to reduce the proliferation of erythrocytes and platelets. Although myelosuppressive drugs such as busulfan[101] and chlorambucil[85] have proven effective in some cases, they have been associated with an increased incidence of acute leukemia and may cause the transformation of PV to acute leukemia. Hydroxyurea, on the other hand, appears to be less leukemogenic and therefore may be the myelosuppressive drug of choice at this time.[9,45]

Ideally, blood counts should approach normal within a short time. The ideal HCT is 0.45 to 0.50 L/L. The leukocyte count will usually approach normal, but the platelet count may remain in the high-normal range (350–500 × 10⁹/L).[41] Granulocytes may be hypogranular. Some giant platelets may be present, and the patient may experience continued bleeding because of platelet hypofunction. If phlebotomy is continued, microcytic, hypochromic erythrocytes may be seen. An iron-deficient state is the desired effect, actually, because it limits the expansion of the RCM. The more expanded the RCM, the higher the chance of hemorrhage or thromboembolic episode leading to a stroke or myocardial infarction.[94]

Course of the Disease

The most obvious change in the peripheral blood in long-term PV (other than a decreasing MCV and MCHC) is the appearance of teardrop red cells on the blood film.[87] This change heralds the most common transition of PV, that of a secondary, reactive response that causes increasing irreversible myelofibrosis and myeloid metaplasia, sometimes referred to as the "spent phase" (Plate 49) of PV or post-polycythemic myeloid metaplasia (PPMM).[24] The latter is demonstrated in the bone marrow by increased reticulin content (marrow fibrosis).

Hepatosplenomegaly becomes more severe as the rate of extramedullary hematopoiesis accelerates. Splenectomy usually is recommended if splenic irradiation is ineffective and splenic enlargement causes increased red cell destruction and platelet sequestration. This operation does not eradicate the myeloid metaplasia, which continues in the liver and other extramedullary sites.

As myelofibrosis and extramedullary hematopoiesis become more advanced, the blood film exhibits dramatic changes. Nucleated red blood cells increase out of proportion to the anemia and the low number of circulating reticulocytes. The differential shows a left shift in myeloid cells, including blast forms. Giant abnormal-appearing platelets increase in numbers, as do the numbers of micromegakaryocytes, micromegakaryoblasts, and megakaryocytic fragments (see Plate 49). The leukocyte count is only moderately increased once corrected for NRBCs and megakaryocytes. The majority of patients in this phase have a poor prognosis. In some patients, platelet numbers increase to more than 1000 × 10⁹/L with only an occasional

TABLE 35–3. Findings in Primary and Secondary Polycythemia

	B_{12} (ng/L)	LAP SCORE	IRON (μg/dL)	RBC MASS (mL/kg BODY WT)	PLASMA VOLUME (mL/kg BODY WT)	ARTERIAL O_2 SATURATION
Reference range*	150–1500	11–95	40–140	Men: 25–35 Women 20–30	Men & women: 40–50	≥92% of pO_2 (arterial)
Primary	>1500	Usually >100	<40	Men: >36 Women: >32	Men & women: Nl to ↑	≥92% of pO_2 (arterial)
Secondary	Nl	Nl	Nl	Nl to ↑	↓	<92% of pO_2 (arterial)

* Note that exact reference values for various tests may differ according to procedure used. However, the tendency toward abnormal values is apparent from this table. Nl = normal; ↑ = increased; ↓ = decreased.

normal form seen, whereas megakaryocytic fragments and micromegakaryocytes reach high numbers.

Ultimately, normal forms of polymorphonuclear leukocytes, erythrocytes, and platelets may be eliminated with either concurrent increases in NRBCs coupled with increasing anemia (ineffective erythropoiesis) or a slow decrease in the number of NRBCs as abnormal megakaryocytes increase. In still other patients, the disorder transforms into a megakaryoblastic crisis, with platelet counts severely reduced. In any case, hemorrhage or infection is the usual cause of morbidity. Thrombosis and acute leukemia were reported as the most common causes of death in one study.[102] In a significant number of patients, PV transforms into AML and in a few patients, to acute lymphoid leukemia. The increased numbers of acute leukemia transformations may be related, not to the MPD, but to its treatment with leukemogenic drugs such as ^{32}P or the alkylating agents such as busulfan (Myleran) or chlorambucil.[10]

The Polycythemia Vera Study Group reported median survival times from diagnosis as 11.8 years for ^{32}P-treated patients, 8.9 years for those receiving chlorambucil, and 13.9 years for those treated by therapeutic phlebotomy.[9]

CHRONIC MYELOGENOUS LEUKEMIA

Chronic myelogenous leukemia is a malignant disorder characterized by leukocytosis with an increase in mature and immature cells of the granulocytic series. Thrombocytosis is common. Splenomegaly, most likely attributable to extramedullary hematopoiesis, is frequent. An abnormal chromosome known as the Philadelphia chromosome (Ph[1]) may be found in cells of the malignant proliferating clone. Other chromosomal abnormalities have also been described. Ph[1] has been found in granulocytes, erythrocytes, megakaryocytes, and lymphocytes (B cells).

Chronic myelogenous leukemia is primarily a disease of adults, although it has been reported at all ages. The term "juvenile CML" is usually reserved for Philadelphia-negative (Ph[1](-)) CML of infants and very young children, usually below the age of 2 years.

Clinical Presentation

Symptoms

The earliest and most common symptoms of CML are fatigue, shortness of breath after mild exertion, malaise, and fullness in the upper abdomen caused by hepatosplenomegaly. Patients often lose their appetite because of a sensation of fullness after they ingest even small quantities of food. This usually leads to anorexia and weight loss. Priapism (persistent penile engorgement) is another symptom associated with an extremely elevated leukocyte or platelet count. Signs of platelet abnormalities may be seen, such as retinal hemorrhage, hematuria, or epistaxis. Platelet abnormalities may occur because of functional or quantitative platelet disturbances.[38,93]

Physical Findings

Sternal tenderness; warm, moist skin; pallor; and a palpable spleen and liver are often detected. Occasionally, lymphadenopathy is present. In juvenile CML, patients usually present with severe splenomegaly and lymphadenopathy. Laboratory tests usually confirm an increased metabolic rate.[103] In adult CML, low-grade fever is common, although many patients have no fever until the terminal disease phase.[23]

Laboratory Findings

Peripheral Blood

A marked leukocytosis is the obvious feature in the peripheral blood (Plate 50). Generally, leukocyte counts range from 50 to 600×10^9/L prior to treatment. However, much higher counts have been reported: this author recalls a CML patient (who refused treatment) who had leukocyte counts exceeding 1500×10^9/L just prior to death.

If anemia is present, it is usually normocytic, normochromic. Platelet counts may be increased (approximately 600×10^9/L) or decreased with occasional giant forms. Frequently, the leukocyte and platelet counts are inversely related: the higher the leukocyte count, the lower the platelet count. This effect is probably attributable to a "squeezing out" of marrow megakaryocytes by the overabundance of granulocytic cells. Leukocyte differential results approach the following: blasts 1% to 5%; promyelocytes 1% to 10%; myelocytes 10% to 20%; metamyelocytes 10% to 30%; bands 20% to 40%; neutrophils 30% to 50%; eosinophils 2% to 15% (including young forms); basophils 2% to 10% (including young forms); and normoblasts 2 to 4 per 100 leukocytes (see Plate 50). In the experience of this author, dysplastic granulocytes and bizarre platelets are not characteristic of CML (see Chap. 33 on dysplasia) except under certain circumstances such as impending myeloid blast transformation, Ph[1](-) CML, or in patients first seen (by a physician) with CML in blast transformation (*i.e.*, CML in blast transformation *de novo*).

Bone Marrow

The marrow is markedly hypercellular with minimal fat, in large part because of myeloid hyperplasia. The majority of cells are in the granulocytic series. Marrow and peripheral blood differentials are similar except that the mean stage of maturity in the marrow is shifted to the left. Along with thrombocytosis, megakaryocytes frequently are increased, sometimes markedly. A reticulin stain on a biopsy specimen may demonstrate fibrosis.

Cytogenetics

The Philadelphia chromosome is one of the oldest known cytogenetic abnormalities in hematology. It is found in cells of the malignant proliferating clone in 70% to 90% of patients with CML.[25] The affected cells include granulocytes, erythrocytes, megakaryocytes, and lymphocytes and are said to be "Ph[1](+)." The abnormality is the result of translocation of the long arm of chromosome 22 to the long arm of chromosome 9: t(9q[+]; 22q[-]) (Fig. 35-2). The general procedure for the detection of Ph[1] is outlined in Chapter 5.

The disease of adults and children cells are Ph[1](-) has recently been suggested to be incorrectly classified as CML. One study[72] indicates that on the basis of the recent proposals by the French-American-British (FAB) group regarding the classification of myelodysplastic syndromes[7] (MDS) (Chap. 33), Ph[1](-) CML probably belongs in the MDS group according to peripheral blood and bone marrow morphology. In this study, 17 previously diagnosed cases of Ph[1](-) CML were reclassified as MDS. It was demonstrated that myelodysplasia was rare in Ph[1](+) CML if blast transformation occurred more than 12 months after initial diagnosis. Myelodysplasia was seen only when blast transformation occurred less than 12 months from initial diagnosis. Conversely, myelodysplasia occurred in all but

one of the Ph[1](-) group. Basophilia was not present in the Ph[1](-) group but was consistently present in the Ph[1](+) group. Finally, monocytosis seemed to be present in the majority of Ph[1](-) cases but not in the Ph[1](+) CML cases.

Other data describe a group of patients with Ph[1](-) CML who have a clinical picture indistinguishable from that of Ph[1](+) CML, both in survival and in disease characteristics.[55] New findings in molecular genetics regarding Ph[1](-) CML may explain this phenomenon. A study of 19 Ph[1](-) CML cases at the molecular level revealed that seven patients had chromosome 9 and 22 rearrangement patterns thought to be pathognomonic for Ph[1](+) CML, although the typical Ph[1](+) rearrangement seen by standard cytogenetic techniques was not found. Specifically, these seven patients had a rearrangement of the oncogene *c-abl* (from 9q34) translocating to the *bcr* region of 22q11.[5,32,62] This group of CML patients may be considered Ph[1](+), albeit at the molecular level.

Differential Diagnosis

The most common cause of leukocytosis with a left shift and mild thrombocytosis is infection or reaction to tissue necrosis or neoplasm. Because of confusion in the past between these reactions and CML, the term "leukemoid reaction" was developed to label any condition that mimicked leukemia but was, in fact, benign. However, differentiation between CML and a leukemoid reaction has been greatly simplified, and confusion is now less common. One of the tests used for differentiation is the leukocyte (or neutrophil) alkaline phosphatase (LAP/NAP) test. The LAP is normal or increased in a leukemoid reaction and decreased in CML unless there is a concurrent infection. Splenomegaly usually is absent with a leukemoid reaction but often present in CML (Table 35-4). The other disease most commonly confused with CML is myelofibrosis with myeloid metaplasia (see later discussion).

Effects of Treatment on Laboratory Results

Allopurinol is usually given prior to therapy, coupled with adequate hydration, to ameliorate the hyperuricemia caused by the rapid turnover and destruction of granulocytes by chemotherapy. The majority of CML patients are treated with an alkylating agent such as busulfan. These agents are myelosuppressive drugs used specifically to reduce the numbers of proliferating myeloid elements in an attempt to return the patient to a clinically normal state (*i.e.*, the elimination of anemia, splenomegaly, thrombocytosis, and the marked leukocytosis with a left shift). At least 75% of patients in the chronic phase of CML respond to various single chemotherapeutic agents, such as busulfan, obtaining a peripheral blood remission.[49] Leukocyte counts can fall to and remain as low as 15×10^9/L, often with only a slight left shift remaining. However, it is not uncommon to find occasional myelocytes, promyelocytes, and even a rare blast even though the patient appears to be well. Platelet counts, although not extremely high, may remain in the high-normal range or even be slightly increased. Relative basophilia (as much as 3%) is not uncommon in the treated CML patient. The Ph[1] chromosome seems to persist regardless of treatment. Drugs have little or no effect on cell

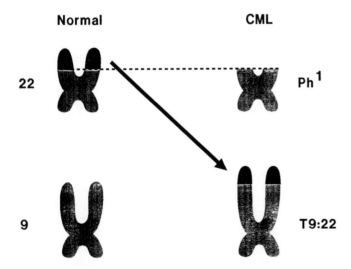

Normal   **CML**

22   Ph[1]

9   T9:22

FIG. 35-2. Philadelphia chromosome results from translocation of long arm of chromosome 22 to long arm of chromosome 9. This is technically written as t(9q[+]; 22q[-]).

TABLE 35–4. Laboratory Features of CML and Leukemoid Reaction

CONDITION	SPLENOMEGALY	WBC	PLATELETS $\times 10^9$/L	LEFT SHIFT	NRBCS PER 100 WBC	BASOPHILS AND EOSINOPHILS	LAP SCORE	Ph^1	ANEMIA
CML	Usually present	$\uparrow\uparrow\uparrow\uparrow$	>600 or <50	Back to blast (1–5%)	0–5	Normal or $\uparrow\uparrow$ with young forms	$\downarrow$ ★	+	Normocytic; normochromic
Leukemoid reaction	Usually absent	$\uparrow\uparrow$	200–450	Blasts seldom >0.5%	0–1	Normal	Nl to $\uparrow$	−	Not present

$\uparrow\uparrow\uparrow\uparrow$ = marked increase; $\uparrow\uparrow$ = moderate increase; $\uparrow$ = slight increase; $\downarrow$ slight decrease; Nl = normal.
★ Except in infection.

morphology *per se,* although granulocytic hypogranulation is sometimes seen.

Today, treatment for CML is not limited to alkylating chemotherapy. Bone marrow transplantation is providing new hope. Because transplantation for CML patients in either the accelerated or the blast crisis phase has shown little therapeutic value,[27,92] transplants are usually performed in the chronic phase or during the patient's first remission. Age is an important variable to transplant success. In patients older than 40 to 50 years of age, common, often fatal, complications include severe graft versus host disease (GVHD), an increase in the incidence of septic complications, and idiopathic interstitial pneumonitis. As a result, 40 to 50 years is frequently the age limit for allogeneic marrow transplantation.[48] Autologous (self), syngeneic (identical human leukocyte antigen [HLA] matched twins), or allogeneic (any HLA-matched person) transplants may be performed. Unfortunately, autologous transplants do not promote long-term remission, because the patient's own marrow is rarely Ph^1(-). Once autologous marrow is infused (when blast crisis develops), only reestablishment of the chronic CML phase can be expected, and this quickly reverts to the blastic phase.[33,51] Many patients have a delay in engraftment, leaving them devoid of platelets and granulocytes, resulting in death from hemorrhage or infection.[34] Of 40 CML patients treated with syngeneic marrow transplants, 65% remained disease free at 6.6 years,[16,17] and 60% to 70% of more than 400 patients receiving allogeneic transplants during the chronic phase were surviving disease free when examined after 3 years.[17,36]

Course of the Disease

Kamada and Uchino proposed a sequential process for CML on the basis of data from 20 patients, 16 of whom had been exposed to nuclear radiation.[44] It was noted that Ph^1(+) patients showed no symptoms when the leukocyte count was less than 50×10^9/L. Increasing symptom severity coincided with disease progression and leukocyte count increases.[12,44] Those investigators concluded that there is a three-stage CML disease process: (1) proliferative and symptomless, lasting an average of 6.3 years; (2) preclinical, lasting approximately 19 months; and (3) terminal, advanced (accelerated), in which patients have symptoms and a 3-year mean survival. Kamada and Uchino therefore deduced that any CML patient who, at diagnosis, had a leukocyte count greater than 100×10^9/L had probably

become Ph^1(+) at least 8 years earlier. More clinical data are needed on a larger and less selected group before statistically valid conclusions can be reached.

Patients whose disease is Ph^1(-) are generally agreed to have a worse prognosis than those with Ph^1(+) disease. One study reported that patients with Ph^1(-) disease were older (median age 66 years compared with 48 years for Ph^1(+) disease), were usually males, had lower initial leukocyte and platelet counts, and responded poorly to therapy.[25] In this study, median survival rate for patients with Ph^1(-) disease was approximately 8 months compared with 40 months for those with Ph^1(+) disease.

For patients ineligible for bone marrow transplantation, the chronic phase generally responds to therapy and continues to do so for several years. However, within 2 to 4 years from the onset of symptoms, increasing marrow fibrosis is evidenced by the presence of approximately 5% teardrops, abnormal platelets, and occasional megakaryocyte fragments. This blood picture is often confused with that of myelofibrosis with myeloid metaplasia.

The terminal accelerated phase is referred to as "blast transformation" or "acute exacerbation blast crisis." Several different patterns seem to emerge that herald blast transformation; these patterns may differ among patients. The patterns may include either evidence of dysplastic myelopoiesis (*e.g.,* hypogranular and hyposegmented granulocytes, giant agranular platelets, and oval macrocytes) or development of an unexpected thrombocytopenia relative to the patient's standard counts during remission. Some patients show minimal dysplasia with the emergence of myeloid blast transformation. The only clue to blast transformation in these patients is a distinct decrease in the platelet count without a corresponding leukopenia and a slight (5%–10%) increase in the blast count over previous numbers.

Not all CMLS transform directly into the myeloblastic phase. Some patients exhibit a marked basophilia (as much as 50%), show evidence of megakaryocytic blast crisis, and then develop a myeloid blast transformation.

No matter how CML blast transformation emerges, the eventual outcome is the same. As transformation progresses, the leukocyte count and blast percentage rise, while thrombocytopenia becomes increasingly severe. The final blood picture may be indistinguishable from that of AML.

Transformation into lymphoblastic leukemia is more common than was once thought possible. In one study,[35] 30% of the subjects in CML blast transformation had a lymphoblastic transformation. Other transformations showed the phenotypes of erythroleukemia, mixed leukemia (having both myeloid and lymphoid blasts), and undifferentiated leukemia.

There are no clear prognostic indicators. However, there is general concurrence that age has no effect on the prognosis and that absence of a Ph^1 chromosome indicates a poor prognosis. All other factors appear to be variable. For example, some studies have agreed that certain findings indicate a poor prognosis: leukocytosis ($>100 \times 10^9/L$); basophilia ($>15\%$–20%); $>1\%$ blasts in the peripheral blood or $>5\%$ in the marrow; thrombocytosis ($>700 \times 10^9/L$); thrombocytopenia ($<150 \times 10^9/L$); splenomegaly; and karyotype abnormalities other than Ph^1 chromosome.[15,91,98] One study demonstrated that an increase in marrow myeloblasts and promyelocytes with a decreased number of mitotic cells also indicates a poor prognosis.[89] On the other hand, some investigators, including JC Marsh from the University of Utah (unpublished data) have reported that the prognosis is not affected by degree of leukocytosis,[43,61,99] a high percentage of blasts,[61] thrombocytosis,[61,99] or thrombocytopenia.[61,99] Likewise, two studies showed that severe anemia had no effect on prognosis[61] (JC Marsh, unpublished data), whereas another found that severe anemia indicated a poor prognosis.[43]

JUVENILE CHRONIC MYELOGENOUS LEUKEMIA

Juvenile CML, although not a chronic MPD, is seen in children who have a CML variant with $Ph^1(-)$ cells. The peak incidence occurs at 1 to 2 years of age.[3] The prognosis is extremely unfavorable. There is a dyserythropoiesis and a marked increase in serum and urine muramidase levels secondary to increased leukocyte destruction. Leukocyte counts are usually below $100 \times 10^9/L$ and typically are lower than those in adult $Ph^1(+)$ CML. Peripheral blood and marrow monocytosis were reported in one study[2] but were not found in another.[75] Increased fetal hemoglobin (Hb F) is common; there are reports of 15% to 50%[2,53] and even 85%[83] Hb F. Other characteristics of fetal erythrocytes are also common, including a decreased Hb A_2 level and low levels of the enzymes G6PD, lactate dehydrogenase (LD), and pyruvate kinase, among others.[22]

Although juvenile CML is very similar to adult $Ph^1(+)$ CML, it is clinically distinguishable. The similarities include a low LAP level, eosinophilia, and basophilia. The difference is that juvenile CML usually presents with a moderate to marked thrombocytopenia and decreased marrow megakaryocytes, resulting in hemorrhagic episodes. The response to standard chemotherapy is poor.[53] See Chapter 33 for another approach to this disease.

AGNOGENIC MYELOID METAPLASIA

"Agnogenic myeloid metaplasia" or "idiopathic myelofibrosis" are terms used to describe a clonal chronic myeloproliferative disorder[42] characterized by fibrosis and granulocytic hyperplasia in the marrow and by proliferation of granulocytes in the spleen and liver.[28] Agnogenic myeloid metaplasia is found mostly in middle-aged to older people.

On rare occasions, it is found in children, either as a primary idiopathic disease or secondary to acute leukemia.[54] The fibrosis is believed to be a secondary reaction to the clonal proliferative disease rather than the direct result of a clonal disorder. This conclusion is based on evidence that fibroblasts in heterozygous patients produce both G6PD isoenzymes A and B (enzyme mosaicism),[21,47] whereas the neoplastic hematopoietic cells of clonal disorders in similar patients produce only one isoenzyme. Megakaryocytes and platelets may contribute to fibrosis.

One of the most consistent findings in AMM is the increase in defective platelets as a consequence of dysplastic megakaryocytopoiesis. This results in premature death of these defective platelets and megakaryocytes and the release of their alpha granules, which contain platelet-derived growth factor (PDGF) (Chap. 58). *In vitro*, the presence of increased alpha granules stimulates fibroblastic growth (scar tissue).[46,56] The substance stimulates collagen secretion, which is required for mending of wounds. It is believed that *in vivo*, alpha granules stimulate marrow fibroblasts, which subsequently increase fibrous tissue, leading to myelofibrosis. The chronic MPDs are closely related; therefore, any of them may demonstrate various degrees of myelofibrosis as a secondary complication (see Fig. 35-1).

There are many synonyms for AMM, the two most common being *myelofibrosis with myeloid metaplasia* and *idiopathic myelofibrosis*. In AMM the marrow may become increasingly dominated by fibroblasts; thus the term *myelofibrosis* is also used in referring to this disorder. *Myeloid metaplasia* indicates that myeloid cells (granulocytes, erythrocytes, and megakaryocytes) are produced in hematopoietic sites outside the marrow. Such production is also referred to as *extramedullary hematopoiesis*. These extramedullary sites are the same as those that formed blood cells *in utero* during the hepatic period of development (Chap. 5), including the liver, spleen, and reticuloendothelial system. "Idiopathic (primary) myelofibrosis" refers to fibrosis arising from an unknown cause.

Clinical Presentation

Symptoms

The most common complaints are those relating to anemia, as well as abdominal pain, indigestion, and a fullness after eating small amounts secondary to splenomegaly. The latter results in anorexia and weight loss. Fever, night sweats, lethargy, and weakness are common complaints.

Physical Findings

Patients may appear ashen. Splenomegaly and sometimes liver enlargement are evident. Petechiae may be present, and epistaxis may occur frequently.

Laboratory Findings

Peripheral Blood

Leukocytes and platelets may be increased, normal, or decreased in number. A mild anemia may be present, and it is usually of the normocytic, normochromic type. Occasionally, a microcytic anemia is found, especially if patients have had repeated episodes of gastrointestinal bleeding. The blood film classically shows *dacryocytes* (i.e., teardrop-shaped red cells) (Fig. 35-3). The teardrops result from the cells' tortuous circulation through the enlarged spleen. Dacryocytes are a significant finding and should immediately alert the morphologist to search for conclusive evidence of myeloid metaplasia. The blood film usually reveals at least one other pathologic finding: (1) an occasional NRBC; (2) a giant, agranular platelet; (3) a rare megakaryocyte fragment; (4) an occasional immature myeloid cell; or (5) a rare myeloblast.

Although a mild reticulocytosis may be found, it is usually not as high as one would expect given the number of NRBCs found. The reticulocyte production index (Chap. 9) usually indicates ineffective erythropoiesis.

As the disease progresses, NRBCs, immature granulocytes (including myeloblasts), megakaryocytic fragments, and micromegakaryocytes increase. Patients may become severely thrombocytopenic with increasing splenic sequestration, or the platelet count may become abnormally high with giant and bizarre forms.

Bone Marrow

Attempts to aspirate bone marrow are usually futile ("dry tap"), and only trephine biopsies are successful. On biopsy, moderate to marked amounts of reticular fibrosis or collagen deposition are found[41] with hypocellularity, although normal or hypercellular areas can be found if, by chance, such an area of the bone marrow is sampled. Usually, increased numbers of megakaryocytes are found. The end stage of AMM usually shows increased osteosclerosis (hardening of the bone), and the marrow spaces are filled with enormous amounts of fibrotic tissue and small groups of megakaryocytes.[8]

Other Laboratory Values

The LAP is normal to increased. Uric acid is increased, but serum albumin and cholesterol often are decreased. The LD is usually increased, probably because of ineffective myelopoiesis.[52,100]

Differential Diagnosis

Agnogenic myeloid metaplasia is most commonly confused with CML because of the similar immaturity of the peripheral blood leukocytes and the presence of all stages of myeloid maturation, including eosinophils and basophils. Several factors may assist in differentiation. The blood film in CML does not have the high numbers of NRBCs or dacrocytes seen in AMM, and although the CML film can have an occasional megakaryocytic fragment and a few abnormal-appearing platelets, the numbers do not even approach those seen in AMM. The Ph[1] chromosome and an extremely low LAP are indicative of CML, whereas Ph[1] is not found in AMM and the LAP in AMM is usually normal or increased (see Table 35-7).

Cell immaturity, basophilia, eosinophilia, thrombocytosis, and the presence of splenomegaly may cause confusion between AMM and PV, particularly in those few AMM patients who are polycythemic rather than anemic.[100] However, the two conditions generally are distinguishable. Significant numbers of dacryocytes and NRBCs with some megakaryocytic fragments indicate AMM. Splenomegaly generally is more pronounced in AMM than in PV, and the degree of fibrosis may be less in PV than in AMM at the time of diagnosis. However, in PV with advanced progression to AMM, the two are indistinguishable.

Confusion also arises when extramedullary hematopoiesis is demonstrated in other MPDs and the bone marrow shows slight fibrosis. In such cases, several characteristics similar to those of the myeloproliferative disorder AMM will be apparent, such as the appearance of a few dacryocytes, an occasional megakaryocytic fragment, and some bizarre platelets. However, none of the changes is as severe as in a moderately advanced AMM, except in PPMM, in which case the changes are indistinguishable. Ferrokinetic studies using ^{52}Fe or ^{59}Fe may be performed to estimate the amount of extramedullary erythropoiesis in the spleen and

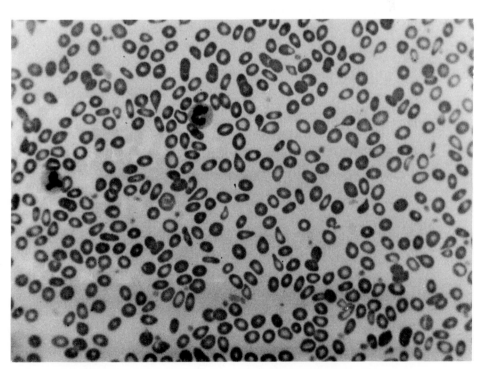

FIG. 35-3. Note teardrop forms on peripheral blood film of patient with agnogenic myeloid metaplasia (original magnification × 500).

liver. Extensive extramedullary erythropoiesis is indicative of AMM.

Agnogenic myeloid metaplasia may also be confused with myelophthisic anemia. The latter condition results from marrow replacement by malignant nonhematopoietic cells and may be accompanied by fibrosis, which leads to compensatory extramedullary hematopoiesis. From a pathogenic standpoint, AMM is a noncompensatory disorder that results from stem cell injury rather than marrow replacement.[77]

Differentiation of AMM from myelophthisic anemia can be difficult when looking at a blood film with no knowledge of the patient. Typically, this anemia demonstrates a leukoerythroblastic blood picture showing the same morphology as an early AMM, namely, normocytic, normochromic anemia with dacryocytes, a few NRBCs, a rare abnormal platelet, and immature granulocytes with an occasional myeloblast. Some conditions that may cause marrow infiltration and result in a leukoerythroblastic blood picture that may be confused with AMM are listed in Table 35–5. Dacryocytes seem to be most commonly associated with breast, bladder, and prostate carcinomas.

A leukoerythroblastic reaction may also be seen without marrow infiltration. This occurs in normal newborns and in conditions where a tremendous bone marrow response is present, such as severe hemolytic crisis (e.g., thalassemia major),[6] hemorrhage (e.g., gastrointestinal bleeding), postsplenectomy, and septicemia. Dacryocytes usually are not found in the leukoerythroblastic reaction associated with hemorrhage or infection but can be found in some congenital hemolytic conditions, such as thalassemia.

Effects of Treatment on Laboratory Results

Treatment generally is aimed at alleviating symptoms, because there is no treatment that will affect the course or outcome of AMM. Patients may remain asymptomatic for long periods, and for them, splenectomy is not advised.

However, once the disease manifests itself, splenectomy is advised early because during the advanced stage, this

TABLE 35–5. Causes of Marrow Infiltration and Leukoerythroblastic Blood Picture that May Be Confused with Agnogenic Myeloid Metaplasia

Hodgkin and non-Hodgkin lymphoma
Infections (miliary tuberculosis, histoplasmosis)
Carcinoma, especially breast, prostate, lung, and bladder
Other neoplasms (neuroblastoma, carcinoma of the gastrointestinal tract, kidney, and thyroid)
Myelofibrosis:
    Primary: agnogenic or idiopathic
    Secondary: cancers or toxins (benzene, radiation)
Other chronic myeloproliferative diseases (PV, CML, ET)
Other hematologic disorders (hairy cell leukemia, ALL, multiple myeloma, acute myelofibrosis, AML)
Lipid storage diseases
Osteopetrosis

Adapted from Sun NCJ: Hematology—An Atlas and Diagnostic Guide, pp 158–163. Philadelphia, WB Saunders, 1983; and Peterson P, McIntyre OR: Myeloproliferative Disorders, pp 24–25. Publication for the ASCP National Meeting, 1987.

operation carries considerable risk because of the possibility of hemorrhage.[63] Splenectomy is particularly helpful if hemolytic anemia or thrombocytopenia persists despite use of chemotherapy and X-rays to reduce splenic size.[88]

Normoblasts, abnormal platelets, and megakaryocyte fragments increase after splenectomy, whereas dacryocytes virtually disappear. This finding upholds the traditional theory that the spleen is responsible for dacryocyte formation. Splenectomy causes the appearance of Howell-Jolly bodies, acanthocytes, spherocytes, and target cells on the blood film. In the absence of the spleen, platelet counts may exceed $1000 \times 10^9/L$, because the intact spleen normally pools many platelets; this increases the risk of thromboembolism. Standard myelosuppressive therapy with busulfan or hydroxyurea is used to decrease the platelet mass. At this point, the blood film is identical to the picture already described as PPMM.

Course of the Disease

At present, bone marrow transplantation is the only hope for reversing myelofibrosis. Three studies have demonstrated that marrow fibrosis is completely reversible, barring complications such as GVHD, after allogeneic transplantation that results in complete marrow engraftment.[57,66,76] In another report, no difference in engraftment time, rate of relapse, or survival was noticed in patients having extensive marrow fibrosis versus those with little or no fibrosis.[67] However, this finding is in complete contradiction to that of another study in which definite adverse effects were reported after bone marrow transplantation for patients with severe fibrosis.[74] Nonetheless, without transplantation, the prognosis is grave. The majority of patients die from complications of total marrow failure. Hemorrhage, infections, or cardiac complications are the immediate cause of death.[8] Approximately 5% to 8% terminate in AML or what appears to be a form of megakaryocytic leukemia. The blood film shows masses of abnormal platelet-producing micromegakaryocytes (Plate 51) with few or no normal myeloid elements. Years ago, Hayhoe and Flemans referred to this pattern as "megakaryocytic myelosis."[39] There are reports, however, of patients who go into remission for periods of as long as 22 months before transformation of the disease into AML.[73]

ESSENTIAL THROMBOCYTHEMIA

Primary or essential thrombocythemia (ET) is a chronic MPD characterized by a thrombocytosis in excess of $1000 \times 10^9/L$ with spontaneous aggregation of functionally abnormal platelets. In this disorder there is no apparent cause for the thrombocytosis, whereas the cause usually is apparent in secondary thrombocytosis associated with splenectomy, chronic infections, and other situations not related to MPDs. Essential thrombocythemia is closely related to PV, the principal difference being that the diagnosis of PV requires an increase in total red cell mass, whereas that of ET requires an increase in platelet mass without accompanying significant erythrocytosis. It is one of the least common of the MPDs, second only to chronic neutrophilic leukemia, which is the least common.

Clinical Presentation

Symptoms

There are frequent episodes of epistaxis, vomiting of blood, easy bleeding after minor dental surgery, and gastrointestinal bleeding. Paradoxically, thrombotic events also are common. Fatigue is a frequent complaint.

Physical Findings

Splenomegaly and, on occasion, hepatomegaly are detected. However, if the splenic blood supply is impeded by platelet aggregates in the microcirculation, the spleen may undergo a slow reduction in size as it atrophies secondary to lack of oxygen and nutrients. In these cases, the spleen is not palpable. There may be arterial or venous thrombosis involving the penile (resulting in priapism), hepatic, mesentric, and portal vessels.[86] Pulmonary emboli and gangrenous toes are not uncommon.

Laboratory Findings

Peripheral Blood

The most striking finding is the persistence of a marked thrombocytosis, with platelet counts exceeding 1100 × 10^9/L. The highest count seen by this author was 8000 × 10^9/L, but there are reports of counts as high as 14,000 × 10^9/L.[26,37] Large masses of platelet aggregates are seen on the blood film, with many abnormal-appearing giant and bizarre forms. Marked platelet anisocytosis (large and small forms) and occasional megakaryocyte fragments are characteristic (Fig. 35-4).

The RBC count is slightly elevated in some cases. In the presence of chronic bleeding, microcytic, hypochromic erythrocytes indicate an iron deficiency anemia. Target cells, acanthocytes, and Howell-Jolly bodies will be found if splenic infarction occurs, causing poor splenic function.

The Polycythemia Vera Study Group[65] reported that the leukocyte count in 37 patients with ET ranged from 6 to 41 × 10^9/L with a median of 11.5 × 10^9/L and a neutrophilic left shift of mostly bands and metamyelocytes.

Bone Marrow

The marrow can be difficult to aspirate because of myelofibrosis; however, it may simultaneously be hypercellular, with a megakaryocytic hyperplasia and masses of aggregated platelets. The megakaryocytes may stick together as well, giving the whole marrow a "glued together" appearance. Some cases have a mild concurrent erythroid and granulocytic hyperplasia.

Coagulation Studies

Platelet function studies are abnormal. Platelet aggregation (Chap. 59) is abnormal with ADP and epinephrine, but, oddly enough, when the platelet count is reduced to normal, platelet function returns to normal.[31] These patients probably have an acquired storage pool disease (Chap. 61), which is a common characteristic of the chronic MPDs.[70]

Differential Diagnosis

The most common condition confused with essential or primary thrombocythemia is a reactive or secondary thrombocytosis. Platelet aggregation studies are useful for differentiation, as they are usually normal in secondary thrombocytosis but abnormal in ET.

A careful clinical evaluation of the patient also is helpful in differentiation. The Polycythemia Vera Study Group has published diagnostic criteria for ET (Table 35-6).[65] Patients with ET usually have some degree of splenomegaly or hepatomegaly or both at initial presentation, whereas this is

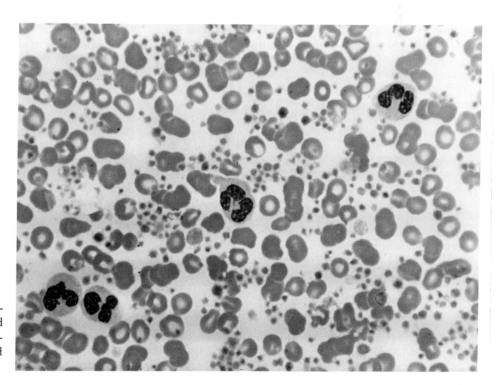

FIG. 35-4. Essential thrombocythemia. Note granulocytosis, marked thrombocytosis, and platelets that appear in clumps in this peripheral blood film (original magnification × 1000).

TABLE 35–6. Diagnostic Criteria for Essential Thrombocythemia

1. Platelet count >600 × 10⁹/L
2. Hemoglobin <13 g/dL or normal red cell mass
   Males <36 mL/kg
   Females <32 mL/kg
3. Stainable iron in marrow or failure of iron trial (<1 g/dL rise in Hb after 1 month of iron therapy)
4. No Ph¹ chromosome
5. Collagen fibrosis of marrow
   Absent OR
   Less than one-third of biopsy area without both splenomegaly and leukoerythroblastic reaction
6. No known cause for reactive thrombocytosis

From Murphy S, Iland H, Rosenthal D, Laszlo J: Essential thrombocythemia: An interim report from the Polycythemia Vera Study Group. Semin Hematol 23:177, 1986, with permission.

unusual for a secondary or reactive thrombocytosis. Bleeding and thrombotic episodes are common with ET but unlikely with reactive thrombocytosis unless the platelet count is higher than 900 × 10⁹/L. Most helpful in differentiation is the platelet count itself, which usually is greater than 1500 × 10⁹/L in ET but rarely above 1000 × 10⁹/L in reactive thrombocytosis.

The most common causes of reactive thrombocytosis are infection, chronic inflammation, neoplasms (including the lymphomas), and acute hemolytic crisis. It may also be found after surgery, including splenectomy, especially after an acute hemolytic crisis or when performed for treatment of idiopathic thrombocytopenic purpura (ITP).[77]

Essential thrombocythemia and PV may also be similar, as both exhibit microcytic, hypochromic red cells and thrombocytosis. By the time either of these disorders reaches this point, however, they usually have already been diagnosed. For the rare occasion when this is not the case, the principal differentiating factor is the erythrocyte count. Generally, if the count is above 6.0 × 10¹²/L and the blood film appears crowded despite the microcytic appearance of the red cells, odds are the disorder is a long-term treated PV. Also, ET rarely demonstrates the severe microcytic, hypochromic state that PV does. The MCVs in PV may fall to 59 fL or lower and the MCHCs to 30.5 g/dL routinely, whereas MCVs in ET usually do not fall below 70 fL. If time permits, iron replacement therapy with observation of patient response is helpful in this differential diagnosis, as indicated in criterion 3 of Table 35-6. No response to therapy (*i.e.*, no increase in Hb) is indicative of ET, whereas a response points to PV.

Effects of Treatment on Laboratory Results

The main objective in the treatment of ET is to reduce the platelet mass. This is most successfully done, for immediate relief, by thrombocytopheresis (a mechanical means of platelet removal from the circulation) and, for the longer term, by myelosuppressive therapy. Thrombocytopheresis alone is not sufficient because it may stimulate thrombopoiesis and formation of blood clots.

Cytotoxic therapy is valuable. However, as in the other chronic MPDs, the cytotoxic agents used are leukemogenic. Although busulfan is still the most common alkylat-

ing agent employed to reduce platelet mass, patients are increasingly being treated with hydroxyurea because it appears less leukemogenic (R Stebbins, personal communication, 1986).

Course of the Disease

As in the other chronic MPDs, the risk of transformation into acute leukemia is high. Whether this transformation is the result of cytotoxic therapy or the natural course of the disease is unclear. There also is a high risk of uncontrolled gastrointestinal hemorrhage, which has been the cause of high mortality rates. Patients whose hemorrhagic tendencies have been kept under control run the risk of acute leukemic transformation, most commonly to AML, although transformation into acute lymphocytic or megakaryocytic leukemia also are strong possibilities. The life expectancy is 1 to 5 years. Young patients (under 30 years of age) have a much better prognosis than older ones.[86] On the other hand, patients who have had multiple splenic infarctions causing autosplenectomy may not fare as well as patients who present with and maintain splenomegaly.[86]

CHRONIC NEUTROPHILIC LEUKEMIA

Chronic neutrophilic leukemia is the rarest of the chronic MPDs, with only 17 cases having been reported.[4,20,29,58,84,95,104] The condition is of special interest because it may be confused, by the novice, with chronic granulocytic (myelogenous) leukemia, although there are many differentiating features. Cells from patients with chronic neutrophilic leukemia have reduced numbers of CFU-C (colony-forming units) when culture is attempted. In contrast, patients with CML or a reactive granulocytosis demonstrate increased CFU-C activity in both the bone marrow and peripheral blood.[58] Cytogenetic studies do not show any abnormal karyotypic pattern in chronic neutrophilic leukemia.

Clinical Presentation

The main complaints are the result of hepatosplenomegaly, including nausea, abdominal pain, and inability to eat normal quantities of food without a full feeling. Patients are afebrile and show no outward signs of infection. However, there may be mild to severe hemorrhagic episodes.

Laboratory Findings

Peripheral Blood

Classically, there is a persistent neutrophilic leukocytosis *without* a left shift. Toxic granulation and a few Döhle bodies are present, and on rare occasions, an NRBC is found. Leukocyte counts may be as high as 100 × 10⁹/L with normal to slightly decreased platelet counts and mild anemia. Hemoglobin is usually around 11 g/dL.

In one patient's case, the granulocytes, although able to phagocytize *Staphylococcus aureus* normally, had a 70% reduction in their ability to destroy the bacteria.[58] Electron microscopic observation of these neutrophils showed a reduction of both azurophilic and specific granulation that was not evident by light microscopy. This could explain why 5 of the 17 patients with chronic neutrophilic leukemia reported thus far have died from overwhelming bacterial infections.[20,29]

The LAP scores are extremely high, ranging from 350 to 400 (Plate 52). The B_{12} levels and B_{12} binding capacity frequently are markedly elevated.[104]

Bone Marrow

The marrow shows a marked cellularity. Although maturation in the granulocytic cell line is normal, there is a neutrophilic hyperplasia (i.e., mature granulocytes generally make up 90% of the marrow's hyperplastic reaction). The marrow shows no signs of myelodysplasia. In contrast, although the marrow in CML also shows a myeloid hyperplasia, this usually consists of increases in both mature and immature myeloid cells. Patients with chronic neutrophilic leukemia are negative for the Ph^1 chromosome.

Differential Diagnosis

The main differential diagnosis to be made is between chronic neutrophilic leukemia and reactive granulocytosis; it is usually made through the process of elimination. There are many causes for neutrophilic granulocytosis (Chap. 26). Infection is one of the more common causes for a neutrophilia, but because patients with chronic neutrophilic leukemia have no fever, infection is an unlikely cause for their disorder. Toxins, certain drugs, metabolic disturbances, and malignancy can all cause a marked neutrophilia.[58] If all possible causative conditions can be ruled out and the neutrophilia persists, then a diagnosis of chronic neutrophilic leukemia should be considered.

Course of the Disease

Because only 17 cases have been reported, any judgment about prognosis is premature. Five patients died from infection[20,29] and two from hemorrhagic episodes.[104] In three patients, the disease advanced to AML blast transformation,[4,84] and one patient was doing well 4 years after diagnosis.[58] Some patients originally believed to have chronic neutrophilic leukemia were found at autopsy to have a previously undiagnosed carcinoma metastatic to the bone marrow.[95]

DRUGS USED IN CHRONIC MYELOPROLIFERATIVE DISORDERS

Most patients with a chronic MPD will suffer from hyperuricemia (increased uric acid), a byproduct of cellular breakdown by cytotoxic agents. To prevent increased uric acid in the kidney, allopurinol, a xanthine oxidase inhibitor, is used.

Busulfan, a dual-function alkylating agent, is given in most cases. It is extremely useful in treating CML, serving to reduce the total granulocyte mass and thus relieving symptoms. There seems to be a better response to busulfan than to ^{32}P, a radioisotope commonly used for myelosuppression. However, busulfan does not appear to be beneficial in cases of juvenile CML, CML in myeloid blast transformation, or $Ph^1(-)$ CML.

Hydroxyurea interferes with DNA synthesis (S-phase drug; see Chap. 5) and seems to work well with patients having ET to reduce the total platelet mass. Because of its properties as an S-phase drug, patients on hydroxyurea may show signs of megaloblastic erythrogenesis.

CHAPTER SUMMARY

The chronic MPDs are a unique group of disorders, each one being independent, although they are similar. To simplify, one could speculate that they are all the same basic disease, each with a slightly different manifestation. In other words the MPDs all develop from the hematopoietic stem cell, all look similar, but each has its own individual idiosyncrasies. These disorders can take on similarities or transform into any other chronic MPD or an acute leukemia or even overlap and take on the characteristics of two diseases. Table 35-7 provides a summary of the laboratory differences and similarities among the disorders.

CASE STUDY 35-1

A 22-year-old man reported to the clinic in January complaining of abdominal discomfort, lethargy, fever, dizziness, anorexia, and painful

TABLE 35–7. General Guide to Peripheral Blood Differences in the Myeloproliferative Disorders

	CML	PV	AMM	ET	CNL
WBC ($\times 10^9$/L)★	>50	15–50	Variable	6–41	30–100
Hb (g/dL)	Nl to ↓	↑↑↑	↓	Variable	↓
Plt ($\times 10^9$/L)★	Up to 800 or <50	>1000; usually not >2000	Variable	>1000	Low Nl to ↓
Marrow fibroblasts	Nl to ↑↑	Nl to ↑↑	↑↑ to ↑↑↑	Nl to ↑↑	No information
LAP	↓↓↓†	↑	Nl to ↑	Nl to ↑	↑↑↑
Ph^1	+(−)	−	−	−	−
Histamine	Nl to ↑	↑	Nl	Nl	Nl
B_{12}	↑↑	Nl to ↑	Nl to ↑	Nl to ↑	↑↑↑
B_{12} binding capacity	↑↑	Nl to ↑	Nl to ↑	Nl to ↑	↑↑↑

★ Reference ranges: WBC $5–10\times10^9$/L; platelet $150–400\times10^9$/L.
† Except when infection is present.
↓ = slight decrease; ↓↓ = moderate decrease; ↑ = slight increase; ↑↑ = moderate increase;
↑↑↑ = marked increase; nl = normal.

swelling in the genital region. Physical examination revealed priapism and moderate splenomegaly. He appeared pale. His skin was damp, and he exhibited sternal tenderness. Blood test results were WBC 587 × 10⁹/L; Hb 9.8 g/dL; HCT 0.305 L/L; platelets 682 × 10⁹/L; vitamin B$_{12}$ 1800 ng/L (increased); histamine 13 μg/dL (increased); uric acid 9.8 mg/dL (increased). The differential revealed 34% neutrophils, 24% bands, 1% monocytes, 2% lymphocytes, 13% metamyelocytes, 9% myelocytes, 5% promyelocytes, 3% blasts, 4% eosinophils, and 5% basophils. There were four normoblasts per 100 WBCs. Red cell morphology was unremarkable. Several abnormal-appearing platelets were noted.

The patient underwent plasmapheresis to relieve his priapism. A bone marrow aspirate showed almost 99% cellularity with myeloid hyperplasia. All forms of granulocytes, both mature and immature, were present in an orderly array. Megakaryocytes were increased, with an occasional uninuclear form. The LAP score was 3. Cytogenetic studies revealed Ph¹(+) cells.

A definitive diagnosis of CML was made, and the patient was started on busulfan and allopurinol. He did well and was released. He maintained a leukocyte count of approximately 25 × 10⁹/L and a platelet count of 175 to 190 × 10⁹/L. In August, his basophil count had risen to 31%, and platelets were 350 × 10⁹/L with several "giant and bizarre" forms seen. In October, several cells like the ones shown in Plate 53 were seen on the blood film, coupled with a rising platelet count. Most platelets were abnormal in appearance. The following January, the patient was admitted for severe epistaxis, petechiae, and gastrointestinal bleeding. His blood film showed a marked granulocytopenia. The majority of cells were of the type seen in Plate 53, all abnormal-appearing platelet precursors. The patient died in March from a cerebral hemorrhage coupled with overwhelming infection.

1. What is the significance of the marked basophilia seen in August?
2. What are the cell types shown in Plate 53?
3. What is the final diagnosis of the disease in this patient? Can this condition usually be treated effectively?

CASE STUDY 35-2

Over a period of several years, four patients presented with severe dysplasia in the granulocytic line, blast counts between 10% and 20%, and markedly dysplastic thrombocytopenia. One patient had a marked increase in the number of eosinophilic myelocytes (>25%). The cells were Ph¹(-). The patients did poorly with standard chemotherapy, and their condition was diagnosed as Ph¹(-) CML.

1. Is the finding of Ph¹(-) cells generally consistent with the diagnosis of CML?
2. Do patients with CML generally do poorly with standard chemotherapy?
3. Is the prognosis less favorable for patients with Ph¹(-) or Ph¹(+) cells?

CASE STUDY 35-3

A 77-year-old woman presented to an ophthalmologist complaining of itchy eyes. The ophthalmologist recommended treatment for allergies, which she received. However, her condition continued to worsen, so she obtained a second opinion. This ophthalmologist referred her to an internist, who, after reviewing the CBC results, referred her to an oncologist. On her first visit to the oncologist, it was noted that her complexion was purple.

Her presenting CBC was WBC 18 × 10⁹/L; RBC 9.04 × 10¹²/L; Hb 20.8 g/dL; HCT 0.64 L/L; MCV 71 fL; MCHC 32.5 g/dL; platelets 406 × 10⁹/L. Treatment first included therapeutic phlebotomy, with four units of blood being removed over approximately 10 days. After this, her Hb was 18.5 g/dL, the HCT was 0.59 L/L, and her platelet count had risen to 514 × 10⁹/L. Blood volume measurement revealed: RCM 43.6 mL/kg (reference range women: 20–30 mL/kg) and plasma volume 30.9 mL/kg. Sixteen months after diagnosis, she was given radioactive phosphorus (³²P) to reduce her RCM. Four

months later, her Hb and HCT had returned to the reference range: 13.6 g/dL and 0.41 L/L, respectively.

1. What is the most likely diagnosis? Why?
2. Were any of the patient's symptoms or physical findings significant in the diagnosis?
3. What other tests might be useful in confirming the diagnosis?
4. Do all of the laboratory criteria fit the classic picture for the most likely diagnosis? If not, which do not and why?
5. Was the treatment unusual in this case?

REFERENCES

1. Adamson JW, Fialkow PJ, Murphy S et al: Polycythemia vera: Stem cell and probable clonal origin of the disease. N Engl J Med 295:913, 1976
2. Altman AJ, Baehner RL: In vitro colony-forming characteristics of chronic granulocytic leukemia in childhood. J Pediatr 86:221, 1975
3. Altman AJ, Palmer CG, Baehner RL: Juvenile "chronic granulocytic" leukemia: A panmyelopathy with prominent monocytic involvement and circulating monocyte colony-forming cells. Blood 43:341, 1974
4. Bareford D, Jacobs B: Chronic neutrophilic leukemia. Am J Clin Pathol 73:837, 1980
5. Bartram CR, Carbonell F: bcr rearrangement in Ph¹ negative CML. Cancer Genet Cytogenet 21:183, 1986
6. Beck WS: Hematology, 3rd ed. Cambridge, MIT Press, 1983
7. Bennett JM, Catovsky D, Daniel MT et al: Proposals for the classification of the myelodysplastic syndromes. Br J Haematol 51:189, 1982
8. Bently SA: Aplasia, hypoplasia, and myelofibrosis. In Koepke JA (ed): Laboratory Hematology, vol 1, p 129. New York, Churchill Livingstone, 1984
9. Berk PD, Goldberg JD, Donovan PB et al: Therapeutic recommendations in polycythemia vera based on Polycythemia Vera Study Group protocols. Semin Hematol 23:132, 1986
10. Berk PD, Goldberg JD, Silverstein MN et al: Increased incidence of acute leukemia in polycythemia vera associated with chlorambucil therapy. N Engl J Med 304:441, 1981
11. Berlin NI: Diagnosis and classification of the polycythemias. Semin Hematol 12:339, 1975
12. Brunning RD: Chronic myelogenous leukemia. In Koepke JA (ed): Laboratory Hematology, vol 1, p 289. New York, Churchill Livingstone, 1984
13. Castro-Malaspina H, Moore MAS: [Pathophysiological mechanisms operating in the development of myelofibrosis: Role of megakaryocytes.] Nouv Rev Fr Hématol 24:221, 1982
14. Castro-Malaspina H, Rabellino EM, Yen A et al: Human megakaryocyte stimulation of proliferation of bone marrow fibroblasts. Blood 57:781, 1981
15. Cervantes F, Roman C: A multivariate analysis of prognostic factors in chronic myeloid leukemia. Blood 60:1298, 1982
16. Champlin R, Mitsuyasu R, Elashoff R et al: The role of bone marrow transplantation in the treatment of chronic myelogenous leukemia. In Gale RP (ed): Recent Advances in Bone Marrow Transplantation, p 141. New York, Alan R Liss, 1983
17. Champlin RE, Gale RP: Role of bone marrow transplantation in the treatment of hematologic malignancies and solid tumors: Critical review of syngeneic, autologous, and allogeneic transplants. Cancer Treat Rep 68:145, 1984
18. Chievitz E, Thiede T: Complications and causes of death in polycythaemia vera. Acta Med Scand 172:513, 1962
19. Dameshek W: Some speculations on the myeloproliferative syndrome. Blood 6:372, 1951
20. Dotten DA, Pruzanski W, Wong D: Functional characterization of cells in chronic neutrophilic leukemia. Am J Hematol 12:157, 1982

21. Douer D, Levin AM, Sparkes RS et al: Chronic myelocytic leukaemia: A pluripotent haemopoietic cell is involved in the malignant clone. Br J Haematol 49:615, 1981

22. Dover GJ, Boyer SH, Zinkham WH et al: Changing erythrocyte populations in juvenile chronic myelocytic leukemia: Evidence for disordered regulation. Blood 49:355, 1977

23. Dutcher JP, Wiernik PH: Leukemia. In Spivak JL (ed): Fundamentals of Clinical Hematology, 2nd ed, p 229. Philadelphia, Harper & Row, 1984

24. Ellis JT, Peterson P, Geller SA et al: Studies of the bone marrow in polycythemia vera and the evolution of myelofibrosis and second hematologic malignancies. Semin Hematol 23:144, 1986

25. Ezdinli EZ, Sokal JE, Crosswhite L et al: Philadelphia chromosome-positive and -negative chronic myelocytic leukemia. Ann Intern Med 72:175, 1970

26. Fanger H, Cella LJ Jr, Litchman H: Thrombocythemia: Report of three cases and review of the literature. N Engl J Med 250:456, 1954

27. Fefer A, Cheever MA, Greenberg PD et al: Treatment of chronic granulocytic leukemia with chemoradiotherapy and transplantation of marrow from identical twins. N Engl J Med 306:63, 1982

28. Feldman F: Myelosclerosis in agnogenic myeloid metaplasia. Semin Roentgenol 9:195, 1974

29. Feremans W, Marceles L, Ardichvili D: CNL with enlarged lymph nodes and lysozyme deficiency. Am J Clin Pathol 36:324, 1983

30. Fialkow PJ: Clonal and stem cell origin of blood cell neoplasms. In Lobue J, Gordon AS, Silber R et al (eds): Contemporary Hematology/Oncology, vol 1, p 1. New York, Plenum Publishing, 1980

31. Franklin DZ, Greaves MF, Grossi CE et al: Atlas of Blood Cells, vol 2, p 605. Philadelphia, Lea & Febiger, 1981

32. Ganesan TS, Rassool F, Guo AP et al: Rearrangement of the bcr gene in Philadelphia chromosome-negative chronic myeloid leukemia. Blood 68:957, 1986

33. Goldman JM, Catovsky D, Goolden AW et al: Buffy coat autografts for patients with chronic granulocytic leukaemia in transformation. Blut 42:149, 1981

34. Goldman JM, Kearney L, Pittman S et al: Haemopoietic stem cell grafting for chronic granulocytic leukaemia: Clinical results and cytogenetic findings. Exp Hematol 10(suppl 10):76, 1982

35. Griffin JD, Todd RF, Ritz J et al: Differentiation patterns in the blastic phase of chronic myelogenous leukemia. Blood 61:85, 1983

36. Grignani F: Chronic myelogenous leukemia. CRC Crit Rev Hematol Oncol 4:31, 1985

37. Gunz FW: Hemorrhagic thrombocythemia: A critical review. Blood 15:706, 1960

38. Hall R, Malia RG: Medical Laboratory Hematology, p 414. Boston, Butterworths, 1984

39. Hayhoe FGJ, Flemans RJ: An Atlas of Hematological Cytology, p 206. New York, John Wiley & Sons, 1970

40. Hennessy TG, Stern WE, Herrick SE: Cerebellar hemangioblastoma: Erythropoietic activity by radioiron assay. J Nucl Med 8:601, 1967

41. Hoffbrand AV, Pettit JE: Myeloproliferative disorders. In Essential Haematology, 2nd ed, p 182. Boston, Blackwell Scientific, 1984

42. Jacobson RJ, Salo A, Fialkow PJ: Agnogenic myeloid metaplasia: A clonal proliferation of hematopoietic stem cells with secondary myelofibrosis. Blood 51:189, 1978

43. Jacquillat C, Chastang C, Tanzer J et al: Facteurs prognostic de la leucémie myéloid chronique. À propos de 798 observations. Nouv Rev Fr Hématol 15:229, 1975

44. Kamada N, Uchino H: Chronological sequence in appearance of clinical and laboratory findings characteristic of chronic myelogenous leukemia. Blood 51:843, 1978

45. Kaplan ME, Mack K, Goldberg JD et al: Long term management of polycythemia vera with hydroxyurea: A progress report. Semin Hematol 23:167, 1986

46. Kaplin DR, Chao FC, Stiles CD et al: Platelet alpha granules contain a growth factor for fibroblasts. Blood 53:1043, 1979

47. Kahn A, Bernard JF, Cottreau D et al: A deficient G-6PD variant with hemizygous expression in blood cells of a woman with primary myelofibrosis. Humangenetik 30:41, 1975

48. Klingemann HG, Storb R, Fefer A et al: Bone marrow transplantation in patients aged 45 years and older. Blood 67:770, 1986

49. Koeffler HP, Golde DW: Chronic myelogenous leukemia—New concepts. N Engl J Med 304:1269, 1981

50. Koeffler HP, Goldwasser E: Erythropoietin radioimmunoassay in evaluating patients with polycythemia. Ann Intern Med 94:44, 1981

51. Körbling M, Burke P, Braine H et al: Successful engraftment of blood derived normal hemopoietic stem cells in chronic myelogenous leukemia. Exp Hematol 9:684, 1981

52. Kough RH: Idiopathic myelofibrosis with myeloid metaplasia of the spleen: A disease entity being recognized with increasing frequency. Med Times 94:489, 1966

53. Lanzkowsky P: Pediatric Hematology Oncology, p 338. New York, McGraw-Hill, 1980

54. Lascari AD: Hematologic Manifestations of Childhood Diseases, p 338. New York, Thieme-Stratton, 1984

55. Lawler SD: Significance of chromosome abnormalities in leukemia. Semin Hematol 10:257, 1982

56. Leeburg WT: Micromegakaryocytes: ASCP Check Sample, Hematology 25:1, 1983

57. McGlave PB, Brunning RD, Hurd DD et al: Reversal of severe bone marrow fibrosis and osteosclerosis following allogeneic bone marrow transplantation for chronic granulocytic leukaemia. Br J Haematol 52:189, 1982

58. Mehrotra DA, Winfield DA, Fergusson LH: Cellular abnormalities and reduced colony-forming cells in chronic neutrophilic leukaemia. Acta Haematol 73:47, 1985

59. Miale JB: Aplastic anemia, myeloproliferative disorders, leukemia, and lymphoma. In Laboratory Medicine, 6th ed, p 699. St Louis, CV Mosby, 1982

60. Mirand EA, Murphy GP, Steeves RA et al: Extra-renal production of erythropoietin in man. Acta Haematol 39:359, 1968

61. Monfardini S, Gee T, Fried J et al: Survival in chronic myelogenous leukemia: Influence of treatment and extent of disease at diagnosis. Cancer 31:492, 1973

62. Morris CM, Reeve AE, Fitzgerald PH et al: Genomic diversity correlates with clinical variation in Ph[1]-negative chronic myeloid leukaemia. Nature 320:281, 1986

63. Mulder H, Steenberger J, Haanen C: Clinical course and survival after elective splenectomy in 19 patients with primary myelofibrosis. Br J Haematol 35:419, 1977

64. Murphy S: Hemopoietic stem cell disorders: Myeloproliferative disorders, polycythemia vera. In Williams WJ, Beutler E, Erslev AJ et al (eds): Hematology, 4th ed, p 193. New York, McGraw-Hill, 1990

65. Murphy S, Iland H, Rosenthal D et al: Essential thrombocythemia: An interim report from the Polycythemia Vera Study Group. Semin Hematol 23:177, 1986

66. Oblon DJ, Elfenbein GJ, Braylan RC et al: The reversal of myelofibrosis associated with chronic myelogenous leukemia after allogeneic bone marrow transplantation. Exp Hematol 11:681, 1983

67. O'Donnell MR, Nademanee AP, Snyder DS et al: Bone marrow transplantation for myelodysplastic and myeloproliferative syndromes. J Clin Oncol 5:1822, 1987

68. Okazaki N, Ozaki H, Arima M et al: Hepatocellular carcinoma

associated with erythrocytosis: A nine year survival after successful chemotherapy and left lateral hepatectomy. Acta Hepato-Gastroenterol 26:248, 1979

69. Ossias AL, Zanjani ED, Zalusky R et al: Case report: Studies on the mechanism of erythrocytosis associated with a uterine fibromyoma. Br J Haematol 25:179, 1973

70. Pareti FI, Mannucci PM, Asti D et al: Acquired storage pool disease in myeloproliferative disorders. Thromb Haemost 42:44, 1979

71. Peterson P, McIntyre OR: Myeloproliferative disorders, p 6. Publication for the ASCP National Meeting, 1987

72. Pugh WC, Pearson M, Vardiman JW et al: Philadelphia chromosome-negative chronic myelogenous leukaemia: A morphological reassessment. Br J Haematol 60:457, 1985

73. Ragni MV, Shreiner DP: Spontaneous remission of agnogenic myeloid metaplasia and termination in acute myeloid leukemia. Arch Intern Med 141:1481, 1981

74. Rajantie J, Sale GE, Deeg HJ et al: Adverse effect of severe marrow fibrosis on hematologic recovery after chemradiotherapy and allogeneic bone marrow transplantation. Blood 67:1693, 1986

75. Rani S, Beohar PC, Mohanty TK et al: Chronic myelogenous leukaemia in infancy and childhood: A 10-year study at New Delhi, India. Acta Haematol 66:233, 1981

76. Rappeport J, Parkman R, Belli J et al: Reversibility of myelofibrosis (MF) after bone marrow transplantation (BM Tx). Blood 52(suppl 1):271,1978

77. Richards JD, Linch DC, Goldstone AH: A synopsis of haematology. In Myeloproliferative and Allied Disorders, p 116. Boston, Wright P.S.G., 1983

78. Ross R, Vogel A: The platelet-derived growth factor. Cell 14:203, 1978

79. Rosse WF, Waldmann TA, Cohen P: Renal cysts, erythropoietin, and polycythemia. Am J Med 34:76, 1963

80. Rowley JD: Nonrandom chromosome changes in hematologic diseases. In Franklin DZ, Greaves MF, Grossi CE et al (eds): Atlas of Blood Cells, vol 2, p 605. Philadelphia, Lea & Febiger, 1981

81. Scher CD, Shepard RC, Antoniades HN et al: Platelet-derived growth factor and the regulation of the mammalian fibroblast cell cycle. Biochim Biophys Acta 560:217, 1979

82. Scott D, Theologides A: Hepatoma, erythrocytosis and increased serum erythropoietin developing in long standing hemochromatosis. Am J Gastroenterol 61:206, 1974

83. Shapira Y, Polliack A, Cividalli G et al: Juvenile myeloid leukemia with fetal erythropoiesis. Cancer 30:353, 1972

84. Shindo T, Sakai C, Shibata A: Neutrophilic leukemia and blastic crisis. Ann Intern Med 87:66, 1977

85. Silverstein MN, Goldberg JD, Balcerzak SP et al: The incidence of acute leukemia in a randomized clinical trial for polycythemia vera. Blood 54 (suppl 1):209a, 1979 (abstract)

86. Silverstein M: Primary thrombocythemia. In Williams WJ, Beutler E, Erslev AJ, Lichtman MA (eds): Hematology, 3rd ed, p 218. New York, McGraw-Hill, 1983

87. Silverstein MN: Postpolycythemia myeloid metaplasia. Arch Intern Med 134:113, 1974

88. Silverstein MN, ReMine WH: Splenectomy in myeloid metaplasia. Blood 53:515, 1979

89. Sjögren U, Brandt L, Mitelman F: Relation between life expectancy and composition of the bone marrow at diagnosis of chronic myeloid leukaemia. Scand J Haematol 12:369, 1974

90. Smith JR, Landaw SA: Smokers' polycythemia. N Engl J Med 298:6, 1978

91. Sokal JE, Cox EB, Baccarani M et al: Prognostic discriminators in "good risk" chronic granulocytic leukemia. Blood 63:789, 1984

92. Speck B, Gratwohl A, Osterwalder B et al: Bone marrow transplantation for chronic myeloid leukemia. Semin Hematol 21:48, 1984

93. Spiers ASD: The clinical features of chronic granulocytic leukemia. Clin Hematol 6:17, 1977

94. Spivak JL: Erythrocytosis and polycythemia. In Fundamentals of Clinical Hematology, 2nd ed, p 115. Philadelphia, Harper & Row, 1984

95. Stein R: Granulocytosis and granulocytic leukemoid reactions. In Koepke JA (ed): Laboratory Hematology, vol 1, p 153. New York, Churchill Livingstone, 1984

96. Sun NCJ: Right lower lung infiltrate with leukoerythroblastosis. In Hematology—An Atlas and Diagnostic Guide, p 158. Philadelphia, WB Saunders, 1983

97. Tso SC, Hua ASP: Erythrocytosis in hepatocellular carcinoma: A compensatory phenomenon. Br J Haematol 28:497, 1974

98. Tura S, Baccarani M, Corbelli G et al: Staging of chronic myeloid leukaemia. Br J Haematol 47:105, 1981

99. Volkova MA: [Analysis of the factor influencing longevity in chronic myeloid leukemia.] Ter Arkh 48:61, 1976

100. Ward HP, Block MH: The natural history of agnogenic myeloid metaplasia. Medicine 50:357, 1971

101. Wasserman LR: The management of polycythaemia vera. Br J Haematol 21:371, 1971

102. Wasserman LR, Balcerzak SP, Berlin NI et al: Influence of therapy on causes of death in polycythemia vera. Trans Assoc Am Physicians 94:30, 1981

103. Wintrobe MM: Chronic myeloid leukemia. In Wintrobe MM, Lee GR, Boggs DR et al: Clinical Hematology, 8th ed, p 1565. Philadelphia, Lea & Febiger, 1981

104. You W, Weisbrot IM: Chronic neutrophilic leukemia. Report of 2 cases and review of the literature. Am J Clin Pathol 72:233, 1979

PART VIII

MALIGNANT

LYMPHOPROLIFERATIVE

DISORDERS

Acute

Lymphoblastic

Leukemias

Anne S. Hobson

Acute lymphoblastic leukemia (ALL) is a malignant disease of the lymphopoietic system that is manifested by the slow but uncontrolled growth of abnormal lymphoid cells in the bone marrow, spleen, and lymph nodes. The DNA synthesis time in the lymphoblast is significantly longer than in normal tissues.[8] In the acute leukemias, the immature blast form predominates, and normal bone marrow elements usually are replaced or displaced by the abnormal cells. Acute lymphoblastic leukemia is predominantly a disease of children, although improved immunologic and cytochemical methods of identification have increased the frequency of diagnosis in adults. Acute lymphoblastic leukemia is the most common malignant disease in children[10] and occurs most frequently between the ages of 2 and 10 years.

This chapter will address the clinical manifestations, laboratory findings, and differential diagnosis of ALL, with a description of the various classification systems. Finally, therapy for ALL and its effects on laboratory results will be discussed.

CLINICAL MANIFESTATIONS

The clinical features of ALL do not differ substantially from those of other types of acute leukemia, but their onset usually is more sudden. Prodromal or preleukemic symptoms are more often associated with nonlymphocytic leukemias. Many of the signs and symptoms of ALL can be related to the replacement of normal hematopoietic elements in the bone marrow by abnormal lymphoid cells. This results in decreases in red cells (anemia), phagocytes (granulocytopenia), and platelets (thrombocytopenia). The most common presenting symptoms for ALL are malaise, fatigue, and pallor that usually are related to the degree of anemia present. Granulocytopenia renders the patient vulnerable to infection that may be accompanied by chills and fever. Easy bruising, petechiae, epistaxis, and other hemorrhagic conditions may also be presenting signs. The severity of the hemorrhagic complications correlates with the degree of thrombocytopenia. Weight loss generally is seen but is not so severe as to cause the patient to see a physician. Bone pain, sternal tenderness and swelling, or tenderness of the large joints may occur. Cranial nerve paralysis, increased intracranial pressure, fundic (eye) hemorrhage, or other neurologic symptoms resulting from meningeal infiltration by leukemic cells may be present. Physical examination usually reveals enlargement of the superficial lymph nodes, as well as splenomegaly and hepatomegaly.

CAUSES OF DEATH

A serious complication in ALL is infection, the incidence of which is directly related to the degree of granulocytopenia. Organisms causing sepsis during induction therapy include *Staphylococcus aureus*, *Pseudomonas aeruginosa*, *Candida albicans*, *Haemophilus influenzae*, *Proteus mirabilis*, and species of *Klebsiella*. Patients in remission after long-term immunosuppressive chemotherapy are at risk for infection by a wide variety of bacteria, viruses, and fungi.

Bleeding is the second significant complication, usually as a result of thrombocytopenia. Spontaneous bleeding can occur when the platelet count falls below $50 \times 10^9/L$ but becomes more likely when the count is less than $20 \times 10^9/L$. The presence of a high leukemic blast count or infection tends to increase the risk of hemorrhage. Salicylates and other drugs that impair platelet function may be contributing factors. Leukemic infiltration of the liver may decrease hepatic function and interfere with the synthesis of the vitamin K-dependent clotting factors.

LABORATORY FINDINGS

The total leukocyte count is elevated ($>10.0 \times 10^9/L$) in approximately 60% of patients. About 15% of patients have markedly increased leukocyte counts ($>100.0 \times 10^9/L$), but approximately 25% are leukopenic ($<5.0 \times 10^9/L$). The leukemic lymphoid blast is the predominant circulating cell except in the leukopenic patients, in whom an aleukemic leukemia may exist with few or no circulating lymphoblasts.

The bone marrow in ALL is almost always hypercellular and heavily infiltrated with, or even replaced by, lymphoid cells. Fibrosis is present in 10% to 15% of cases, particularly in patients with bone pain.[3] Thrombocytopenia and anemia are almost always present at the time of diagnosis, with normal marrow elements usually reduced in number or appearing to have been totally replaced. A detailed description of the morphologic criteria used to distinguish ALL according to FAB classification is found later in this chapter.

Acute lymphoblastic leukemia must be differentiated from other causes of lymphoid leukocytosis in the peripheral blood. Lymphoid leukocytosis or lymphocytosis occurs in pertussis, as well as in infectious lymphocytosis, infectious mononucleosis, and other viral diseases. These reactive disorders may also be accompanied by fever, enlarged superficial lymph nodes, and splenomegaly. In general, however, the bone marrow is minimally affected in these conditions and does not show a predominance of immature cells. Infectious mononucleosis may be associated with an autoimmune anemia and thrombocytopenia with immature-appearing lymphocytes in the peripheral blood; however, the pleomorphic morphology of the variant lymphocytes and serologic tests for the heterophil antibody will help to distinguish this condition.

Adult ALL differs from that seen most frequently in children in that it is more often associated with increased leukocyte counts, a null or unclassified type, the Philadelphia chromosome (Ph[1]), and L2 morphology (see below). The differential diagnosis of ALL in the adult is difficult; the condition must be distinguished from such entities as leukemic lymphoma, subacute or blastic transformation in chronic lymphocytic leukemia, and hairy cell leukemia.

Occasionally, patients with solid tumors that metastasize to bone marrow, such as Ewing's sarcoma, embryonal rhabdomyosarcoma, and neuroblastoma (small cell carcinoma), have bone marrow infiltration by tumor cells that are morphologically similar to those in ALL. The presence of leukoerythroblastic abnormalities in the peripheral blood and clumps or clusters of tumor cells in the marrow preparations may be helpful in identifying metastatic tumor.

In the past the diagnosis of ALL required good bone marrow and peripheral blood preparations and was based solely on morphology in Romanowsky-stained preparations. Today, although these preparations are still important, the use of cytochemical and immunologic markers for the classification or subclassification of ALL has assumed significant if not equal importance. These techniques undoubtedly will have greater clinical application as knowledge of immature cells increases and the ability to target treatment for leukemic diseases is developed more fully.

CLASSIFICATION OF ACUTE LYMPHOBLASTIC LEUKEMIA

Morphologic Classification (FAB)

With the advent in the 1960s of chemotherapeutic drugs for the treatment of acute leukemia and the development of cytochemical stains to identify immature cells, a uniform system for the classification of acute leukemias became necessary. It was necessary to establish uniform criteria for the different types of acute leukemias so as to correlate responses to treatment and prognosis in patients at various medical centers. The French-American-British (FAB) system was developed and has come into general use for the morphologic classification of acute leukemia.[1]

The FAB classification divides lymphoblastic leukemias into three types: L1, L2, and L3.[2] These types are defined according to two criteria: (1) the occurrence of individual cytologic features, and (2) the degree of heterogeneity in distribution among the leukemic cell population of some or all of these cytologic features. The features considered are cell size, chromatin, nuclear shape, nucleoli, degree of basophilia in the cytoplasm, and the presence of cytoplasmic vacuolation. As many as 10% of the cells are allowed to

TABLE 36–1. Features of Acute Lymphoblastic Leukemias

CYTOLOGIC FEATURE	L1	L2	L3
Cell size★	Small cells predominate	Large, heterogeneous	Large and homogeneous
Chromatin	Homogeneous in any one case	Variable: heterogeneous in any one case	Finely stippled and homogeneous
Nuclear shape★	Regular; occasional clefting or indentation	Irregular; clefting and indentation common	Regular, oval to round
Nucleoli★	Not visible or small and inconspicuous	One or more present, often large	Prominent; one or more; vesicular
Amount of cytoplasm★	Scanty	Variable; often moderately abundant	Moderately abundant
Basophilia of cytoplasm	Slight or moderate; rarely, intense	Variable; deep in some	Very deep
Cytoplasmic vacuolation	Variable	Variable	Often prominent

★ Most useful features for differentiating L1 and L2 subtypes.
From Bennett JM, Catovsky D, Daniel MT et al: Proposal for the classification of adult leukaemia. Br J Haematol 33:451, 1976; by permission of Blackwell Scientific Publications Limited.

depart from the characteristics of the proposed cell type (Table 36-1).

It should be emphasized at this point that satisfactory blood films are imperative, because preparations that are too thick or not dried properly can mask the presence of these lymphoblasts, the result being that they are misidentified as lymphocytes.

Type L1: Small Cell, Homogeneous

In L1 the blasts are predominantly small: up to twice the diameter of a small lymphocyte. They are generally uniform, and this lack of variation in size creates a homogenous picture of similar cells. The chromatin is usually finely dispersed but may appear more clumped in smaller cells. Chromatin and cell size may show variation from case to case, but the homogenous features within each particular case are a primary feature. Nuclear shape is regular; however, there may be some degree of clefting, folding, or indentation. Nucleoli often are not visible or, if present, are small and indistinct. The cytoplasm is usually scanty (high nuclear:cytoplasmic ratio) and only slightly to moderately basophilic. Cytoplasmic vacuoles may or may not be present (Plate 54). The L1 type is the acute leukemia common in childhood, and 74% of the cases occur in children 15 years of age or younger.[2] Of the three classes of ALL, L1 generally has the best prognosis, as it responds best to therapy.

Type L2: Large Cell, Heterogeneous

In L2, the majority of immature cells are more than twice the diameter of a small lymphocyte. In many cases, there is a marked heterogeneity of cell size. Chromatin ranges from fine and dispersed to coarse and condensed, thus presenting a mixed picture. Nuclear clefting, indentation, and folding are characteristic, and gross irregularities of nuclear shape are common. Nucleoli are nearly always visible and of various sizes and numbers. The degree of cytoplasmic basophilia is also variable (Plate 55). Approximately 66% of the cases of ALL in patients older than 15 years are of Type L2.

A simple identification system for Types L1 and L2 has been proposed based on four features: (1) nuclear:cytoplas-

mic ratio; (2) presence, prominence, and frequency of nucleoli; (3) regularity of nuclear outline; and (4) cell size (see Table 36-1).[2] Using this system, correct classification of Types L1 and L2 was increased from 63% to 84% among trained hematologists.

Type L3: Burkitt Type

The Burkitt form is a relatively rare type of ALL (3%–5% of cases). The blasts are large and present a characteristically homogeneous picture. They have a dense but rather finely stippled chromatin. The nucleus is oval to round, with a regular contour. One or more prominent vesicular nucleoli are visible in most cells. The cytoplasm is intensely basophilic and moderately abundant. Cytoplasmic as well as nuclear vacuolation is often prominent (Plate 56). These vacuoles stain positively with oil red O, making this stain valuable in the diagnosis of Burkitt leukemia (L3) or lymphoma. By immunologic markers, these are B-cell malignancies. A high mitotic index (approximately 5%) is characteristic. Patients with L3 leukemias generally have a poor prognosis, as their disease responds poorly to chemotherapy.

Cytochemical Classification

In differentiating the ALLs from the nonlymphoblastic leukemias, the myeloperoxidase stain may be helpful. The abnormal lymphoid cells of lymphoblastic leukemia are negative in this study. Very immature myeloid blasts may also be negative; therefore, only positive myeloperoxidase staining is helpful in that it rules out lymphoblasts. Sudan black B may be used instead of myeloperoxidase, because the staining reactions are generally similar; however, some ALLs are weakly positive with Sudan black B.

The periodic acid-Schiff (PAS) stain is very important in the laboratory investigation of L1 and L2 ALL. Staining is strongly positive in L1, being present as chunks or granules in a significant number of blasts. When scored 1 to 4 on the basis of increasing granule size, L1 has a high score. In L2 the degree of positivity and the percentage of cells stained may be quite low—10% or less.

Acid phosphatase is positive in ALL and has a localized

pattern of positivity in the Golgi region in T-cell ALL. Otherwise, it shows a diffuse pattern that also is present in myeloid cells. Thus, the usefulness of this stain is limited.[6]

Nonspecific esterase (NSE) staining produces an area of focal positivity in T lymphocytes. The stain has diagnostic value in distinguishing M5 (acute monocytic leukemia) from L2, because in M5, the cytoplasm is diffusely stained.

Terminal deoxynucleotidyl transferase (TdT) is an intranuclear enzyme that catalyzes the addition of deoxynucleotides to the 3'hydroxy end of oligonucleotides or polydeoxynucleotides without the need of a template. Activity can be detected in human thymocytes, primitive lymphocytes, and a small number of other cells in bone marrow.[4] In hematopoietic malignancies, strong TdT activity is seen in approximately 90% of ALL cases, as well as in lymphoblastic lymphomas. Because this enzyme is not unique to T lymphocytes but is a helpful lymphoid marker, it is especially useful in the "lymphoblastic transformation" of chronic myelogenous leukemia (CML).

Immunologic Marker Classification

Monoclonal antibody techniques that demonstrate immunologic markers on the cell surface are increasing our knowledge of cell differentiation and maturation. The use of surface immunoglobulin (SIg) for the identification of B lymphocytes and of sheep erythrocyte rosettes to detect T lymphocytes reveals that the majority of ALLs are non-B, non-T; that is, they lack these B-cell and T-cell markers. It should be noted, however, that the formation of spontaneous rosettes with sheep erythrocytes may not be totally specific to T cells.[14]

A monoclonal antibody to what is known as common acute lymphoblastic leukemia antigen (CALLA) was produced by immunization of rabbits with SIg- and E-rosette-negative ALL cells.[13] The antigen defined by these antisera has a molecular weight of 98,000 and is present on the leukemic cells of 70% of patients with ALL. The CALLA is not present on normal peripheral blood lymphocytes; however, it is not specific to leukemia, as it has been found on normal bone marrow cells that are positive for TdT and HLA-DR (Ia-like) antigen. Because anti-HLA-DR and other monoclonal antibodies are not specific for a certain cell line but crossreact with cells from other hematopoietic cell lines, a battery of monoclonal antibodies is needed to establish cell lineage[20] (Table 36-2). Using a combination of immunologic and cytochemical markers, ALL can be subclassified into six distinct classes.[9,13]

1. Null or unclassified ALL (uALL) is characterized by the absence of T antigens, SIg, and CALLA. Approximately 10% of all childhood and 40% of adult cases of ALL fall into this category.
2. Common ALL (cALL) is characterized by the presence of CALLA, HLA-DR, and TdT. This type accounts for approximately 75% of childhood and 40% of adult ALL. Common ALL has the highest remission rate and the longest initial remission with chemotherapy. About 1 in 10 adults having common ALL have a tumor chromosome that appears identical to the Ph[1], which places them in a subgroup with a poor prognosis.[17]
3. T ALL has both T-cell antigen and the sheep erythrocyte receptor. This type accounts for about 15% of both childhood and adult ALL. The incidence is much higher in males, with a 5:1 ratio. About half the patients have a mediastinal (thymic) mass. Very high leukocyte counts are more common in this group, and there is a higher incidence of central nervous system (CNS) involvement. This type carries a much poorer prognosis. There is no correlate in the FAB classification for this class of ALL.
4. Pre-T ALL has T-cell antigen but lacks sheep erythrocyte receptors.
5. Pre-B ALL shows the presence of cytoplasmic immunoglobulin (CIg) and the absence of SIg.
6. B ALL has both SIg and the B-cell antigen. This group accounts for less than 5% of ALL cases and corresponds to the FAB classification L3.

Much of the sophisticated subclassification of acute leukemia is done using monoclonal antibodies and cell sorters. Under development are immunocytochemical methods employing immunoperoxidase, avidin-biotin, and immunogold techniques with monoclonal antibodies applied to air-dried blood and bone marrow smears. These methods

TABLE 36–2. Markers Useful for Subclassification of ALL (TdT+, PAS±, OKM1−, Sudan black B−, Peroxidase−)

MARKERS	uALL*	cALL*	PRE-T ALL	T ALL	PRE-B ALL	B ALL
Sheep erythrocyte receptors	−	−	−	+	−	−
SIg	−	−	−	−	−	+
CIg	−	−	−	−	+	+
TdT	+	+	+	+	+	−
HLA-DR†	+	+	−	−	+	+
CALLA†	−	+	±/−	−	+	
T antigen†	−	−	+	+	−	−
B antigen†	−	±	−	−	+	+
Focal acid phosphatase	−	−	+	+	−	−
Acid alpha-naphthyl acetate esterase	−	−	−	±	−	−
Morphology	L1/L2	L1/L2	L1/L2	L1/L2	L1/L2	L3

+, positive; −, negative; ±, may be a positive or negative reaction.
* uALL, unclassified or undifferentiated ALL; cALL, common ALL.
† Antigens demonstrable by immunoalkaline phosphatase stain with monoclonal antibodies for HLA-DR, OKIa1; CALLA, J5; for T antigen, Leu-1; for B antigen, B1. The OK series is produced by Ortho Diagnostic Systems; J5 and B1 by Coulter Immunology; Leu-1 by Becton Dickinson Monoclonal Center.
From Sun T, Li CY, Yam LT: Atlas of Cytochemistry and Immunochemistry of Hematologic Neoplasms. Chicago, ASCP Press, 1985, with permission.

undoubtedly will become more widespread and may eventually become practical for the routine subtyping of ALL.

Cytogenetic Studies

The laboratory evaluation of the karyotype in ALL has not been used to classify subtypes so much as to predict therapeutic outcomes (prognosis). For example, about one-third of cases of ALL have chromosomal translocations that are associated with much poorer prognosis. Also, the lack of normal karyotypes within a population correlates with a poor prognosis.[19] Translocation to chromosome 8 from 2, 14, or 22 is common in L3 ALL.[18] A translocation between 4 and 11 appears to mark a type of ALL that can evolve into a myeloid or monocytic disease.[15]

EFFECTS OF TREATMENT ON LABORATORY RESULTS

Therapy for ALL can be subdivided into chemotherapy and bone marrow transplantation. The goal is eradication of malignant cells. This is usually accompanied by severe pancytopenia.

Chemotherapy

Before the initiation of therapy, any physiologic imbalance is usually corrected. For example, correction of anemia and thrombocytopenia is accomplished by transfusion of packed red cells and platelets, antibiotic treatment is instituted for infection, and intravenous supplements may be given to restore adequate hydration. Any of these measures may cause changes in cell counts and cellular morphology.

Many forms of ALL respond well to treatment (Table 36–3). In the past, approximately 50% of children with ALL who achieved a first remission and remained disease free after 12 months, relapsed with CNS involvement. Such disease is an extension of the leukemic process with infiltration of the leptomeninges by leukemic cells. The importance of being able to detect CNS involvement as soon as possible has been reflected in the clinical laboratory by the use of the cytocentrifuge to concentrate spinal fluid cells for more sensitive detection of blasts. To prevent CNS involvement, patients now receive prophylactic treatment with intrathecal drug injection and cranial irradiation. With this prophylaxis, the incidence of CNS relapse has been reduced to less than 5%, and the continuous first remission has been greatly prolonged. This prolongation of remission has uncovered a previously undetected sex difference for ALL: females respond more favorably to therapy.[7] One possible cause is testicular sanctuary for the malignant cells during chemotherapy.[16]

Morphologic evidence of chemotherapy includes cytoplasmic fragmentation of lymphoid cells (Fig. 36–1), which may artificially elevate the results of electronic platelet counts. Another morphologic feature of chemotherapy is circulating necrotic lymphoid cells exhibiting nuclear lysis or dense pyknotic nuclei.

Purines are metabolized to uric acid. Therefore, hyperuricemia secondary to high purine turnover may result from increased leukocyte proliferation and from the destruction of leukemic cells by chemotherapy and radiation. Renal failure may result because of uric acid nephropathy.

Bone Marrow Transplantation

Marrow transplantation is usually performed during the first remission or relapse. The laboratory must closely monitor the patient's bone marrow and peripheral blood counts. Insufficient time has elapsed to define the role of bone marrow transplants in ALL. Interestingly, patients experiencing graft-versus-host disease (GVHD) seem to have a lower probability of ALL relapse than those without GVHD if the GVHD is controlled.[5]

Newer Approaches

Recent advances in recombinant DNA research have opened a new area for investigation. With the use of DNA probes for immunoglobulin or T-cell receptor genes, it is possible to recognize clonal populations of malignant T and B cells. This technique offers great promise as a highly sensitive means of early detection of lymphoid malignan-

TABLE 36–3. Drugs Used in the Treatment of ALL

DRUG	CLASS	ANTITUMOR ACTION	TOXIC SIDE EFFECTS
Vincristine	Plant alkaloid	Inhibits RNA synthesis	CNS toxicity, peripheral nerve toxicity, reaction at the injection site, baldness, diabetes, increased susceptibility to infection
Prednisone	Corticosteroid	Lysis of lymphoblasts	Personality changes, fluid retention, hypertension, osteoporosis, gastrointestinal ulcerations
Methotrexate	Folic acid antagonist	Inhibits DNA synthesis	Myelosuppression, megaloblastic changes, oral and gastrointestinal ulcerations, liver toxicity
6-Mercaptopurine (6MP)	Purine antagonist	Interferes with purine synthesis, thus inhibiting RNA and DNA synthesis	Myelosuppression, liver toxicity
Cyclophosphamide	Synthetic alkylating agent	Inhibits DNA synthesis; arrests cells in mitosis	Severe myelosuppression, cystitis, baldness, increased susceptibility to infection
Daunorubicin	Antibiotic	Binds to DNA; inhibits DNA and RNA synthesis	Severe myelosuppression, cardiac toxicity, reaction at the injection site, increased susceptibility to infection, baldness
L-Asparaginase	Enzyme (from a strain of E. coli)	Lysis of lymphoblasts; deprives the cells of L-asparagine	Allergic reaction, liver toxicity, acquired coagulation factor deficiencies, diabetes

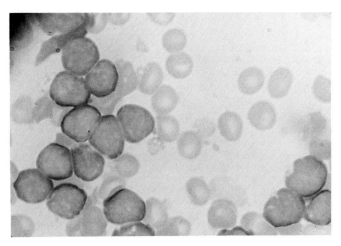

FIG. 36-1.   Cytoplasmic fragmentation in acute lymphoblastic leukemia. Note small, hyaline-like fragments of cytoplasm.

cies. When such probes are combined with the analysis of oncogenes, one can study the relations between events at the DNA–RNA level and the development of neoplasia. This area is now primarily one for investigative research and has not reached the clinical laboratory.

CHAPTER SUMMARY

Acute lymphoblastic leukemia consists of three morphologic types (FAB classification) that can be subclassified into six types using cell-surface markers. The FAB Type L1 is primarily a disease of small children. The cells are small and homogeneous. This type carries a good prognosis. The L2 type is primarily a disease of older children and young adults. Morphologically, the cells are large and heterogeneous. The L3 or Burkitt type is characterized by large cells with very basophilic cytoplasm and numerous vacuoles. Therapy of ALL can cause significant changes in both cell counts and morphology of the predominant cell. Death usually is caused by either infection or bleeding.

CASE STUDY 36-1

A 2.5-year-old girl presented at a primary care clinic with a 1-week history of vomiting, diarrhea, and pallor. Easy bruising and petechiae on her face and trunk had been noted 2 days previously. On the day of admission she felt warm and had been irritable, prompting her parents to bring her to the clinic. Laboratory values were as follows: WBC 105 × 10^9/L; Hb 4.6 g/dL; HCT 0.14 L/L; platelets 23 × 10^9/L; differential: lymphocytes 10%, blasts 90%. The peroxidase stain was negative; acid phosphatase was positive in a diffuse pattern; and PAS was positive. The bone marrow aspirate was heavily infiltrated with lymphoid-appearing blasts. The morphology was described as consistent with L1. Immunologic marker tests showed: CALLA 90%; HLA-DR 93%; and cytoplasmic immunoglobulin positive. E rosette, SIg, IgM, kappa and lambda chains were all less than 10%. The patient responded well to vincristine and prednisone and is in remission.
1. The blasts in this case were said to be "consistent with L1." What does this mean?
2. What might be causing the patient's anemia and thrombocytopenia?
3. Is the child's age consistent with the diagnosis?
4. On the basis of the marker studies, are the cells B, T, pre-B, pre-T, or unclassified?

CASE STUDY 36-2

A 20-year-old man was admitted to a local medical center with a 2- to 3-week history of left upper-quadrant pain and weakness. The patient was noted to have hepatosplenomegaly but no adenopathy. Laboratory data included WBC 37 × 10^9/L; RBC 2.14 × 10^{12}/L; Hb 6.5 g/dL; HCT 0.19 L/L; platelets 112 × 10^9/L; differential: blasts 65%, myelocytes 1%, metamyelocytes 2%, bands 3%, segmented neutrophils 4%, lymphocytes 23%, and monocytes 2%. Occasional NRBCs were seen. The bone marrow aspirate was hypercellular with 74% blast forms. The blasts were consistent with L2; cytochemical stains were consistent with ALL. Marker studies showed SIg 7%, T-cell markers 6% to 14%, CALLA 85%, and HLA-DR 71%.

Despite treatment, the blasts persisted in his peripheral blood. Ten months after diagnosis, he was admitted to the bone marrow transplant unit and given an HLA-identical match from a sister. The patient continues to be well 18 months after transplant.
1. Contrast this case with case 36-1 in terms of FAB classification.
2. What is the prognosis of L2 compared with L1? What treatments have improved survival in ALL?

REFERENCES

1. Bennett JM, Catovsky D, Daniel MT et al: Proposal for the classification of adult leukaemia. Br J Haematol 33:451, 1976
2. Bennett JM, Catovsky D, Daniel MT et al: The morphological classification of acute lymphoblastic leukaemia: Concordance among observers and clinical correlations. Br J Haematol 47:553, 1981
3. Boggs DR, Wintrobe MM, Cartwright CE: The acute leukemias: An analysis of 343 cases and a review of the literature. Medicine 41:163, 1962
4. Bollum FJ: Terminal deoxynucleotidyl transferase as a hematologic cell marker (review). Blood 54:1203, 1979
5. Buckner CD, Cleft RA: Marrow transplantation for acute lymphoblastic leukemia. Semin Hematol 21:43, 1984
6. Catovsky A, Cherchi M, Greaves MF et al: Acid phosphatase reactions in acute lymphoblastic leukaemia. Lancet 1:749, 1978
7. Chessels JM: Acute lymphoblastic leukemia. Semin Hematol 19:155, 1982
8. Dosik GM, Barlogie B, Goehde W et al: Flow cytometry of DNA content in human bone marrow: A critical reappraisal. Blood 55:734, 1980
9. Foon KA, Gale RP, Todd RF III: Recent advances in the immunologic classification of leukemia. Semin Hematol 23: 257, 1986
10. Gale RP: Introduction: Leukemia. Semin Hematol 23: 188, 1986
11. Fraumeni JF Jr, Miller RW: Leukemia mortality: Downward rates in the United States. Science 155:1126, 1967
12. Greaves MF, Brown G, Rapson NT et al: Antisera to acute lymphoblastic leukemia cells. Clin Immunol Immunopathol 4:67, 1975
13. Greaves MF, Janossy G, Peto J et al: Immunologically defined subclasses of acute lymphoblastic leukaemia in children: Relationship to presentation features and prognosis. Br J Haematol 48:179, 1981
14. Guglielmi P, Preud'homme JL, Brouet JC: E-rosette receptor expression by chronic lymphocytic leukemia B lymphocytes. Eur J Immunol 13:641, 1983
15. Kocova M, Kowelezyk JR, Sandberg AA: Translocation 4;11 acute leukemia: Three case reports and review of the literature. Cancer Genet Cytogenet 16:21, 1985
16. Medical Research Council: Testicular disease in acute lymphoblastic leukaemia in childhood. Br Med J 1:334, 1978
17. Rodenhuis S, Smets LA, Slater RM et al: Distinguishing the Philadelphia chromosome of acute lymphoblastic leukemia from its counterpart in chronic myelogenous leukemia. N Engl J Med 313:51, 1985

18. Sandberg A: The chromosomes in human leukemia. Semin Hematol 23:201, 1986

19. Secker-Walker LM, Swanbury GJ, Hardisty RM et al: Cytogenetics of acute lymphoblastic leukaemia in children as a factor in the prediction of long term survival. Br J Haematol 52:398, 1982

20. Sun T, Li CY, Yam LT: Atlas of Cytochemistry and Immunochemistry of Hematologic Neoplasms. Chicago, ASCP Press, 1985

21. Williams WJ, Beutler E, Erslev AJ et al (eds): Hematology, 4th ed, New York, McGraw-Hill, 1990

Chronic

Lymphoproliferative

Leukemic

Disorders

Rita C. East

The hematologic disorders known as chronic lymphoproliferative leukemic disorders (CLLD) are a heterogeneous group from which three distinct disease entities have emerged. Chronic lymphocytic leukemia (CLL), prolymphocytic leukemia (PLL), and hairy cell leukemia (HCL) are generally accepted as separate morphologic and clinicopathologic entities requiring different therapeutic approaches.[12]

Nearly all (99%)[10] of these leukemias are clonal B-lymphocyte diseases; that is, they involve proliferation and accumulation of clones of malignant B lymphocytes in the blood, bone marrow, lymph nodes, or other organs.[21] A much smaller number of the CLLD are caused by T-lymphocyte proliferation. A reduced rate of cell death, rather than an increased rate of cell production, appears to account for the accumulation of these cells.[13] Research with polyclonal and monoclonal antibodies has shown that the B lymphocytes in CLL, PLL, and HCL are malignant equivalents of different stages of normal lymphocyte development, with CLL being the least mature, HCL the most mature, and PLL intermediate in maturity.[1,12,25,29]

It is important to distinguish B-cell malignancies from those caused by T cells, because patients with T-cell disease tend to have a more aggressive disease and a poorer response to therapy.[19,30] It is interesting that cases of CLL[6] and HCL[45] have been reported in which the malignant cells possessed both B- and T-cell markers.

CHRONIC LYMPHOCYTIC LEUKEMIA

The first comprehensive study of CLL was published in 1924 by Minot and Isaacs.[36] This disease has since been recognized as the most common type of leukemia in the Western hemisphere.

Among the important factors in the etiology of CLL are age, male gender, and inherited or acquired immunologic defects that predispose some individuals to disease produced by leukemogenic agents. It appears that ionizing radiation does not cause CLL, but identification of the human T-cell leukemia virus (HTLV) indicates that certain lymphoid malignancies may be viral in origin.[39] Genetic factors may play a significant role in the etiology of some leukemias in man, as multiple instances of leukemia have been reported in some families. Examples of such leukemias are CLL, acute leukemia, and less frequently, other lymphoproliferative diseases.[2,18,28,41,42]

Two relatively common chromosomal abnormalities are found in B-cell CLL. The more frequently encountered is the gain of an extra chromosome 12.[31] The +12 abnormality is a marker for lymphocytic lymphomas in general, not just CLL, and it appears to predict a progressive disease with an early need for treatment.[43] The other cytogenetic abnormality involves various translocations to the end of the long arm of chromosome 14 ($14q^+$) at band 14q32. A number of chromosomes participate in the 14q translocation, but 11;14 with the break in 11q13 seems the most common.[50]

In families in which more than one member has had CLL or another closely related lymphoproliferative disease, some of the apparently healthy kin have immunoglobulin abnormalities or impaired lymphocyte transformation in response to phytohemagglutinin (PHA).[17,18] These immunoglobulin abnormalities may involve qualitative or quantitative changes in serum proteins, abnormal immune responsiveness, and connective tissue vascular diseases.[3,48,54] Because not all individuals who are thus affected develop leukemia, the interaction of environmental and hereditary factors probably is necessary to produce leukemia.

Pathophysiology

Chronic lymphocytic leukemia is the proliferation and accumulation of lymphocytes (usually B cells) that are relatively unresponsive to antigenic stimuli. Consequently, they lie more or less dormant and accumulate in the peripheral blood, bone marrow, lymph nodes, and spleen.[13]

Rarely, CLL is caused by T-cell proliferation. Because T cells are disseminated throughout the circulation, epidermal sites (rash) and the central nervous system (CNS) are more likely to become involved.

Clinical Presentation

Chronic lymphocytic leukemia is a disease primarily of the elderly, with 90% of the patients being over 50 years of age and nearly 65% over 60.[11] Men are affected more than twice as frequently as women.

Symptoms of CLL usually develop so insidiously that the diagnosis often is made unexpectedly during routine or other examinations. Fatigue and reduced exercise tolerance are the most common presenting symptoms. Marked fatigue, bruising, pallor, or jaundice associated with anemia, fever, recurrent or persistent infection, bone tenderness, weight loss, and edema from lymph node obstruction may be seen in those patients with more advanced disease. Erythroderma with pruritus is common with T-cell CLL.

The clinical course of CLL may range from almost completely benign to severe. Approximately 10% to 15% of patients live 10 to 15 years in relatively good health with little or no treatment, whereas a slightly greater percentage have more aggressive disease and die within a year.[27,34] The median survival after diagnosis is 3 to 4 years.[27]

Chronic lymphocytic leukemia is less likely to undergo acute exacerbation than are other leukemias, regardless of whether treatment has been instituted.[38] "Prolymphocytoid transformation" of otherwise typical B-CLL has been reported.[14] However, in cases of transforming CLL, the "prolymphocytes" are not always morphologically typical prolymphocytes, such as are seen in classic PLL, and these cells also are phenotypically different from classic prolymphocytes.[9,14]

Physical Findings

In early presentation of CLL, the most common signs are enlarged lymph nodes and splenomegaly. As the disease progresses, the lymph nodes become larger, and new areas of nodal enlargement appear. Splenomegaly usually increases, and hepatomegaly develops. Lymphoid cells may infiltrate other organs such as the gonads, skin, prostate, kidney, and walls of the gastrointestinal tract.

Laboratory Findings and Correlations with Disease

Chronic lymphocytic leukemia is commonly diagnosed by finding a persistent lymphocytosis in the peripheral blood. An absolute lymphocyte count between 10 and $150 \times 10^9/L$ is usual with CLL, but counts as high as $1000 \times 10^9/L$ may be encountered with untreated aggressive disease.[52]

Morphologically, these lymphocytes may appear virtually normal, especially in patients with mild disease. Usually, however, the lymphocytes are somewhat larger than normal, have nuclei with clumped or condensed chromatin, and may have prominent nucleoli. The cytoplasm may be abundant, nongranular, and moderately basophilic, or it may be relatively scanty. Patients with aggressive disease may have tiny lymphocytes with little cytoplasm and cleft nuclei suggesting a follicular cell origin.[35] The lymphocytes in CLL appear to be somewhat more fragile than normal, and blood films usually contain large numbers of "smudge" cells (lymphocytes broken when the film was made; Plate 57). Although CLL lymphocytes can differ morphologically from patient to patient, they usually are monotonously similar in any given patient. This attests to the clonal origin of the disease.

The percentage of neutrophils is often decreased, but absolute numbers usually are normal or slightly increased, especially in the early stages of the disease.[5]

Patients with aggressive or advanced disease often have granulocytopenia, anemia, or thrombocytopenia when lymphoid tissue fills 50% or more of the marrow space. These cytopenias are especially troublesome after blood loss, treatment with antineoplastic drugs, or infection.

Besides decreased red cell production, anemia is often the result of sequestration of red cells in lymphoid tissue or shortened red cell survival. Autoimmune hemolysis is a third factor, which may account for anemia in 5% to 10% of those patients who have aggressive or advanced disease.[55] Such autoimmune responses may be triggered by viral infections, disease progression, therapeutic agents, or membrane damage by abnormal proteins.[33,34,47,56] Laboratory findings in autoimmune hemolytic anemia include reticulocytosis, often spherocytosis, mild jaundice, shortened red cell survival, bone marrow erythroid hyperplasia, and a positive direct antiglobulin (Coombs) test.

In CLL, the lymphocytes contain more glycogen than usual, thus giving a positive staining reaction with the periodic acid-Schiff (PAS) stain.

Plasma immunoglobulins may be reduced, especially as the disease progresses. Gamma globulin levels may fall to 0.3 to 0.4 g/dL (reference range 0.8–1.6 g/dL), and patients become more susceptible to all types of infection.

Bone marrow aspiration and biopsy usually is not necessary for making the diagnosis of CLL except in those "aleukemic" or "subleukemic" cases with no nodal or splenic involvement and few or no abnormal cells in the peripheral blood. The marrow is sometimes the principal site of involvement in these patients.

Infiltration of the marrow usually occurs slowly with progression of disease, but 30% or more lymphocytes in the marrow, when accompanied by a sustained lymphocytosis in the peripheral blood, is considered diagnostic of CLL. Lymphocytes increase in number until normal marrow cells are crowded out. Eventually, the marrow becomes packed with lymphocytes.

Erythroid cells in the marrow may be megaloblastic, and an erythroid hyperplasia is suggestive of hemolytic complications. Mast cells may be increased in number.

Effects of Treatment on Laboratory Results

At this time, there is no lasting cure for CLL. The two goals of therapy are the relief of symptoms and the prevention of complications.

Basically, there are three modes of therapy: chemotherapy, radiation, and leukapheresis. Chemotherapy involves the use of alkylating agents such as cyclophosphamide or chlorambucil either singly or in a combination with vincristine (a plant alkaloid) and prednisone (a corticosteroid). Unfortunately, no treatment is without its risks to the patient, and one of the main risks with the use of chemotherapy is myelosuppression. Thus, these drugs, which are so effective in reducing both the tumor burden in the tissues and the number of abnormal lymphocytes in the peripheral blood, may also cause anemia, thrombocytopenia, and granulocytopenia.

Radiation is used primarily to treat enlarged lymph nodes and splenomegaly that have proved resistant to chemotherapy. Radiation is an effective means of treating localized disease, but it does nothing to reduce the lymphocytosis in the peripheral blood and bone marrow.

Leukapheresis is especially useful in reducing the number of lymphocytes in the peripheral blood when the patient has symptoms of blood hyperviscosity because of the great number of lymphocytes. Leukapheresis does not reduce the tumor burden elsewhere.

PROLYMPHOCYTIC LEUKEMIA

Prolymphocytic leukemia was first described by Galton and associates in 1974[22] in a study of 15 patients who had a "rare variant" of CLL. Those authors observed that PLL could be distinguished from other lymphoid diseases on the basis of the peculiar morphology of the lymphocytes as seen in blood and bone marrow films. It was also apparent that these patients, in addition to having similar lymphocyte morphology, all had certain other characteristics that differed from those seen in classic CLL.

Pathophysiology

The proliferation and accumulation of abnormal lymphoid cells in the spleen, bone marrow, and to a lesser extent, the liver account for the signs and symptoms of PLL. Immunologic deficiencies, such as low levels of gamma globulins and generally low levels of other immunoglobulin, are frequently found. Additionally, the number of T lymphocytes is below normal.[22]

Clinical Presentation

Prolymphocytic leukemia shows a predilection for men in their sixth decade. Common symptoms are fatigue, weakness, weight loss, sweats, and fever. In direct contrast to CLL, in which the onset may be insidious, the presenting symptoms in PLL are generally acute in onset.[26]

The prognosis for PLL is considerably poorer than for either CLL or HCL. The mean survival is reported to be less than 1 year.[22]

Physical Findings

The most common and most impressive physical sign is enormous enlargement of the spleen and, less often, the liver. Interestingly, lymphadenopathy is uncommon.

Laboratory Findings and Correlations with Disease

The leukocyte count in the peripheral blood typically is high, from approximately 25×10^9/L to 1000×10^9/L.[22] The number of prolymphocytes in the blood differs from patient to patient, and these cells may constitute a small or large percentage of the differential leukocyte count. The prolymphocyte is a relatively large mononuclear lymphoid cell with an oval to round nucleus, coarse-appearing chromatin strands, and one or two large vesicular nucleoli with perinuclear condensations of chromatin. The cytoplasm usually is agranular and is basophilic with Romanowsky stains (Plate 58). Cells of similar morphology generally are not found in normal blood films. It has been suggested on the basis of membrane phenotype that the normal counterpart of the prolymphocyte in PLL can be found in B mantle zones (lymphocyte corona) of the peripheral lymph nodes.[23]

Absolute neutrophil counts can range from low (1 × 10^9/L) to high (20 × 10^9/L).[22] There may be an absolute monocytosis (greater than 0.8 × 10^9/L).[37] Normoblasts and immature granulocytes may be present in the blood film.

Bone marrow examination reveals almost total replacement of the marrow by prolymphocytic infiltration. Usually, only a few residual hematopoietic cells remain. Consequently, it is not uncommon for the patient to be both anemic and thrombocytopenic.

Effects of Treatment on Laboratory Results

The goal of therapy is to reduce the lymphocyte mass in the blood, marrow, and tissues; to reduce symptoms; and to improve hematopoiesis in those patients who are anemic or thrombocytopenic. Unfortunately, PLL responds poorly to the modes of therapy that are successful against CLL, such as alkylating agents and corticosteroids. Alkylating agents do not alleviate the disease symptoms and may, in fact, worsen myelosuppression. Prednisone may cause fluid and sodium retention, as well as increased excretion of calcium and potassium. It also may cause carbohydrate intolerance, glycosuria, and hyperglycemia.[4]

HAIRY CELL LEUKEMIA

Hairy cell leukemia is a relatively rare neoplasm, accounting for only about 2% of all leukemias.[51] In 1923, Ewald[15] described a disease he called "leukemic reticuloendotheliosis." He considered two characteristics commonplace in this disease: a large spleen and the presence in the peripheral blood of mononuclear cells with numerous cytoplasmic projections. Cases bearing similarity to Ewald's original description have appeared under many names, such as reticulosis,[16] aleukemic reticuloendotheliosis,[20] reticulum cell leukemia,[32,49] and others. The term "hairy cell" leukemia, derived from the ultrastructural appearance of the cells, was first suggested by Schrek and Donnelly in 1966[46] and has since become accepted as the name of the disease.

Pathophysiology

Hairy cell leukemia has a rather indolent course in most patients. However, these patients are subject to many medical problems. The growth and accumulation of hairy cells in the spleen, blood, and bone marrow account for the complications, which fall essentially into two groups: those related to cytopenias and splenomegaly, such as anemia, bleeding, and infection, and paraneoplastic complications, including autoimmune syndrome and less often, paraproteinemia.

The mean survival has been said to be 5 years, but one patient has been reported to be alive 27 years after diagnosis.[7]

Clinical Presentation

Men are predominantly affected (4:1–5:1), with the median age at diagnosis being 55 years. Virtually no one under 20 is affected.[53] The symptoms are the same as in many other hematologic neoplasms, namely bleeding, weakness and fatigue, infection, and abdominal discomfort.

Physical Findings

In HCL, the sign found most consistently is splenomegaly: approximately 90% of patients have splenomegaly, and the spleen is often enormous. Lymphadenopathy and hepatomegaly are seen less frequently.

Laboratory Findings and Correlations with Disease

Hairy cells are found in the peripheral blood in greater than 90% of patients, but these cells usually account for fewer than 50% of the cells in the differential leukocyte count.[24] Hairy cells have scant to abundant, agranular, light grayish-blue cytoplasm. The plasma membrane appears irregular with hairlike or ruffled projections, which are seen more easily with phase microscopy on living cells or by electron microscopy. These cells often have a round to oval nucleus; sometimes, the nucleus appears folded or bilobed. The chromatin is loose and lacy, and one or two nucleoli are commonly seen (Plate 59). Surface marker studies using monoclonal antibodies have revealed B-cell markers on these cells.

Pancytopenia is the most consistent laboratory observation. Granulocytopenia and monocytopenia are the most common causes of the leukopenia seen in HCL. Cytopenias result from infiltration of the marrow with malignant cells and fibrous tissue, and the effect is augmented by sequestration of blood cells by an enlarged spleen.

Bone marrow aspiration often results in a "dry tap," because most HCL patients have fibrotic marrows. When an aspirate is obtained, an increase in moderately large (10–15 μ in diameter) lymphoid cells with relatively abundant cytoplasm is observed.

Histologically, the bone marrow biopsy shows a lymphoid infiltrate with greater space between cell nuclei than in non-Hodgkin lymphomas because of the abundant cytoplasm of the hairy cell. Increased reticulin fibers are noted on the marrow biopsy in almost all patients.

The stain for tartrate-resistant acid phosphatase (TRAP) will be positive in hairy cells but negative in most other lymphoid cells. See Chapter 30 for a detailed discussion of this stain.

Effects of Treatment on Laboratory Results

If the patient is asymptomatic, no therapy is needed. In the symptomatic patient, chemotherapy has not been especially effective. Aggressive therapy with alkylating agents, which are so useful in treating many other lymphoid diseases, may reduce the tumor burden very little and, because of their toxicity, may make cytopenias worse.[7,24] Corticosteroids have rarely been helpful in treating HCL because of the association of their use with serious infections.[8]

Splenectomy is the treatment of choice, especially in those patients with severe cytopenias, which are attributable, at least in part, to splenic sequestration of cells. Removal of the spleen allows the volume of cells previously sequestered in the spleen to remain in the circulation and thus raises cell counts.

Hairy cell leukemia is especially problematic in those patients who do not improve after splenectomy. Quesada and associates[40] reported successful treatment with interferons. The results compared favorably with the use of chemotherapy without the toxicity of the latter.

CHAPTER SUMMARY

Most CLLDs are clonal B-lymphocyte diseases, which overall have a rather good prognosis. Surface marker studies using monoclonal antibodies are greatly improving the ability to diagnose these diseases quickly and accurately and to understand their relations to each other, as well as to other lymphoid malignancies. There is reason to be optimistic, because advances are being made in the treatment of CLLDs, as evidenced by the recent approval by the Food and Drug Administration of the use of interferons in the treatment of HCL.

CASE STUDY 37-1

A 72-year-old retired man was seen because of fatigue, weight loss, and fever. He had small nodes palpable in the supraclavicular areas bilaterally, a 3 × 2 cm node in the left axilla, and multiple palpable inguinal nodes. The liver was 3 cm below the right costal margin, and the spleen was enlarged to 8 cm below the left costal margin. Laboratory data included WBC 30.8 × 10⁹/L; Hb 9.0 g/dL; HCT 0.30 L/L; platelets 215 × 10⁹/L; Differential: normal segmentals 18%, lymphocytes 80%, monocytes 2%; and reticulocyte count 9%. The red cells were normocytic and normochromic. The serum bilirubin was 2.1 mg/dL, and the direct antiglobulin (Coombs) test was 4⁺ positive. The bone marrow showed 30% lymphocytes and erythroid hyperplasia. The patient was started on prednisone and was discharged 2 weeks later with a HCT of 0.33 L/L. After 4 weeks of prednisone, his HCT was 0.40 L/L. All medicines were discontinued.

One month later he was readmitted for fatigue and "blackout spells." Physical examination was unchanged. Laboratory data included: WBC 139 × 10⁹/L; HCT 0.20 L/L; platelets 275 × 10⁹/L; and reticulocyte count 30%. The differential showed 88% lymphocytes. The serum bilirubin was 9 mg/dL. The direct antiglobulin (Coombs) test remained 4⁺ positive. The patient was started on chlorambucil and prednisone daily. After 2 weeks in the hospital, his HCT had increased to 0.35 L/L, and his leukocyte count had decreased to 55 × 10⁹/L. Since then, he has been followed in the clinic on a regular basis, being maintained on 2 mg of chlorambucil and 20 mg of prednisone three times weekly. His Coombs test is still positive, although his HCT remains normal. Attempts to taper steroids further have been unsuccessful. Signs of hypercorticism are minimal, and the patient is not Cushingoid.

1. What is the diagnosis?
2. What complication is present?
3. How do we know that hemolysis is occurring in this patient?
4. In the face of a 4⁺ positive antiglobulin (Coombs) test, how can the HCT remain normal?

REFERENCES

1. Aisenberg AC: Cell lineage in lymphoproliferative disease. Am J Med 74:679, 1983
2. Anderson RC: Familial leukemia: A report of leukemia in five siblings, with a brief review of the genetic aspects of this disease. Am J Dis Child 81:313, 1951
3. Axelsson U, Hallen J: Familial occurrence of pathological serum proteins of different gamma globulin groups. Lancet 2:369, 1965
4. Becker TM: Cancer Chemotheraphy: A Manual for Nurses. Boston, Little, Brown and Co, 1981
5. Boggs DR, Sofferman SA, Wintrobe MM et al: Factors influencing the duration of survival of patients with chronic lymphocytic leukemia. Am J Med 40:243, 1966
6. Bona C, Fauci A: In vitro idiotype suppression of chronic lymphocytic leukemia lymphocytes secreting monoclonal immunoglobulin M anti-sheep erythrocyte antibody. J Clin Invest 65:761, 1980
7. Bouroncle BA: Leukemic reticuloendotheliosis (hairy cell leukemia). Blood 53:412, 1979
8. Bouza E, Burgaleta C, Golde DW: Infections in hairy-cell leukemia. Blood 51:851, 1978
9. Caligaris-Cappio F, Janossy G: Surface markers in chronic lymphoid leukemias of B-cell type. Semin Hematol 22:1, 1985
10. Catovsky D: Chronic lymphocytic, prolymphocytic and hairy cell leukemias. In Goldman JM, Preisler HD (eds): Leukemia, p 266. Sevenoaks, England, Butterworths, 1984
11. Cutler SJ, Axtell L, Heise H: Ten thousand cases of leukemia: 1940-62. J Natl Cancer Inst 39:993, 1967
12. Den Ottolander GJ, Schmit HRE, Wayer JLM et al: Chronic B-cell leukemias: Relation between morphological and immunological features. Clin Immunol Immunopathol 35:92, 1985
13. Dormer P, Thelm H, Lau B: Chronic lymphocytic leukemia: A proliferative or accumulative disorder? Leuk Res 2:1, 1983
14. Enno A, Catovsky D, O'Brien M et al: Prolymphocytoid transformation of chronic lymphocytic leukaemia. Br J Haematol 41:9, 1979
15. Ewald O: Die leukmische Reticuloendotheliose. Dtsch Arch Kinderheilkd Med 142:222, 1923
16. Farquhar JW, MacGregor AR, Richmond J: Familial haemophagic reticulosis. Br Med J 2:1561, 1958
17. Fraumeni JF Jr, Vogel CL, DeVita VT Jr: Familial chronic lymphocytic leukemia. Ann Intern Med 71:279, 1969
18. Fraumeni JF Jr, Wertelecki W, Blattner WA et al: Varied manifestations of a familial lymphoproliferative disorder. Am J Med 59:145, 1975
19. Frei E, Sallan S: Acute lymphoblastic leukemia: Treatment. Cancer 42:828, 1978
20. Fukuda T: Malignant reticulosis. Tohoku J Exp Med 94:351, 1968
21. Galton DAG: The pathogenesis of chronic lymphocytic leukemia. Can Med Assoc J 94:1005, 1966
22. Galton DAG, Goldman JM, Wiltshaw E et al: Prolymphocytic leukaemia. Br J Haematol 27:7, 1974
23. Gobbi M, Caligaris-Cappio F, Janossy G: Normal equivalent cells of B-cell malignancies: Analysis with monoclonal antibodies. Br J Haematol 54:393, 1983
24. Golomb HM, Catovsky D, Golde DW: Clinical review: Hairy cell leukemia. Ann Intern Med 89:677, 1978
25. Gordon J, Aman P, Mellstedt H et al: In vitro differentiation of chronic lymphocytic leukemia cells with a small pre-B-like phenotype. Leuk Res 2:133, 1983
26. Gordon MY, Barrett AJ: Bone Marrow Disorders: The Biological Basis of Clinical Problems. Oxford, Oxford Scientific Publications, 1985
27. Green RA, Dixon H: Expectancy for life in chronic lymphatic leukemia. Blood 25:23, 1965
28. Gunz FW, Fitzgerald PH, Crossen PE et al: Multiple cases of leukemia in a sibship. Blood 27:482, 1966
29. Harden EA, Haynes BF: Phenotypic and functional characterization of human malignant T-cells. Semin Hematol 22:13, 1985
30. Heideman R, Falletta J, Mukhopadhyay N et al: Lymphocytic leukemia in children: Prognostic significance of clinical and laboratory findings at time of diagnosis. J Pediatr 92:540, 1978
31. Juliusson G, Robert K-H, Ost A et al: Prognostic information from cytogenetic analysis in chronic B-lymphocytic leukemia and leukemic immunocytoma. Blood 65:134, 1985

32. Lee SL, Rosner F, Rosenthal N et al: Reticulum cell leukemia. NY State J Med 69:422, 1969

33. Lewis FB, Schwartz RS, Dameshek W: X-radiation and alkylating agents as possible "trigger" mechanisms in the autoimmune complications of malignant lymphoproliferative disease. Clin Exp Immunol 1:1, 1966

34. Lockwood K, Stancke B, Clemmesen J: Survival rates for leukemia in various countries. Natl Cancer Inst Monogr 15:341, 1964

35. McKenna RW, Bloomfield CD, Brunning CD: Nodular lymphoma: Bone marrow and blood manifestations. Cancer 36:428, 1975

36. Minot GR, Isaacs R: Lymphatic leukemia: Age incidence, duration, and benefit derived from irradiation. Boston Med Surg J 191:1, 1924

37. Munan L, Kelly A: Age-dependent changes in blood monocyte populations in man. Clin Exp Immunol 35:161, 1979

38. Osgood EE: Contrasting incidence of acute monocytic and granulocytic leukemia in P32 treated patients with polycythemia vera and chronic lymphocytic leukemia. J Lab Clin Med 64:560, 1969

39. Poiesz BJ, Ruscetti FW, Gazdar AF et al: Detection and isolation of type-C retrovirus particles from fresh and cultured lymphocytes of a patient with cutaneous T-cell lymphoma. Proc Natl Acad Sci USA 77:7415, 1980

40. Quesada JR, Hersh EM, Gutterman JU: Hairy cell leukemia. Induction of remission with alpha interferon. Blood 62:207a, 1983

41. Reilly EB, Rappaport SI, Karr NW et al: Familial chronic lymphatic leukemia. Arch Intern Med 90:87, 1952

42. Rigby PG, Pratt PT, Rosenlof RC et al: Genetic relationships in familial leukemia and lymphoma. Arch Intern Med 121:67, 1968

43. Robert K-H, Gahrton G, Friberg K et al: Extra chromosome 12 and prognosis in chronic lymphocytic leukaemia. Scand J Haematol 28:163, 1982

44. Rosenthal MC, Pisciotta AV, Komninos ZD et al: The autoimmune hemolytic anemia of malignant lymphocytic disease. Blood 10:1978, 1955

45. Saxon A, Stevens R, Golde D et al: T-lymphocyte variant of hairy cell leukemia. Ann Intern Med 88:323, 1978

46. Schrek R, Donnelly WJ: "Hairy" cells in blood in lymphoreticular neoplastic disease and "flagellated" cells of normal lymph. Blood 27:199, 1966

47. Schwartz RS, Costea N: Autoimmune hemolytic anemia: Clinical correlations and biological implications. Semin Haematol 3:2, 1966

48. Seligmann M: A genetic predisposition to Waldenström's macroglobulinemia. Acta Med Scand 179(suppl 445):140, 1966

49. Tedeschi LG, Lansinger DT: Sézary syndrome: A malignant leukemic reticuloendotheliosis. Arch Dermatol 92:257, 1965

50. Ueshima Y, Bird ML, Vardiman JW, et al: A 14;19 translocation in B-cell chronic lymphocytic leukemia: A new recurring chromosome aberration. Int J Cancer 36:287, 1985

51. Westbrook CA, Golde DW: Clinical problems in hairy cell leukemia: Diagnosis and management. Semin Oncol 11:514, 1984

52. Williams WJ, Beutler E, Erslev AJ et al (eds): Hematology, 4th ed. New York, McGraw-Hill, 1990

53. Wintrobe MM, Lee GR, Boggs DR et al: Clinical Hematology, 8th ed. Philadelphia, Lea & Febiger, 1981

54. Wolf JK: Primary acquired agammaglobulinemia with a family history of collagen disease and haematological disorders. N Engl J Med 266:473, 1962

55. Young LE, Miller G, Christian RM: Clinical and laboratory observations on auto-immune hemolytic disease. Ann Intern Med 35:507, 1951

56. Zuegler WW, Mastrangelo R, Stulberg CS et al: Autoimmune hemolytic anemia: Natural history and viral immunologic interactions in childhood. Am J Med 49:80, 1970

Charles E. Manner

The lymphomas are a group of malignant diseases that originate from the uninhibited growth of cellular elements normally found in lymphatic tissue. The term "lymphoma" emphasizes the fact that the hallmark of these disorders is abnormal lymph node enlargement, with disruption or replacement of the normal histologic architecture. Although other malignant lymphoproliferative disorders such as acute lymphoblastic leukemia (Chap. 36) and plasma cell dyscrasias (Chap. 39) cause diffuse infiltration of the lymph nodes, the histologic structure of the nodes is still evident. Chronic lymphocytic leukemia can share with the lymphomas the feature of nodal involvement, but lymphomas ordinarily do not have peripheral blood involvement (*i.e.*, abnormal circulating cells) until late in the disease.

PRINCIPAL CLASSIFICATIONS OF LYMPHOMA

Lymphomas have traditionally been divided into two classes: Hodgkin disease (HD) and non-Hodgkin lymphomas (NHL). The cellular infiltrate in the lymph nodes of HD is much more variable or pleomorphic than it is in NHL. Many of the cells in nodes affected by HD are normal in appearance, and only a minor population of cells have neoplastic (*i.e.*, malignant) features.[10] In contrast, the infiltrates of NHL are more uniformly composed of similar-appearing neoplastic cells. To emphasize this distinction, the term "Hodgkin *disease*" is preferred to "Hodgkin *lymphoma*."

In NHL, the B lymphocyte is the neoplastic cell in roughly 95% of the cases; the T lymphocyte is the neoplastic cell in the remaining 5%.[38] In HD, the neoplastic cell generally is considered to be a multinucleated giant cell of distinctive appearance known as the *Reed-Sternberg cell*[29] (Fig. 38-1).

Diagnosis of the lymphomas is based on histologic examination of lymph node tissues. Hodgkin disease and NHL have been further subdivided into subtypes of distinctive histologic appearance, which will be addressed in this chapter. In the case of NHL, the histologic subclass has a much stronger bearing on the biologic behavior of the malignancy, and hence on patient prognosis, than is the case for HD.

Hodgkin disease probably is unifocal in origin. In other words, it starts in one lymph node group and spreads in a predictable fashion to adjacent lymph nodes; in very advanced cases, nonlymphatic tissue can be involved.[41] Non-Hodgkin lymphoma spreads in a much less predictable way. If NHL is ever unifocal, it remains so only briefly, as only 10% of patients present with truly localized disease.[6] Rather, the typical patient with NHL presents with involvement of multiple lymph node groups, which can be noncontiguous. Non-Hodgkin lymphoma also involves nonlymphatic tissue more commonly than does HD. Because of the more predictable biologic behavior of HD compared with NHL, the disease stage (a measure of disease extent) is more important prognostically for the former than for the latter.

HODGKIN DISEASE

History

In 1832 Thomas Hodgkin first described the disease that bears his name.[23] The compound microscope and the histologic methods required to distinguish this disease from

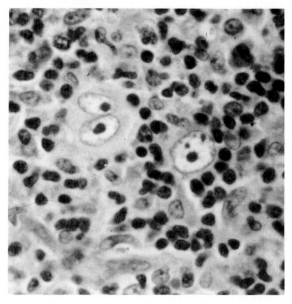

FIG. 38-1. Characteristic Reed-Sternberg cell and mononuclear variant of Hodgkin disease (hematoxylin and eosin, magnification × 400). (From DeVita VT Jr, Hellman S, Rosenberg SA: Cancer Principles and Practice of Oncology, 3rd ed. Philadelphia, JB Lippincott, 1989, with permission.)

other causes of chronic lymph node enlargement were unavailable to Hodgkin. Full appreciation of the histologic features of HD and its characteristic giant cells did not come until the independent publications of Carl Sternberg in 1898[51] and Reed in 1902.[44] From the 1940s to the 1960s, various histologic classifications of HD were proposed. The four-part system in use today was agreed on at a symposium held in Rye, New York, in 1966.[36]

Epidemiology

The cause of HD, as is the case for many neoplasms, is unknown. A number of epidemiologic studies have proposed genetic influences,[18] exposures to environmental hazards,[19] or an infectious agent such as Epstein-Barr virus[39] as part of the pathogenesis. However, none of these hypotheses has been proven.

Taken together, HD and NHL are the seventh most common cause of death from cancer in the United States. Hodgkin disease accounts for roughly 25% of the cases, with NHL making up the remainder.[11] In economically developed countries, HD has a unique bimodal incidence curve.[37] The incidence begins to rise after the age of 10 years and peaks in the 20s, then declines to age 45, after which the incidence rises steadily with advancing age, as it does for NHL. Hodgkin disease is more common in men than in women, with a sex ratio of 3:2.[57]

Clinical Features

The most common presentation of HD is a painless enlarging lymph node, usually in the neck. In some cases, a routine chest radiograph discloses a mediastinal mass (one in the intervening space between the right and left lungs). Further examination may reveal enlarged cervical nodes. Occasionally, rapid enlargement of lymph nodes creates a painful mass.

The more ominous symptoms are fever, night sweats, or weight loss, or a combination thereof, which are referred to as the "B" symptoms. Such symptoms are important in disease staging. The stages of HD and NHL (discussed later in this chapter) can be denoted with the suffix "A" to indicate that the patient has no symptoms or "B" to indicate that the patient has one or more of the B symptoms. For example, Stage IVB is the most advanced stage of HD, the B denoting that the patient is suffering from one or more of the classic symptoms.

Over the course of weeks to months, the involved lymph nodes continue to enlarge. The disease spreads in an orderly fashion to adjacent lymph node chains. This orderliness of spread is reflected in the HD staging system (discussed below). In advanced cases, nonlymphatic tissue can be involved, presumably by metastases via the peripheral blood. Untreated patients die from recurrent infections or organ failure within a year or two of the onset of illness.

Laboratory Findings and Correlations with Disease

The only definitive test for HD is the lymph node biopsy. Other laboratory abnormalities are often nonspecific.

Peripheral Blood

Early in the course of the disease, there may be an absolute increase in monocytes and eosinophils. Usually, there is no anemia, and platelets are normal in number. A transitory increase in lymphocytes may be noted. The blood film may show large, abnormal-appearing lymphocytes, which have very little cytoplasm and irregular nuclear chromatin.[54]

As the disease progresses, there often is a leukocytosis. Granulocytosis occurs in roughly 25% of patients, usually in the more advanced stages. In some cases, this change is extreme and mimics leukemia ("leukemoid reaction") (Chap. 26). Peripheral blood lymphocytopenia may develop with almost the same frequency as granulocytosis. Lymphocytopenia is a sign of a poor prognosis, as it is associated with advanced stages of disease and with histologic subtypes that have poor prognoses.[53]

In advanced disease, granulocytes often display toxic granulation. The disease process may cause the production of large, bizarre platelets observable on the blood film.[4]

Plasma cells sometimes are observed on the peripheral blood film,[8] as, rarely, are Reed-Sternberg cells[48] (see Diagnostic Evaluation of Lymph Node Biopsy). Occasionally, another large (40 μm diameter) abnormal-appearing cell is seen.[20] It has moderately basophilic cytoplasm, and its nucleus is oval or lobulated with fine, reticular chromatin and one or more large nucleoli. Nonspecific abnormalities such as large monocytes with large vacuoles and large lymphocytes with deeply basophilic cytoplasm may also be seen on the blood film or on specially prepared leukocyte concentrate films.[21,22,48] It should be noted, however, that such abnormal cells may be associated with a number of other diseases such as viral infections.

Normochromic, normocytic anemia is a presenting feature in about 10% of patients.[7,54] Typically, the reticulocyte count is normal or low.

Bone Marrow

The bone marrow is seldom involved except in advanced (Stage IV) disease. Typically, films of the marrow aspirate are negative, and only the biopsy reveals disease, which usually is accompanied by marrow fibrosis. Even in positive marrows, the histologic class often cannot be determined, and it may not be possible to distinguish the condition from NHL. Again, the definitive diagnosis of HD depends on the lymph node biopsy.

Other Laboratory Findings

Commonly, the serum iron and total iron-binding capacity (TIBC) are reduced. These features, along with the anemia found in 10% of patients, are typical of the anemia associated with chronic disease (Chap. 13).[7,54] Rarely, the direct antiglobulin test (DAT) is positive, signifying a hemolytic component to the anemia.[34]

A variety of other laboratory abnormalities correlate with disease activity but are entirely nonspecific. These include elevations of the erythrocyte sedimentation rate, fibrinogen, haptoglobin, serum globulins, ceruloplasmin, and copper. Similarly, a number of serum enzymes have been reported to be elevated, including leukocyte alkaline phosphatase, lysozyme, lactic acid dehydrogenase (LD), and transaminases.[43]

Hyperuricemia may be found because of excessive cell turnover. More importantly, with successful therapy, rapid tumor lysis may cause a marked increase in uric acid production with urate crystal deposition in the kidney tubules and urinary tract. Acute renal failure can result unless preventative measures are taken.

Diagnostic Evaluation of Lymph Node Biopsy: The Reed-Sternberg Cell

The diagnosis and classification of HD can be made only by lymph node biopsy (Fig. 38-2). The essential feature confirming the diagnosis is the presence of the Reed-Sternberg giant cell (see Fig. 38-1) in affected lymph nodes. This is a large cell, generally four to eight times the size of normal surrounding lymphocytes. It can be multinucleated or binucleated or may contain a single bilobed nucleus. Most often, the cell is binucleated with the two halves of the cell appearing as mirror images. The nuclear membrane is thick and well demarcated. The nucleoli are large and eosinophilic with a distinct halo, giving the cell what is typically referred to as an owl-eyed appearance (see Plate 63F). Around the nucleus is an abundant cytoplasm of amorphous consistency with a slight eosinophilia.

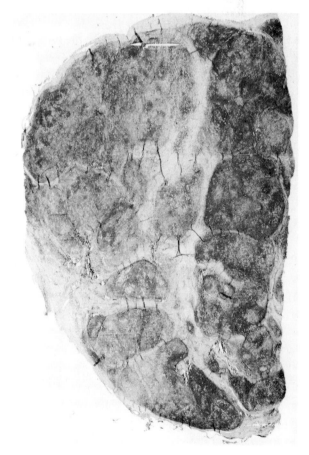

FIG. 38-2. Lymph node, nodular sclerosing Hodgkin's disease. Cellular nodules are surrounded by dense fibrous bands (hematoxylin and eosin, magnification × 8). (From DeVita VT Jr, Hellman S, Rosenberg SA: Cancer Principles and Practice of Oncology, 3rd ed. Philadelphia, JB Lippincott, 1989, with permission.)

Immunohistologic techniques involving monoclonal antibodies have come into increasing use in the identification and classification of lymphomas.[40] The recent ability to isolate and even culture Reed-Sternberg cells from pathologic material has made immunohistologic techniques even more useful in identifying HD.[49]

Table 38-1 profiles the antigenic and enzyme phenotype of the Reed-Sternberg cell. An understanding of the profile provides insight into the origin of this cell. It is apparent that the Reed-Sternberg cell has some features in common with monocytes and T and B lymphocytes. On the other hand, it distinctly lacks some antigens found on other T or B cells. It is no wonder, then, that the origin of the Reed-Sternberg cell has been a matter of controversy! It may be more practical to consider the Reed-Sternberg cell as a malignant cell with aberrant genetic expression that has no true counterpart among normal cells of the immune system.

Classification

Rye Classification

Hodgkin disease usually is classified into four histologic groups, as first proposed at the Rye Conference in 1965 (Table 38-2).[32,35,36] The classification is based primarily on the extent of lymphocyte infiltration and the abundance of Reed-Sternberg cells. Even apart from disease stage, the histologic class correlates with prognosis: the lymphocyte-predominant class has the best outlook, whereas the lymphocyte-depleted class has the worst. Part of the relation of histologic class to prognosis has to do with the age of the patient and the stage of disease at the time of diagnosis. Younger patients and patients with earlier stages clearly do better, and these clinical features are seen in the two best prognostic patterns: lymphocyte predominant and nodular sclerosis.

Ann Arbor Staging System

Hodgkin disease has a universally accepted staging system that was delineated at the Ann Arbor Conference in 1971.[5] The only modification that has been made to this scheme since 1971 has been a further breakdown of Stage III into Stage III$_1$ and Stage III$_2$. Stage III$_1$ represents disease confined to the upper abdomen above the renal artery. Stage III$_2$ signifies disease below this structure.[9] Table 38-3 outlines the modified Ann Arbor Staging System.

Stages may be given the additional suffix letters A or B. Suffix A denotes no symptoms. Suffix B indicates the presence of symptoms, specifically fever greater than 100.4°F, night sweats, or unexplained loss of 10% or more of body weight occurring within the preceding 6 months. Each stage also may be given a subscript of either E or S. Subscript E designates extralymphatic disease and S, splenic involvement (see Table 38-3).

One of the difficulties that can present when using this system is distinguishing either Stages II$_E$ or III$_E$ from Stage IV when a patient has only one extralymphatic site involved. Generally patients are classified as having E disease

TABLE 38–1. Immunohistologic Phenotype of Reed-Sternberg (RS) Cell

ANTIGENIC PROPERTY TESTED*	RS CELL REACTION	OTHER CELLS DEMONSTRATING THE PROPERTY	COMMENTS ON ANTIGENIC PROPERTY	REFERENCES
CD15 (Leu M1)	+	Monocytes, granulocytes	Antigen	24
Fc receptors	+	B and T lymphocytes, monocytes	Receptors for Fc portion of immunoglobulins	29
C3 receptors	+	B and T lymphocytes, monocytes	Receptors for C3, the third component of complement	29
Ia†	+	B lymphocytes, monocytes, activated T lymphocytes	Immune response antigen	52
HLA-DR	+	B lymphocytes, monocytes, activated T lymphocytes	Major histocompatibility complex (MHC) Class II antigen	25, 52
CD25 (Tac)‡	±	T lymphocytes, monocytes, B lymphocytes	Receptor for the lymphokine interleukin-2 (IL-2)	25, 50
CIg	+	B lymphocytes	Cytoplasmic immunoglobulin	49
SIg	+	B lymphocytes	Surface immunoglobulin	49
CD20 (B1)	±	Immature B lymphocytes, B-cell malignancies	Antigen	50
CD19 (B4)	±	Immature B lymphocytes, B-cell malignancies	Antigen	50
CD22 (Leu 14)	−	B lymphocytes	Antigen found on 95% of B lymphocytes	50
CD3 (OKT3)	±	T lymphocytes	Antigen found on all T lymphocytes	50
Lysozyme	+	Monocytes, granulocytes	Enzyme	29
Esterase	+	Monocytes, granulocytes	Enzyme	28

* Note that antigenic properties have been grouped according to common cell types with which they are associated. Where appropriate, the new cluster designation (CD) is given; these designations were established by an international panel and reflect reactivity with similar monoclonal antibodies.
† Ia is most abundant on B lymphocytes but can be found on monocytes and activated T lymphocytes.
‡ Tac is predominant on T lymphocytes but can be found on monocytes and B lymphocytes.

TABLE 38–2. Rye Classification of Hodgkin Disease

PATTERN	DESCRIPTION	REED-STERNBERG (RS) CELLS	PERCENT OF TOTAL CASES	PATIENT AGE	5–YEAR SURVIVAL (%)
Lymphocyte predominant	Diffuse pattern of abundant lymphocytes; sparse granulocytes and plasma cells. No fibrosis	Scarce	5–10	Young	95
Nodular sclerosis	Nodularity with birefringent collagen bands; moderate lymphocytes, granulocytes, and plasma cells; RS cells sit in clear zones (lacunar RS cells)	Occasional	35–65	Young	85
Mixed cellularity	Moderate lymphocytes, granulocytes, and plasma cells in diffuse pattern	Many	20–40	Middle-aged to elderly	65
Lymphocyte depleted	Diffuse fibrosis with few lymphocytes	Abundant	1–5	Middle-aged to elderly	20

TABLE 38–3. Modified Ann Arbor Staging System for Hodgkin Disease and Non-Hodgkin Lymphoma*

STAGE	DESCRIPTION
I	Involvement of a single lymph node region (Stage I) OR Involvement of a single extralymphatic organ or site (Stage I_E)
II	Involvement of two or more lymph node regions on the same side of the diaphragm alone (Stage II) OR With involvement of a contiguous extralymphatic organ or site (Stage II_E)
III	Involvement of lymph node regions on both sides of the diaphragm (Stage III). Stage III_S indicates splenic involvement; Stage III_E indicates involvement of an extralymphatic organ or site; Stage III_{SE} indicates involvement of both spleen and an extralymphatic organ or site
	III_1 Abdominal disease limited to the upper abdomen, spleen, splenic hilar nodes, celiac nodes, or porta hepatis nodes
	III_2 Abdominal disease including para-aortic, mesenteric, iliac, or inguinal involvement with or without involvement of upper abdomen
IV	Diffuse involvement of one or more extralymphatic organs or sites not contiguous with lymphatic tissue

* Any stage can be given the additional suffix letters A or B or subscript letters E or S: A, no symptoms present; B, fever over 100.4°F, night sweats, or 10% weight loss in the preceding 6 months; E, extralymphatic involvement; S, splenic involvement.

if the extent of the disease is limited enough that radiation therapy can most likely cure the patient. If this is not the case, the patient is considered to be in Stage IV.

Diagnosis and Treatment

Proper staging is essential for formulating the best treatment plan for a patient, as well as for evaluating the success of that treatment on followup examinations. The diagnostic methods employed are a mixture of clinical and pathologic methods (Tables 38-4 and 38-5). Implicit in the division of these tables is the fact that not every test needs to be done in each patient to stage the disease and plan treatment properly. The one fundamental principle that guides the use of diagnostic tests in a particular patient is that a procedure should be done if detection of disease by that method would change the stage assignment and therefore the treatment plan.

Effects of Treatment on Laboratory Results

Table 38-6 summarizes the treatments of choice for the various stages of HD according to the modified Ann Arbor staging system. It also lists their approximate cure rates.[13]

Physical Effects

Effective therapy can dramatically reduce bulky adenopathy in a matter of days to weeks. Some patients will have no clinical evidence of disease within a month or so.

TABLE 38–4. Staging Procedures Essential in Hodgkin Disease and Non-Hodgkin Lymphomas Diagnosis

Thorough history and physical examination
Adequate surgical biopsy reviewed by a hematopathologist
Routine laboratory tests
   CBC including platelet count
   Erythrocyte sedimentation rate
   Serum alkaline phosphatase
   Liver function tests
   Serum uric acid
   Blood urea nitrogen
   Serum creatinine
Chest radiograph (posteroanterior and lateral views)
Bilateral core biopsy of marrow from posterior iliac crests
Bilateral lower extremity lymphangiogram
Computed tomographic (CT) scan of abdomen or equivalent study
Needle aspiration biopsy or surgical biopsy of any suspect extranodal lesions
Cytologic examination of any pleural effusion

TABLE 38–5. Ancillary Staging Procedures in Diagnosis
of Hodgkin Disease and Non-Hodgkin Lymphomas

Bone scan with plain skeletal radiographs of suspect areas
Laparoscopy and biopsies
Liver biopsy
Staging laparotomy and splenectomy
Intravenous pyelography
Radionuclide liver–spleen scan
Whole-body gallium-67 scan
CT scans of thorax

Hematologic Effects

Both radiation and chemotherapy are myelosuppressive. Thus, the main effect of treatment on laboratory values is reflected in the CBC. Generally, the effect of radiation in terms of myelosuppression depends on the size of the field treated. Treatment of the disease at an early stage, with radiation limited to the chest, neck, and upper thorax (the area known as a "mantle field") has a much milder effect on blood counts than does the total nodal radiation used in the treatment of intermediate stages of disease.

Combination chemotherapy has the most profound effect on blood counts, particularly the granulocyte and platelet counts. Generally, the lowest counts occur 10 to 15 days after the start of therapy. Granulocytopenia, often with absolute counts in the 0.5 to $1.0 \times 10^9/L$ range (approximate reference range 1.8 to $7.7 \times 10^9/L$), is common. Platelet counts between 50 and $100 \times 10^9/L$ are frequently seen; platelet counts below $20 \times 10^9/L$ can be associated with spontaneous hemorrhage, which can be life-threatening, and usually are an indication for platelet transfusion. Depending on the regimen of chemotherapy used, recovery of granulocyte and platelet counts occurs by day 21 to 28 of the cycle, at which time more chemotherapy is given. Generally, the return of granulocyte counts to normal is heralded by a relative monocytosis 3 to 5 days earlier.

Because the erythrocyte is a much longer-lived cell than the granulocyte or platelet, the temporary cessation of production secondary to chemotherapy does not cause a significant decrease in erythrocytes during a single course of therapy. However, with repeated treatments, it is not unusual for patients to develop anemia severe enough to necessitate red cell transfusions. On achievement of remission of lymphoma and completion of chemotherapy or radiation therapy, the complete blood count returns to and remains normal.

Chemical Effects

Rapid tumor lysis by chemotherapy or radiation or both results in a release of intracellular substances such as uric acid, phosphate, and potassium, which can cause metabolic abnormalities (hyperuricemia, hyperphosphatemia, and hyperkalemia). High serum phosphate levels can lead to hypocalcemia because of precipitation of calcium phosphate salts. Renal failure, with elevated BUN and serum creatinine, can ensue because of uric acid and calcium phosphate deposition in the renal tubules. Management of this problem is preventive, with forced fluids, urine alkalination with bicarbonate, and blockade of uric acid production with allopurinol.

NON-HODGKIN LYMPHOMAS

History

A few decades after the work of Thomas Hodgkin, Rudolph Virchow, the great pathologist, recognized the lymphomas.[55] Enlarging on his knowledge of leukemias, Virchow divided the lymphomas into two types: leukemic and aleukemic. The aleukemic lymphoma was called *lymphosarcoma*. This term was used by others in the latter part of the 19th century and came ultimately to designate a separate lymphoma subtype once specific histologic types were described.

The first comprehensive classification system for lymphomas was introduced by Gall and Mallory in 1942.[15] The true forerunner of modern schemes in use today was described by Rappaport and coworkers in 1956.[42] This system had two criteria, which are still in use in classifying lym-

TABLE 38–6. Treatments of Choice for Hodgkin Disease by Stage and Approximate
Cure Rates

STAGE (ANN ARBOR SYSTEM)	TREATMENT OF CHOICE	APPROXIMATE CURE RATE (%)	COMMENTS
IA, IB, IIA	Radiotherapy	85–90	Early stages of disease respond well to radiotherapy alone (*i.e.*, chemotherapy is not needed)
IIIB, IVA, IVB	Combination chemotherapy	80	Using modern aggressive chemotherapy regimens, 55% to 70% of all patients with advanced disease can expect to be free of disease 5 years after diagnosis
IIB, IIIA₁, IIIA₂	Radiation alone or radiation plus chemotherapy	65–75	Radiation alone is associated with a higher relapse rate than that found in Stages IA, IB, and IIA. Chemotherapy is valuable in relapsing patients

From Fisher RI: Hodgkin's disease. In Wittes RE (ed): Manual of Oncologic Therapeutics 1989/1990, pp 370–373. Philadelphia, JB Lippincott, 1989.

phomas: the presence or absence of nodularity and the size of the cell involved in the infiltrates. This system was simple and prognostically relevant. Several other systems have been proposed to reflect our growing knowledge of lymphocytes and the origin of lymphomas. The most recent, the International Working Classification of Non-Hodgkin's Lymphomas, was proposed in 1982.[46]

Epidemiology

In the United States, NHL is three times as common as HD, with about 25,000 new cases diagnosed annually.[11] The incidence rises steadily with age starting around age 40. Non-Hodgkin lymphoma, like HD, is more common in men than in women, with a ratio of 3:2.

Congenital immunodeficiency diseases such as ataxia telangiectasia, the Wiskott-Aldrich syndrome, IgA deficiency, common variable immunodeficiency, and severe combined immunodeficiency have been associated with a 10,000-fold increase in the risk of developing cancer, of which the vast majority are NHL.[16] Acquired conditions of immune dysfunction also have been associated with an increased predisposition to NHL. Rheumatoid arthritis, Sjögren's syndrome, and systemic lupus erythematosus are rheumatologic conditions associated with a 3- to 40-fold increase in the risk of lymphoma.[26,31,56] Organ transplant recipients taking immunosuppressive drugs to prevent graft rejection have a 40- to 100-fold increase in the risk of lymphoma.[33] This predisposed presentation is shared by the lymphoma associated with acquired immunodeficiency syndrome (AIDS).[17]

Viral agents may also be related to the development of NHL. The Epstein-Barr virus, the etiologic agent of infectious mononucleosis, which infects B lymphocytes, has been closely linked to the development of African Burkitt lymphoma (see below for definitions),[30] a form of small noncleaved-cell lymphoma. Human T-cell lymphocytotrophic virus (HTLV-1), a retrovirus that infects helper T cells, has been closely associated with the development of acute T-cell leukemia and lymphoma.[1]

One must recognize that for every virus-infected individual who has lymphoma, there are many more infected persons who do not develop lymphoma. Thus, any hypothesis of a viral etiology of lymphoma must invoke cocarcinogens. In summary, the exact etiology of NHL remains unknown.

Physical Findings

Painless lymph node enlargement is the most common presenting symptom. The cervical nodes are most often involved.

Symptoms

Systemic symptoms such as fever, weight loss, and night sweats are reported by approximately 30% of patients, particularly those with diffuse histologic patterns and advanced stages. It is more common for patients with NHL to present with more advanced stages (III or IV) than is the case in HD.

Laboratory Findings and Correlations with Disease

Blood counts are normal in most patients with NHL, even in those cases in which the bone marrow is involved.[47] Other laboratory findings often depend on the classification of the lymphoma (see next section for classifications). Some patients with small-cell or follicular lymphomas have a positive direct antiglobulin test and occasionally a consequent autoimmune hemolytic anemia. Sometimes, an autoimmune thrombocytopenia occurs as well.[27] Leukemic phases of disease can be seen with diffuse small-cell lymphocytic lymphoma and in lymphoblastic lymphoma.[14]

Serum chemistry abnormalities such as alkaline phosphatase, LD, and uric acid, as discussed for HD, may also occur in NHL.

Classification

The clinical pace of NHL depends heavily on the histologic pattern. In this regard, the histologic subtypes that make up the International Working Classification can be divided into three groups, ranked according to their aggressiveness as low, intermediate, and high (Table 38-7).

Low Grade

The low-grade lymphomas typically affect patients between the ages of 45 and 60 years. These are slow-growing lymphomas, and lymph node enlargement can be present for years before diagnosis. Often, patients can do well without treatment for 2 to 3 years. Most disease is in Stage III or IV at the time of diagnosis. Although the bone marrow frequently is involved, the peripheral blood often is normal. The median survival ranges from 5 to 7 years. In approximately 30% of these patients, the disease evolves into a diffuse large-cell lymphoma, which worsens the prognosis.[45]

Intermediate Grade

The intermediate-grade lymphomas, like the low-grade varieties, affect individuals in later middle age. Patients present with a much more rapid lymph node enlargement, and extranodal disease is more common. The only exception to this is the bone marrow, which is much less frequently involved than is the case in the low-grade lymphomas. Median survival ranges from 1.5 to about 3 years, although diffuse large-cell lymphoma is a potentially curable disease in as many as one third of the patients.[11]

High Grade

The high-grade lymphomas cause the most rapid enlargement of the lymph nodes and the fastest developing malignancies. Thus, if left untreated, these lymphomas are rapidly fatal.

Immunoblastic sarcoma usually occurs in adults over the age of 50. Advanced stage and systemic symptoms are common at presentation. Primary NHLs that arise in the central nervous system (CNS) are most often immunoblastic sarcoma. This disease responds poorly even to the most aggressive therapy, and short survivals (months to a year) are typical.

TABLE 38–7. International Working Classification of Non-Hodgkin Lymphoma

GRADE	LYMPHOMA TYPE	MITOSES IN MICROSCOPIC FIELDS	PATIENT MEDIAN AGE (YEARS)	PERCENT OF CASES WITH BONE MARROW INVOLVEMENT	SURVIVAL MEDIAN (YEARS)	5 YEAR (%)
LOW	Small lymphocytic	Rare	60	71	5.8	59
	Follicular, small cleaved cell	Infrequent	54	51	7.2	70
	Follicular, mixed (small cleaved and large cells)	Infrequent	56	30	5.1	50
	Follicular, large cell	Usually numerous	55	34	3.0	45
INTERMEDIATE	Diffuse, small cleaved cell	Variable	58	32	3.4	33
	Diffuse, mixed (small cleaved and large cell)	Few to moderate	58	14	2.7	38
	Diffuse, large cell	Moderate	57	10	1.5	35
	Immunoblastic (large cell)	Moderate	51	12	1.3	32
HIGH	Lymphoblastic	Numerous	17	50	2.0	26
	Small noncleaved cell (Burkitt and non-Burkitt types)	Numerous	30	14	0.7	23

From Rosenberg SA, Berard CW, Brown BW et al: National Cancer Institute sponsored study of classification of non-Hodgkin's lymphomas: Summary and description of a working formulation for clinical usage. Cancer 49:2112, 1982.

Lymphoblastic lymphoma is a T-cell malignancy typically seen in men in their teens or twenties. About half of these patients present with a large mediastinal mass, which disseminates rapidly to the bone marrow, peripheral blood, and CNS. This tumor may respond initially to chemotherapy, but relapse and a poor outcome are common.

Small noncleaved-cell lymphoma is an aggressive tumor of B lymphocytes. This disease affects a broad age range, from children to about age 30. It is further subdivided into the Burkitt type (which is common in African blacks) and the non-Burkitt type, depending on the cells found in the lymph node biopsy or bone marrow. There is a high rate of dissemination to bone marrow and the CNS. Patients often have bulky organ involvement with potential obstruction of the respiratory, gastrointestinal, or genitourinary tracts. This tumor is exquisitely sensitive to chemotherapy, but early relapse after a complete remission foretells a poor prognosis.

Diagnostic Evaluation of Lymph Node Biopsy

The lymph node biopsy is the key diagnostic test in NHL. The histologic pattern has a much greater influence on the clinical course and treatment than is the case with HD. The International Working Classification organizes lymphomas by the pattern of lymph node infiltration—follicular (nodular) or diffuse—as well as by the types of cells involved in the infiltrate: small, large, or both. As can be appreciated from Table 38–7, the follicular lymphomas on the whole are less aggressive than the diffuse lesions, as shown by the median and 5-year survival rates.

Table 38–8 presents the characteristics of the various types of malignant cells that may be found in the lymph node biopsy. These are further described here.

Small lymphocytes are associated with low-grade small lymphocytic lymphoma. The nodal biopsy shows a diffuse pattern of small round lymphocytes with clumped chromatin, inconspicuous nucleoli, and scant cytoplasm; rare cells are in mitoses. This infiltrate is identical to that of chronic lymphocytic leukemia, and these cells are indistinguishable from normal peripheral blood lymphocytes. Roughly 95% of these infiltrates are B cell.[38]

The *small cleaved cell* is the same size to slightly larger than a normal peripheral blood lymphocyte (Fig. 38-3). Its cytoplasm is scant to almost nonvisible. The nucleus has coarsely condensed chromatin and prominent clefting or indentation.

The *large cell, cleaved* or *noncleaved*, is two to three times the size of a normal peripheral blood lymphocyte (Fig. 38-4). The nuclei are large and round to oval. The chromatin condensation is spotty such that the nucleus appears to have a lot of clear space. The nucleoli are large and prominent, numbering one to three per cell. The cytoplasm forms a distinct but thin rim around the nucleus.

The *immunoblastic large cell* is four to five times the size of a normal lymphocyte. The cytoplasm is abundant but stains much fainter than the large cell described above. The nucleus is large and round with prominent nucleoli.

The *lymphoblastic cell* has a large round or convoluted nucleus. The chromatin pattern is very fine, and nucleoli are indistinct. There are frequent mitotic forms in infiltrates involving these cells, and the majority are T cells. These cells are identical to those of T-cell acute lymphocytic leukemia.

The *small noncleaved cell* is misnamed. At 15 to 30 μm in diameter, it is a large cell but intermediate in size between the small cleaved lymphocytes (8–12 μm) and large lymphocytes (greater than 20 μm) described above. The cy-

TABLE 38–8. Classification of Non-Hodgkin Lymphoma: Characteristics of Malignant Cells Found Predominantly in Lymph Node Biopsy

LYMPHOCYTE TYPE	CELL SIZE (μm)	NUCLEUS			CYTOPLASM
		CONTOUR	CHROMATIN	NUCLEOLI	
Small	8–12	Round, regular	Dense to coarse	Inconspicuous	Scanty to almost nonvisible
Small cleaved	8–12	Angulated, folded	Coarse	Inconspicuous	Scanty to almost nonvisible
Large, noncleaved	>20	Round to oval	Spotty (vesicular to fine)	Prominent	Distinct but thin rim of cytoplasm
Large, cleaved	>20	Angulated, folded	Vesicular to fine	Inconspicuous	Distinct but thin rim of cytoplasm
Immunoblastic	>20	Round to oval	Fine	Prominent and central	Abundant, faint
Lymphoblastic	>20	Round to folded	Fine	Inconspicuous	Scanty
Small, noncleaved	15–30	Round to oval	Delicate to coarse	2–5 per cell; basophilic	Scanty, basophilic, vacuolated

toplasm is scant, deeply basophilic, and often vacuolated. The chromatin is coarse, and there are two to five prominent basophilic nucleoli. In the Burkitt type small noncleaved-cell lymphoma, the cells are uniform in size and shape, and mitotic figures usually are seen. In the non-Burkitt type small noncleaved-cell lymphoma, there is more heterogeneity in size and shape. The cells usually are larger than the Burkitt lymphocytes, and there usually are numerous mitotic figures.

These basic cell types are summarized in Table 38-8. In various patterns and mixtures, they account for all the subtypes described in the working formulation of Table 38-7.

Diagnosis and Treatment

The Ann Arbor staging system outlined in Table 38-3 is also used for NHL, and the diagnostic studies useful in staging are the same as those in Tables 38-4 and 38-5.

Generally, the sequence of tests performed represents an attempt to demonstrate advanced disease, when present, early in the workup in order to spare the patient unnecessary tests. The bone marrow biopsy is especially useful in this regard because of the high frequency of positivity in the low-grade lymphomas and its effect on the staging of the intermediate- and high-grade lymphomas.

Effects of Treatment on Laboratory Results

As in HD, radiation and chemotherapy are used to treat NHL. The effects of these treatments on the laboratory results are the same as in HD, as discussed in the corresponding section earlier in this chapter.

Radiation therapy generally is given with curative intent for Stages I and II low-grade lymphomas and Stage I intermediate-grade lymphomas. Chemotherapy, usually with a combination of drugs, is used for all other types and

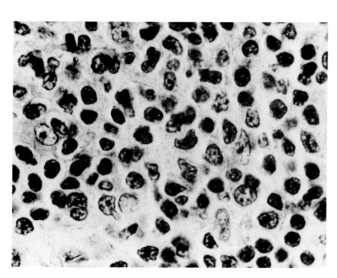

FIG. 38-3. Follicular lymphoma, predominantly small cleaved cell. Atypical lymphocytes are indented and angular (hematoxylin and eosin, magnification × 1000). (From DeVita VT Jr, Hellman S, Rosenberg SA: Cancer Principles and Practice of Oncology, 3rd ed. Philadelphia, JB Lippincott, 1989, with permission.)

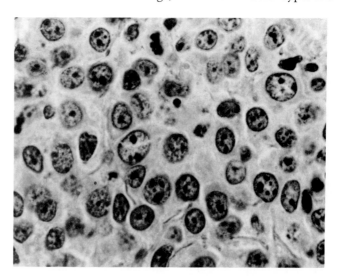

FIG. 38-4. Malignant lymphoma, diffuse, large cell type. Cells resemble large, noncleaved follicular center cells and have multiple prominent, often membrane-bound nucleoli (hematoxylin and eosin, magnification × 1000). (From DeVita VT Jr, Hellman S, Rosenberg SA: Cancer Principles and Practice of Oncology, 3rd ed. Philadelphia, JB Lippincott, 1989, with permission.)

stages. The prognosis with chemotherapy varies greatly, depending on the histologic subtype of the lymphoma.

Stages III and IV low-grade lymphomas readily go into remission with chemotherapy, but relapses are common. No currently available treatment is curative, but years of survival are nonetheless possible. The same applies to Stages III and IV follicular large-cell, diffuse small cleaved-cell, and diffuse mixed lymphomas within the intermediate grades. Stages III and IV diffuse large and diffuse small noncleaved-cell lymphomas, on the other hand, are potentially curable with aggressive chemotherapy regimens.

MYCOSIS FUNGOIDES AND SÉZARY SYNDROME

Mycosis fungoides and Sézary syndrome are rare lymphomas that represent different stages of a single neoplastic disorder. The neoplastic cell involved is the mature T-helper lymphocyte, which is produced in lymphatic tissue and migrates to the skin, which is the early primary site of involvement.

Epidemiology

It has been estimated that only 400 to 600 new cases of the conditions are diagnosed each year in the United States; thus, they account for only 2% of the annual incidence of lymphoma.[2] The typical patient is a man who is in late middle age or elderly.

Clinical Findings

The predominant early symptom is pruritus (severe itching), and the earliest lesions often are misdiagnosed as eczema, psoriasis, or other skin conditions. As the disease progresses, well demarcated reddened plaques form, or the skin can become diffusely thickened, especially about the face and in body folds. In some cases, most of the skin surface is involved, as it becomes red, thickened, and wrinkled; this process is referred to as "generalized erythroderma." In these cases, the skin desquamates in large, dead flakes.

Diagnostic Evaluation of Skin and Lymph Node Biopsy

When the patient presents with the symptoms described above, and in some cases even prior to such a presentation, skin biopsy is diagnostic and will show the upper dermis to be involved with a dense, bandlike infiltrate of lymphocytes close to the epidermis. Characteristically, the epidermis is involved as well, with clusters of lymphocytes forming the so-called "Pautrier's microabcesses." Such a primary skin presentation is referred to as "mycosis fungoides" (although fungal infection is not present) and may exist for months to years before further progression occurs. As this condition evolves, lymph node infiltration and visceral involvement (liver, spleen, and lung) occurs, and a leukemic phase can be seen. This involvement beyond the skin with peripheral blood manifestations is referred to as

Sézary syndrome. At this stage of the disease, the prognosis is worse, with survival between 12 to 15 months.[3]

Laboratory Findings and Correlations With Disease

Patients with mycosis fungoides or Sézary syndrome have laboratory abnormalities similar to those seen in other NHLs.

Peripheral Blood

The laboratory scientist may be asked to search for cells thought to be pathognomonic of this condition. The lymphocyte involved is larger than normal with scanty cytoplasm, and the nucleus is large with clefting. Nuclear folding can be so extensive as to suggest an image of the brain, and these nuclei are thus described as cerebriform. The nuclear chromatin is fine with little condensation. There may or may not be visible nucleoli. These cells can be seen on the peripheral blood film in 15% to 20% of patients with plaque disease and in as many as 90% of those with generalized erythroderma.[2]

Special Laboratory Tests

Monoclonal antibody to surface markers will indicate the CD4$^+$ subtype of helper lymphocyte. Because these disorders are fundamentally an excess of T-helper cells, it is common to see a polyclonal or monoclonal increase in immunoglobulins on serum protein electrophoresis.

Effects of Treatment on Laboratory Results

The skin infiltrative manifestation of this disorder can be treated with superficial electron-beam radiation, topically applied chemotherapy, or phototherapy with a combination of oral methoxsalen and long-wave ultraviolet light. These therapies are directed at alleviating skin symptoms and do not have the systemic effects previously described for radiation and chemotherapy of other lymphomas. Systemic combination chemotherapy is reserved for the treatment of lymph node, visceral, and leukemic manifestations. With current technology, these two conditions are treatable but not curable.

CHAPTER SUMMARY

Lymphomas are a group of malignant diseases associated with abnormal lymph node enlargement that disrupts the normal histology. Peripheral blood abnormalities are not a hallmark of these disorders until the more advanced stages of disease.

Lymphoma is divided into two principal classes: Hodgkin disease (HD) and non-Hodgkin lymphomas (NHLs). The diseases are diagnosed by lymph node biopsy. The cells from biopsies of NHLs generally are uniformly malignant B lymphocytes. The biopsy in HD usually reveals a mixture of normal cells and malignant Reed-Sternberg cells, with normal cells predominating.

The Reed-Sternberg cell is often binucleated, and its prominent nucleoli are eosinophilic with a perinucleolar halo, giving the cell its "owl-eyed" appearance (see Fig. 38-1).

Hodgkin disease usually is an orderly disease in that it starts in one area and spreads in a uniform fashion. It is often diagnosed by the finding of an enlarged, painless lymph node in the neck. Patients may complain of fever, night sweats, or weight loss, known as the B symptoms.

Hodgkin disease is usually classified according to the Rye scheme (see Table 38-2). The more abundant the lymphocytes and the less abundant the Reed-Sternberg cells in the lymph node biopsy, the better the prognosis. Also, the younger the patient and the less advanced the disease, the better the prognosis. The Ann Arbor staging system (see Table 38-3) is used to formulate the treatment plan.

Laboratory abnormalities in HD are often nonspecific; there usually is no anemia, and platelets generally are normal. Leukocytosis may come with advancing disease, and abnormal-appearing lymphocytes with little cytoplasm and irregular chromatin may be found on the peripheral blood film. Lymphocytopenia signals a poor prognosis. The bone marrow is seldom involved except in advanced stages. Treatment with radiation and chemotherapy can have profound suppressive effects on the marrow.

Non-Hodgkin lymphomas are classified according to the International Working Classification of Non-Hodgkin's Lymphomas (see Table 38-7). Characteristics of the malignant cells found in lymph node biopsies from the various diseases within each group are shown in Table 38-8. The blood counts in NHLs generally are normal, and no other laboratory findings are particularly classic. The modified Ann Arbor staging system is also used for NHLs to plan effective treatment, which, as in HD, includes radiation and chemotherapy, with the same effects on the bone marrow and peripheral blood.

Mycosis fungoides and Sézary syndrome are rare lymphomas caused by a neoplastic T lymphocyte that migrates to the skin, causing skin abnormalities. Skin biopsy is the diagnostic tool. The laboratory abnormalities are similar to those of NHLs. The classic cell is a lymphocyte that is larger than normal with scant cytoplasm and a cerebriform nucleus with or without nucleoli and with fine chromatin. The conditions are treatable but not curable.

CASE STUDY 38-1

A 63-year-old woman was admitted with the chief complaint of fever to 102°F for 2 weeks associated with drenching night sweats. In the 4 months preceding admission, the patient had lost approximately 40 pounds. Her medical history was significant only for appendectomy, cholecystectomy, and three normal childbirths. The family history and review of organ systems were not remarkable.

On physical examination, she was obese and ill appearing. Her neck was obviously asymmetric, with a generalized fullness on the left that had gone unnoticed by the patient and her family. This fullness was attributable to a matted mass of cervical lymph nodes approximately 6 cm in diameter underlying the left sternocleidomastoid muscle. There were firm 3-cm lymph nodes under both axillae. The chest was clear. The abdomen was without liver or spleen enlargement. There were no enlarged inguinal nodes.

A complete blood count revealed: WBC 15.5 × 10⁹/L with 6% eosinophils; platelets 475 × 10⁹/L; Hb 12.6 g/dL; and HCT 0.36 L/L. Blood chemistry studies showed an elevated LD and alkaline phosphatase but were otherwise normal.

A routine chest radiograph was normal. Computed tomographic (CT) scans of the chest and abdomen showed mediastinal, mesenteric, and para-aortic adenopathy.

A bone marrow film was normal, but the biopsy core demonstrated an infiltrate of lymphocytes compatible with lymphoma. Biopsy of the left cervical nodes demonstrated mixed-cellularity HD. Because of her symptoms and the involvement of bone marrow, the disease was staged IVB, and no further workup was done.

The patient started on chemotherapy, and within the first week, the fever and night sweats abated. At 1 month, the patient was free of

adenopathy on clinical examination. After 3 months of treatment, repeat CT scans were normal. The patient received a total of six cycles of chemotherapy, with alternating combinations of eight drugs, which lasted 12 months. Three years after diagnosis, the patient remains free of disease.

1. Is this patient anemic? Are her Hb and HCT unusual for such a diagnosis?
2. What granulocyte count level (i.e., elevated, normal, or decreased) might be expected in this patient's condition?
3. Is it common to find a normal bone marrow aspirate but an abnormal biopsy core in patients with HD? Explain.
4. What effect might her chemotherapy have had on her platelet, granulocyte, and erythrocyte counts?
5. If the patient's platelet count had declined to 35 × 10⁹/L during chemotherapy, would a platelet transfusion have been appropriate even if there were no signs of bleeding?
6. Which leukocyte usually increases in relative numbers to herald the coming increase of peripheral blood granulocytes? Approximately how long before the granulocyte recovery does this signal occur?

CASE STUDY 38-2

A 32-year-old homosexual man with AIDS was admitted to the hospital with the chief complaint of fevers to 103°F daily for 2 weeks with night sweats and a 30-pound weight loss over the previous 2 months. The patient also noted gradual enlargement of the left side of his neck, which had been painful for 1 week prior to admission.

On physical examination, there was bilateral adenopathy of the cervical node chains. A 5 × 7-cm mass was palpable on the left side of the neck and a 6 × 2-cm mass on the right side. There was no enlargement of the liver or spleen.

A chest radiograph demonstrated a normal mediastinum and hilar structures. Abdominal CT scan and a magnetic resonance imaging (MRI) scan of the brain were normal.

The CBC, differential, and bone marrow biopsies were normal. Serum chemistry studies were within reference ranges except for the LD, which was highly elevated. The cerebrospinal fluid was acellular with normal protein and glucose but was positive for human immunodeficiency virus (HIV) antibody. Biopsy of the neck mass on the left demonstrated diffuse large-cell lymphoma. The disease was clinically staged IIB.

The patient was started on chemotherapy with a combination that included methotrexate, a drug that crosses well into the brain tissue and cerebrospinal fluid. Intrathecal and intravenous methotrexate were given concurrently to further boost cerebrospinal drug levels. This approach was taken in light of the patient's B symptoms and the lymphoma histology, which, in the context of AIDS, is an aggressive tumor that has great potential to involve the CNS. Within 1 one week, the patient became afebrile and was much better. The neck masses regressed dramatically. Within 1 month, he was normal on physical examination and returned to work.

The patient completed 4 months of therapy and remained free of lymphadenopathy. During this interval, he felt good and gained back all previously lost weight. At this time, the patient's marrow was hypocellular secondary to chemotherapy. He developed fever with negative blood cultures but did not respond to broad-spectrum antibiotics. However, he did respond to antifungal therapy with amphotericin B and was discharged improved.

Three days later, the patient was readmitted for recurrent fever, lethargy, severe headaches, and slurred speech. Reexamination did not disclose adenopathy or any cranial nerve deficits. By the second hospital day, the patient was confused and more lethargic and had experienced nerve paralysis. A CT scan of the brain demonstrated masses in the right cerebellum and cerebrum. An MRI scan of the brain disclosed multiple lesions compatible with tumors or abcesses. Toxoplasmosis serology studies were positive. Antibiotic therapy for toxoplasmosis was given. The day before brain biopsy was scheduled, the patient had a convulsion and respiratory arrest. By the sixth hospital day, he was brain dead secondary to uncal herniation caused by massive cerebral edema. The patient was taken off life support, and he died.

Autopsy confirmed that the patient was free of lymphoma. The cause of death was disseminated toxoplasmosis involving the brain, lungs, liver, stomach, small bowel, and kidneys, probably resulting from the effects of both chemotherapy and AIDS.

REFERENCES

1. Blayney DW, Jaffe ES, Blattner WA et al: The human T-cell leukemia/lymphoma virus (HTLV) associated with American adult T-cell leukemia/lymphoma (ATL). Blood 62:401, 1983

2. Bunn PA Jr, Poiesz BJ: Cutaneous T-cell lymphomas (mycosis fungoides and Sézary syndrome). In Williams WJ, Beutler E, Erslev AJ, Lichtman MA (eds): Hematology, 3rd ed, p 1056. New York, McGraw-Hill, 1983

3. Bunn PA Jr, Huberman MS, Whang-Peng J et al: Prospective staging evaluation of patients with cutaneous T-cell lymphomas. Ann Intern Med 93:223, 1980

4. Bunting CH: The blood picture in Hodgkin's disease. Bull Johns Hopkins Hosp 22:369, 1911

5. Carbone PP, Kaplan HS, Musshoff K et al: Report of the Committee on Hodgkin's Disease Staging. Cancer Res 31:1860, 1971

6. Chabner BA, Johnson RE, Young RC et al: Sequential nonsurgical and surgical staging of non-Hodgkin's lymphoma. Ann Intern Med 85:149, 1976

7. Cline MJ, Berlin NI: Anemia in Hodgkin's disease. Cancer 16:526, 1963

8. Crowther D, Fairley GH, Sewell RL: Significance of the changes in the circulating lymphoid cells in Hodgkin's disease. Br Med J 2:473, 1969

9. Desser RK, Golomb HM, Ultmann JE et al: Prognostic classification of Hodgkin's disease in Stage III, based on anatomic considerations. Blood 49:883, 1977

10. DeVita VT Jr: Lymphocyte reactivity in Hodgkin's disease: A lymphocyte civil war. N Engl J Med 289:801, 1973

11. DeVita VT Jr, Jaffe ES, Hellman S: Hodgkin's disease and the non-Hodgkin's lymphomas. In DeVita VT Jr, Hellman S, Rosenberg SA (eds): Cancer: Principles and Practice of Oncology, 2nd ed, p 1623. Philadelphia, JB Lippincott, 1985

12. DeVita VT Jr, Chabner B, Hubbard SP et al: Advanced diffuse histiocytic lymphoma, a potentially curable disease. Lancet 1:248, 1975

13. Fisher RI: Hodgkin's disease, p 370. In Wittes RE (ed): Manual of Oncologic Therapeutics 1989/1990. Philadelphia, JB Lippincott, 1989

14. Foucar K, McKenna RW, Frizzera G et al: Bone marrow and blood involvement by lymphoma in relationship to the Lukes-Collins classification. Cancer 49:888, 1982

15. Gall EA, Mallory TB: Malignant lymphoma: A clinical pathologic survey of 618 cases. Am J Pathol 18:381, 1942

16. Gatti RA, Good RA: Occurrence of malignancy in immunodeficiency disease. Cancer 28:89, 1971

17. Gill PS, Levine AM, Meyer PR et al: Primary central nervous system lymphoma in homosexual men: Clinical, immunologic, and pathologic features. Am J Med 78:742, 1985

18. Grufferman S, Cole P, Smith PG et al: Hodgkin's disease in siblings. N Engl J Med 296:248, 1977

19. Gutensohn N, Cole P: Childhood social environment and Hodgkin's disease. N Engl J Med 304:135, 1981

20. Halie MR, Huiges W, Nieweg HO: Abnormal cells in the peripheral blood of patients with Hodgkin's disease: I. Observations with light microscopy. Br J Haematol 28:317, 1974

21. Halie MR, Eibergen R, Nieweg HO: Observations on abnormal cells in the peripheral blood and spleen in Hodgkin's disease. Br Med J 2:609, 1972

22. Halie MR, Splett-Romascano M, Molenaar I et al: Abnormal cells in the peripheral blood of patients with Hodgkin's disease: II. Ultrastructural studies. Br J Haematol 28:323, 1974

23. Hodgkin T: On some morbid appearances of the absorbent glands and spleen. Med-Chir Trans 17:68, 1832

24. Hsu SM, Jaffe ES: Leu M1 and peanut agglutinin stain the neoplastic cells of Hodgkin's disease. Am J Clin Pathol 82:29, 1984

25. Hsu SM, Yang K, Jaffe ES: Phenotypic expression of Hodgkin's and Reed-Sternberg cells in Hodgkin's disease. Am J Pathol 118:209, 1985

26. Isomaki HA, Hakulinen T, Joutsenlahti U: Excess risk of lymphomas, leukemias, and myeloma in patients with rheumatoid arthritis. J Chronic Dis 31:691, 1978

27. Jones SE: Autoimmune disorders and malignant lymphoma. Cancer 31:1092, 1973

28. Kadin ME: Possible origin of the Reed-Sternberg cell from an interdigitating reticulum cell. Cancer Treat Rep 66:601, 1982

29. Kaplan HS, Gartner S: "Sternberg-Reed" giant cells of Hodgkin's disease: Cultivation in vitro, heterotransplantation, and characterization as neoplastic macrophages. Int J Cancer 19:511, 1977

30. Kaplan HS, Goodenow RS, Gartner S et al: Biology and virology of the human malignant lymphomas. Cancer 43:1, 1979

31. Kassan SS, Thomas TL, Moutsopoulos HM et al: Increased risk of lymphoma in sicca syndrome. Ann Intern Med 89:888, 1978

32. Keller AR, Kaplan HS, Lukes RJ et al: Correlation of histopathology with other prognostic indicators in Hodgkin's disease. Cancer 22: 487, 1968

33. Kinlen LJ, Sheil AGR, Peto J et al: Collaborative United Kingdom-Australasian study of cancer in patients treated with immunosuppressive drugs. Br Med J 2:1461, 1979

34. Levine AM, Thorton P, Forman SJ et al: Positive Coombs' test in Hodgkin's disease: Significance and implications. Blood 55:607, 1980

35. Lukes RJ, Butler JJ, Hicks EB: Natural history of Hodgkin's disease as related to its pathologic picture. Cancer 19:317, 1966

36. Lukes RJ, Craver LF, Hall TC et al: Report of the Nomenclature Committee. Cancer Res 26:1311, 1966

37. MacMahon B: Epidemiologic evidence on the nature of Hodgkin's disease. Cancer 10:1045, 1957

38. Mann RB, Jaffe ES, Berard CW: Malignant lymphomas: A conceptual understanding of morphologic diversity. Am J Pathol 94:105, 1979

39. Munoz N, Davidson RJL, Witthoff B et al: Infectious mononucleosis and Hodgkin's disease. Int J Cancer 22:10, 1978

40. Nadler LM, Ritz J, Griffin JD et al: Diagnosis and treatment of human leukemias and lymphomas utilizing monoclonal antibodies. Prog Hematol 12:187, 1981

41. Peters MV, Alison RE, Buch RS: Natural history of Hodgkin's disease as related to staging. Cancer 19:308, 1966

42. Rappaport H, Winter WJ, Hicks EB: Follicular lymphoma: A reevaluation of its position in the scheme of malignant lymphomas, based on a survey of 253 cases. Cancer 9:792, 1956

43. Ray GR, Wolf PH, Kaplan HS: Value of laboratory indicators in Hodgkin's disease: Preliminary results. Natl Cancer Inst Monogr 36:315, 1972

44. Reed DM: On the pathological changes in Hodgkin's disease, with special reference to its relation to tuberculosis. Johns Hopkins Hosp Rep 10:133, 1902

45. Risdall R, Hoppe RT, Warnke R: Non-Hodgkin's lymphoma: A study of the evolution of the disease based upon 92 autopsied cases. Cancer 44:529, 1979

46. Rosenberg SA, Berard CW, Brown BW, and the Non-Hodgkin's Lymphoma Pathologic Classification Project Committee: National Cancer Institute sponsored study of classification of non-Hodgkin's lymphomas: Summary and description of a working formulation for clinical usage. Cancer 49:2112, 1982

47. Rosenberg SA, Diamond HD, Jaslowitz B et al: Lymphosarcoma: A review of 1269 cases. Medicine 40:31, 1961

48. Schiffer CA, Levi JA, Wiernik PH: The significance of abnormal circulating cells in patients with Hodgkin's disease. Br J Haematol 31:177, 1975

49. Silar G, Brusamolino E, Bernasconi C et al: Isolation of Reed-Sternberg cells from lymph nodes of Hodgkin's disease patients. Blood 73:222, 1989

50. Stein H, Mason DY, Gerdes J et al: The expression of the Hodgkin's disease associated antigen K_i-1 in reactive and neoplastic lymphoid tissue: Evidence that Reed-Sternberg cells and histiocytic malignancies are derived from activated lymphoid cells. Blood 66:848, 1985

51. Sternberg C: Über eine Eigenartige unter dem Bilde der Pseudoleukämie verlaufende Tuberculose des lymphatichen Apparates. Ztschr Heilk 19:21, 1898

52. Stuart AE, Jackson E, Morris CS: The reaction of xenogenic and monoclonal antisera with Reed-Sternberg cells. J Pathol 137:129, 1982

53. Tubiana M, Attie E, Flamant R et al: Prognostic factors in 454 cases of Hodgkin's disease. Cancer Res 31:1801, 1971

54. Ultmann JE, Moran EM: Clinical course and complications in Hodgkin's disease. Arch Intern Med 131:332, 1973

55. Virchow R: Gesammelte Abhandlungen zur wissenschaftlichen Medizin. Frankfurt, Meindinger, 1856

56. Wyburn-Mason R: SLE and lymphoma. Lancet 1:156, 1979

57. Young JL, Percy CL, Asire AJ (eds): Surveillance, Epidemiology, and End Results: Incidence and Mortality Data, 1973-77, Natl Cancer Inst Monogr 57. Washington DC, US Government Printing Office, 1981

Plasma Cell

Dyscrasias

(Paraproteinemias)

Lynne H. Lyons

Malignant transformation may occur at any point during the maturation and differentiation of lymphocytes. Earlier chapters have described leukemias resulting from neoplastic disorders of lymphoid stem cells (acute lymphoid leukemias) and of immature lymphocytes (chronic lymphoproliferative disorders). This chapter will address malignant disorders of the differentiated end cells of B lymphocytes: plasma cells and plasmacytoid lymphocytes. (See Chap. 24 for schema of normal B-lymphocyte maturation.) These disorders are sometimes referred to as "monoclonal gammopathies," because the malignant plasma cells all produce identical proteins.

REVIEW OF IMMUNOGLOBULINS

Plasma cells are capable of synthesizing heterogeneous proteins—immunoglobulins (Igs)—with the capacity to bind the particular antigens that stimulated their production. Each cell produces a particular, specific Ig.

All Igs are composed of a basic structural unit of four polypeptide chains—two symmetrically arranged, heavy (H) chains and two light (L) chains, which are linked with disulfide bonds (Fig. 39-1). There are two antigen-binding sites per unit. The variable regions on both the H and the L chains are specifically coded for antibody function and share this activity. The Fc portion of the H chains directs the biologic activity of the molecule, such as complement activation or adherence to surfaces of neutrophils, macrophages, and certain lymphocytes.

Although all Igs share a basic structural unit, there are five classes which differ in the amino acid sequence of their H chains and in their structural arrangement, giving them functional uniqueness. The different H chains are designated gamma (γ), alpha (α), mu (μ), delta (δ), and epsilon

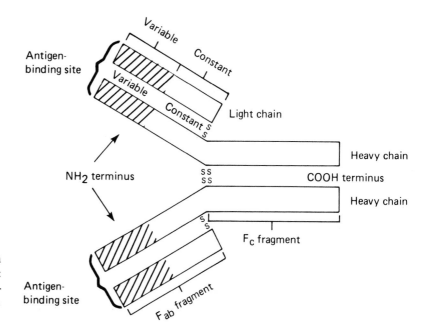

FIG. 39-1. Immunoglobulin structure. (From Bishop ML, Duben–Von Laufen JL, Fody EP (eds): Clinical Chemistry: Principles, Procedures, Correlations, p 154. Philadelphia, JB Lippincott, 1985, with permission.)

(ϵ), and correspond to the five immunoglobulin classes IgG, IgA, IgM, IgD, and IgE. There are only two classes of L chains: kappa (κ) and lambda (λ). Any given molecule of an H-chain class will have either kappa or lambda L chains, never one of each.

Types

IgG exists as a monomer with a molecular mass of 150,000 daltons. It accounts for approximately 80% of the total Ig found in the blood and extravascular space. IgG is responsible for the secondary immune response, precipitating antibodies, virus-neutralizing antibodies, hemagglutinins, hemolysins, and activators of the classical complement pathway.

IgA often exists as a dimer, but monomers as well as polymers are found. Although IgA is the second most abundant Ig, it constitutes only 10% to 15% of the total amount. A slightly larger molecule than IgG (180,000 daltons), it is synthesized by plasma cells in the epithelium of the respiratory and gastrointestinal tracts and in most excretory glands. IgA provides the first line of defense on mucosal surfaces.

IgM, the largest Ig with a molecular mass of 900,000 daltons, has a circular pentameric arrangement. It makes up 5% to 10% of the total Igs and is localized in the blood. IgM is the first antibody to appear in response to antigenic challenge.

IgD is a monomer with the lowest molecular mass (140,000 daltons) of the Igs. Only trace amounts are found in serum. Rather, IgD is a surface Ig on blood lymphocytes and may have lymphocyte activation and suppression activity.

IgE is a monomer with a molecular mass of 200,000 daltons, only slightly greater than IgG and IgA. This is the "reaginic antibody" found mostly in the respiratory and gastrointestinal tracts. IgE attaches to mast cells and basophils. It mediates allergic reactions and plays a role in the response to parasitic infections.

Laboratory Measurement

Igs make up approximately 12% to 20% of the total serum protein of normal individuals. Because of the physical and chemical properties of proteins, Igs in serum and body fluids can be separated from other proteins in an electric field by a process called electrophoresis. These separated serum fractions, namely albumin, alpha-1, alpha-2, beta, and gamma, are then stained, the supporting medium is rendered transparent, and the stained zone is scanned densitometrically to obtain the relative percentage of each fraction. Addressing strictly the gamma region where Igs migrate, a polyclonal increase is noted as a band uniformly larger than normal, representing an increase in heterogeneous Igs. A monoclonal peak occurs when molecules traveling at the same rate concentrate at the same point, suggesting activity of a particular clone of plasma cells (a "paraprotein"). Figure 39-2 demonstrates examples of normal, polyclonal, and monoclonal patterns.

To detect an imbalance of Ig or the presence of free H or L chains, immunotechniques such as immunoelectrophoresis (IEP) or immunofixation electrophoresis (IFE) are used. Detailed discussions of these techniques may be found in immunology or clinical chemistry texts.

The following is a discussion of the more common monoclonal gammopathies. Table 39-1 summarizes the laboratory findings for each of these disorders.

MULTIPLE MYELOMA (PLASMA CELL MYELOMA)

Pathophysiology

Multiple myeloma is the most common malignant disease of plasma cells and generally affects older individuals (50–75 years). Although the etiology is unknown, both genetics and chronic antigenic stimulation have been suggested as predisposing factors. Clonal proliferation of malignant plasma cells begins in the bone marrow, and multi-

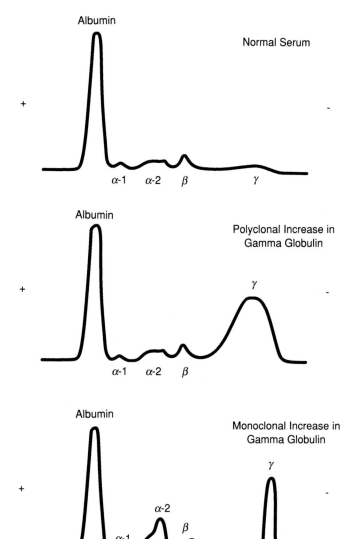

FIG. 39-2. Electrophoretic patterns showing separated serum fractions for normal serum and for polyclonal and monoclonal increases in gamma globulins.

ple tumors appear as patchy infiltrates in skeletal structures, producing osteoporosis and lytic bone disease. As the neoplastic mass grows, pathologic bone fractures and vertebral collapse may occur. Infiltration can spread to lymph nodes, spleen, and other organs. The homogeneous protein synthesized by the abnormal clone may be complete Igs or an L-chain subunit (i.e., kappa or lambda). However, myeloma cells have decreased ability to synthesize normal Igs against specific antigen. In fact, these cells suppress normal lymphocytic function.[10]

More than 50% of the myelomas produce proteins of the IgG class. The second most frequent monoclonal protein is IgA, seen in about 20% of cases. This incidence roughly correlates with the amount of each class of Ig synthesized by healthy individuals. IgD and IgE myelomas are rare, and IgM paraprotein is mostly associated with macroglobulinemia (to be described later), although IgM myelomas have been described.[17] Clones producing only an L chain, the so-called Bence-Jones protein, are a third significant group, about 15%. Free L chains, more frequently kappa, can be detected in about 80% of all myelomas.

Imbalance in plasma proteins with an absolute increase in monoclonal Ig sometimes increases plasma viscosity. The lower molecular weight L chains (Bence-Jones protein) are readily filtered by the renal glomeruli. Early in the disease, the L chains are reabsorbed and catabolized by the proximal tubules. With increasing reabsorptive load, catabolism decreases, permitting Bence-Jones protein to reenter the circulation. As renal impairment progresses, L-chain reabsorption decreases; the amount of L chains exceeds the renal tubule threshold, and they spill into the urine. It is suggested that nephrotoxicity is limited to only some types of L chains.[2] Amyloid deposition is a further complication for about 25% of patients; this topic is discussed later in this chapter.

As the tumor mass grows, the marrow cannot continue normal production of other cellular components. Likewise, there is decreased production of normal Ig. What normal Ig is produced often is destroyed in the catabolism of excessive amounts of abnormal protein. Circulating leukocytes with surface Fc receptors are overwhelmed by the amount of

TABLE 39–1. Laboratory Findings in Plasma Cell Dyscrasias

| | MULTIPLE MYELOMA | PLASMA CELL LEUKEMIA | WALDENSTRÖM's MACROGLOBULINEMIA | HEAVY CHAIN DISEASES | | |
				ALPHA	GAMMA	MU
Peripheral blood	Rouleaux; rare abnormal plasma cells	Rouleaux; >2.0×10⁹/L abnormal plasma cells	Rouleaux; rare plasmacytoid lymphocytes or plasma cells	–	–	–
Bone marrow	10%–15% myeloma cells	Small-type abnormal plasma cells	Plasmacytoid lymphocytes		Variant lymphocytes and plasma cells	Vacuolated plasma cells
Serum proteins	Monoclonal peak	Monoclonal peak	Monoclonal IgM (15%)	——————— Hypogammaglobulinemia ———————		
Urine protein	L chains (80%)	–	L chains (33%)	α H chains	γ H chains	μ H chains
Radiography	Significant osteoporosis; bone lesions	Slight osteolysis	–	α H chains	γ H chains	L chains
				–	–	–
Other	Amyloidosis (15%)	–	Increased plasma viscosity; cryoglobulins	H chains in jejunal fluid	–	Assoc. with CLL

monoclonal Ig; therefore, functional cellular immunity is lost along with the humoral response.

Clinical Presentation

The chief complaint of many myeloma patients is skeletal pain. Initial back pain and that associated with centrally located bones progresses to the severe pain of spontaneous (pathologic) bone fracture. Accompanying anemia and renal insufficiency cause patients to experience weakness and fatigue. There may be episodes of bleeding secondary to thrombocytopenia, as well as a greater susceptibility to infection.

Laboratory Findings and Correlations with Disease

Peripheral blood findings include normochromic, normocytic anemia with Hb levels between 7 and 12 g/dL. As expected, the erythrocyte sedimentation rate (ESR) is increased because of elevated serum globulins. The blood film shows rouleaux, and the differential may show a slight neutropenia with little or no evidence of abnormal plasma cells in the early stages. Later, a few abnormal plasma cells may be seen in the blood (Fig. 39-3). It should be noted that a benign reactive plasmacytosis may also result in a few circulating plasma cells and must be differentiated from multiple myeloma. Overpopulation of the marrow with abnormal plasma cells may produce pancytopenia and elicit a leukoerythroblastic response.

Bone marrow aspirate from an osteolytic site commonly reveals more than 10% to 15% abnormal plasma cells.[4] Within a specific specimen, most myeloma cells will have a particular morphology, thus demonstrating their clonal na-

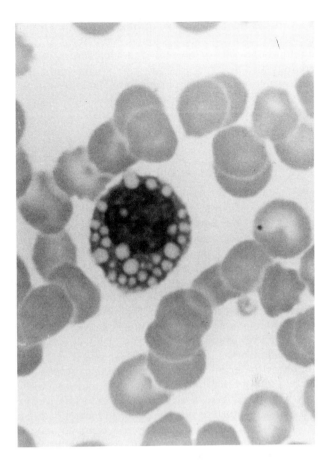

FIG. 39-4. Abnormal plasma cell with immunoglobulin trapped in cisternae of endoplasmic reticulum. This cell has been referred to as a Mott cell, morula cell, or plasma cell with Russell bodies.

ture. From specimen to specimen, however, there may be great diversity (see Plate 60A and B). Myeloma cells may be large with immature-appearing chromatin or small with clumped chromatin and may be pale or dark, depending on the amount of cytoplasmic RNA. Occasionally, bizarre multinucleated plasma cells are encountered, whereas other cases present lobulated nuclei, which adds to the already confusing morphologic possibilities.[11] Cellular inclusions such as intranuclear (Dutcher) bodies, crystalline structures of abnormal Ig, or rounded accumulations of Ig in the cisternae (Russell bodies) are associated with plasma cell myeloma[7] (Fig. 39-4). A few IgA myelomas present flame cells characterized by abundant cytoplasm with a reddish tinge of ribosomal protein (Plate 61).

Routine urinalysis may not determine the extent of proteinuria accurately, as the reagent strip and sulfosalicylic acid tests are more sensitive to albumin than to globulin and L chains. Microscopic examination of urine sediment may reveal hyaline casts and evidence of renal tubular degeneration such as tubular epithelial cells embedded in the hyaline casts.

Protein electrophoresis reveals monoclonal Ig in both serum and concentrated urine. Immunotechniques using sensitive antisera are necessary to ascertain the Ig class and L-chain type. Either IEP or IFE of concentrated urine not

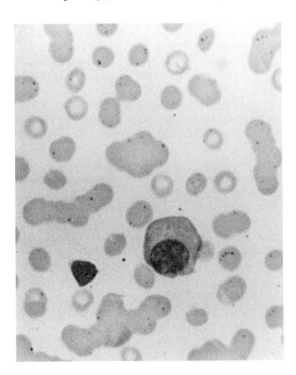

FIG. 39-3. Peripheral blood of patient with multiple myeloma showing rouleaux and circulating plasma cell in center of field.

only identifies the L chain but, of more diagnostic importance, detects Bence-Jones myelomas in the event of hypogammaglobulinemia or normal-appearing serum protein. There may also be hyperuricemia and hypercalcemia from bone destruction. Alkaline phosphatase levels are normal, because compensation for osteoporosis usually does not occur. Radiologic evidence of osteoporosis and lytic bone lesions is of great diagnostic importance.

Effects of Treatment on Laboratory Results

Alkylating agents in combination with prednisone have proved effective in the treatment of multiple myeloma. Complete remissions are uncommon; however, shorter survival has been reported when Bence-Jones proteinuria is present, and Bence-Jones myeloma has the worst prognosis.[8] The median survival can be from 1 to 5 years, depending on the extent of the disease, including the degree of renal impairment, at the time of treatment.[16] In addition to corticosteroids, analgesics and localized radiotherapy may be used to control pain. Steps must be taken to prevent skeletal fractures. Supportive therapy for infection and renal impairment also is indicated. The response to treatment is monitored by serum and concentrated urine protein studies, CBC, and radiographs. Further bone marrow studies usually have little value in therapeutic monitoring. Ideally, serum proteins return to normal levels with a concomitant decrease in the ESR. Likewise, bone lesions should decrease, reflecting decreased tumor cells, with associated resolution of cytopenias.

PLASMA CELL LEUKEMIA

A patient is said to have plasma cell leukemia when circulating plasma cells exceed 2×10^9/L.[4] A leukemic blood picture can occur as a late manifestation of plasma cell myeloma, but plasma cell leukemia has been reported as a discrete entity.[15]

Clinical Presentation

The patient with plasma cell leukemia is usually younger than one with multiple myeloma, complains less of bone pain, and shows less osteolysis. There is a greater incidence of lymphadenopathy and hepatosplenomegaly.

Laboratory Findings and Correlations with Disease

Greater than 2×10^9 abnormal plasma cells/L, pancytopenia with leukoerythroblastic findings, and an elevated ESR are found in the peripheral blood. Morphologically, the abnormal plasma cells are small with little cytoplasm and with pronounced nuclear:cytoplasmic asynchronism. Bone marrow infiltration is diffuse, and the proliferating cells exceed 45% of the population.[15] Serum and urine protein studies will differentiate this disorder from the more common lymphatic leukemias.

WALDENSTRÖM MACROGLOBULINEMIA

Pathophysiology

In 1944, Waldenström described a lymphoproliferative disorder characterized by a large concentration of monoclonal IgM. The abnormal B lymphocytes involved in this rare malignancy are primarily in the extramedullary nodes and have the ability to differentiate into large plasmacytoid lymphocytes and plasma cells.[11] In classic Waldenström macroglobulinemia, IgM exceeds 15% of the gammaglobulin concentration. It is the increased concentration of these macromolecules that is responsible for the principal clinical manifestations. Unlike multiple myeloma, Waldenström macroglobulinemia rarely causes osteolytic lesions. Renal consequences are primarily glomerular lesions caused by deposition of IgM complexes of amyloid.[3]

Clinical Presentation

There appears to be a gradual onset of symptoms as the IgM concentration mounts. Patients are predominantly men and are older than 50 years of age and complain of fatigue, weight loss, blurred vision, and bleeding episodes, especially epistaxis. Physical findings include hepatosplenomegaly, lymphadenopathy, and retinal abnormalities preceding retinal hemorrhage.

Laboratory Findings and Correlations with Disease

Hemorrhage, hemodilution from hypervolemia, and decreased red cell survival contribute to the development of normochromic, normocytic anemia. The reticulocyte count usually is normal or decreased. The numbers of platelets and leukocytes are usually within normal ranges. An increased ESR secondary to rouleaux formation is expected. Bone marrow examination or biopsy reveals a morphologic picture of plasmacytoid lymphoma. There may be considerable variation (small lymphocytes, plasmacytoid lymphocytes, or plasma cells) among patients.[11] Mast cells may be increased, a helpful diagnostic feature if present. Malignant cells circulate in the peripheral blood only in the terminal stages.

Macromolecules at this concentration coat platelets and inhibit normal function, leading to increased bleeding time and abnormal platelet aggregation studies. Also, abnormal IgM can interact with coagulation factors and frequently produces prolonged thrombin times and artifactually low fibrinogen values.

Differential diagnostic data for Waldenström macroglobulinemia are obtained from serum protein electrophoresis and immunoelectrophoresis. An identifiable monoclonal peak frequently migrates in the beta–gamma region and constitutes greater than 15% of the total gammaglobulin. Specific antisera verify the IgM class and L-chain type. About one fourth of the patients produce free L chains in the urine.

Other serum studies show greatly increased plasma viscosity. Significantly, monoclonal IgM may exhibit cryoglobulin activity demonstrated by precipitation or gel formation during refrigeration at 4°C. Some of these IgM proteins possess antigenic specificity associated with Raynaud phenomenon (anti-G) and cold agglutinin disease (anti-i) manifested by an autoimmune hemolytic anemia. Difficulties may occur with electronic cell counts on such specimens. Spuriously elevated platelet counts may indicate that serum precipitates are being counted as platelets.[13]

Effects of Treatment on Laboratory Results

Treatment depends on the degree of marrow infiltration. Early in the course of the disease, a patient might be maintained by plasmapheresis to reduce serum hyperviscosity. Alkylating agents, possibly in combination with prednisone, are effective,[3] and successful interferon treatment has been reported.[9] A good response would consist of decreased IgM with a subsequent decline in hyperviscosity, size of the spleen and lymph nodes, and correction of anemia. Median survival of as long as 6 years is dependent on early diagnosis and treatment.

HEAVY CHAIN DISEASES

The heavy chain diseases are rare immunoproliferative disorders characterized by abnormal synthesis of the Fc portion of a particular H chain. Incomplete H chains of three major classes of Igs are produced by the tumor cells: alpha, gamma, and mu. The tumor cells involved resemble activated lymphocytes and plasma cells and present a clinical picture similar to that of malignant lymphoma.

Clinical Presentation

Alpha HCD, the most common of this group of gammopathies, is characterized by infiltration of plasmacytoid lymphocytes into the duodenal or jejunal wall, producing symptoms of malabsorption and abdominal distress. The respiratory tract, also a site for secretory IgA, is involved in a few cases, leading ultimately to pulmonary insufficiency. Gamma HCD is found mostly in older men and presents like a malignant lymphoma with fever, erythema, lymphadenopathy, and hepatosplenomegaly. Mu HCD, the rarest in this group, has been associated with chronic lymphocytic leukemia in more than half the known cases.[1]

Laboratory Findings and Correlations with Disease

Alpha HCD produces anemia, leukocytosis with eosinophilia, and possibly, thrombocytopenia. Abnormal lymphoid and plasma cells may be found in the peripheral blood during the final stages of the disease. A broad component migrating between the alpha-2 and beta regions may be found by serum electrophoresis. However, serum protein electrophoresis is not helpful in more than half the cases.[12] Analysis of jejunal fluid or respiratory secretions by immunoelectrophoresis using H-chain-specific antisera produces more reliable evidence for alpha HCD.

In gamma HCD, there is mild to moderate anemia and leukopenia with eosinophilia. Thrombocytopenia is often marked. Variant (atypical) lymphocytes and plasma cells can be seen on peripheral blood films. Malignant proliferation usually can be demonstrated from bone marrow, lymph nodes, and sometimes, the spleen. Generally, there is a mixed population of lymphocytes, immunoblasts, and plasma cells, morphologically similar to the picture in Waldenström macroglobulinemia.[12]

A broad heterogeneous-appearing band or a sharp peak can be seen in the beta–gamma region of the electrophoretogram. Hypoalbuminemia and marked hypogammaglobulinemia are responsible for a poor immune response and thus frequent infections. Demonstration of gamma H chains by immunoelectrophoresis is diagnostic. There is no reaction with L-chain antisera.

Detection of mature, vacuolated plasma cells in bone marrow provides a clue to mu HCD in two-thirds of the cases. These large vacuoles do not contain Ig.[12] Serum electrophoresis shows a state of hypogammaglobulinemia. If an abnormal fraction appears, it is small and migrates in the alpha-2 region. Immunoelectrophoresis demonstrates free mu chains in the serum but not in the urine. This is the only HCD where L chains, usually kappa, are secreted in the urine. The abnormality on the H chain prevents H- and L-chain assembly.

Treatment and prognosis are relatively unsatisfactory. Life expectancy ranges up to 5 years from the onset of symptoms.

AMYLOIDOSIS

Amyloidosis is a condition in which proteinaceous deposits (amyloid) occur throughout the body, producing symptoms and clinical disease. *Primary* amyloidosis is closely associated with monoclonal gammopathies such as plasma cell myeloma, although a few patients with polyclonal plasma cells have been described.[14] The proteinaceous material amyloid is composed of L-chain fragments from the variable region of Ig. Lambda chains have a better potential for amyloid formation than kappa chains.[6] Amyloidosis is the byproduct of proteolysis by macrophages that are overwhelmed by excessive amounts of protein. *Secondary* amyloidosis is associated with chronic illness, and the amyloid protein is unrelated to Ig.

Diagnosis is made after biopsy of involved tissue. With electron microscopy and X-ray diffraction, fibrils of amyloid are shown to be organized in a beta-pleated sheet. Because of this fibril configuration, amyloid material stained with Congo red dye can be demonstrated by a green birefringence in polarized light.

Treatment addresses the associated plasma cell dyscrasia or underlying disease to control further amyloid deposition and subsequent loss of organ function.

CHAPTER SUMMARY

Alterations of normal B-lymphocyte maturation by malignant transformation are responsible for the group of dyscrasias described in this chapter. In addition to morphologic identification, essential diagnostic information is obtained by detecting and identifying the monoclonal immunoglobulin by protein studies using electrophoresis and immunotechniques.

CASE STUDY 39-1

A 51-year-old woman was admitted through the emergency room with complaints of fever, chills, photophobia, nucha rigidity, and neck pain. Her medical history was unremarkable. The following laboratory data were obtained: CBC—WBC 4.7×10^9/L; RBC 2.77×10^{12}/L; Hb 8.5 g/dL; HCT 0.23 L/L; platelets 67×10^9/L; differential: segmented neutrophils 38%; neutrophil bands 18%; lymphocytes 37%; monocytes 4%; metamyelocytes 1%; plasma cells 2%; NRBC/100 leukocytes 2; RBC morphology: marked rouleaux formation. The CSF showed RBC 5.2×10^9/L; WBC 0.6×10^9/L; mononuclear cells 18%; polynuclear cells 82%. The ESR was 72 mm/hour. The serum chemistry findings were albumin 2.8 g/dL (reference range 3.5–5.0 g/dL) and total protein 13.2 g/dL (reference range 6.0–7.8 g/dL). Protein electrophoresis showed:

	SERUM PROTEIN ELECTROPHORESIS (g/dL)	URINE PROTEIN ELECTROPHORESIS (mg/dL)
Albumin	2.8	23
Alpha-1	0.3	4
Alpha-2	0.61	2
Beta	0.92	8
Gamma	0.57	74

Haemophilus influenzae was cultured from the cerebrospinal fluid. Serum electrophoresis demonstrated a monoclonal spike in the gamma region. On the urine electrophoretogram two sharp peaks were observed in the gamma region. An IFE study identified the monoclonal protein and the second urine peak. The patient, who was deteriorating rapidly, was given plasmapheresis and antibiotics and packed cells. Two days later, 13% plasma cells were reported in the patient's leukocyte differential.

1. Why were CSF and radiologic studies ordered at admission?
2. From the admission data, what prompted further serum and urine protein studies?
3. What plasma cell dyscrasia should be ruled out and why?

REFERENCES

1. Brouet J, Seligmann M, Danon F et al: μ-Chain disease: Two new cases. Arch Intern Med 139:672, 1979
2. Coward RA, Mallick NP, Delamore IW: Tubular function in multiple myeloma. Clin Nephrol 24:180, 1985
3. Deuel TF, Davis P, Avioli LV: Waldenström's macroglobulinemia. Arch Intern Med 143:986, 1983
4. Dick FR: Plasma cell myeloma and related disorders with monoclonal gammopathy. In Koepke JA (ed): Laboratory Hematology, vol 1, pp 449, 464. New York, Churchill Livingstone, 1984
5. Galian A, Lecestre M, Scotto J et al: Pathological study of alpha-chain disease with special emphasis on evolution. Cancer 39:2081, 1977
6. Glenner GG: Amyloid deposits and amyloidosis: The β-fibrilloses. N Engl J Med 302:1283, 1980
7. Hsu SM, Hsu PL, McMillan PN et al: A light and electron microscopic immunoperoxidase study. Am J Clin Pathol 77:26, 1982
8. Merlini G, Waldenström JG, Jayakar SD: A new improved clinical staging system for multiple myeloma based on analysis of 123 treated patients. Blood 55:1011, 1980
9. Ohno R, Kodera Y, Ogura M et al: Treatment of plasma cell neoplasm with recombinant leukocyte A interferon and human lymphoblastoid interferon. Cancer Chemother Pharmacol 14:34, 1985
10. Paglieroni T, MacKenzie MR: Studies of the pathogenesis of an immune defect in multiple myeloma. J Clin Invest 59:1120, 1977
11. Reed M, McKenna RW, Bridges R et al: Morphologic manifestations of monoclonal gammopathy. Am J Clin Pathol 76:8, 1981
12. Seligmann M, Mihaesco E, Preud'homme J et al: Heavy chain diseases: Current findings and concepts. Immunol Rev 48:145, 1979
13. Waldenström JG, Raiend U: Plasmapheresis and cold sensitivity of immunoglobulin molecules. I: A study of hyperviscosity, cryoglobulinemia, euglobulinemia, and macroglobulinemia vera. Acta Med Scand 216:449, 1984
14. Wolf BC, Kumar A, Vera JC et al: Bone marrow morphology and immunology in systemic amyloidosis. Am J Clin Pathol 86:84, 1986
15. Woodruff RK, Malpas JS, Paxton AM et al: Plasma cell leukemia (PCL): A report of 15 patients. Blood 52:839, 1978
16. Woodruff RK, Wadsworth J, Malpas JS et al: Clinical staging in multiple myeloma. Br J Haematol 42:199, 1979
17. Zarrabi MH, Stark RS, Kane P et al: IgM myeloma, a distinct entity in the spectrum of B-cell neoplasia. Am J Clin Pathol 75:1, 1981

40

Systematic Laboratory Evaluation of Leukocyte Abnormalities

John A. Koepke

The chapters in the preceding two sections of this book provide detailed discussions of malignant myeloproliferative and lymphoproliferative disorders. They also discuss benign conditions that may mimic these diseases because the former become part of the differential diagnosis. This concluding chapter seeks to put these diseases and conditions into perspective by focusing on laboratory methods used to evaluate the various leukocyte abnormalities when such a disorder is first discovered but not yet definitively diagnosed. Ideally, the physician and the laboratory scientist have a similar systematic approach to the evaluation of these disorders and work together to diagnose and monitor them most efficiently.

The value of laboratory studies, including bone marrow and lymph node biopsy, in the diagnosis of these diseases is probably best exemplified by the clinical staging of their extent and gravity. Proliferation of clones of abnormal cells in the marrow or lymph nodes, at times with a spilling over into the peripheral blood, is the characteristic feature of these disorders. This proliferation may be either myeloid or lymphoid.

REACTIONS AND DISORDERS

The term *reaction* is used here to designate a normal or physiologic proliferation of either myeloid or lymphoid elements in response to a stimulus such as infection or inflammation. The term *disorder* is reserved for malignant proliferation of these cells. Thus, four types of leukocyte responses are seen clinically: benign reactions and malignant disorders of myeloproliferation and benign reactions and malignant disorders of lymphoproliferation.[6] Dr. William Dameshek must be credited with the initial popularization of these unifying concepts of modern hematology.[3]

MYELOPROLIFERATION

At times, the myeloid cell compartment produces either increased numbers of normal myeloid cells as a response or reaction to some stimulus[7] or increased numbers of abnormal myeloid cells as part of a malignant process or disorder.[3] This process can involve any or all of the myeloid elements—granulocytic, megakaryocytic, or erythrocytic. The process frequently evolves over time. Most often, the bone marrow is the first organ involved, but extramedullary tissues (*i.e.*, the liver, spleen, or lymph nodes) may subsequently participate in this proliferation. Hepatosplenomegaly more often signals the progression of a malignant process, although it may indicate a benign infectious process.[3]

LYMPHOPROLIFERATION

Increased production of lymphoid cells, either abnormal numbers or abnormal types of lymphocytes, can occur as a response to certain agents (*e.g.*, viruses) or conditions. This proliferation is evident in lymph nodes as well as in lymphoid tissue in the liver, spleen, or bone marrow. The process can be either benign or malignant. Lymphoproliferation may be confined to the tissues (*i.e.*, lymphoma), with little if any peripheral blood involvement, or it can be manifested primarily by peripheral blood changes (*i.e.*, leukemia).[5]

Malignant lymphoproliferation can be a continuum from frank lymphocytic leukemia to tissue lymphoma and any blend of these two extremes. Late in the disease process, lymphomas sometimes evolve into a frankly leukemic picture. These interrelations are understandable if one appreciates the broad scope of the term *lymphoproliferative disorder*. It therefore follows that the apparent evolution of the disease from primary tissue involvement to evident leukemia is not unusual; in fact, it occurs frequently.

MONOCYTOSIS AND EOSINOPHILIA

Increased numbers of monocytes are a feature of a number of infections as well as a harbinger of several premalignant conditions (Chap. 26). In addition, acute and chronic monocytic leukemias have evident increases in monocytes. Morphologic differentiation of benign from malignant monocytes may be difficult unless the cells are frankly malignant.[8]

Eosinophilia is associated with infestations with parasitic helminths and protozoa, especially during the visceral (tissue) phases of the infestation. The intensity of the eosinophilic response is variable but tends to decrease as the disease becomes more chronic. A wide variety of additional diseases have been associated with eosinophilia, such as acute and chronic allergic reactions. Rarely, increased eo-

sinophils are found in malignant conditions such as eosinophilic leukemia.

THE PHYSICIAN'S ROLE IN THE DIAGNOSTIC PROCESS

Determination of the etiology of leukocyte abnormalities is made by integrating clinical information and laboratory data.[3] In addition to ordering appropriate tests initially, the physician plays a key role in evaluating the information obtained from a medical history and a physical examination of the patient and in interpreting laboratory data. These studies include the leukocyte count and differential, sometimes leukocyte cytochemical or monoclonal antibody studies, and a bone marrow examination or lymph node biopsy when necessary.

The etiology of the patient's problem is not always obvious. Table 40-1 presents examples of clues from the patient's history or physical examination that may help to make the diagnosis or at least suggest helpful laboratory tests. For instance, the patient may recount a history of an infection, which becomes a stimulus for granulocyte production. On the other hand, leukemia manifests itself as anemia or bleeding tendencies, both reactions being secondary to the primary leukemic process. A patient with agranulocytosis often may be unaware of exposure to toxic drugs or chemicals. Thus, the patient's history may or may not be helpful.

The most important abnormal physical findings in patients with leukocyte disorders are related to liver and spleen size and lymph node size and consistency. Lymphadenopathy (palpable lymph nodes) may be generalized or localized. Hepatic or splenic enlargement or both also provide clues to the cause of leukocyte changes.

Laboratory evidence of anemia and thrombocytopenia usually indicates significant bone marrow replacement by neoplastic cells. Thrombocytopenia without significant evidence of anemia is characteristic of an acute and rapid growth of neoplastic cells in the marrow.

LABORATORY EVALUATION OF LEUKOCYTE ABNORMALITIES

In Chapter 21, the "anemia tree" was introduced as a logical approach to the laboratory evaluation of anemia. The decision tree for leukocyte abnormalities in Figure 40-1 can be

TABLE 40–1. Examples of Common Signs and Symptoms Associated with Leukocyte Reactions and Disorders

SIGNS AND SYMPTOMS	ASSOCIATED WITH
Lymph node enlargement	Lymphoma, metastatic tumor, chronic leukemia
Hepatosplenomegaly	Chronic leukemia, lymphoma
Fever	Infection; less often, malignancy
Petechiae	Acute leukemia
Rashes	Viral infection
Swollen gums	Monocytic leukemia
Bone pain	Acute leukemia, myeloma
Ruddy complexion	Polycythemia vera or reactive

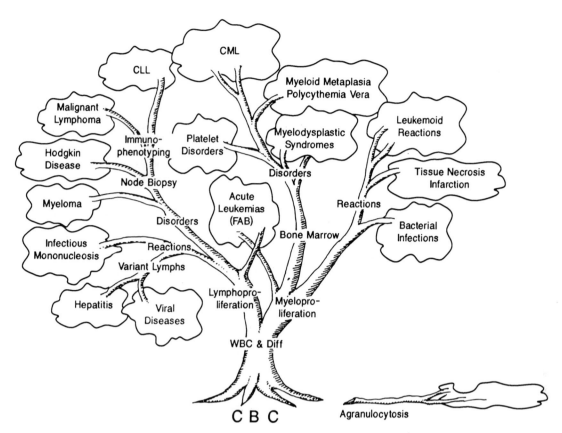

FIG. 40-1. Decision tree for leukocyte reactions and disorders, both myeloproliferative and lymphoproliferative. Evaluation of peripheral blood film is the primary test, but additional studies such as bone marrow or lymph node biopsy frequently are necessary for diagnosis.

applied in a similar fashion. This tree is based on the division of benign and malignant proliferation of leukocytes. It illustrates these subgroups with some of the more common clinical entities involving leukocytes. Although monocytic and eosinophilic proliferative responses are not rare, they are omitted primarily for the sake of clarity in the presentation of the principal theme.

THE BLOOD FILM EVALUATION

The CBC is the basic and primary laboratory test. To "climb the tree," the blood film is examined thoroughly in an effort to discover additional clues, with emphasis on leukocytes, both number and morphology.

Other tests may be useful to the diagnosis. Special studies may be required to differentiate the various leukemias. The FAB classification scheme for myeloid as well as lymphoid leukemias has made a great contribution to the exact diagnosis of leukemia.[1] Cytochemical stains also contribute greatly to the diagnosis of leukemias.[2]

THE BONE MARROW EXAMINATION

Patients with leukocyte reactions or disorders may be candidates for a marrow study. The cause of an unexplained

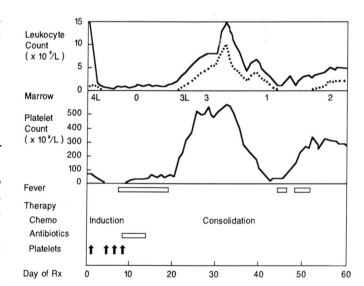

FIG. 40-2. Characteristic clinical course of patient with acute myelogenous leukemia receiving induction and consolidation chemotherapy. Note leukopenia and thrombocytopenia after therapy. Solid line, total white cell count; dotted line, granulocyte count. Platelet transfusions were given when count was below $10 \times 10^9/L$. Marrow examinations show estimated cellularity, 4 being packed marrow and 0 being acellular; L indicates presence of leukemic infiltrate.

leukocytosis may become evident during careful study of the bone marrow. The diagnosis of leukemia and the assessment of the response to therapy rely heavily on the status of the marrow compartment. In Figure 40-2 for example, six marrow biopsies or aspirates were obtained during the course of diagnosis and treatment of acute myelocytic leukemia.

LYMPH NODE BIOPSY

In lymphoproliferative disorders as well as reactive conditions that may mimic malignant lymphoma or non-Hodgkin lymphoma, the lymph node biopsy is a key study in the differential diagnosis. In addition to the usual hematoxylin and eosin-stained histologic sections, various special preparations (*e.g.*, immunoperoxidase or monoclonal antibodies) are helpful in differentiating these diseases. The exact role of some newer procedures (*e.g.*, DNA probes) is still being determined, but the techniques appear promising.

REFERENCES

1. Bennett JM, Catovsky D, Daniel MT et al: Proposals for the classification of acute leukaemias. Br J Haematol 33:451, 1976
2. Bennett JM, Catovsky D, Daniel MT et al: Proposed revised criteria for the classification of acute myeloid leukemia. Ann Intern Med 103:626, 1985
3. Dameshek W: Some speculations on the myeloproliferative syndromes. Blood 6:372, 1951
4. Dacie JW, Lewis SM: Use of haematological techniques in clinical work. In Practical Haematology, 6th ed, p 132. Edinburgh, Churchill Livingstone, 1984
5. Dick FR: Chronic lymphocytic leukemia, prolymphocytic leukemia and leukemic non-Hodgkin's lymphoma. In Koepke JA (ed): Laboratory Hematology, p 325. New York, Churchill Livingstone, 1984
6. Koepke JA, Koepke JF: Leukemia and leukemoid reactions. In Guide to Clinical Laboratory Diagnosis, 3rd ed, p 189. Norwalk, CT, Appleton and Lange, 1987
7. Stein RB: Granulocytosis and granulocyte leukemoid reactions. In Koepke JA (ed): Laboratory Hematology, p 153. New York, Churchill Livingstone, 1984
8. Stein RB, Linder J: Mononuclear leukocytosis and infectious mononucleosis. In Koepke JA (ed): Laboratory Hematology, p 189. New York, Churchill Livingstone, 1984

PART IX

INSTRUMENTATION

FOR

HEMATOLOGIC

EVALUATION

41

Introduction

to

Hematologic

Automation

E. Anne Stiene-Martin

The concept of counting blood cells automatically began in the mid-1930s with a report describing a photoelectric method for counting cells passing through a capillary tube using darkfield optics.[10] Later, darkfield optics or light scatter were proposed to scan hemocytometer chambers in an attempt to bypass human error.[6] Endeavors to correlate the RBC count with the turbidity of cell suspensions were also proposed.[13] However, instruments manufactured on these principles did not gain wide acceptance at that time because of their inaccuracy, lack of sensitivity, or lack of practicality.

In the late 1940s and early 1950s, two instruments were introduced that proved to be accurate as well as practical. The first was a modification of the original capillary method using darkfield optics. A suspension of cells was pumped through a narrow capillary tube in the path of darkfield lighting.[3] Light pulses reflected by the cells were collected with a series of mirrors and lenses into a photomultiplier tube. This information was then converted to cells per microliter. The original instrument (Fisher Autocytometer) is no longer in production, but the principle of darkfield optical scan or light scatter is still used today in other instruments.

The second instrument was based on a completely new nonoptical principle of cell counting: electrical gating or electrical impedance.[9] This instrument was introduced by Coulter Electronics, Inc., and the counting principle was patented, so no other manufacturer in the United States could produce such an instrument for 17 years. The patent restrictions were not applicable outside this country, however, and several European companies developed similar instruments (Celloscope, Microscal), and at least one Japanese instrument (TOA) appeared.[5]

Electrical impedance measurement is based on the fact that cells are relatively poor conductors of electricity. If two electrodes conducting an electrical current through an electrolyte solution such as saline are separated so that the only connection is through a tiny aperture, any interference (such as a blood cell) will change the conductance. As cells are pulled through the aperture, the changes in voltage that occur as the cells increase resistance to the current are sensed by the instrument. This is a good illustration of Ohm's Law: voltage = current × resistance. The magnitude of the voltage pulses produced by cells is directly related to their size, a fact that has been used in subsequent clinical instruments for direct measurement of cell volume.

In order for these instruments to count and size particles accurately, a means of discriminating between particle sizes had to be developed. Thus, the concept of "thresholds" was born. A threshold is a voltage limit with which a pulse is compared. Only pulses that exceed the threshold are sized or counted. Both a lower and an upper threshold can be set. Increasing the lower threshold eliminates unwanted small pulses such as those caused by debris. An upper threshold eliminates large pulses. By manipulating the upper and lower thresholds, it is possible to produce a "window," a specific particle size range. Because these instruments have adjustable thresholds, they are capable of being calibrated to eliminate spurious counts and produce clinically accurate cell counts. Thus, they can be considered to be reference methods. As such, they are unique and will be covered in Chapter 42.

Up to this point, automated cell counters were not capable of counting erythrocytes, leukocytes, and platelets simultaneously. Hence, these instruments are sometimes referred to as "single-parameter" instruments. In the mid

1960s, Coulter Electronics introduced a new instrument capable of simultaneous RBC and WBC counts, as well as determinations of Hb concentration and mean red cell volume (MCV). Using these data, the instrument calculated the HCT, mean cell Hb (MCH), and mean cell Hb concentration (MCHC). This instrument is an example of a "multiparameter" instrument and has since undergone several modifications leading to increased capacity, new determinations, and subsequent decreased cost per determination. These instruments will be discussed in Chapter 43.

At about the same time Technicon Instruments Corporation introduced a multiparameter instrument based on darkfield optical scanning using the same continuous-flow mechanisms that had become popular in the clinical chemistry laboratory. This instrument was referred to as a sequential multiple analyzer (SMA). A problem soon surfaced relative to the method Technicon had chosen to determine HCT (electrical resistance of a suspension of blood cells) in that it was discovered that inaccurate results were obtained in certain patients with plasma conductivity abnormalities. The SMA instruments remained in production only a few years and were replaced by a new instrument called the Hemalog, that was capable of performing a CBC and platelet count. Prothrombin times and partial thromboplastin times were also included in early models. A centrifuged HCT as well as one based on electrical conductivity was available with this instrument. Technicon also produced an instrument that determined leukocyte differential counts based on cellular cytochemistry, which was named the Hemalog D. Subsequent models, the most recent called the H·2, have combined the blood cell counts with the leukocyte differential count. These instruments will be discussed in Chapter 43.

Automation of the leukocyte differential has since been dominated by three principles: (1) colorimetric cytochemical differentiation; (2) computer pattern-recognition; and (3) a newer concept, known as the "histogram differential," based on volumetric cytochemistry. Automated leukocyte differentials will be discussed in Chapter 44.

The late 1960s also saw a new entry into the multiparameter instrument market. Ortho Diagnostic Systems introduced a cell-counting instrument based on laser light scatter. In addition to the use of a laser beam as a means of cell detection, this instrument introduced the concept of hydrodynamic focusing to routine cell counting. Hydrodynamic focusing generates an extremely narrow channel through which cells may proceed in single file, thus avoiding a problem that had plagued cell counters until that time: the inability to size individual cells accurately because of the random coincidental passage of more than cell through the orifice simultaneously. Hydrodynamic focusing or a modification thereof has since been adopted by many manufacturers. The laser cell counter will be discussed in Chapter 43.

The first years of the 1970s witnessed a significant event in that the Coulter Electronics patent on electrical impedance counting expired. There followed throughout the 1970s and 1980s a large number of cell counters introduced to the marketplace by several companies, some of which have since been purchased by other companies. The result has been a bewildering array of multiparameter and single-channel cell counters based on electrical impedance. The situation is so fluid that it would be impractical to list the companies involved: such a list would be outdated within months. The resulting competition in the market has been beneficial, yielding a wide range of instruments with various capacities that are able to fit the needs of laboratories ranging from large high-volume laboratories to physician offices.

Recently, a fourth, unique principle of cell counting and differentiation based on expansion and analysis of the stained buffy coat in a centrifuged specimen has been introduced. This will be described in Chapter 43.

Chapter 45 describes the flow cytometer, a new instrument that has not yet reached the routine, clinical laboratory but has great potential. The flow cytometer is capable of analyzing single cells for a particular characteristic using monoclonal antibodies.

In summary, the majority of instruments produced today are multiparameter, although a few instruments have been marketed that are capable of counting only one cell type (usually platelets). Instruments with adjustable thresholds that can be calibrated without the use of a reference method are very few in number.

REFERENCES

1. Ansley H, Ornstein L: Enzyme histochemistry and differential white cell counts on Technicon Hemalog D. Automated Analysis, vol 1. Tarrytown, NY, Mediad, Inc, 1971
2. Brittin GM, Dew SA, Felwell EK: Automated optical counting of blood platelets. Blood 38:422, 1971
3. Gagon TE, Atherns JW, Boggs DT et al: An evaluation of the variance of leukocyte counts as performed with the hemacytometer, Coulter and Fisher instruments. Am J Clin Pathol 46:684, 1966
4. Haberman T, Cox C, Pierre R: Evaluation of the Coulter S-Plus IV three-part differential as a screening tool (abstract). Blood 62:80a, 1983
5. Helleman PW, Benjamin CJ: The TOA micro cell counter. Scand J Haematol 6:69, 1969
6. Langerkranz C: Photoelectric counting of individual microscopic plant and animal cells. Nature 161:25, 1948
7. Lewis SM: Hemacytometry by laser beam optics: Evaluation of the Hemac 630L. J Clin Pathol 30:54, 1977
8. MacFarlane RG, Payne AM, Poole JCF et al: An automatic apparatus for counting red blood cells. Br J Haematol 5:1, 1959
9. Mattern CFT, Bracket FS, Olson BJ: Determination of number and size of particles by electrical gating: Blood cells. J Appl Physiol 10:56, 1957
10. Moldavan A: Photoelectric technique for the counting of microscopical cells. Science 80:188, 1934
11. Pinkerton PH, Spence I, Oglivie JC et al: An assessment of the Coulter counter model "S." J Clin Pathol 23:68, 1970
12. Wardlaw SC, Levine RA: Quantitative buffy coat analysis: A new laboratory tool functioning as a screening complete blood count. JAMA 249:617, 1983
13. Whitlock JH: The use of photoelectric turbidimetry in the determination of red blood count, hematocrit and hemoglobin. Blood 2:463, 1947

42

Single-Parameter Particle-Counting Instruments

Marshall E. Bowman

There are a few instruments on the market today that are semiautomated single-parameter counting instruments, as defined in the previous chapter. They may be categorized into two main groups: those that have adjustable threshold settings and known dilution volumes, and those that have fixed thresholds and relative dilution volumes. Instruments with adjustable thresholds can be used to check the calibration of instruments having fixed thresholds. According to a 1982 College of American Pathologists Survey,[4] the most commonly used single-parameter instruments in this country are Coulter single-channel instruments (Coulter Electronics, Inc., Hialeah, FL). Therefore, this chapter describes a representative series of such instruments with adjustable thresholds—the Coulter Electronics Series Z—their operation and calibration and the errors that can occur during their operation.

PRINCIPLE OF OPERATION

Cell counters manufactured by Coulter Electronics operate on the principle of electrical impedance.[3] Cells are suspended in an electrolyte such as saline. The electrolyte is a good conductor of electrical current, whereas cells are relatively poor conductors. Electrical current is applied to the cell suspension between two electrodes. One electrode (external) is in the cell suspension, and the second electrode (internal) is within a tube made of inert material (glass). The only connection between the two electrodes is a small aperture (orifice) in the side of the tube (Fig. 42-1). A measured volume of diluted cells is pulled through the aperture. Differences in electrical resistance between the two electrodes occur as the cells pass through the aperture, causing changes in voltage (voltage pulses) that are amplified and counted. Because the size of the voltage pulse is directly proportional

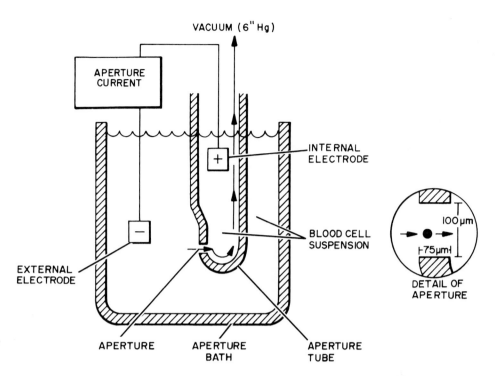

FIG. 42-1. Aperture tube. (Courtesy of Coulter Electronics, Inc.)

to the size of the cell, voltage pulses caused by cells of a specific size can be amplified, discriminated, and counted through the use of threshold circuits (Fig. 42-2).

Before proceeding to a description of the instrument, the concept of "critical volume" must be discussed. The critical volume of a standard aperture may be defined as the sensing zone of the aperture and is equivalent to the volume of the aperture plus approximately 75% of the aperture volume on each side of the aperture (Fig 42-3). A cell entering the critical volume will generate a voltage pulse *regardless of whether it passes through the aperture*. The critical volume is produced by resistance to electrical current at the aperture.

INSTRUMENT COMPONENTS

In order to understand the operation of these instruments, it is necessary to describe the various components and their functions[2] (Fig. 42-4).

Aperture Tube

The aperture tube is a hollow glass tube with an open upper end that is shaped to permit an airtight seal between the aperture tube and the stopcock assembly described below. The lower end is closed except for a small aperture (orifice). The size of the aperture is indicated on the tube; several sizes

are available (*e.g.*, 200, 100, 70, and 50 μM). When properly positioned, the aperture tube is suspended from the stopcock assembly and contains an internal electrode as well as a tube that may be used to deliver electrolyte solution into the aperture tube.

Stopcock Assembly

The stopcock assembly connects the aperture tube to the manometer to be described below. Its two ends are shaped to provide airtight seals. It contains two stopcocks (vacuum control and filling or flushing). When the vacuum stopcock is opened, vacuum is applied to the manometer. When both stopcocks are opened, the aperture tube can be filled and flushed with electrolyte solution. The stopcock assembly contains two inlets: one from the vacuum pump and the other from a reservoir of electrolyte solution.

Aperture Current Electrodes

There are two platinum electrodes. The internal electrode is within the aperture tube. The external electrode is suspended by a wire next to the aperture tube. Their function is to generate current across the aperture. Current polarity alternates with each count.

Manometer

The manometer is a specialized glass U-tube containing mercury. One end is connected to the aperture tube through the stopcock assembly, and the other end is open. Electrodes are placed in the manometer that are activated by the passage of mercury. When vacuum is applied to one side of the manometer tube, mercury is pulled up, creating a simultaneous drop in the mercury level on the other side of

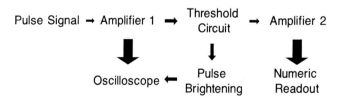

FIG. 42-2. Amplification of signal.

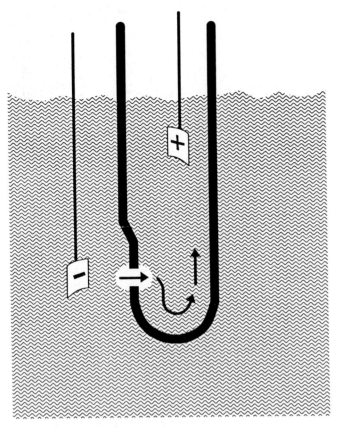

FIG. 42-3. Magnified diagram of aperture. Nonshaded area with arrow (pointing right) represents critical volume.

the U-tube. When the manometer is isolated from the vacuum supply, mercury will seek to equilibrate its levels in the two sides of the U-tube. Two things then happen simultaneously. First, because the manometer is connected directly to the aperture tube, the dropping mercury column pulls the cell suspension through the orifice at the bottom of the aperture tube. Second, the rising mercury on the other side activates the electrodes within the manometer. The first electrode causes the instrument to start counting, and the second electrode stops the counting. The electrodes are placed in the manometer tube so that during the time it takes the mercury to travel from the start to the stop electrodes, a specified amount of cell suspension is pulled through the aperture. (Most manometers have one "start" electrode and two "stop" electrodes). By means of a toggle switch, the operator can determine whether 100 or 500 μL of cell suspension will be counted (Fig. 42-5). Leukocytes and erythrocytes generally are counted in 500 μL whereas platelet counts require 100 μL.

Vacuum System

The vacuum system consists of a simple rotary pump (see Fig. 42-5) connected to a trap, which in turn is connected to the stopcock assembly. Because excessive vacuum is produced by the pump, a regulator valve capable of bleeding off excessive vacuum is placed within the system. By adjusting this regulator valve, the operator can control how

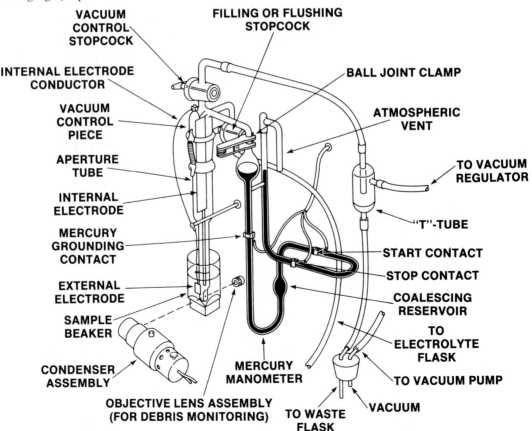

FIG. 42-4. Sample stand glassware. (Courtesy of Coulter Electronics, Inc.)

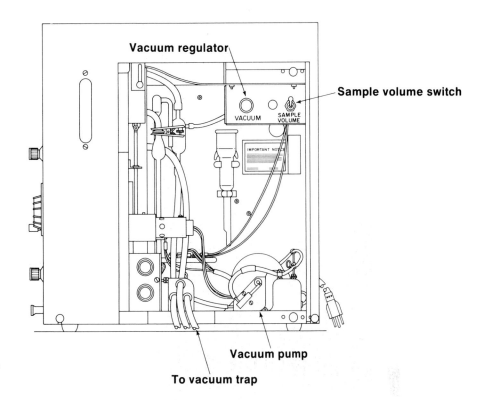

Vacuum regulator

Sample volume switch

VACUUM

SAMPLE VOLUME

IMPORTANT NOTE

Vacuum pump

To vacuum trap

FIG. 42-5.   Vacuum system. (Courtesy of Coulter Electronics, Inc.)

far the mercury will be pulled: the valve is adjusted so that mercury on the other side of the U-tube drops just past the start electrode and stabilizes.

Oscilloscope

An oscilloscope on the front of the instrument displays a visual representation of voltage pulses caused by cells as they pass through the critical volume (Fig. 42-6). This depiction is a visual guide to the size and number of particles being counted. Various controls for adjusting the focus, brightness, and distinction of image, and the position of the pattern are located on the side of the instrument.

Threshold Dials

One or two threshold controls are located on the front of the instrument (Fig. 42-7). If only one is present, it will control the lower threshold; if two are present, both lower and upper thresholds may be manipulated. These dials are marked in units of 0 to 100. By moving the lower control up or the upper control down, the operator can place increasing limits between the voltage pulse and the detector and thus determine the size of particle to be counted.

Aperture Current Setting

A rotary switch on the front of the instrument controls the amount of current passing between the internal and external aperture electrodes (through the aperture) (see Fig. 42-7). Increases in aperture current will increase the voltage pulse amplitude caused by individual cells. The first four settings double the current at each increment; the following settings provide increments of roughly 1.5.

Amplification Switch

The amplification switch, referred to on some models as the attenuation switch, is located on the front of the instrument and controls the first amplification of the pulse signal (see Fig. 42-7). Each increment roughly doubles the amplification.

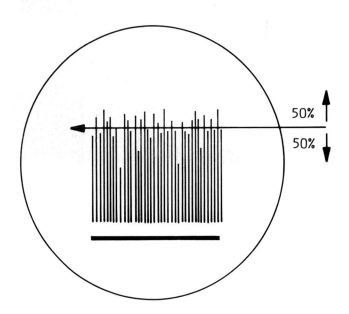

50% ↑

50% ↓

RBC PULSE PATTERN
ON OSCILLOSCOPE

FIG. 42-6.   Diagram of oscilloscope pulse pattern generated by red cells as they pass through critical volume. (Courtesy of Coulter Electronics, Inc.)

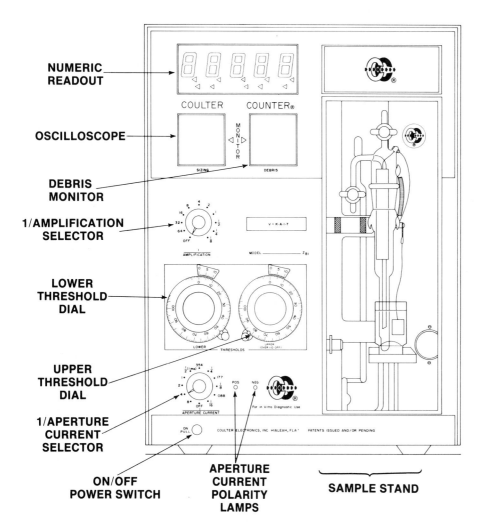

NUMERIC READOUT

OSCILLOSCOPE

DEBRIS MONITOR

1/AMPLIFICATION SELECTOR

LOWER THRESHOLD DIAL

UPPER THRESHOLD DIAL

1/APERTURE CURRENT SELECTOR

ON/OFF POWER SWITCH

APERTURE CURRENT POLARITY LAMPS

SAMPLE STAND

FIG. 42-7. Front panel of Coulter ZBI showing threshold and aperture current controls. (Courtesy of Coulter Electronics, Inc.)

Digital Readout

A five-digit numerical display records cells as they are counted (see Fig. 42-7). An audible click is emitted as each thousand is counted. These clicks create the cadence or rhythm of the count; by listening to this cadence, the operator can detect malfunctions without having to watch the instrument constantly.

Debris Monitor

The debris monitor consists of a modified microscope lens system and back light focused on the aperture (see Fig. 42-7). The image of the aperture is transmitted to a small viewing screen so the operator can detect any debris interfering with the aperture during a count.

Other Settings

There is a series of four controls on the side of the instrument that generally are set once prior to calibration and not used thereafter in the routine clinical laboratory. These are the gain trim control, matching switch, bandwidth selector, and separate/locked switch. An operator's manual that accompanies the instruments will describe these in detail.

INSTRUMENT OPERATION
Reagents and Supplies

1. The *electrolyte* is a buffered isotonic salt solution that may contain one or more preservatives. Azides were used in the past as antimicrobials but have been discontinued because of the explosion hazards. The electrolyte reagent must be particle free. It is used to dilute cells and to flush the instrument.
2. The *lysing reagent* is a detergent solution. It is used to lyse erythrocytes by dissolving their stroma when leukocyte counts are to be performed. The reagent should be particle free.
3. The *cleaning agents* should be used at regular intervals to remove protein buildup from the aperture tube and electrodes. Both dilute sodium hypochlorite solutions and detergents made specifically for this purpose may be used.
4. The *sample container* may range from small glass beakers to plastic vials manufactured for this purpose. The principal criteria are that the containers be particle free and that their internal surfaces not react with or attract cells.
5. Other supplies, such as brushes to remove debris from the aperture, are commercially available.

Specimen Requirements

Both whole venous blood and diluted capillary blood may be used. The recommended anticoagulant is EDTA, because it has the least adverse effect on cells. Venous blood should be checked for clots before use. Capillary blood may be utilized if proper methods are followed to prevent coagulation (*i.e.,* immediate dilution or use of heparinized capillary pipets).

Specimen Dilution

Leukocyte and erythrocyte counts require different dilutions of whole blood. Leukocyte counts generally are performed on a 1:500 dilution (40 μL blood in 20 mL of electrolyte). If an erythrocyte count is to be performed, a 1:50,000 dilution may be made by diluting 200 μL of the 1:500 dilution in an additional 20 mL of electrolyte. Dilutions may be done manually or with specially designed automatic dilutors. It should be remembered that diluted blood cells are vulnerable to lysis, especially the 1:50,000 dilution. Therefore, dilutions should be made just before performing the cell count. When a leukocyte count is to be performed, six drops of a lysing agent are added to the cell suspension and mixed gently just prior to the count.

Cell Counting Procedure

1. Turn instrument power on. Check instrument settings (aperture current, amplification, threshold) to ensure their appropriateness for the cell type being counted. For counting red and white blood cells, the 100 $\times$ 75 μM aperture tube is used, and a volume of 500 μL is sampled.
2. Perform a background count on the electrolyte solution and lysing reagent to determine the number of particles in the diluent-vial system, which will become part of a final sample count. The maximum allowable background count will differ according the laboratory, but acceptable values generally are between 50 and 100 particles.

    Possible problems include microbial growth in the diluent reservoir or within the instrument tubing, bubbles in the diluent, contaminated stock reagents, or particles in the sample containers.
3. Perform cell counts in a similar manner. Erythrocyte counts should be performed first, as these cells are the most vulnerable to lysis. At least two counts should be made of each cell suspension. These counts should agree within specified tolerance ranges according to the cell type being counted (*e.g.,* within 200 cells for leukocytes or within 50,000 cells for red cells). Lack of reproducibility indicates instrument malfunction, the most common cause being aperture plugging.

Calculation and Reporting

1. Leukocyte count. The usual dilution is 1:500, and 500 μL is counted. Therefore, no calculations are necessary: the count is recorded directly from the readout. Some laboratories require leukocyte counts to be rounded to the nearest 50 cells.
2. Erythrocyte count. The usual dilution is 1:50,000, and 500 μL is counted. Therefore, the count on the readout is multiplied by 100.
3. Most erythrocyte counts must be corrected for coincidence counting, defined as the presence of more than one cell in the critical volume (or sensing zone) at the same time. When this happens, only one voltage pulse is generated, resulting in a negative error (failure to count an RBC). The degree of coincidence counting is a function of both the concentration of cells in the suspension and the size of the aperture, and the magnitude of the error is mathematically predictable. Coincidence correction tables are available from the instrument manufacturer, a different table being necessary for each aperture size. Generally, when a 100-μM aperture is used, any count over 10,000 must be corrected for coincidence. With a 70-μM aperture, counts exceeding 3000 need to be corrected.

INSTRUMENT CALIBRATION
Preliminary Instrument Settings

Calibration of a single-parameter Coulter counter with an adjustable threshold consists of determining the volume (femtoliters) screened out by each unit on the threshold control. Once this is determined, the proper threshold settings to count erythrocytes or leukocytes can be calculated. Threshold calibration for platelets using a 70-μM aperture and a 100-μL manometer is based on the same principle but will not be described here.

Before performing a threshold calibration, all instrument settings other than threshold must be set. Some of these are set as recommended by the manufacturer based on the nature of the electrolyte used for all cell counts and the fact that the calibration is for leukocytes and erythrocytes.

Aperture current setting (AC), amplification or attenuation control (A), and the gain trim (GT) should be set so that the pattern of pulses on the oscilloscope screen are between one-third and one-half the height of the screen. To accomplish this, perform the following:
1. Set the controls as recommended by the manufacturer (*i.e.,* AC = 1, A = 1/2, and GT = 6.5).
2. Dilute a blood sample 1:50,000 with electrolyte and initiate a count.
3. Examine the oscilloscope. If the pattern of pulses does not occupy one-third to one-half of the screen, adjust either the AC or the A control by one increment.
4. Continue to make single adjustments and observe the pattern after each adjustment until the pattern is satisfactory.
5. If the AC or A adjustments do not correct the pattern satisfactorily, adjust the GT control and then readjust the AC or A control as necessary.
6. Once the oscilloscope pattern is satisfactory, record all instrument settings.

RBC Half Count Procedure

1. Choose a blood specimen from a normal healthy subject whose characteristics are similar to the routine patients whose specimens are to be counted by the instrument.
2. Determine the MCV of the erythrocyte population in the specimen. This may be done using a spun microhematocrit and an RBC count performed on another calibrated instrument (either in-house or by another laboratory). For purposes of discussion and to illustrate the calculations, an example of the data that might be generated will be provided for each step. Example: MCV = 90 fL.
3. Make an approximately 1:50,000 dilution of the normal specimen. Once this dilution has been made, the remainder of the procedure should be done within 10 minutes to minimize cell lysis. Set the lower threshold dial to 10. If the instrument has an upper threshold, it is not used for this procedure and should be set as high as possible (*i.e.,* off scale). Mix the dilution gently but thoroughly and allow it to stand for approximately 1 minute to disperse as many microbubbles as possible. Perform five counts. Average and record. Example: The average cell count at threshold 10 is 40,700.
4. Open the vacuum stopcock to clear the digital readout. While observing the oscilloscope pattern, quickly adjust the lower threshold setting upward until it appears to reach about the midpoint of all the peaks. Close the stopcock, and recount the specimen. Make further adjustments to the threshold setting, upward or downward, until a count is reached that is approximately one-half the count at a setting of 10. Ensure that the sample is well mixed before each counting cycle. Perform five counts at this higher threshold,

average, and record. Example: An average cell count of 20,350 might be obtained at a threshold of 30.5 using the hypothetical specimen.

5. Calculate the threshold factor and setting as follows. Sample MCV (Example: 90 fL) divided by the threshold setting where the half count was obtained (Example: 30.5) shows the femtoliters screened out by each threshold unit: Example: 90/30.5 = 2.95 fL. Once the number of fL screened out by each threshold unit is determined, it is divided into the smallest cell volume that is likely to be encountered in routine practice (*e.g.*, 25 fL). Example: 25/2.95 = a threshold setting of 8.5 for RBC and WBC counts.

Validation of Threshold

1. The entire procedure may be repeated with different blood samples. The half count threshold should occur at the same threshold setting plus or minus 0.5 units.

2. Plateau check for WBC (Fig. 42-8). Prepare a 1:500 dilution of blood, and add lysing reagent according to manufacturer instructions. Count the cells at threshold increments of 2 starting at a threshold of 2. Continue until there is a marked drop in the leukocyte count. Plot count versus threshold setting on linear graph paper. The steep fall in the first portion of the graph is an indication of the amount of debris and electrical interference detected at very low thresholds. The level portion of the graph (plateau) indicates the threshold range over which blood cells can be counted accurately. The next portion of the graph should exhibit a drop, because smaller nucleated cells are being screened out. Determine the midpoint of the plateau. A threshold setting to the left of the midpoint should ensure that all small leukocytes and nucleated RBCs will be counted and should coincide with the calculated threshold setting for leukocytes described above.

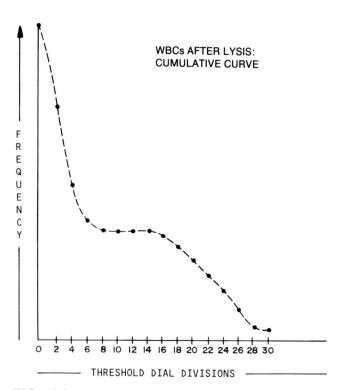

FIG. 42-8.   Threshold curve illustrating plateau. (Courtesy of Coulter Electronics, Inc.)

QUALITY CONTROL

The accuracy of cell counting instruments may be monitored on a day-to-day basis using whole blood specimens having known values or with various kinds of commercially available fixed whole blood specimens. (See Chapter 47 for a detailed discussion of this topic.)

The intent of these calibration and quality control procedures is to ensure that the instrument is properly set to detect and count either RBCs, WBCs, or platelets. Even in the best of circumstances, there is some question about how absolute this counting method is, because it is impossible to control all aspects of the procedure or to check the calibration of some parts of the instrument accurately. The inherent problems include: (1) some RBCs may lyse after dilution; (2) microbubbles (caused by vigorous mixing) introduce a positive error; (3) manometers cannot easily be calibrated or checked for calibration in the routine laboratory; and (4) coincidence tables are difficult to validate (Brian S. Bull, M.D. personal communication). However, even with all these factors playing a part in the counting procedure, one can be reasonably assured that reliable cell counts are possible if the setup, calibration, and quality control procedures are performed with care.

COMMENTS AND SOURCES OF ERROR

Potential errors from the cell counting instruments described in this chapter can be categorized into two types: instrumental errors and errors caused by the nature of the specimen.

Instrumental Errors

Aperture plugs are probably the most common problem in cell counting. They will produce a positive error because a plug has essentially decreased the volume of the aperture, and with the decreased aperture size, there is a corresponding effective increase in aperture current. This change causes some particle sizes that previously were below the lower threshold limit to be included in the count. Plugs can be detected in several ways: an increase in the pulse size on the oscilloscope screen, a change in the cadence of counting (either faster or slower during a single count), a detectable increase in the time necessary to produce a count (inspection of the mercury manometer will reveal the mercury traveling at a slower rate), and visible debris on the aperture image. The problem can be solved either by gently brushing the orifice (special brushes are available for this purpose) or by lowering the sample stand and allowing air to be pulled through the orifice. The latter maneuver results in bubbles within the aperture tube. When this occurs, the aperture tube should be flushed several times by opening and closing the vacuum and flushing stopcocks simultaneously.

Extraneous electrical pulses from improperly grounded or shielded equipment may be picked up by the instrument electrodes. This will cause fluctuations in the instrument detection of particles, giving rise to positive errors. This type of error usually can be detected by examination of the oscilloscope screen (Example: pulses on the screen when no count has been initiated).

Improper settings of aperture current or threshold will cause either a positive or a negative error. These errors should be detectable through the use of control samples.

Bubbles in the sample caused by too vigorous mixing will cause a positive error. The problem is detectable in sequential counts on the same cell suspension that decrease as the bubbles rise to the top of the suspension. The counts should stabilize after the third or fourth count.

Excessive lysing of RBCs because of delay either in making the larger dilution or after addition of the lysing reagent will cause a negative error. This problem is present if sequential counts on the same cell suspension continue to decrease rather than stabilize.

Problems in the electronic circuitry of the instrument are usually detectable through controls. Because the polarity of the internal and external electrodes alternates with every count, circuitry problems sometimes are detectable when alternate counts on the same cell suspension are reproducible but sequential counts are not (*e.g.*, 7500, 8900, 7400, 9000).

Errors Caused by the Nature of the Specimen

Physiologic conditions may create circumstances that make accurate enumeration of cells difficult if not impossible.[1] Giant platelets may be counted as RBCs or WBCs. Fragments of leukocyte cytoplasm, such as may be present during leukemia therapy, may be counted as platelets or RBCs. Increased numbers of schistocytes may make accurate erythrocyte and platelet counts impossible; for example, in severely burned patients.

Agglutination of erythrocytes, leukocytes, or platelets will cause false-negative results for each of the respective cell counts. Agglutinated red cells or platelets may also cause false-positive leukocyte counts.

Carryover from sample to sample normally is not a problem. However, an especially high count may cause sufficient carryover to affect the next specimen, particularly if the next specimen has a low count. This problem can be solved by rinsing off the aperture tube with a portion of the specimen dilution to be counted before it is analyzed.

Platelet satellitism will result in falsely low platelet counts.

Some abnormal RBCs tend to resist lysis, which may result in falsely high WBC counts. Examples include sickle cells, extremely hypochromic cells, and target cells. The problem usually can be solved by delaying 2 to 3 minutes between the addition of the lysing reagent and counting.

The moral of the story of errors caused by physiologic conditions (the nature of the sample) is that careful morphologic evaluation of a well prepared, properly stained blood film is essential in all cases. Such an examination will alert the technologist to possible discrepancies, so corrective action can be taken. Adjustment of the threshold may help solve some of the problems, or manual hemocytometer counts may be required.

General Comments

A cell counter will function optimally if it is kept clean and properly maintained. Every laboratory should establish preventive maintenance procedures to ensure cleanliness and absence of contamination by extraneous particles. It should be noted that the saline solutions used with these instruments may cause the tubing (used to make the various connections within the instrument) to harden and split after a period of time. Consequently, the tubing should be checked regularly and changed when necessary.

The instruments utilize mercury, and proper handling of this toxic heavy metal is necessary. In order for the instrument to function properly, the mercury needs to be kept reasonably clean at all times. Spilled mercury must be properly disposed of and the working area adequately decontaminated according to OSHA guidelines.

CHAPTER SUMMARY

Single-parameter cell counters are those instruments not capable of producing more than one cell count at a time. This chapter has discussed a representative of single-parameter cell counters having adjustable thresholds that is commonly used in this country, namely, the Coulter Electronics instruments designated as the Z series. The instrument has been described, its proper operation has been discussed, the calibration procedures have been described, and potential errors have been enumerated.

REFERENCES

1. Cornbleet J: Spurious results from automated hematology cell counters. Lab Med 14:509, 1983
2. Coulter Electronics, Inc: Instrument Operator's Manual (ZBI). Hialeah, FL, 1982
3. Coulter WH: High speed automatic blood cell counter and cell size analyzer. Proc Natl Electron Conf 12:1034, 1956
4. Koepke JA (ed): Laboratory Hematology. New York, Churchill Livingstone, 1984

43

Multiparameter Hematology Instruments

Judith S. Watson
Mary Ann Dotson

Instruments capable of measuring more than one hematologic parameter at a time were introduced in the mid-1960s by two manufacturers who used different principles of cell counting. Technicon Instruments offered the SMA 4, capable of providing simultaneous WBC and RBC counts as well as Hb and HCT determinations. Coulter Electronics introduced a seven-parameter instrument, the Model S, which was capable of performing the four studies listed above plus the three red cell indices (MCV, MCH, MCHC). In 1966 Technicon added the three indices to their system to produce the SMA 7. The Technicon instruments were based on darkfield optical scanning, whereas the Coulter instruments utilized electronic impedance for cell counting. Other manufacturers soon followed with their own seven-parameter instruments. Ortho Diagnostic Systems introduced a laser-based optical instrument in 1975.

Today's marketplace has a variety of multiparameter instruments from several manufacturers. These instruments may be subdivided into two basic principles of operation: electronic impedance (or resistance) and light scatter (both laser and nonlaser light). A new instrument using centrifugal force was introduced in the early 1980s, but it does not count individual cells. Most manufacturers offer several instruments of increasing complexity and sophistication. These instruments differ in the number of tests available and the degree of automation, ranging from discrete analyzers to walkaway instruments.

In this chapter the development of various technologies will be covered, and the evolution of the CBC as it is done today will be described. The general principles of cell counting and characterization will be detailed. The particular characteristics of each of the principal systems will be described with consideration given to interferences and review criteria. Several illustrations of histograms from the principal systems are discussed. Guidelines and considerations helpful in selecting instruments are reviewed for various types of laboratories.

DEVELOPMENT OF AUTOMATED ANALYZERS

The development of the automated hematology analyzer has been continuous, with each step increasing the number of tests performed simultaneously, increasing the speed, and decreasing the required sample size. The first multiparameter instruments expanded the CBC from WBC and RBC counting and Hb and HCT measurements to include an electronic MCV measurement with automatic calculation of MCH and MCHC. Automation of some measurements, such as the addition of platelet enumeration in the presence of RBCs, came in response to diagnostic needs. Of the laboratories reporting in the 1986 CAP Comprehensive Hematology Survey, 92% were using an automated method for platelets,[6] up from 12% in 1977.[4] Other new tests followed engineering developments and advances in computerization. An example is the measurement of the coefficient of variation (CV) of volume distribution within a population of RBCs, which is variously reported as the red cell distribution width (RDW) or red cell morphology index (RCMI). This value is proposed as an indicator of anisocytosis. Together with the MCV, the RDW or RCMI has been used as a means of classifying anemias.[3] Similar volume measurements and calculations have been extended to platelets as a mean platelet volume (MPV) and platelet distribution width (PDW). Studies have linked platelet measurements to clinical states,[2] but to date such measures have not been widely used.

Oscilloscope displays have been part of clinical instruments since the time of the first Coulter counters. This display of the pulses that are created by the cells as they interrupt the current is a real-time display that ceases when counting ends. However, by identifying the size channel in which each pulse occurs, one can count the pulses and store them in memory in their appropriate channel. Plotting the number of pulses on the Y axis and the cell size (channel number) on the X axis produces a histogram (Fig. 43-1) that depicts the volume distribution of the cell population. The first histogram provided by an instrument was the platelet histogram, but RBC and WBC histograms soon followed. Cytograms and Hb reaction curves are more recent additions. Two-dimensional cytograms represent two cell properties, and cell types appear as clusters, the number of dots in each cluster denoting the concentration of that cell type. Figure 43-2 compares a cytogram and a histogram of unstained normal WBCs. The X axis of the cytogram is internal cell complexity, and the Y axis is relative size.

The ability to produce histograms brought with it the ability to count the number of cells within selected size ranges. This capability, in concert with new lysing agents, has allowed more recent instruments to generate data on relative and absolute numbers of small, medium, and large leukocytes: the "three-part differential." The result of all of these advances has been a redefinition of the CBC, which may now include more than 20 measurements and calcula-

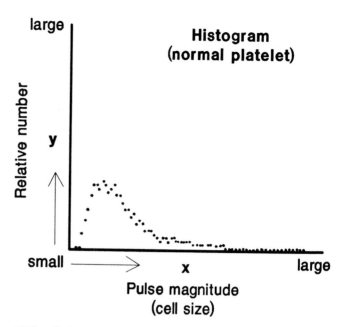

FIG. 43-1. Visual display of one cell characteristic and cell frequency as a histogram with X axis being pulse magnitude (cell size) and Y axis in this case being relative number (cell concentration).

tions that characterize the red cell, white cell, and platelet populations in approximately 60 seconds using 100 μL of whole blood. The latest technological developments analyze cells simultaneously using two or more methods. These advancements in technology produce a "five-part differential."

Automation brought significant improvement in counting precision; and, as each method was automated, it became a more valuable diagnostic tool. Volume distribution histograms have been available since 1979; these offer useful tools for detecting certain conditions and interferences, as will be demonstrated later.

With increasing microprocessor development, computer programs direct the instrument to perform diagnostic self-checks on the electronic and optical systems. Extensive quality control (QC) files are available that automatically accept, calculate, graph, and store the data. On many instruments, it is possible to store and retrieve patient results, some with additional data manipulation. Startup, shutdown, and maintenance procedures are automated on some models, requiring just a touch on the keypad. Software permits relatively simple conversion of a system to reporting in SI units or to a selected language in some cases.

GENERAL PRINCIPLES OF INSTRUMENT OPERATION

Electronic Impedance

The basic principle developed by Coulter in the 1950s of electronic impedance is the basis for the method of operation used by a number of manufacturers, including TOA Medical Electronics Co., Ltd., Instrumentation Laboratory, J. T. Baker Instruments, Unipath Company (formerly

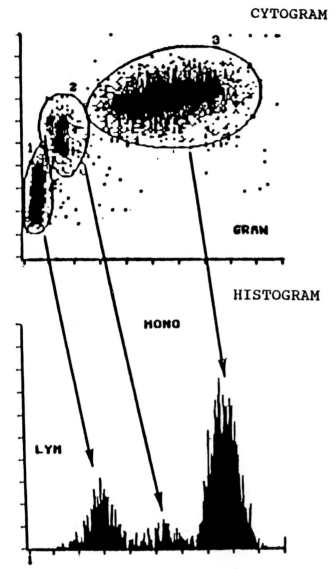

CYTOGRAM

GRAN

HISTOGRAM

MONO

LYM

FIG. 43-2. Visual display of two cell characteristics as cytogram and histogram. This example is a normal unstained whole blood sample from ELT. Normal human leukocytes scatter light into three distinct regions (referred to as clusters) on the forward *v* right-angle scatter cytogram. By mathematically transforming this information into a one-dimensional histogram, three peaks (arrows) are derived, corresponding uniquely to each of the three clusters. Peaks, left to right, are lymphocytes, monocytes, and granulocytes. (Courtesy of Ortho Diagnostic Systems Inc.)

Sequoia-Turner Corporation), Clay Adams, and others. The principle is discussed in detail in Chapter 42. Briefly, cells suspended in an electrically conductive diluent increase the resistance between two electrodes when passing through a sensing aperture. The impedance creates measurable pulses.

The change in electrical resistance, or the size of the pulse generated by the cell is proportional to its volume. The cell count is determined by the number of pulses generated. Separate channels are used for WBC and RBC counting. The WBCs are counted in a dilution in which the RBCs have been lysed. In the RBC channel, the dilution is great enough to make the number of WBCs negli-

gible and thus not a source of interference except when they are present in extremely high numbers. In the more advanced models, platelets and RBCs generally are counted together and the counts separated by computer analysis of pulse heights.

In first-generation electrical impedance instruments, several things were found to affect volume measurements. The "coincidence" of more than one cell arriving at the orifice at a time or the position of the cell with respect to the center of the orifice may make the cell appear larger and create an artificially large pulse. Also, cells recirculating back into the sensing zone can create erroneous pulses. These problems have been addressed in the newer generation of instruments. To deal with orientation and coincidence, Coulter Electronics employed more sophisticated circuitry to "edit" out anomalously shaped pulses electronically. A back-wash of diluting fluid is used to prevent recirculation of cells into the counting zone. To increase platelet counting sensitivity, the RBC/PLT aperture size was decreased. The TOA instrument uses hydrodynamic focusing to force the cells into single-file-passage through the sensing zone. The fluid aperture produced through hydrodynamic focusing minimizes the protein buildup and plugs inherent in small rigid apertures.

In recent generations of instruments employing electronic impedance, the method has been extended to leukocyte differential analysis. With the aid of lysing agents that strip away or shrink the cells' plasma membrane and cytoplasm, leaving "bare" nuclei, the cells are counted and sized as they pass through the aperture. The various size determinations have been related to WBC types. The instruments report three subpopulations of cells, which can be used as screening differentials. Counts and information for five different cell populations are provided in the newest instruments, which use a more controlled (reagent) alteration of the cell nucleus and cytoplasm. These instruments employ multiple analytic methods to characterize each population of cells. The automated differential count is discussed at length in the next chapter.

Light Scattering

Great strides have been made in just a few years in the development of cell analysis using light scattering methodology. Cells are detected and counted as they pass through a focused beam of light instead of through an electrical field. Instruments using light scatter methodology that are capable of making multiple measurements of individual cells processed in a flowing fluid are termed "flow cytometers." Many new terms used to describe the characteristics of flow cytometers are defined here.

The word *laser* is an acronym for **l**ight **a**mplification by **s**timulated **e**mission of **r**adiation. Laser light differs in character and effectiveness from a beam of ordinary light in that it is emitted as a single wavelength (monochromatic light). Laser light is also coherent: it travels in phase (wave peaks and valleys are together) from its source and thus enables detection of the effects of interference. Laser light has little spread (*i.e.,* low divergence). The fourth characteristic of laser light is its brightness (high power per solid angle). *Noncoherent light* sources are present in some instruments that use filters to obtain appropriate wavelengths instead of the more expensive lasers.

Light scatter by cells is the summation of the three independent processes: *diffraction* (bending around corners),[27] *refraction* (bending because of a change in speed),[26] and *reflection* (light rays turned back by the surface or boundary of an obstruction).[24,25] Cells scatter light in all directions, with diffraction generally dominating at small angles relative to the incident light, reflection dominating at larger angles, and refractive index generally dominating at intermediate angles.[15,22]

Flow cells are made of quartz rather than glass because quartz is transparent and does not bend the light that passes through it. It also allows ultraviolet (UV) light to pass, whereas glass blocks the passage of UV light. The flow cell is where counting is done and cell characteristics are measured. The light source is focused on a small area of the flow cell, and the sample stream is directed through this area (sensing zone for analysis).

Sheath fluid is the fluid that fills a flow cell and surrounds the sample stream as it passes through the flow cell. It prevents the flow cell from being coated by reagents, cell stroma, or any other substance that would bend the rays of light as they entered the flow cell. Sheath fluid also facilitates laminar flow and hydrodynamic focusing.

Laminar flow is the physics term that describes the flow properties of a fluid moving relatively constantly through a long channel or pipe. Particles within this fluid follow paths or streamlines. When laminar flow conditions exist, all particles flow in parallel lines as they travel through the channel (flow cell). Under these conditions, a second fluid (sample) does not mix with the surrounding fluid (sheath). Laminar flow is dependent on flow velocity, channel diameter, fluid density, and the fluid viscosity coefficient. These factors plug into a formula to give a value called the "Reynolds number," which must be below the critical value of

2300 for laminar conditions to exist. Flow is more laminar as the Reynolds number gets further below the critical value, whereas flow becomes turbulent when the critical value is exceeded.[10,22] Figure 43-3 depicts laminar flow and the region of hydrodynamic focusing.

Hydrodynamic focusing of the sample stream is produced by symmetrically decreasing the cross sectional area of the fluidic channel in the flow cell and reducing the area in which the fluid is flowing. This results in faster-flowing central fluid with narrowing of the central sample stream. The design is such that the sample stream is sufficiently narrowed to separate and align the cells into a single file for passage through the sensing zone.[10,22]

Light scattered by a particle in the sensing zone of the flow cell is detected by appropriately placed *photodetectors (scatter detectors)*. Photodiodes and photomultiplier tubes (PMT) are commonly used for this purpose. Photodiodes are light detectors that are not very sensitive but are sufficient to detect forward scatter, which has a relatively strong light level. On the other hand, PMT are sensitive to weak light levels and, as the name implies, multiply weak signals into stronger, useful signals.

Blocker bar or *darkfield stop* are the names given to the barriers that prevent direct (unscattered) light from reaching (and "blinding") the light scatter detectors. A labeled blocker bar is shown in Figure 43-3.

Forward low-angle light scatter correlates with cell volume primarily because of diffraction of light (bending by the outside surface of a cell).[15] Figure 43-3 depicts photodetectors in an optical system. *Forward high-angle light scatter* measurements depict the degree of structure inside the cell.[9] *Differential scatter* is the combination of low- and high-angle forward scatter. This scatter analysis is used to analyze RBC (volume versus Hb concentration) and WBC (volume

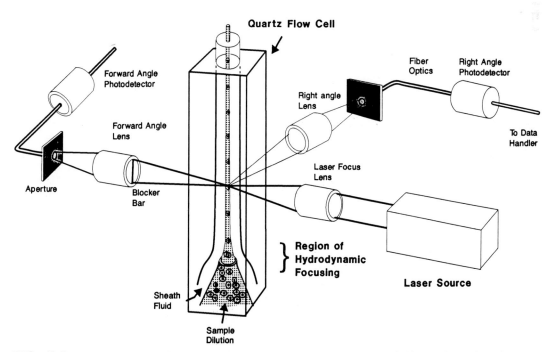

FIG. 43-3.   ELT optics bench. Labels identify laser source, quartz flow cell, blocker bar, photodetectors (forward and right-angle), sheath, sample stream, region of hydrodynamic focusing in flow cell, and concept of laminar flow. (Courtesy of Ortho Diagnostic Systems Inc.)

versus nuclear lobularity) properties[12] (Fig. 43-4). The intensity of light scatter at larger angles (90°) is attributable primarily to refraction and reflection of light from larger structures inside the cell. Structures such as nuclei and cytoplasmic granules determine the intensity of light scattering at 90° (right-angle scatter).

A *beam splitter* separates different wavelengths of light for collection by different photosensing devices and for analysis. *Mia analysis* is a light scattering technique in which RBC volume and Hb concentration are determined by analyzing scattered monochromatic light from individual sphered RBCs at two carefully chosen angular intervals[21] (Fig. 43-5).

Theory of Light Scatter

Cells pass through a flow cell on which a beam of light is focused. As the cells interrupt the beam, light is scattered in all directions. Photodetectors sense and collect the scattered rays at specific angles as individual cells pass through the sensing zone. Analysis and conversion into digital form provides cell counts and size information. Hemoglobin is determined by a modified cyanmethemoglobin measurement with colorimetric analysis. Red cell and platelet counts are performed on the same portion of the diluted sample, whereas WBC counts are performed on a different diluted portion in which the RBCs have been lysed. Hematocrit determination methods differ depending on the specific instrumentation (see next section). Indices (MCV, MCH, MCHC) and RBC size variation generally are calculated parameters. White cell population percentages also are calculated.

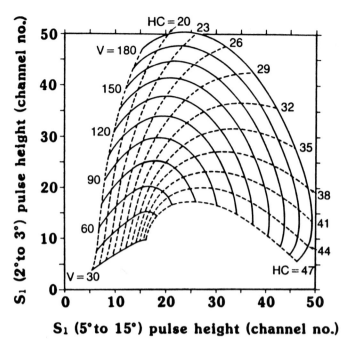

FIG. 43-5.   Mia analysis of red cells. Transformation between scatter angles 2°–3° and 5°–15° permits separate measurements of cell volume (V) and Hb concentration (HC). (Copyright 1986 by the Technicon Instruments Corporation; reproduced with permission.)

Absorbance Combined with Light Scatter

The darkfield optical method of light scatter combined with light absorbance measurements used by Technicon counts and classifies the leukocytes for differentials. With this method, when no cells are present in the scatter channel, the darkfield disk prevents the light from hitting the photodetector. As each cell passes through the sensing zone, light is scattered through the opening around the darkfield disk, hitting the photodetector and generating signals or pulses, which are summed for the cell counts. In the absorbance channel, when either unstained cells or no cells are passing, there is no light lost because of staining; therefore, the photodiode receives maximum light. As a stained cell passes, it absorbs a portion of the light, decreasing the amount hitting the photodetector (photodiode). The amount of light absorbed is proportional to the amount of staining. The cell types are differentiated on this basis.[17] Table 43-1 summarizes the use of light scatter for cell analysis by Ortho and Technicon hematology instruments.

Centrifugal

The innovative centrifugal method does not actually count cells but rather analyzes the buffy coat layer (leukocytes and platelets) in centrifuged whole blood samples. The technique was first described in the early 1980s.[23] Whole blood, when centrifuged, will layer according to the specific gravity of each component (from bottom to top: RBCs, WBCs, platelets, plasma). Quantitative analysis of the buffy coat is performed in a modified microhematocrit tube and provides an HCT value, total WBC count, platelet count, and

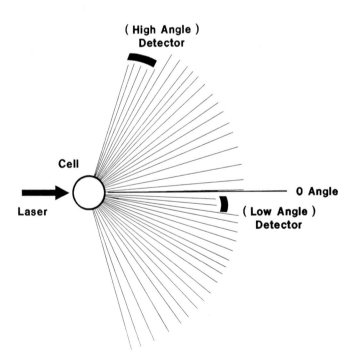

FIG. 43-4.   Differential scatter detection. High forward-angle scatter and low forward-angle scatter detection used by H·1 for red cell and white cell analysis. (Copyright 1986 by the Technicon Instruments Corporation; reproduced with permission.)

TABLE 43–1. Data Obtained from Light Scatter Cell Analysis

	ANGLE 1		ANGLE 2
ORTHO			
Cell counts	Low forward scatter (size) 2°–9°		
Differential	Low forward scatter (size)	AND	Internal complexity 90° scatter
TECHNICON			
Cell counts	Low forward scatter (size)		
Differential	Low forward scatter (size)	AND	Absorbance (stain) Right-angle scatter (90°)
RBC analysis	Low forward scatter (RBC vol.) 2°–3°		High-angle forward scatter (Hb conc.) 5°–15°
Lobularity index	Low forward scatter (size) 2°–3°		High-angle forward scatter (internal complexity) 5°–15°

the separation of the white cells into two populations: granulocytes and nongranulocytes.

Precisely manufactured glass capillary tubes are precoated with acridine orange, which acts as a supravital stain. The dye is taken up by nucleoproteins of WBCs and fluoresces green when excited by violet light. Granulocytic cells have numerous granules that contain glycosaminoglycans. Acridine orange absorbed on these molecules fluoresces at a different wavelength than that of the nucleoproteins and when combined with nuclear fluorescence, makes this part of the white cell layer appear bright orange. The granulocytic cell layer is the heaviest component of the buffy coat and layers immediately on top of the RBCs. Cells lacking granules with glycosaminoglycans (lymphocytes and monocytes) remain above the granulocytes in a single layer and fluoresce a brilliant emerald green. Platelets, fluorescing yellow, form the top cell layer. The cell-free plasma fluoresces green.

Analysis of each layer is possible because of a solid cylindrical plastic float that expands the buffy coat layer (Fig. 43-6). The plastic cylinder has a specific gravity between that of plasma and red cells. It becomes positioned at the top of the RBC layer during centrifugation and is surrounded by the expanded buffy coat layers. These layers are expanded by a factor of 10.71 and are only two to three cells thick, which is optimum. A viewer with a UV light source, appropriate filters, and a micrometer is used to measure the length of each layer. The operator identifies each of the interfaces between the cell layers with the aid of a cursor and an entry key. Precise measurements of the tube's longitudinal movement are made from interface to interface, and the band (layer) lengths are converted into count equivalents.

This instrument was designed primarily for use in physician offices. Successful operation does not require extensive training or a background in laboratory techniques. The instrument provides accurate and rapid screening CBC results, with less than 5% unreadable samples from populations seen in an outpatient setting. A study comparing buffy coat analysis results and standard hematology testing methods showed good correlation.[23] The authors of this study recommend that platelet values less than $80 \times 10^9/L$ be confirmed by an independent method such as blood film

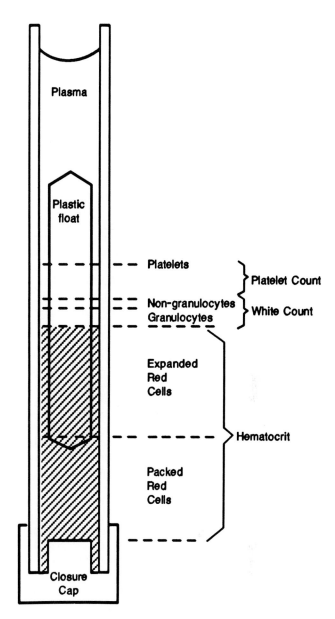

FIG. 43-6. Whole blood layers in centrifugal analyzer tube. Cell counts are derived from expanded and nonexpanded layers as indicated.

examination. If a hematologic dyscrasia is suspected, referral for a blood film examination is essential, and cell counts may need to be determined by another method. Buffy coat analysis provides rapid results but is not designed to detect red cell abnormalities (e.g., hypochromia), increases in cell types (e.g., eosinophils), or abnormal (leukemic) white cells. Samples from inpatient populations tend to have more frequent streaming problems (poor separation of layers) in the instrument than samples from an outpatient setting.

PRINCIPAL INSTRUMENT SYSTEMS

To date, Coulter instruments account for the majority of the instruments in laboratories of all sizes, with instruments of the S-Plus series accounting for approximately 62% of the systems in American laboratories in 1986.[5]

Electronic Impedance Instruments

The basic components of a hematology instrument such as the Coulter S-Plus series are the power unit, the analyzer module, the diluter, and a data terminal. A ticket printer prints the determined values, and a matrix printer-plotter provides a hard copy of the data displayed on the terminal.

The pneumatic portion of the power unit consists of vacuum and pressure pumps, which move liquid through the diluter. The electronic portion of the power unit provides regulated voltages for the circuitry of the system. The diluter portion contains the pipeters, mixing chambers, WBC and RBC sensing apertures, and the hemoglobinometer. The analyzer module contains electronic and computing circuitry. This module controls the sequence of operations in the diluter and processes the data generated. The information from the analyzer is received by the data terminal, where results and histograms are displayed.

The aspirated whole blood sample is divided into two aliquots, and each is mixed with isotonic diluent. One dilution is delivered to the RBC aperture bath for information about RBCs and platelets. The other is delivered to the WBC bath, where a lytic reagent is added to break down the RBC stroma and release Hb. There are three sensing apertures in each of the counting baths. Count and size information is generated in triplicate in the form of pulses. After the leukocyte information is obtained, the diluted specimen is delivered to the hemoglobinometer for Hb reading. This information is sent to the analyzer.

Three values are considered to be measured directly. The RBCs and WBCs are counted directly. Hemoglobin concentration is measured by the amount of light transmittance at a wavelength of 525 nm. Other values are calculated.

The platelet count is determined from a segment of the RBC histogram within the range of 2 to 20 fL. The pulses obtained in this range are classified as platelets for the raw count. To obtain an accurate platelet count in the presence of red cells, a mathematical model is applied to the raw data. Histograms of the raw count (data) are fitted to a lognormal curve ranging from 0 to 70 fL. The extended curve eliminates particles interfering at both ends, such as debris (low end) or microcytic RBCs (high end). The final platelet count is derived from this fitted curve. If certain criteria for curve fitting and platelet data are not met, the count is flagged and not reported.[7]

Size distribution histograms of WBC, RBC, and platelet populations are established by pulse height analysis. When a histogram does not reach one half scale (Y axis), it is automatically scaled to one half height on the Y axis for evaluation of the cell distribution pattern. Thus, cell counts cannot be estimated from these histograms. (Fig. 43-8A illustrates patterns from a normal sample.) The MCV and RDW are derived from the RBC histogram, whereas the MPV and PDW are derived from the platelet histogram. The HCT, MCH, and MCHC are calculated from measured and derived values.

With newer models the sample size is reduced to 100 μL, and correspondingly less reagent is required. Also, the microprocessing capabilities have been expanded, permitting two-part and three-part leukocyte subpopulation analysis. Increased computer memory accommodates as many as 3000 patient records plus 300 selected histograms. The user also has the option of sorting files by parameters, such as all samples with abnormal platelet values. The QC package includes files for commercial and patient controls (with Levey-Jennings charts) (Chap. 47), the use of the Bull algorithm for moving averages (Chap. 47), and an automated calibration procedure. An automated cap-piercing sampler is available on some models. Daily startup, including controls, takes 30 to 40 minutes.

In more recent instruments (e.g., STKS), the volumetric method of cell sizing is combined with laser light scatter and conductivity measurements. The laser light is used to scan each cell to determine characteristics of the surface such as structure, shape, and reflectivity. Conductivity measurements of each cell provided by a high-frequency electromagnetic probe give measurements of internal contents. High-frequency current passing through a cell changes in response to the cell's nuclear composition, granular (cytoplasmic) makeup, and interior chemical composition. The cell wall itself acts as a conductor when exposed to high-frequency current. The addition of scatter and conductivity characteristics to volumetric measurement provides precise mapping of cellular characteristics in the form of scatterplots and histograms. This "three-dimensional" analysis of each cell's characteristics produces percent and absolute counts for neutrophils, lymphocytes, monocytes, eosinophils, and basophils (a five-part differential).

Electronic Resistance (Impedance) Counters

There is a full line of Sysmex instruments (TOA Medical Electronics Co., Ltd.) with up to 15 parameters based on the electronic resistance (impedance) detection method for counting and sizing the WBCs, RBCs, and platelets. These instruments have three hydraulic subsystems: WBC, RBC/PLT, and Hb. There are two unique features: (1) the use of hydrodynamic focusing in the RBC/PLT subsystem to narrow the sample stream to single file, preventing off-center cell passage, and (2) a discrimination circuit that eliminates signals above and below certain thresholds and automatically determines the optimum level for each sample, allowing for precise discrimination of cell types. In the RBC sample, this feature is used to separate small RBCs from platelets.[20]

The E-5000 model is fully automated with a sampler and bar-code ID reader and is capable of processing 116 samples per hour using 200 μL of sample. Special features include warming of the RBC diluent to 37°C and the option to relocate the threshold (discriminator) levels to isolate a special population of cells such as separating two RBC populations to measure number and volume of native and transfused red cells. In addition, computer memory stores complete data, including histograms, from 300 samples. Data manipulation, such as retrieval of selected abnormals, also is possible. Extensive QC options include a program that adopts the Bull moving average formula for patient samples, multiple files for Levey-Jennings or duplicate sample analysis, and automatic calibration.

New technology has been added to the instrument just described to produce the NE-8000, which gives a five-part differential count. New lysing reagents slightly alter the WBC size. Radiofrequency (RF) analysis has been combined with direct current (DC) volumetric sizing to measure each white cell simultaneously. The DC method sizes the entire cell, including the nucleus and the cytoplasm, whereas the RF method detects and sizes the cell on the basis of the overall density. Changes in the RF signal correlate primarily with the nuclear size and density. In cells having heavy cytoplasmic granulation, the RF signal correlates with the overall cell density, including the heavy granulation. Eight floating discriminators automatically adjust to each individual sample to separate the cell populations (lymphocyte, monocyte, granulocyte). Separate cell-specific lysing reagents permit eosinophil and basophil counts. Scatterplots and histograms are displayed and may be printed.

J.T. Baker, Clay Adams, Instrumentation Laboratory, and Unipath Company are other companies that manufacture instruments based on electrical impedance with parameters and features similar to those of the two instruments just described. The strengths and weaknesses of each line, and a particular system within a line, will have to be determined by each potential user. A guide for this process of determination will be described later in the chapter.

Laser Optical Counters

The Hemac (Ortho Diagnostic Systems Inc.) was the first laser-based clinical cell counter. Changing from light extinction to light scatter detection, enhancing computer programming, and redesigning resulted in the later ELT series of instruments (ELT is an acronym for **e**rythrocyte, **l**eukocyte, **t**hrombocyte). The ELT-8 and -800 produce results for eight parameters, the 800 instruments having a faster throughput time. Similarly, the ELT-15 and -1500 produce 15 results at two rates of speed. The higher throughput is derived mostly from changes in mechanical design and fluidic improvements, including less reagent consumption. The sample size (100–120 μL) remains the same. The instrument system is made up of two units (a data handler and a sample handler) and an optional plotter. The sample handler is the diluting and counting unit and houses the printer. The data handler consists of a computer that is programmed to interpret, analyze, and display the results in numeric and histogram forms on a CRT. The operator interacts with the computer via the data handler keypad. A hard copy of numeric data is printed by the ticket printer. A hard copy of histograms and numeric data display can be plotted by the page printer/plotter.

Samples progress through instrument tubing with two cams driving slide valves and various-size pumps, which, along with poppet valves, direct samples to the flow cell for analysis. Slide valves direct the fluid along appropriate pathways, while poppet valves simply control fluid movement (stop and go). Pumps provide the drive for fluidic movement through the system, as well as reagents for dilutions. Sample (100 μL) is aspirated into the ELT and split into two equal portions (far left of Fig. 43-7). One portion (lower half of same figure) is for the WBC count. The ELT-15 also performs a three-part WBC differential. The reagent used to lyse the red cells does not alter the white cells,

so size and internal complexity are measured simultaneously to determine WBC count and distribution by type (lymphocyte, monocyte, and granulocyte) in absolute numbers and percentages. Counting takes place in the flow cell (far right of Fig. 43-7).

The second portion of the sample is utilized for Hb, RBC count, platelet count, HCT, red cell indices, and morphology index. The top half of Figure 43-7 shows fluidics that pertain to red cell analysis. Hemoglobin reagent is added to a portion of the first red cell dilution and destroys white cells in the process of Hb color development. Most other cell counters count WBCs and read the Hb concentration from the same sample dilution. A second red cell dilution is made in final preparation for counting of RBCs and platelets. Red cell size is determined from the electrical pulse integrals (area under each pulse), and HCT is determined by summing these integrals. Red cells and platelets are counted simultaneously, with three variables (volume, refractive index, and time of flight) being used to distinguish these two cell types. Time of flight is the number of microseconds it takes a cell to pass through the sensing zone. At a constant speed, cells with a larger diameter have a longer time of flight than cells with a smaller diameter.[15] Platelet counts by this method are superior to those dependent on size alone because the refractive index of the red cell, due to the presence of Hb, plays a role in determining the distinctive signals that distinguish RBCs from platelets (without Hb). The extremely small sensing zone greatly reduces the amount of interference. This portion of the sample also provides information about RBC size distribution variation called RCMI (red cell morphology index), which is determined from the red cell histogram. The RCMI is determined for each sample by calculating and comparing the histogram area coefficient of variation of the sample with that expected in an average normal population. The calculation is done on the single-cell population, whereas the doublet RBC population is excluded from the determination unless the doublet population exceeds the mathematically predictable concentration, in which case it is included in the calculations. Thus, a sample with two RBC populations will have a large RCMI.[8]

Counting takes place in a quartz flow cell on which a helium-neon laser beam is focused. The flow cell is large (250 μm in diameter), with the sample stream occupying only the center portion of the flowing fluid. This is accomplished (aided) by hydrodynamic focusing and laminar flow (see Fig. 43-3). The concentrated sample (WBC dilution 1:19, RBC/PLT dilution 1:600) is injected into the center of the sheath fluid under laminar flow conditions. The sheath fluid and flow cell design hydrodynamically focuses the sample into a stream of cells in single file separated sufficiently to allow one-by-one passage through the sensing zone of the laser beam, which is 20 $\times$ 7 μm. Each particle passing the sensing zone scatters the laser beam. Photodetectors at low forward and 90° angles collect the scattered light. The blocker bar prevents direct light from reaching the low-angle forward scatter detector. The "optics bench" includes the flow cell, laser, and photodetectors, as shown in Figure 43-3. Computer analysis of the signals generated by cells scattering light provides digital printouts of cell counts, as indicated earlier.

The Ortho ELT series of instruments does not permit

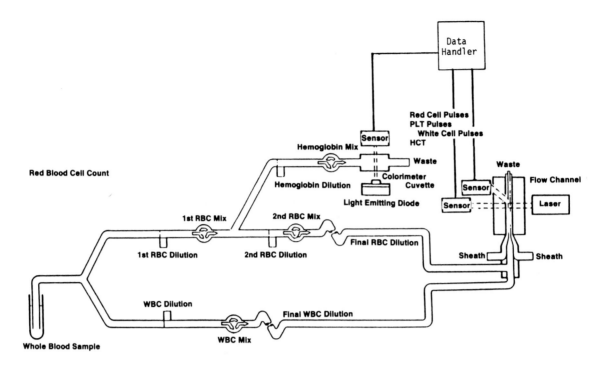

Red Blood Cell Count

White Blood Cell Count

FIG. 43-7. Fluidic diagram of Ortho ELT 15. At far left is whole blood aspiration and split. Colorimeter for Hb analysis is in top center. Red cell dilutions follow upper pathway of sample split; white cell dilution follows lower pathway to flow cell (far right), where red cells, platelets, and then white cells are counted. All measurement signals are sent to data handler (top right) for conversion to digital form for printout or display. (Courtesy of Ortho Diagnostic Systems Inc.)

carryover from one sample to the next. The 60-second cycle consists of three equal time divisions in which dilution, counting, and rinsing and refilling take place. Thorough rinsing of the sample probe prevents sample carryover.[13]

Features of the computer programming include alarms and messages of linearity limits, the laboratory's own panic value alerts, a low reagent-level alarm, several QC storage files (libraries), automatic updating of mean, SD, and CV with each addition to the data file, Bull moving average program, Levey-Jennings charts of all QC data, and printing-plotting capabilities. Other features include storage of 3700 patients' results, an ID worklist program, and a test-options program for diagnostic self-testing of electronics and optical alignment. Calibration may be done using commercial material or whole blood with reference count values and selected calibration of all measures or a single measure. Quality control data may be edited any time; the results that are edited out are marked with a caret and remain in the database but are excluded from the calculation of means, SDs or CVs. Edited data may also be restored when desired. This feature permits rapid manipulation of data without loss of documentation of a problem and its solution.

The startup time depends on the extent to which laboratories go to verify calibration each day. Twenty to thirty

minutes is sufficient when recalibration is not required. The time depends on the number of (1-minute) cycles performed in the startup procedure. Visual inspection of pumps, valves, and tubing for evidence of leaks takes only a few seconds. Background checks, reagent level checks, and other routine maintenance may add to startup time or be scattered over three shifts. Although each maintenance procedure is done every 24 hours, the block of time identified as "start up" will vary depending on the calibration verification and maintenance schedules.

Histograms of RBC and platelet size distribution are displayed for each patient sample. The WBC histogram display uses a combination of size and internal complexity measurements for the X axis, with the Y axis being relative number (see Fig. 43-2). The kinetics of the Hb reaction are also available for display or plotting. A composite of WBC, RBC, and platelet histograms may be displayed on the CRT for each sample, and may be printed for interpretation or permanent record.

Figure 43-8B is a composite from the ELT (with three-part screening differential) of a normal sample. Single full-page individual histograms may be viewed for detailed pattern analysis, and single histograms with very low counts (flat display) or counts high enough to reach the upper limits of the display may be scaled for pattern interpretation. The utility of histograms and their interpretation

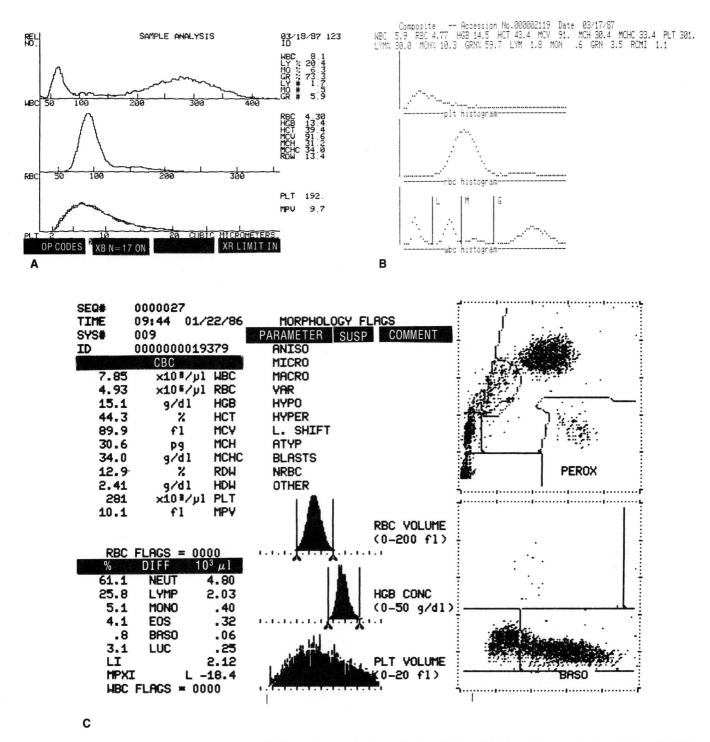

FIG. 43-8. Normal composite printouts. (A) Normal example from Coulter S-Plus. (B) Normal example from Ortho ELT-15. (C) Normal example from Technicon H·1.

are discussed later in this chapter. Three-part WBC differential displays and results will be discussed in Chapter 44.

Optical Plus Cytochemical Counters

The darkfield optical method of cell analysis employed by Technicon Instruments Corporation has been modified through several generations of instruments. The H6000 combines the leukocyte differential analysis of the earlier

D-90 and the CBC of the Hemalog 8 into one operation in a continuous-flow analyzer. On this instrument, an automated sampler aspirates whole blood, dilutes it, and divides it into three streams. The sample streams travel through the system separated by bubbles of air to minimize carryover. Three analytical manifolds provide a means of combining reagents and sample in the proper proportions. In the RBC/PLT manifold, the sample is diluted and directed to each of two channels, RBC/PLT and Hb. In the Hb channel, reagents convert released Hb to cyanmethemoglobin. The resulting solution is measured in a colorimeter at 550 nm. In the RBC channel, reagents "sphere" and fix the cells.[11] The sample is then routed to the RBC/PLT optic system, where the cells are enumerated and sized according to their light-scattering properties. A PMT permits quantitation of platelets, which scatter light at low levels. The HCT is the sum of the signals for the detected RBC population. In the peroxidase and basophil manifolds, the RBCs are lysed. The remaining cells are fixed and stained for myeloperoxidase in one channel and with alcian blue in the other (basophil) channel. The samples are then routed to their respective optics for analysis.

A peroxidase cytogram (Fig. 43-9) is generated by plotting size versus staining intensity. On the basis of these properties, and the count from the basophil channel, the WBCs are differentiated into the five traditional categories plus large unstained cells (LUCs) and cells with high peroxidase activity (HPX). The LUCs correspond to variant lymphocytes, blast cells, or any large cell devoid of peroxidase activity. The HPX relates to immature neutrophils, although not necessarily to morphology.[1] Several thousand cells are analyzed in both the peroxidase and the basophil channels, but the signals from the peroxidase channel are used for the WBC count. Cytograms provide characteristic "pictures" of the WBC populations and are useful in suggesting disease states.

Four optical assemblies are positioned around a common tungsten-halogen light source. Sheath fluid is added around the sample stream to achieve single-file passage of cells, both to prevent clogging and to eliminate coating or staining of the flow cell. Signals generated in each of the optics assemblies are converted to digital form and sent to a microprocessor for output on a printer or into a laboratory information system. In addition to the 15-parameter re-

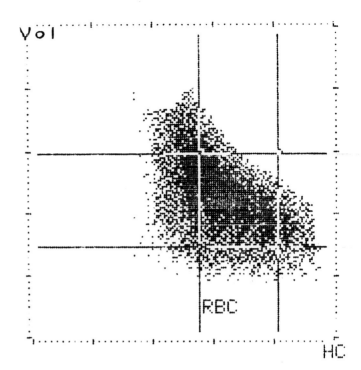

FIG. 43-10.   Linear analysis display. Cytogram from the RBC channel of H·1 plotting RBC volume v Hb concentration. Majority of cells in this example are normocytic and normochromic. (Copyright 1986 by the Technicon Instruments Corporation; reproduced with permission.)

sults, size distribution histograms of RBCs and platelets are developed.

The startup time for this system is close to 1 hour, with calibration required once per shift. This system is fully automated with a barcode reader, and once it is under way, 90 samples can be processed per hour. Routine maintenance is extensive, as the series of pump tubes requires replacement every 200 hours of use.

The QC package is similar to those discussed earlier that are found on other instruments. The system will store results from 250 patients, which can be retrieved individually or in a batch. Also available with this system is a unique slide-making assembly that prepares a monolayer of cells on a film, stains it, and then transfers the stained film to a glass microscope slide.

The H·1 extends the technology of previous systems while greatly simplifying the operation of the hydraulics. The instrument is a discrete analyzer in three modules: the electronics and analytic modules and the data terminal. A whole-blood sample of 100 μL is aspirated and split four ways. One portion is analyzed for Hb concentration by a cyanmethemoglobin method in a colorimeter; a second portion is used for RBC and platelet information; a third is cytochemically stained for myeloperoxidase for leukocyte differential analysis, in principle much the same as in previous models[14]; and the final portion is analyzed in a basophil and lobularity channel. Figure 43-8C illustrates a composite of a normal sample.

The main feature of this new cytometer is based on differential light scattering (defined earlier). With this laser-

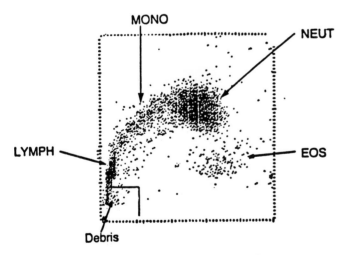

FIG. 43-9.   Cytogram (normal stained whole blood sample). Peroxidase channel display showing clusters of unstained lymphocytes, slightly stained monocytes, moderately stained neutrophils, intensely stained eosinophils, and unstained debris (platelets and red cell stroma). (Copyright 1986 by the Technicon Instruments Corporation; reproduced with permission.)

based method, there are two detectors, which are sensitive to light scattered at two separate angles (see Fig. 43-4). Analyzing the RBC sample in this channel, a two-dimensional cytogram is produced, plotting volume versus Hb concentration (Fig. 43-10). Computer analysis of this cytogram enables RBC enumeration plus independent measurements of RBC volume and individual red cell Hb concentration. The reported MCHC value is calculated in the traditional manner from the Hb and HCT, whereas the direct measurement of concentration, termed the "CHCM" (*c*ellular *h*emoglobin *c*oncentration *m*ean), is unaffected by lipemia and icterus. The instrument performs an internal cross-check of these two measures and flags any discrepancy. Histograms of both RBC volume and the Hb concentration distribution are generated. The dispersion of each distribution curve is reported as RDW and HDW, respectively. Further computer analysis of this information provides morphology flags for microcytosis, macrocytosis, anisocytosis, hypochromia, hyperchromia, and anisochromia. Figure 43-11 is an example of an abnormal patient sample and shows the independent variation of the RBC volume and concentration and the morphology reports.

The peroxidase cytochemistry test is similar to that in the H6000, with a shortened reaction time and more sophisticated analysis.[18] The computer establishes floating thresholds that fit around the population clusters, identifying the cell types. The thresholds differ for each individual sample. Total leukocyte, neutrophil, lymphocyte, monocyte, and eosinophil counts are determined in this channel.

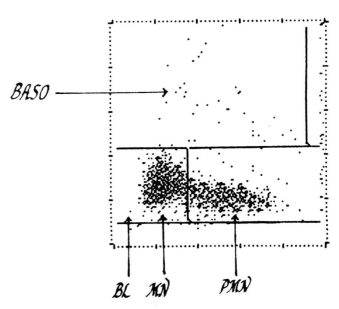

FIG. 43-12. Basophil/lobularity cytogram. This cytogram generated by H·1 shows detection of cell types using laser optics with differential light scatter. Locations of blasts (BL), mononuclear cells (MN), and combination of neutrophils and eosinophils (PMN) are identified. (Copyright 1986 by the Technicon Instruments Corporation; reproduced with permission.)

In the new basophil channel, the WBCs are selectively stripped of their cytoplasm, leaving the nuclei intact. Only the basophils are resistant to the lysing agent. Using the RBC laser optics with the two-angle light scatter to analyze the effluent, leukocyte subpopulations can be identified on the basis of the scatter information from the nuclei.[19] In the basophil/lobularity cytogram (Fig. 43-12) the polymorphonuclear cells (neutrophils and eosinophils) fall to the right on the X axis and the mononuclear cells (lymphocytes and monocytes) to the left. Blasts fall to the far left. This information, in conjunction with that obtained in the peroxidase channel, greatly expands the information available concerning leukocytes. Special indicators include such data as blasts, left shift, and atypical lymphocytes. A total WBC count is performed in this channel as well as in the peroxidase channel, providing an internal cross-check. Discrepancies are flagged for review, and when necessary, the WBC count from the basophil channel is reported. For example, platelets are completely lysed in the basophil channel, so the WBC count from this channel is unaffected by platelet clumps or giant platelets, which would alter the WBC count from the peroxidase channel.

The system has a less than 5-minute menu-driven startup. It can process 60 samples per hour in the CBC plus differential mode. There is a data storage buffer for results from 200 patient samples. Also included is a QC package similar to those on other instruments.

Additionally, the peroxidase cytometer can be used for an immunoperoxidase method of lymphocyte subset analysis which is of interest in certain laboratories. This feature allows the laboratory to extend its testing capability to lymphocyte T- and B-cell analysis without investing in a second flow cytometer.

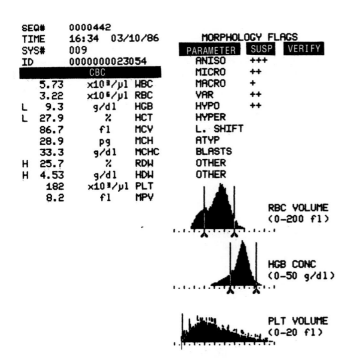

FIG. 43-11. Technicon H·1. Data display demonstrating independent measurements of RBC volume and Hb concentration. Morphology flags are generated by computer analysis of numeric and histogram data. (Copyright 1986 by the Technicon Instruments Corporation; reproduced with permission.)

GENERAL CONSIDERATIONS

Interferences and Limitations

Each system or methodology has its own unique set of limitations. Although a laboratory with instruments based on differing methodologies has problems of reconciling calibration, there are interesting possibilities for cross-checks on abnormal values.

Unusual samples may cause erroneous results. The operator must be familiar with the instrument operation and recognize those factors leading to error to prevent incorrect results from being reported. Table 43-2 summarizes the interferences or limitations of the principal systems.

Instrument Selection

The last 10 years have seen a proliferation of instruments on the market, which may be overwhelming to the prospective buyer. How does one sort through this plethora? First, outline the priorities. Consider the patient mix the laboratory will deal with and the need for screening versus diagnosis. For example, a large oncology service may require an instrument that can identify abnormal cells within low WBC counts, not merely flag these for the less precise and tedious microscopic counts. Second, the throughput requirements will differ depending on the percentage of emergencies (STATs) and on whether analysis is performed in batches. A throughput of 90 samples an hour will not be important if only 200 samples are analyzed a day. Third, evaluate the values to be measured. Some of the more esoteric, such as the MPV, may have little relevance to the particular laboratory. Weigh the optional functions: are computer interface capabilities needed? Consider the technical skills needed to operate the instrument and interpret the results. Communicate directly with users of a system. A careful review of the professional literature can provide valuable information about instrumentation currently on the market, as well as studies or reviews of new products. Finally, be wary of salespeople who downgrade a competitor rather than sell their system on its own merits. Care-

ful selection will save money and reduce headaches in the long run.

Calibration

There are a few instances with all systems when performance of calibration procedures is imperative. Initial installation of the instruments will require calibration. Adjustments to optical alignment and replacement of lamps, apertures, critical length tubing, or other parts that directly affect calibration may necessitate recalibration. However, because of the imperfection of calibration methods in hematology, a general rule for an instrument is the less calibration performed, the better. The final calibration achieved is not going to be any better than the reference method used. If the reference instrument has not been maintained and properly controlled, the instrument being calibrated will be off correspondingly. Widespread use of commercial products such as S Cal introduce a bias[16]; however, that may be tolerable if a reference instrument is lacking. Methods of calibration will be discussed in detail in Chapters 46 and 47.

Film Review Criteria

The goal in setting blood film review criteria for an instrument is to ensure the accuracy of the patient result while fully utilizing the potential of automation. This requires a hard look at the strengths and limitations of the instrument and the imprecision of the microscopic method. For instance, most of the more sophisticated instruments count several thousand cells for a WBC count and differential. Thus, no purpose would be served in trying to recheck the precise numbers generated solely on the basis of a count outside normal limits. Normal samples can be screened out, and the technologist's time can be spent more productively in examining blood films that require an experienced morphologist's interpretations of abnormalities. Scrutinize all data: values, histograms, cytograms, and instrument function flags. Flagging limits on specific parameter data in

(text continues on page 511)

TABLE 43–2. Interferents Causing Error in Automated Systems

EXAMPLES	IMPEDANCE COUNTERS		LASER LIGHT SCATTER		CYTOCHEMICAL AND LIGHT SCATTER	
Microcytes, schistocytes	PLT	↑	PLT	↑	PLT	↑
	RBC	↓	RBC	↓	RBC	↓
	MCHC	↑	MCHC	↑	MCHC	↑
Platelet clumps, giant platelets	PLT	↓	PLT	↓	PLT	↓
	WBC	↑	WBC	↑	WBC–Perox	↑
					WBC–Baso unaffected	
Platelet satellitism	PLT	↓	PLT	↓	PLT	↓
Agglutinated RBCs	RBC	↓	RBC	↓	RBC	↓
	MCV	↑	MCV	↑	MCV	↑
	MCH	↑	MCH	↑	MCH	↑
	MCHC	↑	MCHC	↑	MCHC	↑
Increased or abnormal plasma proteins	WBC	↑	WBC ↑ ↓ (PLT ↑)		WBC	↑
Lysis resistant RBCs			WBC ↑ (ELT-15)		WBC	↑
Lipemia	Hb	↑			Hb	↑
	MCHC	↑			MCHC	↑
					CHCM unaffected	
NRBCs	WBC	↑	WBC ↑ (ELT-8)		WBC	↑
WBC ↑ ↑ ↑ (leukemia)	Hb	↑			Hb	↑

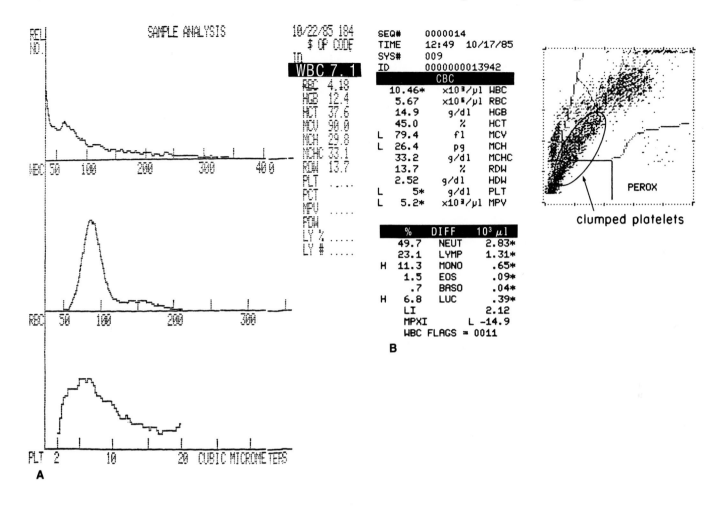

B

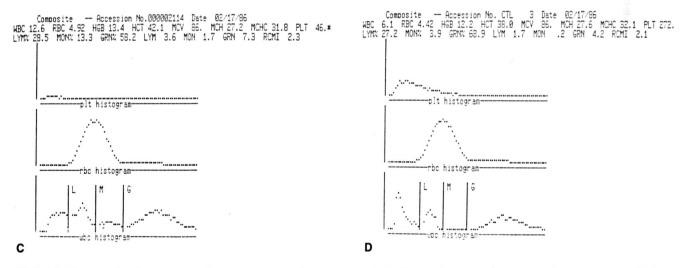

FIG. 43-13.   Platelet clumping interference apparent in histograms. (*A*) Coulter S-Plus: WBC histogram, showing increased debris at 50 on X axis; clumped platelets falsely elevating total WBC count and causing vote-out of platelet and differential measures. Platelet histogram shows tailing up at 20 on X axis. (*B*) Technicon H·1: clumped platelets on peroxidase cytogram (arrow) causing characteristic pattern and falsely elevating WBC count. White count measurement in basophil channel is unaffected by platelet clumping and can be used to replace peroxidase channel WBC (affected) count. (*C*) Ortho ELT-15: Interference at debris : lymphocyte threshold (L). Pattern should return to baseline but is high above baseline here. Nearly flat platelet (PLT) Histogram with very low PLT count. Film estimation of PLT count = 300 × 10^3/L and of WBC count = 6.8 × 10^3/L. (*D*) Ortho ELT-15: new sample from same patient as in *C* with sodium citrate as anticoagulant. No platelet clumping in this sample; counts now match file estimates.

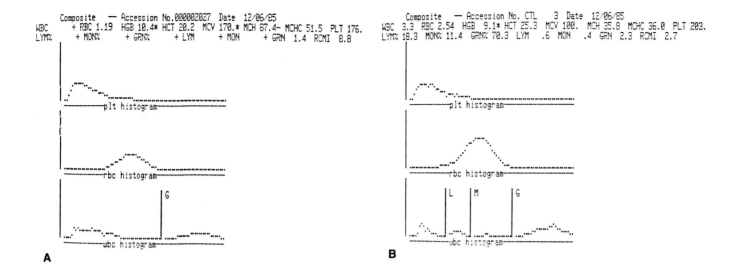

Composite   — Accession No.000002027 Date 12/06/85
WBC   + RBC 1.19 HGB 10.4* HCT 20.2 MCV 170.* MCH 87.4- MCHC 51.5 PLT 176.
LYM%   + MON%   + GRN%   + LYM   + MON   + GRN 1.4 RCMI 8.8

plt histogram

rbc histogram

G

wbc histogram

A

Composite   — Accession No. CTL   3 Date 12/06/85
WBC 3.3 RBC 2.54 HGB 9.1* HCT 25.3 MCV 100. MCH 35.8 MCHC 36.0 PLT 203.
LYM% 18.3 MON% 11.4 GRN% 70.3 LYM .6 MON .4 GRN 2.3 RCMI 2.7

plt histogram

rbc histogram

L   M   G

wbc histogram

B

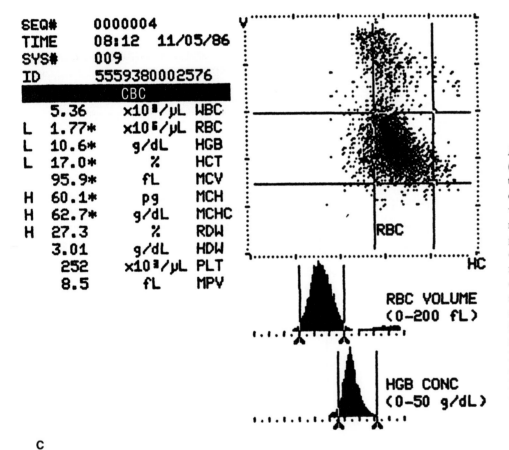

SEQ#   0000004
TIME   08:12   11/05/86
SYS#   009
ID   5559380002576

	CBC		
	5.36	×10³/µL	WBC
L	1.77*	×10⁶/µL	RBC
L	10.6*	g/dL	HGB
L	17.0*	%	HCT
	95.9*	fL	MCV
H	60.1*	pg	MCH
H	62.7*	g/dL	MCHC
H	27.3	%	RDW
	3.01	g/dL	HDW
	252	×10³/µL	PLT
	8.5	fL	MPV

RBC

HC

RBC VOLUME
(0–200 fL)

HGB CONC
(0–50 g/dL)

C

FIG. 43-14. Cold agglutination. (*A*) Sample tested on ELT 15 at room temperature indicates low RBC count, low HCT that does not agree with Hb value, very high MCV, abnormal indices, and low RBC histogram with abnormal RCMI; WBC count flagged with plus (+), because no threshold was placed between debris and lymphocytes. (*B*) Same sample after warming; RBC count and HCT increased, MCV lower, indices normal, total WBC count and three-part differential given, and RCMI near normal. (*C*) H·1 and cold agglutination; agglutinated RBCs form second population on far right of volume histogram. Same population falls above normal population in cytogram display of volume *v* Hb concentration.

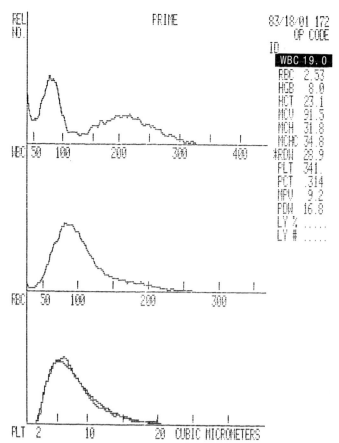

FIG. 43-15. Nucleated red blood cells interfering with WBC count in Coulter S-Plus. White cell histogram shows interference at 50 on X axis, which is where debris and white cells are separated. Total white cell count must be corrected for presence of nucleated red cells.

combination with instrument limits and histogram and cytogram pattern flags allow for detection of samples that may have significant morphologic findings. Once identified, an abnormality can be reviewed periodically. If a significant morphologic change is identified during a film review, a manual differential count may be performed and added to the final laboratory report. Each laboratory must establish its own rules and limits to be used in the flagging system that prompts blood film review and, at times, the addition of a manual differential.

To a greater extent, with each generation of instruments the laboratory scientist is required to be more expert in interpretation of computer-analyzed electronic data. Once it is accepted that this information is a valuable adjunct to the blood film, the information made available to the clinician is greatly expanded.

UTILIZATION OF COMPUTER DATA: HISTOGRAMS AND CYTOGRAMS

Histogram analysis provides valuable information. Normal histogram pattern examples for Coulter, Ortho, and Technicon are shown in Figure 43-8; refer to these normal pat-

terns to help in recognizing the abnormal pattern examples that are discussed in this section.

Abnormal histogram patterns suggest anomalous cell distributions. Problems with the sample or the instrument may be suggested by histogram patterns. Careful blood film examination of samples with abnormal histogram patterns may explain the abnormal pattern. For example, platelet clumping in EDTA usually produces a very low platelet count, a distinctive WBC histogram pattern with increased debris, and a falsely elevated WBC count (Fig. 43-13). Giant platelets may also affect histogram patterns and counts. Another sample problem reflected in histogram patterns is RBC cold agglutination (Fig. 43-14). Also, increased abnormal plasma proteins may precipitate with lysing reagent and produce abnormal WBC histograms (increased debris) and give invalid white cell counts. Nucleated RBCs (Fig. 43-15) and red cell fragments (Fig. 43-16) may produce invalid counts and recognizable histogram patterns affecting the WBC and platelet counts, respectively. Red blood cells that resist lysis, such as sickle cells, can produce falsely elevated WBC counts and falsely increase the number of lymphocytes (Fig. 43-17). Specific unusual histogram patterns that occur repeatedly on sequential patient samples strongly suggest an instrument problem that needs to be identified and fixed. Thus, information provided by histogram patterns can be used as a QC tool in the identification of sample or instrument problems. White cell histograms and cytograms provide the information to produce three-part WBC differential screens and the traditional five-parameter differentials as well. Figures 43-13 through 43-17 are examples of the data interpretation required of laboratory scientists operating complex multiparameter hematology instruments.

CHAPTER SUMMARY

Continued improvements in precision and speed and addition of new measures have come about with advances in computer programming and analysis. Built-in quality control programs, such as the Bull moving average program (Chap. 47), have greatly enhanced QC monitoring and reduced manual documentation.

With the development of laser technology and advances in fluidic processes such as hydrodynamic focusing and laminar flow management came the ability to count platelets accurately and precisely at extremely low concentrations ($1.0 \times 10^9/L$). Continuing advances have provided more information about cell maturity and RBC morphology. The most popular instruments now provide visual as well as numeric information about each sample. Histogram and cytogram patterns can be valuable when an experienced eye analyzes them for suggestions of cellular abnormality or sample or instrument problems. Instrumentation has gone beyond the point where an operator simply processes samples with the touch of a button. A sound background in instrument theory and clinical hematology is necessary to analyze and interpret the numeric and graphic data provided by these sophisticated instruments.

Screening blood samples rapidly for suggestions of clinically significant morphologic and numeric abnormalities is possible with these multiparameter instruments. The newest screening instrument, which is based on centrifugation of whole blood, does not actually count cells, yet is small, inexpensive, rapid, and quite useful in settings such as physician offices or outpatient clinics. When choosing a new instrument for a hematol-

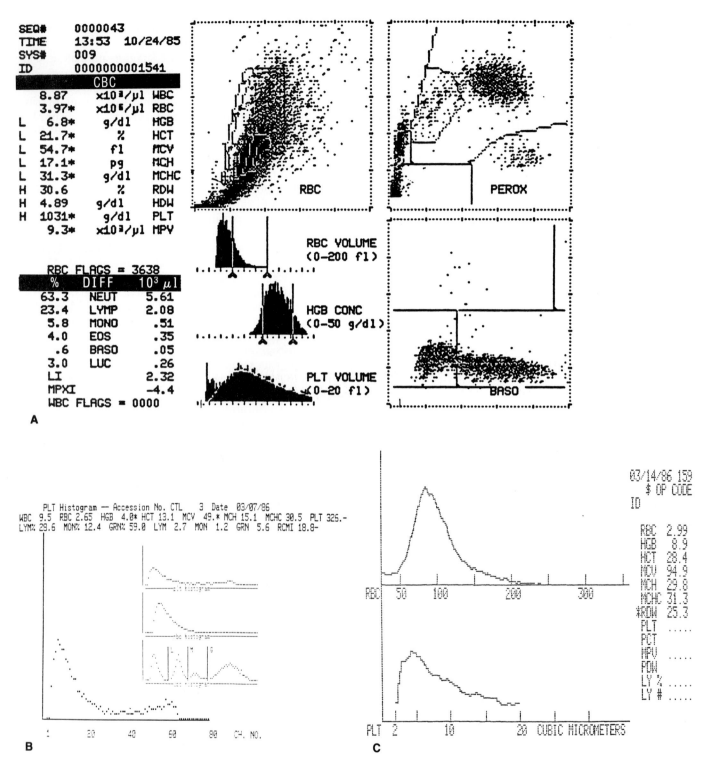

FIG. 43-16. Platelet interference caused by red cell fragments (schistocytes). (*A*) Technicon H·1: low MCV with schistocytes on blood film examination. Schistocytes falsely increase platelet count and reduce red cell count; RBC indices calculated from red cell count are also affected. All of these measures are flagged. Alternate methods are necessary to determine correct (reportable) count. (*B*) Ortho ELT15: single platelet histogram (and composite insert); platelet histogram shows far-right upward tail (arrow) with instrument alert (minus sign by platelet count) of 20% platelet interference. Red cell histogram (composite insert) is shifted far left with MCV of 49 fL. Blood film reveals schistocytes, platelet estimate of 200×10^9/L. Reported platelet count was 220×10^9/L (phase). (*C*) Coulter S-Plus: platelet count omitted ("no fit"). Red cell histogram has far-left activity, and blood film examination confirms presence of schistocytes. Alternate method count for platelets is necessary.

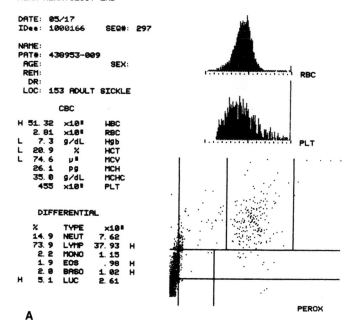

NCMH HEMATOLOGY LAB

DATE: 05/17
IDoo: 1000166   SEQ#: 297

NAME:
PAT#: 438953-009
 AGE: SEX:
 REM:
 DR:
 LOC: 153 ADULT SICKLE

CBC

H 51.32	x10³	WBC
2.81	x10⁶	RBC
L 7.3	g/dL	Hgb
L 20.9	%	HCT
L 74.6	µ³	MCV
26.1	pg	MCH
35.8	g/dL	MCHC
455	x10³	PLT

DIFFERENTIAL

%	TYPE	x10³	
14.9	NEUT	7.62	
73.9	LYMP	37.93	H
2.2	MONO	1.15	
1.9	EOS	.98	H
2.0	BASO	1.02	H
H 5.1	LUC	2.61	

A

Composite -- Accession No.000002016 Date 10/10/86
WBC 40.9* RBC 2.00 HGB 6.6* HCT 18.7 MCV 94. MCH 33.0 MCHC 35.3 PLT 230.
LYM%   + MON%   + GRN%   + LYM   + MON   + GRN   + RCMI 6.7

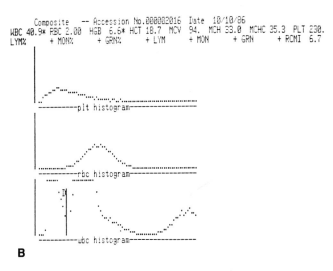

B

Composite -- Accession No. CTL   3 Date 10/10/86
WBC 6.5 RBC .87 HGB 3.3* HCT 8.3 MCV 95. MCH 37.9 MCHC 39.8 PLT 263.
LYM% 33.9 MON% 13.8 GRN% 52.3 LYM 2.2 MON .9 GRN 3.4 RCMI 6.9

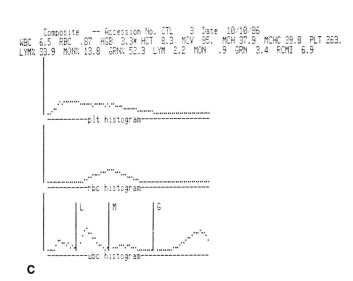

C

FIG. 43-17.   Lysis-resistant RBCs. (*A*) Technicon H6000: sickled RBCs resist lysis in WBC (peroxidase) channel, falsely elevating total WBC and lymphocyte counts. Usually clean separation between debris and lymphocytes is filled in by unlysed red cells; this picture indicates need for WBC count evaluation. (*B*) Ortho ELT-15: incomplete lysis of sickled red cells results in falsely elevated WBC count and, in this case, no three-part differential. Histogram pattern of WBCs suggests interference, because valley between debris and lymphocytes does not return to baseline. (*C*) Ortho ELT-15: sample prediluted with ammonium oxalate, which promotes red cell lysis and return of debris–lymphocyte valley to baseline. Compare dilution-corrected Hb value with original value to check dilution technique, then correct WBC count and absolute differential counts for final report. Do not apply dilution factor to WBC differential percentages.

ogy laboratory, ask what information is needed in this setting? Do not buy an instrument with additional features or information that will not be used by the purchasing laboratory. Unused features are expensive, and the medical community and government regulations leave little room for extravagance.

REFERENCES

1. Bentley SA, Pegram MD, Ross DW: Diagnosis of infective and inflammatory disorders by flow cytometric analysis of blood neutrophils. Am J Clin Pathol 88:177, 1987
2. Bessman JD: New parameters on automated hematology instruments. Lab Med 14:488, 1983
3. Bessman JD, Gilmer PR, Gardner FH: Improved classification of anemias by MCV and RDW. Am J Clin Pathol 80:322, 1983
4. College of American Pathologists: Comprehensive Hematology Survey: Limited Coagulation Module. Participant Summary, Set H-1A. Skokie, IL, CAP, 1977
5. College of American Pathologists: Comprehensive Hematology Survey; Limited Coagulation Module. Participant Summary, Set H-1A. Skokie, IL, CAP, 1986
6. College of American Pathologists: Comprehensive Hematology Survey; Limited Coagulation Module. Participant Summary, Set H-1C. Skokie, IL, CAP, 1986
7. Coulter Electronics, Inc: Coulter Counter Model S-Plus IV Operator's Manual, PN 4235360. Hialeah, FL, September 1983
8. Hoffman RA: Red Cell Morphology Index. Orthority, Ortho Diagnostic Systems Inc (410 University Ave, Westwood, MA 02090), October 1985
9. Jovin TM, Morris ST, Striker G et al: Automated sizing and separation of light scattering intensities. J Histochem Cytochem 24:269, 1976

10. Kachel V, Menke E: Hydrodynamic properties of flow cytometric instruments. In Melamed MR, Mullaney PF, Mendelsohn ML (eds): Flow Cytometry and Sorting, p 41. New York, Wiley Medical, 1979

11. Kim YR, Ornstein L: Isovolumetric sphering of erythrocytes for more accurate and precise cell volume measurement by flow cytochemistry. Cytometry 3:419, 1983

12. Mohandas N, Kim YR, Tyeko DH et al: Accurate and independent measurement of volume and hemoglobin concentration of individual red cells by laser light. Blood 68:506, 1986

13. Ortho Diagnostic Systems Inc: Ortho ELT 15 Advanced Hematology Analyzer with Screening Differential: Operator Reference Manual. Clinical and Research Laboratory Instrument Systems (410 University Ave, Westwood, MA 02090), December 1985

14. Ross DW, Bardwell A: Automated cytochemistry and the white cell differential in leukemia. Blood Cells 6:455, 1980

15. Salzman GC, Mullaney PF, Price BJ: Light scattering approaches to cell characterization. In Melamed MR, Mullaney PF, Mendelsohn ML (eds): Flow Cytometry and Sorting, p 106. New York, Wiley Medical, 1979

16. Savage RA: Calibration bias and imprecision for automated hematology analyzers. Am J Clin Pathol 84:186, 1985

17. Technicon Instruments Corp: Technicon H6000 System Product Labeling. Technicon Publications No. UA81-443-00. Tarrytown, NY, May 1981

18. Technicon Instruments Corp: Technicon H·1 System Operator's Guide. Technicon Publications No. TA8-5588-10. Tarrytown, NY, October 1985

19. Technicon Instruments Corp: Proceedings of the Technicon H·1 Hematology Symposium. Tarrytown, NY, October 1985

20. TOA Medical Electronics Co., Ltd: Sysmex Operator's Manual Model E-5000, Code No 461-2104-2. Kobe, Japan, April 1985

21. Tycko DH, Metz MH, Epstein EA, Grinbaum A: Flow-cytometric light scattering measurements of red blood cell volume and hemoglobin concentration. Appl Optics 24:1355, 1985

22. Van Dilla MA, Mendelsohn ML: Introduction and resume of flow cytometry and sorting. In Melamed MR, Mullaney PF, Mendelsohn ML (eds): Flow Cytometry and Sorting, p 14. New York, Wiley Medical, 1979

23. Wardlaw SC, Levine RA: Quantitative buffy coat analysis. JAMA 249:617, 1983

24. Williams JE, Trinklein FE, Metcalfe HC (eds): The nature of light: Waves and particles. In Modern Physics, p 279. New York, Holt, Rinehart and Winston, 1979

25. Williams JE, Trinklein FE, Metcalfe HC (eds): Reflection. In Modern Physics, p 313. New York, Holt, Rinehart and Winston, 1979

26. Williams JE, Trinklein FE, Metcalfe HC (eds): Refraction. In Modern Physics, p 329. New York, Holt, Rinehart and Winston, 1979

27. Williams JE, Trinklein FE, Metcalfe HC (eds): Diffraction and polarization: Interference and diffraction. In Modern Physics, p 357. New York, Holt, Rinehart and Winston, 1979

44

Instruments

for Automation

of the

Differential

Barbara A. Payne

Over the years the microscopic examination of leukocytes, erythrocytes, and platelets on a blood film, better known as the manual differential count, has been recognized as the foundation for diagnosis of hematologic abnormalities. However, the manual study has the reputation of being expensive and tedious, requiring a highly skilled technologist and having a relatively high inherent error rate.[2,3] Its high variability is an outgrowth of preparation techniques, sample size, and operator subjectivity.[20,23] Not until companion technologies of integrated circuits, computers, artificial intelligence, cytochemical techniques, flowthrough systems, and computer-assisted image analysis were developed could automated differential systems be realized.[2,20] A fortunate byproduct of the automation of the differential count has been the standardization of blood film processing, as well as more nationally recognized definitions of standard cell types.

AUTOMATED DIFFERENTIALS

In the early 1970s, two different techniques for automating differentials were refined sufficiently to be acceptable for clinical laboratory use.[2,20] One approach was computer-assisted image analysis, the pattern recognition system. This technique consists of detecting cell images electronically and then interpreting them with a computer programmed with descriptions. The other approach was a flowthrough system based on light scatter and cytochemical staining for the identification of leukocytes. Recent years have seen the addition of lasers, differential lysing agents, discrete sampling, and cellular histogram analysis. These additions and modifications have improved the separation of normal and abnormal cells in suspension while using less costly reagents and smaller samples. These newer flowthrough systems are included in several instrument packages and will be described later in this chapter.

Pattern Recognition

Pattern recognition instruments are no longer available on the market; however, numerous such instruments are still in use in laboratories across the country and therefore will be described here. The pattern recognition instruments are most closely related to the manual method for performing differentials. The sample is a stained blood film and the instrument has an adjustable sample size setting from 100 to 500 leukocytes. Classification is based on color, size, density of nucleus, nuclear:cytoplasmic ratio, cytoplasm color, and granules.

Automated blood cell classification instruments based on the pattern recognition principle have included the LARC (leukocyte automatic recognition computer), manufactured by Corning Medical and Scientific Company; Hematrak (Geometric Data Corporation); Coulter Diff 3 (Diff 350 and Diff 4), produced by Coulter Electronics; and the ADC-500 (Abbott Laboratories).[2,20] The Hematrak system will be described as representative of the group.

The Hematrak is capable of automatically providing normal and some abnormal leukocyte classifications, numerical platelet estimates, and graded erythrocyte morphologic abnormalities (based on user-defined percentages). An optional program provides a reticulocyte count from a properly prepared slide. The Hematrak is based on the use of a "flying spot scanner" to generate a stream of light directed through a stained blood film. Three primary color filters are used to sort the light beam from the image. Three photomultiplier tubes (PMT) collect the filtered light beams and convert the light into electrical energy to be digitized into a cell image. This digitized image is passed on to an image memory. A morphologic analyzer measures the cell mathematically, looking first at the nuclear morphology (mononuclear versus segmented), the nuclear:cytoplasmic ratio, and the chromatin pattern (for textural openness as recognition of nucleoli). Finally, the cytoplasm is analyzed for color, granularity, and vacuoles. All of these data are passed to the recognition computer, where they are compared with a reference memory. The cell type is identified by a process of matching. Cells are tallied and displayed on the monitor at the conclusion of the differential (Fig. 44-1).[16,22]

This system classifies leukocytes into six normal and six abnormal categories. Morphology comments of slight, moderate, and marked are used in describing RBC size, shape, and color. Also displayed is the Price-Jones curve with the red cell mean and standard deviation. Suspected target or spherocytic RBCs are flagged for review. The user determines the numbers of RBCs and WBCs to be counted and the type of smear to use (wedge versus spinner). Additional features are storage and display of neutrophil and lymphocyte profiles, a quality control (QC) program with Levey-Jennings plots, a self-checking electronic system, and the ability of the user to examine microscopically specific cell types that have been flagged by the instrument as abnormal. The maximum data storage is 200 counts before operator review is necessary.[10] One new direction for this instrument has been its use in classifying T and B lymphocytes using an immunogold procedure.

Pattern recognition systems eliminate the subjective error inherent in the manual method while not becoming "tired"; however, they retain the sampling error inherent in the manual differential. Their processes imitate the manual method, making them more familiar to the laboratorian.

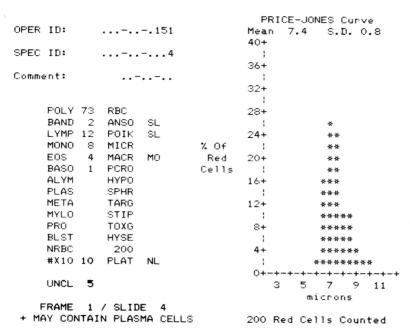

FIG. 44-1.   Example of result display of Geometric Data Hematrak 590 system. A 100-cell leukocyte differential and 200-red cell evaluation have been performed. Red cell abnormalities appear as comments, and Price-Jones curve has been plotted. Leukocytes are within reference values.

Cytochemical Flowthrough

In 1975 the Hemalog D was introduced by Technicon Instruments. This system was able to perform a seven-part leukocyte differential and leukocyte count using volume determination based on light scatter and light absorbency of stained cells. Granulocytes and eosinophils were stained for peroxidase, monocytes for lipase/esterase, and basophils for heparin (by alcian blue).[14,20] Small cells that did not take up stain were categorized as lymphocytes, whereas large cells that did not take up stain were called "large unstained cells" (LUC) and might include reactive lymphocytes as well as blast forms.

Since that time, three more generations of instruments have been introduced. The H-6000 eliminated the lipase channel for monocytes and incorporated two stain channels: alkaline peroxidase for differentiation of lymphocytes, neutrophils, eosinophils, and monocytes and toluidine blue for basophils. Cells flowed through a 250-μm aperture in a sheath flow system and were counted and differentiated for approximately 16 seconds, resulting in counts of between 5000 and 15,000 cells, depending on the total number present.[11,17,20] In addition the machine produced an automated blood smear preparation (autoslide). Both percentages and absolute numbers were reported (Fig. 44-2).

The instrument did not provide quantitative counts of immature neutrophils such as band forms or juvenile forms but had been found to be superior to manual counts in quantifying minority populations such as eosinophils and basophils.[26] It also was capable of detecting neutrophil populations having partial or complete myeloperoxidase deficiency, an inherited disorder that is more common than previously thought. The autoslide automatically made, stained, labeled, and permanently fixed a wedge smear to a glass slide while the CBC was performed on a separate portion of the blood.[20] The autoslide provided a blood film for review whenever a specimen was flagged as abnormal.

Because of its sample volume requirements (2 mL minimum) and its dwell time (9.5 minutes), this system was not practical in a laboratory where there was a need to process microsamples or emergency samples.[11,25] A second drawback was reagent cost because the instrument took the same amount of reagents to process 1 sample or 15 samples. One benefit was that a cytochemical differential could be performed on whole blood as late as 30 hours after specimen collection when the specimen was stored at room temperature.

The third-generation developed by Technicon was the H·1. The peroxidase reaction time was shortened from 10 minutes to 33 seconds by increasing the temperature to 65°C. The thresholds were floating rather than fixed, and the computer used cluster analysis algorithms to fit thresholds around the cell population based on the individual characteristics of each patient sample.[26] The H-1 uses two sources of light: a helium laser, which is used for counting RBCs and platelets and for detecting nuclear lobularity (see below), and a tungsten lamp, which is used in the counting of leukocytes and for differentiating the granulocyte population in the alkaline peroxidase channel.

The basophil channel not only detects basophils but also examines cells for the complexity of their nuclear shape (lobularity). This is done by stripping the cytoplasm from all cells except basophils using an acid with a buffer that enhances the natural resistance of the basophils. Basophils thus are much larger than the other particles remaining (the nuclei of other leukocytes) and can be detected as those cells above a set scatter threshold. The use of a laser light source with scatter detection at two angles separates the nuclei of the remainder of the leukocytes according to their degree of lobulation. Segmented neutrophils, which have a large

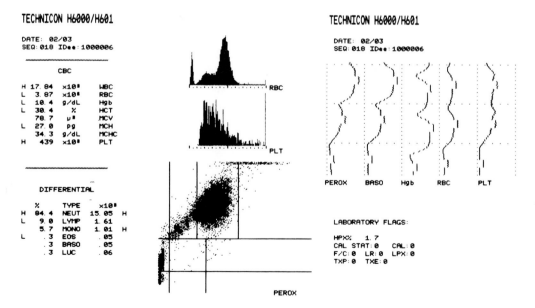

FIG. 44-2. Technicon H-6000 result display showing numerical results with high (H)/low (L) flags (left column); distribution graphs for leukocyte peroxidase (perox), red blood cells (RBC), and platelets (PLT) (center column); phasing of each channel, including basophil (BASO), hemoglobin (Hgb); etc., and additional instrument function flags (right column).

amount of high-angle scatter, fall to the right on the X axis, and mononuclear cells fall to the left. When neutrophils are less mature (band and juvenile forms), their scatter signature is different, and the cells move to the left on the X axis. Blasts give an even lower amount of high-angle forward scatter based on their chromatin texture and are separated from the mononuclear cells at the extreme left of the X axis. The instrument keeps track of the ratio of highly lobulated nuclei to nonlobulated nuclei and reports a lobularity index (LI). Theoretically, as the ratio approaches 1, the proportion of less mature neutrophils increases; however, the reliability of the LI as an indication of increased neutrophilic immaturity must be further evaluated.

The presence of this basophil/lobularity channel allows a considerable number of internal checks. For example, the number of neutrophils detected according to lobularity is compared with the same cell count in the peroxidase channel. If there is a discrepancy between the two counts that exceeds preset tolerance limits, a flag appears. Such discrepancies can occur in the presence of clumped platelets and nucleated or lysis-resistant RBCs.[31] In addition, the number of blasts detected according to nuclear shape is compared with the LUC in the peroxidase channel, and a flag appears if the presence of blasts is likely.

The H·1 operates in a discrete mode; therefore, reagents are consumed only when the test is performed. It uses a 100-μL sample and produces 60 tests per hour, with the dwell time being less than 1 minute and sample stability being 24 hours.[26] The data printout includes a six-part differential in both percent and absolute values, the LI, and population cytograms for the different channels (Fig. 44-3).

The abnormal flagging systems consist of high and low limits determined by the user and an internal four-digit leukocyte flag. Other options available are a closed tube feeder (for single-tube stopper piercing), a cathode ray tube (CRT) screen printer, and a lymphocyte subset analysis package.[26]

With experience in interpreting the cytograms generated by this instrument, the operator can detect a large number of abnormalities that may require further investigation using stained blood films. For example, distinctive cytogram patterns are produced in the presence of clumped platelets, as well as in certain disease states such as chronic lymphocytic leukemia. In some cases, the presence of reactive lymphocytes can be deduced by careful interpretation of the cytograms. A further advantage of this system is the identification of leukocytes by means of enzymes that reflect their functional activity; size and Romanowsky staining characteristics do not indicate whether the cell is functionally normal.

The fourth-generation Technicon instrument is the H·2. This newest instrument has almost doubled the number of tests per hour (100+), has an autosampler, and provides positive patient identification.

SCREENING DIFFERENTIAL SYSTEMS

The concept of a screening differential was first realized in the early 1980s. With pressures for increased efficiencies (*e.g.*, the DRG system of standard payments for disease-related groups), there was a need for the laboratory to

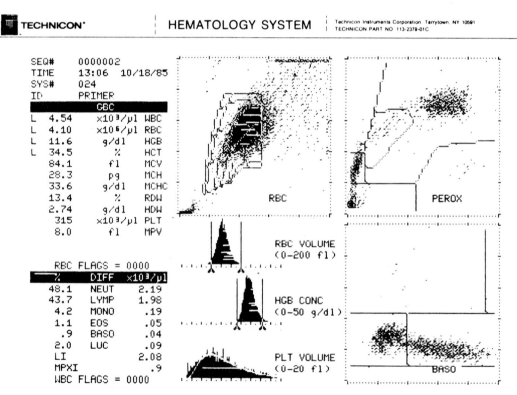

FIG. 44-3. Result display on CRT from H·1 system with peroxidase scattergram and added scattergram for basophils (top section of square labeled BASO), red blood cells, Hb concentration (HGB CONC), and lobularity index (LI) (bottom section of square labeled BASO).

become cost effective. One way to meet this demand was to use new technology to modify multiparameter instruments already on the market. Changes were made in reagent systems, electronic measurements, and internal flagging systems to allow the measurement and display of new features.

The goal of the screening differential was to have an effective means, at no additional cost in time or reagents, to identify samples that have a high probability of being abnormal. These samples would then be given additional attention, which might include a manual differential, a blood film evaluation, or both.

Screening differentials consist of a two- or three-part differential that separates leukocytes into large versus small cells or lymphocytes versus granulocytes versus mononuclear cells or monocytes. Screening differential systems sense particles in two different ways: laser scatter or impedance-resistance methods.

Laser Types

The Ortho Diagnostic Systems for determining erythrocytes, leukocytes, and thrombocytes (ELT) are based on hydrodynamic focusing and laser scatter technology. Those instruments that can perform an automated screening differential contain a photodetector placed at a 90° angle from the laser source. In addition, the lysing reagent was altered so that RBCs are lysed, but leukocytes are not altered. The internal complexity of each leukocyte (nucleus and cytoplasmic characteristics such as granularity) determines the amount of light scattered at a 90° angle. The forward-scatter signals (i.e., cell size) and the right-angle scatter signals (i.e., internal complexity) are plotted in cytogram form, and the data from these clusters of cells (lymphocytes, monocytes, and granulocytes) are mathematically transformed into a histogram.

Peak (cell population), valley (separation between cell populations), and overlap analysis are performed to determine placement of thresholds for cell type separation. Thresholds are not placed if analysis is not acceptable. When lymphocyte-monocyte separation is not acceptable according to internally preset tolerances, a debris threshold and a granulocyte threshold are placed so that total leukocyte and granulocyte counts are reported. A plus (+) sign appears on the report form when a count cannot be determined. Otherwise, leukocyte, lymphocyte, monocyte, and granulocyte absolute counts are made, and the percentages for each are calculated.[13,16,17,27,30] A typical display is seen in Figure 44-4.

The system was not designed to identify immature cells or other abnormal features of morphology such as toxic granulation and RBC inclusions. The presence of increased numbers of immature granulocytes, eosinophils, or variant lymphocytes is not recognized, because there are only three categories in which to place the differentiated leukocytes. Blast forms generally are categorized with lymphocytes as well as between lymphocytes and monocytes, which may increase the interference at the lymphocyte-monocyte interface (threshold). Increased numbers of eosinophils may blend in with granulocytes or fall between monocytes and granulocytes, thereby increasing the interference at that interface. Increased numbers of immature granulocytes (bands, metamyelocytes, myelocytes) generally fall with the granulocytes and may interfere at the monocyte-granulocyte interface. Other interferences include lysis-resistant RBCs (e.g., sickled red cells), which increase total lymphocyte counts, and clumped platelets, which likewise increase total lymphocyte counts. An extensive built-in flagging system that places a combination of limits on various results and histogram patterns such as the threshold interferences described above indicates which samples are normal and which need further evaluation using a stained blood film. All flags (user or manufacturer set) result in a printed warning and an audible alarm.[13,16,27]

The main disadvantage of this system is the lack of de-

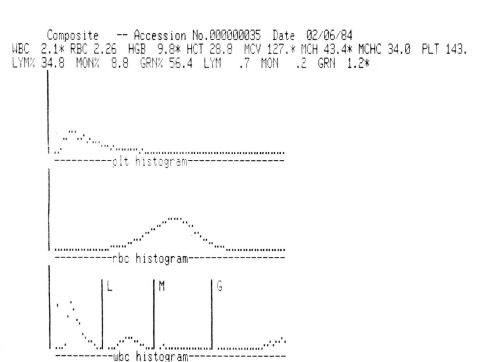

FIG. 44-4.   Example of Ortho ELT series histograms and numerical results plot. Note left-to-right display of results and absence of units on X/Y axis of histograms.

fined particle size on the X axis of the generated histogram causing difficulty in visual evaluation of the histogram for shifts in cell population volumes.

Impedance Types

The Coulter Counter S-Plus series (Models IV through VI) provide (in addition to the routine 10-parameter profiles) percentage and absolute values of lymphocytes, mononuclear cells, and granulocytes, as well as leukocyte, erythrocyte, and platelet histograms (Fig. 44-5A). Leukocytes are sized electronically after they have had their cytoplasm and nucleus differentially shrunk by a special lysing agent and reagent system.[4] The cells are then categorized into lymphocytes (small cells), mononuclear cells (medium cells), and granulocytes (large cells).

A relative-size histogram is constructed and smoothed, and mathematical equations are applied to it looking at peaks and valleys. Internal flags such as region (R) codes (see Fig. 44-5B), backlighting of values, or instrument data rejection (dotting out or dashing out) may occur if the values or shapes of the curves are not acceptable to the instrument according to preset tolerances.[4,21]

The R_1 flag denotes interference in the valley to the left of the lymphocyte subpopulation at approximately 35 fL. This interference could be caused by clumped or giant platelets, nucleated RBCs, nonlysed red cells (e.g., sickled red cells), malarial parasites, fibrin strands, cryoglobulin, or fat globules attributable to total parenteral nutrition.[21] The R_2 flag indicates excessive overlap of cell populations at the lymphocyte-mononuclear boundary (approximately 90 fL). Abnormal cell types or numbers that could be present are variant lymphocytes, abnormal lymphocytes (e.g., plasma or hairy cells), blasts, eosinophilia, monocytosis, and basophilia.[21] The R_3 flag indicates an overlap of cells at the mononuclear-granulocyte boundary (approximately 160 fL). Many of these are false-positive flags, but they may indicate neutrophilia, neutrophilic left shift, eosinophilia, or a sample processed less than 30 minutes after collection. An R_4 flag indicates truncation of the distribution at the upper leukocyte threshold (450 fL) and is most often triggered when granulocyte numbers are increased.

Each flag will appear simultaneously next to the percentage and the absolute values of the cell type(s) in question. "RM" indicates interference at more than one region. Incomplete computation (...) may or may not appear in place of the numerical value simultaneously with R flags.

Backlighting of the leukocyte count indicates that the histogram curve does not start on the baseline below 35 fL (the lower leukocyte threshold). This flag can be caused by the same interferences as the R_1 flag. When backlighting occurs behind the total leukocyte count, it will also appear behind all the absolute numbers for each cell type, because the total leukocyte count is used to calculate them. Such backlighting indicates a possible erroneous value. Backlighting can sometimes occur only on relative and absolute numbers of mononuclear cells. This event is automatic when the absolute mononuclear number exceeds 1500 cells/μL.[4,7]

The disadvantages of this system include the lack of a barcode-positive identification system for autosampling (still needs worklists) and limited patient data storage (only 15 histograms can be stored).

Resistance Types

The Sysmex cell counting instruments from TOA Medical Electronics Co. Ltd. use a single transducer capacitance detection method. This method takes advantage of the difference in the conductivities of the blood cell and the diluent. In 1984, TOA introduced the E series. The E-5000 uses a single transducer (aperture) for leukocytes and provides a three-part differential (small, middle, and large cell ratios) in both percentages and absolute numbers. The three-part differential, as described for other systems, is developed by treating the leukocytes with special lysing agents. Strips of leukocyte cytoplasm are lysed, and a sophisticated logic system "looks" at the leukocyte populations. Automatic floating discrimination function (to threshold and flag abnormal histogram curves) is included. Fewer channels (50) count the treated leukocytes,[8,18,28] resulting in a condensed-appearing histogram compared with those generated by other instruments (Fig. 44-6).

The TOA E-5000 has internal flags similar to the R_1 to R_4

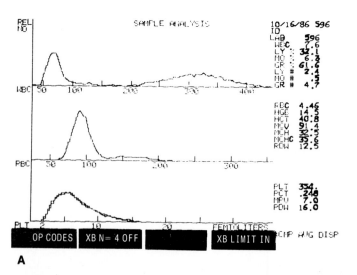

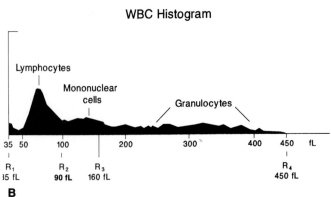

WBC Histogram

A

B

FIG. 44-5.   Example of display of Coulter S-Plus series. (A) Histogram display using reagent system for three-part differential display. (B) Close-up view of leukocyte histogram, indicating approximate locations of region (R) flags.

flags generated by Coulter instruments. The types of abnormalities that trigger flags in this system correspond to those described above for the Coulter instruments. The E-5000 uses a lower threshold of 30 fL and an upper threshold of 300 fL compared with Coulter's 35 fL and 450 fL. The only disagreement between the two manufacturers seems to be in their definition of where the five normal cell types fall in the three-part differential. Both agree that lymphocytes are in the small cell category. However, TOA states that eosinophils and basophils fall with the mononuclear or middle cell group, whereas Coulter states that eosinophils and basophils are grouped with neutrophils in the granulocyte or large cell group. There is documentation that eosinophils and basophils may fall in either population but more often fall in the mononuclear or middle cell group.[21,22]

Other flags produced by the TOA instrument are ABN, *, +/-, and * accompanying a number. ABN indicates that there has been a distribution error, and population thresholds have been exceeded. An asterisk replaces a number when the number is beyond the display or there is a leukocyte plug in the transducer or an analysis error. The +/- flag designates values that are outside the numerical limits preset by the user. An asterisk *with* a number occurs when the value exceeds the linearity of the system (*e.g.*, RBC count greater than 20×10^{12}/L or platelets greater than 3000×10^9/L).[28]

Another feature of the TOA system is the ability to set thresholds manually instead of allowing the machines to scan and set them automatically. This feature allows the operator to count the cell population, move the thresholds, and count again to break down abnormal curves and interferences from other particle channels (*e.g.*, large platelets or nucleated RBCs).

The disadvantages include the lack of a closed sampling system (stoppers are removed manually), a reagent system that must be temperature controlled to keep volume measurements from changing, and a sample MCV stability of only 12 hours.[17]

The year 1990 saw the introduction of the Sysmex NE-8000, which boasts a five-part differential. The WBCs are counted and differentiated in a precisely measured volume of prediluted specimen. The NE-8000 uses a combination of direct-current resistance (to measure cell size and number) and high radiofrequency wave impedance (to measure nuclear size and density). The instrument produces a scattergram and histograms.

Other Types

The years 1984 through 1986 have brought three additional hematology systems from companies who have previously offered instruments geared to the small laboratory or physician office. These instruments not only produce histograms and sort out granulocyte-lymphocyte-middle cells but are available at substantially lower prices ($40,000 to $100,000 versus >$100,000). These systems are the Diagnostic Technology Inc. PHA-3D, the Cell-Dyn 2000 (Fig. 44-7) from Unipath Company, and the CELLECT 8 from Instrumentation Laboratory Inc.[9,12,14]

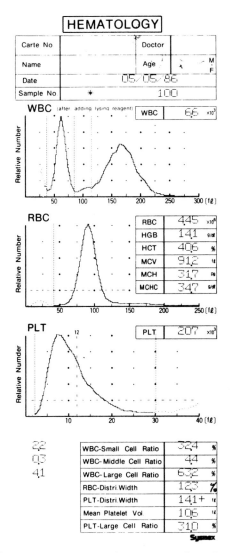

FIG. 44-6. The TOA E-5000 histogram and result printout. Note three peaks in leukocyte channel between 30 and 250 fL. Also note vertical dotted lines denoting discriminator settings. Three-part differential cell ratios in percentage are shown in box at bottom. Absolute values for each cell count ($\times 10^3/\mu$L) are displayed to left of cell ratios.

SCREENING DIFFERENTIAL EVALUATION

In all the systems described, the user has the option of inspecting all histograms visually for any unusual shapes and of requesting that a stained blood film be reviewed.

One important aspect of the screening differential is its stability. In terms of the three-part differential, the specimen is somewhat unstable in comparison with the other hematology group parameters.[7,17] In fact, many of the systems have very specific minimum and maximum time limits. For example, Coulter Electronics suggests greater than 30 minutes but less than 4 hours[4] from the time of the blood collection. It seems that the leukocytes need time to equilibrate with the EDTA anticoagulant before the lysing agent is added. On the other hand, cells may age to the point that their reaction to the lysing agent can cause a curve where the peaks shift to a smaller size. It has been our experience

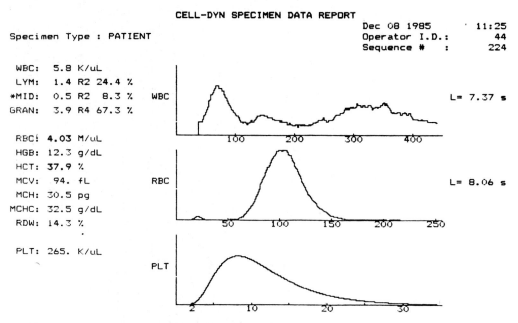

FIG. 44-7.   Unipath Cell-Dyn 2000 histogram display showing slightly different three-part differential terminology and units for red cells, platelets, etc.

that the time limits could be expanded (from 15 minutes to 12 hours) without significant change to the numerical results. However, there is a slight increase in the number of region flags (Mayo Clinic, unpublished data). This specific time limit restricts the length of time a sample can be stored or how far a sample can be shipped. Thus, a three-part screening differential would be an unacceptable alternative to a slide differential in a reference or regional laboratory where specimens are not run until they are more than 12 hours old. These time limitations are not applicable to the six-part cytochemical differential described earlier in this chapter.

The three-part differential can accurately identify leukocyte abnormalities, either distributional or morphologic. As stated in the NCCLS standard, the automated differential systems must prove that they are at least as good as the manual method in flagging or identifying abnormalities.[15] In earlier studies, the false-positive and false-negative rates for manual differentials were found to be as high as 14.5% and 11.5%, respectively.[14] In recent comparisons using the NCCLS standard, [15] the three-part differential was found to, have a false-positive range of 7.4% to 21.7% and a false-negative range of 1.7% to 7.8 % depending on the study and instrument.[7,17] Both results are within acceptable handling limitations of the laboratory, with the false-negative rates being well below those of the manual method.

NEW DIRECTIONS

An interesting new development in screening blood counts is the QBC (quantitative buffy coat analysis) centrifugal

hematology system manufactured by the Clay Adams Company. A precision-bore capillary tube internally coated with acridine orange is used. The tube is filled with 40 to 100 μL of whole blood, one end is sealed, and a plastic float with a specific gravity identical to that of the buffy coat layer (1.005) is placed inside the tube. After the tube has been spun, the float visually expands the buffy coat linearly. The buffy coat then is shown in layers differentially stained by acridine orange. With an ultraviolet light source, granulocytes appear bright orange, mononuclear cells are emerald green, platelets are yellow, and plasma is clear green. With the aid of a special reading device, six interfaces separating plasma, erythrocytes, platelets, granulocytes, and nongranulocytes are identified. A microprocessor translates these readings into a packed cell volume (hematocrit) and total leukocyte, granulocyte, nongranulocyte, and platelet counts. Published comparisons show good correlation with established methods.[29] This system is being marketed as an inexpensive hematology screening system that may be useful in a physician office or other outpatient setting.

Coulter Electronics has recently introduced two new systems (Coulter VCS Flow Cytometer and Coulter STKS).[5] Five cell populations are identified by subjecting cells to three kinds of measurement. The first is the familiar impedance of cell volume, the second is conductivity, and the third is light scatter. The three results are compared and plotted against one another to display a five-part scattergram. The STKS incorporates the VCS technology to produce a five-part differential. In addition, it has a comprehensive QC program, a results management program (delta checks), and walkaway operation (Fig. 44-8).

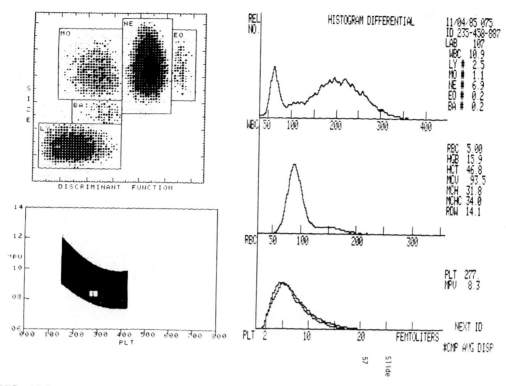

FIG. 44-8. Example of Coulter STKS display using five-part differential format. Histogram differential (right) and scattergram differential (upper left) from multidimensional analysis provide crosschecks for each other.

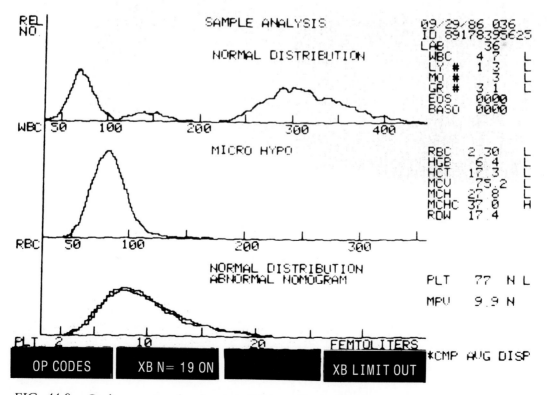

FIG. 44-9. Coulter counter plot showing addition of interpretative comments about cell population histogram.

TABLE 44–1. Comparison of Instrument Specifications

	HEMATRAK 590	TECHNICON H-6000	TECHNICON H·1 (H·2)	ORTHO ELT SERIES	UNIPATH CELL-DYN 2000	TOA E-5000	COULTER S-PLUS SERIES	COULTER STKS
DETECTION METHOD	Pattern recognition	Light scatter, sheath, cytochemical, tungsten lamp	Laser & tungsten lamp, cytochemical sheath	Laser, sheath	Resistance	Resistance, sheath	Impedance	Impedance, light scatter, sheath, conductivity, cytochemical
NO. OF PARAMETERS								
RBC	1–10	7	8	7	7	7	7	7
WBC	6–14	13	15	7	7	4	7	7–11
PLT	1	1	2	1	1	4	4	2
SAMPLE SIZE (μL)	Blood film	700	100 or 150	100–1000	100–250	200	100–750	100 or 175
WBCs SAMPLE	100–500	10×10^3	10×10^3	$7–14 \times 10^3$	Varies with WBC count	Varies with WBC count	20×10^3	8.2×10^3
SAMPLING SYSTEM	Blood film	Open auto	Open or auto cork piercing	Open or auto cork piercing	Open	Open, manual, or auto	Open or auto cork piercing	Open or auto cork piercing
THROUGHPUT/HR	90	90	60 (100+)	60–100	90–100	119	119–135	109
GRAPHICS	Price-Jones	Scattergram	Cytogram/ histogram	Histogram	Histogram	Histogram	Histogram	Cytogram, histogram, nomogram
STARTUP TIME (MIN)	0	5–30	40–160 sec	0–5	0–3	0–5	0–5	0–5
BARCODE	Yes	Yes (not same as patient ID)	No	Only with sampling device	No	Yes	No	Yes
DATA STORAGE								
PATIENT	200	Yes	Yes	Yes	320	300	257	1000
QC	Yes	Yes	Yes	Yes	Yes	60×9 files	Yes	Yes

FUTURE NEEDS

As technology advances, we can expect greater sophistication and ease of handling of hematology instruments. Some of these machines include programming to interpret histograms automatically and enclosed automatic sampling systems with barcode identification (Fig. 44-9).

It is important to voice concerns or needs (with ideas) to manufacturers about items that should be changed or included in instrument systems. This is how practical instrumentation developed.

CHAPTER SUMMARY

Two basic approaches to automation of the leukocyte differential count have been developed: image processing and flow-through instruments based on cytochemical or volume criteria or both. Image recognition and processing instruments are gradually being phased out. Flow systems have branched out into several approaches for counting leukocytes in suspension and into different numbers of categories for leukocyte classification (i.e., two part, three part, seven part). Both basic concepts have developed into a variety of practical and effective instruments (Table 44-1). Currently, available hematology instruments for the clinical laboratory can perform the routine differential or screening differential on large numbers of leukocytes accurately with greater speed and precision than is possible with manual techniques. The screening differential, in conjunction with the CBC, appears to be an effective means to identify patient specimens that do not require more extensive testing and to flag specimens on which more testing is valuable.

Thus, the laboratory can more readily meet the needs of cost containment and efficiency.

Lastly, as technology develops, so does the sophistication of laboratory equipment. New advances seem to be in the direction of extended leukocyte classification, more sophisticated sample handling systems, and patient data integration and processing systems.

REFERENCES

1. Alexander BC: New hematology analyzers. Am Clin Prod Rev, Oct 1984
2. Bacus JW: The development of automated differential systems. In Koepke JA (ed): Differential Leukocyte Counting, p 95. Skokie, IL, College of American Pathologists, 1978
3. Connelly DP, McClain MP, Crowson TW et al: Use of the differential leukocyte count for inpatient casefinding. Hum Pathol 13:294, 1982
4. Coulter Electronics, Inc: Coulter Counter Model S-Plus IV with Three-Population Differential and Auto Transfer: Product Reference Manual 4235328B. Hialeah, FL, November 1983
5. Coulter Electronics, Inc: Coulter Scattergram Differential from Multidimensional Cytometry. Hematology Analyzer Publication, vol 6. Hialeah, FL, December 1985
6. Coulter Electronics, Inc: Coulter Counter Analyzer Model S-Plus STKR Manual, PN4235547. Hialeah, FL, June 1986
7. Cox CJ, Habermann TM, Payne BA et al: Evaluation of the Coulter Counter Model S-Plus IV. Am J Clin Pathol 84:297, 1985
8. DeCresce R: The E-5000. Lab Med 17:6, 1986
9. Diagnostic Technology Inc: PHA-3D Product Brochure. Hauppauge, NY 11788 (240 Vanderbilt Motor Parkway), 1986

10. Geometric Data Corporation: Hematrak 590 Operator's Manual. Wayne, PA 19087 (999 West Valley Road)

11. Hosty TA, Harris LG, Stonacek SM et al: Evaluation of an automated continuous flow hematology instrument: The Technicon H6000. J Clin Lab Autom 2:408, 1982

12. Instrumentation Laboratory Inc: CELLECT 8 Hematology System Brochure No.H201. Lexington, MA 02173-3190

13. Johnson CL, Brockwell P: Evaluation of the leukocyte screening capabilities of the Ortho hematology analyzer with screening differential. Westwood, MA, Ortho Diagnostic Systems Inc, 1985

14. Koepke JA (ed): Differential Leukocyte Counting. Skokie, IL, College of American Pathologists, 1978

15. National Committee for Clinical Laboratory Standards: Tentative standard for leukocyte differential counting. NCCLS H20-T, vol 4 (11), Villanova, PA, 1984

16. Ortho Diagnostic Systems Inc: Ortho ELT8/ds Operator Reference Manual. Westwood, MA 02090, 1984

17. Payne BA, Pierre RV, Morris MA: Use of instruments to obtain red blood cell profiles. J Med Technol 2:379, 1985

18. Payne BA, Pierre RV: TOA E-5000 multiparameter automated hematology analyzer. Am J Clin Pathol 88:51, 1987

19. Pierre RV: Automation of blood film preparation and staining utilizing the Technicon Autoslide. Blood Cells 6:471, 1980

20. Pierre RV: Differential counting. In Koepke JA (ed): Laboratory Hematology. New York, Churchill Livingstone, 1984

21. Pierre RV: Seminar and case studies: The automated differential (medical education program). Hialeah, FL, Coulter Electronics, Inc, 1985

22. Pierre RV, Payne BA, Lee WK et al: Comparison of four leukocyte differential methods with the National Committee for Clinical Laboratory Standards (NCCLS) reference method. Am J Clin Pathol 87:201, 1987

23. Rumke CL: The statistically expected variability in differential leukocyte counting. In Koepke JA (ed): Differential Leukocyte Counting. Skokie, IL. College of American Pathologists, 1978

24. Sequoia-Turner Corporation (now Unipath Company): Cell-Dyn 2000 Automated Hematology Analyzer Operators Reference Manual, P/N 9140170B. Mountain View, CA 94043, November 1985

25. Technicon Instruments Corp: Technicon H6000 System (90.h): Technical Publication No. UA8-3515-00. Tarrytown, NY, April 1983

26. Technicon Instruments Corp: Technicon H·System Operators Guide, Technical Publication No. TAB-5588. Tarrytown, NY, October 1985

27. Tisdall PA: Evaluation of a laser-based three-part leukocyte differential analyzer in detection of clinical abnormalities. Lab Med 16:228, 1985

28. TOA Medical Electronics Co, Ltd: Sysmex E-5000 Multiparameter Fully Automated Hematology Analyzer E-Series Particle Size Distribution Handbook, Sysmex Document No. 0114H/07.84. Kobe, Japan

29. Wardlaw SC, Lerune RA: Quantitative buffy coat analysis: A new laboratory tool furnishing a screening complete blood count. JAMA 249:617, 1983

30. Wardlaw SC, Rathbone R, McPhedran P: An instrument for white blood cell subclassification. Am Clin Prod Rev, June 1985

31. Watson JS, Davis RA: Evaluation of the Technicon H·1 Hematology System. Lab Med 18:316, 1987

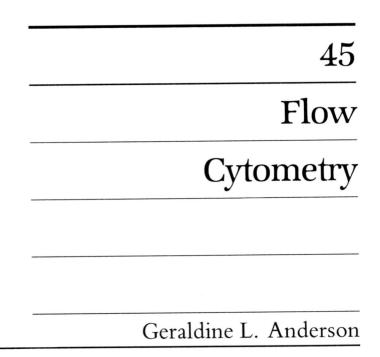

45

Flow

Cytometry

Geraldine L. Anderson

Flow cytometry is a technology that analyzes thousands of cells individually and rapidly for various physical or other properties. By using flow cytometry, one is able to obtain quantitative measurements of multiple individual cellular properties. Through computer analysis of the data generated, detection of specific subpopulations of cells is possible. This technology has produced significant diagnostic and prognostic information and has had a major impact on basic immunology and hematology. It also has increased our understanding of the normal development of human blood cells.

DEVELOPMENT

The basic principle of flow cytometry was incorporated into the first Coulter counter. In this instrument, individual cells were counted and sized as they flowed in a conductive liquid through a small orifice between two chambers. The change in voltage that occurred as each cell passed through the sensing zone was detected and counted.[4]

In 1953 Crossland-Taylor described a technique capable of directing cells to the center of a flow stream in single file.[5] This technology is variously known as laminar sheath flow or hydrodynamic focusing and is the foundation on which most flow cytometers operate today. In 1965, a flow cytometer based on light scattering and capable of measuring more than one property of each cell was introduced.[12] The technology was further advanced by the introduction of the first instrument able to separate and sort cells using electrical charge.[6] The use of an argon laser as the light source provides an intense, nondiverging, monochromatic beam of light with sufficient power at selected wavelengths to enable fluorescence measurements. Flow cytometry grew in concert with advances in electronics, computers, and reagents such as monoclonal antibodies.[3,10,11] Today, cytometers measure cellular properties such as size, cytoplasmic granularity, and fluorescence.

PRINCIPLE

Flow cytometry measures the features of a single cell in suspension as it enters a flow chamber. The cell suspension is introduced through a specimen needle under pressure. The specimen is surrounded by a sheath of particle-free saline. Both the sample and the sheath fluid must exit through an orifice whose size is selected according to the type of cell population being analyzed. The sheath and specimen fluid pressures may be adjusted to produce the desired stream diameter, which usually is between 10 and 30 μm when measuring leukocytes. The specimen passes between the light source and stationary light detectors. Illuminated cells scatter light in all directions. The low-angle forward-scattered light discriminates the size of cells, and the 90° (right-angle) scatter discriminates their internal structure such as granularity.

Cells usually are stained in suspension with either a fluorochrome-tagged antibody, a dye that stains the DNA, or another fluorochrome with specific reactivity. Fluorescent light is collected through an optical detector system located orthogonally (at right angle) to the laser beam. If more than one fluorochrome is present in or on the cell, the fluorescence is analyzed by selective optical filters into constituent wavelengths. Each wavelength may be directed to a different detector (Fig. 45-1). The detectors are connected to photomultiplier tubes (PMTs) that convert light photons to an electrical impulse or analog signal. This signal is further converted to a digital signal or a number that is recorded by the computer as a data point in a frequency distribution or histogram. In combination, these signals enable one to differentiate lymphocytes from other leukocytes on the basis of light scatter, volume, and fluorescence. Monocytes and granulocytes can be analyzed in a similar manner, because each cell type has distinct properties.

Cells may be analyzed while in the flow chamber or, in some cases, outside the flow chamber. The sample stream carrying cells directed along a precise path is analyzed as it traverses the sensing zone (see Fig. 45-1).

Some flow cytometers are capable of sorting cells after they pass through the sensing area. The fluid stream is broken into charged droplets when an electrical charge is applied to the individual droplets. Computer software determines whether the droplet is positively or negatively charged. The charged droplet containing a single cell with predetermined attributes is directed into appropriate collection vessels as it passes between two charged deflection plates (see Fig. 45-1).

Lasers are used to intensify the monochromatic properties of light at desired wavelengths. The argon laser, which is most frequently chosen for cellular studies, usually operates in the region of blue light (i.e., 488 nm). Some flow cytometry systems use a mercury arc lamp as the light source. Although this latter system is less expensive to operate, it does not offer the flexibility or power of a laser.

An electronic window or "gate" around an area of cells within a mixed population permits data collection or sorting for further tests. Figure 45-2 shows a histogram from a sample of whole blood in which the RBCs have been lysed. Figure 45-3 shows a computer-drawn map of the same sample enclosing the lymphoid cells, which are close to the forward angle of light scatter (FALS) axis. One or more computer systems are used to control the instrument's op-

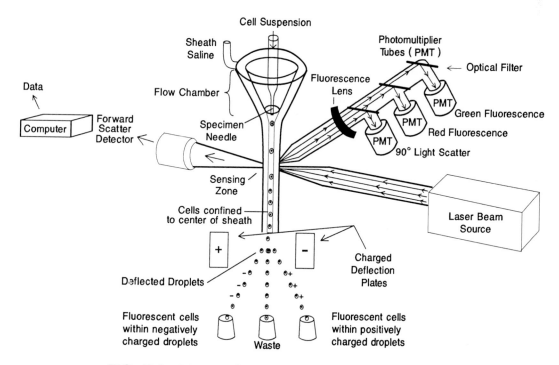

FIG. 45-1.   Diagram of operation of flow cytometer and cell sorter.

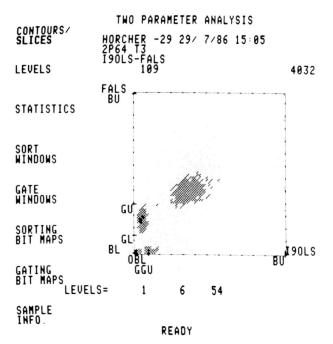

FIG. 45-2. Flow cytometric histogram of normal blood after RBC lysis.

eration, data collection, and analysis. Newer computer software permits analysis of cells at rates of 20,000 per second and allows the sorting of 10,000 cells per second.

CLINICAL APPLICATIONS

The identification of specific hemopoietic cell subsets using immunofluorescent reagents has become increasingly important in the study of lymphoid malignancies (Table 45-1).

Monoclonal antibodies are most commonly labeled with fluorescein and phycoerythrin dyes that excite at the same wavelengths. When a specific monoclonal antibody conjugated to the fluorescent dye is bound by an antigen on a cell surface, the antigen can be detected by the instrument by the antibody fluorescence. The World Health Organization nomenclature for several of these human leukocyte antigens, called the cluster designation (CD), along with the antibody and disease state, are listed in Chapter 24. This recommended terminology based on differentiation clusters is an effort to establish standardized nomenclature for the various lymphocyte species.

Labeling of DNA and RNA in cells with fluorescent dyes

was one of the earliest clinical uses of flow technology. Vital dyes for DNA allow its measurement in living cells. The dye can be removed by washing to allow further studies of the same cells. Individual cell content of DNA and RNA can be measured, and populations can be identified. The DNA content reflects the stage of the cell cycle and thus allows an estimate of the proportion of cells in different stages of division. These methods have been applied to estimate the growth fraction of malignant cells such as blasts from leukemic bone marrow.

Flow technology can also detect small populations of cells containing abnormal numbers of chromosomes, a process that is being explored in clinical studies.[1] Such information might be of value in planning chemotherapy and in following the results of therapy.

In summary, commercial flow cytometers are capable of producing rapid, accurate, and reproducible results and are becoming important tools in the diagnosis of lymphomas and leukemias. The general association of cell-surface markers (phenotypic features) with functional properties and the numerical and maturation changes can reflect significant alterations in the immune system. Those conditions in which phenotypic typing may be useful are listed in Table 45-2. Several helpful articles review this field.[8,9,13,14,19]

EMERGING TECHNIQUES

Some emerging clinical applications for flow cytometry are listed in Table 45-3.[8,16,17]

Flow cytometers are being tested in research for selection of proper therapeutic regimes. A new application employs the use of appropriate reagents to distinguish monoclonal proliferations of malignant cells from reactive (polyclonal) immunologic processes and distinguishing between benign and malignant lymphoid proliferations.[2]

New techniques involving the extraction of single cells from preserved paraffin sections are being perfected for comparative surface antigen and DNA analysis.[7] When combined with standard morphologic studies of the same sections, significant new information concerning well-

TABLE 45–1. Cellular Features Measured by
Flow Cytometry

Cell size or volume
DNA content
Cytoplasmic granularity
Cell-surface antigens
Intracellular enzymes
RNA content

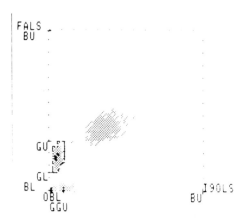

FIG. 45-3. Histogram of sample in Figure 45-2. Computer-drawn map has delineated lymphocyte population.

TABLE 45–2. Conditions in Which Leukocyte Phenotyping May Be Useful

Lymphoproliferative disorders
Persistent unexplained lymphadenopathy
Autoimmune diseases
Immune deficiency syndromes
Bone marrow transplantation
Immunosuppressive drug regimes for organ transplantation
Immune regeneration
Viral, fungal, or protozoal infections

TABLE 45–4. Complementary Advantages of Flow Cytometry and Fluorescent Tissue Microscopy

Flow cytometry
  High statistical significance of analysis
  Population distribution of features rather than averages
  Abnormal cells detected and quantitated in very low numbers
  Sorting of subpopulations for functional, biochemical, or morphologic analysis
Fluorescent tissue microscopy
  Retention of intercellular (histologic) relations
  Ease of correlation with known morphology
  Single cell quantitation
  Significantly lower capital investment

known diseases will be forthcoming. The advantages of each technique are listed in Table 45-4.

An immunomonitoring system for the analysis of leukocyte cell surface markers that combines monoclonal antibody technology and flow cytometry is available. In this system, monocytes are labeled with two fluorescent dyes so they can be differentiated from single-color cells and can be used in the differential diagnosis and immune monitoring of a variety of disease states.

Improved stain specificities allow three-dye combinations to be analyzed with a single argon laser. Mechanisms of intracellular pH regulation in tumor cells, where lower pH could point to early tumor growth and metastasis, are becoming important research settings. Cell activation, endocytosis into acid compartments, and internalization of surface markers can be detected with pH-sensitive dyes. Likewise, large calcium ion movements across cell membranes that most likely generate changes in membrane potential are being investigated using dye molecules as probes.

New research applications continue to appear, and this list serves only as a hint of the procedures that are emerging for flow cytometry use.

SELECTING A COMMERCIAL INSTRUMENT

The instruments available are constantly being improved; therefore, the possibility of upgrading is an important feature. Projected uses and hardware costs, maintenance and service contract fees, installation requirements and related costs, as well as operator ease of learning and use must be considered when purchasing this equipment.[15]

The instrument that uses a mercury arc for the light source requires only bench top space, is easy to operate, is simple to maintain, produces inexpensive dual-color fluorescence analysis, and is less expensive to install than the larger water-cooled laser flow cytometers. On the other hand, these instruments are not as versatile as the laser flow cytometers. The larger, 2 or 5 W argon laser instruments require flowing water to cool them. Their installation therefore must include proper water filters and drain hookup. Some of the newer flow cytometers, however, are capable of sorting individual cells or can be fitted with a second laser for multiple color analysis. The newest laser flow cytometers are smaller, air cooled, fit on a bench top, contain 15- to 25-mW lasers, and come with user-friendly software for analysis.

TABLE 45–3. Emerging Clinical Applications of Flow Cytometry

Detection of small populations of cells or organisms
  Reticulocyte counts
  Small numbers of circulating blasts
  Fetal cells in maternal circulation
  Bacteria or intracellular parasites
Determination of cell-surface phenomena
  Drug uptake
  Membrane potential (mitochondrial effects)
  Tumor markers (e.g., estrogen receptors)
Evaluation of leukocyte function
  Assessment of phagocytosis
  Autofluorescence (e.g., oxidative burst)
Evaluation of intracellular metabolism
  pH (cell activation, internalization of surface markers)
  Cellular enzymes
  Calcium transport (T-cell proliferation)
  Total protein content of fixed cells
  Cytoplasmic antigens
Cytogenetics
  Chromosome analysis
  Oncogene analysis
Semen Analysis
  Identification of normal and abnormal sperm (e.g., DNA content)
  X:Y sperm sorting
Other
  Detection of autoantibodies
  Measurement of cytotoxicity
  Analysis of platelet function

TECHNICAL PRECAUTIONS AND SUGGESTIONS

It is not within the scope of this textbook to detail the operational features of these instruments. In order for them to perform at their maximum accuracy, precision, and efficiency, several precautions should be observed. Proper alignment, setting for maximum scatter and fluorescence sensitivity, and careful calibration are of the utmost importance. This alignment and fine-tuning needs to be performed before and after each run. The experienced cytometer operator will select the proper gates around the area of interest in a frequency distribution, install the correct filters, discriminately set gain and PMT voltages, correct fluidic problems as encountered, recognize interference from poor cell preparation, and perform analyses. Samples should be checked using a fluorescent microscope to ensure that cells are monodispersed such that very few doublets are present. Further, the suspensions must be free of damaged cells or cell debris, and the medium should not contain an excess of unbound fluorescent material.

Each laboratory needs to establish its own reference values.[18] Correlation with conventional hematology morphology helps evaluate phenotyping with therapeutic response, remission, and relapse. The operator should understand cell biology and be well trained in sample preparation and labeling.

CHAPTER SUMMARY

The rapid development of flow cytometry makes the use of these instruments important additions to the clinical laboratory. Newer systems measuring both fluorescent intensity and light scatter, combined with computer analysis, allow detection and characterization of functionally and biologically important subpopulations of leukocytes. Many systems are flexible, and new applications await only the creative imagination of the user.

REFERENCES

1. Ault K: Detection of small numbers of monoclonal B lymphocytes in the blood of patients with lymphoma. N Engl J Med 300:1401, 1979
2. Ault K: Clinical applications of fluorescence-activated cell sorting techniques. Diagn Immunol 1:2, 1983
3. Bonner WA, Hulett HR, Sweet RG et al: Fluorescence activated cell sorting. Rev Sci Instr 43:404, 1972
4. Coulter WH: High speed automatic blood cell counter and cell size analyzer. Proc Natl Electron Conf 12:1034, 1956
5. Crossland-Taylor PJ: A device for counting small particles suspended in a fluid through a tube. Nature 171:37, 1953
6. Fulwyler MJ: Electronic separation of biological cells by volume. Science 150:910, 1965
7. Friedlander ML, Hedley DW, Taylor IW: Clinical and biological significance of aneuploidy in human tumors. J Clin Pathol 37:961, 1984
8. Horan PK: Single cell analysis enters the space age. Diagn Med Special Issue on Technology, p 1, 1981
9. Horan PK, Wheeless LL: Quantitative single cell analysis and sorting. Science 198:149, 1977
10. Hulett HR, Bonner WA, Barrett J et al: Cell sorting: Automated separation of mammalian cells as a function of intracellular fluorescence. Science 166:747, 1969
11. Hulett HR, Bonner WA, Sweet RG et al: Development and application of a rapid cell sorter. Clin Chem 19:813, 1973
12. Kamentsky LA, Melamed MR, Derman H: Spectrophotometer: New instrument for ultrarapid cell analysis. Science 150:630, 1965
13. Laerum OD, Farsund T: Clinical application of flow cytometry: A review. Cytometry 2:1, 1981
14. Lovett EJ, Schnitzer B, Keren DF et al: Application of flow cytometry to diagnostic pathology. Lab Invest 50:115, 1984
15. Measel JW Jr: Clinical Applications of Flow Cytometry. Diagn Clin Test 27:25, 1989
16. Miller RG, LaLande ME, McCutcheon MJ et al: Usage of the flow cytometer-cell sorter: Review article. J Immunol Meth 47:13, 1981
17. Murihead KA, Horan PK, Poste G: Flow cytometry: Present and future. Biotechnology 3:337, 1985
18. National Committee for Clinical Laboratory Standards: Clinical Applications of Flow Cytometry: Immunophenotyping of Peripheral Blood Lymphocytes—Proposed Guideline, NCCLS, Document H42. Villanova, PA, CCLS, 1989
19. Shapiro HM: Multistation multiparameter flow cytometry: A critical review and rationale. Cytometry 3:227, 1983

SUGGESTED READING

Andreeff M (ed): Clinical Cytometry. Ann NY Acad Sci 468, 1986

Colvin RB, Preffer FI: New technologies in cell analysis by flow cytometry. Arch Pathol Lab Med 111:628, 1987

Giorgi JV: Lymphocyte subset measurements: Significance in clinical medicine. In Rose NR, Friedman H, Fahey JL (eds): Manual of Clinical Laboratory Immunology, 3rd ed, Chap 33. Washington, DC, American Society for Microbiology, 1986

Marti GE, Fleisher TA (eds): Clinical applications of flow cytometry symposium. Pathol Immunopathol Res 7(5), 1988

Vogt RF, Cross G, Henderson LO et al: Model system evaluating fluorescein-labeled microbeads as internal standards to calibrate fluorescence intensity on flow cytometers. Cytometry 10:294, 1989

PART X

QUALITY CONTROL AND QUALITY ASSURANCE IN HEMATOLOGY

46

Introduction to Quality Control and Quality Assurance in Hematology

Pamela B. Bollinger

The clinical hematology laboratory is an integral part of contemporary medical practice because its comprehensive analyses of body fluids are utilized in diagnosis and treatment. As the utility of laboratory tests and the reliability of the results improve, clinicians have become dependent on these hematologic results in making critical decisions on therapeutic interventions for their patients. This reliance has greatly increased the responsibility of the clinical laboratory to ensure the quality of its analyses.

The methods used to assure reliable test results are collectively referred to as a *quality assurance program*. The term *quality assurance* (QA) encompasses comprehensive concepts, including components of *quality control* (QC), which are primarily quantitative and statistical, and those aspects of laboratory management that impart perceptions of credibility and medically useful results to the clinician. The goal of QC is the reduction of both systematic and random errors to zero. In Japan, this concept is called *zero defect*.[30] Although QC is invaluable in the laboratory setting, it serves only as a foundation for a comprehensive program of assuring high-quality patient care. The Joint Commission on Accreditation of Healthcare Organizations (JCAHO) defines QA as a "well-defined, organized program designed to enhance patient care through the ongoing objective assessment of important aspects of patient care and the correction of identified problems."

HISTORY OF QUALITY CONTROL

The concept of the quality of workmanship of any kind has always been present, but it was not until the emergence of industries and mass production that the term quality control was used.[14] In the late 1920s and early 1930s, Dodge and Shewhart of the Bell Telephone Company originated a systematic approach to QC utilizing statistics.[14,31] It was a few decades later, however, that clinical laboratories adopted similar programs for their routine analyses. Before 1950, there were few QC programs established in the clinical laboratory. The first reported survey, by Belk and Sunderman in 1947, revealed enormous disagreement in the results of different clinical chemistry laboratories.[5] This finding triggered a great deal of interest in devising methods for producing high-quality analytical results. In 1950 the idea of analyzing a control serum daily and plotting the results graphically was introduced by Levey and Jennings.[27] In 1953 control sera for use in clinical chemistry laboratories were made available commercially.

Several years passed before any type of commercial control material or QC program was utilized in the clinical hematology laboratory. A standard cyanmethemoglobin solution certified by the College of American Pathologists (CAP) was available in 1959 for standardization of spectrophotometers used in the measurement of hemoglobin (Hb) concentration.[25] However, control of this test procedure was achieved only by utilizing a normal donor blood or hemolysate specimen for comparison with the patient specimens. Commercial control materials for all hematologic measures were not readily available until the first automated hematology analyzers were introduced in the late 1960s. Furthermore, it was not until 1967 that the hemiglobincyanide (HiCN) standard solution and methodology, described in 1961,[36] was adopted as a reference procedure by the International Committee for Standardization in Haematology (ICSH).[22]

Unfortunately, in contrast to the clinical chemistry laboratory, where the approach to QC is relatively well established and straightforward, many areas of QC in hematology still lack clear-cut standardized approaches, to a great extent because the measurements in hematology involve living cellular components. This fact results in specific problems, such as a lack of stable materials for use as standards or controls.

This chapter will deal with several strategies and statistical tools available for use in hematology QA and QC programs. If these tools are diligently applied, reliable test results can be obtained.

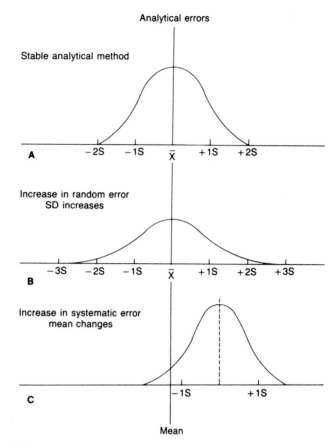

FIG. 46-1.   Schematic representation of distributions of control data. (A) Situation with no analytical error. (B) Increased random error, which causes increased standard deviation (s or SD). (C) Systematic error causing shift in mean ($\bar{x}$). (From Cembrowski GS, Sullivan AM: Quality control and statistics. In Bishop ML, Duben–Von Laufen JL, Fody EP (eds): Clinical Chemistry: Principles, Procedures, Correlations, p 77. Philadelphia, JB Lippincott, 1985, with permission.)

CONCEPTS AND STATISTICAL METHODS USED IN QUALITY CONTROL

Variations and Errors in Laboratory Measurements

Every measurement performed in the hematology laboratory contains an inherent variability. These variations result in two types of errors—*random* and *systematic* (Fig. 46-1). Random (indeterminate) errors affect precision, as repeated measurements increase the scatter of values about the true value. Random errors are the result of chance and sampling errors; they generally do not affect an entire batch of specimens and therefore cannot be detected by testing control specimens. In contrast, systematic or determinate errors (sometimes referred to as bias) affect all determinations in a batch equally and usually can be detected by testing control specimens. Systematic errors are attributable to causes other than chance, such as deteriorating reagents or an instrument that has lost calibration. Random errors introduce increased *variability* into an analysis, whereas systematic errors introduce a *bias*. Both types of analytical errors and the methods used to control them are discussed in detail in Chapters 47 and 48.

Assessments of the Quality of Laboratory Measurements—Precision and Accuracy

Two terms used in conjunction with laboratory measurements to define the quality of the analyses are *precision* and *accuracy*. The precision of a test is its reproducibility or the variation among duplicate or replicate measurements of the same analyte; for example, the consistency of a cell count between the first and second measurement or on two different days. The statistical means by which the precision of a quantitative analysis is expressed is described later in this chapter under Frequency Distributions and Associated Statistical Terms. Accuracy, on the other hand, refers to the closeness with which measured values agree with the true values. Accuracy has been defined by the ICSH as "agreement between the best estimate of a quantity and its true value."[35]

Precision is possible without accuracy. The difference between the two is graphically represented in Figure 46-2, where 10 gunshots are shown on each of three targets. Just like the performance of the hypothetical marksman shooting at the targets in Figure 46-2, the quality of an analysis can be described one of three ways: (1) neither accurate nor precise; (2) precise but lacking accuracy; or (3) both accurate and precise.

Initial Establishment of Accuracy in Hematology by Calibration

Establishment of the accuracy or true value of an analysis begins with calibration of the method using a standard or calibrator. Ideally, a stable material of precise concentration and purity of the analyte to be measured is used to prepare a *primary standard* for use in the calibration procedure. For example, in the chemistry laboratory, a sample of chemically pure glucose may be carefully weighed and dissolved in chemically pure water to make a primary glucose standard.

There are no primary standards in hematology. Instead, reference methods are utilized to measure the analyte in a whole blood sample, and that whole blood sample then becomes a *secondary standard*. A reference method is defined as one that is specific for the analyte and which quantitates the true concentration of the analyte. It may require instrumentation not available in many laboratories.[34] The International Federation of Clinical Chemistry defines a reference method as one which, after exhaustive investigation, has been found to have negligible inaccuracy in comparison with its degree of random analytical variation.[34]

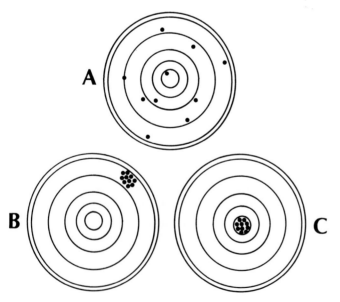

FIG. 46-2. Accuracy *v* precision. Bullseye represents accurate shot. (*A*) Shots are neither accurate nor precise. (*B*) Shots are precise (all clustered in one area) but not accurate. (*C*) Shots are both precise and accurate.

The only reference method in hematology that has been formally accepted nationally and internationally is the photometric measurement of hemiglobincyanide for determination of Hb concentration in human blood.[23] This method is calibrated using a hemiglobincyanide secondary calibration standard. Reference methods for other hematologic measures are discussed in Chapter 47.

Because in hematologic testing, only the Hb measurement has an approved and commercially available reference material, other hematologic procedures must be calibrated using commercial calibrators or fresh whole blood samples on which reference tests have been performed.[6,18,26] Chapter 47 provides more details.

Use of Controls for Monitoring Precision and Accuracy

Once accuracy has been established for a particular method, precision and accuracy are monitored with stabilized control materials. The ICSH definition states that a control material is "a substance used in routine practice for checking the concurrent performance of an analytical process or instrument. [Controls] must be similar in properties to, and be analyzed along with, patient specimens."[35] Commercial control products, patient specimens, or both can be used in many ways for this purpose,[6] as discussed later in this chapter under Establishment of Control Procedures and also in more detail in Chapters 47 and 48.

Frequency Distributions and Associated Statistical Terms[1]

Gaussian Distribution

When a number of analytical values or observations are plotted against the frequency of their occurrence, a distribution curve is obtained. A common distribution curve is a normal, or Gaussian, distribution, which is symmetric about the center and bell shaped (Fig. 46-3). The distribution can be described in terms of where its center (mean) value is, how dispersed it is, how symmetric or skewed it is, and how broad it is. Precision is measured by data dispersion, whereas bias (accuracy) is measured by the agreement of the mean value with the true value.

Median, Mode, and Mean

Median, mode, and mean are the three measures generally used to indicate the midpoint of a distribution (Table 46-1).

MEDIAN.   The median is simply the middle value of a set of numbers arranged according to size; therefore, 50% of the observations lie below the median and 50% above it. When the number of observations is even, the median is the average of the two values closest to the middle.

MODE.   The mode is the value occurring most frequently. When a distribution has two values with the same frequency, indicating two populations, the distribution is termed *bimodal*.

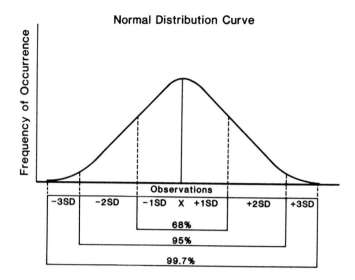

Normal Distribution Curve

Frequency of Occurrence

Observations

| -3SD | -2SD | -1SD | X | +1SD | +2SD | +3SD |

68%

95%

99.7%

FIG. 46-3. Normal curve known as Gaussian distribution. It is characteristically symmetrical about the center and bell shaped.

in the data set, but it is markedly affected by extreme values. In contrast, the median is not affected by extreme values. In a normally distributed set of data, the mean (average value), the median (central value), and the mode (most frequent value) are identical.

Skewness

When the values are not distributed evenly about the mean, the lack of symmetry is known as skewness. Frequency distributions that are not symmetric extend farther in one direction than in the other. A distribution with extreme values on the high side is skewed to the right and is said to have positive skewness. It has a mean larger than the median and a median greater than the mode. A distribution with extreme values on the low side is skewed to the left and said to have negative skewness. It has a mean smaller than the median and a median smaller than the mode. Examples of both types of skewness are shown in Figure 46-4.

Range, Variance, and Standard Deviation

Just as there are three measures of the middle of a distribution, there are three measures of variation or dispersion of a distribution: range, variance, and standard deviation. Measures of variation are used to indicate the spread of the curve.

MEAN. The arithmetic mean ($\bar{x}$) is the average value of a group of observations. It equals the sum (Σ) of all the values (Σx) divided by the number of observations (n), as shown in Table 46-1. The mean is the most reliable measure of the center of a distribution and uses all of the information

RANGE. The range is the difference between the largest and the smallest values in a data group (see Table 46-1).

TABLE 46-1. Calculation of Various Values from a Hypothetical Reference Range Study of Hemoglobin Values

VALUE	$(x - \bar{x})$*	$(x - \bar{x})^2$				
14.5	-0.9	0.81				
14.5	-0.9	0.81				
14.6	-0.8	0.64				
14.6	-0.8	0.64				
14.7	-0.7	0.49				
14.8	-0.6	0.36				
14.8	-0.6	0.36				
14.8	-0.6	0.36				
14.9	-0.5	0.25				
15.0	-0.4	0.16				
15.2	-0.2	0.04	VARIANCE (s^2)	$\dfrac{\Sigma(x - \bar{x})^2}{n - 1}$	$= \dfrac{11.58}{(30 - 1)}$	$= 0.4$
15.3	-0.1	0.01				
15.3	-0.1	0.01				
15.4	0.0	0.00				
15.5	0.1	0.01	STANDARD	$\sqrt{\dfrac{\Sigma(x - \bar{x})^2}{n - 1}}$	$= \sqrt{0.4}$	$= 0.63$
15.5	0.1	0.01	DEVIATION (s)			
15.5	0.1	0.01				
15.6	0.2	0.04				
15.6	0.2	0.04	COEFFICIENT OF	$\dfrac{s}{\bar{x}} \times 100\%$	$= \dfrac{0.63}{15.4} \times 100$	$= 4.1\%$
15.6	0.2	0.04	VARIATION (CV)			
15.6	0.2	0.04				
15.9	0.5	0.25	STANDARD ERROR	$\dfrac{s}{\sqrt{n}}$	$= \dfrac{0.63}{\sqrt{30}}$	$= 0.12$
16.1	0.7	0.49	OF THE MEAN			
16.2	0.8	0.64	(SEM)			
16.2	0.8	0.64				
16.3	0.9	0.81				
16.3	0.9	0.81				
16.3	0.9	0.81				
16.4	1.0	1.00				
16.4	1.0	1.00				
Σ (sum) = 463.4		$\Sigma = 11.58$				

* Mean ($\bar{x}$) = $\dfrac{\Sigma x}{n}$ = $\dfrac{463.4}{30}$ = 15.4; median (middle value) = 15.5; mode (most common value) = 15.6; range 14.5–16.4

Skewness Curves

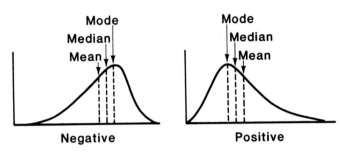

Test 1	Test 2	d	d²	2n − 1
11.5	11.4	0.1	0.01	2(5) − 1 = 9
11.6	11.7	−0.1	0.01	
11.4	11.6	−0.2	0.04	
11.2	11.3	−0.1	0.01	
11.5	11.2	0.3	0.09	
			0.16 = Σd^2	

FIG. 46-4. Distribution curves with extreme values on high side have positive skew (right). Curves with extreme values on low side have negative skew (left).

This is a simple but weak measure, because it fails to give any consideration to the array of values between the two extremes and is greatly influenced by extremely large or small values.

VARIANCE. The variance (s^2), another measure of variability, is computed as the sum of the squared deviation of each observation (x) from the mean ($\overline{x}$) divided by the number of observations (n) minus 1. Table 46-1 provides an example of the calculation of variance. The deviations of each observation from the mean are squared before summation to resolve the problem of cancellation by the equal number of positive and negative deviations which could result in a meaningless value.[16]

STANDARD DEVIATION. Although the variance is an accurate measure of dispersion, it is still the square of the deviations. The square root of the variance is called the standard deviation (s or SD). The formula, shown in Table 46-1, is used to calculate the SD when replicate determinations are performed on the same sample and, in some cases, for determining the population reference range. As with the formula for variance, the denominator can be represented by either n or n − 1, depending on the number of observations. If fewer than 30 replicates are tested, the n − 1 denominator is used.

STANDARD DEVIATION IN DUPLICATE SAMPLE TESTING. When one or more samples in a batch are tested in duplicate, a second equation is used to calculate s. The summation of the square of the differences between the duplicate analyses (Σd^2) is divided by the number of analyses, and the square root of this number is determined. The following formula is used, where n - 1 is the number of samples minus 1, 2n - 1 represents the actual number of analyses minus one, and Σd^2 is the summation of the difference between duplicate measurements of each sample:[12]

$$s = \sqrt{\frac{\Sigma d^2}{2n - 1}}$$

For example, five samples were run in duplicate in testing the prothrombin time, with the following results:

For this example:

$$s = \sqrt{\frac{0.16}{9}} = 0.13$$

In the clinical hematology laboratory, the standard deviation is an extremely helpful measure, and it is used more extensively than the variance. When the standard deviation is used together with the mean, the shape of the normal distribution curve is completely defined. When the normal curve is drawn on the standard deviation scale in positive and negative directions from the mean (see Fig. 46-3), 68.27% of the values fall within the area under the curve that is enclosed by lines ± 1 SD from the mean, 95.45% of the values fall within the area that is ± 2 SD from the mean, and 99.73% of the values fall within the area ± 3 SD from the mean. This principle is embodied in a large portion of all QC programs in the clinical laboratory. Analytical values outside ± 3 SD are statistically unacceptable; they should be within ± 3 SD when the analysis is properly performed and in control.

Coefficient of Variation

Standard deviation is expressed in the same units of measurement as the value being analyzed. It can be expected to increase as the concentration of analyte increases. It is therefore impossible to compare the variation between methods that use different units for reporting results. It is likewise impossible to compare the variation between methods if specimens of different concentration are used to evaluate the methods. For example, an SD of $5.0 \times 10^9/L$ does not give any idea of the quality of the measurement unless one knows the mean cell count for the measurements from which the SD was derived. If the mean were $7 \times 10^9/L$, an SD of $5.0 \times 10^9/L$ would indicate poor precision for the method evaluated, whereas if the mean were $300 \times 10^9/L$, the SD of $5.0 \times 10^9/L$ would be excellent. For example, in the hematology laboratory, an SD of $5.0 \times 10^9/L$ would be acceptable for platelet counts but not for leukocyte counts. This dilemma is solved by expressing the SD as a fraction of the mean; that is, by converting the SD into percentage form.

The coefficient of variation (CV) is calculated as the SD (s) divided by the mean ($\overline{x}$) and expressed as a percentage (see Table 46-1). The CV gives a more understandable picture of the deviation regardless of the nature of the measurement or method.

Standard Error of the Mean

Commonly, the standard deviation of a sampling distribution of a statistic is referred to as the standard error of that statistic. When a sample is taken of a population to make an inference about that population, the standard error of the sample mean is referred to as the standard error of the mean (SEM) and is calculated as shown in Table 46-1. Note that as the standard deviation (s) decreases and the number of observations in the sample (n) increases, the SEM decreases. The lower the SEM, the less a sample mean varies due to chance. Thus, it is advisable to have as large a sample as possible in any statistical study of this nature.

With a sample size of at least 30, the SEM may be used to calculate the 95% confidence limits (approximately ±2 SD of the mean) commonly used for determining reference ranges. This range is calculated as:

$$\bar{x} \pm \frac{2s}{\sqrt{n}}$$

For the study in Table 46-1, the 95% confidence limits based on the SEM would be 15.2 to 15.6 g/dL according to the following calculations:

$$15.4 - \frac{2(0.63)}{\sqrt{30}} = 15.2 \text{ and } 15.4 + \frac{2(0.63)}{\sqrt{30}} = 15.6$$

The 95% confidence limits predict a range of values within which the true population mean will fall 95% of the time.

Determining Population Reference Ranges

The purpose of most statistical studies is to make accurate and unbiased generalizations about measurements on the basis of samples taken from certain populations. A population is the whole group about which specific information is required, whereas the sample is any portion of the fully defined population. Most of the time, a sample is the only means by which inferences about the population as a whole can be made.

In hematology and hemostasis testing, the most important application in selecting a population sample is in the determination of reference ranges, which is required in all laboratories to establish what is "normal" for healthy persons in the population from which the patients come. The concept of a reference range is now used in laboratories to indicate that a reported patient value falling within this range corresponds with those values in a reference group that is presumed to be free of any condition that might distort the measurement. The use of reference ranges is important to both clinicians and laboratorians, especially in hematology, where multiple values are measured simultaneously and the coordinated interpretation of more than one test frequently is used in diagnosis and treatment. Reference ranges include the expected intraindividual and interindividual nonpathologic sources of variation and help to discern whether a patient's value is pathologic or simply indicative of the usual physiologic variations of the analyte in that patient population.

It is recommended that each laboratory establish its own reference ranges for all tests performed, both when tests are introduced and when they are modified. In designing a statistical study to obtain reference ranges based on samples, it is important to establish the method of sampling to be used prior to data collection. Once data are collected, the frequency distribution curve of that data indicates the type of statistical analysis required. Unfortunately, the process of obtaining and characterizing reference values is fraught with problems both in selecting the population samples and in the methods of statistical analysis. These problems can be overcome for the most part, however, and valid reference ranges can be determined.

Selecting and Testing Samples from the Population to Determine the Reference Range

Ideally, one should use at least 40 subjects, and preferably more, who provide the necessary variety of demographic factors (*e.g.*, sex, age, and race) and who do not have any conditions that might influence the measurement under study. Of course, data from populations that are expected to be different, such as adults and children, should not be mixed, because the reference ranges are expected to be different. It often is difficult for a laboratory to obtain a suitable subject population.

All personnel normally responsible for specimen analysis should be involved in determination of the reference range, and the samples collected for this determination should be treated just the same as the patient specimens. Only five to ten samples should be drawn and tested per day; if all samples are drawn and analyzed at the same time, an erroneous reference range may be determined because of transient instrument or reagent differences, which cannot be accounted for when analyzing samples over a short period of time. The reader is referred to Chapter 62 for a discussion of factors that must be considered in selecting subjects for a reference range study for hemostasis tests and for further details on the general rules for testing specimens in a reference range study.

Selecting Statistical Methods to Determine the Reference Range

Once sufficient data have been obtained, the frequency distribution histogram may be plotted (Fig. 46-5) to determine whether the data have a Gaussian (normal) (see Fig. 46-3) or skewed (lognormal) (see Fig. 46-4) distribution. In addition, if any outliers are found among the data, these should be investigated further to see if there is any explanation for them, such as a previously undiagnosed abnormal hematologic condition. If an explanation is found, these data should not be used in the determination of the reference range.

From the distribution curve, the method of statistical analysis may be chosen. In the unusual event that the curve is Gaussian, as is the case in Figure 46-5, the mean ±2 SD may be calculated, as explained earlier in this chapter, to obtain the reference range. If a frequency histogram is only slightly skewed, the reference range may be determined simply by excluding 2.5% of the values at the lower end and 2.5% of the values at the upper end of the range of values obtained.[19] Thus, in this procedure, the 95% range of values is taken as representing the reference range. Table 46-2 presents an eosinophil reference range study for which this procedure was used to determine the population reference range, even though the data are skewed (see Fig. 46-7).

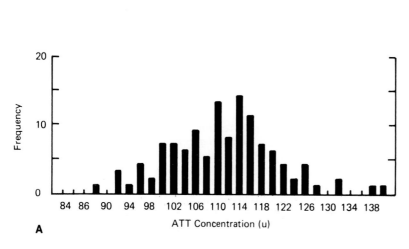
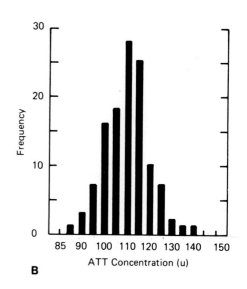

FIG. 46-5.   Frequency distribution histograms show number of results falling at various intervals across range of values obtained in any given reference range study. In this example, study of antithrombin III was performed to obtain reference range for local patient population. (*A*) Data have been grouped in intervals of 2 units. (*B*) Data have been grouped in intervals of 5 units; note how same data can look different graphically although both form normal Gaussian curve. $(\bar{x})$ = 111.6; standard deviation (s) = 9.5 units. (From Cembrowski GS, Sullivan AM: Quality control and statistics. In Bishop ML, Duben–Von Laufen JL, Fody EP (eds): Clinical Chemistry: Principles, Procedures, Correlations, p 59. Philadelphia, JB Lippincott, 1985, with permission.)

TABLE 46–2. Eosinophil Reference Range Data for Frequency Histogram* and Cumulative Frequency Histogram**

EOSINOPHIL INTERVAL (%)	# OF SUBJECTS	CUMULATIVE NUMBER	CUMULATIVE PERCENT
0.0	5	5	2.9—2.5%
0.5	10	15	8.8
1.0	28	43	25.3
1.5	21	64	37.6
2.0	25	89	52.4
2.5	16	105	61.8
3.0	14	119	70.0
3.5	19	138	81.2
4.0	9	147	86.5
4.5	7	154	90.6
5.0	6	160	94.1
5.5	4	164	96.5
6.0	0	164	96.5
			—97.5%
6.5	3	167	98.2
7.0	0	167	98.2
7.5	0	167	98.2
8.0	0	167	98.2
8.5	0	167	98.2
9.0	1	168	98.8
9.5	1	169	99.4
10.0	0	169	99.4
10.5	1	170	100.0

Reference range is determined by the eosinophil interval % closest to 2.5% and 97.5% cumulative percent. In this study, the population reference range is 0.0 to 6.0% eosinophils. Cumulative number represents a running total of the number of subjects. Cumulative percent represents the cumulative number divided by the number of subjects in the study (n = 170). For example, 10 subjects had an average of 0.5 eosinophils per 100 leukocytes differentiated. The cumulative number at that point is 15 (10 + 5 subjects who had 0% eosinophils on the differential) and the cumulative percent is 8.8 ((15/170) × 100%). Courtesy of Duke University Department of Laboratory Medicine, Durham, NC.

* See Figure 46-7.
** See Figure 46-8.

If the curve is skewed calculation of the reference range is a little more complicated. Most biologic measurements do not fit Gaussian frequency distributions;[2] rather, they often form a skewed curve (see Fig. 46-4).[15] If the mean and SD are calculated from data that are not Gaussian, the results may be nonsensical. For example, the mean ±2 SD may give a reference range with a lower limit that is a negative number, whereas no hematologic measure is expected to have a negative value. In a study of the mean ±2 SD for the ESR reference range, the calculation might well yield a range of –6 to 18 mm/hour, whereas the lowest possible true result is 0. Therefore, in order to apply parametric statistical analysis (*e.g.*, mean, median, mode, SD, CV), the raw data must be transformed to fit a distribution that is Gaussian.

Such a transformation of data may be performed in several ways. One method, applicable for slightly skewed distribution curves, requires plotting a cumulative frequency histogram on probability paper, as shown in Figure 46-6. Note that this method makes the Gaussian distribution linear and allows drawing of the best fit line. From this curve, the values that correspond to 2.5% and 97.5% cumulative frequency determine the 95% confidence limits and thus the reference range for that measure. For the antithrombin III study in Figure 46-6, the 95% limits for the reference range are 92.5 and 129 U.

For significantly skewed distributions, such as that in Figure 46-7 (for which the raw data are shown in Table 46-2), which result in a curved cumulative frequency histogram when plotted on probability paper (Fig. 46-8), it is difficult to draw a best fit line. However, determination of the 95% confidence limits using this probability plot is still valid because the percentiles are unaffected by the curved form of the graph. From Figure 46-8 and Table 46-2, the 2.5 and 97.5 percentile limits that establish the overall 95% confidence limits are 0 to 6 eosinophils.

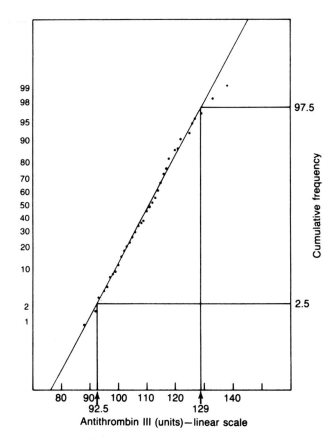

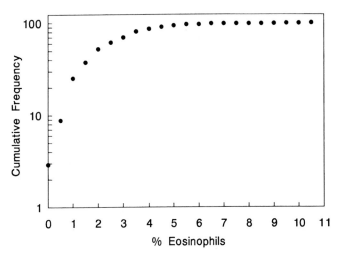

FIG. 46-8.   Linear scale probability plot for eosinophil reference range study. (Courtesy of Duke University Department of Laboratory Medicine, Durham, NC.)

FIG. 46-6.   Cumulative frequency histogram or probability plot for antithrombin III using linear scale. Line represents best fit; 92.5 and 129 represent the 2.5 and 97.5 percentiles, respectively, and indicate the 95% reference range values. (From Cembrowski GS, Sullivan AM: Quality control and statistics. In Bishop ML, Duben–Von Laufen JL, Fody EP (eds): Clinical Chemistry: Principles, Procedures, Correlations, p 66. Philadelphia, JB Lippincott, 1985, with permission.)

As an alternative, skewed data distributions can, in some cases, be transformed to normal distributions using a lognormal data transformation. This may be accomplished by using graph paper with a logarithmic scale on one axis and a normal-probability scale on the other. Because a skewed distribution curve is not always indicative of a lognormal distribution, the assumption of a lognormal distribution must be tested. On testing the data from Figure 46-8, there was no significant improvement in the linearity of the data. The 95% reference range using the lognormal transformation method was 0.5 to 7, not a clinically significant difference from the range determined by the probability plot in Figure 46-8.

Lognormal data transformation may also be performed by converting all data to logarithmic form, then plotting the cumulative frequency against these values on a linear scale. If the resulting best fit line is linear, the log values of the 2.5 and 97.5 percentiles indicating the 95% reference range may be determined. The antilog of these values is then taken to obtain the final reference range.

In many cases, transformation by any of the above methods still cannot change the data enough to fit a Gaussian distribution. Alternatively, nonparametric statistics may be used, which are not as dependent on the distribution of the data being normal or Gaussian as are the parametric statistics such as mean and standard deviation. Refer to standard statistical texts for further information on nonparametric analysis.

The choice of statistical analysis method can greatly affect the reference range. Thus, it can be seen that reference ranges do not provide final definitive diagnostic guidelines; rather, they provide 95% interval estimates for biological measures.

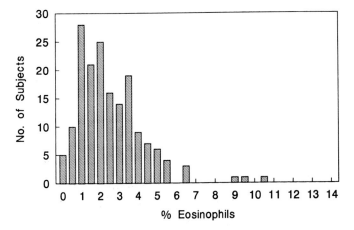

FIG. 46-7.   Skewed frequency histogram from eosinophil reference range study. Corresponding probability plot is shown in Figure 46-8. (Courtesy of Duke University Department of Laboratory Medicine, Durham, NC.)

Statistical Measures of Correlation Between Two Methods

Part of laboratory QA and QC involves the evaluation and selection of satisfactory instrumentation and methodologies for measurement of one or more values. For example, a new instrument may be advertised to be faster, less expensive, more precise, and more accurate than other instruments for performing CBCs. Many aspects must be considered in such an evaluation, and these are discussed in more detail later in this chapter. At this point, the statistical tools for evaluation of a new method or instrument will be discussed.

Statistical analysis is required for the comparison-of-methods study, which is one of the last steps in the method or instrument evaluation process. If all other aspects of an instrument or method are found to be satisfactory, such as precision and accuracy, then the laboratory must compare the new method with the current method, or, if possible, a reference method, to determine whether the two methods agree.

The recommended statistical tools for comparison of methods are regression analysis and $s_{y/x}$, the standard deviation of the regression line, sometimes abbreviated as $s_{y \cdot x}$ (Table 46-3). Regression analysis measures the strength of association or correlation between two methods. The $s_{y/x}$ measures intermethod imprecision by calculating the deviation of sample points from the estimated regression line. Another commonly used statistic to be discussed in this section is the correlation coefficient; however, it has been suggested that this statistic may not be useful for determining agreement between two methods.[21]

Regression Analysis

When two methods are compared, the strength of the association between their results is indicated in terms of correlation. The same variables from each method are represented by paired data points. Traditionally, data from the current or reference method are plotted on the x axis and data from the new method on the y axis to produce a scatter plot (Fig. 46-9). Although the best fit line may be drawn visually to estimate the agreement between the two methods, a more accurate calculation of the agreement may be obtained through *regression analysis*. A straight line through the points is obtained called the *linear regression line* or *least-squares line*. This line of best fit is calculated so that the sum of the squares of the deviations from the points to the line is the least. This line may be represented by the formula:

$$y = y_o + bx$$

where y_o is the y intercept (the value of y at x = 0) and b is the slope of the line.

The y intercept is an indication of one form of systematic error called *constant error*. The slope determines the other type of systematic error, called *proportional error*. Both of these errors are discussed below and shown in Figure 46-9.

Calculation of the regression line slope (b) usually is performed by a computer using the following formula:

$$b = \frac{n\Sigma x_i y_i - \Sigma x_i \Sigma y_i}{n\Sigma x_i^2 - (\Sigma x_i)^2}$$

The y intercept is calculated based on the slope (b) and the means of all observations in each method:

$$y_o = \frac{\Sigma y_i}{n} - \frac{b\, \Sigma x_i}{n}$$

OR

$$y_o = \bar{y} - b\bar{x}$$

Figure 46-9 demonstrates the hypothetical results of six comparison-of-methods regression analysis studies that illustrate various kinds of error. Figure 46-9B through F should be compared with Figure 46-9A which shows perfect agreement between two methods because the y intercept is 0 and the slope is 1.0. Figure 46-9B illustrates a test method with a constant systematic error: it has consistently higher measurements than the reference method, as indicated by the y intercept of 5.0. Figure 46-9C shows a y intercept of 0 but a slope of 1.1, indicating that unless the analyte being measured has a value of 0, the test method measures are higher than those of the reference method. Figure 46-9D illustrates a test method where the measures are lower than those of the comparative method for all nonzero values, as the y intercept is again 0, but the slope is 0.9 (*i.e.*, less than 1). Both Figures 46-9C and 46-9D reflect proportional systematic error because the difference between the test and the reference method is proportional to the analyte value.

Standard Deviation of the Regression Line (Standard Error of Estimate)

One statistical measure of the degree of scatter about the regression line is the standard error of estimate, which is denoted $s_{y/x}$. This is defined as the average SD of the y values for a given x in a comparison of methods experiment (*i.e.*, the standard deviation around the regression line in the y direction) and is expressed in the units of measurement contained in the data groups. It is calculated as follows:

$$s_{y/x} = \sqrt{\frac{1}{n-2}\left[\left[\Sigma y_i^2 - \frac{(\Sigma y_i)^2}{n}\right] - \frac{\left[\Sigma x_i y_i - \frac{(\Sigma x_i)\,(\Sigma y_i)}{n}\right]^2}{\Sigma x_i^2 - \frac{(\Sigma x_i)^2}{n}}\right]}$$

The $s_{y/x}$ is a measure of random error (*i.e.*, error attributable to chance). It measures intermethod imprecision.

Figure 46-9E and F graphically demonstrate the effects of a nonzero $s_{y/x}$. When this value is 0 as it is in Figure 46-9A through 46-9D, there is no scatter about the regression line.

TABLE 46-3. Statistical Analysis of Paired Samples Recommended in Method Comparison*

ANALYTICAL METHOD	COMMENTS
Scatter plot	Graph results of each specimen using reference (or currently used) method and new test method (Fig. 46-9)
Linear regression analysis	Use 100 samples, if possible, 5 per day over 20 days
Slope	Proportional systematic error
y intercept	Constant systematic error
$s_{y/x}$ (SD of regression line)	Intermethod random error

* These tests are a part of the total procedure required for comparison of a new test method with a reference method or the method currently in use in a laboratory, as outlined in Table 46-4.

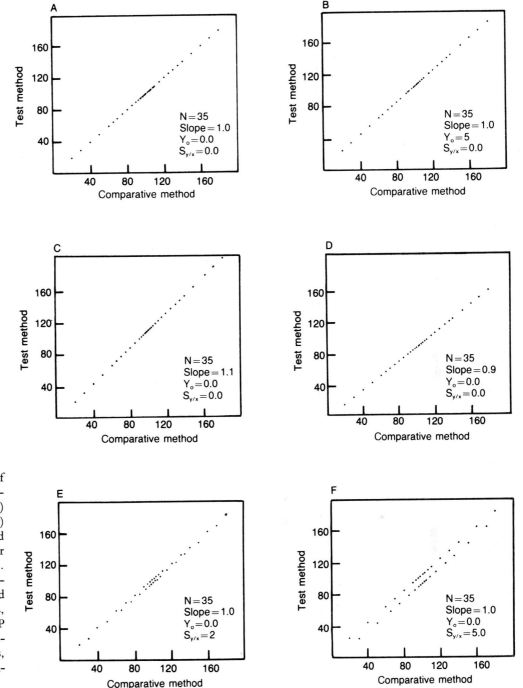

FIG. 46-9. Comparison of methods experiments using simulated data. (A) No error. (B) Constant error ($Y_o = 5$). (C, D) Proportional error (slope 1.1 and 0.9). (E, F) Random error ($S_{y/x} = 2$ and 5, respectively). (From Cembrowski GS, Sullivan AM: Quality control and statistics. In Bishop ML, Duben–Von Laufen JL, Fody EP (eds): Clinical Chemistry: Principles, Procedures, Correlations, p 62. Philadelphia, JB Lippincott, 1985, with permission.)

In Figure 46-9E and 46-9F, the values of 2 and 5, respectively, were alternately added and subtracted from each value in Figure 46-9A, where there was a perfect correlation between methods, causing the scatter shown on each graph and increased $s_{y/x}$ values.

Correlation Coefficient
The Pearson correlation coefficient (r) may be used in method comparisons for measuring how closely the points cluster about the regression line.
The calculation is:

$$r = \frac{n\Sigma x_i y_i - \Sigma x_i \Sigma y_i}{\sqrt{(n\Sigma x_i^2 - (\Sigma x_i)^2) \times (n\Sigma y_i^2 - (\Sigma y_i)^2)}}$$

The r value has been popular because it is a straightforward measure of correlation between two methods with values ranging from -1 (perfect negative correlation) through 0 (no correlation) to +1 (perfect positive correlation). Although the r often has been used in method comparisons, it is not advisable to rely on this value alone for conclusive information. Other statistical measures such as $s_{y/x}$ and visual inspection of the regression line also should be used to make valid conclusions in method comparisons.

The disadvantages of the correlation coefficient include its sensitivity to random error, outliers, and the range of concentration of the analyte.[38] Sensitivity to these factors can be considered a drawback in method comparison. Furthermore, the correlation coefficient is not sensitive to constant or proportional error,[21] which are important factors in a method comparison. The correlation coefficient may, however, be helpful in determining when an alternate method of regression analysis is necessary, such as weighted regression or transformation of the data (*e.g.*, logarithmic transformation or square root transformation).[13]

T-Tests and F Ratios

The *t*-test and F ratio are two inferential values that are discussed in most standard statistical texts. These values have been and continue to be used by some investigators in comparing methods; however, their real value in such comparisons is questionable.[21]

The *t*-test is used to determine whether there is a statistically significant difference between the actual means of two groups of data.[10] The *paired t*-test is used to compare the mean of the differences between positively correlated pairs of results such as the results in a comparison-of-methods study, the results being obtained on the same blood specimen using the two methods or instruments. An important reason that the *t*-test is not recommended for use in comparative studies is that it may show a statistically significant bias between two methods that may not be clinically significant.

The F ratio is used in method comparison to determine whether there is a statistically significant difference between the standard deviations of two methods. Like the *t*-test, it does not indicate clinical significance. Indeed, Westgard and Hunt state that the F ratio should not be used to determine whether a test or method is acceptable.[38]

Comments on Statistical Analysis in Comparison of Methods

Regression analysis frequently is used in method comparisons, because it quantitates the correlation between two data groups and can indicate the positive or negative bias of one group compared with the other. It is important to note, however, that *all* summary statistics (*i.e.*, y intercept, slope, and $s_{y/x}$) obtained from the linear regression analysis should be used to describe the association between two methods to prevent an erroneous interpretation of the data.

A set of guidelines for method comparisons has been proposed by the National Committee for Clinical Laboratory Standards (NCCLS).[28]

COMPONENTS OF A QUALITY ASSURANCE PROGRAM

Basic Requirements

Meaningful QA in hematology, as in all other areas of the laboratory, requires an appreciation that a good portion of the activities occur away from the laboratory. Monitoring the processing of test measurements therefore is only a part of the program. The laboratory must design a program that encompasses all activities rather than limiting its scope to data acquisition. These activities can be divided into two basic types, nonanalytic control and analytic QC, both of which are important in QA.

Nonanalytic Control Functions

Nonanalytic activities encompass all those not directly related to the performance of the clinical assay itself. These include control procedures for preanalytic functions such as test ordering; patient preparation and identification; and specimen collection, identification, transport, accession, and handling prior to analysis.[20] Also included are control procedures for such postanalytic functions as reporting results and test charging mechanisms. A procedure manual concerning all nonanalytic activities should be available to appropriate laboratory personnel.

Analytic Quality Control Functions

Analytic activities and their control are discussed in detail in the remainder of this chapter and in Chapters 47 and 48.

Method and Instrument Evaluation and Selection

An analytic method is defined as "a set of instructions which describe the procedure, materials, and equipment which are necessary for the analyst to obtain a result."[9] A well-conceived QA program should include procedures to be used in the evaluation and selection of analytic instruments and methods. In this manner, a consistent and objective evaluation can be performed, resulting in selection of methods of the highest quality and reliability. The evaluation results show the laboratory both the strengths and the weaknesses of each method or instrument, and provide standards for comparing alternatives. Information about the performance of an analytic method or instrument should be obtained prior to purchase or use in the processing of patient specimens. This performance is judged on both the *feasibility* and *analytic reliability* of the method. Table 46-4 summarizes the factors for consideration in method and instrument evaluation and selection.

Feasibility

Feasibility is evaluated on the basis of speed, cost, technical skill required, dependability, and safety. *Speed* encompasses both turnaround time (the time needed for analysis of one specimen) and throughput (the number of specimens that can be analyzed per unit of time under routine conditions). Time spent on required maintenance, reagent preparation, calibration, and troubleshooting also must be considered. The *cost* per assay includes both the cost of all materials and an established value for technologist time. *Dependability* is assessed by the average frequency and duration of breakdowns or method failure.

Analytic Reliability

The reliability of a proposed method is judged on the basis of many factors (see Table 46-4). The magnitude of analytic variation also reflects reliability and requires further explanation.

ANALYTIC VARIATION: PRECISION. Analytic variation can be divided into two types: random and systematic. The term *precision* is often used when referring to random analytic variation. It is assessed by performing replicate analyses of a biologic specimen containing stable amounts

TABLE 46–4. Factors to be Considered in Method and Instrument Evaluation and Selection

FEASIBILITY	Speed	Turnaround time; throughput
	Cost	Materials; technologist time
	Technical skill required	Higher skill levels cost more money
	Dependability	Average frequency and duration of breakdowns
	Safety	
ANALYTIC RELIABILITY	Sensitivity	Minimum concentration of constituent method is capable of measuring; reliability of test being positive when condition to be detected IS present
	Specificity	Extent to which test measures only single constituent; reliability of test being negative when condition to be detected is NOT present
	Dynamic range	Range of test linearity without specimen dilution
	Freedom from interference	Effects of interfering substances and factors (*e.g.*, hemolysis, lipemia, cold agglutinins, platelet clumps)
	Magnitude of analytic variation	Random variation (precision); systematic variation (accuracy)

of a constituent and is expressed as the magnitude of error inherent in the method. The NCCLS has described a protocol for establishing the precision of automated analytic systems[4] in which a distinction is made between the total random analytic variation and the within-run or within-day variation (short-term imprecision). The total variation includes all components that affect method performance, including within-run, run-to-run, and day-to-day variation, as well as the stability of materials and calibration factors.

Hackney and Cembrowski[21] have made recommendations for measurement of within-day and day-to-day imprecision. Both measurement types may be performed during the same period. For measurement of within-day imprecision, those authors recommend ten replicate analyses of five to ten samples that represent the various levels of medical interest. The samples should be a mixture of patient and control specimens. Tests of within-day imprecision should be run over a 3-to 5-day period (using different samples) to avoid bias on any given day. For measurement of day-to-day imprecision, those same authors recommend that two or three levels of control material be analyzed three or four times per day, these levels being normal, low abnormal, and high abnormal.[21] Because such a study should extend over at least 7 days and if possible, 20 days using the same material, stabilized control material is used: patient specimens are stable for only 24 hours at best. Hackney and Cembrowski[21] recommend analysis of each control level four times per day for the 7- to 20-day period.

To evaluate the data for imprecision, the mean value of the data for the within-day and day-to-day categories is calculated, and the associated dispersion is calculated as the SD and CV. These values may then be compared with the known SD and CV for the reference or current method.

ANALYTIC VARIATION: ACCURACY. The systematic analytic variation is the accuracy of a proposed method and is defined as the extent to which measurements approach the "true value" of the constituent being analyzed. This analytic bias may be measured in several ways.

Assessing the Magnitude of Analytic Bias
Different methods have been suggested for assessing the magnitude of bias of any given laboratory procedure in-

cluding the use of control specimens assayed by different methods, comparison of the new method with a proven method using both "normal" donor specimens and patient specimens, and the use of recovery experiments.[2,37,38] Recovery experiments are rarely, if ever, used in hematology and so will not be discussed.

In the first approach, commercial control samples are obtained that have a stated value for the constituent in question. The control specimens should cover a broad range of values and must be compatible with the manual or automated methods in use. With linear regression analysis, the relation between the observed values and the stated control values may be assessed for all methods and the magnitude of any bias determined. Both constant (y intercept) and proportional (slope of the regression line) biases can be detected by this method (see Fig. 46-9).

When using the technique of comparison with a proven method, a number of specimens are assayed using the new method and a comparison method. About 40 patient specimens spanning the entire analytic range are assayed by the two methods. If the study is to be published in a medical journal, at least 100 specimens should be analyzed to ensure adequate data.[21] The selection of the comparison method is important.

Selection of Instrumentation and Reagents
An integral part of method evaluation is the use of high-quality materials. These include everything from expendables used for specimen collection, processing, storage, and preservation to reagents and standards to miscellaneous equipment, such as centrifuges and thermometers, to the instruments themselves.

The selection of reagents and instrumentation should be made according to the unique requirements of the individual laboratory, as well as the general performance characteristics of the product. In the case of reagents and controls, these general characteristics are included in the manufacturer's data sheet. If an in-house evaluation is not possible, it is best to base the decision on results obtained at a well known, reliable institution. The results from a widely used comprehensive proficiency survey may be helpful as well. But remember, surveys use stabilized specimens, which may introduce other problems. Selection of analytic instrumentation is particularly important and usually is based on a number of factors, including those listed in Table 46-4 and manufacturer support and reputation. Certain intangible factors relating to how the proposed system fits with existing space, personnel, preferences, and equipment (*e.g.*, computer information systems) cannot be ignored.

Establishment of Control Procedures

When a new analytic test is introduced to the clinical laboratory, it is imperative that its performance reliability be maintained under day-to-day operating conditions. Various control protocols should be established to involve all laboratory personnel responsible for performing the procedure. The purpose of these control procedures is threefold: (1) to assess the laboratory's usual analytic performance realistically and establish acceptable limits of error; (2) to identify significant problems or errors; and (3) to document all QC results and any corrective action taken. With these objectives in mind, the statistical control procedures should be designed so that the expected frequency of analytic errors is taken into consideration for each individual method or instrument. Ideally, a control procedure should be designed to have a very low probability for false rejections (rejection of a run with no errors) and a very high probability for error detection.

Biologic Controls

The widely accepted practice of running whole blood controls along with patient samples provides the most common means by which clinical laboratories maintain performance reliability and identify significant problems. These biologic control materials can be used in a number of ways (Chaps. 47 and 48) and can be of two types, either commercial stabilized control products or retained patient specimens.

Control Result Limits Requiring Staff Action

Control procedures establish the means by which abnormal, erroneous, or out-of-control results can be detected. When control limits are exceeded (*i.e.*, the control value falls outside of the 3 SD range), action by the staff is mandatory. Tolerance limits must be established for each of the following aspects of a QC program: biologic control materials (commercial controls and retained patient specimens), instrument function checks, interlaboratory comparisons, and proficiency testing. If the tolerance limits are too narrow, an inordinate amount of time and effort will be spent pursuing insignificant problems. If the limits are too broad, significant problems may go uncorrected. Specific methods utilized for these different aspects of a QC program are discussed in Chapters 47 and 48.

Once out-of-control situations or abnormal patient results have been identified, action must be taken according to an established mechanism. This protocol should delineate the steps to be followed by personnel to differentiate the specimens involved in an out-of-control situation from those that are clinically abnormal. If the test system is out of control, procedures must be in place either to rectify the problem or to utilize an alternative method to obtain accurate results on the samples incorrectly analyzed. Likewise, in the case of an abnormal specimen or one containing interfering substances, specific procedures should be written that include the abnormal indicators to identify such a specimen as well as the action to be taken to obtain accurate results.

Monitoring and Documenting Control Results

A monitoring program should be established to evaluate, display, organize, summarize, and document statistically the results obtained from control procedures. This type of program usually involves one or more charting techniques, sophisticated statistical analyses and data management systems, multirule QC algorithms, and the Bull algorithm.[8] These are discussed in Chapter 47.

CHAPTER SUMMARY

In the last 15 years the clinical hematology laboratory has seen tremendous change in all aspects with the advent of fully automated, multiparameter, high-speed hematology analyzers. Nationwide, standardization techniques have been increasingly accepted, and significant improvements have been made in reagent and control stability.

Although many powerful techniques and procedures have been developed recently for assessing and monitoring the quality of all these changes, a complex job still exists for the laboratorian within the hematology area. The supervisor is well challenged when establishing a QC program for formative instrumentation and new analytic measurements to ensure the highest-quality results. To increase that challenge, the laboratory may be forced to develop such a program within narrow financial constraints. To meet this challenge the laboratory scientist must be constantly aware of new developments in laboratory hematology and be prepared to implement innovative techniques in a constantly evolving, dynamically changing QA program.

REFERENCES

1. Bahn AK: Basic Medical Statistics. New York, Grune & Stratton, 1972
2. Barnett RN: Clinical Laboratory Statistics, 2nd ed. Boston, Little, Brown and Co, 1979
3. Barnett RN, Youden WJ: A revised scheme for the comparison of quantitative methods. Am J Clin Pathol 54:454, 1970
4. Bauer S, Fowle GD Jr, Levine JB et al: Protocol for establishing the precision and accuracy of automated analytic systems PSEP-1. Villanova, PA, National Committee For Clinical Laboratory Standards, 1975
5. Belk WP, Sunderman FW: A survey of the accuracy of chemical analyses in clinical laboratories. Am J Clin Pathol 17:853, 1947
6. Bollinger P, Drewinko B: A quality control program for a computerized, high-volume, automated hematology laboratory. Am J Med Technol 49:9, 1983
7. Brittin GM, Brecher G, Johnson CA et al: Stability of blood in commonly used anticoagulants. Am J Clin Pathol 52:690, 1969
8. Bull BS, Elashoff RM, Heilbron DC et al: A study of various estimators for the deviation of quality control procedures from patient erythrocyte indices. Am J Clin Pathol 61:473, 1974
9. Buttner J, Borth R, Boutwell JH et al: Provisional recommendations on quality control in clinical chemistry. 2: Assessment of analytical methods for routine use. Clin Chim Acta 69:F1, 1976
10. Castle WM: Statistics in Small Doses. New York, Churchill Livingstone, 1977

11. College of American Pathologists: Summing Up: A publication of the Surveys Committee of the College of American Pathologists 14(3):6, Fall 1984

12. Dharan M: Total Quality Control in the Clinical Laboratory. St Louis, CV Mosby, 1977

13. Dixon WJ, Massey FJ: Introduction to Statistical Analysis, p 323. New York, McGraw-Hill, 1969

14. Dodge HF: Using inspection data to control quality. Manufacturing Industries 16:517, 1928

15. Flynn FV, Piper KA, Garcia-Webb P et al: The frequency distribution of commonly determined blood constituents in healthy blood donors. Clin Chim Acta 52:163, 1974

16. Freund JE: Statistics—A First Course. Englewood Cliffs, NJ, Prentice-Hall, 1970

17. Gilmer PR Jr, Williams LJ: The status of methods of calibration in hematology. Am J Clin Pathol 74:600, 1980

18. Gilmer PR Jr, Williams LJ, Koepke JA et al: Calibration methods for automated hematology instruments. Am J Clin Pathol 68:185, 1977

19. Golob JK: Normal ranges in clinical work: Their uses and methods of determination. Am J Med Technol 26:167, 1960

20. Gulati GL, Hyun BH: Quality control in hematology. Clin Lab Med 6:675, 1986

21. Hackney JR, Cembrowski GS: Need for improved instrument and kit evaluations. Am J Clin Pathol 86:391, 1986

22. International Committee for Standardization in Haematology: Recommendation for haemoglobinometry in human blood. Br J Haematol 13(suppl): 71, 1967

23. International Committee for Standardization in Haematology: Recommendations for reference method for haemoglobinometry in human blood. J Clin Pathol 31:139, 1978

24. International Committee for Standardization in Haematology: Recommended Methods for the Determination of Packed Cell Volume. Geneva, World Health Organization, 1980

25. King JW, Willis CE: Cyanmethemoglobin certification program of the College of American Pathologists. Am J Clin Pathol 54:496, 1970

26. Koepke JA: The calibration of automated instruments for accuracy in hemoglobinometry. Am J Clin Pathol 68:180, 1977

27. Levey S, Jennings ER: The use of control charts in the clinical laboratory. Am J Clin Pathol 20:1059, 1950

28. National Committee for Clinical Laboratory Standards: User comparison of quantitative clinical laboratory methods using patient samples, EP9-P, Vol 6, p 1. Villanova, PA, NCCLS, 1986

29. Savage RA: Calibration bias and imprecision for automated hematology analyzers: An evaluation of significance of short-term bias resulting from calibration of an analyzer with S-Cal. Am J Clin Pathol 84:186, 1985

30. Schonberger RJ: Japanese Manufacturing Techniques: Nine Hidden Lessons in Simplicity. New York, Free Press, 1982

31. Shewhart WA: Economic Control of Quality of Manufactured Products. New York, Van Nostrand Reinhold, 1931

32. Skendzel LP, Barnett RN, Platt R: Medically useful criteria for analytic performance of laboratory tests. Am J Clin Pathol 83:200, 1985

33. Statland BE, Westgard JO: Quality control: Theory and practice. In Henry JB (ed): Clinical Diagnosis and Management by Laboratory Methods, 17th ed, p 74. Philadelphia, WB Saunders, 1984

34. Statland BE, Winkel P: Sources of variation in laboratory measurements. In Henry JB (ed): Clinical Diagnosis and Management by Laboratory Methods, 16th ed. Philadelphia, WB Saunders, 1979

35. van Assendelft OW, England JM: Terms, quantities and units. In: Advances in Hematological Methods: The Blood Count. Boca Raton, FL, CRC Press, 1982

36. van Kampen EJ, Zijlstra WG: Standardization in hemoglobinometry. II: The hemiglobincyanide method. Clin Chim Acta 6:538, 1961

37. Wakkers PJM, Hellendoorn HB, Op-de-Weegh GJ et al: Applications of statistics in clinical chemistry: A critical evaluation of regression lines. Clin Chim Acta 64:173, 1975

38. Westgard JO, Hunt MR: Use and interpretation of common statistical tests in method comparison studies. Clin Chem 19:49, 1973

47

Methods to Monitor and Control Systematic Error

Mary Ann Dotson

A systematic error affects all samples equally in a proportionate or constant manner. Improper instrument calibration or loss of calibration secondary to malfunction are causes of systematic errors. Such errors are detected and corrected by a quality control (QC) program, a series of activities performed to ensure accuracy and precision of results and include calibration, internal and external monitoring of accuracy, documentation, preventive maintenance, and troubleshooting—all of which are essential.

CALIBRATION

Calibration involves any adjustments made to an instrument to correct the results recovered so that they match "truth," which is defined by standards or reference procedures.

Standards: Primary Versus Secondary

A primary standard is a pure chemical substance that can be weighed and placed in solution. A glucose standard of 50 mg/dL is an example of a primary standard. A secondary standard is a biologic specimen in which the analyte in question is measured by an accurate reference method. A cyanmethemoglobin standard is an example of a secondary standard. The cyanmethemoglobin standard is also an example of an international standard in that the International Committee for Standardization in Haematology (ICSH) certifies well-characterized physical and chemical properties of this reference material. Secondary standards may be used to make instrument calibration adjustments. Fresh whole blood samples drawn from healthy donors become secondary standards when tested by reference methods.

Reference Methods

Reference methods that are acceptable for instrument calibration have been selected by the ICSH and by the National Committee for Clinical Laboratory Standards (NCCLS). A reference method is one whose accuracy has been well established over the years by independent means. When a reference method is used on a sample of blood, that sample becomes a secondary standard with a known value that is a reasonable estimate of "truth." However, the reference method is accurate only if it is performed correctly. The NCCLS has published detailed documents outlining the correct procedures for hematologic methods, including proper calibration. These documents are also referred to as standards (written standards). Selected committees of the NCCLS may spend as long as 3 years in the development of a document or standard. Each standard goes through three consensus levels of development: proposed, tentative, and approved. Approved documents undergo periodic review and updating. An up-to-date list of these documents can be obtained on request from the NCCLS.*

Calibration by Reference Methods Using Fresh Whole Blood

The ideal method for first time calibration of hematology cell counters uses fresh whole blood and reference methods. Hemoglobin reference values are obtained through photometric measurement of cyanmethemoglobin using a spectrophotometer that has been calibrated with a cyanmethemoglobin standard.[5] Reference erythrocyte and leukocyte counts are determined using a single-channel semiautomated electronic counter that has been calibrated by threshold curve methods.[6] Packed cell volume (PCV) or hematocrit (HCT) is determined using the microhematocrit method without correction for trapped plasma.[8] Reference platelet counts may be performed on a calibrated electronic whole-blood counting instrument.[1]

The numbers of fresh normal whole blood samples and of replicate tests required are given in each reference method procedure. Calibration of multiparameter cell counters using reference methods and fresh whole blood specimens usually is reserved for the initial calibration of a new instrument when no other calibrated multiparameter instrument is available. Other simpler and less time-consuming methods to be described below are utilized to recalibrate instruments and for the calibration of second- or third-generation instruments.

Preserved Cells as Calibrators for Cell Counters

In the past, a common calibration procedure for cell counters was to adjust the instrument to target values on the insert sheet of a commercial *control* product. This practice is no longer acceptable. Although calibration and control procedures share much in the way of materials and methods, they are fundamentally different. If reference method results on fresh whole blood are not available or another calibrated instrument does not exist in the setting, commercial *calibration* material is available for purchase. Commercial calibration material has assigned values for each parameter. These values are obtained by the manufacturer under strictly controlled conditions using instruments calibrated by whole blood reference methods and are specific for individual instrument-reagent systems. The manufacturers monitor their calibration products throughout the dating period of each lot number. *Control* material, on the other hand, is not as carefully monitored and does not have assigned values. Rather, controls have *ranges* for each measurement.

If commercial calibrating material is used to calibrate an instrument, the following precautions are recommended:

1. The manufacturer of the calibrating material should be *different* from the manufacturer of the control material to be used.
2. The directions from the manufacturer must be followed carefully.
3. The purchase of calibrating material should be handled differently from that of control material because calibration adjustments are not made daily, and the material may inadvertently be kept past its expiration date.

Statistical System for Calibration of Cell Counters

A statistical formula referred to as the Bull algorithm[3] has been proposed as capable of acting as a calibrator. The algorithm is programmed into computers to perform a statistical analysis on patient red cell indices. The predictability and stability of patient indices are resulting in the development of methods to use this algorithm for instrument calibration.

Calibration and Control of Other Equipment

Other equipment used in the hematology laboratory, such as centrifuges, balances, and dilutors, must also be properly calibrated and controlled. It is beyond the scope of this chapter to describe these procedures. Calibration of microscopes is covered in Chapters 4 and 25, HCT centrifuge and spectrophotometer calibration are discussed in Chapter 9, and detailed calibration and control methods for dilutors and balances may be found in standard reference texts for clinical chemistry.

The College of American Pathologists (CAP) publishes the *Laboratory Instrument Verification and Maintenance Manual*, which includes information on requirements, regulations, and standards of the CAP, the Joint Commission on Accreditation of Healthcare Organizations (JCAHO), and NCCLS.[10] Sample forms for documentation, frequency,

---

* National Committee for Clinical Laboratory Standards (NCCLS), 771 East Lancaster Avenue, Villanova, PA 19085.

and type of maintenance for all laboratory equipment are outlined in this publication.

USE OF CONTROLS

Any material used as a "control" for a test procedure should be as nearly identical as possible to the material that will be tested. Fresh whole blood is stable for only a short period before cell deterioration, and death alters the results. Many routine hematology procedures can be performed on blood samples for up to 24 hours if the samples are refrigerated. Sample requirements, storage instructions, stability, and limitations should be written into the laboratory procedure manual.

Commercial Control Material

Automated cell counters prompted the development of commercially prepared control materials, which subsequently became the backbone of most QC systems in hematology. Controls are also available commercially for sickle cell testing and Hb electrophoresis. Commercial controls and QC methods for coagulation are discussed in Chapter 62.

Commercial control material consists of blood cells (human, avian, porcine, and others) that have been "fixed," "buffered," "stabilized," or "preserved," in other words, altered to delay deterioration. Nucleated avian red cells are frequently used as "white" cells in control material. Each manufacturer provides an expiration date for each lot number of control material, which refers to stability of the *unopened* bottle or vial. The information sheet that comes with each package indicates how long a vial should be stable once it has been opened, but this time will be greatly decreased if the material is not handled or stored properly. Evaporation and contamination should also be avoided.

The primary function of commercial controls is to monitor the performance of automated cell counters on a continuing basis. The principal drawback of these materials is their relatively short shelf life. Month-to-month continuity in monitoring is difficult. Most hematology controls have a shelf life of at least 4 weeks. Attempts are being made through modification of the manufacturing process to extend the shelf life beyond a 4- to 6-week period.

Control Levels

Most commercial hematology controls are available at three levels: normal, low, and high, based primarily on red cell parameters. These three levels are a conceptual carry-over from the chemistry laboratory, where it is necessary to check for appropriate substrate availability in enzyme testing, and are relevant in the hemostasis laboratory. However, substrate concentration is not a concern in cell counting or colorimetric tests such as Hb measurement. For these tests, a single level of control material, preferably within the normal range, should be sufficient. The linearity limits of each measurement are published by the manufacturer of the instrument, and the ranges of linearity extend well beyond the values encountered in most samples tested.

In fact, the use of three levels of control material for cell counts increases the chance of error secondary to improper handling or storage of the control. Questions that are raised include: What is done when one control is "out" and the others are "in"? How many times does an abnormal control detect a problem with the instrument that is not detected by the normal-level control? Moreover, a high- or low-level control value that is beyond acceptable limits frequently is attributable to production problems of the control, especially when the normal-level control is within range.[7] Statistically, only 5% of test results should fall beyond two standard deviations from the mean. This number will be greater if three levels of control are tested than if a single level is used.

Target Values in Commercial Control Material

Producers of commercial controls supply an insert or assay sheet with statistical data for each lot number. The mean and range for each measurement are usually listed by instrument type regardless of the reagent system in use. Some companies determine the assay or target values in-house using their own reference methods, whereas other companies send their material to reference laboratories to gather a consensus for each instrument type represented on the assay sheet. The values that are recovered for each measurement differ from instrument to instrument of the same model, from one model to another (same company), and among instruments from different companies. In addition, the values may be reagent system dependent. Each individual instrument "sees" the altered blood product in its own manner, resulting in the generation of different target values and ranges. The method for target value assignment should be noted. Control limits are usually ± 2 standard deviations (SD) from the mean, but this should be confirmed.

Commercial material does deteriorate even though we want to think that it is perfectly acceptable until the expiration date. Shipping conditions and delivery can affect the status of the cells, and original target values may no longer be recovered.

Procedures for Ensuring Validity with Commercial Controls

It is appropriate to overlap the use of old and new control lots when changing lots because most control products change lots every 4 to 6 weeks. New lots should be validated before the old lot becomes outdated. Product changes attributable to shipping and delivery, as well as inaccurate target value assignment, may be detected during this overlap period. Assuming the new lot evaluation is performed using an instrument that is "in control," the mean of the control samples represents the laboratory's target value for the new lot of control. The new control lot is acceptable as long as this value is within the range printed on the manufacturer's assay sheet.

The laboratory's target values do *not* have to match the manufacturer's target or mean values, but if target values outside the manufacturer's suggested ranges are recovered, either the new lot has deteriorated, it is incorrectly labeled, or the instrument is malfunctioning. The manufacturer should always be notified when control material is suspect, and that lot should not be used. If the laboratory's target values are within the specific range but are not the same as the mean specified by the manufacturer, the laboratory should adopt its own target values obtained during the control overlap testing period plus or minus the manufacturer's standard deviation range for that control. Instrument recalibration is not required.

Additionally, a microhematocrit test should be performed on a random bottle from a new shipment to evaluate the amount of color in the "plasma." A pale pink color is not uncommon, but without a baseline color evaluation, it is difficult to tell later if hemolysis caused by red cell destruction has occurred. Another clue to the acceptability of the control product is the histogram pattern produced on many multiparameter instruments. Abnormal patterns may indicate deterioration. The platelet value of a control product that does not contain platelets is actually representative of "debris," which is an indication of control deterioration. All the above information, taken together, is useful in evaluating each bottle as well as the entire lot of control material.

Use of Unassayed Control Products

Some companies offer unassayed control products, although these products are not yet widely used. A concept being evaluated by the NCCLS and the manufacturing community proposes that the manufacturer stop assaying and including target means and ranges with control materials. This change has been suggested because every laboratory should establish its own values on each new lot number of control material when it is received.

Fresh Whole Blood Controls

In recent years, some innovative methods of monitoring instrument stability have been developed using data from samples of fresh whole patient blood. In addition, fresh (less than 1 hour old) whole blood is used as a control in the osmotic fragility and autohemolysis tests. Other examples of special tests that use fresh blood as controls are the Kleihauer Betke stain for fetal Hb and the heat precipitation test for demonstration of Heinz bodies. Special staining procedures use normal blood slide preparations as controls.

Fresh whole blood is the ideal control, because it is identical to the material being tested. Hemoglobin is stable for several days, but platelet and leukocyte counts are affected quickly by aging unless the sample is refrigerated, in which case fresh whole blood can safely be used as a control for 24 hours. It should be noted, however, that leukocyte subpopulations in fresh whole blood (5-part differentials) are stable for only 4 to 8 hours, depending on the instrument used. The reproducibility of the 5-part differential will deteriorate as the sample ages. Sample age is critical because leukocyte subpopulations are identified according to how they are altered by the reagent system.

Within-day Monitoring

A small number of patient blood specimens are tested repeatedly throughout the day to monitor the reproducibility of all values, particularly those for leukocytes and platelets. Standard deviation and coefficient of variation (CV) information must be interpreted according to the number of observations (n) over the 24-hour period (all shifts) and the level or concentration of the measure. Repeat testing at least every 4 hours provides a minimum n of six. If time permits, duplicate testing is encouraged to provide paired data, as well as to increase n to 12.

The concentration of cells greatly influences the SD and CV recovered for leukocyte and platelet counts. For example, if the CV limit is 3.0% for the leukocyte count precision check, this limit may be exceeded with a very low leukocyte count while the SD is well within the acceptable limits. A solution for this problem is to use only the SD for evaluation of low mean values. A second choice is to establish another set of limits for SD and CV for low values.

Day-to-Day Monitoring

Fresh patient specimens that are tested, refrigerated for 24 hours, returned to room temperature, mixed, and tested again can also serve as a check on instrument reproducibility. These samples may be split and a portion used for within-day testing while the other portion is used for 24-hour testing. Five samples should be tested, and a mean for each determination should be established before refrigeration. The 24-hour mean is calculated and compared with the original mean. Differences between the two means are dependent on concentration. The original mean, plus or minus a variable percentage of the mean (which is determined by the laboratory), establishes the limits of acceptability. Plus or minus 0.5 g/dL should be the maximum limit of acceptability for Hb, which changes minimally over 24 hours. Deterioration of leukocyte or platelet counts is not uncommon and should be taken into account to avoid the incorrect conclusion that the instrument is out of control or has lost calibration. Leukocyte subpopulations (5-part differential) are *not* stable for 24 hours.

Frequency of Control Testing

Controls are used to monitor the calibration of instruments from day to day. Repeat testing of patient samples can be used to check instrument function from batch to batch, especially if an hour or more elapses between batches. In laboratories that have large workloads, repeat testing of the same patient sample (so-called secondary controls) should be done every 2 to 3 hours. More frequent checks are provided when a laboratory uses a moving average program (see below). Commercial material is too expensive to use as a batch-to-batch check. Testing of control material (both commercial and patient) may be as frequent as each batch, every 2 to 3 hours, every shift, and from one 24-hour period to the next. When more than 100 patient samples are tested every 24 hours, the moving average program can provide sufficient information to allow commercial control testing to be done once per shift.

Procedures Without Controls

Despite all the technical advances of the last decade, there remain hematology procedures that are difficult to control because appropriate control materials are not available.

These include the erythrocyte sedimentation rate, manual reticulocyte counts, manual leukocyte differential counts, eosinophil counts, and spinal fluid cell counts. In such cases, accuracy and reproducibility are maintained through strict attention to procedure and adequate education of personnel.

QUALITY CONTROL CHARTS AND THEIR INTERPRETATION

Many of the multiparameter hematology instrument systems include computer programs that automatically store and chart data for control materials. This is done for each control level, lot number, and test value. Instruments without QC computer programs require manual charting of the data. The mean and 2 SD ranges of a specific control lot are drawn on manually prepared charts. Every time values are determined on the control material, the results are plotted. The results and the charts should be reviewed regularly. Each lot of control must have its own set of charts.

Levey-Jennings Charts

Levey-Jennings charts are the most commonly used and consist of parallel lines representing the mean ± 1, 2, and 3 SD limits for a single control parameter (Fig. 47-1). Time is plotted along the horizontal axis and analyte concentration along the vertical axis. New charts must be prepared each time a new lot is placed in service.

When a particular determination is "in control," the data points fall within the 2 SD limits and are scattered equally above and below the mean. Five percent of the data points are expected to fall between the 2 SD and 3 SD limits. When this occurs, repeating the control once should bring it back within the 2 SD limits as long as an in-control situation exists. When two or more consecutive values fall between the 2 SD and 3 SD limits, the instrument is considered to be out of control. Any single value beyond 3 SD is out of control. The problem and all corrective action taken must be recorded in a problem log, and controls should be tested after completion of repair work to confirm that the problem has been resolved.

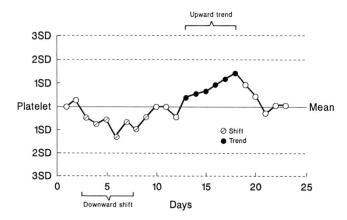

FIG. 47-2. Levey-Jennings control chart of platelet data with downward shift and upward trend indicated. Shift is indicated by six successive data points on same side of mean. Trend is indicated by six successive data points with increasing (or decreasing) values relative to mean.

Out-of-control situations also are identified by reviewing control charts for trends or shifts, either of which suggests a change in instrument function or calibration. An example of a Levey-Jennings chart with acceptable results is shown in Figure 47-1. A downward shift is shown in Figure 47-2. An upward trend is also shown in the same figure (47-2) with the successive data points being increasingly farther from the mean. Some situations that may cause a determination to be out of control are mechanical failure, power surges, improper equipment calibration, technical error, and reagent deterioration or contamination.

Youden Plots

Youden plots may be appropriate when two levels of controls are used; however, these plots are not easily done without a computer program. A modified Youden plot displays single-parameter results from two different levels of control. The chart design is shown in Figure 47-3: a

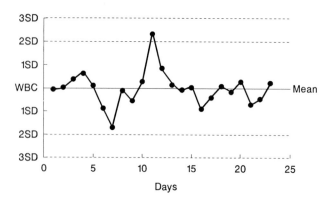

FIG. 47-1. Levey-Jennings chart of WBC control results for 23 days with mean and 1, 2, and 3 SD limits indicated. Distribution is normal and in control.

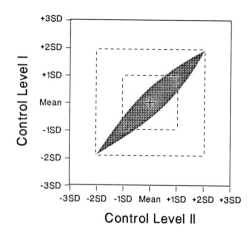

FIG. 47-3. Modified Youden plot for two levels of control material, one plotted on X axis (abscissa) and the second plotted on Y axis (ordinate). Mean and 1, 2, and 3 SD are indicated. Shaded area indicates where results should fall to be in control.

square with the center being the mean of both levels of control. The scaling is difficult to do manually. When both control results are acceptable, the data points will fall along a diagonal line from the lower left (2 SD) corner, shown by the shaded area in Figure 47-3.

Plots that fall in the upper right or the lower left corner suggest random error, which usually is corrected by a single repeat of the control material. Plots falling in the upper left or lower right corners of the chart need immediate attention, because one control is reading too high, whereas the other is reading too low. Patient results should not be reported until corrective action has fixed the problem and the patient samples have been retested under an in-control situation. Control results that fall in any of the four corners indicated as shaded areas on Figure 47-4 also mandate immediate corrective action on the instrument, as results in these areas indicate that both control results are beyond 2 SD. Only 1 in 20 test results is allowed to fall between the 2 SD and 3 SD limits.

Upward shifts and trends are identified on the Youden plot by the accumulation of dots above horizontal line A and to the right of vertical line B (see Fig. 47-4). Downward shifts and trends would be indicated by most dots falling below line A and to the left of line B.

Cumulative Sum Charts

A cumulative sum chart is another monitoring technique consisting of the summation of the differences of each test value from the expected value. This charting technique, commonly called *Cusum*, is not widely used. Once a target value or mean is established for a measurement, this value is subtracted from each subsequent value obtained. The difference is then added to the total of the previous days' differences to calculate the cumulative sum of the differences from the mean. Table 47-1 demonstrates the Cusum technique using a WBC control with a mean value of 4.7×10^9/L. This value may be plotted daily on a chart with a zero line and the Cusum plotted as shown in Figure 47-5. Ideally, the Cusum of the differences remains around zero,

TABLE 47-1. Calculation of Cumulative Sum (Cusum) During First 18 days of January for normal WBC Count Control*

DATE	WBC CONTROL RESULTS ($\times 10^9$/L)	DIFFERENCE FROM MEAN ($\bar{x} = 4.7 \times 10^9$/L)	CUMULATIVE SUM CUSUM OF DIFFERENCES FROM MEAN
1	4.8	0.1	0.1
2	4.7	0.0	0.1
3	4.7	0.0	0.1
4	4.5	−0.2	−0.1
5	4.6	−0.1	−0.2
6	4.7	0.0	−0.2
7	4.6	−0.1	−0.3
8	4.9	0.2	−0.1
9	4.8	0.1	0.0
10	4.8	0.1	0.1
11	4.7	0.0	0.1
12	4.5	−0.2	−0.1
13	4.5	−0.2	−0.3
14	4.6	−0.1	−0.4
15	4.9	0.2	−0.2
16	4.6	−0.1	−0.3
17	4.5	−0.2	−0.5
18	4.7	0.0	−0.5

* Results are plotted in Figure 47-5.

as the Cusum will alternate in sign (positive and negative). An out-of-control situation may be indicated when the Cusum constantly falls on one side of the zero line, indicating a shift or trend. A statistically significant difference is not necessarily medically significant. In addition, the Cusum chart is very sensitive to systematic errors but not to random errors. Therefore, another monitoring device such as the Levey-Jennings chart should be used in conjunction with the Cusum.

Monthly Control Performance Reports

Monthly control performance reports should be generated for each lot number of commercial control to summarize its performance. The report should include charts for each

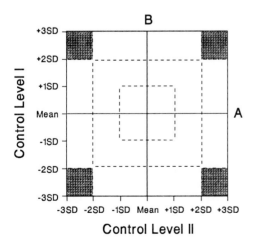

FIG. 47-4.   Youden plot with shaded areas indicating where both control values are beyond 2 SD; such a result means stop immediately and troubleshoot to correct instrument problem before resuming patient testing.

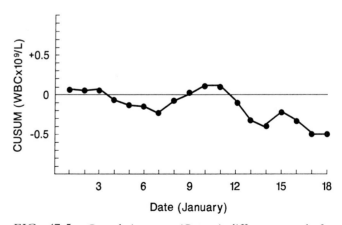

FIG. 47-5.   Cumulative sum (Cusum) difference graph for WBC count control for first 18 days of month. (Calculations are shown in Table 47-1.) Days 12 through 18 show downward shift, indicating that WBC is out of control. Problem must be determined and corrected before running any more patient samples.

measurement and level of control material tested and the final mean, SD, and CV for each parameter. Many vendors provide a computer service for their customers that generates monthly reports that include all of this information plus comparisons with other laboratories using the same lot number and instrumentation.

STATISTICAL SYSTEMS FOR QUALITY CONTROL

A statistical formula known as the Bull algorithm was developed by Bull and colleagues in 1974[3] as an alternate method for monitoring instrument accuracy. Other names for this algorithm include: moving average indices, moving averages, and $\overline{X}_B$ (pronounced x-bar-b). The development of the Bull algorithm was based on the following findings.

Analysis of indices from various hospitals in different regions of the United States and the world revealed that the mean MCV, MCH, and MCHC are similar for the various population groups. The average indices from acute care facilities were shown to be stable from day to day, week to week, and month to month, and the mean values of the indices were found to be the same in a study of acute care centers in the US, Japan, and Wales. The "international" means are MCV = 89.5 fL, MCH = 30.5 pg, and MCHC = 34% (or 34 g/dL).[2] The mean values may differ if the patient population mix is not similar to that found in an acute care center. For example, oncology or pediatric patient populations may have different mean values than those predicted for an acute care center.

Once the mean value for each red cell index has been established for a given laboratory's patient population, the Bull algorithm is applied to evaluate the indices of consecutive groups of specimens as they are processed. The algorithm analyzes the data and provides the operator with an error message or flag when abnormalities in the moving averages are detected.

The Bull algorithm provides a sensitivity of 1% to changes in instrument calibration or patient population when the batch size is set at 20 samples.[9] The principal functions of the algorithm are to "smooth" and "trim" the data in each new batch. Smoothing is accomplished by incorporating previous batch data in the formula, giving it a weight of 40%, and giving new batch data a weight of 60% on the new mean. Trimming is accomplished by using the square root function. This proportionately decreases the effect of outliers within a batch, thus reducing the incidence of abnormal samples causing the moving averages to be out of control.

The beauty of the moving average program is that the control material IS the tested material (*i.e.,* patient samples are also control samples) making this control material *identical* rather than *similar* to the tested material. Laboratories that test more than 100 patient samples daily should consider the purchase of a hematology cell counter that incorporates the Bull program. The purchase of a computer into which patient data can be transferred is an alternate means for a laboratory with sufficient workload but an instrument that is not already programmed for moving average indices.

The target values of the indices should be established using an instrument whose calibration is carefully controlled. One thousand patient samples is ideal, but as few as 250 will suffice to establish the mean index values *if* the resulting values correspond to the international mean index values. Once target values for the MCV, MCH, and MCHC have been established for the moving average program, patient samples will provide a continuing check of instrument RBC count calibration.

The limits of acceptable operation are set at ± 3% of the mean. Sample testing must stop and corrective action must be taken when two consecutive batch calculations are beyond the limits on two determinations simultaneously. Figure 47-6 is an example of moving average indices charts representing data analyzed by an instrument computer program over 10 days of sample testing. The pattern displayed for MCH is the expected normal pattern, with all dots within the 3% limit and also bounding above and below the mean.

Calculation of each RBC index is based on two measurements, including the RBC count, Hb or HCT, as shown in Table 47-2. This pairing, combined with the narrow range of indices compatible with life, leads to the unique monitoring system described by Bull.

In Figure 47-6 the patterns represented for MCV and MCHC both show a drift toward the 3% limit. The MCV has remained within the limit; however, the most recent

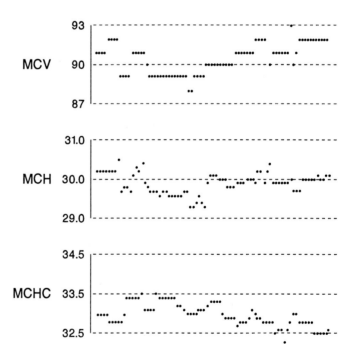

FIG. 47-6. Charts of moving average indices (Bull moving averages). New moving average calculation of each batch of 20 patients is represented by successive dots. Only one dot (MCHC chart) is out of limits, but a pattern that warrants investigation is developing with MCV and MCHC. Situation is still in control, as only one dot of one indice has gone beyond 3% of mean limit. Measure of concern is HCT, because it is common to MCV and MCHC formulas (see Table 47-2). Retesting a few samples from earlier in-control batch may help confirm or rule out instrument problem involving HCT.

TABLE 47–2. Erythrocyte Indices Formulas*

$$MCV = \frac{HCT \times 10}{RBC}$$

$$MCH = \frac{Hb \times 10}{RBC}$$

$$MCHC = \frac{Hb \times 100}{HCT}$$

* Note that each index is calculated from two measured parameters: either HCT, RBC count, or Hb. These formulas are used both in the diagnosis of hematologic abnormalities and as a monitoring system for instrument malfunction.

plots were above the mean rather than both above and below it, reflecting an upward shift. One dot on the MCHC chart has dropped below the lower limit, and the MCHC plots reflect a downward shift. The upward shift of the MCV, combined with the downward shift of the MCHC, points to a problem with the measurement that is common to both of these indices—the HCT. Looking again at Table 47-2, it would appear from the formulas for MCV and MCHC that the HCT value has shifted upward, causing the MCV to shift upward. In other words, because the HCT is in the numerator of the MCV formula and in the denominator of the MCHC formula, a change in HCT calibration will cause these indices to respond in opposite directions.

The RBC count is common to the MCV and MCH formulas, and because it is the denominator in both formulas, a change in RBC measurement will result in changes in the same direction for MCV and MCH. For example, an upward shift in the calibration of RBC would cause both the MCV and the MCH to show a downward shift. If the Hb calibration changes, the MCH and MCHC patterns should respond together in the same direction.

Pattern interpretation must include review of instrument function checks as well as the distribution of patient type. Once the measure at fault is determined, troubleshooting the instrument begins. Targeting a specific parameter makes such troubleshooting easier, because certain reagents, pumps, tubing, or other parts that are related to that specific determination may be inspected for malfunction. The general procedures listed in Table 47-3 should be followed to examine the reasons for the abnormal moving averages and to determine whether corrective action is required.

Finally, as mentioned in the section on calibration, it should be noted that although the Bull algorithm was developed as a monitoring (control) device, the mean target values of the indices program are so predictable and stable that it has been proposed that they can also be used for instrument calibration. In conjunction with reference Hb or HCT determinations, they are proposed for calibration of red cell parameters.

INSTRUMENT MAINTENANCE

Routine maintenance procedures are outlined in each manufacturer's instrument manual. Proper routine maintenance of all instruments such as cell counters, stainers, centrifuges, refrigerators, and pipets is essential to keep a laboratory functioning smoothly and to ensure reporting of accurate results. The key to the longevity and proper functioning of any instrument is good routine preventive maintenance. This point cannot be overemphasized. The best way to ensure proper care of an instrument is to follow the recommendation of the manufacturer for cleaning, lubrication, and replacement of expendable parts. This maintenance will minimize instrument down time and decrease the frustration of personnel. The CAP also publishes guidelines for routine maintenance of laboratory instruments.[10]

TROUBLESHOOTING PROCEDURES

Difficulties encountered in troubleshooting an instrument problem are greatly reduced when a comprehensive preventive maintenance program and a reliable and sensitive QC program are in place. Problems must be approached calmly and in an orderly manner. Quick identification of the true nature of the problem is essential. All symptoms must be recognized, and the order in which the events occurred must be established and documented. A sixth sense, intuition, should not be ignored; some individuals develop a sense for how an instrument is working. Familiarity with the instrument and experience are the best training available for instrument troubleshooting.

Diagnosis of a problem will be easier if the step-by-step approach outlined in Table 47-4 is taken.[4] All of these observations and, especially, the exact sequence of events are crucial to a successful and rapid solution to an instrument problem. All of this information documented in a problem log can be used by company engineers to solve problems and as a reference when a problem recurs.

TABLE 47–3. Procedures for Determining Cause of Abnormal Moving Averages

1. Check type of samples run in batch in question
2. Check instrument calibration and precision with a control
3. Visually inspect reagents and instrument
4. Troubleshoot instrument
5. Rerun samples from batch with moving averages error flag

TABLE 47–4. Steps for Troubleshooting a Malfunctioning Instrument

1. Rerun last sample tested
2. Rerun previously run normal control specimen
3. Review maintenance log
4. Inspect visually for leaks, disconnected tubes, wires, reagent depletion
5. Observe for persistent abnormality
6. Review QC data (e.g., look for shifts or trends)
7. Identify specific nature of problem
   a. Search problem log book for similar problems in past
   b. Check troubleshooting section of instrument manual
8. Notify supervisor and manufacturer's service department as needed
9. Complete all necessary adjustments to correct problem(s)
10. Document all symptoms and corrective action taken; note duration of down time
11. Repeat controls to ensure return to proper functioning state

QUALITY CONTROL DOCUMENTATION

Laboratories must maintain records in accordance with accreditation requirements. Documentation is the backbone of QC programs. Procedure, safety, and laboratory policy manuals must be complete, reviewed yearly, and updated periodically. Patient result records, QC results, charts, and summaries with timely reviews documented are necessary for accreditation. Instrument maintenance records should include documentation of routine maintenance, periodic manufacturer preventive maintenance, and instrument problems, as well as the corrective actions taken. An instrument problem log is a vital part of a complete QC program. Step-by-step documentation of a problem is critical to the quick solution of an instrument problem. The following information should be included:[4]

1. Record nature and frequency of problem. The exact nature of the problem must be detailed, along with its frequency: is it consistent or sporadic?
2. Record sequence of events. The sequence is important, especially when a second problem develops.
3. Identify measurements involved in the problem: are the cell counts involved, the Hb, the HCT, or the indices? If all measurements are affected, this may indicate a dilution malfunction, whereas a problem with a single measurement can eliminate certain difficulties from consideration.
4. Identify the segment of the instrument cycle involved. Is the problem in the diluting, counting, or calculating phase of the cycle?
5. Record all corrective actions. If several things need to be "fixed," fix one at a time to observe the effect on specimen results before fixing another. If several items are changed simultaneously, it is difficult to tell what solved the problem. Jumping in and "fixing" everything without documentation can lead to further problems.

A written record of all QC measures taken must be available for evaluation by accreditation inspectors. If a review or action taken is not documented, it did not take place, and the inspector will cite the laboratory for a deficiency.

INTERNAL LABORATORY MONITORING

Exchanges of patient samples and blood films between laboratories within the same institution or at nearby institutions constitute internal laboratory monitoring of hematology instruments. Exchange of samples from instrument to instrument within any given institution's laboratory and with other laboratories in the local area provides valuable QC information. Any laboratory that has at least two similar instruments in operation can set up an exchange of samples, which provides cross comparison of results. The frequency of exchanging samples will differ depending on the distance separating the instruments, the type of transport system available, and the overall QC program that is in place.

Blood film exchange on a weekly or bimonthly basis will identify areas of disagreement in cell type identification.

This should prompt establishment of continuing education sessions that standardize the criteria for cell identification such as segmented versus band neutrophils, normal versus variant lymphocytes, or variant lymphocytes versus monocytes. The preparation of extra films and their subsequent exchange provides interesting, unusual, and stimulating cases from which individuals from several laboratories or shifts can learn.

When evaluating the results of sample exchange, it must be realized that results will differ somewhat from instrument to instrument. How much variation is normal must be determined when all instruments are in control. There will be more variation among instruments from different manufacturers than among instruments of the same type and model. The main purpose of monitoring patient cell counts is to identify clinically significant changes. Within-instrument and instrument-to-instrument variation must remain below the clinically significant variation that prompts physician intervention. Normal cell counts differ depending on the time of sample collection in relation to meals, physical activity, hydration, and other variables. Surgical trauma and medications also will affect cell counts. A good QC program attempts to minimize the variations between instruments so that they do not mask these physiologic and pathologic variations.

EXTERNAL LABORATORY MONITORING

Regional Programs

Most large manufacturers of commercial controls offer free QC programs that monitor data from program participants. These data are analyzed, and a monthly report is distributed to the participating laboratories. The report usually includes mean, SD, and CV based on the laboratory's data. It also compares results from laboratories using the same instrumentation or methods. This peer group comparison provides one more piece of the puzzle for the overall picture of the QC program being used.

State Programs

Regulations concerning laboratory testing and personnel differ widely from state to state. Requirements range from none to proficiency testing or licensing requirements for laboratory personnel.

The terms *proficiency testing* or *proficiency survey* refer to the practice of sending aliquots of the same sample (plasma, serum, preserved cells, blood films, or pictures of cells) to all participating laboratories and collecting data for analysis and evaluation. Regulations differ according to the type of laboratory being evaluated (*i.e.*, state, independent or commercial, physician's office, or hospital). The state department of health usually is the branch of state government that provides proficiency testing, continuing education programs, and enforcement of existing regulations.

Federal Programs

The US Centers for Disease Control (CDC) offers continuing education programs and workshops for laboratory personnel but no longer provide interlaboratory survey programs.

Professional Programs

Hospital and laboratory accreditation is voluntary, but accreditation by the JCAHO is required for a hospital to receive Medicare and Medicaid payments. A JCAHO hospital inspection includes the laboratory unless it is accredited by the CAP, as JCAHO accepts CAP accreditation as comparable. Accredited laboratories participate in a proficiency survey program, in which results from each laboratory are compared with those of other laboratories using the same methods. These surveys provide laboratories with an accuracy check. The mean of all participants is considered to be "truth."

Evaluation of External Laboratory Monitoring Results

State-of-the-art information is provided by regional, state, federal, and professional programs. These data analyses provide valuable information about the performance of the various clinical laboratory services throughout the United States. Good and acceptable performance by a laboratory on unknown samples includes all reported values that are within 2 SD of the method mean. Data that fall between ± 2 and 3 SD are judged as unacceptable performance. It is very important that one keep in mind the fact that statistically, 1 in 20 values should fall within this range. For the most part, the statistical limits are much tighter than the limits of variation that constitute a clinically significant change in the condition of a patient.

One important disadvantage of these surveys is the manner in which laboratories handle them. Many laboratories handle survey samples with special care that does not reflect routine testing conditions under which patient samples are tested. Thus, peak rather than routine performance may be represented by survey data.

CHAPTER SUMMARY

Procedures to monitor and control systematic error in hematology differ widely. Two fundamental areas of quality control (QC) for systematic error are calibration of instruments so they generate accurate data and monitoring (controlling) the instruments over time to be sure they remain accurate. Three monitoring methods are frequently used. The first involves commercial control material. Relatively high cost, short shelf life, and constituents different from those in patient samples limit the usefulness of this material, but it offers readily available control systems, especially for laboratories with a small workload. The second method utilizes blood samples from patient sources. This material is identical to that routinely tested and is readily available. However, it is stable for only 24 hours. The third method utilizes a statistical system called the Bull algorithm, which incorporates patient data into a statistical formula and updates the data after every batch of 20 patient samples. Combinations of these three procedures provide most laboratories with an effective and cost-manageable means of detecting the systematic error (a QC system).

If a computerized system for maintaining records of control material results is not available, the laboratory may choose to plot control results using the Levey-Jennings charting method, which may be supplemented by charts using the cumulative sum (Cusum) method. A more difficult manual charting system is the Youden plot, which is used to plot a normal and abnormal control on the same chart. Study of the patterns of these charts indicates whether or not the instrument is in control. When it is out of control, instrument troubleshooting is required before patient samples may be run.

Documented instrument maintenance is a critical component of any QC program. Records of instrument performance and troubleshooting incidents are invaluable tools in maintaining complex instruments in top running order for reliable reporting of results.

Internal and external monitoring systems provide the final component of a total QC program. Frequent exchanges among laboratories within the same or closely located institutions constitute internal systems; subscription external programs at the state, regional, and federal levels provide information regarding accuracy among laboratories across the continent.

REFERENCES

1. Bull BS: Quality assurance strategies. In Koepke JA (ed): Laboratory Hematology, vol 2, p 1007. New York, Churchill Livingstone, 1984
2. Bull BS, Hay KL: Are red cell indices international? Arch Pathol Lab Med 109:604, 1985
3. Bull BS, Elashoff RM, Heilbron DC et al: A study of various estimators for the derivation of quality control procedures from patient erythrocyte indices. Am J Clin Pathol 61:473, 1974
4. Dotson MA: Troubleshooting multichannel hematology instruments. Lab Perspect 1:9, 1982
5. International Committee for Standardization in Haematology: Recommendations for reference method for haemoglobinometry in human blood, ICSH Standard EP 6/2, 1977, and Specifications for international hemiglobincyanide reference preparation, ICSH Standard EP 6/3, 1977. J Pathol 31:139, 1978
6. Koepke JA: Instruments for quantitative hematology measurements. In Koepke JA (ed): Laboratory Hematology, vol 2, p 915. New York, Churchill Livingstone, 1984
7. Levy WC, Bull BS, Koepke JA: The incorporation of red blood cell index mean data into quality control programs. Am J Clin Pathol 86:193, 1986
8. National Committee for Clinical Laboratory Standards (NCCLS): Procedure for Determining Packed Cell Volume by the Microhematocrit Method, Approved Standard H7-A, vol 5, no 5. Villanova, PA, NCCLS, 1985
9. Skonie V: Hematology quality control—A continuing education course in print. Lab World 29:14, 1978
10. Sodeman TM, Floering DA, Mozdzem JJ Jr et al: Laboratory Instrument Verification and Maintenance Manual, 4th ed, Skokie, IL, College of American Pathologists, 1989

RECOMMENDED READING

College of American Pathologists: CAP Survey Manual. Skokie, IL, 1986
Gilmer PR, Williams LJ: The status of methods of calibration in hematology. Am J Clin Pathol 74:600, 1980
Gilmer PR, Williams LJ, Koepke JA et al: Calibration methods for automated instruments. Am J Clin Pathol 68:185, 1977

48

Methods to Monitor and Control Random Error

Charles E. Stewart

Errors can be defined simply as mistakes; random errors are mistakes that occur without a definable pattern or frequency. In a perfect world, no errors are made, and the results of a laboratory analysis are always accurate and precise. Unfortunately, we do not live in a perfect world. Random as well as systematic errors always occur to various degrees. Systematic errors (Chap. 47) differ from random errors in that the former are regularly occurring deviations in a test "system," in contrast to the haphazard nature of large random errors. Each error has a different impact on patient care. This chapter will focus on random error and its prevention.

DEFINITION

Each laboratory procedure has intrinsic imprecision or, in other words, *minor random errors* caused by factors beyond the laboratory scientist's control, which therefore cannot be avoided. These imprecisions are continuously operative and are caused by small fluctuations in the analyzing system. Examples include the inherent unpredictable motion of particles in a suspension (*e.g.*, blood cells in a diluting fluid) moving rapidly in a flowing stream through a flow cell or over the surface of a glass slide.

A test method's inherent imprecision or random error is numerically demonstrated when a specimen is analyzed many times and a standard deviation (SD) is calculated. The SD describes the dispersion of individual values around the mean value and is indicative of the method's precision. A large SD indicates poor precision and a large amount of inherent random error. It is the goal of the laboratory scientist to be sure that the amount of error is limited to the method's inherent imprecision and is not increased by other errors.

TABLE 48–1. Some of the Random Errors Observed in Clinical Laboratories

1. Specimen is labeled with wrong name, and results are reported on wrong patient.
2. Results are recorded on wrong requisition and reported on wrong patient.
3. Air bubble is trapped in bottom of sample cup of an analyzer that samples from bottom, resulting in a short sample.
4. EDTA-anticoagulated specimen is not mixed well at the time of collection, resulting in formation of a fibrin clot and platelet clumping. Specimen is not checked for fibrin and is used for a platelet count.
5. While a specimen is held for sampling on an automated cell counter, the sample probe is not placed deep enough during aspiration, resulting in a short sample.
6. An EDTA-anticoagulated specimen is not mixed well prior to sampling, resulting in a concentration of cells in the lower portion of the collection tube. The aliquot for counting is collected from the upper portion of the tube.
7. While recording a prothrombin time from the printout of an automated coagulation instrument, the technologist reads 12.8 seconds but writes 18.2 seconds.
8. While performing a manual WBC count on a serous fluid, the technologist misreads the meniscus in the pipet and underdilutes the specimen by 10 μL.

Major random errors are mistakes or accidents that occur haphazardly and can have a significant impact on patient care. These errors cause a greater loss of precision and accuracy than normal and occur in an unpredictable fashion that differs from one sample to the next. Some examples are listed in Table 48-1.

QUALITY CONTROL AND RANDOM ERROR

Controlling Minor and Major Random Error

Although most quality control (QC) procedures in hematology adequately measure the amount of small inherent random error and systematic error in a test procedure, they do not detect or control the random errors or mistakes discussed in the preceding paragraphs. Because systematic errors are more consistent than random errors, systematic errors are routinely detected and measured using commercially prepared control materials and patient samples that are analyzed periodically and compared with established control ranges. Random errors, by their unpredictable nature, will not be detected with control samples unless the error happens to occur while analyzing the control. Therefore, other strategies must be employed to prevent and detect potentially harmful random error.

Strategies for the Prevention of Random Error

Technologist Awareness

The best defense against a significant random error is an alert laboratory scientist. If the investigator knows where the pitfalls and problems may be in a procedure and is vigilant in guarding against their occurrence, the chance of an accident or error greatly decreases. There can be no substitute for this, nor can its importance be overemphasized. All of the quality assurance and QC programs that have been and will be instituted to prevent errors and mistakes are no better than the investigators who perform the analyses and produce the results. Continuing education programs are useful in keeping levels of awareness of potential problems high and should be regularly scheduled.

Specimen Awareness

The flow chart in Figure 48-1 outlines a simple strategy for evaluating whether an individual test result is reasonable. The following list details additional actions that can be taken at the time of analysis to reduce random errors.

1. Reaffirm the patient's identification at the time of specimen collection.
2. Double check the name on the specimen requisition against the name label on the specimen at the time of analysis to avoid sample mixups, one of the more common random errors.
3. Use a wooden applicator stick or toothpick to stir all specimens prior to analysis on an automated cell counter. The wood will pick up small pieces of fibrin. If fibrin clots are present, the sample is unacceptable. Cell counts accidentally performed on partially clotted samples will be falsely decreased because of entrapment of cells in the clot. Also, small fibrin clots aspirated into the analyzer could clog sample tubing, causing the analyzer to go out of control.
4. Inspect all pipeted specimens visually to see if it appears that the appropriate volume of sample has been delivered and that inappropriate air bubbles have not been trapped in sample cups, cuvettes, reagent tubing, or mixing chambers. For example, check cuvettes after pipeting plasma for coagulation testing to see if there has been a gross short sampling. If possible, watch the samples as they go through the analyzer to see if all dilutions look right.
5. Check to see if the test results are reasonable. For each sample, the operator should review the result to consider whether it is a reasonable value, one that is compatible with life or at least with the patient's state of health.[1] For example, an erythrocyte count of 0.70×10^{12}/L should be investigated to see if there was short sampling, if the specimen was diluted with intravenous fluid, or if this is not a peripheral blood specimen but some other type of fluid such as a bloody abdominal or cerebrospinal fluid incorrectly labeled and processed as whole blood. Simply evaluating the reasonableness of a value is the first step in detecting error.

Current Procedure Manuals

Clearly written and comprehensive specimen collection and technical procedure manuals provide the blueprints for a well-structured error prevention program. Procedure manuals outlining the materials required in a technical procedure and the step-by-step instructions for performing it will help to reduce errors caused by ignorance. Careful adherence to instructions by the staff is a must for consistent performance.

Proper Instrument Maintenance

Properly maintained instruments are less likely to be the source of random and systematic errors than are marginally maintained instruments. The manufacturer's instructions

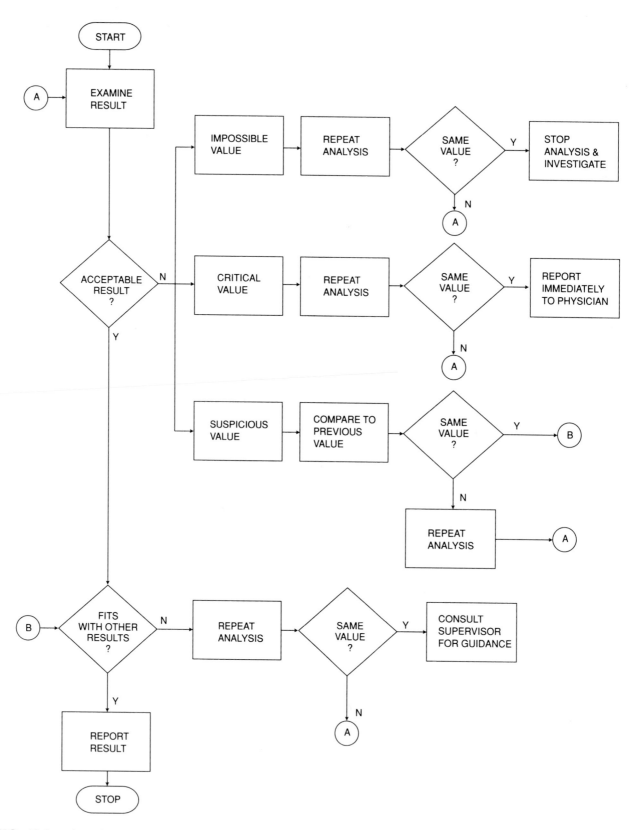

FIG. 48-1.   Flow chart for evaluation of test result for random error: A simple strategy for determining whether individual test result is reasonable and correlates with other results. Y, yes; N, no. Symbols A and B show interconnection between results of evaluation of repeat testing and where decision-making strategy should resume (far left). For example, if an impossible value is obtained, and repeat analysis does not show same value, uppermost horizontal line of chart says that testing procedure should return to symbol A, where the steps are begun again with EXAMINE RESULT. Adapted from Cembrowski GS: Use of patient data for quality control. Clin Lab Med 6:715, 1986, with permission.

and recommendations for routine preventive maintenance should be developed into a documented daily, weekly, and monthly schedule. All auxiliary equipment such as pipets, dilutors, and waterbaths should also be maintained to deliver reliable service. Well-maintained instrumentation will increase the confidence of the operator in its abilities to produce error-free results.

Strategies for the Detection of Random Error

Duplicate Specimen Testing

A straightforward method for detecting random error is duplicate specimen testing. This method was formerly employed in laboratory medicine when more of the testing was performed manually, which was subject to a greater incidence of random technical error. For example, in coagulation studies, prothrombin times and activated partial thromboplastin times were performed in duplicate using the fibrometer. Some electronic cell counters perform counts in duplicate or triplicate using two or three orifices. The counts are compared, and if there is variation outside a specified range, the result is rejected, and no answer is given. If there is agreement, an average is calculated and reported.

Whereas duplicate testing may be a good way to discover a significant random error, it can be expensive and time consuming and may not be justified with the current highly precise analyzers. When considering duplicate testing, weigh the time and effort involved in relation to the number of random errors detected by duplicate testing and look for alternative methods for eliminating the chance of random error.

Multivariate Checks

Multivariate checks are a form of QC in which the interrelations between different tests and the measurements within a test are compared with acceptable limits to detect random errors. Certain hematologic tests lend themselves to comparison with others, and when these comparisons are performed on a routine basis, many spurious results can be detected. Some of these comparisons can be performed at the bench as the specimen is analyzed, whereas others require either access to the medical record, the patient's physician, or other laboratory work as available through a computer information system.

COMPARISON OF AUTOMATED BLOOD COUNT WITH BLOOD FILM. One of the simplest correlations is accomplished by comparing the automated leukocyte, platelet, and differential (if available) counts with the blood film. This method is discussed in Chapter 25 in detail. Every time an investigator performs a manual leukocyte differential or peripheral blood film review, the steps outlined in Chapter 25 for the verification of blood film adequacy should be followed to ensure that the blood film accurately reflects the blood sample. An unacceptable film quality can result in disagreement between the film and automated results and can lead to extra time and effort in repeating tests with results that were correct in the first place. In cases where there is disagreement between the automated blood count and the film estimate, the film should be prepared and

evaluated again, and the automated count should be repeated.

RULE OF THREE. Another correlation that can be checked is that of the erythrocyte count, Hb, and HCT agreement for each specimen. This is accomplished by applying the "Rule of Three," which is described in Chapter 9 and Table 9-3. With few exceptions, erythrocyte size, shape, and Hb content do not change during an infection or after the loss of blood. The Rule of Three should be applied to every blood count; however, it generally applies only to normocytic, normochromic erythrocytes, which can be verified by a blood film check. If the erythrocytes are found to be abnormal, the automated values cannot be expected to conform to these rules.

CORRELATION OF ERYTHROCYTE INDICES. The erythrocyte count, Hb, and HCT relations are also demonstrated in the RBC indices mean corpuscular volume (MCV), mean corpuscular hemoglobin (MCH), and mean corpuscular hemoglobin concentration (MCHC). The calculations and sample reference ranges for these are reviewed in Chapter 9, and sample reference ranges are given in Table 9-1. If a random error occurs during the counting of erythrocytes or the measurement of Hb or HCT, the indices will be significantly outside the reference ranges, and the results are suspect. The count should be repeated and the blood film inspected for abnormalities that might point to the problem.

CORRELATION OF OTHER HEMATOLOGY VALUES. Correlation of results with other hematology values can be helpful. For example, an increased reticulocyte count should correspond with increased polychromasia on the blood film. If there is a computer information system that can supply other clinical data, or if there is good communication with the physician, correlations such as this can be established with other clinical information.

Delta Checks

The *delta check* is a technique for the detection of random errors in individual samples. This method has been greatly advanced with the improvement of laboratory computer information systems. One of the first manual delta check systems was described in 1974.[2] Today delta checks involve either a manual or a computer determination of the difference between consecutive measurements of an analyte or blood component for a specific patient and comparison of this difference with a predefined maximum allowable difference limit for that component.

When calculating the difference between consecutive measurements, the time that has elapsed between the measurements must be taken into consideration. For example, the operator or computer must consider whether the time lapse has been only hours, days, or months. The computer may be programmed to consider the time factor and compare the difference with a certain maximum allowable difference set by the laboratory on the basis of a given time lapse between consecutive measurements. In this way, results that are correct usually will not be flagged as possible errors. If various time frames and maximum allowable difference limits for the delta check are properly assigned, then the most frequent causes of delta check rejection of an individual specimen will be specimen mixup or random sampling and processing errors.

When the delta check is exceeded, the operator should first review the specimen to ensure that it is definitely the specimen of the patient in question. Next, the patient's cumulative results record should be reviewed. If necessary, the specimen should be retested, if possible using a different method.[1] If both the specimen identification and the retesting yield no clues to the delta check failure, improper collection of the specimen should be suspected, and another sample should be requested. If no errors are found, the results should be reported with a comment on the requisition indicating that the unusual result has been checked and verified to ensure the physician of the result's validity.

The delta check difference between consecutive measurements can be determined as either the difference in absolute units or in percent: (1) delta check as a difference in the absolute value: result 2 − result 1 = delta in test units or (2) delta check as a percentage difference: ([result 2 − result 1] /result 1) × 100 = delta percent. Once determined, this difference must be compared with a predefined maximum allowable difference.

There are two methods to determine the maximum allowable difference for the delta check. The more analytic approach is to collect a minimum of 20 paired consecutive test runs on the analyte in question and determine the deltas (differences between each consecutive test) for each pair. The deltas are then plotted as a frequency histogram, and either a 95% or a 99% confidence limit is determined. The other approach is to estimate the delta limit on the basis of clinical experience and expected intraindividual variation. This approach is less empirical but is less strenuous to determine. Regardless of the method used, the delta limit should be adjusted so that the majority of the real changes in patient test values are not flagged as failure of the delta limits.

Hematology tests that lend themselves to delta checks have little intraindividual variation over a short period of time. Red cell parameters, platelet counts, prothrombin time, and other coagulation studies are more adaptable to delta checking than are leukocyte counts and WBC differentials, which can have significant physiologic variation over short time periods.

USE OF COMPUTERS AND LABORATORY INFORMATION SYSTEMS FOR THE DETECTION OF RANDOM ERRORS

Computers can perform many of the functions that the laboratory scientist uses for detecting random error. The computer follows a series of defined rules and instructions and will apply these calculations and instructions with equal vigor to every result given to it. A computer does not know boredom and distraction, nor is it tempted to take short cuts when it is busy.

The key to having a computer system search for random error is to define the program in such a manner that random error is detected with equal if not greater probability than the probability by human detection. Much of the same logic used to contemplate the validity of a test result can be used in defining the program instructions. However, a word of caution: computer detection of random error is no better than the thought and logic put into the program. Computers will be just as consistent in not detecting errors as they are in detecting errors if the programming is not comprehensive.

Detection of Unusual Results

The computer can check each result to establish whether it is reasonable: to see if the value falls within the physiologic range compatible with life. If not, the value is flagged to alert the operator, and automatically the value is rejected. For example, a Hb of 1.0 g/dL for a whole blood specimen would be rejected because it is not compatible with life. This practice should be extended, not only to computer-interfaced analyzers, but also to results entered manually on the computer. The individual responsible for entering a rejected result after it has been verified as correct must take some distinct action to force acceptance of the value by the computer system if it falls outside the specified limits.

Detection of Data Entry Errors

To detect random data entry errors, the laboratory information system can be programmed to check the validity of entered data by performing a variety of calculations and other checks. For example, a search for correct decimal placement in the entries can be performed on each blood count. A manual differential count can be checked by the computer to see if it equals 100%. Many other calculations can be used to detect data entry errors.

A laboratory information system can perform sophisticated multivariate checks. Samples with a low MCV can be flagged, and the erythrocyte morphology report from an accompanying differential can be checked to see if the cells are indeed microcytic. A specimen with low serum iron levels can be checked to see if the Hb and RBC indices are also low. Because of access to a larger database and the computer's ability to process information rapidly, the computer-generated multivariate check is more sophisticated than a human one. Multivariate checks are more useful when reviewing the patient's cumulative laboratory report than when reviewing any individual laboratory result.

Performance of Delta Checks

Perhaps the most dramatic impact of the laboratory computer in detecting random error is in the performance of delta checks. By accessing the laboratory patient database, the computer can rapidly perform a delta check on the measurements of each sample for each patient. Test-specific rules can be defined that spell out the maximum allowable differences in consecutive results on a single patient based on various defined time limitations between analytical runs. These rules determine when the computer will flag a result.

Computer-Generated Reports

Computers can generate a variety of reports from their accumulated databases. For example, an "abnormal patient" report can list all patient results that exceed defined limits, such as alert or panic values. This report can be generated on a next-day basis for review by the pathologist or laboratory supervisor. This procedure will detect random errors whose magnitude would not cause rejection by a reasonable value rule but for which there were no previous results with which to perform a delta check. The report permits comparison of exception results with the patient's chart and clinical symptoms.

CHAPTER SUMMARY

Random error is unpredictable and is not always detected by conventional quality control methods using commercial controls or patient specimens. An alert and vigilant laboratory scientist is the best insurance against random error. A variety of strategies can be used to detect its occurrence, including checking test results to ensure that they are reasonable and performing duplicate analysis, multivariate checks, and delta checks. The use of laboratory computers and information systems can increase the efficiency of random error detection,

because computers can perform truly consistent analysis of results, thus preventing most mistakes.

REFERENCES

1. Cembrowski GS: Use of patient data for quality control. Clin Lab Med 6:715, 1986
2. Nosanchuk JS, Gottmann AW: CUMS and delta checks. Am J Clin Pathol 62:707, 1974

SUGGESTED READING

Iizuka Y, Kume H, Kitamura M: Multivariate delta check method for detecting specimen mix-up. Clin Chem 28:2244, 1982
Ladenson JH: Patients as their own controls: Use of the computer to identify "laboratory error." Clin Chem 21:1648, 1975
Sheiner LB, Wheeler LA, Moore JK: The performance of delta check methods. Clin Chem 25:2034, 1979
Stewart CE, Koepke JA: Basic Quality Assurance Practices for Clinical Laboratories. Philadelphia, JB Lippincott, 1987
Van Kampen EJ: Throwing a curve at laboratory error. Diagn Med 3:54, 1980

PART XI

HEMOSTASIS

49

Introduction

to

Hemostasis

Cheryl A. Lotspeich-Steininger

Hemostasis is derived from Greek meaning "the stoppage of blood flow." The subject of hemostasis is interesting but sometimes complex. This chapter provides a brief preparatory introduction to the concepts of hemostasis. The coagulation and fibrinolytic mechanisms, as well as platelets, will be introduced. In addition, the contribution of blood vessels to hemostasis and the vessel abnormalities that interfere with hemostasis will be addressed, because they will not be covered at length in any other chapter.

The next 13 chapters in this section of the text will address the theories of coagulation and fibrinolysis (Chap. 50), as well as disorders related to abnormalities of the coagulation and fibrinolytic mechanisms (Chaps. 55 and 56). Laboratory procedures for the evaluation of hemostatic abnormalities will be discussed in detail (Chaps. 51–54 and 57). The production and function of platelets, qualitative and quantitative abnormalities of plateles, and the laboratory evaluation of platelets will also be discussed (Chaps. 58–61). The final chapter in this section (Chap. 62) will present concepts of instrumentation and quality control (QC) as they relate uniquely to the hemostasis laboratory.

THE THREE HEMOSTATIC COMPONENTS

There are three basic components of hemostasis: the extravascular component (the tissues surrounding blood vessels), the vascular component (the blood vessels through which blood flows), and the intravascular component (the platelets and plasma proteins that circulate within the blood vessels).

Extravascular Component

The extravascular hemostatic component involves the tissues surrounding a vessel, which become involved in hemostasis when a local vessel is injured. Extravascular mechanisms play a part in hemostasis by providing back pressure on the injured vessel through swelling and the trapping of escaped blood. The increased tissue pressure tends to collapse venules and capillaries. The ability of the surrounding tissues to aid in hemostasis depends on the following factors:

1. The bulk or amount of surrounding tissue. A wound in the fleshy part of the thigh will not bleed as profusely as an identical wound in the scalp.
2. The type of tissue surrounding the injured vessel. For example, skeletal muscle is more absorbent and effective in arresting hemorrhage than is loose connective tissue.
3. The tone of the surrounding tissue. The amount of tissue elasticity correlates with the amount of bleeding, so that identical wounds in a 17 year old with great tissue elasticity and in a 71 year old with less tissue elasticity tend to have different bleeding characteristics.

Vascular and Intravascular Components

The vascular hemostatic component involves the vessels through which blood flows. The role played by vessels in hemostasis depends on their size, the amount of smooth muscle within their walls, and the integrity of the endothelial cell lining.

The key components in intravascular hemostasis are platelets and biochemicals (procoagulants) in the plasma. These components are involved in coagulation (clot or thrombus formation) or fibrinolysis (clot or thrombus dissolution), the two essential processes of hemostasis.

CONCEPTS OF NORMAL HEMOSTASIS, HYPOCOAGULATION, AND HYPERCOAGULATION

Normal Hemostatic Balance

Prior to the many advances in biomedical research and laboratory techniques of recent decades, hemostasis was understood simply as the normal process by which bleeding from injured blood vessels was stopped through blood coagulation. Today, hemostasis is more thoroughly understood as a complex interaction between blood vessels, platelets, and biochemical reactants or factors in the plasma (Fig. 49-1). These interactions not only create clots that stop bleeding through the coagulation process but also dissolve clots through the fibrinolytic process as injured vessels are healed.

Under normal conditions, the formation and dissolution of thrombi is maintained in a delicate balance, as shown in Figure 49-1. Without this balance, an individual may experience either excessive bleeding (as a result of poor clot formation or excessive fibrinolysis) or vasoocclusion (as a result of uncontrolled formation of thrombi in the vascular system, occluding vessels and depriving organs of blood). Conditions associated with excessive bleeding are referred to as *hypocoagulable* states. Conditions in which there is uncontrolled thrombosis are called *hypercoagulable* states. Both abnormal states can be fatal if not controlled promptly.

Hypocoagulation

Many clinical conditions, both inherited and acquired, are associated with hypocoagulation or abnormal bleeding. Several of these conditions are readily diagnosed by laboratory tests, particularly coagulation factor assays that measure the activity of coagulation reactants (factors). Hemophilia is a well-known example of an inherited hypocoagulable disorder (Chap. 55). Patients with hemophilia have a defective coagulation mechanism that is unable to form adequate clots, resulting in excessive bleeding from cuts. Classic hemophilia (type A) is caused by a deficiency in one of the plasma coagulation proteins, factor VIII. Acquired conditions associated with hypocoagulation generally involve many clinical problems in addition to bleeding (Chap. 55). Examples include disseminated intravascular coagulation (DIC), as well as liver and kidney disease.

Hypercoagulation

Hypercoagulation or thrombosis is associated with the inappropriate formation of thrombi in the vasculature that occlude normal blood flow. Thrombi generally consist of leukocytes, platelets, and erythrocytes held together by fibrin. Thrombi can be painful and cause a number of symptoms and abnormal physical findings, as well as ab-

FIG. 49-1. Balance of hemostasis. Vessels, coagulation and fibrinolytic proteins, and platelets work together toward thrombus formation in well-orchestrated, carefully balanced process. Platelets are the center of clot formation (thrombogenesis). Swing of balance to the right (*i.e.,* excessive fibrinolysis or inadequate coagulation) can result in bleeding; shift of balance to the left (*i.e.,* excessive coagulation or inadequate fibrinolysis) can result in pathologic clotting (thrombosis). (From Corriveau DM, Fritsma GA (eds): Hemostasis and Thrombosis in the Clinical Laboratory, p 9. Philadelphia, JB Lippincott, 1988, with permission.)

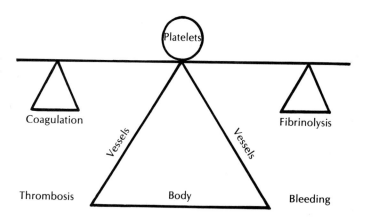

normal laboratory results. Thrombi can even be life-threatening if the blood supply to a vital organ is cut off. Hypercoagulation is caused by a defect in or lack of activation of the fibrinolytic system.

Most hypercoagulable states are associated with acquired diseases or altered physiologic states (see Table 56-2). Most often, a malignancy[17] or surgical procedure[13,19] is the stimulus for hypercoagulation. Unfortunately, it is difficult to predict the risk of thrombosis by the more common laboratory tests. Hypercoagulable states are discussed in Chapter 56.

HISTORICAL BACKGROUND OF HEMOSTASIS

The study of hemostasis dates to the time of Aristotle and Plato.[26] The bleeding disorder "hemophilia" was the first coagulation disorder to be recognized, being described during the second century A.D., although, its pathophysiology was not understood. In the twelfth century Moses Maimonides[20] described two male children who had died from excessive bleeding after circumcision. It was recommended that any male child born subsequently to the mother of an infant who had died from such a bleeding problem not be circumcised; otherwise, he was also likely to die.

Clinical descriptions of families with the hemophilia disorder were first published in 1803.[25] The disorder was given the name hemophilia, which means "love of hemorrhage," by Schönlein.[33] The disorder was first described as hemophilia in a thesis by Hopff published in 1828.[10]

HISTORICAL DEVELOPMENT OF CLINICAL HEMOSTASIS

It was not until 1913 that a laboratory test to evaluate the clotting mechanism was described in the literature. This test was the Lee-White whole blood coagulation (clotting) time (WBCT).[14] The WBCT is an *in vitro*, visual, qualitative assessment of blood clotting capability. It is seldom performed today because it is qualitative, it is sensitive only to severe factor deficiencies, and it is subjective and time consuming. A prolonged WBCT (*i.e.*, prolonged time for whole blood to clot compared with that of a "healthy" population) indicates a bleeding disorder.

As recently as the 1940s, there were only a few routine tests for evaluating the hemostatic mechanism: the platelet count, bleeding time, WBCT, and the prothrombin time (PT). The PT was developed by Quick in the 1930s.[28] Even though it is somewhat misnamed, being dependent on more than prothrombin, slightly modified versions are still in use today.[29] Because of the paucity of hemostasis tests in the past, the few PT, WBCT, and bleeding time tests ordered were historically performed in the hematology laboratory.

THE HEMOSTASIS LABORATORY TODAY

Over the past few decades, many tests of the coagulation and fibrinolytic system have been developed and automated, and test reagents have been made commercially available. Consequently, many clinical hemostasis laboratories now operate independent of the hematology laboratory. Visual examination of clot formation has been replaced in large part by mechanical or turbidimetric clot detection as well as by spectrophotometric measurement of synthetic substrates. Automation has considerably improved the precision and accuracy of coagulation testing.

The PT and activated partial thromboplastin time (APTT) are the two most commonly performed tests in the hemostasis laboratory. These tests are used to assess the activity of the reactants involved in the coagulation mechanism. Other plasma proteins involved in fibrinolysis can also be evaluated in the laboratory.

OVERVIEW OF THE HEMOSTATIC MECHANISM

Primary and Secondary Hemostasis

Hemostasis involves the interaction of blood vessels, platelets, the coagulation mechanism, fibrinolysis, and tissue repair. Hemostasis occurs in two phases, primary and secondary (Table 49-1). Primary hemostasis involves the vascular and platelet response to vessel injury. Secondary hemostasis includes the response of the coagulation process to such injury. These processes ultimately lead to the formation of a stable fibrin-platelet plug at the site of injury, which permits vessel healing. At the same time, fibrinolysis is initiated, allowing for gradual clot dissolution.

Role of Blood Vessels in Hemostasis

Intact Vessels

Blood flows through the vascular system to and from all parts of the body. The vascular system consists of capillaries, arteries, and veins (Fig. 49-2).

CAPILLARIES.   Metabolic exchange between the blood and tissues takes place in thin-walled capillaries, which are lined with a single continuous endothelial cell layer that is attached to a supportive basement membrane (see Fig. 49-2). In the figure note the large nucleus in the endothelial cell. The capillary lumen is just large enough for a single

TABLE 49-1. Basic Sequence of Events in Primary and Secondary Hemostasis After Vessel Injury

	EVENT	COMMENTS
Step 1	Vasoconstriction	Controlled by vessel smooth muscle; enhanced by chemicals secreted by platelets
Step 2	Platelet adhesion	Adhesion to exposed subendothelial connective tissue
Step 3	Platelet aggregation	Interaction and adhesion of platelets to one another to form initial plug at injury site
Step 4	Fibrin–platelet plug formation	Coagulation factors interact on platelet surface to produce fibrin; fibrin–platelet plug then forms at site of vessel injury
Step 5	Fibrin stabilization	Fibrin clot must be stabilized by coagulation factor XIII

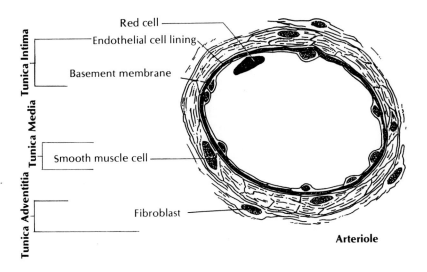

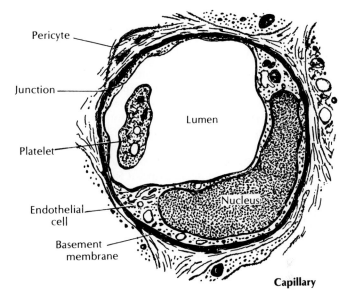

FIG. 49-2.   Comparison of capillary and arteriole structure viewed through vessel lumen. Capillary is shown at higher magnification than arteriole to display details. (From Corriveau DM, Fritsma GA (eds): Hemostasis and Thrombosis in the Clinical Laboratory, p 15. Philadelphia, JB Lippincott, 1988, with permission.)

erythrocyte or leukocyte to pass. There are openings called *junctions* along the capillary wall that allow the passage of leukocytes, oxygen, and nutrients into and out of the blood as necessary. Also, waste may pass from the tissues into the blood through these junctions. Erythrocytes and platelets usually do not leave the intravascular system. Pericytes are cells that lie beneath the endothelium of capillaries as well as arteries and veins. Pericytes may differentiate into vessel-related cells when needed.

ARTERIES AND VEINS.   The arteries and veins are larger than capillaries (see Fig. 49-2). Their structure includes three layers: (1) the *tunica intima* or inner endothelial lining, which comes into contact with blood cells and separates them from a subendothelium composed of a basement membrane, elastic connective tissue, and collagen fibers; endothelial cells deposit von Willebrand factor (vWF—a protein required for normal platelet function) in the subendothelial matrix where vWF binds to collagen; (2) the *tunica media*, composed of smooth muscle cells and connective

tissue, including collagen fibers and occasional fibroblasts; and (3) the *tunica adventitia* or outer part of the vessel wall, which consists of connective-tissue fibroblasts and collagen fibers.

Blood is normally carried within vessels whose physical capabilities include constriction and dilation, which are controlled by the smooth muscle of the vessel media. Vasoconstriction and vasodilation provide the means for control of blood flow rate and blood pressure. Substances released from the endothelial cells and subendothelial smooth muscle also contribute to normal blood flow and prevent abnormal formation of clots. Endothelial cells secrete several important substances, which are briefly described in Table 49-2. These substances influence coagulation, fibrinolysis, and platelets (Chap. 50).

The intact endothelial lining of blood vessels is antithrombotic: it does not activate platelets or promote coagulation. This lining provides a smooth surface that facilitates blood flow and reduces turbulence, which can promote thrombosis.

Damaged Vessels

Blood is maintained in a fluid state as it flows through intact vessels. On vessel injury, vasoconstriction occurs as a neurogenic response. Injury breaks the smooth endothelial lining, exposing collagen, a surface that promotes thrombus formation by causing the adherence of platelets to the area of injury. Collagen exposure also initiates the *contact phase* of coagulation, which begins a series of biochemical reactions known as the *intrinsic coagulation pathway*. Tissue thromboplastin is released from the injured vessel, which promotes coagulation through a different series of reactions known as the *extrinsic coagulation pathway*.

In addition to coagulation promotion, vessel injury initiates fibrinolysis through endothelial cell release of tissue plasminogen activators (tPAs). This response provides one of the necessary checks and balances on the coagulation system to ensure that excessive coagulation does not occur. The physiologic responses to vessel injury are summarized in Figure 49-3.

Role of Coagulation in Hemostasis

Coagulation is the process whereby, on vessel injury, plasma proteins, tissue factors, and calcium interact on the surface of platelets to form a fibrin clot. Platelets not only provide a surface for the coagulation reaction; they also interact with fibrin to form a stable platelet-fibrin clot.

Table 49-3 lists the coagulation factors. Most are referred to both by Roman numerals and by names assigned by the International Committee on Nomenclature of Blood Coagulation Factors.[39] These factors (except calcium and tissue thromboplastin) normally circulate in the plasma as inactive proteins. On activation, some factors form enzymatic proteins known as *serine proteases* that activate other specific factors in the coagulation sequence.

Basically, there are three interrelated pathways of coagulation, each representing a unique series of biochemical reactions, as shown in Figure 49-4. These pathways are the intrinsic, the extrinsic, and the common. Each pathway is activated by a different mechanism. The extrinsic and intrinsic pathways ultimately come together to initiate the common pathway, which leads to stable fibrin clot formation. There is a great deal of interaction among these pathways, which will be discussed in Chapter 50.

The Extrinsic Pathway

The extrinsic coagulation pathway is activated by the release of tissue thromboplastin into the plasma from injured tissue cells. Tissue thromboplastin activates factor VII to the serine protease factor VII_a (see Fig. 49-4); the subscript "a" indicates the activated state of the factor. Factor VII_a, with calcium and platelet phospholipid (PL), activates factor X to factor X_a in the common pathway.

The Intrinsic Pathway

Activation of the intrinsic pathway occurs when a vessel is injured, exposing the subendothelial basement membrane and collagen, both surfaces that promote coagulation. When the subendothelial surface is contacted by the coagulation contact factors XII, XI, high-molecular-weight kininogen (HMWK), and prekallikrein, the contact activation of the intrinsic pathway is begun (see Fig. 49-4). The contact factors XII and XI are converted to the serine proteases XII_a and XI_a. Factor XI_a, with calcium, in turn converts factor IX to the serine protease IX_a. Factor IX_a, with platelet PL, calcium, and a cofactor, factor VIII_a, con-

TABLE 49–2. Antithrombotic, Fibrinolytic, and Coagulant Substances Released from or Found on the Surface of Intact Endothelial Cells

SUBSTANCE	ACTION	HEMOSTATIC ROLE
Prostacyclin (PGI$_2$)	Inhibits platelet activation	Anticoagulant
	Stimulates vasodilation	Reduces blood flow rate
Adenosine (metabolic product of ATP and ADP)	Stimulates vasodilation	Reduces blood flow rate
Thrombomodulin	Endothelial surface receptor for thrombin	Anticoagulant
	Binds and inactivates thrombin and enhances anticoagulant and fibrinolytic action of protein C found in the plasma (see Fig. 56-1)	Fibrinolytic
Heparan sulfate	Coats the endothelial cell surface and weakly enhances activity of antithrombin-III, a plasma anticoagulant	Anticoagulant
Tissue plasminogen activator (tPA)	Converts plasminogen to plasmin, which plays important role in fibrinolysis	Fibrinolytic
	Released only on appropriate stimulus, such as vessel injury, to prevent excessive clot formation at the site of injury and begin slow clot dissolution as the injured vessel heals	
von Willebrand factor (vWF)	Protein secreted by endothelium into subendothelium; required for platelet adhesion to site of vessel injury	Coagulation

The endothelium plays multiple roles to promote normal blood flow and prevent thrombotic episodes and to prevent excessive clot formation at the site of vessel injury. On the other side of the hemostatic spectrum, endothelial cells produce vWF, which promotes platelet adhesion to exposed collagen on vessel injury.

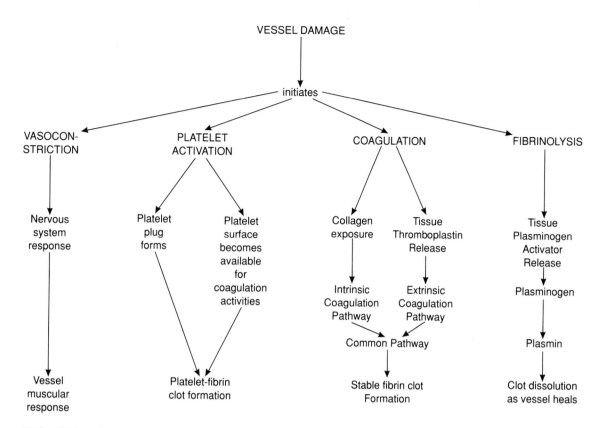

FIG. 49-3. Physiologic response to vessel damage. Platelet activation causes platelet plug formation and makes platelet surface conducive to coagulation factor activation. Activation of coagulation initiates intrinsic and extrinsic coagulation pathways.

verts factor X to the serine protease factor X_a in the common pathway.

The Common Pathway

The common pathway begins with activation of factor X to factor X_a by either the intrinsic or the extrinsic pathway (see Fig. 49-4). Factor X_a with a cofactor, factor V_a, and calcium, converts factor II, prothrombin, to factor II_a, thrombin. Factor II_a converts factor I, fibrinogen, to fibrin. Factor XIII then stabilizes the fibrin clot.

TABLE 49–3. Coagulation Factor Nomenclature with Preferred Names★

FACTOR	PREFERRED NAME
I	Fibrinogen
II	Prothrombin
III	Tissue factor
IV	Calcium
V	Proaccelerin
VII	Proconvertin
VIII:C	Antihemophilic factor
IX	Plasma thromboplastin component
X	Stuart-Prower factor
XI	Plasma thromboplastin antecedent
XII	Hageman factor
XIII	Fibrin stabilizing factor
HMWK	High-molecular-weight kininogen
Prekallikrein	Prekallikrein

★ See Table 50–1 for preferred names and their synonyms.

Role of Platelets in Hemostasis

History of Clinical Recognition and Investigation

Platelets were described by several investigators in 1842,[1,3,5,35] although no one at that time knew the origin of platelets. In 1878, it was recognized that platelets, like erythrocytes and leukocytes, are unique elements of the blood.[8] Soon thereafter, it was discovered that platelets originate from large cells in the bone marrow called megakaryocytes.[40] In the 1940s, researchers were first able to study platelet structure using the electron microscope. It has become clear that platelets play a vital role in hemostasis and that qualitative or quantitative platelet abnormalities can cause hypocoagulation or hypercoagulation disorders. Normal hemostatic function requires peripheral blood platelets that are normal in number (approximate reference range $150–400 \times 10^9/L$) and function.

Quantitation of platelet numbers has been performed since the early part of the 20th century using a hemocytometer, microscope, and stain specific for platelets. In 1950 a method for counting platelets was described that utilizes phase-contrast microscopy[2] (Chap. 59). Today, platelets are routinely enumerated using automated methods.

Qualitative (functional) platelet evaluation was first available with the introduction of the *bleeding time test* by Duke in the early 1900s.[4] A prolonged bleeding time can indicate either a thrombocytopenia (decreased platelet count; Chap. 60) or thrombocytopathy (abnormal platelet function; Chap. 61). Although the bleeding time is still the best

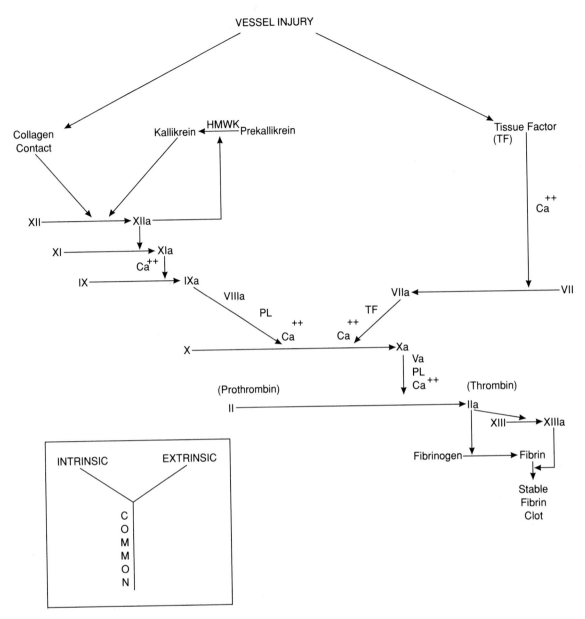

FIG. 49-4.   Intrinsic, extrinsic, and common pathways of coagulation. Vessel injury initiates intrinsic pathway through contact activation by exposed collagen. Extrinsic pathway is initiated by endothelial release of tissue factor (*i.e.*, tissue thromboplastin). Extrinsic and intrinsic pathway each initiate common pathway to create stable fibrin clot. A more extensive picture of these pathways and their interactions with one another and other systems is presented in Figure 50-1.

screening test for platelet function, more specific tests such as *platelet aggregation studies* (Chap. 59) are now available.

Platelet Morphology and Function in Hemostasis

As shown in Table 49-1 and Figure 49-3, platelets play a central and immediate role in the response to vessel injury. Platelets are the smallest microscopically visible element observed on the peripheral blood film. They are 2 to 4 μm in diameter and approximately 7 fL in volume and have a discoid shape. With Wright stain, platelets have a light violet-purple granular appearance and look like specks of dust. Platelets are small fragments of megakaryocyte cytoplasm. They have a lifespan of 9 to 10 days.[7] The platelet

maturation cycle and platelet function are presented in Chapter 58. Platelets play the following important roles in hemostasis: (1) they adhere to injured vessels; (2) they aggregate at the injury site; (3) they promote coagulation on their phospholipid surface (Fig. 58-11); (4) they release biochemicals important to hemostasis; and (5) they induce clot retraction.

SUBSTANCES SECRETED BY PLATELETS.   Platelets secrete substances stored on their surface membrane and within cytoplasmic granules called dense granules (or dense bodies) and alpha granules. The important substances for this discussion are listed in Table 49-4 along with their source and function. These are discussed further in Chapter 58.

PLATELET INDUCTION OF CLOT RETRACTION. The last act of platelets within a platelet–fibrin clot is contraction of the clot, which is associated with a tremendous consumption of energy (ATP). Calcium also is required for retraction. This phenomenon can be observed *in vitro* when blood clots in a test tube. The clot contracts after a few hours, leaving clear serum adjacent to the test tube walls. This is an *in vitro* phenomenon that is subjectively indicative of normal platelet function *in vivo* but requires verification using tests of platelet function.

The retraction process involves stabilization of platelet–platelet and platelet–fibrin attachments. The pulling forces are provided by contractile platelet elements in a process similar to muscle tissue contraction. The exact purpose of clot retraction is unclear; hypotheses include participation in the vascular constrictive response to injury, the stabilization of the fibrin clot network, and debulking of the clot to help reestablish blood flow.

Fibrinolysis in Hemostasis

History of Investigation

In the late 1700s John Hunter reported the unexplained finding that blood from people who had died in accidents or while in some traumatic situation did not clot.[12] In 1937 MacFarlane reported that damaged tissues release a substance (plasminogen activator) that activates the inert precursor called plasminogen, which normally circulates in the plasma, to its active form, plasmin.[18] Plasmin is a nonspecific proteolytic enzyme capable of degrading fibrin as well as fibrinogen and factors V and VIII. The process of factor degradation by plasmin provides some explanation for the lack of clotting in deceased accident and trauma victims. The process of fibrinolysis has since been elucidated extensively (Chap. 50) and its laboratory evaluation greatly advanced (Chap. 54).

Function of Fibrinolysis in Hemostasis

Fibrinolysis is the system whereby the temporary fibrin clot is systematically and gradually dissolved as the vessel heals in order to restore normal blood flow.

TABLE 49–4. Summary of Most Important Substances Secreted by Platelets and Their Role in Hemostasis

ROLE IN HEMOSTASIS	SUBSTANCE	SOURCE	COMMENTS ON PRINCIPAL FUNCTION*
Promote coagulation	HMWK	Alpha granules	Contact activation of intrinsic coagulation pathway
	Fibrinogen	Alpha granules	Converted to fibrin for clot formation
	Factor V	Alpha granules	Cofactor in fibrin clot formation
	Factor VIII:vWF	Alpha granules	Assists platelet adhesion to subendothelium to provide coagulation surface
Promote aggregation	ADP	Dense bodies	Promotes platelet aggregation
	Calcium	Dense bodies	Same
	Platelet factor 4	Alpha granules	Same
	Thrombospondin	Alpha granules	Same
Promote vasoconstriction	Serotonin	Dense bodies	Promotes vasoconstriction at injury site
	Thromboxane A_2 precursors	Membrane phospholipids	Same
Promote vascular repair	Platelet-derived growth factor	Alpha granules	Promotes smooth muscle growth for vessel repair
	Beta thromboglobulin	Alpha granules	Chemotactic for fibroblasts to help in vessel repair[34]
Other systems affected	Plasminogen	Alpha granules	Precursor to plasmin, which induces clot lysis
	α_2-Antiplasmin	Alpha granules	Plasmin inhibitor; inhibits clot lysis
	Cl esterase inhibitor	Alpha granules	Complement system inhibitor

* Functions other than those indicated also exist for some substances.

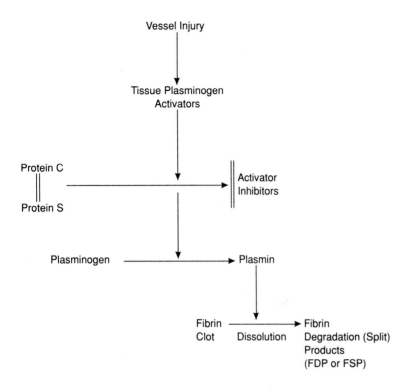

FIG. 49-5.   Simple overview of fibrinolytic pathway. Tissue plasminogen activators activate plasminogen within clot to plasmin, which slowly dissolves fibrin clot. Inhibitors are neutralized by protein C–S complex, thus enhancing fibrinolysis.

There are a number of substances responsible for fibrinolysis (Fig. 49-5). The proteolytic enzyme *plasmin* is the primary substance responsible. *Tissue plasminogen activators*, which convert plasminogen to plasmin, are released from injured vessel walls. Plasmin is trapped within the clot, and clot lysis begins slowly as soon as the clot is formed, with fibrin degradation (split) products (FDP or FSP) being released in the plasma. Lysis is slow because of fibrin clot stabilization by factor XIII, fibrin-stabilizing factor. Proteins C and S are two hemostatic substances that further enhance fibrinolysis and inactivate tPA inhibitors.

BASIC TERMINOLOGY FOR CLINICAL FINDINGS IN BLEEDING DISORDERS

The reader should be familiar with the meanings of the terms describing the clinical findings associated with bleeding disorders caused by abnormal vessels or platelets or an abnormal coagulation or fibrinolytic mechanism. The following is a short list of basic clinical terms that will be used in this and later chapters to describe such clinical findings.

Petechiae are purplish red, pinpoint hemorrhagic spots in the skin caused by loss of capillary ability to withstand normal blood pressure and trauma. Poor capillary integrity allows erythrocytes to leak out of capillary beds into tissue. Many petechiae close together can create purpura (see below). Petechiae are more indicative of a vascular or platelet disorder than of coagulation or fibrinolytic defects.

Purpura is produced by hemorrhage of blood into small areas of skin, mucous membranes, and other tissues (see Fig. 49-8). At first these areas appear red but later turn purple and finally brownish yellow. The colors of hemorrhagic areas coincide with the degradation of the Hb deposited there. The heme molecule causes a reddish purple or black color; conversion to biliverdin causes the greenish yellow color. As the color fades, biliverdin is converted to bilirubin, which is removed from the area and processed in the liver.

Ecchymosis is a form of purpura in which blood escapes into large areas of skin or mucous membranes, but not into deep tissue. The area turns black and blue and later, greenish brown or yellow (see Fig. 49-7). The term *easy bruisability* is used to describe individuals with extensive or repeated occurrences of purpura and ecchymoses.

Epistaxis is a nosebleed.

Hemarthrosis is leakage of blood into a joint cavity.

Hematemesis designates vomiting of blood.

Hematoma is a swelling or tumor in the tissues or a body cavity that contains clotted blood.

Hematuria is intact red cells in the urine.

Hemoglobinuria refers to Hb (no intact red cells) in the urine.

Hemoptysis is expectoration of blood secondary to hemorrhage in the larynx, trachea, bronchi, or lungs.

Melena is stool containing dark red or black blood. The black color is caused by the action of intestinal juices on blood that has escaped into the gastrointestinal tract from the vascular system.

Menorrhagia is excessive menstrual bleeding.

BLEEDING DISORDERS CAUSED BY VASCULAR DEFECTS

Many types of vascular defects result in hemostatic abnormalities. Often these defects are initially diagnosed because a patient has a bleeding tendency or a specific type of skin lesion, although platelet quantities and function and coagulation factor activity are found to be normal. Diagnosis of these defects generally is not based on laboratory results, because there are no characteristic laboratory findings;

however, the finding of normal results can help to rule out some possible diagnoses. Fortunately, there usually is some clinical sign or symptom that assists in the diagnosis.

Vascular defects may be categorized by a variety of methods. Table 49–5 divides vascular abnormalities into hereditary and acquired defects causing bleeding secondary to vascular defects of several types.

Hereditary Connective Tissue Defects

Connective tissue is found in all three layers of the vessel wall; thus, hereditary connective tissue defects affect vessels in all three layers of their structure. Connective tissue provides support for vessels as well as other structures of the body. Such tissue may be damaged by either hereditary or acquired disorders (discussed in the next section of this chapter).

Ehlers-Danlos Syndrome
The Ehlers-Danlos syndrome has an autosomal dominant pattern of inheritance.[21] The affected individual has hyperextensible joints and hyperplastic skin, which can be stretched much more than normal skin but which returns to normal on release. The connective tissue of the skin, vasculature, and bones is adversely affected, causing a lack of structural support in these tissues and great tissue fragility. The defect may lie in a peptidase enzyme that converts procollagen to collagen.[27]

PHYSICAL FINDINGS.   There may be large skin ecchymoses and hematomas, bleeding from the gums, excessive postpartum bleeding, and gastrointestinal bleeding. Patients often report easy bruisability.

LABORATORY FINDINGS.   Coagulation test results and platelet function studies usually are normal.

TREATMENT.   In spite of the complications, these patients generally have a normal life span. There is no known therapy.

Pseudoxanthoma Elasticum
Pseudoxanthoma elasticum is a rare connective tissue disorder. The inheritance pattern is autosomal recessive. The cause of this disorder is unclear, although it is recognized that the connective tissue elastic fibers in small arteries are calcified and structurally abnormal. Many symptoms and physical findings relating to hemorrhagic episodes are common. Subarachnoid and gastrointestinal bleeding are the most common causes of death.

LABORATORY FINDINGS.   Tests usually are not helpful in the diagnosis except to rule out other causes of the clinical abnormalities.

TREATMENT.   There is no known therapy for the disorder.

Acquired Connective Tissue Defects

Vitamin C Deficiency (Scurvy)
Scurvy is an acquired disorder caused by dietary deficiency of vitamin C (ascorbic acid), which is required for

TABLE 49–5. Principal Hereditary and Acquired Bleeding Disorders Associated with Vascular Abnormalities

ABNORMALITY	HEREDITARY	ACQUIRED
Connective tissue defects	Ehlers-Danlos syndrome Pseudoxanthoma elasticum	Vitamin C deficiency (scurvy) Senile purpura Corticosteroid purpura Aging Cushing's disease Others
Altered vessel wall structure	Hemorrhagic telangiectasia Hemangiomata— congenital (Kasabach-Merritt syndrome)	Diabetes mellitus Amyloidosis Others
Endothelial damage		Infectious purpura Bacterial: tuberculosis, scarlet fever, typhoid fever, diphtheria, endocarditis, others Viral: smallpox, influenza, measles, others Rickettsial: Rocky Mountain spotted fever, others Protozoal: malaria, others Autoimmune vascular purpura Allergic purpuras: Henoch-Schönlein purpura Drug-induced purpuras: quinine, procaine penicillin, aspirin, sulfonamides, sedatives, coumarins
Miscellaneous abnormalities causing purpura secondary to vessel damage		Waldenström's macroglobulinemia Kaposi's sarcoma Certain skin diseases Hemochromatosis Snake venom Others

Modified from Wintrobe MM: Clinical Hematology, 8th ed, p 1073. Philadelphia, Lea & Febiger, 1981.

the formation of the intact structure of the vascular basement membrane. The RDA for ascorbic acid is 60 mg.[24] Without vitamin C, hydroxylation of the amino acids proline and lysine cannot take place and collagen cannot be formed properly. This deficiency can cause serious bleeding problems because collagen is necessary to the structural integrity of vessels and their connective tissue.

Dietary deficiency was historically identified on a large scale in British sailors, who developed bleeding gums and other hemorrhagic manifestations secondary to lack of dietary vitamin C while at sea for lengthy periods. On the basis of observations of James Lind, sailors began eating limes to relieve the symptoms; thus, the sailors' nickname "Limies."

PHYSICAL FINDINGS. Gingival (gum) bleeding and hemorrhage into subcutaneous tissues and muscles are characteristic. Petechiae often develop on the thighs and buttocks, particularly around the hair follicles (perifollicular petechiae). Large hemorrhagic areas may develop just below the eyes, particularly in affected infants. In some cases, splinter-like hemorrhages appear in the fingernail beds.

LABORATORY FINDINGS. There may be anemia and a low plasma ascorbic acid level. Measurement of ascorbic acid in the platelet-leukocyte layer of centrifuged peripheral blood[15] is a more reliable indicator of vitamin C deficiency and body stores than the plasma or whole blood levels, which more closely reflect recent dietary intake. However, vitamin C measurement in the platelet–leukocyte layer is technically difficult and requires more than 2 mL of blood; therefore, it is seldom performed in the laboratory. The reference range for leukocyte vitamin C is 15 to 30 mg/dL.[11] Other methods are available for quantitation of vitamin C in the plasma, leukocytes, and urine.[31] Reference values for plasma range from 0.5 to 1.0 mg/dL.[11]

The *tourniquet test* for capillary fragility is usually positive (*i.e.*, petechiae are found on the skin after the test). This test is an inexact, qualitative test in which a blood pressure cuff is inflated on the arm to between 70 to 90 mm Hg and left in place for 5 minutes.[6] After removal of the cuff, the arm, wrist, and hand are inspected for petechiae. In healthy normal adults, only occasional petechiae are found or none at all.[22] If vitamin C deficiency is severe, the petechial hemorrhages may be extensive. Therefore, the time of tourniquet application should be shortened if extensive petechiae are noticed before the end of the usual 5-minute interval. This test can be painful for the patient, and it is therefore rarely performed.

A modification of the tourniquet test for capillary fragility involves the use of controlled suction, which is applied using an instrument called a petechiometer. It is normal for an adult to have 0 to 10 petechiae in the area where suction is applied for a short time at 15 to 20 mm Hg.

The bleeding time and coagulation tests usually are normal in patients with scurvy.

TREATMENT. Administration of ascorbic acid usually brings the serum level of vitamin C and the vascular integrity back to normal.

Senile Purpura

Senile purpura is an acquired and chronic disorder of the elderly causing abnormalities in connective tissue. The aging process brings about a degeneration of collagen, elastin, and subcutaneous fat.

PHYSICAL FINDINGS. Characteristically, patients demonstrate red to purple ecchymotic areas on the forearm and on the backs of the hands and neck secondary to loss of skin and vascular elasticity.[37] Often the area retains a permanent brownish color, possibly because the Hb is not properly removed by the aging macrophage system.

Corticosteroid therapy and Cushing disease can induce formation of purpura similar to that seen in senile purpura.

LABORATORY FINDINGS. The tourniquet test is positive in some of these patients; however, this test is rarely necessary to make the diagnosis. The bleeding time is normal or only slightly prolonged, and other coagulation tests are normal.

TREATMENT. No measure of any real value has been found.[38]

Hereditary Alterations of Vessel Wall Structure

Hereditary Hemorrhagic Telangiectasia

An autosomal dominant trait, hereditary hemorrhagic telangiectasia is characterized by vascular malformations and surface skin lesions called telangiectasias. The small blood vessels are focally disorganized and dilated throughout the body, their wall support is poor, and their ability to contract is diminished.

DEMOGRAPHICS. This disorder is found most often in Anglo-German, Latin, Scandinavian, and Jewish populations.[38] Although relatively uncommon, it is the most common vascular disorder with a hemorrhagic diathesis (predisposition to hemorrhage).

PHYSICAL FINDINGS. Telangiectasias are thin, dilated vessels. The lesions range from pinpoint size to 3 mm and are red to violet. They may bleed either spontaneously or from minor trauma. They appear most commonly on the face, lips (Fig. 49-6), tongue, mucous membranes of the mouth and nose, the ears, conjunctivae, and the palms of the hands and soles of the feet. Although they may be detected in childhood, the number of lesions increases with advancing age. Telangiectasias are permanent: they do not disappear with time like ecchymoses or purpura. Ecchymoses and purpura are not seen in this disorder.

Patients may report frequent epistaxis and symptoms of anemia.

LABORATORY FINDINGS. Anemia is seen in many cases, depending on the degree of bleeding. An iron deficiency anemia may develop from either gastrointestinal bleeding or other chronic blood loss. There are no unusual or characteristic laboratory findings. Usually the bleeding time, platelet function tests, tourniquet test, and coagulation tests are normal. The diagnosis is based largely on the finding of telangiectasias.

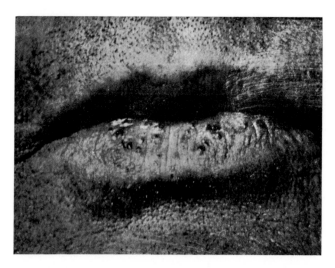

FIG. 49-6.   Hereditary hemorrhagic telangiectasia; characteristic lesions on lips. (From Wintrobe MM: Clinical Hematology, 8th ed, p 1080. Philadelphia, Lea & Febiger, 1981, with permission.)

TREATMENT.   The oral administration of iron may be used to alleviate anemia. A number of therapeutic drugs and surgical techniques may be required to stop or prevent bleeding episodes.

Congenital Hemangiomata
(Kasabach-Merritt Syndrome)

The congenital hemangiomata or Kasabach–Merritt syndrome is a disorder associated with tumors composed of vessels that commonly swell and bleed at the surface. The tumors range in size from small to enormous lesions that protrude from the skin surface. They generally require surgical removal.

Formation of fibrin clots, platelet consumption, and red cell destruction secondary to vascular obstruction occur at the site of the tumor. This leads to laboratory test results indicative of diffuse intravascular coagulation (DIC) (Chap. 55), which is found in a variety of disorders.

Acquired Alterations of Vessel Wall Structure

A number of other disorders may damage the vessel wall structure. In *diabetes mellitus* the large vessels may become atherosclerotic, and the capillary basement membrane may thicken, thus blocking the normal flow of blood. Most often affected are the capillaries of the renal glomeruli (causing proteinuria and renal failure) and the retina (which may cause blindness). There are no characteristic hematologic or hemostatic abnormalities associated with diabetes.

Amyloidosis also alters vessel structure. It can involve and obstruct the function of many organs, including the vascular system, in which there is deposition of the fibrillar protein called amyloid, which causes various degrees of vessel obstruction. Purpura may result from amyloid deposition in small vessels at the skin surface. There generally are no hematologic or hemostatic abnormalities, although some may be caused by the underlying disorders.

Endothelial Damage

Many autoimmune or infectious agents (*e.g.*, rickettsia) are responsible for damage to the endothelial lining of the vessels. Damage may be caused by the agent directly or by its byproducts or toxins. This damage can lead to either hypocoagulation or hypercoagulation. Autoimmune and infectious processes that damage endothelium are discussed below. Hypertension may also damage the endothelium, resulting in a microangiopathic hemolytic anemia.

Autoimmune Vascular Purpura

Autoimmune vascular purpura may be caused by an allergic reaction, or it may be drug induced.

DRUG-INDUCED PURPURA.   Table 49-5 lists some of the more common drugs that induce purpura in susceptible patients. Such purpura disappears on discontinuance of the drug.

ALLERGIC PURPURA.   This purpura includes a broad group of disorders resulting from an autoimmune process that is not clearly understood. Patients with allergic purpura develop characteristic purpuric eruptions on the skin surface. The tissues below the surface are also affected to some degree. The lesions may be accompanied by swelling, and in some cases ulcers develop at the lesion sites. Most commonly, lesions develop on the arms and legs (see Fig. 49-7). The lesions begin as small round, raised, pink areas that within hours turn to a darker red and begin to coalesce

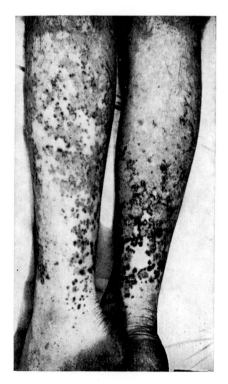

FIG. 49-7.   Henoch-Schönlein purpura; note ecchymoses and erythematous lesions on both legs. (From Wintrobe MM: Clinical Hematology, 8th ed, p 1076. Philadelphia, Lea & Febiger, 1981, with permission.)

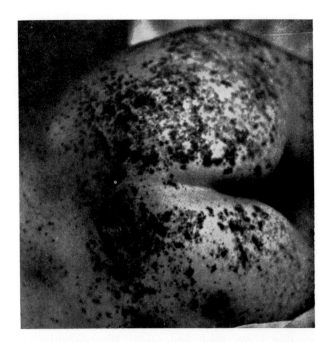

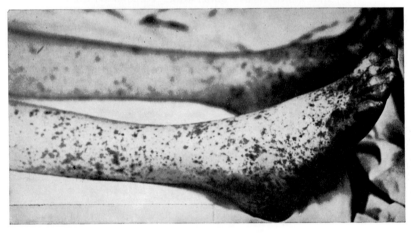

FIG. 49-8. Purpura in patient with scarlet fever. Note purpuric lesions on both legs. Thrombocytopenia was ruled out. (From Fox MJ, Enzer N: A consideration of the phenomenon of purpura following scarlet fever. Am J Med Sci 196:321, 1938.)

into larger patches. In the healing process the area turns purple and then brown.

Children are the most frequently affected by allergic purpura. Adolescents are affected less often and adults rarely.[16,38] Patients may complain of headaches, abdominal or joint pain, anorexia, or fever. They may also report an itching, tingling, or numb sensation at the lesion sites.

HENOCH-SCHÖNLEIN PURPURA. Two specific types of allergic purpura have been recognized since the 1800s, although their etiology was not well understood. Purpura associated with abdominal pain secondary to gastrointestinal hemorrhaging is called Henoch's purpura.[9] When associated with joint pain, especially in the knees, ankles, and wrists,[30] the disorder is called Schönlein's purpura.[32] Abdominal and joint pain related to allergic purpura may occur together, thus the designation Henoch-Schönlein purpura (Fig. 49-7).

LABORATORY FINDINGS. Usually, there is no anemia, but there may be a modest neutrophilia or eosinophilia.[38] The tourniquet test may be positive, but other tests of coagulation, platelet number, and platelet function usually are normal. The stools may be positive for blood.

The diagnosis can be difficult because purpura is not always obvious, and other disorders may produce similar symptoms, particularly joint and abdominal pain, which are associated with a number of conditions.

TREATMENT. Treatment usually is limited to symptomatic therapy, as the purpuric episodes begin and subside spontaneously. Any recognized allergen should be avoided. There generally is a favorable prognosis.

Infectious Purpura

As listed in Table 49-5, endothelial damage can be caused by several agents, which may produce purpura as well as petechiae. The purpura may form for several reasons: as a result of an inflammatory response to the infectious process, an autoimmune response, bacterial products, toxins, or direct injury by the infectious agent. Figure 49-8 shows a patient with marked purpura. In some disorders, there is concurrent thrombocytopenia and DIC that contribute to the formation of purpura.

The most significant laboratory findings are microbiologic identification of the infectious agent and tests to select appropriate antibiotic treatment. Treatment centers on elimination of the infectious agent through the use of antibiotics when possible.

CHAPTER SUMMARY

The hemostatic process involves an interaction among blood vessels, platelets, and biochemical substances in the plasma (the procoagulants). Abnormalities in any of these components may result in hemostatic abnormalities that lead to mild, moderate, or life-threatening bleeding or clotting.

When the vascular system is injured, four steps in hemostasis are initiated sequentially (see Fig. 49-3): (1) vasoconstriction; (2) platelet activation, including platelet adhesion, aggregation, and release of substances that promote hemostasis (see Table 49-4); (3) coagulation, in which inactive coagulation factors (see Table 49-3) are converted to serine proteases, which activate other factors (see Fig. 49-4); and (4) fibrinolysis. The delicate balance of the hemostatic system is required to prevent hypocoagulation (excessive bleeding) and hypercoagulation (excessive clotting—*i.e.*, thrombus formation) (see Fig. 49-1).

Arteries and veins are composed of three layers (see Fig. 49-2). The tunica intima comes into contact with blood cells and is antithrombotic. That is, it does not ordinarily promote coagulation or platelet adherence. Secreted substances from the endothelium also promote normal blood flow and influence coagulation, fibrinolysis, and platelets (see Table 49-2). On vessel injury and exposure of the collagen of the tunica media and tunica adventitia, contact activation of the intrinsic system of coagulation is initiated (factors XII, XI, IX, VIII, calcium, platelet phospholipid) (see Fig. 49-4). Tissue thromboplastin released from the damaged vessel wall initiates extrinsic coagulation (factor VII, calcium). Both the intrinsic and the extrinsic system initiate the common coagulation pathway that leads to fibrin clot formation (factors X, V, calcium, platelet phospholipid, factors II, I, XIII).

Normal hemostatic function requires peripheral blood platelets that are normal in number ($150–400 \times 10^9$/L) and function. Platelets are usually quantitated today by automated methods. Decreased platelet counts are referred to as thrombocytopenia and increased counts as thombocytosis; abnormal counts are associated with a number of disorders. Thrombocytopathies are disorders associated with platelet function abnormalities.

Fibrinolysis is required to dissolve clots on vessel healing. Plasmin, the active form of plasminogen, is responsible for clot dissolution (see Fig. 49-5). Without normal fibrinolysis, clots remain in the vessels or form uncontrollably and obstruct blood flow.

Hereditary and acquired defects of vessels (see Table 49-5), as well as of coagulation factors, fibrinolytic components, and platelets, can cause serious imbalance of the hemostatic mechanism and lead to uncontrolled bleeding or clotting, depending on the component affected. Whereas vessel defects usually cannot be detected by laboratory tests, defects of the other hemostatic components often can be.

CASE STUDY 49-1

A small group of physicians, laboratory scientists, and nurses had set up a clinic in a developing country plagued by famine. In one particular village the group noticed that many of the children, as well as adults, had bleeding gums and petechiae on the buttocks. A few of the children had hemorrhagic areas below their eyes.

1. What is the most likely cause of these abnormal physical findings?
2. What is the name of this disorder, and how does it affect the vascular system?
3. To assist in the diagnosis, what test could be performed easily in this primitive environment? What are the expected results of such a test given the likely diagnosis?
4. Is this test qualitative or quantitative?
5. What equipment is required for the test, and how is it used?
6. What constitutes a positive or negative test result?
7. What results would you expect if coagulation tests or a bleeding time test were performed on these patients? Why?
8. What would be the physician's treatment of choice?

REFERENCES

1. Addison W: On the colorless corpuscles and on the molecules and cytoblasts in the blood. London Med Gaz (New Series) 30:144, 1842
2. Brecher G, Cronkite EP: Morphology and enumeration of human blood platelets. J Appl Physiol 3:365, 1950
3. Donné AD: L'origine des globules der sang de leur mode de formation et de leur fin. Comp Rend Acad Sci 14:366, 1842
4. Duke WW: The pathogenesis of purpura haemorrhagica with especial reference to the part played by the blood platelets. Arch Intern Med 10:445, 1912
5. Gerber F: Elements of General and Minute Anatomy of Man and Mammals. London, G Gulliver, 1842
6. Hare FW Jr, Miller AJ: Capillary resistance tests. Arch Dermatol Syph 64:449, 1951
7. Harker LA: Platelet survival time: Its measurement and use. In Spaet TH (ed): Progress in Hemostasis and Thrombosis, p 321. New York, Grune & Stratton, 1978
8. Hayem G: Recherches sur l'évolution des hématies dans le sang del'homme et des vertébrés. Arch Physiol Norm Pathol 5:692, 1878
9. Henoch E: Über eine eigenthümliche Form von Purpura. Berlin Klin Wochenschr 11:641, 1874
10. Hopff F: Über die Hämophilie oder die erbliche Anlage zu todtlichen Blutungen [thesis]. Würzburg, Germany, 1828
11. Howard L, Meguid MM: Nutritional assessment in total parenteral nutrition. Clin Lab Med 1:611, 1981
12. Hunter J: A Treatise on the Blood, Inflammation, and Gun-Shot Wounds, 3rd ed. London, Sherwood, Gilbert, and Piper, 1828
13. Kakkar VV: The diagnosis of deep vein thrombosis using the ^{125}I-fibrinogen test. Arch Surg 104:152, 1972
14. Lee RI, White PD: A clinical study of the coagulation time of blood. Am J Med Sci 145:495, 1913
15. Lee W, Hamernyik P, Hutchinson M et al: Ascorbic acid in lymphocytes: Cell preparation and liquid-chromatographic assay. Clin Chem 28:2165, 1982
16. Lewis IC: The Schönlein-Henoch syndrome compared with certain features of nephritis and rheumatism. Arch Dis Child 30:212, 1955
17. Lipinska I, Lipinski B, Gurewich V et al: Fibrinogen heterogeneity in cancer, in occlusive vascular disease, and after surgical procedures. Am J Clin Pathol 66:958, 1976
18. MacFarlane RG: Fibrinolysis after operation. Lancet 1:10, 1937
19. Madden JL, Hume M: Venous Thromboembolism: Prevention and Treatment. New York, Appleton-Century-Crofts, 1976
20. Maimonides M: Laws of Circumcision. Book of Adoration (Sefer Ahavah). In Code of Maimonides (Mishneh Torah), Chapter 1, Paragraph 18. Jerusalem, Pardes, 1957
21. McKusick VA: Multiple forms of Ehlers-Danlos syndrome. Arch Surg 109:475, 1974
22. Miale JB: Laboratory Medicine Hematology, 6th ed, p 916. St Louis, CV Mosby, 1982

23. Muller JY, Michailov T, Izrael V et al: Maladie de Rendu-Osler dans une grande famille saharienne. Presse Med 7:1723, 1978

24. National Academy of Sciences: Recommended Dietary Allowances, 9th rev ed. Washington, DC, Food and Nutrition Board of the National Research Council, 1980

25. Otto JC: An account of an hemorrhagic disposition existing in certain families. Med Resposit 6:1, 1803

26. Plato: Timaeus. In Jewett B (ed): The Dialogues of Plato, 3rd ed, vol 3, p 339. New York, Macmillan, 1982

27. Prokop DJ, Kivirikko KI, Tudeman L et al: Biosynthesis of collagen and its disorders. N Engl J Med 301:77, 1979

28. Quick AJ: The prothrombin in hemophilia and obstructive jaundice. J Biol Chem 109:73, 1935

29. Quick AJ: The development and use of the prothrombin tests. Circulation 19:92, 1959

30. Rogers PW, Bunn SM Jr, Kurtzman NA et al: Schönlein-Henoch syndrome associated with exposure to cold. Arch Intern Med 128:782, 1971

31. Sauberlich HE: Ascorbic acid (vitamin C). Clin Lab Med 1:673, 1981

32. Schönlein JL: Allgemeine und specielle. Patholgie und Therapie 2:45, 1837

33. Schönlein JL: Hämorrhaphilie (erbliche Anlage zu Blutungen) in Allgemeine und specielle Pathologie und Therapie. In Nach JL: Schönleins Vorlesungen niedergeschrieben und herausgegeben von einem seiner Zuhörer, 2nd ed, vol 2, p 88. Würzburg, Germany, Etlinger, 1832

34. Senior RM, Griffin GL, Huang JS et al: Chemotactic activity of platelet alpha granule proteins for fibroblasts. J Cell Biol 96:382, 1983

35. Simon JF: Physiologische und pathologische Anthropochemie mit Berücksichtigung der eigentlichen Zoochemie. Handbuch der angewandten medizinischen Chemie nach dem neuesten Standpunkte der Wissenschaft und nach zahlreichen eigenen Untersuchungen, part II. Berlin, A Förstner, 1842

36. Smith JL, Lineback MI: Hereditary hemorrhagic telangiectasia. Am J Med 17:41, 1954

37. Tattersall RN, Seville R: Senile purpura. Q J Med 19:151, 1959

38. Wintrobe MM: Bleeding disorders caused by vascular abnormalities. In Wintrobe MM: Clinical Hematology, 8th ed, pp 1073, 1075, 1078, 1083. Philadelphia, Lea & Febiger, 1981

39. Wright IS: The nomenclature of blood clotting factors. Thromb Diath Haemorrh 7:381, 1962

40. Wright JH: The origin and nature of the blood platelet. Boston Med Surg J 154:643, 1906

50

Mechanisms of Coagulation and Fibrinolysis

Muriel I. Jobe

Blood extravasation (the escape of blood from vessels into surrounding tissues) normally is controlled or prevented by the delicate balance among at least five components and their biochemical reactions: (1) the blood vessels (Chap. 49); (2) platelets (Chap. 58); (3) plasma coagulation proteins; (4) physiologic and naturally occurring protease inhibitors; and (5) the fibrinolytic system. The emphasis in this chapter is on the coagulation proteins, inhibitors, and fibrinolysis. In addition, the kinin and complement systems will be discussed as they relate to coagulation.

Blood is prevented from leaving the vascular system by the lining of endothelial cells in the blood vessels. This endothelial lining can be disrupted by mechanical trauma (*e.g.,* surgery), physical agents (*e.g.,* heat), or chemical injury (*e.g.,* bacterial endotoxins or drugs).

HEMOSTASIS OVERVIEW

Hemostasis can be divided into two stages: primary and secondary. *Primary hemostasis* includes the platelet and vascular response to vessel injury. *Secondary hemostasis* includes the coagulation factor response to such injury. Together, platelets, vessels, and coagulation factors combine to stop bleeding and allow for vessel repair through formation of a stable fibrin-platelet plug at the site of injury.

Primary Hemostasis

Primary hemostasis is initiated by the exposure of platelets to the subendothelial connective tissue components of blood vessels (collagen, microfilaments, basement membranes). If acute injury occurs, the small vessels constrict, and platelets immediately adhere to the exposed surfaces and release ADP and ATP (see Table 49-1). Thromboxane A_2 also is released, which promotes further vasoconstriction (see Table 49-4).

Next, a reversible primary platelet aggregation takes place during which platelets adhere to one another. Platelets also change shape, and their organelles become centralized. At this point, platelets may disaggregate in the absence of further stimulation. However, with continued stimulation, secondary, irreversible, platelet aggregation characteristically occurs. Important substances released during platelet aggregation include ADP, ATP, and serotonin. The ADP promotes secondary platelet aggregation and recruits additional platelets to the site of injury. The role of ATP is not clear. Serotonin promotes further vasoconstriction. During aggregation, phospholipid (PL) becomes available on the platelet membrane surface (Chap. 58), providing a site for fibrin formation and thrombogenesis (the formation of blood clots).

Secondary Hemostasis—The Intrinsic and Extrinsic Coagulation Pathways

In Chapter 49 the intrinsic and extrinsic pathways of coagulation, involving various proteins and other substances, were introduced. To review, the intrinsic system is activated *in vivo* by the contact of certain coagulation proteins with subendothelial connective tissue, which sets the secondary hemostatic mechanism into motion (Fig. 50-1). The extrinsic coagulation pathway, in contrast, is initiated with the release of *tissue factor* from injured vessel endothelial cells and subendothelium into the vessel lumen. Tissue factor, a high-molecular-weight lipoprotein, is found in most organs, including the lungs, kidneys, liver, brain, placenta, and spleen, as well as in large blood vessels such as the vena cava and aorta. Both the intrinsic and the extrinsic coagulation pathways lead to secondary hemostasis, namely, the formation of the stable fibrin clot. The clot thus includes both fibrin formed in secondary hemostasis and the platelet plug formed in primary hemostasis. This chapter will provide a detailed explanation of the factors and reactions of the intrinsic and extrinsic coagulation pathways.

THE COAGULATION PROTEINS— ZYMOGENS AND SERINE PROTEASES

The intrinsic and extrinsic coagulation pathways are a series of reactions that involve coagulation factors known as enzyme precursors *(zymogens),* nonenzymatic cofactors, and calcium (Ca^{++}). A fourth component is PL. All coagulation factors normally are present in the plasma, with PL being provided by platelets. The zymogens are factors II, VII, IX, X, XI, XII, and prekallikrein; the cofactors are factors V, VIII, tissue factor, and high-molecular-weight kininogen (HMWK). Zymogens are substrates that have no biologic activity until converted by enzymes to active enzymes called *serine proteases,* which have exposed, serine-rich, active enzyme sites. Serine proteases selectively hydrolyze arginine- or lysine-containing peptide bonds of other zymogens, thus converting them to serine proteases.[23]

Zymogen activation may involve either a conformational change (*e.g.,* twist, turn, or bend) in the zymogen molecule or hydrolytic cleavage of a specific zymogen peptide bond through a converting enzyme, the serine protease, in the presence of a platelet PL surface. Initially, coagulation reactions occur on the injured, exposed endothelial surfaces of blood vessels and consist of conformational changes in the zymogens that convert them to serine proteases. Later, coagulation reactions occur on the PL surfaces of aggregated platelets and involve hydrolytic cleavage of the next sequential zymogen to an active enzyme.

The activation of zymogen factors X and II requires the presence of the nonenzymatic cofactors, VIII and V, respectively. To perform their functions, these cofactors must be activated (VIII_a and V_a) by small amounts of thrombin. Thrombin enhances their ability to assist in the activation of factors X and II, respectively, although high concentrations of thrombin inhibit VIII and V activity. Cofactors assist in activation of zymogens by either altering zymogen conformation to permit more efficient cleavage by the serine protease, or binding the zymogen and appropriate serine protease on a platelet PL surface to enhance and accelerate the zymogen activation process, or both.

The transformation of zymogens to active serine proteases causes biochemical amplification of the coagulation process; that is, the production of serine proteases increases the rate of further transformation of zymogens and the activity levels of cofactors. For example, traces of thrombin increase the activity of factor VIII 80-fold.[92]

In contrast the hemostatic process also provides amplification of the control mechanisms that prevent excessive clotting and thrombosis. Inhibitors and thrombolytic factors maintain a balance in the system between clotting and clot lysis. While tissue is being repaired, the fibrinolytic system slowly dissolves the clot with the glycoprotein plasmin (also called fibrinolysin). Although plasmin is capable of digesting many proteins (fibrin, fibrinogen, factors V and VIII), it is also held in check by several inhibitors.

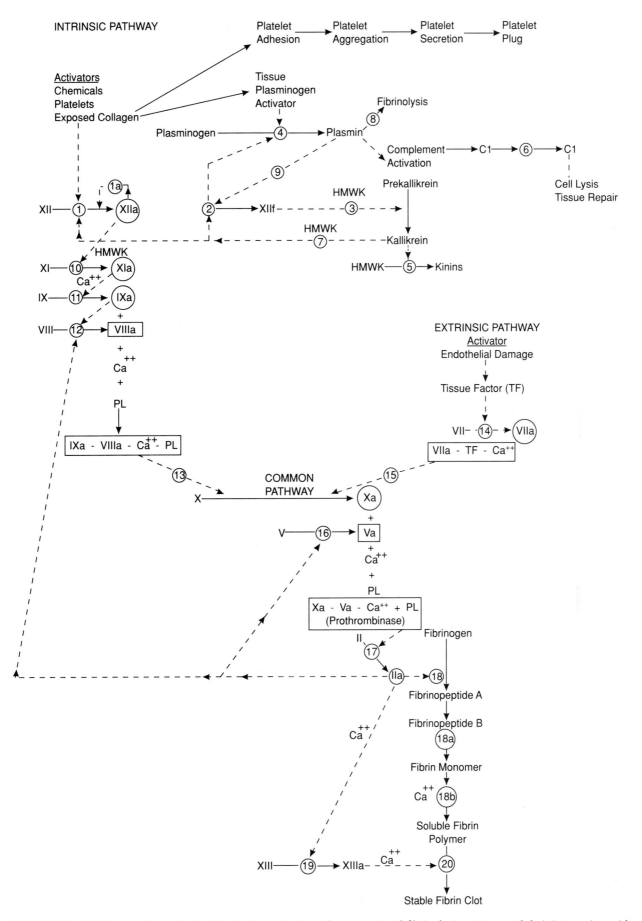

FIG. 50-1.   Pathways of coagulation (intrinsic, extrinsic, and common) and fibrinolytic systems and their interaction with kinin and complement systems. Circles containing Roman numeral factor numbers are serine proteases. Factors within a square are cofactors (V$_a$ and VIII$_a$). Rectangles are coagulation complexes. Numbers for various reactions indicated within arrows in small circles are referred to in text as reaction (Rxn) numbers. Solid arrows indicate factor transformation. Dashed arrows indicate action. PL, platelet phospholipid.

COAGULATION AND THE KININ SYSTEM

Kinins are peptides of low molecular weight composed of a series of amino acids. The *kinin system* contains factors that are activated by the coagulation and fibrinolytic systems. Kinins are involved in chemotaxis and the sensation of pain. They mediate inflammatory responses, increase vascular permeability, cause vasodilation and hypotension, and induce contraction of smooth muscle. They also are important in the contact activation phase of the intrinsic coagulation pathway, as well as in complement activation.

The kinin system factors do not have assigned Roman numerals. They include: (1) prekallikrein (Fletcher factor); (2) kallikrein (the serine protease or activated form of prekallikrein); (3) kininogen, including the low-molecular-weight (LMWK) and high-molecular-weight (HMWK [Fitzgerald factor]) forms; and (4) the kinins, including bradykinin and other substances produced through conversion of kininogens by the enzyme kallikrein.[47,48]

Prekallikrein circulates in plasma as a complex with the cofactor HMWK, and both also are a part of the "contact group." Prekallikrein is converted to the serine protease kallikrein in the presence of factor XII_a and HMWK. Kallikrein is in turn responsible for the conversion of HMWK to kinins. Kallikrein also accelerates factor XII activation.

Kallikrein is also involved in the fibrinolytic system. Kallikrein and activated factor XII (XII_a) form a complex known as the "plasminogen activator," which converts plasminogen to its active form, *plasmin*. Plasmin is necessary for the degradation of the fibrin clot (fibrinolysis). Indirectly or directly, plasmin can also activate Cl in the complement system of immune reactions, as discussed below.

COAGULATION AND THE COMPLEMENT SYSTEM

The complement system is activated during coagulation and fibrinolysis. Complement is important in the mediation of immune and allergic reactions. Of particular importance in hematology is its function in lysing antibody-coated cells (Chap. 19). Plasmin activates the first complement component in the cascade, Cl, and it causes cleavage of C3 to C3a and C3b. C3a is an anaphylatoxin, causing increased vascular permeability, and C3b causes immune adherence of red cells to neutrophils and macrophages, thus enhancing their phagocytosis. Complement system activation is held in check by an inhibitor known as C'l inactivator, which also inhibits factors XII_a, XII_f, XI_a, plasmin, and kallikrein.

THE COAGULATION FACTORS

Factor Nomenclature

The nomenclature of coagulation factors covers those referred to by Roman numerals and the two factors in the kinin system, prekallikrein and HMWK, which are referred to by name only. Each factor was assigned a Roman numeral by the International Committee on Nomenclature of Blood Coagulation Factors[122] in the order of its discovery, not its place in the reaction sequence. These factors are listed in Table 50-1 with their preferred names and other synonyms.

An important aspect of coagulation factor nomenclature is the "a" that sometimes accompanies a Roman numeral (*e.g.,* factor XII_a). It denotes the activated serine protease form of that factor rather than the zymogen (except in the case of factors V and VIII, discussed earlier). An "f" refers to fragmented factor XII (XII_f).

Tissue factor is sometimes referred to as factor III and calcium ions, as factor IV (see Table 50-1). However, *tissue factor* and *calcium* (Ca^{++}) are the generally accepted terms today, and these terms will be used in the various figures in this chapter demonstrating the coagulation process. What was once called factor VI was discovered to be activated factor V; therefore, "factor VI" is nonexistent.

Characteristics of the Coagulation Factors

Table 50-2 provides information concerning the characteristics of the active form of each clotting factor.

TABLE 50–1. Coagulation Factor Nomenclature with Preferred Names and Synonyms

NUMERAL	PREFERRED NAME	SYNONYMS
I	Fibrinogen	
II	Prothrombin	Prethrombin
III	Tissue factor	Tissue thromboplastin
IV	Calcium	
V	Proaccelerin	Labile factor Accelerator globulin (aCg)
VII	Proconvertin	Stable factor Serum prothrombin conversion accelerator (SPCA) Autoprothrombin I
VIII:C	Antihemophilic factor (AHF)	Antihemophilic globulin (AHG) Antihemophilic factor A Platelet cofactor l
IX	Plasma thromboplastin component (PTC)	Christmas factor Antihemophilic factor B Platelet cofactor 2
X	Stuart-Prower factor	Stuart factor Prower factor Autoprothrombin III
XI	Plasma thromboplastin antecedent	Antihemophilic factor C
XII	Hageman factor	Glass factor Contact factor
XIII	Fibrin stabilizing factor	Laki-Lorand Factor Fibrinase Plasma transglutamimase Fibrinoligase
—	Prekallikrein	Fletcher factor
—	High-molecular-weight kininogen (HMWK)	Fitzgerald factor Contact activation cofactor Williams factor Flaujeac factor

The presence or absence of factors in barium sulfate (BaSO₄)-adsorbed plasma is an important characteristic of all coagulation factors, as it permits laboratory testing using mixing studies (Chap. 53) in which patient plasma and adsorbed plasma or serum are mixed to help diagnose factor deficiencies. Prekallikrein and HMWK are also present in adsorbed plasma but at slightly reduced levels because they are partially adsorbed by BaSO₄.

Genetics of the Coagulation Factors

Factor deficiencies may be inherited or acquired. Table 50-3 presents an overview of the mode of inheritance for each factor deficiency. It also gives the names of the coagulopathies associated with both inherited and acquired deficiencies of each factor (see Chap. 55 for details).

THE COAGULATION GROUPS

The properties of the coagulation and kinin factors have similarities that can divide these factors conveniently into three groups: (1) the contact group; (2) the prothrombin or vitamin K-dependent group; and (3) the fibrinogen group. The features common to each group are listed in Table 50-4. The reader should become familiar with the properties that distinguish the three coagulation groups.

Contact Group

Prekallikrein and HMWK of the kinin group, along with factors XII and XI, make up the contact group. The contact group is adsorbed by contact with a negatively charged surface such as collagen or the subendothelium *in vivo* (see Fig. 50-1). This contact causes slow conversion of factor XII to XII$_a$, which initiates both intrinsic system coagulation and fibrinolysis. Factor XII$_a$ and HMWK together activate factor XI to XI$_a$ and convert prekallikrein to kallikrein. Kallikrein and HMWK together play a role in intrinsic coagulation activation, activation of fibrinolysis, kinin formation, and activation of the complement system (see Fig. 50-1).

Prothrombin (Vitamin K-Dependent) Group

The prothrombin group contains the vitamin K-dependent coagulation factors II, VII, IX, and X. These factors are synthesized in the liver in the presence of vitamin K, which acts as a cofactor. Vitamin K is fat soluble. It is normally ingested in the diet and also is manufactured by the gut flora. There is no substantial storage of vitamin K in the body.

Vitamin K is necessary to γ-carboxylate the preformed enzyme precursors of factors II, VII, IX, and X. This reaction brings about γ-carboxylation of the glutamic acid residues at the N-terminal or amino- (NH$_2$) end of the factor polypeptide chains,[110] thus allowing the factors to bind Ca^{++} and form *calcium bridges* with the acidic PL surface of activated platelets. Both Ca^{++} and platelet surface PL are essential for enzyme and substrate functions in the coagulation pathways.[60,61,78]

Vitamin K-dependent γ-carboxylation reactions may be inhibited by several mechanisms: (1) dietary vitamin K deficiency; (2) administration of antibiotics that sterilize the intestinal tract, where normal flora usually synthesize vitamin K; or (3) oral anticoagulant therapy, such as with the coumarin drug warfarin, which interferes with γ-carboxylation.[8,79] Any of these mechanisms can cause the formation of nonfunctional vitamin K-dependent coagulation factors. When such factors are released to the circulation, they cannot bind to the platelet PL surface and ultimately prevent prothrombin activation, causing a deficiency in the coagulation pathway.[39,40,44]

TABLE 50–2. Characteristics of Clotting Factors

FACTOR	ACTIVE FORM	MOLECULAR WEIGHT (× 10³)	PATHWAY PARTICIPATION	SITE OF PRODUCTION	VITAMIN K DEPENDENT?	IN VIVO HALF-LIFE (HOURS)	PLASMA CONCENTRATION (mg/dL)	MINIMUM HEMOSTATIC LEVEL (%)*	PRESENT IN BaSO₄-ADSORBED PLASMA?
I	Fibrin clot	340	Common	Liver	No	90	300–400	100 mg/dL	Yes
II	Serine protease	72	Common	Liver	Yes	60	10–15	20–40	No
V	Cofactor	330	Common	Liver	No	12–36	0.5–1.0	10–25	Yes
VII	Serine protease	63	Extrinsic	Liver	Yes	4–6	0.2	5–10	No
VIII:C	Cofactor	70–240 (VIII/vWF > 1000)	Intrinsic	Uncertain for (VIII:C)**	No	12 22–40†	1–2 (VIII/vWF)	25–30	Yes
IX	Serine protease	62	Intrinsic	Liver	Yes	24	0.3–0.4	15–25	No
X	Serine protease	58.9	Common	Liver	Yes	48–72	0.6–0.8	10–20	No
XI	Serine protease	160	Intrinsic	Liver	No	48–84	0.4	10–20	Yes
XII	Serine protease	80	Intrinsic	Liver	No	48–52	2.9	0–5	Yes
XIII	Transglutaminase	320	Common	Liver	No	3–5 days	2.5	2–3	Yes
Prekallikrein	Serine protease	85	Intrinsic	Liver	No	35	5.0	?‡	Yes
HMW Kininogen	Serine protease	120	Intrinsic	Liver	No	6.5 days	4.7–12.2	?	Yes

* Approximate minimum plasma concentration required for normal coagulation. Note that minimum hemostatic level for factor XII is 0–5% (*i.e.*, factor XII may not be required for normal coagulation).

** vWF portion synthesized by endothelial cells and megakaryocytes.

† 22–40 hours for high-molecular-weight subunit of factor VIII.

‡ None reported.

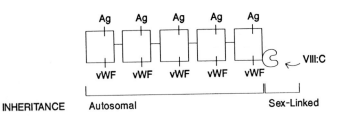

INHERITANCE   Autosomal   Sex-Linked

MOLECULAR   High   Low
WEIGHT

FUNCTION   VIIIR:Ag → molecule's   VIII:C → coagulation in
                           antigenic   intrinsic pathway
                           properties

               VIII:vWF → von Willebrand
                           factor activity
                           required for
                           platelet adhesion

FIG. 50-2. Factor VIII molecule (VIII/vWF) consists of multiple subunits composed of VIIIR:Ag and VIII:vWF and small coagulant unit known as VIII:C. See Table 50-5 for detailed explanation of nomenclature of factor VIII molecule.

Fibrinogen Group

The fibrinogen group includes fibrinogen (factor I) and factors V, VIII, and XIII. These have the highest molecular weights of all the factors, are the most labile, are consumed in coagulation, and are the only group that act as substrates for the fibrinolytic enzyme plasmin. Only the factors found in the fibrinogen group are found in platelets, specifically in the alpha granules, with two exceptions: (1) factor XIII is found in the general platelet cytoplasm, not in alpha granules; and (2) factor VIII:C, the coagulant portion of factor VIII, is not found in platelets.

TABLE 50–3. Disorders of Coagulation Causing Clotting Factor Deficiencies

| FACTOR | INHERITED COAGULOPATHIES | | ACQUIRED COAGULOPATHIES |
	INHERITANCE PATTERN	COAGULOPATHY	
I	Autosomal recessive	Afibrinogenemia	Severe liver disease Diffuse intravascular coagulation Fibrinolysis
	Autosomal dominant	Dysfibrinogenemia	
II	Autosomal recessive	Prothrombin deficiency	Liver disease Vitamin K deficiency Anticoagulant therapy
V	Autosomal recessive	Factor V deficiency	Severe liver disease Diffuse intravascular coagulation Fibrinolysis
VII	Autosomal recessive	Factor VII deficiency	Liver disease Vitamin K deficiency Anticoagulant therapy
VIII	X-linked recessive	Hemophilia A	Diffuse intravascular coagulation Fibrinolysis
	Autosomal dominant	von Willebrand's disease	
IX	X-linked recessive	Hemophilia B	Liver disease Vitamin K deficiency Anticoagulant therapy
X	Autosomal recessive	Factor X deficiency	Liver disease Vitamin K deficiency Anticoagulant therapy
XI	Autosomal recessive	Hemophilia C	?*
XII	Autosomal recessive	Factor XII deficiency	?
XIII	Autosomal recessive	Factor XIII deficiency	Liver disease Diffuse intravascular coagulation Fibrinolysis
Prekallikrein	Autosomal recessive	Fletcher trait	?
HMWK	Autosomal recessive	Fitzgerald trait	?

* It is unclear whether any acquired disorders cause factor XI or XII deficiencies or prekallikrein or HMWK deficiency.

Factor VIII (VIII/vWF) is a large multimeric molecule that has two principal parts: the coagulant portion (VIII:C), which acts as a cofactor in the intrinsic coagulation pathway, and the von Willebrand portion (VIII:vWF), which is important to normal platelet function. *In vitro* the molecule can be separated into low-molecular-weight and high-molecular-weight parts (Fig. 50-2). Factor VIII:C, which probably is produced in the liver, has also been called *antihemophilic factor,* because it is defective in patients with hemophilia A, the best known of all bleeding disorders (Chap. 55). The high-molecular-weight portion of factor VIII is synthesized by the endothelial cells and megakaryocytes and is composed of two parts, the antigenic portion (factor VIIIR:Ag) and the von Willebrand portion (VIII:vWF). If either of these factors is decreased along with decreased factor VIII:C, von Willebrand's disease results (Chap. 55).

The International Committee on Thrombosis and Haemostasis has proposed a nomenclature for factor VIII and its various parts, which is shown in Table 50-5. This nomenclature reflects the different laboratory methods used to detect functional and physical abilities of the high- and low-molecular-weight parts of the factor VIII molecule.

PHOSPHOLIPIDS CONTRIBUTING TO COAGULATION

Tissue Factor

The existence of a lipoprotein called thromboplastin (a complex of two parts, a PL and a protein) was first recognized in 1905, when Paul Morawitz presented his classic theory of coagulation.[73] Morawitz theorized that blood remained fluid because a thromboplastic factor was not found in plasma. This factor was believed to remain inside cells until tissue injury occurred.

Today, Morawitz's proposed thromboplastic factor is known as *tissue factor* or *tissue thromboplastin*. This substance initiates the extrinsic coagulation pathway by binding its PL portion to factor VII, converting factor VII to VII_a. The term *extrinsic* was applied to this pathway because of the necessity of adding a tissue extract (PL) to plasma samples *in vitro* to initiate and evaluate this coagulation pathway in the laboratory. The prothrombin time (PT) test, which evaluates the extrinsic system, is performed using a reagent containing rabbit brain or lung tissue thromboplastin as

TABLE 50-4. Properties of the Coagulation Groups

	CONTACT	PROTHROMBIN	FIBRINOGEN
FACTORS	XII, XI, prekallikrein, HMWK	II, VII, IX, X, protein C, protein S	I, V, VIII, XIII
FUNCTION	Serine proteases: XII, XI, prekallikrein	Serine proteases: II, VII, IX, X, protein C	Precursor of fibrin: I
	Cofactor: HMWK	Cofactor: protein S	Cofactors: V, VIII Transamidase: XIII
MOLECULAR WEIGHT ($\times 10^3$)	Medium (80–200)	Low (55–70)	High (> 250)
STABILITY	Fairly stable	Heat labile: VII, IX, X Well preserved in stored plasma	Heat labile: I, V, VIII Storage labile: V, VIII
VITAMIN K DEPENDENT FOR SYNTHESIS?	No	Yes	No
ADSORBED BY $BaSO_4$, $Al(OH)_3$ AND OTHER SALTS?	Partially	Yes	No
CONSUMED IN COAGULATION?	Partially	No (except II)	Yes
SITE	Plasma or serum	Plasma or serum (except II is not present in serum)	Plasma
DESTROYED BY PLASMIN OR HIGH CONCENTRATIONS OF THROMBIN?	No	No	Yes
FOUND IN PLATELETS?	No	No	α granules: I, V, VIIIR:Ag General cytoplasm: XIII Not present: VIII:C
ACUTE-PHASE REACTANTS?	No	No	Yes
PRODUCTION REDUCED BY ORAL ANTICOAGULANTS?	No	Yes	No

TABLE 50–5. Nomenclature for Factor VIII of the International Committee on Thrombosis and Haemostasis

VIII/vWF	The entire molecule as it circulates in the plasma. Composed of VIII:C and VIII:vWF portions noncovalently bound
VIII:vWF	Portion of molecule responsible for binding to endothelium and supporting normal platelet adhesion and function. Tested by bleeding time (Chap. 59)
VIII:C	Portion of molecule acting in intrinsic system as cofactor to factor IXa (with Ca^{++}) in the conversion of factor X to X_a. Tested by partial thromboplastin time (Chap. 52)
VIIIC:Ag	Antigenic property of procoagulant portion as measured by immunologic monoclonal antibody techniques
VIIIR:Ag	Factor VIII-related antigen, which is a property of the large vWF portion of the molecule and measured by immunologic techniques of Laurell rocket or immunoradiometric assay (Chap. 53)
VIIIR:RCo	Ristocetin (an antibiotic no longer used therapeutically) cofactor activity, which is factor VIII-related activity required for aggregation of human platelets with ristocetin (Chap. 59) in in vitro aggregation studies

well as Ca^{++} to activate factor VII and initiate the extrinsic pathway.

Partial Thromboplastin and Platelet Phospholipid

Partial thromboplastin is a reagent used as a platelet substitute in evaluating the intrinsic coagulation system with a test appropriately called the "partial thromboplastin time" ("partial" because the reagent consists only of the PL portion of tissue thromboplastin; Chap. 52). The intrinsic system requires platelet membrane PL for factor X activation in vitro. In vitro tests of the intrinsic system require the use of platelet-poor plasma to avoid test variation attributable to the patient's platelets. Without dependence on the patient's platelets, the test may be run independently of the number of platelets available, as partial thromboplastin provides the necessary platelet substitute.

PHYSIOLOGIC VARIATIONS OF THE COAGULATION FACTORS

Newborns

The concentration of various coagulation factors depends on the patient's age and physical condition. At birth, infants normally are deficient in vitamin K; therefore, a moderate deficiency exists in the vitamin K-dependent factors.[1,84] Newborn infants are frequently given vitamin K supplements to correct this deficiency.

Adults

Among adults, physiologic variations of coagulation factors are most commonly associated with increases in the concentrations of various coagulation factors (Table 50-6). These variations generally do not cause coagulation abnormalities. A few conditions are associated with decreases in coagulation factor concentrations that are not clinically significant, as they do not cause abnormal hemostasis. When factor abnormalities are the primary cause of clinical disorders, not simple physiologic variations, they are considered acquired (e.g., liver disease) or inherited (e.g., hemophilia) coagulation disorders, which are discussed in Chapters 55 and 56 and summarized in Table 50-3.

THE PROCESS OF FIBRIN CLOT FORMATION

Earlier Theories

Many theories were proposed to explain the mechanisms of blood clotting during the past three centuries. In 1905, Morawitz's classic coagulation theory was widely accepted. He proposed that coagulation takes place in two stages. In the first stage, prothrombin was thought to be converted to thrombin by a factor known as thrombokinase in the presence of Ca^{++}. The second stage was thrombin converting fibrinogen to fibrin.

TABLE 50–6. Conditions Most Often Associated with Physiologic Variations in Coagulation and Fibrinolytic Factors

CONDITION	RELATED FACTOR INCREASES	RELATED FACTOR DECREASES
Stress[121]	I	
Tissue necrosis[121]	I	
Inflammation[121]	I	
Pregnancy[19,33,46,88]	I, VIII, IX, X	XIII, XI, AT-III
Oral contraceptives[13,20]	I, VIII, VII, IX, X	
Hypermetabolism (e.g., hyperthyroidism)[9,41]	I, VIII, plasminogen	
Vigorous exercise[43,95]	VIII, XI, XII	
Chronic thrombocytopenia[53]	VIII	
Hypothyroidism[9,104]		IX, XI, plasminogen
Childbirth[53,55]★	I, VIII	
Surgical procedures[53,55]★	I, VIII	
Trauma[53,55]★	I, VIII	
Myocardial infarction[53,55]★	I, VIII	
Acute illness[53,55]★	I, VIII	

★ Temporary elevations associated with acute conditions. Once the acute reaction has subsided, factor concentration usually declines to normal.

Modern Theory

In 1964 two theories were presented, the "cascade"[56,57] and the "waterfall,"[22] which have today become the accepted models for the coagulation mechanism. The difference in the intrinsic and extrinsic coagulation pathways is in the mechanism of initial activation and their mechanism of activation of factor X. Both pathways consist of a group of zymogens, which are inert when they enter the plasma but when activated are enzymes. These enzymes act as substrates for the next coagulation factor in the pathway. Figure 50-1 provides a detailed explanation of the intrinsic and extrinsic pathways and their interactions with the kinin, complement, and fibrinolytic systems as well as platelets. All reaction numbers in circles on the figure correspond to reaction (Rxn) numbers in the text for easy reference as the various parts of each pathway are described. This model is still valid; however, modifications are made as necessary when new information becomes available.

Intrinsic Coagulation Pathway

The intrinsic system is considered to be dominant. The term *intrinsic* was used to describe this pathway of coagulation because all of the components in the system are found in circulating blood. *In vitro* initiation of the intrinsic pathway occurs by exposure of the coagulation factors to negatively charged surfaces such as glass. *In vivo* the initiation mechanism is believed to be associated with damaged vascular endothelium.

Initiation of the intrinsic coagulation pathway begins with what is called the *contact phase of coagulation*. The factors involved are the contact factors: factor XII, HMWK, prekallikrein, and factor XI.

Factor XII Activation

Factor XII is a single polypeptide chain zymogen.[29,94] The contact phase begins with factor XII absorption to the negatively charged surface of vascular collagen exposed by vessel wall damage. Prekallikrein, a single-chain polypeptide, circulates as a complex with the cofactor HMWK. This complex is absorbed *in vivo* to the negatively charged surface with factor XII. Factor XI also complexes with HMWK on the surface.

Once the contact group is assembled, factor XII undergoes a conformational change (Rxn 1—see Fig. 50-1) in the presence of kallikrein, which accelerates the conversion rate to factor XII$_a$ with enhancement by HMWK (Rxn 7). Factor XII can autoactivate (*i.e.*, be activated without stimulation from HMWK); however, this is an extremely slow reaction (Rxn 1a). Enzymes in basophils and endothelial cells also appear to activate factor XII.

Factor XII$_a$ is cleaved into fragments called XII$_f$ (Rxn 2). This is achieved by a number of proteolytic enzymes, including plasmin and, probably most importantly, kallikrein. The HMWK enhances the proteolytic effect of kallikrein on factor XII$_a$ (Rxn 2). Both factors XII$_a$ and XII$_f$ activate prekallikrein to kallikrein (Rxn 3).

Factor XII$_a$ plays several roles in contact activation.[12,38,103]

1. *It initiates the intrinsic pathway of coagulation.* In the presence of HMWK, XII$_a$ converts the zymogen factor XI to the serine protease XI$_a$ (Rxn 10).
2. *It initiates fibrinolysis.* Factor XII$_a$ and kallikrein together (Rxn 2) form the complex required for conversion of the zymogen plasminogen to the serine protease plasmin (Rxn 4), which is fibrinolytic.
3. *It initiates kinin and complement systems.* The formation of kallikrein by XII$_f$ and HMWK (Rxn 3) causes the conversion of HMWK to kinins (Rxn 5) such as bradykinin. The plasmin formed as a result of kallikrein can also initiate the complement system (Rxn 6).

To summarize, *kallikrein* plays four important roles in contact activation (see Fig. 50-1).

1. It perpetuates factor XII activation and its own production (Rxns 7, 2, and 3).
2. It initiates the kinin system (Rxn 5).
3. It initiates the fibrinolytic and complement systems (Rxns 2 and 4) together with factor XII$_a$.
4. It directly activates factor IX. Kallikrein can, on its own, activate factor IX to IX$_a$, thus completing the contact activation phase (not shown in Fig. 50-1).

Plasmin, which is formed as a result of contact activation, plays three important roles (see Fig. 50-1)

1. It promotes clot dissolution (Rxn 8). Plasmin begins the fibrinolytic process of gradual blood clot dissolution, which limits the coagulation process.
2. It activates the complement system (Rxn 6).
3. It cleaves factor XII$_a$ to XII$_f$ (Rxn 9).

Factor XI Activation

Factor XII$_a$, with HMWK, activates factor XI to XI$_a$ (Rxn 10). Factor XI$_a$ is the enzyme that cleaves the substrate factor IX to form the serine protease factor IX$_a$. This reaction requires Ca^{++} as a cofactor (Rxn 11). It appears that factor XI can be activated directly by contact activation like factor XII[116] and that factor XI$_a$ also activates plasminogen;[58] thus, both XI$_a$ and XII$_a$ are involved in initiation of the fibrinolytic and complement systems.

Factor IX Activation

The activation of factor IX to IX$_a$ by factor XI$_a$ and Ca^{++} (Rxn 11) completes the contact activation phase of coagulation. Kallikrein is also capable of activating factor IX. Factor IX$_a$ combines with the factor VIII cofactor, VIII$_a$, and Ca^{++} on the platelet PL surface to activate factor X (Rxn 13). The coagulation cascade continues on the platelet surface (see Chap. 58, Fig. 58-11).

Extrinsic Coagulation Pathway

The extrinsic pathway is much less complex than the intrinsic. It was named "extrinsic" because factors other than those normally found in the plasma are required for initiation. This pathway consists only of tissue factor, factor VII, and Ca^{++}.

Tissue factor (also called tissue thromboplastin) is a lipoprotein that is released from cell membranes into the plasma on vascular endothelial injury. Factor VII is vitamin K dependent and circulates as a single-chain glycoprotein. The γ-carboxyglutamic acid residue of factor VII binds the PL portion of tissue factor in the presence of Ca^{++} which acts as a bridge between factor VII and tissue factor. Thus, factor VII is converted to factor VII_a (Rxn 14). The factor VII_a-Ca^{++}-tissue factor complex on the platelet PL surface (see Fig. 58-11) converts factor X to X_a in the common pathway (Rxn 15).

Alternate Pathways Linking the Extrinsic and Intrinsic Pathways

In the past, the extrinsic and intrinsic systems were thought of as separate entities. However, research has revealed interdependence and interaction between the two.[49,100] These interactions have been termed "alternate pathways." Figure 50-3 highlights the alternate pathways of coagulation activation.

It has been reported that factor XII_a (intrinsic system) can activate factor VII (extrinsic system).[90] In fact, the factor VII_a formed in this reaction is a two-chain form rather than the single chain formed in the usual extrinsic pathway. The two-chain factor VII_a has a greater effect on factor X activation than does the single-chain form.[3] In addition, factor IX_a and kallikrein have been reported to activate factor VII in plasma that has been exposed to glass or other surfaces.[3]

Intrinsic pathway activation by way of the extrinsic pathway has been shown to occur in vitro and is thought to occur in vivo. The complex of Ca^{++}-factor VII_a-tissue factor at the site of injury can slowly activate factor IX to IX_a with subsequent activation of X to X_a (see Fig. 50-3).[60,65,68,85] This alternate pathway allows the coagulation system to bypass the contact activation phase and could be the key to the lack of bleeding associated with hereditary deficiencies of the contact activation factors XII, prekallikrein, and HMWK.

In another feedback pathway, factor X_a can hydrolyze factor VII to produce a two-chain form that is reported to have 85 times the procoagulant activity of the normal single-chain factor VII_a.[89] A further control mechanism exists in that large concentrations of factor X_a cleave factor VII into a three-chain molecule that is inactive in coagulation.[89]

Common Coagulation Pathway

The activation of factor X begins the common coagulation pathway, so called because it is common to the intrinsic and extrinsic pathways. Equal amounts of factor X_a are generated by activation through either pathway.[80,81]

Extrinsic Pathway Activation

Extrinsic activation of the common pathway occurs when factor VII_a, tissue factor, and Ca^{++} form a complex on the platelet PL surface. This complex acts on the common coagulation pathway to convert factor X to X_a (see Fig. 50-1, Rxn 15; see also Fig. 58-11).

Intrinsic Pathway Activation

Figure 58-11 displays the many intrinsic pathway factors present on the platelet PL surface during coagulation and the multimolecular complexes formed in the coagulation process.

Factor VIII, although only a cofactor, must be modified to its functional form (VIII_a) by thrombin (Rxn 12) to take part in the activation of factor X.

The platelet provides a surface for the formation in the intrinsic pathway of the multimolecular complex of factor IX_a-Ca^{++}-factor VIII_a, which binds with platelet PL and together converts factor X to X_a (Rxn 13). This complex causes the conversion rate of factor X to X_a to be accelerated several thousand times beyond the reaction rate associated with factor IX_a acting alone.[21,42,114] With the γ-carboxyglutamic acid residue of factor X_a and in the presence of Ca^{++}, factor X_a also binds to the platelet PL surface and is thus prevented from diffusing away from the complex.

On formation of factor X_a a multimolecular complex known as the *prothrombinase complex* (see Fig. 58-11) is formed in the common pathway. The complex includes X_a-V_a-Ca^{++}-platelet PL. Factor V requires modification to factor V_a by thrombin to be active in this complex (Rxn 16). The prothrombinase complex converts prothrombin to thrombin (Rxn 17).[59,61] The common pathway reactions are completed with thrombin activation of fibrinogen to fibrin through a series of steps that stabilize the fibrin clot.

The Thrombin Feedback Mechanism

Thrombin (factor II_a) has many roles in hemostasis. Most importantly, it acts to control and balance the hemostatic mechanism by providing feedback mechanisms to achieve control of the coagulation process (i.e., to prevent excessive bleeding and clotting). Table 50-7 summarizes the various roles and divides them into two groups: activator and inhibitor of coagulation.

Thrombin's Role as Coagulation Activator

Thrombin is a strong serine protease generated through the action of the prothrombinase complex on the platelet surface. It is said to be autocatalytic; that is, once it is generated, thrombin enhances the rate of prothrombinase production and is thus, to some extent, self-perpetuating. This activity is thought to relate to the effects of thrombin on factors V and VIII (Rxns 12 and 16). When present in plasma in small amounts, thrombin enhances the reactivity of factors V and VIII and stimulates platelet aggregation.

TABLE 50–7. Roles of Thrombin as Both Activator and Inhibitor of Coagulation

ROLE AS ACTIVATOR	ROLE AS INHIBITOR
Low levels of thrombin "activate" V to V_a and VIII to VIII_a	High levels of thrombin inhibit V and VIII activation
Activates XIII to XIII_a	Initiates fibrinolysis by converting plasminogen to plasmin
Induces platelet aggregation	Activates protein C (a potent anticoagulant)

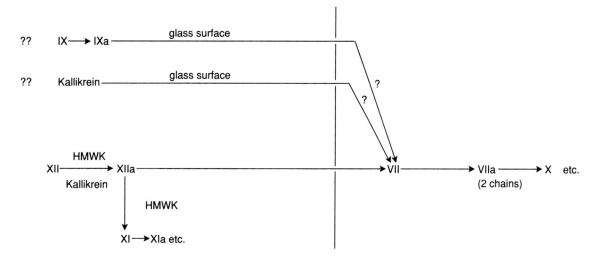

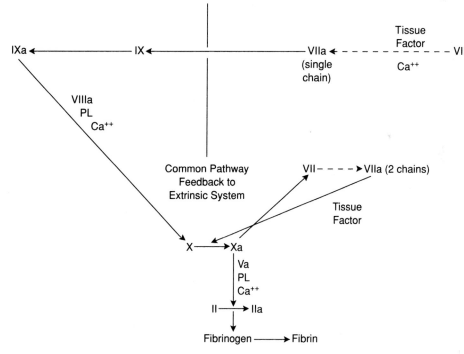

FIG. 50-3.   Alternate pathways of coagulation activation. Intrinsic and extrinsic systems are no longer thought of as separate entities but as being intertwined in a complex coagulation mechanism. Note that when factor VII is activated, either by intrinsic system (factor XIIa) or by common pathway (factor Xa), two-chain form of VIIa is produced, which has much greater procoagulant effect on factor X than does single-chain form of VIIa. Factor IXa and kallikrein activation of factor VII has been reported[3] in *in vitro* studies of plasma exposed to glass; therefore, it may be a mode of alternate pathway activation *in vitro*. PL, platelet phospholipid.

Thrombin is also a trypsin-like enzyme, which acts on fibrinogen, causing its conversion to soluble fibrin monomers (Rxns 18 and 18a). Factor XIII, the clot-stabilizing factor, must be activated by thrombin (Rxn 19) to permit conversion of soluble fibrin to a stabilized fibrin clot (Rxn 20).

Thrombin's Role as Coagulation Inhibitor

Thrombin controls coagulation by acting also as an inhibitor to prevent excessive clotting. In higher concentrations, thrombin has the opposite effect on factors V and VIII—it can destroy them. The mechanism for this action is unclear.

Thrombin also activates protein C, which is a potent anticoagulant. Such activation is enhanced by calcium, a cofactor called *thrombomodulin* on the endothelial surface,[26] and the cofactor protein S. Enhanced activation of protein C takes place on the endothelial surface. The protein C-S complex inhibits factors V_a and VIII_a, thus acting as a coagulation inhibitor (see Chap. 56, Fig. 56-1). Protein C-S also stimulates fibrinolysis by increasing plasminogen activator activity. Activated protein C also inhibits tissue plasminogen activator inhibitor (TPAI). The net effect is prevention of interference with plasmin production (*i.e.,* enhanced fibrinolysis). Once thrombin has formed a complex with thrombomodulin, it can no longer enhance factor V or VIII activity, stimulate platelet aggregation, or convert fibrinogen to fibrin.

Final Clot Formation and Stabilization

The action of thrombin on fibrinogen begins the final steps of coagulation (Rxn 18). Fibrinogen is a glycoprotein composed of three nonidentical but intricately interwoven paired chains called Aα, Bβ, and γ, which are linked by disulfide bonds near the terminal ends. Both the α and β chain pairs have a small fibrinopeptide at their terminal ends known as fibrinopeptides A and B (16 and 14 amino acids, respectively) for a total of four fibrinopeptides (two A and two B).

Conversion of Fibrinogen to Fibrin

The conversion of fibrinogen to fibrin involves three steps (see Fig. 50-1).

STEP 1. First, there is cleavage of the four fibrinopeptides from the fibrinogen molecule α and β ends by the enzymatic action of thrombin. The γ chains remain intact and do not hydrolyze during the formation of fibrin. Once the A and B fibrinopeptides are removed, the structure is referred to as a *soluble fibrin monomer* or *unstable gel* (Rxn 18a), which is essential for the second step, polymerization of fibrin.

STEP 2. The fibrin monomers aggregate spontaneously end to end and side to side to form weak (electrostatic bonds only) fibrin polymers or strands given the correct environment, including *p*H and ionic concentration (Rxn 18b). However, fibrin polymers are soluble and can be dissolved *in vitro* in 5 M urea or weak acids such as 1% monochloracetic acid. At this point, the fibrin polymer also is vulnerable to the fibrinolytic enzyme plasmin.

STEP 3. The third step provides clot stabilization. It requires factor XIII, Ca^{++}, and thrombin. Thrombin activates factor XIII (Rxn 19), which then functions as a transamidase, crosslinking adjacent fibrin monomers through formation of covalent bonds. Both α and γ chains are involved in the formation of the stabilized fibrin clot (Rxn 20). The stabilized clot is insoluble in 5 M urea and weak acid. Laboratory tests may be performed with these reagents to screen for factor XIII deficiency (Chap. 53).

THE FIBRINOLYTIC SYSTEM

Physiologic Fibrinolysis

Many similarities exist between the coagulation and fibrinolytic systems. Just as there are checks and balances in the formation of a clot, there are similar mechanisms for dissolution of the clot to promote wound healing. Fibrinolysis is the body's defense against occlusion of blood vessels, but it is also important that bleeding does not recur because of premature lysing of the clot.

Activation of Plasminogen to Plasmin

Fibrinolysis is dependent on the enzyme plasmin, which normally is not present in the blood in an active form. Plasmin, a serine protease like many of the coagulation factors, can digest or destroy fibrinogen, fibrin, and factors V and VIII. Plasmin also promotes coagulation and activates the kinin and complement systems (see Fig. 50-1). Table 50-8 summarizes the roles of plasmin in hemostasis.

A zymogen known as plasminogen, which normally is present in plasma, is converted to plasmin by the action of specific enzymes called plasminogen activators. Plasminogen is a single-chain glycoprotein that is synthesized in the liver and has a molecular weight of 90,000. It is stored and transported in eosinophils. Increased concentrations are found in association with inflammation.

Activation of plasminogen to plasmin may occur because of substances normally present in the plasma. Such activation is referred to as "intrinsic activation." Extrinsic activation occurs through substances that enter the plasma from an outside source (Fig. 50-4).

TABLE 50–8. Multiple Roles of Plasmin in Hemostasis

PLASMIN'S ROLES	COMMENTS
Activates fibrinolysis	Cleaves fibrin and fibrinogen to fibrin (ogen) degradation products X, Y, D, E
Activates intrinsic coagulation system	Factor XII --->XII$_a$ is amplified indirectly by plasmin
Interferes with intrinsic and common pathways	Destroys factors VIII and V
Blocks thrombin conversion of fibrinogen to fibrin	Fibrin(ogen) degradation products interfere with thrombin influence on fibrinogen
Activates kinin system	Enhances conversion of prekallikrein to kallikrein and subsequently of kininogen to kinin
Activates complement system	Cleaves C3 into fragments C3a and C3b and activates C1, the first component in the complement system

ACTIVATION OF THE FIBRINOLYTIC SYSTEM

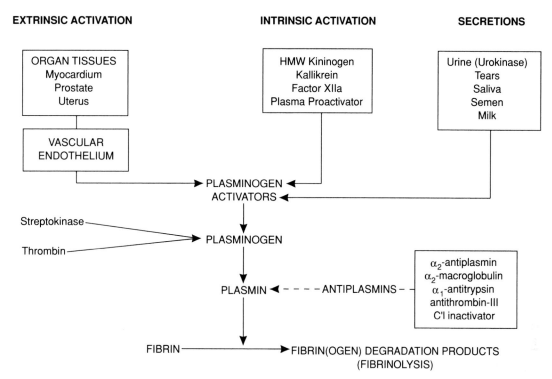

FIG. 50-4.   Fibrinolytic system may be activated by plasminogen activators from extrinsic sources such as vascular endothelium or by intrinsic sources such as factor XII$_a$ and others as shown. These plasminogen activators convert plasminogen to plasmin. Thrombin also activates plasminogen; streptokinase, administered therapeutically in thrombotic disorders, acts in same way. Plasmin promotes fibrinolysis. Antiplasmins control (inhibit and neutralize) excess plasmin, thus preventing excessive and premature fibrinolysis.

Intrinsic Plasminogen Activation

Factor XII$_a$, kallikrein, HMWK, and a specific plasma protein (proactivator) can activate plasminogen to plasmin intrinsically by one or more pathways.[51,58] The plasma proactivator is activated by kallikrein during coagulation contact activation.

Extrinsic Plasminogen Activation

The extrinsic plasminogen activation pathway involves plasminogen activators present in organ tissues (see Fig. 50-4). Tissue plasminogen activators also have been found in endothelial cells in the form of proteases,[118] particularly in the veins.[113]

Plasminogen Activators in Secretory Ducts

Plasminogen activators are also present in body fluids (see Fig. 50-4). These activators may keep the secretory passages functioning properly.[72]

Exogenous Plasminogen Activation

For therapeutic destruction of thrombi, urokinase, a trypsin-like protease purified from urine, may be administered to a patient to activate plasminogen (see Fig. 50-4) to plasmin and induce fibrinolysis.[102,119] Streptokinase is another therapeutic agent used to activate plasminogen to plasmin[112] (Chap. 57).

A new agent, tissue plasminogen activator (tPA), is now being used for the treatment of thrombosis[87] (Chap. 57). It is released *in vivo* on endothelial cell damage and can be manufactured *in vitro* through recombinant DNA techniques.

Role of Plasminogen and Plasmin in Normal and Abnormal Fibrinolysis

Under normal circumstances, plasminogen is a part of any clot because of the tendency of fibrin to absorb plasminogen from the plasma. When plasminogen activators perform their function, plasmin is formed within the clot, which gradually dissolves the clot while leaving time for tissue repair. Free plasmin also is released to the plasma; however, antiplasmins there immediately destroy any plasmin released from the clot (see Fig. 50-4).

When pathologic coagulation processes are involved, excessive free plasmin is released to the plasma. In these situations, the available antiplasmin is depleted, and plasmin begins destroying components other than fibrin, including fibrinogen, factors V and VIII, and other factors. Plasmin acts more quickly to destroy fibrinogen because of fibrinogen's instability. The covalent bonds of fibrin slow the fibrin degradation process by plasmin.

Fibrin(ogen) Degradation by Plasmin

In the process of fibrinogen or fibrin degradation by plasmin within a clot, specific molecular fragments are produced called *fibrin(ogen) degradation products* (FDP) or *fibrin(ogen) split products* (FSP). Plasmin cannot distinguish between fibrinogen and fibrin; therefore, it degrades both. This results in the appearance of essentially the same fragments for fibrinogen and fibrin degradation, although the Aα and Bβ chains may remain intact in fibrinogen fragments.[111] These degradation products are removed by the reticuloendothelial system and other organs.

Figure 50-5 shows the sequence of reactions in the degradation of fibrin(ogen) by plasmin and the four principal products, fragments X, Y, D (D-D dimer), and E. Note that plasmin acts on specific sites of each fragment to create smaller fragments throughout the reaction sequence. Fragments X and Y are referred to as *early* degradation products; fragments D and E are *late* degradation products.

Fragment X is the first and largest fragment formed (MW 250,000). Fragment X is the result of plasmin cleav-age of the terminal portions of the alpha chains from a fibrin polymer, leaving isolated fibrin strands. Fragment X is then cleaved by plasmin (P) to form two fragments called Y (YY)[63] and an intermediate complex, DXD (see Fig. 50-5). This complex is further cleaved into intermediate complexes DED and DY/YD until finally, fragments E and D (D-D dimer) are formed. A single fragment D has a molecular weight of approximately 90,000, and that of the D-D dimer is approximately 180,000.[63] It is now thought that the presence of the D-D dimer is a specific indicator of *in vivo* fibrinolysis, namely, intravascular thrombin formation leading to fibrin formation and its subsequent degradation. In the past, laboratory tests for FDP were incapable of distinguishing fibrin degradation products and fibrinogen degradation products.[30] Now, tests specific for the D-D dimer (Chap. 54) permit verification of *in vivo* fibrinolysis, because the presence of the D-D dimer is indicative only of fibrin (not fibrinogen) degradation products.[34,117]

Pathologic Effects of Fibrin Degradation Products

The FDPs are significant because of their hemostatic effects, which include antithrombin activity, interference with polymerization of the fibrin monomer, and interference with platelet activity. The early and larger fragments X and Y, along with the intermediate FDPs, appear to be the most important in exerting anticoagulant effects. Fragments Y and D inhibit fibrin polymerization.[2,7] Fragment E is a powerful inhibitor of thrombin.[7] In general, most FDPs inhibit coagulation and also form incoagulable or slowly coagulable complexes with fibrin monomers or fibrinogen. These complexes in pathological fibrinolytic states are detectable by the protamine sulfate and ethanol gel tests (Chap. 54). Recently, the fibrin monomer test has been introduced, which is a more accurate test for detection of these complexes.

All four fragments, but particularly low-molecular-weight FDP,[106] have an affinity for coating platelet membranes and therefore cause a clinically significant platelet dysfunction by inhibiting aggregation.

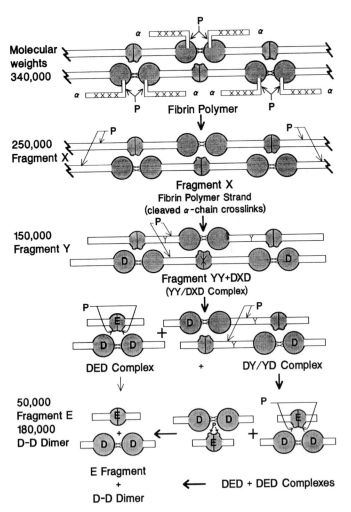

FIG. 50-5. Degradation of fibrin by plasmin. P indicates sites where plasmin cleaves fibrin polymer, fibrin strand, and various complexes. (From Thompson AR, Harker LA: Manual of Hemostasis and Thrombosis, p 38. Philadelphia, FA Davis, 1983, with permission.)

NATURALLY OCCURRING COAGULATION AND FIBRINOLYTIC INHIBITORS

A regulatory system must exist within the body to control coagulation and fibrinolysis. This system includes both naturally occurring biochemical inhibitors and physiologic control mechanisms.

The counterforces of the naturally occurring biochemical coagulation and fibrinolytic inhibitors are necessary to achieve a balance between activated clotting factors and fibrinolytic enzymes.[4,5] Some inhibitors quickly neutralize activated factors in the circulation, thus localizing coagulation to the sites where it is required, whereas others perform a similar function that limits fibrinolysis. Table 50-9 summarizes the features of the well-characterized inhibitors of coagulation and fibrinolysis.

Naturally Occurring Inhibitors of Coagulation

Antithrombin III

Antithrombin III (AT-III) is an important coagulation inhibitor. It is a protein (α_2 globulin) synthesized in the liver; some studies suggest that endothelial cells may be a source as well. It has a half-life of approximately 2.7 days.

Antithrombin III inhibits thrombin, XII$_a$, XI$_a$, X$_a$, and IX$_a$ by forming enzyme inhibitor complexes with these activated factors, thus neutralizing them and preventing their action on other zymogens (Chap. 56, Fig. 56-1).[123] It also has an inhibitory effect on plasmin and kallikrein. Thus, AT-III plays a vital role in monitoring the coagulation, fibrinolytic, kallikrein-kinin, and complement systems. If these four systems are allowed to function without inhibition because of decreased levels of AT-III, the result can be severe, even fatal (Fig. 50-6).

The action of the AT-III anticoagulant is enhanced by the cofactor heparin,[99] which attaches to AT-III, causing a conformational change that makes the arginine residue of the AT-III reactive site more accessible to the active site of serine proteases (Fig. 50-7).[4,11,28] Heparin appears to increase the rate of factor inactivation, not the magnitude.[96]

A heparin-like substance is normally present *in vivo*. It is an acidic mucopolysaccharide that acts as an anticoagulant similar to the action of commercially prepared heparin used in anticoagulant therapy. Naturally occurring heparin has been isolated from a variety of organs and also is present in mast cells and basophils. It is reported to enhance AT-III activity.[96] Heparan sulfate, a naturally occurring chemical relative of heparin and likewise an anticoagulant, has been identified on the surface of platelets and the vascular endothelium. Heparan sulfate on these surfaces, together with AT-III, protects uninjured vessels against abnormal thrombus formation by neutralizing serine proteases.

Without heparin, AT-III neutralizes thrombin by forming a 1:1 complex with thrombin slowly over a period of minutes. If heparan sulfate is added to the reaction complex, neutralization of thrombin occurs instantaneously, and the rate is accelerated from 2000 to 10,000 times that when AT-III alone neutralizes thrombin.[62] A small decrease in the concentration of AT-III may cause a faster clotting reaction because of the lack of control and inhibition by AT-III.

Ironically, AT-III can be decreased by the therapeutic use of heparin as an anticoagulant (Chap. 57). Because heparin accelerates the rate of binding of AT-III with serine proteases, treatment with heparin over several days may deplete available plasma AT-III.

Hereditary deficiencies of AT-III, both qualitative and quantitative, have been reported (Chap. 56).[69,70,98]

Alpha-2-Macroglobulin

Alpha-2-macroglobulin is a large, naturally occurring plasma glycoprotein.[45] This inhibitor binds with various proteolytic enzymes including thrombin, but does not completely inhibit them.[83] Its rate of thrombin inhibition is slower than that of AT-III. In addition, α_2-macroglobulin seems to protect its bound enzymes against other circu-

TABLE 50–9. Naturally Occurring Inhibitors of Coagulation and Fibrinolysis

INHIBITOR	MOLECULAR WEIGHT ($\times 10^3$)	PLASMA CONCENTRATION (mg/dL)	RATE OF INHIBITION	RATE ACCELERATED BY HEPARIN?	SYSTEM INHIBITED	FUNCTION INHIBITED
Antithrombin III	67	23–40	Slow	Yes	Coagulation	Thrombin, XII$_a$, XI$_a$, X$_a$, IX$_a$, and kallikrein
					Fibrinolytic	Plasmin and kallikrein
α_2-Macroglobulin	725	190–330	Variable	No	Coagulation	Thrombin and kallikrein
					Fibrinolytic	Plasmin and kallikrein
α_1-Antitrypsin	40–50	245–335	Slow	No	Coagulation	Potent inhibitor of XI$_a$; weak inhibitor of thrombin
					Fibrinolytic	Plasmin
C'1 Inactivator	135	14–30	Slow	No	Coagulation	XII$_a$, XII$_f$, XI$_a$, and kallikrein
					Fibrinolytic	Plasmin
					Complement	C'1 Esterase
Protein C	62	0.5	Slow	No	Coagulation	Complexed with protein S, inhibits V$_a$ and VIII$_a$
					Fibrinolytic (enhanced)	Complexed with protein S, *enhances* fibrinolysis by inactivating inhibitors of plasminogen activators
Protein S	69	1.5 (free form)	Slow	No	Coagulation	Complexed with protein C, inhibits V$_a$ and VIII$_a$
					Fibrinolytic (enhanced)	Complexed with protein C, *enhances* fibrinolysis by inactivating inhibitors of plasminogen activators
α_2-Antiplasmin	65–70	9.6–13.5	Rapid	No	Fibrinolytic ONLY	Principal inhibitor of plasmin

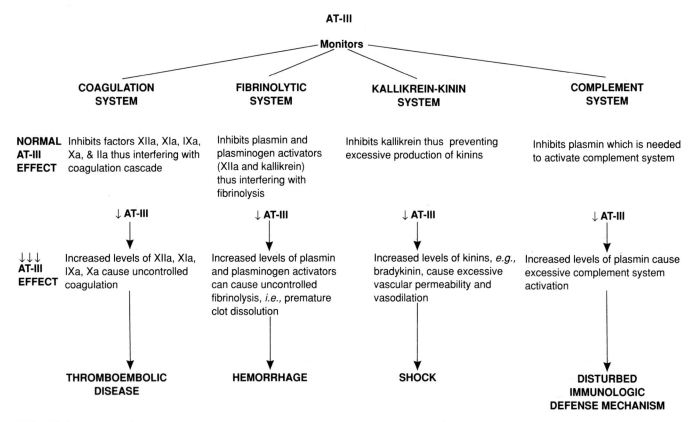

	COAGULATION SYSTEM	FIBRINOLYTIC SYSTEM	KALLIKREIN-KININ SYSTEM	COMPLEMENT SYSTEM
NORMAL AT-III EFFECT	Inhibits factors XIIa, XIa, IXa, Xa, & IIa thus interfering with coagulation cascade	Inhibits plasmin and plasminogen activators (XIIa and kallikrein) thus interfering with fibrinolysis	Inhibits kallikrein thus preventing excessive production of kinins	Inhibits plasmin which is needed to activate complement system
↓↓↓ **AT-III EFFECT**	Increased levels of XIIa, XIa, IXa, Xa cause uncontrolled coagulation	Increased levels of plasmin and plasminogen activators can cause uncontrolled fibrinolysis, *i.e.*, premature clot dissolution	Increased levels of kinins, *e.g.*, bradykinin, cause excessive vascular permeability and vasodilation	Increased levels of plasmin cause excessive complement system activation
	THROMBOEMBOLIC DISEASE	**HEMORRHAGE**	**SHOCK**	**DISTURBED IMMUNOLOGIC DEFENSE MECHANISM**

FIG. 50-6. Antithrombin III is important in controlling four physiologic systems. Thus, if there is a decrease in the concentration of AT-III, serious clinical abnormalities can result.

lating inhibitors. For example, thrombin bound to α_2-macroglobulin may still activate small amounts of factors V and VIII.

Alpha-2-macroglobulin also inhibits fibrinolysis by inhibiting, although not totally eliminating, plasmin's function in fibrinolysis. Alpha-2-macroglobulin inhibits the kinin system by inhibiting kallikrein.

Two families have been reported with decreased α_2-macroglobulin levels equivalent to 20% to 40% of the normal levels in pooled plasma. Nevertheless, these persons were asymptomatic.[10,105]

Alpha-1-Antitrypsin

Alpha-1-antitrypsin is an alpha globulin[82] that is a potent inhibitor of factor XI$_a$.[37] It may also inactivate thrombin

at a slow rate, although this is still uncertain.[31] The fibrinolytic system is inhibited by α_1-antitrypsin by its inactivation of plasmin,[31] although it is the least significant of the three naturally occurring fibrinolytic system inhibitors.

Hereditary deficiencies have been found in conjunction with liver cirrhosis (possibly because of its production by the liver) and pulmonary disease (*e.g.*, emphysema), because α_1-antitrypsin is important to normal pulmonary function. Hereditary deficiencies have not been associated with thrombotic disorders.

C'l Inactivator (C'l Esterase Inhibitor)

The C'l inactivator is a glycoprotein[71] that was initially identified in the complement system as an inhibitor of C'l esterase. It is now known that the coagulation, fibrinolytic,

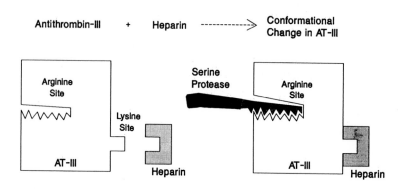

FIG. 50-7. Antithrombin III (AT-III) inhibits serine proteases by binding them in an arginine site that is not easily accessible. If heparin is available, it binds to AT-III at lysine site, causing conformational change in AT-III that makes arginine site more accessible to bind and inhibit serine proteases. With heparin cofactor, AT-III can inhibit serine proteases instantaneously.

kinin, and complement systems are all affected by this inhibitor. In the coagulation system, C'1 inactivator is an important inhibitor of factor XII_a and the fragments of factor XII (XII_f). It also inhibits factor XI_a. In the fibrinolytic system, it inhibits plasmin,[36] and in the kinin system, kallikrein.

Proteins C and S

Protein C and protein S are vitamin K-dependent glycoproteins, but unlike the vitamin K-dependent serine proteases, activated protein C and its cofactor protein S are potent inhibitors of coagulation.[27] Protein C is activated slowly by thrombin circulating in the plasma (see Chap. 56, Fig. 56-1). Protein C activation is greatly enhanced when thrombin binds to thrombomodulin on the surface of endothelial cells and forms a 1:1 stoichiometric complex with the protein C cofactor called protein S (Fig. 56-1).[25,86] Thrombin's specificity is altered when it complexes with thrombomodulin on the endothelial surface. It appears that a structural change occurs that activates protein C but inhibits thrombin's other functions. Structurally altered thrombin will not activate factors V and VIII or platelets, nor will it convert fibrinogen to fibrin. In addition, protein C and its cofactor protein S actually destroy factors V_a and VIII_a (Fig. 56-1).[66]

The protein C-S complex also enhances fibrinolysis[67] by inactivating inhibitors of plasminogen activators. This enhances the formation of plasmin and thus fibrinolysis. A protein C inhibitor has been reported that regulates activated protein C.[32,64,115]

Protein C deficiencies are clinically similar to AT-III deficiencies[14] in that thromboembolic episodes present before 30 years of age.[15]

Naturally Occurring Inhibitors of Fibrinolysis

Fibrinolysis must be controlled to maintain a delicate balance between wound healing and clot dissolution. Fibrinolysis is controlled by both the affinity of formed fibrin for plasminogen and the opposition affinity of fibrinolytic inhibitors for formed plasmin known as antiplasmins, which are discussed in this section.

Alpha-2-Antiplasmin

Alpha-2-antiplasmin is an α_2-glycoprotein.[120] It acts as the principal inhibitor of fibrinolysis by binding in a 1:1 stoichiometric complex with any plasmin that is free in the plasma,[74] thus neutralizing plasmin. This prevents plasmin from binding to fibrin and prevents plasmin's premature and uncontrolled digestion of fibrin, fibrinogen, and factors V and VIII. It also permits a slow and orderly dissolution of the clot and adequate time for repair of damaged tissues.[6,17,74]

The complex formed between plasmin and α_2-antiplasmin is similar to the thrombin-AT-III complex. Both inhibitors bind to the active serine site of their respective enzyme targets, thus inactivating the serine protease and preventing its enzymatic action on its usual substrates.

Alpha-2-antiplasmin inhibits the serine proteases XII_f, XI_a, II_a,[97] and X_a.[75] It also inhibits the clot-promoting activities of plasma kallikrein.[97] The conversion of plasminogen to plasmin is also suppressed by α_2-antiplasmin through inhibition of tissue plasminogen activator.[50,91]

Studies have shown that α_2-antiplasmin is the most important naturally occurring inhibitor of fibrinolysis,[17,77] as it is the first to bind with plasmin in the plasma. When α_2-antiplasmin stores are depleted, the naturally occurring inhibitor α_2-macroglobulin binds plasmin. When it too is depleted, α_1-antitrypsin is the last major naturally occurring defense against plasmin and uncontrolled fibrinolysis. In vitro, α_2-antiplasmin can decrease the normal binding rate of plasminogen to fibrin 30 times as effectively as a synthetic fibrinolytic inhibitor called epsilon-aminocaproic acid (EACA),[35,76] which is used to treat bleeding disoders,[93] particularly urinary tract bleeding, by inhibiting plasminogen activation.

Hereditary deficiencies of α_2-antiplasmin have been associated with a severe hemorrhagic tendency. In pathologic conditions involving excessive clotting (e.g., diffuse or disseminated intravascular coagulation [DIC]) or excessive fibrinolysis (Chap. 55), the α_2-antiplasmin levels may be depleted secondary to excessive conversion of plasminogen to plasmin.

Alpha-2-Macroglobulin

Alpha-2-macroglobulin is a large naturally occurring plasma glycoprotein that inhibits components in both the fibrinolytic and the coagulation systems (see Table 50-9). It effectively inhibits plasmin after α_2-antiplasmin depletion.

Alpha-1-Antitrypsin

Alpha-1-Antitrypsin is the third most important naturally occurring inhibitor of the fibrinolytic system. It inactivates plasmin slowly and does not bind plasmin until both α_2-antiplasmin and α_2-macroglobulin are saturated.[18,83] This inhibitor plays a more important role in the inhibition of coagulation by its potent inhibitory effects on factor XI_a.

Other Fibrinolytic Inhibitors

Antithrombin-III also functions to inhibit fibrinolysis by inhibiting plasmin and kallikrein. The C'1 inactivator also inhibits plasmin.

Physiologic Coagulation Control Mechanisms

Physiologic control mechanisms work together with biochemical control mechanisms to maintain blood fluidity. These mechanisms include inhibiting processes at the site of clot formation as well as hepatic and other clearance mechanisms for coagulation components.

Inhibiting Processes at the Site of Clot Formation

Rapid blood flow through the vessels is important to prevent excessive propagation of a thrombus and dilute any excess procoagulants or profibrinolytic components at sites of injury.

Fibrin itself restricts the active coagulants to the interior of the fibrin clot. The platelets and endothelium also restrict coagulation to the site of injury.

Hepatic and Other Clearance Mechanisms for Coagulation Components

The hepatic clearance of soluble components such as plasminogen activators and activated serine proteases, including factors IX_a, X_a, and VII_a,[24,108,109] prevents them from circulating in the venous system.[107] Consequently, liver impairment by conditions such as cirrhosis or hepatitis may cause systemic fibrinolysis or thrombosis.

Finely particulate procoagulants such as soluble fibrin components[52] and early FDPs[16] are removed in the pulmonary vascular bed.

Peripheral blood leukocytes and tissue macrophages may also participate in the clearance of coagulation components.[101]

CHAPTER SUMMARY

The mechanism of hemostasis begins with injury to the endothelium, which triggers the release of components by platelets, the endothelium, and tissues and the interaction of these components with those in the plasma. Extrinsic and intrinsic coagulation pathways (see Fig. 50-1) and fibrinolysis each exist to control hemostasis (i.e., prevent excessive bleeding or clotting).

The *intrinsic system* is initiated when factor XII is exposed to damaged endothelium. Subsequently, the contact factors XII, XI, prekallikrein, and HMWK play a complex role in initiating coagulation intrinsically as well as extrinsically through alternate pathways in which factor VII is activated by factor XII_a. The contact phase of coagulation also initiates the fibrinolytic system, the kinin system, and the complement system. The contact phase is completed with activation of factor IX, which binds with the cofactor VIII_a and Ca^{++} to activate factor X.

The *extrinsic system* is initiated when tissue factor released from damaged endothelium causes activation of factor VII. The factor VII_a-Ca^{++}-tissue factor complex activates factor X.

Factor X_a, the nonenzymatic cofactor V_a, and Ca^{++} form a complex on the platelet phospholipid surface (see Fig. 58-11) known as the *prothrombinase complex,* which is responsible for prothrombin activation to thrombin.

Thrombin is a central regulatory component of coagulation, as it can accelerate or inhibit coagulation. *Endothelial cells* also regulate by providing: (1) the vascular plasminogen activator that initiates fibrinolysis; (2) the site of protein C activation, which can neutralize major cofactors in coagulation; (3) the site of AT-III adherence, allowing for its inhibitory effects on thrombin and other serine proteases; and (4) a site for thrombomodulin adherence, which binds thrombin, preventing thrombin's coagulant effects on platelets and factors V, VIII, and fibrinogen.

Fibrinolysis is the breakdown of fibrin by plasmin contained within the fibrin clot from its formation. Plasmin is formed as a result of plasminogen activation (see Fig. 50-4). Fibrin(ogen) degradation results in the formation of *fibrin(ogen) degradation products (FDP)* of high and low molecular weights (see Fig. 50-5). Laboratory tests for the D-D dimer, a fibrin degradation product, provide an indication of abnormal *in vivo* fibrinolysis.

In normal plasma, *naturally occurring inhibitors* of coagulation and fibrinolysis (see Table 50-9) include *AT-III* (see Figs. 50-6 and 50-7), α_2-*macroglobulin,* α_1-*antitrypsin, and C'1 inactivator.* *Protein C* and its co-factor *protein S* inhibit coagulation by inhibition of factors V_a and VIII_a and enhance fibrinolysis. The principal inhibitor of fibrinolysis is α_2-*antiplasmin,* which inhibits plasmin.

REFERENCES

1. Aballi AJ, DeLamerens S: Coagulation changes in the neonatal period and in early infancy, Pediatr Clin North Am 9:785, 1962; Pediatrics 42:685, 1968
2. Alkjaersig N, Fletcher AP, Sherry S: Pathogenesis of the coagulation defect developing during pathological plasma proteolytic ("fibrinolytic") states: II. The significance, mechanism and consequences of detective fibrin polymerization. J Clin Invest 41:917, 1962
3. Altman R, Hemker HC: Contact activation in the extrinsic blood clotting system. Thromb Diath Haemorrh 18:525, 1967
4. Aoki N: Natural inhibitors of fibrinolysis. Prog Cardiovasc Dis 21:267, 1979
5. Aoki N, Moroi M, Matsuda M et al: The behavior of α_2-plasmin inhibitor in fibrinolytic states. J Clin Invest 60:361, 1977
6. Aoki N, Saito H, Kamiya T et al: Congenital deficiency of α_2-plasmin inhibitor associated with severe hemorrhagic tendency. J Clin Invest 63:877, 1979
7. Arnesen H: The effect of products D and E on the thrombin induced conversion of fibrinogen to fibrin. Scand J Haematol 12:166, 1974
8. Bajaj SP, Butkowski RJ, Mann KG: Prothrombin fragments: Ca^{++} binding and activation kinetics. J Biol Chem 250:2150, 1975
9. Bennett NB, Ogston CM, McAndrew GM: The thyroid and fibrinolysis. Br Med J 4:147, 1967
10. Bergqvist D, Nilsson IM: Hereditary α_2-macroglobulin deficiency. Scand J Haematol 23:433, 1979
11. Bjork I, Jackson CM, Jornvall H et al: The active site of antithrombin. J Biol Chem 257:2406, 1982
12. Bouma BN, Griffin JH: Human blood coagulation factor XI. J Biol Chem 252:6432, 1977
13. Brakman P, Albrechtsen OK, Astrup T: Blood coagulation, fibrinolysis, and contraceptive hormones. JAMA 199:69, 1967
14. Broekmans AW, Veltkamp JJ, Bertina RM: Congenital protein C deficiency and venous thromboembolism. N Engl J Med 309:340, 1983
15. Broekmans AW, Bertina RM, Loeliger EA et al: Protein C and the development of skin necrosis during anticoagulant therapy. Thromb Haemost 49:251, 1983
16. Budzynski AZ, Marder VJ: Degradation pathway of fibrinogen by plasmin. Thromb Haemost 38:793, 1977
17. Collen D: Identification and some properties of a new fast-reacting plasmin inhibitor in human plasma. Eur J Biochem 69:209, 1976
18. Collen D, Wiman B: Fast-acting plasmin inhibitor in human plasma. Blood 51:563, 1978
19. Coopland A, Alkjaersig N, Fletcher AP: Reduction in plasma factor XIII (fibrin stabilizing factor) concentration during pregnancy. J Lab Clin Med 73:144, 1969
20. Crowell EB Jr, Clatanoff DV, Kiekhofer W: The effect of oral contraceptives on factor VIII levels. J Lab Clin Med 77:551, 1971
21. Davie EW: Introduction to clotting in blood plasma. Methods Enzymol 80:153, 1981
22. Davie EW, Ratnoff OD: Waterfall sequence for intrinsic blood clotting. Science 145:1310, 1964
23. Davie EW, Fujikawa K, Kurachi K et al: The role of serine proteases in the blood coagulation cascade. Adv Enzymol 48:277, 1979
24. Deykin D, Cochios F, DeCamp G et al: Hepatic removal of activated factor X by the perfused rabbit liver. Am J Physiol 214: 414, 1968
25. Esmon CT: Protein C: Biochemistry, physiology, and clinical implications. Blood 62:1155, 1983

26. Esmon CT, Owen WG: Identification of an endothelial cell cofactor for thrombin-catalyzed activation of protein C. Proc Natl Acad Sci USA 78:2249, 1981

27. Esmon CT, Stenflo J, Suttie JW et al: A new vitamin K-dependent protein: A phospholipid-binding zymogen of a serine esterase. J Biol Chem 251:3052, 1976

28. Feinman RD, Li EHH: Interaction of heparin with thrombin and antithrombin III. Fed Proc 36:51, 1977

29. Fujikawa K, Davie EW: Human factor XII (Hageman factor). Methods Enzymol 80:198, 1981

30. Gaffney PJ, Perry MJ: Unreliability of current serum fibrin degradation product (FDP) assays. Thromb Haemost 53:301, 1985

31. Gans H, Tan BH: α_1-Antitrypsin, an inhibitor for thrombin and plasmin. Clin Chim Acta 17:111, 1967

32. Giddings JC, Sugrue A, Bloom AL: Quantitation of coagulant antigens and inhibition of activated protein C in combined factor V VIII deficiency. Br J Haematol 52:495, 1982

33. Gjonnaess H, Fagerhol MK: Studies on coagulation and fibrinolysis in pregnancy. Acta Obstet Gynecol Scand 54:363, 1975

34. Greenberg CS, Devine DV, McCrae KM: Measurement of plasma fibrin D-dimer levels with the use of a monoclonal antibody coupled to latex beads. Am J Clin Pathol 87:94, 1987

35. Griffin JD, Ellman L: Epsilon-aminocaproic acid (EACA). Semin Thromb Hemostas 5:27, 1978

36. Harpel PC: C′1 inactivator inhibition by plasmin. J Clin Invest 49:568, 1970

37. Heck LW, Kaplan AP: Substrates of Hageman factor: I. Isolation and characterization of human factor XI and inhibition of the activated enzyme by α_1-antitrypsin. J Exp Med 140:1615, 1974

38. Heimark RL, Davie EW: Bovine and human plasma prekallikrein. Methods Enzymol 80:157, 1981

39. Hemker HC, Muller AD, Loeliger EA: Two types of prothrombin in vitamin K deficiency. Thromb Diath Haemorrh 23:633, 1970

40. Hemker HC, Veltkamp JJ, Loeliger EA: Kinetic aspects of the interaction of blood clotting enzymes: III. Demonstration of an inhibitor of prothrombin conversion in vitamin K deficiency. Thromb Diath Haemorrh 19:346, 1968

41. Hoak JC, Wilson WR, Warner ED et al: Effects of triiodothyronine-induced hypermetabolism on factor VIII and fibrinogen in man. J Clin Invest 48:768, 1969

42. Hultin MB, Nemerson Y: Activation of factor X by factors IX_a and VIII: A specific assay for factor IX_a in the presence of thrombin-activated factor VIII. Blood 52:928, 1978

43. Iatridis SG, Ferguson JH: Effect of surface and Hageman factor on the endogenous or spontaneous activation of the fibrinolytic system. Thromb Diath Haemorrh 6:411, 1961

44. Jackson CM, Brenckle GM: Biochemistry of the vitamin K-dependent clotting factors. In Menache D, Surgenor DM, Anderson HD (eds): Hemophilia and Hemostasis, p 27. New York, Alan R Liss, 1981

45. Jones JM, Creeth JM, Kekwick RA: Thiol reduction of human alpha 2-macroglobulin. Biochem J 127:187, 1972

46. Kasper CK, Hoag MS, Aggeler PM et al: Blood clotting factors in pregnancy: Factor VIII concentrations in normal and AHF-deficient women. Obstet Gynecol 24:242, 1964

47. Kato H, Nagasawa S, Iwanaga S: HMW and LMW kininogens. Methods Enzymol 80:172, 1981

48. Kerbiriou DM, Griffith JH: Human high-molecular-weight kininogen. J Biol Chem 254:12020, 1979

49. Kisiel W, Fujikawa K, Davie EW: Activation of bovine factor VII (proconvertin) by factor XII_a (activated Hageman factor). Biochemistry 16:4189, 1977

50. Korninger C, Collen D: Neutralization of human extrinsic (tissue-type) plasminogen activator in human plasma: No evidence for a specific inhibitor. Thromb Haemost 46:662, 1981

51. Laake K, Vennerod AM: Factor XII-induced fibrinolysis: Studies on the separation of prekallikrein, plasminogen proactivator, and factor XI in human plasma. Thromb Res 4:285, 1974

52. Lewis JH, Szeto ILF: Clearance of infused fibrin. Fed Proc 24:840, 1965

53. Libre EP, Cowan DH, Watkins SP Jr et al: Relationships between spleen, platelets and factors VIII levels. Blood 31:358, 1968

54. Loeliger EA, van der Esch B, Mattern MJ et al: The biological disappearance rate of prothrombin, factors VII, IX, and X from plasma in hypothyroidism, hyperthyroidism, and during fever. Thromb Diath Haemorrh 10:267, 1964

55. Lombardi R, Mannucci PM, Seghatchian MJ et al: Alterations of factor VIII von Willebrand factor in clinical conditions associated with an increase in its plasma concentration. Br J Haematol 49:61, 1981

56. MacFarlane RG: An enzyme cascade in the blood clotting mechanism, and its function as a biochemical amplifier. Nature 202:498, 1964

57. MacFarlane RG: The basis of the cascade hypothesis of blood clotting. Thromb Diath Haemorrh 15:591, 1966

58. Mandle RJ Jr, Kaplan AP: Hageman-factor-dependent fibrinolysis: Generation of fibrinolytic activity by the interaction of human activated factor XI and plasminogen. Blood 54:850, 1979

59. Mann KG: Membrane-bound enzyme complexes in blood coagulation. Prog Hemost Thromb 7:1, 1984

60. Mann KG, Pendergast FG, Bloom JW: The metal ion and phospholipid interactions of the vitamin K-dependent factors. In Mann KG, Taylor FB Jr (eds): The Regulation of Coagulation, pp 3–9. New York, Elsevier North-Holland, 1980

61. Mann KG, Nesheim ME, Hibbard LS et al: The role of factor V in the assembly of the prothrombinase complex. Ann NY Acad Sci 370:378, 1981

62. Marciniak E: Thrombin-induced proteolysis of human antithrombin III: An outstanding contribution of heparin. Br J Haematol 48:325, 1981

63. Marder VJ, Budzynski AZ: Data for defining fibrinogen and its plasmic degradation products. Thromb Diath Haemorrh 33:199, 1975

64. Marlar RA, Griffin JH: Deficiency of protein C inhibitor in combined factor V/VIII deficiency disease. J Clin Invest 66:1186, 1980

65. Marlar RA, Griffin JH: Alternative pathways of thromboplastin-dependent activation of human factor X in plasma. Ann NY Acad Sci 370:325, 1981

66. Marlar RA, Kleiss AJ, Griffin JH: Human protein C: Inactivation of factors V and VIII in plasma by the activated molecule. Ann NY Acad Sci 370:303, 1981

67. Marlar RA, Kleiss AJ, Griffin JH: Mechanism of action of human activated protein C, a thrombin dependent anticoagulant enzyme. Blood 59:1067, 1982

68. Marlar RA, Kleiss AJ, Griffin JH: An alternative extrinsic pathway of human blood coagulation. Blood 60:1353, 1982

69. Matsuo O: Incidence of thrombosis in inherited antithrombin III deficiency. Thromb Res 24:509, 1981

70. Matsuo T, Ohki Y, Kondo S et al: Familial antithrombin III deficiency in a Japanese family. Thromb Res 16:815, 1979

71. McConnell DJ: Inhibitors of kallikrein in human plasma. J Clin Invest 51:1611, 1972

72. McNicol GP, Fletcher AP, Alkjaersig N et al: Impairment of hemostasis in the urinary tract: The role of urokinase. J Lab Clin Med 58:34, 1961

73. Morawitz P: Die Chemie der Blutgerinnung. Ergebn Physiol Biol Chem Exp Pharmakol 4:307, 1905. Available in the English translation as: "The chemistry of blood coagulation," translated by Hartman RC, Guenther PF. Springfield, IL, Charles C Thomas, 1958

74. Moroi M, Aoki N: Isolation and characterization of α_2 plasmin inhibitor from human plasma: A novel proteinase inhibitor which inhibits activator-induced clot lysis. J Biol Chem 251:5956, 1976

75. Moroi M, Aoki N: Inhibition of proteases in coagulation, kinin-forming and complement systems by α_2 plasmin inhibitor. J Biochem 82:969, 1977

76. Moroi M, Aoki N: Inhibition of plasminogen binding to fibrin by α_2-plasmin inhibitor. Thromb Res 10:851, 1977

77. Mullertz S, Clemmensen I: The primary inhibitor of plasmin in human plasma. Biochem J 159:545, 1976

78. Nelsestuen GL: Role of calcium and phospholipid in in vitro thrombin generation. In Mann KG, Taylor FB Jr (eds): The Regulation of Coagulation, p 31. New York, Elsevier North-Holland, 1980

79. Nelsestuen GL, Suttie JW: The purification and properties of an abnormal prothrombin protein produced by dicumarol-treated cows: A comparison to normal prothrombin. J Biol Chem 247:8176, 1972

80. Nemerson Y: Biological control of factor VII. Thromb Haemost 35:96, 1976

81. Nemerson Y, Bach R: Tissue factor revisited. Prog Hemost Thromb 6:237, 1982

82. Ogston D, Bennett B: Naturally occurring inhibitors of coagulation. In Ogston D, Bennett B (eds): Haemostasis: Biochemistry, Physiology and Pathology, p 202. London, John Wiley & Sons, 1977

83. Ogston D, Bennett B: Biochemistry of naturally occurring inhibitors of the fibrinolytic enzyme system. In Ogston D, Bennett B (eds): Haemostasis: Biochemistry, Physiology and Pathology, p 230. London, John Wiley & Sons, 1977

84. Oski FA, Naiman JL: Hematologic Problems in the Newborn, p 236. Philadelphia, WB Saunders, 1972

85. Osterud B: Activation pathways of the coagulation system in normal haemostasis. Scand J Haematol 32: 337, 1984

86. Owen WG, Esmon CT: Functional properties of an endothelial cell cofactor for thrombin catalyzed activation of protein C. J Biol Chem 256:5532, 1981

87. Pennica D, Holmes WE, Kohr WH et al: Cloning and expression of human tissue-type plasminogen activator cDNA in E. coli. Nature 301:214, 1983

88. Phillips LL, Rosano L, Skrodelis V: Changes in factor XI (plasma thromboplastin antecedent) levels during pregnancy. Am J Obstet Gynecol 116:1114, 1973

89. Radcliff RD, Nemerson Y: Mechanism of activation of bovine factor VII: Products of cleavage by factor X_a. J Biol Chem 251:4797, 1976

90. Radcliff R, Bagdasarian A, Colman R et al: Activation of bovine factor VII by Hageman factor fragments. Blood 50:611, 1977

91. Ranby M, Bergsdorf N, Nilsson T: Enzymatic properties of the one- and two-chain form of tissue plasminogen activator. Thromb Res 27:175, 1982

92. Rapaport SI, Schiffman S, Patch MJ et al: The importance of activation of antihemophilic globulin and proaccelerin by traces of thrombin in the generation of intrinsic prothrombinase activity. Blood 21:221, 1963; Scand J Clin Lab Invest Suppl 84:88, 1965

93. Reid WO, Hodge SM, Cerutti ER: The use of EACA in preventing or reducing haemorrhages in the haemophiliac. Thromb Diath Haemorrh 18:179, 1967

94. Revak SD, Cochrane CG: Hageman factor: Its structure and modes of activation. Thromb Haemost 35:570, 1976

95. Rizza CR: Effect of exercise on the level of antihaemophilic globulin in human blood. J Physiol 156:128, 1961

96. Rosenberg RD: Heparin, antithrombin, and abnormal clotting. Annu Rev Med 29:367, 1978

97. Saito H, Goldsmith GH, Moroi M et al: Inhibitory spectrum of α_2-plasmin inhibitor. Proc Natl Acad Sci USA 76:2013, 1979

98. Sas G, Peto I, Banhegyi D et al: Heterogeneity of the "classical" antithrombin III deficiency. Thromb Haemost 43:133, 1980

99. Seegers WH, Warner ED, Brinkhous KM et al: Heparin and the antithrombic activity of plasma. Science 96:300, 1942

100. Seligsohn U, Osterud B, Brown SE et al: Activation of human factor VII in plasma and in purified systems: Roles of activated factor IX, kallikrein, and activated factor XII. J Clin Invest 64:1056, 1979

101. Sherman LA, Lee J: Specific binding of soluble fibrin to macrophages. J Exp Med 145:76, 1977

102. Sherry S, Fletcher A, Alkjaersig N: Fibrinolysis and fibrinolytic activity in man. Physiol Rev 39:343, 1959

103. Silverberg M, Nicoll JE, Kaplan AP: The mechanism by which the light chain of cleaved HMW-kininogen augments the activation of prekallikrein, factor XI and Hageman factor. Thromb Res 20:173, 1980

104. Simone JV, Abildgaard CF, Schulman I: Blood coagulation in thyroid dysfunction. N Engl J Med 273:1057, 1965

105. Slenbjerg S: Inherited α_2 macroglobulin deficiency. Thromb Res 22:491, 1981

106. Solum NO, Rigollot C, Budzynski AZ et al: A quantitative evaluation of the inhibition of platelet aggregation by low molecular weight degradation products of fibrinogen. Br J Haematol 24:419, 1973

107. Spaet TH: Hemostatic homeostasis. Blood 28:112, 1966

108. Spaet TH: Studies on the in vivo behavior of blood coagulation product I in rats. Thromb Diath Haemorrh 8:276, 1962

109. Spaet TH, Cintron J: Clearance of blood coagulation product I in rabbits. Proc Soc Exp Biol Med 104:498, 1960

110. Stenflo J: Vitamin K, prothrombin and γ-carboxyglutamic acid. N Engl J Med 296:624, 1977

111. Thompson AR, Harker LA: Manual of Hemostasis and Thrombosis, 3rd ed, p 38. Philadelphia, FA Davis, 1983

112. Tillett WS, Garner RL: The fibrinolytic activity of hemolytic streptococci. J Exp Med 58:485, 1933

113. Todd AS: The histological localization of fibrinolysin activator. J Pathol Bacteriol 78:281, 1959

114. van Dieijen G, Tans G, Rosing J et al: The role of phospholipid and factor VIII_a in the activation of bovine factor X. J Biol Chem 256:3433, 1981

115. Walker FJ: Regulation of activated protein C by a new protein. J Biol Chem 255:5521, 1980

116. Walsh PR, Biggs R: The role of platelets in intrinsic factor X_a formation. Br J Haematol 22:743, 1972

117. Whittaker AN, Elms MJ, Masci PP et al: Measurement of crosslink fibrin derivatives in plasma: An immunoassay using monoclonal antibodies. J Clin Pathol 37:882, 1984

118. Wiggins RC, Loskutoff DJ, Cochrane CG et al: Activation of rabbit Hageman factor by homogenates of cultured rabbit endothelial cells. J Clin Invest 65:197, 1980

119. Williams JRB: The fibrinolytic activity of urine. Br J Exp Pathol 32:530, 1951

120. Wiman B, Collen D: Purification and characterization of human antiplasmin, the fast-acting plasmin inhibitor in plasma. Eur J Biochem 78:19, 1977

121. Wintrobe MM et al: Blood coagulation. In Wintrobe MM et al: Clinical Hematology, 8th ed. Philadelphia, Lea & Febiger, 1981

122. Wright IS: The nomenclature of blood clotting factors. Thromb Diath Haemorrh 7:381, 1962

123. Yin ET, Wessler S, Stoll PJ: Biological properties of the naturally occurring plasma inhibitor to activated factor X. J Biol Chem 246:3703, 1971

51

Specimen Collection and Processing for Hemostasis Testing

Reaner G. Shannon

A nontraumatic venipuncture is the goal any time blood is drawn, but probably in no other area of laboratory testing is the quality of the sample as important to the accuracy of test results as in studies related to hemostasis. A prime concern is premature activation of the clotting process, before the sample can be evaluated in the test procedures. The causes of such activation include contamination of the specimen with tissue thromboplastin, contact with the surface of an inappropriate specimen container, improper temperature, and hemolysis.

Tissue thromboplastin is a potent clot-activating substance found in fluids that escape from injured cells and tissue spaces. When tissues are traumatized or blood vessels are disrupted or cut, this substance activates the extrinsic pathway of clotting and causes erroneous test results. Even slight contamination with tissue thromboplastin is enough to affect the results obtained in both normal and abnormal specimens.

The effect of *glass surfaces* on hemostasis is well known. The contact factors (prekallikrein [Fletcher], XII, and XI) will be activated prematurely by contact with glass, causing a shortening of both the intrinsic and the extrinsic pathway. The recommended materials for collecting, transporting, and storing blood specimens for hemostasis testing are plastic, polystyrene, or silicone-coated glass.

Temperature has long been known to affect hemostasis testing in that the labile factors (V and VIII) will deteriorate if left at room temperature for an extended period of time. The last decade has brought about the realization that cold tends to activate factors VII and XI prematurely.[16]

Hemolysis is the release of hemoglobin from ruptured red cells into the plasma. Hemolyzed red cells act like tissue thromboplastin in activating plasma clotting factors. When hemolysis occurs in the blood-drawing process, technical problems are usually the cause. Some of the most common technical errors are listed in Table 51-1.

A poor venipuncture can cause erroneous test results. The fact that blood obtained by defective collection techniques often is satisfactory for biochemical or cytologic studies can mislead clinical laboratory workers such as phlebotomists into believing that the same applies to studies for blood coagulation. Ideally, a person familiar with coagulation tests obtains the blood for clotting studies or a member of the coagulation laboratory supervises its collection. Another option is to draw such blood separately rather than as part of a large collection for other tests. Because these approaches are often impractical, it is acceptable for the samples for coagulation testing to be drawn by well-trained personnel and as a part of large blood samples provided specific standards and guidelines for such drawings are followed.[14,15] General techniques for obtaining blood samples are described in Chapter 2 of this book. Only the areas that specifically apply to obtaining and processing blood samples for hemostasis studies will be discussed in this chapter.

EQUIPMENT

Venous occlusion or stasis occurs in the blood-collecting process when the tourniquet is applied too tightly or for an extended period of time (more than 1 minute). When arterial flow or venous return is interrupted, there is activation of the fibrinolytic system and clotting factors.[19] To minimize such stasis and the hemoconcentration that also develops, the tourniquet should be released as soon as the vein is entered and blood appears in the syringe or evacuated tube. Many types of flexible rubber tubing may be used as tourniquets, but because increased stasis is the concern, the Seraket tourniquet (Propper Manufacturing Co, Inc, Long Island, NY) is recommended. Venous pressure created when this tourniquet is applied can be partially released by lifting a lever without totally releasing the tourniquet from the arm.[13] If the flow of blood should decrease or stop while blood is being drawn, the pressure can be reapplied.

The use of the appropriate needle size is important. It is generally believed that needles with small bores are more likely to cause hemolysis. In collecting blood for coagulation tests, the 20-gauge needle is most commonly used, but when more than 20 mL of blood is to be drawn, a 19-gauge needle may be preferred. For pediatric patients or those with narrow or small veins a smaller size (21 gauge) might be selected. Needles should be of the disposable type and

TABLE 51-1. Technical Errors that May Cause Hemolysis

Excessive stasis through prolonged application of the tourniquet
Moisture or contamination in the needle, syringe, or blood container
Using needles with too small a bore
Frothing of sample due to entry of air
Expelling blood from the syringe through the needle
Excessive and vigorous mixing of blood with the anticoagulant

coated with polymeric silicone. These needles make skin penetration and vein entry smooth and easy with minimal pain, trauma, and activation of coagulation factors.

Samples for coagulation tests should be collected in plastic syringes or silicone-coated evacuated tubes to minimize the effect of contact activation. Silicone-coated evacuated tubes containing the anticoagulant trisodium citrate may be used whenever citrated plasma is required. Samples drawn into these tubes are satisfactory for both coagulation and platelet function studies.[19]

ANTICOAGULANTS

Citrate

The anticoagulant used in the collection of specimens for coagulation testing is important. Both oxalate and citrate have been used in the past; however, the anticoagulant of choice today is trisodium citrate, as citrate has several features that make it desirable. Citrated plasma preserves the labile clotting factors V and VIII better, and it is the most satisfactory for platelet aggregation studies. Citrated plasma samples also are more sensitive to the effects of heparin and therefore preferred for tests to monitor heparin therapy.[19] Sodium oxalate and sodium citrate both function as anticoagulants by binding ionized calcium, but when oxalated plasma is recalcified in the test system, insoluble complexes or precipitates are formed that may interfere with endpoint detection by instruments that measure changes in optical density. This reaction is critically important because more than 70% of routine coagulation tests are performed on instrumentation based on the turbidimetric principle of clot detection.[3]

Ratio of Anticoagulant to Blood

The ratio of blood to anticoagulant is critical for valid coagulation test results. The standard ratio for citrate is nine parts of blood to one part of anticoagulant (9:1). This ratio is satisfactory for specimens with relatively normal hematocrits. However, if the hematocrit value exceeds 0.50 L/L, as in polycythemia, or if there is incomplete filling of the sample tube, the amount of unbound citrate in the citrate:plasma mixture causes a false prolongation of clotting times, particularly in the prothrombin time (PT) and the activated partial thromboplastin time (APTT) tests. This occurs because the fixed or standard amount of calcium used to recalcify the plasma in these coagulation procedures must inactivate excess unbound citrate in addition to initiating clotting of the specimen.[6]

To prevent spurious prolongations of clotting times associated with elevated hematocrits, at least three techniques have been proposed. One is to adjust the volume of anticoagulant used on the basis of the patient's hematocrit value.[9,24] This process can be time consuming and almost always means a second venipuncture for the patient, because the problem usually is identified after the first sample is drawn. The second method is to increase the amount of calcium used to recalcify the plasma in the test system. However, because excess concentrations of calcium ions inhibit coagulation, clotting times may be significantly increased instead of decreased, as one would expect.[12]

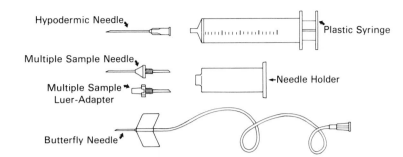

FIG. 51-1. Different types of blood-drawing equipment labeled according to terminology used in this chapter.

The third and most practical means of correcting the prolongation problem is by decreasing the concentration of the anticoagulant. Coagulation tests are more sensitive to an excess of citrate in the plasma, which occurs with high hematocrits, than to an excess of calcium, which occurs with low hematocrits or an overfilled tube.[10,17] Because probably only half of the 3.8% (0.129 M) concentration of sodium citrate is required to anticoagulate normal blood samples, it is possible routinely to use a lower concentration such as 3.2% (0.109 M) sodium citrate and eliminate the testing problem associated with elevated hematocrits. This concentration has no apparent effect on the test values from samples with low hematocrits. Although 3.8% sodium citrate solution is still used, 3.2% buffered sodim citrate has been adopted as the standard anticoagulant for coagulation studies by the National Committee for Clinical Laboratory Standards (NCCLS). Buffering of the citrate solution has the added effect of stabilizing the *p*H of blood samples and increasing the stability of the labile clotting factors.[23]

EDTA

Sequestrene or ethylenediaminetetraacetic acid (EDTA) is not a satisfactory anticoagulant for coagulation testing because it inhibits the fibrinogen-thrombin reaction. Also, factor V is not stable in its presence.

Heparin

Heparin is an organic acid that acts with anti-thrombin III and inhibits the reactions of all stages of coagulation. Because of its many anticoagulant actions, heparin is not used for collecting blood for coagulation studies. However, it may be the anticoagulant of choice when blood is collected for the platelet retention test.

COLLECTION OF BLOOD

A clean rapid venipuncture prevents tissue thromboplastin or air from entering the sample. If there is any difficulty in performing the venipuncture, the attempt should be aborted, a new site should be chosen, and fresh blood-drawing equipment should be used. For common coagulation tests such as the PT and APTT tests, routine vacuum tube collection is satisfactory so long as contamination with tissue juices is avoided. If difficulties in drawing blood are anticipated or if blood is being drawn for special procedures, a two-syringe technique using either syringes or evacuated tubes is recommended (Fig. 51-1).

Two-Syringe Technique

Figure 51-2 illustrates the blood-drawing apparatus assembled for a two-syringe technique and how both syringes and evacuated tubes may be used to draw blood when a variety of tests has been requested. The butterfly needle may be used instead of the standard disposable needle and is recommended when blood must be drawn directly into syringes containing an anti-

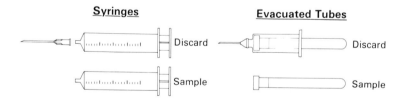

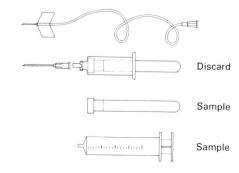

FIG. 51-2. Blood-drawing apparatus for two-syringe technique may be either syringes, evacuated tubes, or a combination. Use of butterfly needle and Luer adapter is recommended, especially if it is necessary to change from evacuated tube needle holder to syringe.

coagulant or some other toxic solution, such as the formalin used in some procedures to evaluate platelet hyperactivity. The long connecting tubing prevents accidental infusion of such a solution into the vein.

Procedure Using Syringes

When a sample is being drawn into a syringe, the tourniquet is released and 1 to 3 mL of blood is withdrawn into the first syringe after the vein is entered. This blood may be discarded or used for tests requiring serum. Before syringes are switched, sterile gauze is placed beneath the hub of the needle to absorb any blood that escapes when the syringe is switched. With the needle in the vein, the first syringe is carefully detached from the needle and replaced with the second syringe. Blood for coagulation tests is drawn into this syringe and transferred without delay into the appropriate tubes. To avoid air bubbles and frothing of the sample, the needle should be securely fitted on the syringe. When blood is being aspirated with a syringe, the plunger should be withdrawn at a rate equal to the flow of blood. If the rate is in excess of that needed to aspirate the blood, air bubbles will enter the syringe and cause hemolysis.[22] Forced aspiration may also cause the vein to collapse and result in a sudden release of gases from red cells, resulting in hemolysis.[5]

Procedure Using Evacuated Tubes

The evacuated system of collecting blood is generally preferable to that using syringes because blood goes directly from the vein into the tube and is immediately mixed with anticoagulant, thus reducing the likelihood of clotted samples.[20] This is an important factor when collecting blood for hemostatic workups that include the evaluation of platelets and clotting factors and require as much as 30 to 50 mL of blood. Figure 51-3 shows how blood for such studies can be drawn and the recommended order in which the samples should be collected. Should a specimen anticoagulated with EDTA be required, the EDTA tube should be drawn after the citrate tubes to avoid contaminating the citrated plasma with EDTA.[2,13]

A multiple-sample Luer adapter, which fits into the hub of a standard disposable or butterfly needle, is screwed into a needle holder and used for the initial venipuncture. After the needle enters the vein, the tourniquet is released and the system cleansed of tissue thromboplastin by drawing blood into a red-stoppered evacuated tube. This blood may be used for other tests requiring serum, or it may be discarded. Samples for tests requiring citrated plasma are drawn next; the last evacuated tube to be filled should be the EDTA tube. While the needle is still in the vein, the needle holder is removed with the Luer adapter still attached, and a plastic syringe is attached to the needle. Blood is drawn into this syringe and dispensed into appropriate tubes for any additional platelet function tests.

Drawing blood from an indwelling catheter is not recommended. However, if this is unavoidable, the first blood should be drawn into a syringe or evacuated tube and discarded before the specimen is obtained for coagulation tests. The volume discarded is dependent on the length and diameter of the catheter. It may be necessary to discard as much as 30 mL, especially if the thrombin clotting time is to be determined.

TRANSFERRING AND MIXING SAMPLES

To avoid frothing and hemolysis of the sample, blood should not be expelled through the needle. Immediately after the venipuncture is completed, the needle should be removed from the syringe and the blood allowed to run down the side of the tube.[21] Samples transferred into tubes containing anticoagulants should be stoppered and thoroughly mixed by gently inverting the tubes five to ten times. Blood drawn into evacuated tubes is partially mixed with the anticoagulant when the blood enters the tube, but to assure that mixing is thorough, the tubes should be inverted several times immediately after removal from the needle holder. Vigorous shaking must be avoided.

CAPILLARY BLOOD

Sometimes, only capillary blood can be obtained from a patient. The PT test done on such blood probably is reliable provided the sample is obtained rapidly and anticoagulated immediately. It is recommended, however, that capillary blood be avoided for coagulation studies. Certainly, it would be unwise to make a firm diagnosis of a congenital bleeding disorder, such as hemophilia, unless a satisfactory venous sample is available.[4,18]

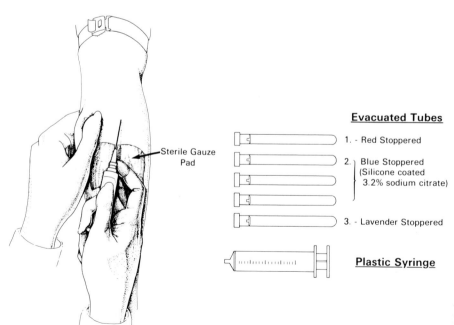

Sterile Gauze
Pad

Evacuated Tubes

1. - Red Stoppered

2. } Blue Stoppered
   (Silicone coated
   3.2% sodium citrate)

3. - Lavender Stoppered

Plastic Syringe

FIG. 51-3. Recommended order of sample collection when multiple samples are necessary.

PROCESSING AND HOLDING SAMPLES BEFORE TESTING

Once blood is drawn, changes begin to occur in the sample. These changes range from surface activation, which results in shortened clotting times, to increased lability of factors V and VIII, which may lengthen clotting times. Such changes become significant sources of errors in testing if measures are not taken to minimize and control them when processing and holding samples.

Effect of pH

Changes in the pH of samples can affect values by causing prolongation of clotting times. Changes in pH are mediated by the loss of carbon dioxide (CO_2) from the sample. As CO_2 is lost, the pH of the sample increases. The buffered citrate solution contained in evacuated tubes protects samples against such loss for a period of time. Also, red blood cells have a buffering effect that helps to stabilize the pH of blood samples. To maintain this effect, samples should remain in unopened tubes if testing is not done immediately. Normal samples collected in evacuated tubes and stored unopened at room temperature for as long as 6 hours show no significant changes in PT or APTT results.[10]

Effect of Temperature

If samples are left at room temperature for an extended time, factors V and VIII are likely to deteriorate. Factors VII and XI tend to be prematurely activated at refrigerator temperatures (4°C).

Centrifugation

For most coagulation testing, platelet-free plasma is required. Platelet-poor plasma (PPP) is prepared by centrifuging anticoagulated blood at $2000 \times g$ for 10 minutes. Plasma should be removed immediately with a plastic or siliconized pipet and stored in a stoppered plastic or siliconized tube. Only the upper three-fourths of the plasma layer should be aspirated. For some tests, centrifugation of the sample at a temperature of 2° to 4°C is advisable. For this process, a refrigerated centrifuge or a small centrifuge placed in a refrigerator is required.

The buffering effect of the red cells is lost once the sample is centrifuged and the plasma exposed to air.[1,25] Testing should be done immediately on centrifuged samples, or the plasma should be stored at 4°C for a time not to exceed 2 hours.

Frozen Samples

Samples should not be frozen if testing can be done within 2 hours after collection. If freezing is necessary, it should be done rapidly at −20°C or lower. With slow freezing, ice particles form that may denature the clotting proteins.[11] If frozen properly, fibrinogen is stable for at least 4 hours after thawing and survives refreezing and thawing.[8]

SAMPLES FOR PLATELET FUNCTION TESTING

Collection

The same care taken in performing the venipuncture and drawing blood samples for other hemostatic testing should be exercised in obtaining samples for platelet function studies. Hemolysis should be avoided at all times because red cells contain ADP, which, if released into the plasma, may prematurely activate the platelets. Citrate is the anticoagulant of choice for platelet function testing except for the glass bead retention test, which requires heparin. The pH of the sample is critical and is best controlled with the buffered sodium citrate previously recommended for anticoagulating hemostasis samples.

Centrifugation

Samples drawn for platelet function studies should be processed immediately. To prepare platelet-rich plasma (PRP), the anticoagulated sample is centrifuged at 60 to $100 \times g$ for 10 minutes at room temperature. The plasma is removed immediately with a plastic or siliconized pipet and transferred to stoppered plastic or siliconized test tubes. Red cell contamination should be avoided by removing carefully only as much PRP as necessary from the upper portion of the sample.

Platelet aggregation studies also require PPP. This is obtained by recentrifuging the sample remaining from the PRP at $2000 \times g$ for 10 minutes. The upper three-fourths of the plasma layer is aspirated and stored in stoppered plastic or siliconized tubes.

For some platelet function tests, such as the beta-thromboglobulin (βTG) and platelet factor 4 (PF4) determinations, the samples should be centrifuged at 2° to 4°C.

Influence of Time

Platelets are stable and most responsive between 30 minutes and 3 hours after blood is drawn.[7] Thereafter, platelet function diminishes significantly, so that testing is unsatisfactory. The responses of platelets to the various aggregating agents are different and vary as a function of time. When platelet aggregation tests are performed, Ristocetin aggregation testing should be done immediately after the sample is processed because the response of platelets to Ristocetin decreases as the pH of the plasma changes. On the other hand, aggregation with epinephrine should be performed last because the response of platelets to this agent continues to increase with time. Consistent or maximum aggregation with epinephrine is reached after PRP has been at room temperature for about 60 minutes.

Influence of Temperature

The storage temperature of PRP prepared for platelet function studies has a significant influence on the rate and degree of platelet response in the test. Platelets prepared for aggregation studies and stored at room temperature are more sensitive to various aggregating agents than platelets stored at 37°C. The storage of platelets at low temperatures (0°–4°C) increases the tendency for platelets to aggregate spontaneously.[26] Because of the variability of platelet activity at these temperatures, samples collected and prepared for platelet function studies, particularly platelet aggregation, should remain at room temperature until testing.

CHAPTER SUMMARY

This chapter presents the proper methods for collecting specimens to be used in hemostasis testing. With an understanding of all the factors that can influence the test results (*i.e,* technique, *p*H, and temperature), the phlebotomist can obtain the best possible specimen for each test performed in the hemostasis laboratory.

REFERENCES

1. Bandi ZL: Estimation, prevention and quality control of carbon dioxide loss during aerobic sample processing. Clin Chem 27:1676, 1981
2. Calam RR, Cooper MH: Recommended "order of draw" for collecting blood specimens into additive containing tubes. Clin Chem 28:1399, 1982
3. Corriveau DM: Chemical assessment of coagulation. In Bishop ML, Duben-Von Laufen JL, Fody EP (eds): Clinical Chemistry: Principles, Procedures, Correlations, p 512. Philadelphia, JB Lippincott, 1985
4. Dacie JV: Practical Haematology, 5th ed, p 326. London, Churchill Livingstone, 1975
5. Diggs LW: Hematological techniques. In Miller SE (ed): A Textbook of Clinical Pathology, 8th ed, p 3. Baltimore, Williams & Wilkins, 1971
6. Hardisty RM, Ingram GIC: Bleeding Disorders: Investigation and Management, p 162. Oxford, Blackwell Scientific Publications, 1965
7. Harms CS: Routine laboratory procedures. In Triplett DA (ed): Platelet Function: Laboratory Evaluation and Clinical Application, p 214. Chicago, American Society of Clinical Pathologists, 1978
8. Hoffman M, Koepke JA, Widman FK: Fibrinogen content of low volume cryoprecipitate. Transfusion 27:356, 1987
9. Ingram GIC, Hills M: The prothrombin time test: Effect of varying citrate concentration. Thromb Haemorrh 36:230, 1976
10. Koepke JA, Rodgers JL, Ollivier MJ: Pre-instrumental variables in coagulation testing. Am J Clin Pathol 64:591, 1975
11. Lenahan JG, Smith K: Hemostasis, 16th ed, p 13. Morris Plains, NJ, General Diagnostics, 1982
12. Lovelock JE, Porterfield BM: Blood clotting: The function of electrolytes and calcium. Biochemistry 50:415, 1952
13. Lotspeich CA: Specimen collection and processing. In Bishop ML, Duben-Von Laufen JL, Fody EP (eds): Clinical Chemistry: Principles, Procedures, Correlations, p 42. Philadelphia, JB Lippincott, 1985
14. National Committee for Clinical Laboratory Standards: Standard Procedures for the Collection of Diagnostic Blood Specimens by Venipuncture. Villanova, PA, NCCLS, 1977
15. National Committee for Clinical Laboratory Standards: Proposed Standard Procedures for Handling and Processing of Blood Specimens. Villanova, PA, NCCLS, 1981
16. Palmer RN, Gralnick HR: Cold induced contact activation of the prothrombin time in whole blood. Blood 59:38, 1981
17. Peterson P, Gollfried EL: The effects of inaccurate blood sample volume on prothrombin time (PT) and activated partial thromboplastin time (APTT). Thromb Haemorrh 47:101, 1982
18. Raphael SS: Lynch's Medical Laboratory Technology, 4th ed, p 734. Philadelphia, WB Saunders, 1983
19. Sirridge MS, Shannon R: Laboratory Evaluation of Hemostasis and Thrombosis, 3rd ed, pp 58, 60, 170. Philadelphia, Lea & Febiger, 1983
20. Slockbower JM: Blood drawing techniques. In Seligson D, Schmidt RM (eds): Handbook Series in Clinical Laboratory Science, p 22. Boca Raton, CRC Press, 1979
21. Slockbower JM, Blumenfeld TA: Collection and Handling of Laboratory Specimens: A Practical Guide, p 43. Philadelphia, JB Lippincott, 1983
22. Tocantins LM: Processing of blood, preparation of glassware and reagents. In Tocantins LM, Kazal LA (eds): Blood Coagulation, Hemorrhage and Thrombosis, p 3. New York, Grune & Stratton, 1964
23. Todd M: Buffered citrate tubes offer advantages, pose no problems. Lab Note Number 3. Rutherford, NJ, Becton Dickinson VACUTAINER Systems, 1978
24. Triplett DA: Obtaining good specimens for coagulation testing. Lab Notes 3:7. Rutherford, NJ, Becton Dickinson VACUTAINER Systems, 1978
25. Triplett DA, Smith C: Routine testing in the coagulation laboratory. In Triplett DA (ed): Laboratory Evaluation of Coagulation. Chicago, American Society of Clinical Pathologists, 1982
26. Zucker MB, Borrelli J: Reversible alterations in platelet morphology produced by anticoagulants and by cold. Blood 9:602, 1954

52

Routine

Laboratory

Evaluation

of Coagulation

Cheryl S. Cook

REFERENCE RANGES

TESTS FOR THE INTRINSIC AND COMMON PATHWAYS
  Lee and White Whole Blood Coagulation Time
  Plasma Recalcification Time
  Activated Clotting Time
  Partial Thromboplastin Time

TESTS FOR THE EXTRINSIC AND COMMON PATHWAYS
  Prothrombin Time
  Other Tests

For centuries, man has been intrigued by the process of blood coagulation and has strived to perfect accurate and precise methods for evaluating the complex process. Since William Henson's discovery in the late 1700s that blood ligated in the veins of a living animal clotted much more slowly than blood that has been shed from the body,[32] investigators have been avidly experimenting with ways to measure the blood's capacity to clot.

In 1905, knowledge of coagulation took a significant step forward when Paul Morawitz, a young German scientist, published a comprehensive explanation of the chemistry of coagulation.[23] His observations that coagulation did not occur when plasma was placed in containers with "nonwettable" surfaces, such as paraffin-lined tubes, but did so rapidly when placed in contact with "wettable" surfaces such as glass tubes led to the development of methods for the measurement of coagulation.[2]

Among the first researchers to expand on the theory of Morawitz were Drs. Roger Lee and Paul White.[18] Modifying the numerous procedures described in the literature in the early 1900s, these investigators developed a procedure known as the Lee and White whole blood clotting time (L-W). Today, more sensitive and precise procedures have replaced this test in most institutions. It was not until the mid 1930s that the next breakthrough in coagulation testing came about. At this time, Dr. Armand Quick[31] described a procedure called the prothrombin time (PT) test. With minor modifications, this test has become a routine coagulation procedure for evaluating the extrinsic coagulation system. In the 1950s, studies of blood from hemophiliacs, whose blood yielded normal prothrombin times despite its

Extrinsic System

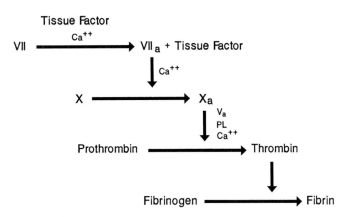

FIG. 52-1.   Extrinsic system of coagulation that is monitored by prothrombin time. PL, phospholipid; Ca^{++}, calcium ions.

inability to clot normally, led to the development of the partial thromboplastin time (PTT) test.[17] Although procedural modifications have since been made, this test is still one of the best available for evaluating the intrinsic coagulation system.

Separating the coagulation process into the extrinsic and intrinsic systems evolved from observations made in the laboratory.[3] The extrinsic system requires the addition of a tissue extract to the plasma to induce coagulation. Damaged tissue will stimulate the extrinsic system by releasing a lipoprotein substance commonly referred to as *tissue thromboplastin*. This lipoprotein, in conjunction with factor VII, activates factor X in the common pathway and leads to the production of a fibrin clot. The extrinsic and common pathways include factors I, II, V, VII, and X (Fig. 52-1).

The intrinsic system is stimulated by activating blood or plasma with negatively charged surfaces in the presence of phospholipid supplied by platelets or other reagents. The intrinsic and common pathways include all factors except VII and XIII. The intrinsic pathway is recognized to be the dominant one, with the extrinsic pathway having auxiliary status.[36] Figure 52-2 depicts the intrinsic and common pathways.

In this chapter, laboratory methodologies routinely used today will be discussed. The tests are grouped into two general categories: those measuring the intrinsic and common pathways of coagulation and those measuring the extrinsic and common pathways. The background of each test will be presented, along with a general discussion of the procedure. Reference ranges (see discussion below), interpretation of results, sources of error, and comments also will be presented.

REFERENCE RANGES

Although approximate reference ranges will be given for each of the tests discussed in this chapter, it must be stressed that reference ranges in hemostasis are significantly affected by patient populations, methodology, reagent systems, instrument systems, and combinations thereof. Consequently, every laboratory *must* establish its own reference ranges. This will involve the performance of 20 to 40 determinations on plasma from healthy volunteers in the same manner as patient samples are to be tested. Calculation of the mean and 95% confidence limits produces a reference range, which must be reevaluated any time changes are made in the method (*e.g.*, changes in reagents or instruments). Refer to Chapters 46 and 62 for further details on establishing reference ranges.

Intrinsic System

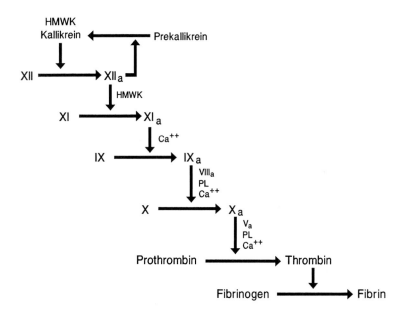

FIG. 52-2.   Intrinsic system of coagulation that is monitored by whole blood clotting time or partial thromboplastin time (either activated or nonactivated). HMWK, high-molecular-weight kininogen.

TESTS FOR THE INTRINSIC AND COMMON PATHWAYS

Lee and White Whole Blood Coagulation Time

With the development in the early 1900s of safe and easy ways to obtain blood by venipuncture, many variations on the whole blood coagulation time were tried. In 1913, Lee and White described a procedure for the whole blood coagulation time that was a modification of the numerous methods described in the literature at that time.[18] The L-W test is based on the fact that when venous blood is put into a glass tube (foreign surface), it will form a solid clot. The time required for this response is a measure of the overall intrinsic and common pathways of coagulation.

The L-W is insensitive to factor deficiencies, and moderate defects may be present in the face of normal results.[4] Only 1% to 2% of the normal level of factor VIII will result in a normal L-W clotting time when mixtures of normal and hemophiliac plasmas are tested. Technical errors, such as excessive agitation of the tube when checking for a clot, cause shortened times. Moreover, there is no suitable quality control measure for this procedure.[16] For these reasons, the L-W is no longer considered an adequate test.

Plasma Recalcification Time

A modification of the L-W is the recalcification time of plasma, using citrated plasma (instead of whole blood), $CaCl_2$, glass or siliconized tubes, and either platelet-rich plasma (PRP), platelet-poor plasma (PPP), or both.[14] This test is based on the fact that except for calcium, normal PRP contains all the components of the coagulation mechanism necessary for generating a fibrin clot. Removal of red cells makes the clot easier to see. The time required for blood to clot after Ca^{+2} is added is a general measure of the intrinsic and common pathways. By using a parallel test on PPP, screening for a platelet function defect may also be accomplished. Reference ranges for PRP and PPP are 100 to 150 seconds and 130 to 240 seconds, respectively. Platelet-rich plasma should clot at least 20 seconds faster than platelet-poor plasma.[9]

The principal disadvantages of the plasma recalcification time are the difficulty in standardizing the number of platelets in the PRP and the length of time necessary to perform the test, which moreover is insensitive to moderate factor deficiencies. In addition, errors in collection technique can significantly affect the results, as will the amount of glass contact. It is important that the same size tube always be used for testing and that the specimens be tilted uniformly. Because the procedure cannot be standardized, it is important to keep as many variables constant as possible. The sensitivity of this test is somewhat improved by diluting the plasma. This accomplishes three things: (1) it adjusts the PRP closer to the actual *in vivo* platelet count; (2) it increases the sensitivity of the test system to factor deficiencies; and (3) it dilutes the natural inhibitors to coagulation that are present. A normal control should be run with each test.

ACTIVATED CLOTTING TIME

By the mid 1960s, the lack of sensitivity and precision of the L-W and the plasma recalcification test had led researchers to look for better methods of monitoring heparin therapy (Chap. 57). Although by 1964, the PTT test was recognized to be sensitive to heparin, the test had not yet gained widespread acceptance as the heparin-monitoring procedure. Devising a new procedure based loosely on the L-W test, Dr. Paul Hattersley developed the activated clotting time (ACT) test.[6,7] The ACT uses diatomaceous earth (diatomite) as an activator of the contact factors and requires the blood to be kept warmed to a constant 37°C by taking a special incubator to the patient's bedside.

Principle

Whole blood contains all the components necessary to produce a clot when removed from the veins and put into a glass tube. By adding an activator and keeping the blood at a constant 37°C, a more reliable and rapid screen of the intrinsic and common pathways is achieved.

Reagents

Two evacuated tubes containing 12 mg of diatomite are needed.

Equipment

A portable heat block, thermometer, and two stopwatches are used.

Procedure

The two tubes containing diatomite are brought to 37°C in a heat block at the patient's bedside. Using good venipuncture technique, at least 2 mL of blood is drawn into a tube and discarded. The tourniquet is removed, and the first tube with diatomite is attached to the needle. When blood starts to flow into the tube, the first stopwatch is started. The tube is filled, mixed, and placed in the heat block. The procedure is repeated with the second tube, and the second stopwatch is started. After 60 seconds, the first tube is observed by tilting it at 5-second intervals until a clot is formed, at which time the second tube is observed using the same procedure. The appropriate stopwatch is stopped at the first appearance of a clot in each tube. The duplicates should agree within 10 seconds. The average time is reported.[6]

Reference Range

The reference range is 75 to 120 seconds. The target range during heparin therapy is 140 to 185 seconds.

Interpretation

Prolongation of the ACT is indicative of one or more factor defects in the intrinsic or common pathways or the presence of a circulating anticoagulant such as heparin.

Comments

Temperature control is critical: all testing must be maintained at 37°C. The primary use of the ACT is during extracorporeal circulation, where frequent testing and rapid turnaround time is required.[8] Other than the duplicate testing, there is no suitable method of quality control for this procedure.

PARTIAL THROMBOPLASTIN TIME

Several researchers observed that blood samples from classic hemophiliacs have a prolonged clotting time, but that when tissue thromboplastin is added, as in the PT, the plasma clots just as normal plasma does.[17] Expanded studies showed that thromboplastins, which are lipoproteins (protein + phospholipid), may be classified as complete or partial (only phospholipid). From these conclusions, investigators developed the nonactivated PTT. This test is more sensitive to abnormalities in the early stages than were previous tests of the intrinsic system. An important refinement of the PTT was the addition of negatively charged activators to the system, resulting in significantly shorter clotting times.[22] This modification is the activated partial thromboplastin time (APTT), the method now used exclusively. It is the test of choice to screen for factor deficiencies of the intrinsic and common pathways and also for monitoring heparin therapy. It also is the basis for assays of factors of the intrinsic system (see Fig. 52-2).

The APTT reagent consists of two components: a platelet substitute (phospholipid), prepared from brain or plant phospholipids, and an activator. Kaolin, Celite, micronized silica, or ellagic acid are used as the activator, depending on the manufacturer.

Principle

The APTT measures all factors except VII and XIII. Maximum activation of the contact factors is accomplished by addition of the activator. Phospholipid is supplied to substitute for platelet factor 3 (PF3). From this point, the APTT is essentially the same as a recalcification time of plasma.

Specimen Requirements

Citrated platelet-poor plasma should be collected according to the guidelines in Chapter 51.

Reagents

Phospholipid with activators (APTT reagent) and 0.025 M $CaCl_2$ (or as recommended by reagent manufacturer) are used.

Controls

Commercial lyophilized controls are available in normal, midrange, and extended ranges. It is recommended that a normal control and at least one abnormal control be used.[24] In-house preparations of pooled/frozen plasma may be used as controls. Each laboratory must specify when controls are to be tested, what the satisfactory control limits are, and, if duplicates are run, how closely the values should agree.

Equipment

For the manual method, 12 × 75-mm glass tubes, a heat block, and pipets are needed. For the fibrin strand method, an instrument for electromechanical fibrin strand detection and appropriate cups and pipets, as recommended by the manufacturer, are required. For the photo-optical method, the specialized instrument and appropriate accessories as listed by the manufacturer, are needed.

Procedure

Platelet-poor plasma (0.1 mL) is added to 0.1 mL of APTT reagent and incubated at 37°C for the period of time specified by the reagent manufacturer (approximately 3 to 5 minutes). After incubation, 0.1 mL of warmed $CaCl_2$ is added, and the time for clotting to occur is recorded.

Reporting

The APTT is reported in seconds, to the nearest tenth, along with the reference range.[24]

Reference Range

The ranges differ according to the reagent, method, and instrument used. The reference ranges may extend from a lower limit of 20 seconds to an upper limit of 45 seconds.

Interpretation

When properly performed, the APTT is an excellent screening test for the intrinsic and common coagulation pathways. A prolonged APTT in the absence of heparin use indicates a factor deficiency, an acquired circulating anticoagulant such as the lupus inhibitor, or an antibody to a specific factor such as factor VIII. Most commercial reagents will demonstrate a prolonged

APTT if any factor measured by the APTT is less than 40% to 50% of normal.

Comments

Sources of error in the APTT may be grouped into three categories: sample collection and preparation, reagent preparation, and instrumentation. Improper collection and processing of specimens may significantly affect the results. The anticoagulant volume should be adjusted for individuals with hematocrits greater than 0.55 L/L and less than 0.20 L/L to avoid error caused by an incorrect anticoagulant-to-plasma ratio (Chap. 51). Hemolysis may cause a falsely shortened APTT. Platelets in the plasma sample may cause erratic results or falsely shorten the APTT. Unexpected heparin contamination (e.g., from heparin locks) can spuriously lengthen the APTT.

Reagents may be affected by improper storage, water impurities, or incorrect dilution. Reagent systems should be tested for sensitivity to factor deficiencies by performing the APTT on serial dilutions of plasma.

A failing light source, fluctuations in temperature, loss of calibration of tubing, or contamination will cause instrument error. A good quality control program should reveal any instrumental or reagent-related error. Refer to Chapter 62 for a discussion of instruments and quality control.

TESTS FOR THE EXTRINSIC AND COMMON PATHWAYS

PROTHROMBIN TIME

Early experiments by the French physiologist de Bainville[1] showed that blood could be made to clot quickly by adding tissue factors. The discovery that oxalate and citrate inhibit coagulation[33] led to the assumption that clotting was dependent on calcium.

The one-stage PT, as described by Dr. Armand Quick in 1935, was believed to be an indirect measure of prothrombin in plasma, dependent on the presence of fibrinogen. Subsequent discoveries of factors V, VII, and X showed that the PT is a reflection of the activities of several factors.[30] Thus, the PT used in today's laboratory screens for deficiencies of factors I, II, V, VII, and X.

Although the PT is no longer considered a measure of prothrombin itself, it is still the test of choice for monitoring anticoagulant therapy by vitamin K antagonists (Chap. 57). Three of the five factors measured by the PT (II, VII, X) are sensitive to and depressed by these anticoagulants.[29] Only factor IX, the other factor depressed by vitamin K antagonists, is not detected by the PT.

Principle

When tissue extract or thromboplastin is added to PPP along with calcium, it reacts with factor VII_a to convert factor X to X_a. Factor X_a, along with factor V_a, phospholipid, and Ca^{+2} converts prothrombin to thrombin. Thrombin subsequently converts fibrinogen to fibrin (see Fig. 52-1). The time from the addition of thromboplastin/$CaCl_2$ to the formation of a clot is reported as the PT.[9]

Specimen Requirements

Citrated platelet-poor plasma is collected according to the guidelines in Chapter 51.

Reagents and Equipment

Thromboplastin/$CaCl_2$ (PT reagent) and controls (see discussion under APTT controls) are needed. The equipment is the same as that used for the APTT.

Procedure

Aliquots of control and patient plasma are warmed according to the method being used. The PT thromboplastin reagent is warmed by incubating it at 37°C for 3 to 5 minutes, and 0.2 mL of PT reagent is added to 0.1 mL of plasma (patient or control). The clotting time is recorded.

Reference Range

Normal values differ with the reagent and method. These values may range from 10 to 12 seconds in some photo-optical systems to 12 to 14 seconds with manual methods.

Reporting

Prothrombin times may be reported in several ways: (1) patient time (in seconds) with the reference range[24]; (2) patient time with the control time (in seconds); (3) prothrombin ratio (the PT of the patient divided by the mean of the reference range and multiplied by 100—rarely used in the United States); and (4) percent activity (outdated and not recommended). The use of an international normalized ratio (INR) has been proposed as the standard method of reporting. It is popular in Europe but not widely used in the United States (see Chap. 62).

Interpretation

Prolongation of the PT indicates an abnormality of one or more common or extrinsic coagulation factors. This abnormality may be hereditary or acquired. Prolongation may also occur with factor inhibitors. Using most commercial reagents, the PT is sensitive to factor deficiencies of less than 40% to 50% of normal.

Comments

Reporting of percent activity is no longer recommended because the dilution curve used to determine percent activity dilutes all factors, not just those affected by anticoagulant therapy, and is therefore an inaccurate representation of therapy. The preferred method of reporting in the US is patient PT along with the reference range. The British and Dutch have established standardized national systems for PT. They use a standardized reference reagent (e.g., the British Comparative Thromboplastin) and a national system of reporting PT results that have proved to be highly successful.[26,28,37] The sources of error in this test are similar to those discussed for the APTT.

Other Tests

Two other laboratory determinations related to the extrinsic and common pathways are the Stypven time and prothrombin–proconvertin time. Neither test has enjoyed widespread popularity, and they are rarely performed today. Therefore, they will be discussed in a historical sense only.

The Stypven time utilizes the powerful coagulant properties of Russell's viper venom, obtained from the snake *Vipera russelli*. This venom is capable of bypassing the action of factor VII and directly activating factor X to X_a. When it is combined with dilute thromboplastin, a fibrin clot will form through the reaction of factors X_a and V_a, phospholipid, factor II, and fibrinogen. In one of many modifications of Quick's original PT, Witts and Hobson believed the venom to be a convenient substitute for the thromboplastins used in the PT system. This substitution caused problems in managing patients on anticoagulant therapy, as the Stypven time produced shorter clotting times than did the PT and led to serious overdosing, with resultant bleeding. Because of the discrepancy, the Stypven

time was abandoned as unreliable. The discovery of factors VII[25] and X[34] explained the discrepancy between the Stypven time and the PT.[21] The Stypven time was reinstated, and until factor assays became more routine, it was used to help differentiate between factor VII and factor X deficiencies. Today, the Stypven time is ordered occasionally.

In 1951, Drs. Owren and Aas[27] developed the prothrombin and proconvertin (P & P) test based on earlier observations that minor deficiencies can be more pronounced when test plasma is diluted. Plasma is tested at 1:10 dilution,[13] and a reagent containing dilute thromboplastin extract from bovine brain, $CaCl_2$, and an excess of bovine factors V and I (fibrinogen) is used.[28] The addition of labile factor V made the test more sensitive to those factors in the extrinsic and common pathways that are affected by vitamin K antagonists (i.e., factors II, VII, and X). Owren later developed a freeze-dried, commercially available reagent (Thrombotest) based on the original P & P procedure. Its sensitivity was adjusted to give reliable determinations in the therapeutic range.[35] Thrombotest is most commonly used in the Netherlands and Scandinavia for monitoring vitamin K antagonist therapy. In this country, the P & P test was particularly favored at the time when sodium oxalate was used as an anticoagulant, as this material failed to hold factor V stable. Today, the test has little value as an overall screen for the extrinsic system because of its insensitivity to factor V and fibrinogen. Also, with the current use of sodium citrate as the anticoagulant of choice, the instability of factor V is no longer a great problem.

CHAPTER SUMMARY

In this chapter, the development of some of the procedures used routinely in coagulation testing was discussed. General procedures were described, along with reference ranges, the significance of abnormal results, and potential sources of error. Utilizing these procedures, general screening for basic coagulation abnormalities may be performed. In addition, many of these tests are suitable for monitoring anticoagulant therapy.

Quality control in the coagulation laboratory is imperative because of the numerous variables that affect test results. If not controlled, they can have adverse consequences for those patients being monitored on anticoagulant therapy. Chapter 62 discusses in detail quality control for the coagulation laboratory.

Two other procedures that have become routine coagulation tests in recent years were not discussed in this chapter: fibrinogen measurement and quantitation of fibrinogen/fibrin degradation products. These two procedures are covered in Chapters 53 and 54, respectively.

REFERENCES

1. de Bainville HMD: Injection de matière cérébrale dans les veines. Gaz Med Paris 2:524, 1834
2. Brandt J: Principles of Coagulation—1982. Symposium sponsored by General Diagnostics Corporation, Lexington, KY, 1982
3. Davie EW, Ratnoff OD: Waterfall sequence for intrinsic blood clotting. Science 145:1310, 1964
4. Giddings JC: Hereditary coagulation disorders: Laboratory techniques. In Thomson JM (ed): Blood Coagulation and Hae-

mostasis: A Practical Guide, 2nd ed, p 117. Edinburgh, Churchill Livingstone, 1980

5. Giddings JC: The investigation of hereditary coagulation disorders. In Thomson JM (ed): Blood Coagulation and Haemostasis: A Practical Guide, 2nd ed, p 48. Edinburgh, Churchill Livingstone, 1980

6. Hattersley P: Activated coagulation time of whole blood. JAMA 196:436, 1966

7. Hattersley P: Progress report: The activated coagulation time of whole blood (ACT). Am J Clin Pathol 66:899, 1976

8. Hill J: A simple method of heparin management during extracorporeal circulation. Ann Thorac Surg 17:129, 1974

9. Hougie C: Recalcification time test and its modifications (partial thromboplastin time, activated partial thromboplastin time and expanded partial thromboplastin time). In Williams WJ, Beutler E, Erslev A et al (ed): Hematology, 3rd ed, p 1662. New York, McGraw-Hill, 1983

10. Hougie C: One stage prothrombin time. In Williams WJ, Beutler E, Erslev AJ et al (eds): Hematology, 3rd ed, p 1665. New York, McGraw-Hill, 1983

11. Jackson CM, Nemerson Y: Blood coagulation. Annu Rev Biochem 49:765, 1980

12. Kahan J: Regional quality control of coagulation assay procedures. Thromb Diath Haemorrh 32:79, 1974

13. Keyser JW: Control of anticoagulant therapy by Thrombotest method. Br Med J 2:1514, 1963

14. Korsan-Bengsten K: Routine tests as measures of the total intrinsic blood clotting potential. Scand J Haematol 8:359, 1971

15. Korsan-Bengsten K: Comparison of Thrombotest and simplastin A (a modified P&P test) in the detection of prolonged clotting times of whole blood and plasma during anticoagulant therapy. Scand J Haematol 8:369, 1971

16. Langdell RD: Coagulation and hemostasis. In Davidsohn I, Henry JB (eds): Clinical Diagnosis by Laboratory Methods, 15th ed, p 414. New York, WB Saunders, 1974

17. Langdell RD, Wagner RH, Brinkhous KM: Effect of antihemophilic factor on one-stage clotting tests. J Lab Clin Med 41:637, 1953

18. Lee RI, White PD: A clinical study of the coagulation time of blood. Am J Med Sci 145:495, 1913

19. Loeliger EA: Reliability of laboratory tests for the control of oral anticoagulation. Thromb Diath Haemorrh 32:483, 1974

20. Loeliger EA, van den Besselaar AMHP: Introduction. In van den Besselaar AMHP, Gralnick HR, Lewis SM (eds): Thromboplastin Calibration and Oral Anticoagulant Control, p 1. The Hague, Martinus Nijhoff, 1984

21. MacFarlane RG: The theory of blood coagulation. In Biggs R (ed): Human Blood Coagulation, Haemostasis and Thrombosis, 2nd ed, p 1. Oxford, Blackwell Scientific, 1976

22. Marlar RA, Bayer PJ, Endres-Brooks JL et al: Comparison of the sensitivity of commercial APTT reagents in the detection of mild coagulopathies. Am J Clin Pathol 82:436, 1984

23. Morawitz P: Die Chemie der Blutgerinnung. Ergebn Physiol Biol Chem Exp Pharmakol 4:307, 1905

24. National Committee for Clinical Laboratory Standards (NCCLS): Tentative Guidelines for the Standardized Collection, Transport and Preparation of Blood Specimens for Coagulation testing and Performance of Coagulation Assays, vol 2, p 102. Villanova, PA, NCCLS, 1982

25. Owren PA: The prothrombin activating complex and its clinical significance. In Report of 3rd International Congress of Hematology, p 379. New York, Grune & Stratton, 1950

26. Owren PA: Standardization of thromboplastin reagents and control plasmas. Haematologia (Budapest) 8:441, 1974

27. Owren PA, Aas K: The control of Dicumarol therapy and the quantitative determination of prothrombin and proconvertin. Scand J Clin Lab Invest 3:201, 1951

28. Platt WR: Laboratory diagnosis of coagulation defects. In Color Atlas and Textbook of Hematology, p 222. Philadelphia, JB Lippincott, 1969

29. Poller L, Thomson JM, Alderson MR: The British system for anticoagulant control and Thrombotest. J Clin Pathol 24:143, 1971

30. Quick AJ, Hussey CV, Geppert M: Prothrombin: Analytical and clinical aspects. Comparison of the one- and two-stage methods. Am J Med Sci 1:517, 1963

31. Quick AJ, Stanley-Brown M, Bancroft W: Study of coagulation defects in hemophilia and jaundice. Am J Med Sci 190:501, 1935

32. Ratnoff OD, Saito H: Surface mediated reactions. Curr Top Hematol 2:1, 1979

33. Sabbatini L: Le calcium-ion dans le coagulation du sang. C R Soc Biol (Paris) 54:716, 1902

34. Telfer TP, Denson KWE, Wright DR: A "new" coagulation defect. Br J Haematol 2:308, 1956

35. Thomson JM: Laboratory control of anticoagulant therapy. In Thomson JM (ed): Blood Coagulation and Haemostasis: A Practical Guide, p 279. Oxford, Churchill Livingstone, 1980

36. Triplett DA: The extrinsic system. Clin Lab Med 4:221, 1984

37. van den Besselaar AMHP: Standardization of the prothrombin time in oral anticoagulant control. Haemostasis 15:271, 1985

53

Special Laboratory Evaluation of Coagulation

Janis Schaeffer Dixon
Kim A. Musgrave

This chapter continues the subject of laboratory assessments of coagulation. Whereas the previous chapter described routine tests for the extrinsic and intrinsic pathways, this chapter focuses on the more specialized procedures performed in the coagulation laboratory. The general principles of the methods are presented, followed by a discussion of the problems and pitfalls of specific assays. Older tests involving coagulation are presented from a historical perspective, whereas the more commonly used assays are discussed at some length, although space does not permit inclusion of all the details. Step-by-step procedures can be obtained from other texts or laboratory operating procedure manuals. The next chapter is devoted to those laboratory determinations related to evaluation of the dissolution of a clot (fibrinolysis).

TESTING METHODOLOGIES

Traditionally, coagulation studies have been performed using the detection of clot formation as an endpoint. In recent years, technologic advances have increased the scope of special coagulation testing. The development of monoclonal antibodies has made highly specific antisera available for immunologic testing, and synthetic substrates have made it possible to view coagulation from an enzymatic perspective. In addition, new instruments and methods have been developed to keep pace with the expanding knowledge of hemostasis.

Fibrin Endpoint

Fibrin endpoint methodologies depend on detection of a fibrin clot as it is formed through proteolytic cleavage of fibrinogen. Methods for clot detection commonly used are the manual tilt-tube techniques, electromechanical (fibrin strand), and optical density (turbidity). (See Chap. 62 for a detailed discussion of the instruments used in hemostasis.) Optical systems measure the rate of change of optical density, and thus the results are potentially more reproducible than those of manual or electromechanical methods. Coagulation times will differ significantly depending on the instrument, reagent, and instrument–reagent combination being used. Thus, it is imperative that each laboratory establish the reactivity of its reagent–instrument combination or system to the various factors and its own reference ranges for each determination.

Immunologic Methods

Immunologic assays are gaining importance because of the recent discovery that there are hereditary variants of coagulation proteins that have normal antigenic properties but lack functional activity. Such a protein is termed *crossreactive material* (CRM), and plasma containing such a protein is called CRM[+]. It is important to identify these variants in order to understand the pathophysiology of coagulation disorders.[49] Several immunologic techniques are available; the more commonly used procedures will be described very briefly below.[33,35,94] Refer to immunology tests for greater detail.

Ouchterlony Double Diffusion

The Ouchterlony technique is based on the principle that antigen and antibody specific to that antigen placed in separate wells cut in agar will diffuse toward each other in a radial manner and precipitate as immune complexes when they meet. The resultant precipitate can be seen as a transverse line (straight or curved) between the two wells. This method is not quantitative but will establish whether two antigens are serologically identical or different.

Radial Immunodiffusion

In radial immunodiffusion (RID) studies, specific antibody is incorporated into agar, and antigen is placed in wells cut in the agar. As the antigen diffuses, it precipitates with the antibody, forming a halo around the well. A linear relation exists between the square of the diameter of the ring and the concentration of antigen in the well.

Laurell Rocket Electrophoresis

Agarose containing antibody specific for the antigen to be measured is poured on a glass plate. Antigen is placed in wells cut on one side of the plate, and direct electric current is applied. As the antigen migrates and contacts antibody molecules, a rocket-shaped precipitate is formed (Fig. 53-1). The area of the rocket or, more commonly, the height is proportional to the antigen concentration.[14,57,58]

Crossed Immunoelectrophoresis

Crossed immunoelectrophoresis (CIE) is a two-dimensional method. In the first dimension, plasma is electrophoresed through plain agarose to separate the antigens. Agar containing antibody specific to the antigen being mea-

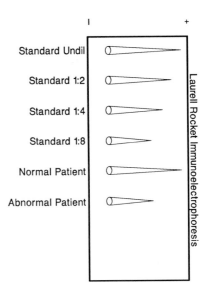

FIG. 53-1.   Laurell rocket electrophoresis. Height of "rocket" is proportional to antigen concentration.

sured is then poured on the plate, and a second electrophoresis is performed at right angles to the first. As the antigen-antibody complexes form, they create bell-shaped precipitin lines. Abnormalities can be detected by abnormal migration patterns or abnormally shaped precipitin areas (Fig. 53-2).

Radioimmunoassay

In a radioimmunoassay (RIA), a known concentration of radiolabeled antigen and an unknown concentration of antigen in a test sample compete for binding sites on a known amount of antibody. The bound antigen is separated from the free antigen, and the ratio of radioactivity associated with the bound antigen to the free antigen is determined.[98]

Enzyme-Linked Immunosorbent Assay

An enzyme-linked immunosorbent assay (ELISA) is an adaptation of the RIA. The antigen-specific antibody in this case is linked to an enzyme, and a substrate for that enzyme is then added. Color formed by cleavage of the substrate is read spectrophotometrically. The amount of color is directly proportional to the concentration of antigen being measured.[68,84]

Synthetic Substrates

Synthetic substrates are small peptide chains consisting of amino acid sequences that mimic the natural substrate of an enzyme. An indicator group, either a chromophore or a fluorophore, is attached to the synthetic substrate, which is cleaved by the enzyme for which the substrate has specificity (Chap. 62). Synthetic substrate assays allow coagulation testing to be approached as a series of enzymatic reactions in an accurate and sensitive manner. A sound knowledge of enzyme kinetics is necessary for optimal use of synthetic substrate assays. Endpoint or initial rate analysis may be performed, and many assays have been adapted for use on automated instrumentation.[32,40]

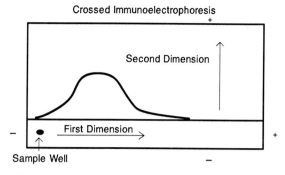

Crossed Immunoelectrophoresis

Second Dimension

First Dimension

Sample Well

FIG. 53-2.   Precipitin lines formed during crossed immuno-electrophoresis.

INDIRECT TESTS FOR COAGULATION PROTEINS OR SYSTEMS

Early Tests for Coagulation Abnormalities

The *two-stage prothrombin time*[95,96] is of historic interest, as it was the first method to measure the prothrombin concentration indirectly in plasma.[13,83] Test plasma is defibrinated by the addition of thrombin. After the clot is removed, all prothrombin in the plasma is converted to thrombin by adding thromboplastin, calcium, and a source of factors V, VII, and X. The thrombin formed is then measured by adding aliquots of the activation mixture to standard fibrinogen solutions and recording the clotting time. The results are expressed in prothrombin units/mL of plasma. This test is rarely used today, as it has been replaced by other methods such as factor assays for prothrombin.

The *prothrombin consumption test* is a prothrombin time study performed on serum from blood that has been allowed to clot for 60 minutes.[72] Severe deficiencies of factors V, VIII, IX, X, XI, or XII, as well as platelet deficiencies or abnormalities, will slow the rate of prothrombin conversion,[87] thus leaving significant amounts of prothrombin in the serum. The prothrombin consumption time will be short in such cases. The test is unique in that normal serum will have a long time (usually greater than 20–25 seconds).

This test has largely been replaced by more sensitive and specific assays.

The *thromboplastin generation test* (TGT) was based on the observation that barium sulfate or aluminum hydroxide will adsorb to certain coagulation factors. If $BaSO_4$ or $Al(OH)_3$ is added to normal plasma, factors II, VII, IX, and X will be adsorbed and thus can be removed by centrifugation. Likewise, if blood is allowed to clot, the remaining serum will not contain fibrinogen, factor II, the labile factors V and VIII, or XIII. Therefore, if normal adsorbed plasma, normal serum, platelets, and $CaCl_2$ are mixed, the mixture cannot form a clot until prothrombin (factor II) is supplied by the addition of normal plasma. The assay was devised to identify deficiencies of specific factors.[5] The TGT is labor intensive and takes a significant amount of time to perform. It is not a popular test in most hemostasis laboratories today.

However, the TGT reagents (*i.e.,* normal adsorbed plasma and normal serum) can be used in either the PT or the APTT systems (sometimes referred to as mixing studies or substitution studies). For example, if the patient has a normal PT and prolonged APTT, factors I, II, V, VII, and X are assumed to be normal. If the patient's APTT is corrected by addition of normal adsorbed plasma (containing factors I, V, VIII, XI, XII, and XIII) but not by addition of normal serum, factor VIII is presumed to be abnormal. If the patient's APTT is corrected by normal serum (containing factors IV, VII, IX, X, XI, and XII) but not by adsorbed plasma, factor IX probably is abnormal. The third possibility is for both serum and adsorbed plasma to correct the APTT. In this case, factors XI or XII may be abnormal. See Table 53-1 for a summary of the use of substitution studies in conjunction with other coagulation determinations to define factor deficiencies.

THROMBIN CLOTTING TIME
Principle

Addition of thrombin to plasma bypasses all coagulation reactions except polymerization of fibrinogen. The thrombin clotting time measures the conversion of fibrinogen to fibrin and is not influenced by deficiencies of the other coagulation factors.[54] Dysfibrinogenemia, hypofibrinogenemia, fibrin split products,

TABLE 53–1. Use of Substitution Studies in Conjunction with PT, APTT, and Thrombin Time to Define Factor Defects

DEFICIENCY	PT*	APTT†	THROMBIN TIME‡	SUBSTITUTION STUDIES		
				NORMAL PLASMA**	ADSORBED PLASMA‖	AGED SERUM¶
I	Abn	Abn	Abn	C	C	NC
II	Abn	Abn	Nor	C	NC	NC
V	Abn	Abn	Nor	C	C	NC
VII	Abn	Nor	Nor	C	NC	C
VIII	Nor	Abn	Nor	C	C	NC
IX	Nor	Abn	Nor	C	NC	C
X	Abn	Abn	Nor	C	NC	C
XI or XII	Nor	Abn	Nor	C	C	C
Heparin	Abn	Abn	Abn	NC	NC	NC

* Screens extrinsic pathway (I, II, V, VII, and X).
† Screens intrinsic pathway (I, II, V, VIII, IX, X, XI, and XII).
‡ Identifies presence of heparin and fibrinogen abnormalities.
** Contains all factors.
‖ Contains I, V, VIII, XI, XII, and XIII.
¶ Contains VII, IX, X, XI, and XII.
Abn = abnormal, Nor = normal, C = corrected, NC = not corrected.

immunologic antithrombins, and the presence of abnormal globulins will prolong the thrombin clotting time. The thrombin clotting time also is prolonged by heparin and may be used to monitor heparin therapy.[48,71,73]

Procedure

A standardized thrombin solution is added to citrated platelet-poor plasma. The clotting time is a measure of the rate of conversion of fibrinogen to fibrin.

Comments

Platelets contain platelet factor 4, which is a heparin-neutralizing substance. Therefore, the specimen must be obtained and handled carefully to avoid platelet disruption. The plasma tested must be platelet free.

Thrombin times should not be performed on heparinized plasma samples that have been frozen.[71]

Thrombin is highly unstable. To preserve its activity, it is diluted to 100 NIH units/mL with a solution of equal parts 0.15 M NaCl and glycerol. Aliquots are then frozen. Just prior to use, an aliquot of the stock thrombin is thawed and diluted with 0.15 M NaCl to give a control value established by each laboratory. Thrombin activity decreases after 20 minutes at 37°C.

Protamine can be added to determine if the thrombin time is prolonged because of heparin or other antithrombin activity, as protamine neutralizes heparin.[71]

Some procedures utilize a thrombin–$CaCl_2$ reagent.[54] Calcium ions enhance the rate of polymerization of fibrin monomers.[54]

Plastic or siliconized glass should be used to pipet thrombin, as it will adhere to glass surfaces.[13]

A normal control sample must be run. Control and patient plasmas are tested in duplicate (duplicates should agree within 1.5–2.0 seconds). Each laboratory must establish its own control values based on the type of thrombin, reagents, and equipment used.

Reference Ranges

Depending on the thrombin concentration selected, reported reference ranges are 8 to 9 seconds,[71] 15 to 20 seconds,[13] less than 24 seconds,[91] and 20 to 25 seconds.[73]

REPTILASE TIME
Principle

Reptilase is a thrombinlike enzyme isolated from the reptile *Bothrops atrox*. Reptilase cleaves fibrinopeptides from the alpha chain of fibrinogen, whereas thrombin releases fibrinopeptides from both the alpha and the beta chains. Fibrin monomers formed by the action of Reptilase polymerize only end to end, whereas monomers formed by thrombin polymerize both side to side and end to end. The Reptilase time is not influenced by heparin or immunologic antithrombins. Fibrin(ogen) split products will prolong the Reptilase time to a lesser degree than the thrombin time, whereas dysfibrinogenemia will more greatly affect the Reptilase time. Therefore, if both the Reptilase and the thrombin time tests are performed, the cause of the

prolonged thrombin time can be identified more easily[34] (Table 53-2).

Procedure

Reptilase is added to citrated platelet-poor plasma. The time necessary for clot formation is proportional to the amount and quality of fibrinogen present.

Comments

Platelet-poor plasma is required because, like thrombin, Reptilase is capable of aggregating platelets. If thrombin is present in the specimen, it may interfere with Reptilase. This problem can be eliminated by adding heparin, which will inhibit thrombin but not Reptilase.

After reconstitution with water Reptilase is stable for 6 hours at 37°C and for 5 days at 4°C.

Clotting may be observed with either manual or automated techniques.

A normal plasma control is run in the same manner as the test plasma. Reptilase times should be determined in duplicate for each specimen.

Reference Range

The reference range is approximately 18 to 20 seconds.

Fibrinogen

Many methods for the measurement of fibrinogen have been described. Five are most commonly performed.

1. Precipitation or denaturation methods,[36,45,86] in which heat, salt, or another agent is used to denature fibrinogen to an insoluble state. The suspended fibrinogen precipitate may be measured turbidimetrically, or the precipitated fibrinogen may be isolated and measured by colorimetric or ultraviolet protein quantitation. These methods generally are semiquantitative and are subject to many technical problems.

2. Turbidimetric or fibrin clot density procedures[24] are based on photo-optical measurement of the change in turbidity of plasma as fibrinogen is converted to fibrin by thrombin. The kinetics of this conversion have been used to measure the fibrinogen concentration.[46] Turbidimetric procedures are the basis for some automated fibrinogen methods that have been introduced.[88,99] Modifications of the original procedure have improved sensitivity at lower fibrinogen levels and have eliminated heparin interference.[80,81,88]

3. Coagulable protein assays are performed by clotting the plasma sample using thrombin or $CaCl_2$, isolating the fibrin clot, and then measuring the fibrin by weight, chemically, or by ultraviolet absorbance.[45,74,86] Ancrod, a thrombinlike enzyme that is specific for fibrinogen and not influenced by heparin, also has been used to clot

TABLE 53–2. Comparison of Thrombin Times and Reptilase Times in Various Conditions

	THROMBIN TIME	REPTILASE TIME
HEPARIN THERAPY	Prolonged	Normal
FIBRIN SPLIT PRODUCTS	Greatly prolonged	Prolonged
HYPOFIBRINOGENEMIA	Prolonged	Prolonged
DYSFIBRINOGENEMIA	Prolonged	Greatly prolonged
IMMUNOLOGIC ANTITHROMBINS	Prolonged	Normal

plasma.[28] The coagulable protein assay is considered the reference procedure for fibrinogen measurement. The principal disadvantage of this type of assay is the time required to perform the test.[86]

4. Immunologic assays utilize antibodies to fibrinogen in assays such as radial immunodiffusion,[12,16] kinetic latex agglutinometry,[2] measurement of turbidity,[28] or rocket immunoelectrophoresis. Immunologic assays are time consuming and also measure fibrin(ogen) degradation products. Because immunologic assays measure dysfunctional as well as functional fibrinogen, performing an immunologic fibrinogen assay along with a functional fibrinogen assay is a useful tool in diagnosing dysfibrinogenemia.

5. The modified thrombin time fibrinogen determination is the most widely performed clinical fibrinogen assay[51] and is discussed below. This assay was first described by Clauss in 1957.[18] The clotting time of diluted plasma to which a high concentration of thrombin has been added is inversely proportional to the fibrinogen concentration. This procedure is relatively insensitive to heparin and fibrin(ogen) degradation products.[47,62,86] A thrombokinetic procedure in which the maximal rate of change in optical density is measured during the modified thrombin time has been described.[63]

It is vital to realize that there may be discrepancies in the fibrinogen concentration as measured by the various methods described above on the same specimen. A dysfibrinogenemia will generally result in a low fibrinogen level as measured by the modified thrombin clotting time,[8] whereas immunologic techniques (or other techniques that do not depend on the formation of a clot) will yield normal or above normal results in such specimens.

MODIFIED THROMBIN CLOTTING TIME ASSAY FOR FIBRINOGEN
Procedure

A high concentration of thrombin is added to diluted, citrated, platelet-poor plasma to convert fibrinogen to fibrin. The clotting time is inversely proportional to the fibrinogen concentration. Quantitation is achieved through the use of standards with known concentrations of fibrinogen.

Comments

Improper specimen collection with the wrong blood:anticoagulant ratio or lack of correction of citrate volume for a low or high hematocrit may cause erroneous results.

A higher dilution of the test plasma must be made if the clotting time is too short. A lesser dilution of plasma is necessary for very long clotting times: however, less than a 1:3 dilution should not be tested. Appropriate dilution factors must be used in calculating results.

Fibrinogen degradation products at a concentration of greater than 100 μg/mL may affect the thrombin clotting time. High levels of the larger degradation products may interfere at lower concentrations.

Heparin concentrations greater than 1 U/mL may result in falsely low fibrinogen concentration measurements. Care must be taken to avoid obtaining specimens through heparinized lines.

If the patient is receiving fibrinolytic therapy, either epsilon aminocaproic acid (EACA) or soybean trypsin inhibitor should be added to the collection tube to prevent *in vitro* clot lysis.

Hemolysis or lipemia may interfere with photo-optical measurements.

Manual, semiautomated, or automated endpoint detection devices may be used, but each will result in a different endpoint.

The thrombin reagent (100 NIH units/mL) is unstable. (See comments under Thrombin Time.)

Known normal and abnormal controls should be run every 20 samples or every shift. Duplicates should agree within 0.5 seconds. A new standard curve must be established for each new lot of reagents. Only the linear portion of the calibration curve should be used to interpret plasma fibrinogen levels.

Reference Range
Each laboratory must establish its own reference range. The range should be approximately 170 to 410 mg/dL.

INHIBITOR STUDIES

SCREENING TESTS
Principle
Coagulation testing abnormalities may be caused by either a factor deficiency or an inhibitor. The inhibitor's action may be confined to a specific factor (*e.g.*, factor VIII inhibitor); it may be nonspecific (*e.g.*, lupus anticoagulant); or it may be global, affecting several factors simultaneously (*e.g.*, heparin). Correction studies with normal plasma are performed to differentiate a factor deficiency from an inhibitor (Table 53-3).

Procedure
Patient plasma is mixed with normal plasma, which will correct the abnormality caused by a factor deficiency, whereas if the abnormality is secondary to the presence of an inhibitor, the abnormality will not be corrected.[23,75] Testing is performed both immediately on mixing and after incubation for 2 hours at 37°C. Testing after incubation will reveal the time and temperature dependency of the inhibitor.

Comments
A citrated blood specimen is centrifuged immediately to prevent interference from platelets.

Normal plasma is preferably obtained from a normal plasma pool, although it may be obtained by drawing blood from a healthy donor. This plasma is treated in the same manner as the patient specimen.

Depending on the system to be tested, prothrombin time (PT) or activated partial thromboplastin time (APTT) reagents will be necessary (Chap. 52).

Fresh pooled normal plasma mixed 1:1 with Owren's Veronal buffer is used as the control and is incubated at 37°C in the same manner as the patient specimen. Additional controls may include undiluted patient plasma and undiluted pooled normal plasma that are treated in the same way as the patient mixture.

The interpretation of this test is based on the correction, if any, of the abnormal test time (see Table 53-3). If the abnormality is attributable to a factor deficiency, the addition of one part normal plasma will correct the abnormal test time close to the normal range. If the abnormality is secondary to an immediate-acting inhibitor (*e.g.*, factor IX inhibitor, heparin), the addition of normal plasma will not correct the abnormal test time. If, however, the inhibitor is time or temperature dependent (*e.g.*, factor VIII inhibitor) an immediate correction will be noted, but on incubation, the test time will become prolonged if the inhibitor titer is high enough. Lupus anticoagulants generally are immediate acting but may be time dependent.[92] Equivocal results may be obtained in borderline or mild abnormalities.[59]

If an inhibitor is indicated, a more sensitive and specific test should be performed to identify and quantify it.

TABLE 53–3. Interpretation in Correction Studies Using Normal Plasma

	IMMEDIATE TESTING	TESTING AFTER 2-HOUR INCUBATION AT 37°C
FACTOR DEFICIENCY	Correction	Correction
INHIBITOR	No correction	No correction
Immediate-acting (*e.g.*, heparin, factor IX inhibitor, most lupus anticoagulants)		
Time-dependent (*e.g.*, factor VIII inhibitor)	Correction	No correction

Reference Range

Depending on the total test system used, the reference range for the PT or APTT will differ. Each laboratory must establish its own reference range.

INHIBITOR IDENTIFICATION AND QUANTITATION

A special type of circulating anticoagulant or inhibitor, the lupus anticoagulant, is generally identified in the laboratory through the tissue thromboplastin inhibition test, the platelet neutralization procedure, or the agarose plasma gel technique. On the other hand, specific factor inhibitors, such as factor VIII inhibitor, may be quantitated by the agarose inhibitor plasma gel technique or, more commonly, the Bethesda inhibitor assay.

Tissue Thromboplastin Inhibition Test

The tissue thromboplastin inhibition test (TTI) is a modified clotting test.[82] Citrated plasma is incubated at 37°C with dilute thromboplastin, $CaCl_2$ is added, and the clotting time is measured. The results are expressed as a ratio of the clotting time (in seconds) of the patient sample to that of the control sample. The TTI is considered normal if this ratio is 1:1 or less; borderline if 1:2 to 1:3; and abnormal if it is greater than 1:3. Despite its popularity, the TTI is neither sensitive nor specific.[93]

Platelet Neutralization Procedure

In the platelet neutralization procedure, freeze-thawed platelets are added to the test plasma, and an APTT is performed. The platelets serve as an additional source of phospholipid and "neutralize" lupus anticoagulant. A significant shortening of the abnormal APTT is indicative of lupus anticoagulant.[93]

Agarose Plasma Gel Technique

Agarose containing fresh normal plasma is poured on a plate. Patient and control plasmas are placed in wells cut into the agar and allowed to diffuse into the gel. After incubation, the plate is flooded with $CaCl_2$ solution. The agarose will turn cloudy or opaque as fibrin is formed in the agarose. In the presence of an inhibitor, a clear area or zone of inhibition will be seen surrounding the well containing that plasma.[7,90]

Bethesda Inhibitor Assay

Factor VIII inhibitor can be quantitated by mixing test plasma with a known amount of factor VIII and incubating the mixture for 2 hours at 37°C. After incubation, the amount of residual factor VIII is measured by specific factor assay. By comparing the factor VIII activity in the patient incubation mixture with that in the control mixture, the amount of inhibitor present in the former can be calculated. The result is expressed in Bethesda units; one Bethesda unit of inhibitor is defined as the amount that will inactivate 50% of the factor VIII activity present.[50]

FACTOR ASSAYS

Currently, a variety of methods are in use for the measurement of factor activity, including one-stage clotting methods,[38,53] two-stage clotting methods,[6] fluorometric methods,[61] and colorimetric methods.[27,85] The fluorometric and colorimetric methodologies are based on the principles that govern synthetic substrates. The one-stage clotting method is widely used because of its simplicity.[4]

ONE-STAGE CLOTTING ASSAYS
Principle

One-stage factor assays are based on a simple modification of the PT or APTT. Assays for factors II, V, VII, and X generally are based on the PT, whereas assays for factors VIII, IX, XI, and XII are based on the APTT.

Procedure

The clotting time of a substrate plasma known to be deficient in the factor to be assayed is shortened or "corrected" by adding diluted factor-containing plasma. By using various dilutions of a known normal plasma or standard, a curve is constructed (Fig. 53–3). Unknown sample values are derived by using an appropriate dilution and converting the clotting time to factor activity from the standard curve.

Comments

Because of the length of this procedure, the citrated platelet-poor plasma obtained from the patient and subsequent dilutions should be kept on slush ice. Plasma should be tested within 1 to 2 hours and dilutions within 30 minutes. Frozen plasma may be used provided the standard liquid reference plasma has likewise been frozen.

Normal reference plasma and factor-deficient plasma may be obtained commercially in lyophilized form. Care should be taken to ensure the accuracy of the stated values.

Known controls should be run simultaneously with the unknown samples. Other quality control measures should parallel those used in PT or APTT testing.

Only the linear portion of the calibration curve should be used. The curve may become flat at the most extreme dilutions if sensitivity is lost. Only a high-quality standard with an accurate value and a high-quality substrate should be used. The following is an example of the calculations for normal and abnormal plasmas using the curve shown in Figure 53-3.

	DILUTION	CLOTTING TIME (SECONDS)	% ACTIVITY FROM CURVE	% ACTIVITY CORRECTED FOR DILUTION*
Normal subject	1:10	46	74	74
	1:20	52.5	37	74
Factor-deficient patient	1:10	68	10	10
	1:20	78	5	10

* Assume 1:10 dilution defines 100% of normal factor assay.

Reference Range

The reference range for most factors is 50% to 150% of normal activity.

Factor VIII Immunologic Assays

In addition to the functional factor assays discussed above, immunologic methods have been developed. Perhaps the coagulation protein most widely studied using immunologic methods is factor VIII-related antigen (factor VIII R:Ag). The methodologies employed in quantitative immunologic assay of this factor include the Laurell rocket technique or rocket electroimmunodiffusion (EID),[57,100] the immunoradiometric assay (IRMA),[21,70,77] and the ELISA.[84] Crossed immunoelectrophoresis and SDS-polyacrylamide gel methods[44,76] are used to characterize qualitative abnormalities of the molecule. The Laurell rocket technique is the most convenient and popular method for the routine laboratory.[10]

RISTOCETIN COFACTOR

In addition to determining the antigenic level of factor VIII R:Ag, it is highly recommended that the functional properties of the von Willebrand factor (vW factor, VIII/vWF, VIII:vWF, VIIR:RCo, ristocetin cofactor) be assayed.

Ristocetin was originally introduced as an antibiotic but was taken from the market because it can cause thrombocytopenia. In the test tube, it will agglutinate platelets in normal platelet-rich plasma.[9] It was subsequently discovered that factor VIII protein is able to bind ristocetin and platelet membranes, causing the platelets to agglutinate. This substance has been called various names, including ristocetin cofactor. In cases of von Willebrand's disease, which is secondary to a deficiency of this cofactor, ristocetin will not agglutinate platelets.[42,43]

Principle

Agglutination of fixed platelets in response to ristocetin depends on the presence of von Willebrand factor in plasma.

Procedure

Plasma dilutions and ristocetin are added to normal fixed platelets, and the rate of agglutination is observed using an aggregometer (Chap. 62). Test plasma and normal standard plasma are treated similarly. A standard curve of the percent of von Willebrand factor versus either the slope or the percent of agglutination is constructed. Patient samples are compared with the standard curve, and percentages of von Willebrand factor are calculated.

Comments

The normal platelet reagent consists of platelets fixed in formalin or paraformaldehyde and must be examined to be sure it is free of clumps before the test. Once reconstituted, formalin-fixed platelets are stable for only a while; generally, they should not be used after 24 hours. Commercial preparations are easier to use and give consistent results.

Citrated platelet-poor normal plasma or a plasma standard with a known value is used in the construction of a standard curve. Known controls are run simultaneously with the unknown samples, and all testing should be done in duplicate.

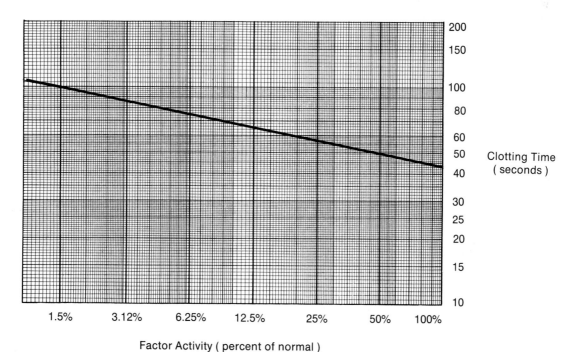

FIG. 53-3. Sample factor activity curve based on dilutions of normal or standard plasma.

Reference Range

The reference range is approximately 50% to 150% of normal activity.

FACTOR XIII

Factor XIII is known as the fibrin-stabilizing factor. It is a transglutaminase that is activated by thrombin in the presence of Ca^{+2} and is essential for the formation of covalent crosslinking between adjacent fibrin monomers to form a stable clot.

Principle

In the presence of activated factor XIII, the fibrin clot that forms is insoluble in urea[52] or monochloroacetic acid.[65]

Procedure

Test plasma is clotted. The clot is immersed in 5 M urea and observed to see if it is dissolved or remains intact.

Comments

A normal control should be run simultaneously with the unknown sample. In addition, a control tube containing both a normal clot and the test clot in 5 M urea should be observed. The normal clot should contain sufficient factor XIII to keep the test clot from dissolving regardless of its factor XIII level. If the clot dissolves in this tube, the presence of abnormal fibrinolytic activity should be investigated.

This procedure should be considered a screening test for the almost total absence of factor XIII, because levels as low as 1% to 2% are adequate for hemostasis and will result in a normal test. To detect individuals with less than 50% but more than 2% activity, immunologic methods are necessary. These include immunoelectrophoresis to measure factor XIII subunit A and S levels[3] or SDS polyacrylamide gel electrophoresis.[97]

Reference Range

In the presence of factor XIII_a, the clot should remain insoluble for 24 hours at 37°C.

Fletcher Factor

Fletcher factor (prekallikrein) participates in the contact phase of the intrinsic system (see Fig. 52-2) and was first described by Hathaway and associates in 1965.[39] Laboratory detection of prekallikrein deficiency is initially made by a simple screening test in which the prolonged APTT is corrected by additional incubation with an activator such as Celite or kaolin.[39] Partial thromboplastins containing ellagic acid as an activator *do not* usually detect this deficiency.[25] Fletcher factor deficiency is confirmed by a quantitative assay using a modified APTT technique and factor-deficient substrate or a synthetic substrate.[29]

REGULATORY PROTEINS

Antithrombin III

Antithrombin III (AT-III), which together with heparin will inactivate many activated serine proteases, may be assayed by either immunologic or functional methods. Immunologic assays commonly used include RIA,[15] RID,[60] and Laurell rocket immunoelectrophoresis.[57] Immunologic methods do not distinguish free-circulating AT-III from that which is complexed and inactive. The results are expressed in milligrams per deciliter. Normal plasma contains between 20 and 50 mg/dL of AT-III, depending on the assay.

Functional assays for AT-III activity may be performed by a clotting technique[17] or by employing synthetic substrates.[1,66] Functional assays are based on the fact that AT-III inhibits activated serine proteases. Exogenous heparin is added to the plasma to accelerate the action of AT-III. Thrombin or factor X_a is added in excess to the plasma. The amount of thrombin or factor X_a not inactivated by AT-III is quantitated by a clotting time or color formation (spectrophotometric). Functional values are expressed as a percentage of normal. Reference values should be established by each laboratory but should lie between 80% and 120% of normal activity.

Protein C

Protein C plays a role in the fibrinolytic and coagulation systems as a regulatory protein and may be assayed immunologically and functionally. Immunologic methods for protein C involve the Laurell rocket immunoelectrophoresis technique,[37] RIA techniques,[26] or ELISA methodology.[11] Normal plasma contains approximately 3 to 4 µg of protein C per milliliter.

Only recently have functional assays become available.[19,31,67,79] A relatively simple automated clot-based method for assaying the functional activity of protein C has been described by Odegard and associates.[67]

Protein S

Protein S, which functions as a cofactor for activated protein C, may likewise be measured immunologically or functionally. Protein S determinations are complicated by the fact that it circulates both as a free protein and in a reversible complex with C4b-binding protein.[22] Protein S levels have been measured by Laurell rocket immunoelectrophoresis.[19] The reference level is approximately 1 µg/mL. Functional assays have recently been developed and are based on the ability of protein S to serve as a cofactor for the anticoagulant effects of activated protein C.[20]

CHAPTER SUMMARY

This chapter has focused on specialized procedures performed in the coagulation laboratory that play a vital role in the assessment of the patient with a bleeding disorder. The methodologies employed by these tests are diverse. The intent has been to describe the principles of the methods and to comment on potential problems.

REFERENCES

1. Abildgaard U, Lie M, Odegard OR: Antithrombin (heparin cofactor) assay with "new" chromogenic substrates (S-2238 and Chromozym TH). Thromb Res 11:549, 1977
2. Babson AL, Opper CA, Crane LJ: Kinetic latex agglutinometry I: A rapid quantitative immunologic assay for fibrinogen. Am J Clin Pathol 77:424, 1982
3. Barbui T, Rodeghiero F, Dini E et al: Subunits A and S inheritance in four families with congenital factor XIII deficiency. Br J Haematol 38:267, 1978

4. Barrowcliffe TW, Ingram GIC, Kirkwood TBL et al: A survey of VIII:C assays in the United Kingdom. Clin Lab Haematol 3:186, 1981

5. Biggs R, Douglas AS: The thromboplastin generation test. J Clin Pathol 6:23, 1953

6. Biggs R, Eveling J, Richards G: The assay of antihaemophilic-globulin activity. Br J Haematol 1:20, 1955

7. Bird P: Coagulation in an agarose gel and its application to the detection and measurement of factor VIII antibodies. Br J Haematol 29:329, 1975

8. Bithell TC: Hereditary dysfibrinogenemia. Clin Chem 31:509, 1985

9. Bouma BN, Wiegerinck Y, Sixma JJ et al: Immunological characterization of purified anti-haemophilic factor A (factor VIII) which corrects abnormal platelet retention in von Willebrand's disease. Nature 236:104, 1972

10. Bowie EJW, Owen CA: Abnormalities of factor VIII. In Triplett DA (ed): Laboratory Evaluation of Coagulation, p 115. Chicago, American Society of Clinical Pathologists, 1982

11. Boyer C, Rothschild C, Wolf M et al: A new method for the estimation of protein C by ELISA. Thromb Res 36:579, 1984

12. Brittin GM, Rafinia H, Raval D et al: Evaluation of single radial immunodiffusion for quantitation of plasma fibrinogen. Am J Clin Pathol 57:89, 1972

13. Brown B: Hematology: Principles and Procedures, 4th ed, p 202. Philadelphia, Lea & Febiger, 1984

14. Cann JR: A phenomenological theory of rocket and crossed immunoelectrophoresis. Immunochemistry 12:473, 1975

15. Chan V, Chan TK, Wong V et al: The determination of antithrombin III by radioimmunoassay and its clinical application. Br J Haematol 41:563, 1979

16. Chen T, Lai CH: Fibrinogen assay by an immunodiffusion plate. Tech Bull Reg Med Technol 39(10):231, 1969

17. Chockly M, Penner J: An improved clinical assay for antithrombin III (heparin cofactor). Am J Clin Pathol 74:213, 1980

18. Clauss A: Gerinnungsphysiologische Schnellmethode zur Bestimmung des Fibrinogens. Acta Haematol (Basel) 17:237, 1957

19. Comp PC, Nixon RR, Cooper MR et al: Familial protein S deficiency is associated with recurrent thrombosis. J Clin Invest 74:2082, 1984

20. Comp PC, Nixon RR, Esmon CT: Determination of functional levels of protein C, an antithrombic protein, using thrombin-thrombomodulin complex. Blood 63:15, 1984

21. Counts RB: A solid-phase immunoradiometric assay of factor VIII protein. Br J Haematol 31:429, 1975

22. Dahlback B, Stenflow J: High molecular weight complex in human plasma between vitamin K-dependent protein S and complement component C4-binding protein. Proc Natl Acad Sci USA 78:2512, 1981

23. Deutsch E, Lechner K: Circulating anticoagulants. In Bang NU, Beller FK, Deutsch E et al (eds): Thrombosis and Bleeding Disorders: Theory and Methods, p 286. New York, Academic Press, 1971

24. Ellis BC, Stransky A: A quick and accurate method for the determination of fibrinogen in plasma. J Lab Clin Med 58:477, 1961

25. Entes K, LaDuca FM, Tourbaf KD: Fletcher factor deficiency, source of variations of the activated partial thromboplastin time test. Am J Clin Pathol 75:626, 1981

26. Epstein DJ, Bergum PW, Bajaj SP et al: Radioimmunoassays for protein C and factor X. Am J Clin Pathol 82:573, 1984

27. Eriksson E, Rosen S, Knos M et al: Chromogenic substrate methods for the determination of factor VIII C, endotoxin and plasminogen activator. Thromb Haemost 46:315, 1981 (abstr)

28. Exner T, Burridge J, Power P et al: An evaluation of currently available methods for plasma fibrinogen. Am J Clin Pathol 71:521, 1979

29. Fisher CA, Schmaier AH, Addonizio VP et al: Assay of prekallikrein in human plasma: Comparison of amidolytic, esterolytic, coagulation, and immunochemical assays. Blood 59:963, 1982

30. Forbes CD, Douglas AS: Thrombin and thromboplastin generation techniques. In Bang NU, Beller FK, Deutsch E et al (eds): Thrombosis and Bleeding Disorders: Theory and Methods, p 82. New York, Academic Press, 1971

31. Francis RB, Patch MJ: A functional assay for protein C in human plasma. Thromb Res 32:605, 1983

32. Friberger P: Chromogenic peptide substrates: Their use for the assay of factors in the fibrinolytic and plasma kallikrein-kinin systems. Scand J Clin Lab Invest 42(suppl 162), 1982

33. Fudenberg HH, Stites DP, Caldwell JL et al (eds): Basic and Clinical Immunology, 2nd ed, p 337. Los Altos, CA, Lange Medical Publications, 1978

34. Funk C, Gmur J, Herold R et al: Reptilase-R: A new reagent in blood coagulation. Br J Haematol 21:43, 1971

35. Garvey JS, Cremer NE, Sussdorf DH (eds): Methods in Immunology: A Laboratory Text for Instruction and Research, 3rd ed p 301. Reading, MA, WA Benjamin, 1977

36. Goodwin JF: An evaluation of turbidimetric techniques for estimation of plasma fibrinogen. Clin Chem 13:1057, 1967

37. Griffin JH, Evatt B, Zimmerman TS et al: Deficiency of protein C in congenital thrombotic disease. J Clin Invest 68:1370, 1981

38. Hardisty RM, Macpherson JC: A one-stage factor VIII (antihaemophilic globulin) assay and its use on venous and capillary plasma. Thromb Diath Haemorrh 7:215, 1962

39. Hathaway WE, Belhasen LP, Hathaway HS: Evidence for a new plasma thromboplastin factor: I. Case report, coagulation studies and physiochemical properties. Blood 26:521, 1965

40. Hemker HC: Handbook of Synthetic Substrates for the Coagulation and Fibrinolytic System. Boston, Martinus Nijhoff, 1983

41. Hicks ND, Pitney WR: A rapid screening test for disorders of thromboplastin generation. Br J Haematol 3:227, 1957

42. Howard MA, Firkin BG: Ristocetin—A new tool in the investigation of platelet aggregation. Thromb Diath Haemorrh 26:362, 1971

43. Howard MA, Sawers RJ, Firkin BG: Ristocetin: A means of differentiating von Willebrand's disease into two groups. Blood 41:687, 1973

44. Hoyer LW, Shainoff JR: Factor VIII-related protein circulates in normal human plasma as high molecular weight multimers. Blood 55:1056, 1980

45. Huseby RM, Bang NU: Fibrinogen. In Bang NU, Beller FK, Deutsch E et al (eds): Thrombosis and Bleeding Disorders: Theory and Methods, p 222. New York, Academic Press, 1971

46. Inada Y, Okamoto H, Kanai S et al: Faster determination of clottable fibrinogen in human plasma: An improved method and kinetic study. Clin Chem 24:351, 1978

47. Jespersen J, Sidelmann J: A study of the conditions and accuracy of the thrombin time assay of plasma fibrinogen. Acta Haematol (Basel) 67:2, 1982

48. Jim RTS: A study of the plasma thrombin time. J Lab Clin Med 50:45, 1957

49. Jolgren VR, Triplett DA: Immunologic methods in the coagulation laboratory. ASCP Check Sample, Thrombosis and Hemostasis, TH 80-4 (TH-10). Chicago, American Society of Clinical Pathologists, 1980

50. Kasper CK, Aledort LM, Counts RB et al: A more uniform measurement of factor VIII inhibitors. Thromb Diath Haemorrh 34:869, 1975

51. Koepke JA, Gilmer PR, Filip DJ et al: Studies of fibrinogen measurement in the CAP survey program. Am J Clin Pathol 63:984, 1975

52. Laki K, Lorand L: On the solubility of fibrin clots. Science 108:280, 1948

53. Langdell RD, Wagner RH, Brinkhous KM: Effect of antihemophilic factor on one-stage clotting tests: A presumptive test for hemophilia and a simple one-stage antihemophilic factor assay procedure. J Lab Clin Med 41:637, 1953

54. Latallo ZS: Thrombin clotting assays. In Bang NU, Beller FK, Deutsch E et al (eds): Thrombosis and Bleeding Disorders: Theory and Methods, p 183. New York, Academic Press, 1971

55. Latallo ZS, Teisseyre E: Evaluation of Reptilase R and thrombin clotting time in the presence of fibrinogen degradation products and heparin. Scand J Haematol 13:261, 1971

56. Laurell CB: Antigen-antibody crossed electrophoresis. Anal Biochem 10:358, 1965

57. Laurell CB: Quantitative estimation of proteins by electrophoresis in agarose gel containing antibodies. Anal Biochem 15:45, 1966

58. Laurell CB: Electroimmunoassay. Scand J Clin Lab Invest 29(suppl 124):21, 1972

59. Lenahan JG, Smith K: Hemostasis, 18th ed. Durham, NC, Organon Teknika, 1986

60. Mancini G, Carbonara AO, Heremans JF: Immunochemical quantitation of antigens by single radial immunodiffusion. Immunochem 2:235, 1965

61. Mitchell GA, Abdullahad CM, Ruiz JA et al: Fluoregenic substrate assays for factors VIII and IX: Introduction of a new solid phase fluorescent detection method. Thromb Res 21:573, 1981

62. Morse EE, Panek S, Menga R: Automated fibrinogen determination. Am J Clin Pathol 55:671, 1971

63. Natelson EA, Dooley DF: Rapid determination of fibrinogen by thrombokinetics. Am J Clin Pathol 61:828, 1974

64. National Committee for Clinical Laboratory Standards: Proposed guidelines for a standardized procedure for the determination of fibrinogen in biological samples, Vol 2(13):404. Villanova, PA, NCCLS, 1982

65. Nussbaum M, Morse B: Plasma fibrin stabilizing factor activity in various diseases. Blood 23:669, 1964

66. Odegard OR, Lie M, Abildgaard U: Heparin cofactor activity measured with an amidolytic method. Thromb Res 6:287, 1975

67. Odegard OR, Try K, Abildgaard U: Protein C: A simplified-automated activity assay. Thromb Res 42:257, 1986

68. O'Sullivan MJ, Bridges JW, Marks V: Enzyme immunoassay: A review. Ann Clin Biochem 16:221, 1979

69. Owen CA, Thompson JH: Soybean phosphatides in prothrombin-consumption and thromboplastin-generation tests: Their use in recognizing "thrombasthenic hemophilia." Am J Clin Pathol 33:197, 1960

70. Peake IR, Bloom AL: The use of an immunoradiometric assay for factor VIII related antigen in the study of atypical von Willebrand's disease. Thromb Res 10:27, 1977

71. Penner JA: Experience with a thrombin clotting time assay for measuring heparin activity. Am J Clin Pathol 61:645, 1974

72. Quick AJ, Favre-Gilly J: The prothrombin consumption test: Its clinical and theoretic implications. Blood 4:1281, 1949

73. Rapaport SI, Ames SB: Clotting factor assays on plasma from patients receiving intramuscular injections of subcutaneous heparin. Am J Med Sci 234:678, 1957

74. Ratnoff OD, Menzie AB: A new method for the determination of fibrinogen in small samples of plasma. J Lab Clin Med 37:316, 1951

75. Rodman NF Jr, Barrow EM, Graham JB: Diagnosis and control of the hemophilioid states with the partial thromboplastin time (PTT) test. Am J Clin Pathol 29:525, 1958

76. Ruggeri ZM, Zimmerman TS: Variant von Willebrand's disease: Characterization of two subtypes by analysis of multimeric composition of factor VIII/von Willebrand factor in plasma and platelets. J Clin Invest 65:1318, 1980

77. Ruggeri ZM, Mannucci PM, Jeffcoate SL et al: Immunoradiometric assay of factor VIII related antigen with observations in 32 patients with von Willebrand's disease. Br J Haematol 33:221, 1976

78. Sabo MG: Coagulation instrumentation and reagent systems. In Triplett DA (ed): Laboratory Evaluation of Coagulation, p 315. Chicago, American Society of Clinical Pathologists, 1982

79. Sala N, Owen WG, Collen D: A functional assay of protein C in human plasma. Blood 63:671, 1984

80. Saleem A, Fretz K, Krieg AF: Comparison of three methods for plasma fibrinogen. Ann Clin Lab Sci 6:65, 1976

81. Saleem A, Krieg AF, Fretz K: Improved micromethod for plasma fibrinogen unaffected by heparin therapy. Am J Clin Pathol 63:426, 1975

82. Schleider MA, Nachman RL, Jaffe EA et al: A clinical study of the lupus anticoagulant. Blood 48:499, 1976

83. Schroer H: Assay for prothrombin. In Bang NU, Beller FK, Deutsch E et al (eds): Thrombosis and Bleeding Disorders: Theory and Methods, p 175. New York, Academic Press, 1971

84. Schuurs AH: Enzyme-immunoassay: A powerful analytical tool. J Immunol 1:229, 1980

85. Seghatchian MJ, Miller-Andersson M: A colorimetric evaluation of factor VIII:C potency. Med Lab Sci 35:347, 1978

86. Shaw ST: Assays for fibrinogen and its derivatives. CRC Crit Rev Clin Lab Sci 8:145, 1977

87. Shulman NR: Prothrombin consumption tests. In Bang NU, Beller FK, Deutsch E et al (eds): Thrombosis and Bleeding Disorders: Theory and Methods, p 79. New York, Academic Press, 1971

88. Siefring GE, Riabov DK, Wehrly JA: Development and analytical performance of a functional assay for fibrinogen on the DuPont aca analyzer. Clin Chem 29:614, 1983

89. Thomas JE, Peake IR, Giddings JC et al: The application of a monoclonal antibody to factor VIII related antigen (VIII R:Ag) in immunoradiometric assays for factor VIII. Thromb Haemost 53:143, 1985

90. Triplett DA, Cassidy PG: The use of plasma-agarose gels in the coagulation laboratory. ASCP Check Sample. Thrombosis and Hemostasis, TH 85-3, (TH-39), vol 7(3). Chicago, American Society of Clinical Pathologists, 1985

91. Triplett DA, Harms CS: Procedures for the Coagulation Laboratory, p 20. Chicago, American Society of Clinical Pathologists, 1981

92. Triplett DA, Brandt JT, Maas RL: The laboratory heterogeneity of lupus anticoagulants. Arch Pathol Lab Med 109:946, 1985

93. Triplett DA, Brandt JT, Kaczor D et al: Laboratory diagnosis of lupus inhibitors: A comparison of the tissue thromboplastin inhibition procedure with a new platelet neutralization procedure. Am J Clin Pathol 79:678, 1983

94. Unanue ER, Benacerraf B: Textbook of Immunology, 2nd ed, p 56. Baltimore, Williams & Wilkins, 1984

95. Ware AG, Seegers WH: Two-stage procedure for the quantitative determination of prothrombin concentration. Am J Clin Pathol 19:471, 1949

96. Warner ED, Brinkhous KM, Smith HP: A quantitative study on blood clotting: Prothrombin fluctuations under experimental conditions. Am J Physiol 114:667, 1936

97. Weber K, Osborn M: The reliability of molecular weight determinations by dodecyl sulfate polyacrylamide gel electrophoresis. J Biol Chem 244:4406, 1969

98. Yalow RS, Berson SA: Immunoassay of endogenous plasma insulin in man. J Clin Invest 39:1157, 1960

99. Zacharski LR, Rosenstein R: Comparison of the reaction-rate and clot-density methods for determination of plasma fibrinogen. Am J Clin Pathol 68:45, 1977

100. Zimmerman TS, Hoyer LW, Dickson L et al: Determination of the von Willebrand's disease antigen (factor VIII related antigen) in plasma by quantitative immunoelectrophoresis. J Lab Clin Med 86:152, 1975.

Laboratory Evaluation of Fibrinolysis

Robert L. Baglini

Laboratory evaluation of fibrinolysis has been evolving for the past 30 years. It began with a simple assay, the whole-blood clot lysis test (WBCLT), and has progressed to assays of fibrin(ogen) degradation products (FDP) and D-dimers by latex particle methodology as well as to plasminogen assays using chromogenic substrates.

This chapter discusses some assays commonly used for the evaluation of the fibrinolytic mechanism. It outlines the principles, expected results, and technical difficulties associated with their performance. The reader should already have a clear understanding of the fibrinolytic mechanism and is referred to Chapter 50 for a detailed discussion.

DETERMINATION OF LYSIS TIME

Historical Aspects

The WBCLT is significant from a historical perspective, even though it has been replaced by more sophisticated methods, which will be discussed later in this chapter. The WBCLT is based on the fact that whole blood will clot spontaneously when collected in a glass tube without anticoagulant. This clot should remain intact for approximately 48 hours at 37°C; clot lysis or dissolution prior to 48 hours is indicative of excessive systemic fibrinolysis. This test detects only grossly increased activity.[7]

Modifications of the WBCLT include the dilute whole-blood clot lysis time, which is said to be a more sensitive assay. It is based on the principle that dilution of blood or plasma with a buffer will decrease the activity of inhibitors to plasmin(ogen), thus leaving plasminogen activator or plasmin free to lyse the fibrin clot.[11] Another modification of the WBCLT is the plasma clot lysis test. In this assay, blood is collected in an anticoagulant, centrifuged, and the plasma is recalcified. The resultant plasma clot is then incubated at 37°C and observed for lysis over a 48-hour period.

The WBCLT, as well as its modifications, are empiric procedures for the detection of lytic activity in the blood. Because of the technical difficulties, as well as the poor correlation of the results with clinical conditions, these tests are not recommended for use in the modern laboratory.

EUGLOBULIN LYSIS TIME

The euglobulin lysis time avoids the problems of plasmin(ogen) inhibitors in the assay system. The result is a more rapid and sensitive assay of lytic activity.

Principle

Euglobulins are proteins that precipitate when plasma is diluted with water and acidified. They include plasminogen, plasmin, fibrinogen, and plasminogen activators. The inhibitors of fibrinolysis (antiplasmin and antiplasminogen activators) remain in the supernatant fluid and therefore can be removed from the plasma.

Procedure

The patient's citrated, platelet-poor plasma is diluted with water, acidified, and refrigerated. The euglobulins will precipitate, whereas inhibitors of fibrinolysis remain in the supernate, which is carefully decanted. The precipitate is then redissolved and clotted with thrombin. If the plasminogen in the euglobulin fraction is converted to plasmin, it will lyse the fibrin clot. The time needed for complete lysis at 37°C is recorded as the euglobulin lysis time.

Quality Control

Parallel testing of a presumed normal specimen can serve as a crude quality control measure. Strict adherence to a standardized procedure is necessary.

Reference Range

The time required for complete clot lysis should be greater than 2 hours.[4] Lysis in less than 2 hours is indicative of increased fibrinolytic activity.

Comments

The procedure will detect increased fibrinolysis as a result of surgery, obstetric complications, various medical problems, and disseminated intravascular coagulation. This test does not detect fibrin(ogen) split products (X, Y, D, E).

The euglobulin lysis time is performed by many specialized coagulation laboratories but has relatively little application in the clinical routine laboratory because of the associated technical problems. For example, the fibrinolytic activity of the euglobulin fraction is greatly influenced by the precipitation procedure, pH, ionic strength, and protein concentration of the test plasma.[2]

If the plasma fibrinogen concentration is less than 80 mg/dL, or if a significant concentration of FDP is present, a poor clot will form, resulting in a false shortening of the lysis time, hence a false positive. In the case of greatly reduced plasminogen concentration, as in disseminated intravascular coagulation, there is insufficient plasminogen in the euglobulin fraction for activation and hence a false-negative result.[21]

Reference ranges will depend to some extent on the anticoagulant used, as sodium citrate enhances fibrinolysis.

Excessive agitation of the tube containing the clot may result in an erroneous endpoint.

The sample must be tested within 1 hour of collection.

DETERMINATION OF LYSIS PRODUCTS

The degradation of either fibrin or fibrinogen by plasmin results in fragments of protein referred to synonymously as either fibrin(ogen) degradation (or split) products (FDP or FSP).

Historical Aspects

For many years, the tanned red-cell hemagglutination inhibition test (TRCHII) was the standard against which all other quantitative assays of FDP were measured.[19] Although the TRCHII is still used in research laboratories, its usefulness in the routine clinical laboratory is limited because of its complexity. Historically, the reagents used to perform the TRCHII assay needed to be prepared by the laboratory; however, today, they are available commercially.

The assay is based on the fact that rabbit-derived antihuman fibrinogen antisera, when mixed with the patient's serum, will combine with FDP. After incubation, formalin-fixed, fibrinogen-coated, human group O red cells (tanned RBC) are added to the mixture. These tanned RBC will then react with the residual antihuman fibrinogen antisera (antisera that has not combined with FDP). The mixture is evaluated for inhibition of red cell agglutination, which is inversely proportional to the amount of FDP in the patient serum. Normally, there should be less than 12 μg of fibrinogen-like antigen per milliliter of plasma.

The staphylococcal clumping test[13] is of little use today even though it is a sensitive assay for detecting the presence of split products X and Y (early breakdown products), soluble fibrin monomers, and fibrinogen. To perform the test, whole blood is collected and allowed to clot, thus removing all fibrinogen. The remaining serum is diluted then mixed with a suspension of *Staphylococcus aureus* strain Newman D2C (coagulase negative) in a microtiter plate. High-molecular-weight split products X and Y as well as monomers will complex with the bacteria, resulting macroscopic agglutination. The highest dilution of patient's serum that induces agglutination is determined. The sensitivity of the bacterial suspension is quantitated using a fibrinogen standard plasma and the final result is reported in fibrinogen equivalents/mL. Normally, there should be 0 to 8 μg of fibrinogen equivalents/mL of serum.

PROTAMINE SULFATE DILUTION TEST

The action of thrombin on fibrinogen results in the formation of fibrin monomers that spontaneously polymerize to form a fibrin mesh. When FDP are present in large amounts, they may interfere with this polymerization reaction, thus forming soluble fibrin monomers. Primary (larger) degradation products X and Y may spontaneously polymerize and are also inhibited by complexing with fibrinogen, as well as with the secondary (smaller) degradation products D and E.[12]

Principle

When protamine sulfate is added to plasma, it displaces the secondary (smaller) degradation products from fibrin monomers and primary (larger) FDP, which will then polymerize spontaneously. This phenomenon is referred to as "paracoagulation."[15]

Procedure

The assay is performed by adding patient's plasma to protamine sulfate in various dilutions. At the end of 30 minutes, the dilutions are examined for gel formation, which indicates polymerization of fibrin monomers and early FDP. The gel is somewhat difficult to detect, and reading of the results requires some experience.

Quality Control

There is no adequate quality control procedure for this method. Positive and negative controls should be run along with the patient sample. A positive control may be obtained from patients with known fibrinolytic activity. Strict adherence to procedure is essential.

Reference Range

Normally, no gel formation is seen.

Comments

If fibrinogen is present in high concentrations, an amorphous precipitate will develop. This should not be mistaken for a positive reaction.[20]

Because this test is insensitive to fibrinogen and its degradation products, it readily distinguishes between primary and secondary fibrinolysis. Primary fibrinolysis (degradation of fibrinogen) results in a negative reaction, whereas secondary fibrinolysis (degradation of fibrin) yields a positive reaction.

A positive result may be expected in disseminated intravascular coagulation, pulmonary embolism, and during thrombolytic therapy, as well as in any other clinical conditions which lead to the formation of FDP. This reaction can be completely inhibited by high levels of plasmin, often found in patients with pulmonary embolism.[23]

False-positive reactions may be seen in healthy women immediately before and during menstruation and in patients with advanced cirrhosis or metastatic cancer.[12]

Generally speaking, this test is of limited value unless frequently performed, because experience in interpretation is of prime importance.

ETHANOL GELATION TEST

The ethanol gel test is said to be less sensitive but more specific than the protamine sulfate dilution test in detecting soluble fibrin monomers and polymers in plasma.[7]

Principle

In the presence of a 50% solution of ethanol, any soluble fibrin monomer complexes present will dissociate, resulting in polymerization of the monomers and subsequent gel formation.[6] This is the same paracoagulation reaction involved in the protamine sulfate test.

Procedure

The test is performed by adding a 50% solution of ethanol to platelet-poor plasma and observing for gel formation.

Reference Range

There should be no gel formation under normal conditions.

Comments

This test has been used in conjunction with, or substituted for, the protamine sulfate dilution test, however, it suffers from similar interpretation problems.

LATEX FDP ASSAY

Because of the need for a convenient, rapid, and sensitive assay for FDP, the latex FDP test was developed.

Principle

Latex particles coated with antibody against either fibrin(ogen) fragments D and E or human fibrinogen are mixed with patient serum. Macroscopic agglutination of the latex particles indicates the presence of degradation products of either fibrinogen or fibrin.

Specimen Requirements

Certain precautions are required during blood collection. First, because trace amounts of fibrinogen will cause false-positive reactions, it is essential that the sample be thoroughly clotted with thrombin. Second, if heparin is present in the sample, a snake venom preparation (Reptilase) must be added to ensure complete clotting.[7] Also, plasma from patients having excessive fibrinolytic activity may develop FDP *in vitro* during the clotting process. Therefore, a trypsin inhibitor should be added to the collection tube to assure the measurement of *in vivo* and not *in vitro* split products. Tubes containing thrombin, a trypsin inhibitor, and venom or a combination of these components are commercially available.

Procedure

The patient's serum in various dilutions is mixed with the latex particles, and the highest dilution in which macroscopic agglutination is present represents the titer of FDP. Depending on which manufacturer's kit is used, the sensitivity of the latex particles may be to degradation products D and E or to high-molecular-weight fragments X and Y.

Quality Control

Positive and negative controls should be run along with the patient specimens. These controls may be supplied by the manufacturer of the kit. If not, a positive control can be made by diluting normal plasma, which contains fibrinogen. A normal serum sample will serve as a negative control. The activity of the latex particles should be checked with dilutions of fibrinogen or plasma.

Comments

Comparisons of these assays have been performed.[8,24,25]

Positive results have been reported in the following: disseminated intravascular coagulation, pulmonary embolism, deep vein thrombosis, acute myocardial infarction, abruptio placentae, preeclampsia, eclampsia, fetal death *in utero*, postpartum hemorrhage, malignant neoplasms, ovarian tumor, polycystic disease, renal failure, hydronephrosis, lupus nephritis, proliferative glomerulonephritis, renal transplantation, cirrhosis, after surgical complications, and during thrombolytic therapy, and in healthy normal women during menstruation. Fluctuating levels have been observed during normal pregnancy.

False-positive results have been observed in samples that have not been clotted properly (*e.g.*, heparin contamination or dysfibrinogenemia) or from patients with circulating rheumatoid factor. Also, if the latex–serum mixture is not read at the prescribed time, a false-positive reaction may result, as prolonged exposure to air will cause evaporation and apparent clumping.

LATEX D-DIMER ASSAY

A more recent development in the evaluation of fibrinolytic activity is the D-dimer (D-D) assay, which measures a specific fragment arising from the degradation of cross-linked fibrin (D-dimer) and not fragments X, Y, D, or E. Because it measures fibrinolysis and not fibrinogenolysis, the presence of D-dimers is specific evidence of intravascular fibrin formation[9] as opposed to primary fibrinolysis (*i.e.*, lysis in the absence of fibrin formation).

Specimen Requirements

This assay may be performed on fresh citrated, heparinized or EDTA plasma specimens as well as serum. It should be noted, however, that D-dimer levels are somewhat lower in serum than in plasma.[26] This needs to be taken into consideration when interpreting test results.

Procedure

There are basically two methods to assay this product: enzyme immunoassay and latex bead. The enzyme immunoassay is useful when levels of D-dimer are low and a very sensitive assay is required. It does, however, require special technique and is expensive and time consuming. A busy clinical laboratory has need for a rapid, simple, yet specific method. For this reason, the latex bead method has gained popularity despite the fact that it is not as sensitive as the enzyme immunoassay.

This method utilizes latex beads coated with monoclonal antibody which is specific for D-dimer but not to fibrinogen degradation products or early degradation products X and Y. The plasma or serum in various dilutions is mixed with a suspension of sensitized latex beads, and the highest dilution of plasma or serum that causes macroscopic agglutination of these beads is determined.

Reference Range

Under normal circumstances, less than 200 ng/mL should be present.

Comments

Positive results may be seen in patients with DIC, pulmonary and cerebral embolism, phlebitis, thrombosis, and postoperatively, prethrombotic risk, sickle cell disease, and clot resolution secondary to thrombolytic therapy.[3] The presence of rheumatoid factor, a heterologous antibody, may cause a false-positive reaction.[16] There is new evidence to suggest the usefulness of the D-dimer assay as a screening test for the diagnosis of venous thrombosis.[14,22]

Fresh citrated, heparinized, or EDTA plasma specimens may be used, as well as serum. It should be noted, however, that D-dimer levels are somewhat lower in serum than in plasma;[24] this needs to be taken into consideration when interpreting test results.

DETERMINATION OF PROTEINS INVOLVED IN LYSIS

Plasminogen Assays

Over the years, many methods have been developed to assay plasminogen, among them are the fibrin plate assay[2] and the caseinolytic method.[1] There exist other methodologies having wider acceptance and application. Assays of plasminogen by radial immunodiffusion (RID)[10] and its modification[18] are available commercially. In these tests, the patient's plasma is added and allowed to diffuse from a well cut into an agarose matrix containing plasminogen antibody. The interaction of patient's plasminogen with the antibody results in an immunoprecipitation reaction, the diameter of which is measured and compared to that caused by control plasma. Although the test is simple to perform, 48 hours are required to obtain results. Also, it measures only the concentration of the plasminogen molecule immunologically, not taking into account its functional capabilities.

Plasminogen should be assayed by both immunologic and functional assays. The functional assays are all based on the same principle: an excess of plasminogen activator, such as streptokinase is added to a plasma sample. The resultant plasminogen–streptokinase complex generates plasmin activity that will react with a synthetic (chromogenic) substrate. The result is a color change proportional to the plasminogen level of the plasma. These assays are commercially available.

The problems inherent to the synthetic substrate procedure are: (1) a spectrophotometer or fluorometer is required (e.g., DuPont aca, Dade Protopath); (2) technique is critical: the timing of specific reactions as well as the narrow temperature range in which the assays are performed must be accurately monitored; and (3) icteric or hemolyzed plasma will interfere with the spectrophotometric measurement.

Plasminogen Activators

Assays of these proteins have been introduced only recently to the clinical laboratory. A method using 125 I alpha-casein has been proposed to be accurate and precise.[17] Chromogenic assays for Tissue Plasminogen Activator (t-PA) and Plasminogen Activator (a modification of the euglobulin lysis time) as well as an enzyme immunoassay (EIA) procedure for t-PA are now available commercially. The kits, however, are expensive and the interpretation of the data derived from the assays is difficult to apply to its relationship to thrombotic risk in the patient.

CHAPTER SUMMARY

The laboratory assays described in this chapter measure some components of the fibrinolytic system. They are divided into three major categories: measurement of the time for lysis to occur, of the products of lysis, or of specific reactants in the fibrinolytic system. The author has selected for discussion those tests most commonly employed in routine hemostasis laboratories.

The most important requirement for any of these tests is that they measure *in vivo* and not *in vitro* lysis. To accomplish this, the instructions pertaining to specimen collection, preparation, and assay must be strictly followed. If carefully performed, these assays will aid in the diagnosis and monitoring of events associated with activation of the fibrinolytic system.

CASE STUDY 54-1

A 35-year-old man was admitted through the emergency department with an anterior-wall myocardial infarction. It was determined that he would be a favorable candidate for clot dissolution with thrombolytic therapy (streptokinase). A coagulation profile was performed before and 2 hours after induction of the therapy. It was later determined in the cardiac catheterization laboratory that the clot was not effectively lysed, and the patient was subsequently treated by conventional therapy using anticoagulants. Coagulation results were as follows:

	PRETHERAPY	POST-THERAPY
PT (9–13 sec)	12.2 sec	17.0 sec
APTT (24–37 sec)	28 sec	55 sec
Fibrinogen (150–400 mg/dL)	300 mg/dL	32 mg/dL
FDP (latex) (< 10 μg/mL)	< 10 μg/mL	> 160 μg/mL
D-Dimer (< 200 ng/mL)	< 200 ng/mL	300 ng/mL
Plasminogen (68%–150%)	70%	22%

1. Explain the elevated FDP level.
2. Explain the decreased plasminogen level.
3. Why is the D-dimer level not elevated in proportion to the greatly elevated FDP level?

REFERENCES

1. Alkjaersig N, Fletcher AP, Sherry S: The mechanism of clot dissolution by plasmin. J Clin Invest 38:1086, 1959
2. Bang NU, Beller FK, Deutsch E et al: Thrombosis and Bleeding Disorders: Theory and Methods. New York, Academic Press, 1971
3. Berberian L, Cercek B, Laramee P et al: The serum level of D dimer, a degradation product of crosslinked fibrin is elevated following intravenous streptokinase but not following conventional management in acute myocardial infarction. Proceedings of the 35th Annual Scientific Sessions of the American College of Cardiology, 1986 (abstr)
4. Blix S: Studies on the fibrinolytic system in the euglobulin fraction of human plasma. Scand J Clin Lab Invest 13(suppl):3, 1961
5. Bowie EJ, Thompson JH, Didisheim P et al: Mayo Clinic Laboratory Manual of Hemostasis, p 131. Philadelphia, WB Saunders, 1971
6. Breen FA, Tullis JL: Ethanol gelation: A rapid screening test for intravascular coagulation. Ann Intern Med 69:1197, 1968
7. Brittin GM: Fibrinolysis. Chicago, American Society of Clinical Pathologists Commission on Continuing Education, 1972
8. Drewinko B, Surgeon J, Cobb P et al: Comparative sensitivity of different methods to detect and quantify circulating fibrinogen/fibrin split products. Am J Clin Pathol 84:58, 1985
9. Elms MJ, Bunce IH, Bundesen PG: Measurement of crosslinked fibrin degradation products: An immunoassay using monoclonal antibodies. Thromb Haemost 50:591, 1983
10. Fahey JL, McKelvey EM et al: Quantitative determination of serum immunoglobulins in antibody-agar plates. J Immunol 94:84, 1965
11. Fearnley GR, Balmforth G, Fearnley E: Evidence of diurnal fibrinolytic rhythm with a simple method for measuring natural fibrinolysis. Clin Sci 16:645, 1957
12. Gurewich V, Hutchinson E: Detection of intravascular coagulation by a serial-dilution protamine sulfate test. Ann Intern Med 75:895, 1971
13. Hawiger J, Niewiarowski S, Gurewich V et al: Measurement of fibrinogen and fibrin degradation products in serum by staphylococcal clumping test. J Lab Clin Med 75:93, 1970
14. Heaton D, Billings J, Hickton C: Assessment of d-dimer assay for the diagnosis of deep vein thrombosis. J Lab Clin Med 110:588–591, 1987
15. Kopec M, Kowalski E, Stachurashi J: Studies on paracoagulation: Role of antithrombin VI. Thromb Diath Haemorrh 5:285, 1961
16. Lane DA, Preston FE, Van Ross ME: Characterization of serum fibrinogen and fibrin fragments produced during disseminated intravascular coagulation. Br J Haematol 40:609, 1978
17. Lewis JG, Pizzo SV, Adams DO: A simple and sensitive assay employing stable reagents for quantification of plasminogen activator. Am J Clin Pathol 76:403, 1981
18. Mancini G, Carbonara AO, Heremans JF: Immunochemical quantitation of antigens by single radial immunodiffusion. Immunochem 2:235, 1965
19. Merskey C, Kleiner GJ, Johnson AJ: Quantitative estimation of split products of fibrinogen in human serum: Relation to diagnosis and treatment. Blood 28:1, 1966
20. Niewiarowski S, Gurewich V: Laboratory identification of intravascular coagulation: The serial dilution protamine sulfate test for the detection of fibrin monomer and fibrin degradation products. J Lab Clin Med 77:665, 1971
21. Penner JA: Blood Coagulation Laboratory Manual. Ann Arbor, University of Michigan Medical Center, 1977
22. Rowbotham B, Carol P, Whitaker A, Bunce I, Cobcroft R: Measurement of crosslinked fibrin derivatives—use in the diagnosis of venous thrombosis. Thrombosis and Haemostasis 57:59–61, 1987
23. Sanfelippo M, Stevens D, Koenig R: Protamine sulfate test for fibrin monomers. Am J Clin Pathol 56:166, 1971
24. Smith L, Kitchens C: Experience with a commercially available kit for determining concentration of serum fibrin degradation products. Lab Med 14:554, 1983
25. Sorenson P, Galluzzo T, Ts'ao C: Evaluation of new latex FDP assay. Lab Med 13:688, 1982
26. Whitaker A, Elms M, Masci P et al: Measurement of crosslinked fibrin derivatives in plasma: An immunoassay using monoclonal antibodies. J Clin Pathol 37:882, 1984

Disorders of Coagulation and Fibrinolysis

Margaret C. Schmidt

The disorders of hemostasis are complex. For purposes of clarity, this chapter will classify them into two major etiologic groups: inherited and acquired. Inherited disorders usually affect one hemostatic component. Acquired syndromes differ in severity and complexity and characteristically involve multiple hemostatic components or pathways. The section describing inherited disorders is arranged to follow the reactive sequence of events in the intrinsic, extrinsic, and common pathways as well as fibrin stabilization processes. The acquired disorders that will be discussed are diverse but represent syndromes frequently encountered in clinical practice.

INHERITED DISORDERS OF COAGULATION

Intrinsic Pathway Disorders

The purpose of the intrinsic pathway is to bring about the activation of factor X (X_a). Three separate proteins in the plasma begin the intrinsic pathway. The interrelated roles of these three proteins are collectively termed the "contact phase" of coagulation. In this context, "contact" denotes a point in time when plasma hemostatic components and tissue or artificial surfaces meet, after which a chain of reactions ensues. The product of the contact phase is the activation of factor XI (XI_a) that carries the intrinsic pathway forward.

Factor XII (Hageman), prekallikrein (Fletcher), high-molecular-weight kininogen (HMWK; Fitzgerald), and factor XI (plasma thromboplastin antecedent or PTA) are the four plasma contact factors and are synthesized by the liver. Patients deficient in any one of the first three proteins generally are hemostatically competent and asymptomatic.

They appear to bypass these contact activation schemes and generate fibrin by other means. The intrinsic system is markedly slowed by a defective contact phase only when tested *in vitro*.

The roles of these four proteins are interdependent, and the proteins are structurally related (Fig. 55-1). Prekallikrein and factor XI (considered substrates for factor XII_a) circulate complexed to HMWK. The role of the catalytic cofactor HMWK is to configure these substrates so that their reactive sites are available for factor XII_a.

The first three contact factors also have roles in the fibrinolytic system, in the activation of factor VII, and in the body's response to systemic infectious agents.[17]

Factor XII (Hageman Factor) Deficiency

Factor XII deficiency is an autosomal recessive trait that can be expressed in homozygous or heterozygous forms. The homozygote, possessing two abnormal alleles, has no factor XII; heterozygotes demonstrate variance in their factor XII plasma concentrations.[8]

CLINICAL FINDINGS. Patients homozygous for factor XII deficiency do not suffer from a bleeding disorder. In fact, they may be vulnerable to excessive clotting (thromboses). It is noteworthy that the index patient, Hageman, succumbed to pulmonary embolism.[8]

LABORATORY FINDINGS. Laboratory findings are normal except for determinations of the intrinsic system such as a prolonged activated partial thromboplastin time (APTT). The APTT is corrected with both adsorbed plasma and aged serum (Chap. 53). Factor XII assays will confirm the deficiency.

THERAPY. Generally, no therapy is necessary for this disorder, as the abnormality is an *in vitro* phenomenon.

Prekallikrein (Fletcher Factor) Deficiency

CLINICAL FINDINGS. Fletcher factor deficiency is believed to be transmitted as an autosomal recessive trait. As in Hageman factor deficiency, prekallikrein-deficient patients generally do not demonstrate clinical bleeding and may be vulnerable to thrombotic events.

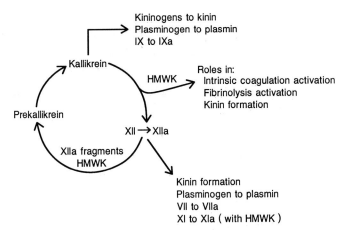

FIG. 55-1. Interdependence of factors of contact activation phase of coagulation.

LABORATORY FINDINGS. The laboratory findings are similar to those in factor XII deficiency. However, the patients' APTT results will shorten if the plasma is incubated with a surface-activating substance such as kaolin.[16]

High-Molecular-Weight Kininogen (Fitzgerald Factor) Deficiency

High-molecular-weight kininogen normally facilitates contact activation of factors XII and prekallikrein. Its absence results in poor contact-phase reactions, a deficiency of kinin formation (active forms derived from kininogen), and defective fibrinolysis reactions.[7]

The autosomal recessive Fitzgerald defect does not produce clinical bleeding. The APTT results typically are mildly prolonged, other tests are within reference limits.

Factor XI Deficiency (Hemophilia C)

Once factor XII is activated during contact-phase reactions, the active form (XII_a), in the presence of HMWK, enzymatically cleaves factor XI (PTA) to XI_a. This reaction takes place on a phospholipid-rich surface, such as platelets.

Factor XI_a behaves as a serine protease and can cleave more factor XII to XII_a to amplify the contact reactions. The other substrate for factor XI_a in the intrinsic system is factor IX.

Originally described in 1953, factor XI deficiency represents the first inherited disorder in the intrinsic cascade to which a clinical bleeding syndrome is attributed. The defect is thought to be a result of decreased synthesis of the protein rather than production of an abnormal molecule[35] and is controlled by an incompletely recessive autosome found largely in Jewish populations.

CLINICAL FINDINGS. The disorder produces a mild bleeding syndrome that responds well to therapy. Most factor XI-deficient patients are symptomatically "silent" until stressed by trauma or surgery. The clinical syndrome may include episodes of epistaxis (nosebleeds), hematuria, and menorrhagia. Surgery or trauma produces exaggerated bleeding. The same patient may differ in the degree of bleeding response from one event to another.

LABORATORY FINDINGS. Deficiencies of factor XI produce prolonged APTT values that are corrected by both adsorbed plasma and aged serum. Factor assay reveals the specific factor deficiency and activity levels. Factor XI increases in concentration on storage. This fact can interfere with laboratory testing for the factor if the test sample is not handled properly. One-stage prothrombin time (PT) values and bleeding time results are not affected. A radioimmunoassay procedure has been developed that correlates positively with assay levels.[30] A two-stage test utilizing a fluorogenic substrate to detect the presence of factor XI_a has been described.[21]

THERAPY. No single specific blood component exists to treat factor XI deficiency. Fresh whole blood, fresh plasma, or fresh frozen plasma have all been used. Plasma concentrations should be raised to 20% to 30% of normal activity to protect the patient.

Factor X Activation Phase Disorders

The activation of factor X is considered the final reaction occurring in both intrinsic and extrinsic pathways. Once activated, factor X_a begins another series of reactions termed the "common" pathway leading to formation of fibrin. Factors VIII:C and IX_a in the intrinsic pathway and factor VII_a in the extrinsic pathway, in conjunction with lipid and Ca^{++}, are required for the activation of factor X.

Deficiencies of the factors necessary for the activation of factor X by way of the intrinsic pathway (VIII:C and IX_a) cause serious bleeding disorders and occur frequently.

Factor VIII:C Deficiency
(Hemophilia A; Classic Hemophilia)

Classic hemophilia is recorded in antiquity. It is sometimes referred to as the "royal disease," as Queen Victoria of England was a carrier, and the condition eventually spread through Europe's royal families. It was first described scientifically in 1803. Much of the current knowledge about hemophilia A has evolved in the last 30 years.

Today, 85% of diagnosed congenital bleeding disorders are hemophilia A or factor VIII:C deficiency. Exact incidence figures are difficult to find, but best estimates in the Western world cite 5 cases per 100,000 population.[23]

Hemophilia A is a sex-linked disorder transmitted on an X chromosome by carrier women to their sons. Carrier women produce clinically normal daughters who *may* carry the chromosomal defect. Sons of affected men are unaffected, but the daughters are obligatory carriers. One-third of new cases occur spontaneously through mutations or variability in the expression of the X chromosome, causing skipped generations.

Factor VIII/vWF (or factor VIII complex) is a macromolecular complex circulating in plasma that consists of two distinct but related components (VIII:C and VIII:vWF). These two components have been characterized experimentally by their genetic, functional, and immunologic properties. Table 55–1 presents the terms applied to this complex molecule. Figure 55–2 depicts the formation of the factor VIII/vWF complex and the pattern of inheritance of the two components.

The functional role of factor VIII:C is as a cofactor in the activation of factor X to X_a. Thrombin is required to modify the structure of factor VIII:C in order for it to fulfill its role in accelerating the proteolytic action of factor IX_a on factor X.

CLINICAL FINDINGS. A bleeding diathesis arises from decreased or defective factor VIII:C. The severity of the disorder is tied to the degree of deficiency. Most severely affected patients possess less than 1% activity of factor VIII:C; moderately affected patients have 2% to 5% activity; and mildly affected patients generally have more than 5% activity. Clinical bleeding necessitating medical intervention occurs most frequently in severely afflicted hemophiliacs. Patients who maintain factor activity levels above 6% may remain clinically silent until traumatized or submitted to surgical procedures without prophylactic preparation. A patient's factor activity level remains fairly constant throughout life.

Typical bleeding episodes result from trauma but may be spontaneous in the most severe cases. Bleeding into soft tissues (hematomas) or joints (hemarthroses), epistaxis, hematuria, gastrointestinal or intracranial hemorrhages, and postoperative bleeding constitute the majority of hemorrhagic events in the hemophiliac. Repeated hemarthroses can cripple and deform over time. The joints of the knee, hip, elbow, ankle, and shoulder are most vulnerable. Taking analgesics such as aspirin during these events is contraindicated, as the drug inhibits platelet function.

LABORATORY FINDINGS. The screening test to detect factor VIII:C deficiency is the APTT. Prolonged APTT results that are corrected by fresh adsorbed plasma but not by serum and results of factor VIII:C assays identify the deficiency and characterize the activity levels. Obligatory carriers have been detected by combined factor VIII:C and VII C:Ag assays. Carrier detection is not without error because of procedure variation and unpredictable X chromosome inactivation (Lyon hypothesis). Levels of factor VIII:C differ in the daughters of carrier females (maternal carriers) and the daughters of hemophiliacs (paternal carriers).[6]

THERAPY. The therapy for hemophilia A involves many issues. Replacement of factor VIII:C by infusion of cryoprecipitate products is done when the goal is to arrest bleeding. The decision to administer prophylactic (preventive) infusions depends on less well-defined criteria: cost, availability, home or hospital setting, age, status of joints, frequency of bleeding episodes, risk of hepatitis or AIDS, and the psychological adjustment of the patient, as well as of family members. In milder cases, pharmacologic agents

TABLE 55–1. Nomenclature for Factor VIII of the International Committee on Thrombosis and Haemostasis

VIII/vWF	The entire molecule as it circulates in the plasma. Composed of VIII:C and VIII:vWF portions noncovalently bound
VIII:vWF	Portion of molecule responsible for binding to endothelium and supporting normal platelet adhesion and function. Tested by bleeding time (Chap. 59)
VIII:C	Portion of molecule acting in intrinsic system as cofactor to factor IXa (with Ca^{++}) in the conversion of factor X to X_a. Tested by partial thromboplastin time (Chap. 52)
VIIIC:Ag	Antigenic property of procoagulant portion as measured by immunologic monoclonal antibody techniques
VIIIR:Ag	Factor VIII-related antigen, which is a property of the large vWF portion of the molecule and measured by immunologic techniques of Laurell rocket or immunoradiometric assay (Chap. 53)
VIIIR:RCo	Ristocetin (an antibiotic no longer used therapeutically) cofactor activity, which is factor VIII-related activity required for aggregation of human platelets with ristocetin (Chap. 59) in *in vitro* aggregation studies

Factor VIII/vWF Complex Formation

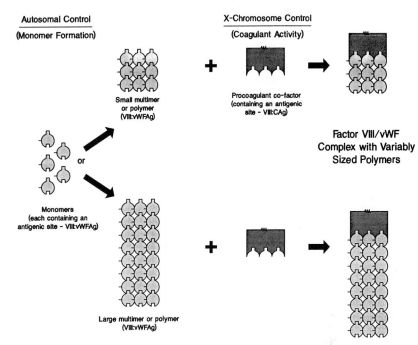

FIG. 55-2.   Factor VIII/vWF complex is composed of (right) procoagulant protein that is coded for by an X-linked gene and (left) a multimer that functions in platelet adhesion and whose synthesis is controlled by an autosomal gene. For proper platelet adhesion, larger multimer complexes are necessary.

such as 1-desamino-8-D-arginine-vasopressin (DDAVP) may be substituted for donor components. This synthetic analogue of the antidiuretic hormone 8-arginine vasopressin increases plasma factor VIII:C by causing its release from endogenous stores.

The incorporation of a siphon technique during plasma thawing has markedly improved factor VIII:C recovery from single-donor plasma.[24] Compared with single-donor cryoprecipitate, commercially prepared and purified concentrates have a lower yield, higher cost, and higher risk of transmitting hepatitis and AIDS. On the other hand, these products are highly purified, they state concentrations on the label, they are stable and store well, and lower volumes are required. The use of single-donor cryoprecipitate pools is common in hospital settings, whereas commercial concentrates generally are used in clinic or home care settings, but practices differ.

Factor assays are used to monitor therapeutic progress. Activity levels of 10% to 20% will stop most bleeding into joints or muscles. Deeper joint bleeding and hematomas mandate 20% to 30% activity levels. Gastrointestinal bleeding, dental extractions, and surgery necessitate 50% to 80% activity levels.

Intravenous administration of DDAVP to mild hemophiliac patients may raise plasma levels of factor VIII:C threefold to sixfold. Baseline plasma levels of factor VIII:C must be sufficient so that an increase invoked by DDAVP will protect the patient.

An estimated 10% of severely affected patients develop antibodies against factor VIII:C. These antibodies appear without regard to the number of transfused products received or the type of product used. No linkage has been established between the major histocompatibility complex and the response to factor VIII:C. There is no method to determine who will develop antibodies and who will not.

The antibodies are IgG with kappa light chains and γ_4 heavy chains.[32] These antibodies are characteristically found in patients who fail to respond to infusions of factor VIII:C products but who previously had responded well. A single patient may respond differently from infusion to infusion.[23]

Patients have been plasmapheresed in an attempt to purge the antibody from plasma, but the procedure has not been strikingly successful. Porcine factor VIII:C concentrates have been used because of the low crossreactivity between human factor VIII:C antibodies and porcine factor VIII. Prothrombin complex concentrates present another option for patients with high titers of antibody. These concentrates bypass the need for factor VIII:C by providing factors II, VII, IX, and X, some of which may be activated. Use of these concentrates usually is reserved for life-threatening situations.

Factor IX Deficiency (Hemophilia B; Christmas Disease)

In 1947, Pavlovsky demonstrated that *in vitro* mixing of plasmas from two "hemophilia" patients resulted in correction of the recalcification time of both plasmas.[27] At that time, all male patients exhibiting hemophilia symptoms were thought to have classic hemophilia; in which case, these results would not have been obtained. In 1952, other investigators found hemophilia patients who possessed factor VIII in their plasma but whose serum did not contain another substance that required vitamin K for synthesis and could be adsorbed to barium salts. The factor was named plasma thromboplastin component (PTC) or Christmas factor for the surname of one index patient.

CLINICAL FINDINGS.   Factor IX deficiency (hemophilia B) is a sex-linked recessive trait and is expressed in mild, moderate, and severe forms. It generally is considered to be a milder form of hemophilia than factor VIII:C deficiency because clinically, these patients are not as prone to hemorrhages in the gastrointestinal tract, abdomen, central nervous system, or genitourinary tract. However, the severely factor IX-deficient patient is clinically indistinguishable from the factor VIII:C-deficient patient.

Three variants of the disease are known on the basis of the antigenic reactivity of factor IX. If the antigen reacts with specific antibody, the patient is termed cross-reactive material positive (CRM[+]); if the antigen is undetectable, the patient is termed CRM[-]; if the antigen reactivity is reduced but detectable, the patient is termed CRM[R] (reduced). Patients who are CRM[+] have been the most extensively studied. No correlation exists between antigen presence and clotting activity of the factor IX molecule.[29] Some CRM[+] variants of factor IX deficiency apparently entail a gene that codes for a defective primary sequence (structure) of the factor IX molecule. Six varieties of CRM[+] factor IX deficiency have been described, each presenting different molecular and behavioral properties.[3] Differentiation of these variants is not clinically useful at this time.

LABORATORY FINDINGS.   Moderate to severe factor IX deficiency is revealed by a prolonged APTT that is corrected with aged serum but not with adsorbed plasma. Mild cases can produce an APTT value within normal limits, yet the patient may exhibit severe bleeding with trauma or surgery. The one-stage PT test using rabbit brain or lung thromboplastin will be within reference limits, but ox brain thromboplastin testing may reveal an abnormal result in a subgroup of these patients. Specific factor IX assay procedures are used for diagnosis and to assess activity levels during therapy. Severely affected patients may have activity levels below 1%. Moderately affected patients possess 1% to 5% of normal activity, and mild affliction is manifest as 6% to 49% activity.[18]

THERAPY.   Therapy involves either commercial concentrate products or human single-donor plasma units. Because of volume considerations, single plasma unit infusions may be unable to increase the activity to a level needed for hemostasis. One unit of factor IX activity is equal to the activity of factor IX in 1.0 mL of normal plasma. Calculations of dosage reveal that infusion of unrealistically large quantities of plasma would be necessary to bring factor IX activity levels to more than 20% of normal in most deficient patients. Commercial concentrates can achieve higher levels of activity in smaller infusion volumes but have the same infection risks discussed for factor VIII concentrates. Heparin is administered with these products to minimize the thrombotic risk, and the timing of the infusion is controlled over a short period. Concentrates are reserved for use in life threatening situations. Plasma exchanges with normal donor plasma have been performed to achieve 50% to 100% activity levels and prevent cardiac overload.

Laboratory monitoring of the patient is achieved by factor IX assays before and after therapy. Factor IX activity levels of 20% to 30% will initially correct minor soft-tissue hemorrhages. Correction of hematuria, body cavity hemorrhage, central nervous system hemorrhage, or gastrointestinal bleeding requires activity levels of 50% to 100%.

Computer tomography scanning has proved valuable in identifying the location and extent of these hemorrhages. Dental extractions may require prophylactic infusions.

Von Willebrand's Disease

In 1926, Eric von Willebrand described the disorder that bears his name as an autosomal dominant trait that produces a prolonged bleeding time and evidence of vascular fragility.[36] These patients are vulnerable to bruising, epistaxis, menorrhagia, and hemorrhage from tooth extraction.

Von Willebrand's disease is now known to be an autosomal trait with either dominant or recessive inheritance. It is caused by defects in both the factor VIII:C and the von Willebrand factor (VIIIR:Ag) of the factor VIII complex described earlier. An important contribution by Zimmerman and associates in 1971 demonstrated that the vWF portion of the VIII complex (VIII:vWF) is reduced or absent in von Willebrand's disease.[38] In this same year, it was demonstrated that platelets in von Willebrand plasma, in contrast to platelets in normal plasma, do not aggregate in the presence of an antibiotic, ristocetin. The ristocetin effect is secondary to a lack of vWF (or factor VIIIR:RCo) in the plasma, as von Willebrand platelets react normally when placed in normal plasma. It is not clear what relation this *in vitro* effect bears to *in vivo* bleeding defects in the patient.

Structural defects in the factor VIII complex in this disorder result in a variety of vWF multimer combinations in plasma (see Fig. 55-2). Although decreased, the factor VIII:C component is nearly always present, as is VIIIR:Ag. Variation in the large multimers of vWF in plasma is the basis for identifying variant types of this disease (Table 55-2).

Von Willebrand's disease is the most frequently inherited coagulopathy. True incidence figures are difficult to locate as many cases are clinically silent and thus undiscovered. No racial or ethnic prevalence is observed. Sometimes, the disorder is not manifested until adulthood and the patient is surgically or traumatically stressed. Cases of acquired von Willebrand's disease have been reported[15,20] and generally are associated with autoimmune or lymphoproliferative disorders, where abnormal antibodies are generated against the vWF. Treatment of the primary disease ameliorates the symptoms of acquired von Willebrand disease.

CLINICAL FINDINGS.   Bleeding appears to be more severe in the child and decreases in severity with age. Muscular hematomas and hemarthroses are rare unless the patient inherits the autosomal recessive form of the disease. There is no real clinical difference in presentation between Type I and Type II disease (see Table 55-2) except in liver disease or pregnancy, in which levels of vWF are increased. Under these circumstances, patients with Type I disease may have correction of the hemostatic defect; patients with Type II disease will not.[25]

LABORATORY FINDINGS.   Typical laboratory data include prolonged bleeding time, equivocal APTT results (depending on plasma levels of factor VIII:C), decreased activity of factor VIII:C, abnormal ristocetin platelet factor VIII related activity (VIIIR:RCo) and decreased levels of large vWF multimers.

TABLE 55–2. Classification of Types of von Willebrand's Disease

TYPE	MODE OF INHERITANCE	EFFECT	RESULTS
Homozygous ("doubly heterozygous")	Autosomal recessive	Severe	VIII:vWF and VIIIR:Ag absent to trace; VIIIR:RCo markedly decreased; VIII:C and VIIIC:Ag present but decreased
Heterozygous I	Autosomal dominant	Variable: mild to moderate	VIIIR:Ag, VIIIR:RCo, and VIII:C variably decreased; VIIIR:Ag present in platelets and endothelial cells; all normal multimers decreased but present
Heterozygous II	Autosomal dominant	Variable	VIIIR:Ag large multimers absent
Subtype IIa	Autosomal dominant	Variable	VIIIR:RCo absent or deficient; VIII:C, VIIIR:Ag, and VIIIR:RCo levels are discrepant
Subtype IIb	Autosomal dominant	Variable	Increased sensitivity of vWF to ristocetin; VIIIR:Ag binds to platelets at lower concentrations of ristocetin than required for normal subjects; VIIIR:RCo is normal, borderline, or reduced

THERAPY. Therapy measures are targeted at increasing levels of factor VIII:C in plasma and shortening the bleeding time. Infusion of cryoprecipitate, the only component that contains all elements of the factor VIII complex, is commonly used. Cryoprecipitate contains the high-molecular-weight multimers of vWF that affect the bleeding time. Commercial factor VIII:C concentrates contain increased levels of factor VIII:C but lack other components of the factor VIII complex (VIII:vWF) necessary to correct the bleeding time. After cryoprecipitate infusion, factor VIII:C levels increase in plasma within 12 to 24 hours and remain elevated for several days. Intravenous DDAVP also has been successful in controlling the hemorrhagic sequelae of surgery, bypassing the patient's dependence on human blood products.

Extrinsic and Common Pathway Disorders

In order for the extrinsic system to become operative, tissue damage and the release of tissue lipoproteins must occur. In the presence of Ca^{+2} and tissue lipoprotein (thromboplastin), plasma factor VII is activated and, in turn, activates factor X to X_a.

The intrinsic and extrinsic systems possess interrelated feedback loops, which are not entirely understood. Examples include the ability of active factor XII (XII_a) fragments to amplify the activity of factor VII, the ability of factor IX_a to activate factor VII, and the ability of factor VII_a to activate both factors IX and X.

Factor X_a begins the common pathway. In combination with phospholipid, Ca^{++}, and cofactor V, factor X_a will convert prothrombin (II) to thrombin (II_a), which in turn converts fibrinogen (I) to fibrin.

Factor VII Deficiency

Factor VII deficiency is an autosomal recessive genetic abnormality with intermediate expression. It is rare, occurring in approximately 1 in 500,000 individuals. Variants exist, labeled CRM$^+$ and CRM^R according to their antigenic reactivity. The behavior of this factor can vary in testing procedures depending on the tissue source of the thromboplastin used. Correlation between clinical bleeding tendency and activity levels in assays are poor.

CLINICAL FINDINGS. Hemorrhage from mucous membranes and into soft tissues occurs most frequently in children. Adult heterozygotes usually tolerate surgery well but may be vulnerable to thrombotic events.

LABORATORY FINDINGS. Diagnosis of factor VII deficiency is based on a family history and demonstrated prolongation of the one-stage PT, while the APTT and thrombin clotting time (TCT) results are within reference ranges. This is the only deficiency in which the PT is the only observed abnormality. Substitution testing procedures exhibit correction of the PT with normal aged serum but no correction with adsorbed plasma. Specific factor VII assay confirms the diagnosis; affected patients demonstrate 10% to 20% of normal activity. Chromogenic substrate procedures exist to measure factor VII's ability to cleave factor X. It should be noted that factor VII levels increase during pregnancy.

THERAPY. Donor plasma and serum components and commercial concentrates containing the prothrombin complex factors are used.

Factor X (Stuart–Prower Factor) Deficiency

Factor X was recognized as unique and given its numeral in 1959. The index patients' surnames (Stuart and Prower) are synonymous with factor X. Deficiency of this factor is inherited as an autosomal trait that is incompletely recessive but shows high penetrance. Immune variants (CRM$^+$, CRM$^-$ and CRM^R) exist. This disorder is uncommon in the general population.

CLINICAL FINDINGS. The symptoms of factor X deficiency are highly variable. Patients may exhibit lifelong histories of bruising, soft-tissue bleeding, or postsurgical or post-trauma hemorrhages. All possible acquired causes, as well as the possibility of multiple factor deficiencies, must be eliminated in making the diagnosis.

LABORATORY FINDINGS. The deficiency produces prolonged PT, APTT, and Stypven time values and a prothrombin utilization abnormality. Specific factor X assay procedures are diagnostic. The PT is corrected by aged serum but not by adsorbed plasma.

THERAPY. Frozen plasma components or prothrombin complex concentrates are used for therapy. Activity levels of 10% to 40% of normal are considered adequate for hemostasis.

Factor V Deficiency (Owren's Disease; Labile Factor Deficiency)

Factor V deficiency was discovered in 1944 in Norway by Professor Owren. He demonstrated that adsorbed normal plasma, when added to his patient's plasma, corrected the prolonged PT. Other investigators subsequently described similar findings.

An autosomal recessive trait, factor V deficiency is demonstrated by homozygotes and is mild to silent in heterozygotes. Factor V also has been described as being deficient in conjunction with factor VIII:C (V–VIII deficiency) in another group of patients.[12,13] A variety of autoimmune disorders is known to produce mixtures of IgG and IgM antibodies to factor V, resulting in an acquired form of the disease.[10]

CLINICAL FINDINGS. Factor V activity less than 10% of normal results in hemorrhagic diatheses. Clinical episodes are similar to those in the mild to moderate hemophilias. Deficiencies of platelet-borne factor V (platelet factor 1) may cause an abnormal bleeding time and seem to precipitate more clinical problems than do decreases in plasma factor V levels. It is suggested that activated platelet-borne factor V is the binding site for activated plasma factor X (X_a) and factor II (prothrombin). Platelet aggregation studies are normal.

LABORATORY FINDINGS. Both the PT and the APTT are prolonged. If the PT is corrected with adsorbed normal plasma, evidence points to factor V deficiency. The possibility of combined (multiple) factor deficiencies must be eliminated. The specific factor V assay is considered diagnostic.

THERAPY. Therapy requires infusion of fresh frozen plasma, as factor V is labile in storage. Plasma activity levels of 25% to 30% of normal are sufficient in most cases to ensure hemostasis. Because of the apparent platelet involvement in this disorder, aspirin products should be avoided. The plasma supernatant fluid removed after cryoprecipitates have formed in component preparations (cryofree plasma) contains adequate levels of factor V when fresh and is used in some locations.

Factor II (Prothrombin) Deficiency

Factor II deficiency may be inherited as either a deficiency or a dysfunction and is rare in the general population. Hypoprothrombinemia is an autosomal recessive trait. Homo-

zygotes have assayed levels of 2% to 25% of normal, whereas heterozygotes maintain levels of 50% or greater. Eleven variants of dysfunctional prothrombin molecules have been reported.[2,22,33]

CLINICAL FINDINGS. Patients with less than 50% activity exhibit mild bleeding tendencies similar to those seen in mild hemophilia. Hemarthroses are rare. Medications containing aspirin may cause bleeding tendencies.

LABORATORY FINDINGS. Laboratory values differ with activity levels of factor II. Both APTT and one-stage PT will be prolonged. The TCT procedures produce normal results. Diagnostic procedures include a two-stage assay for prothrombin activity and immune-based factor assays using antiprothrombin antisera.[34] Dysprothrombinemic patients will produce abnormal results in the two-stage assay but normal immune reactions.

Care should be taken to rule out vitamin K deficiency, liver disease, and multifactor defects.

THERAPY. Therapy depends on which type of disorder is present and on its severity of expression. Fresh frozen plasma is the usual choice. Vitamin K-dependent protein concentrates are also available but carry a risk of thrombosis.

Factor I (Fibrinogen) Deficiency

A defect in fibrin formation may be the result of an inherited lack of fibrinogen (afibrinogenemia), an inherited deficiency of fibrinogen (hypofibrinogenemia), or an inherited production of a dysfunctional fibrinogen molecule (dysfibrinogenemia). The condition is rare. Afibrinogenemic patients have nearly undetectable amounts of fibrinogen; hypofibrinogenemic patients possess less than 100 mg/dL (reference range: 200–400 mg/dL), and in both cases, the molecular structure of fibrinogen is normal. Substitution of amino acids in fibrinogen's polypeptide chains produces a structural change that may result in: (1) the inability to submit to proteolysis by thrombin, because the cleavage sites are inappropriate; (2) peculiar behavior during polymerization stages secondary to aberrant charge distribution across the molecule; (3) the addition of "dangling" (inappropriate) side groups that affect reactivity; or (4) the persistence of fetal fibrinogen into adulthood. All four possibilities are categorized under the term *dysfibrinogenemia,* and many variants have been described.[1] These patients demonstrate abnormal function but have normal levels in antigenic assays.

All three forms of fibrinogen disorder are inherited as autosomal traits. Afibrinogenemia is recessive in expression and clinically severe. Hypofibrinogenemia and dysfibrinogenemia are phenotypically dominant, and bleeding episodes are less severe.

Afibrinogenemic patients' platelets appear affected in that a prolonged bleeding time may be measured. Platelets have a surface receptor for fibrinogen, and fibrinogen apparently is necessary for platelet function *in vivo.*

A host of acquired disorders may reduce the fibrinogen concentration in the plasma. Examples include renal disease, hepatic disease, and "consumptive" disorders such as disseminated intravascular coagulation. The history and clinical features aid in the differentiation between inherited and acquired forms.

CLINICAL FINDINGS. Hemorrhages in afibrinogenemia and hypofibrinogenemia differ in severity. With a complete lack of fibrinogen, spontaneous bleeding has occurred. Mucosal, intestinal, and intracranial sites are most commonly affected. Surgery and trauma present risks commensurate with the concentration of functional fibrinogen available, and poor wound healing has been observed.

LABORATORY FINDINGS. All laboratory test times that depend on fibrin formation will be prolonged in afibrinogenemia, whereas these tests may or may not be prolonged in hypofibrinogenemia. Thrombin clotting times are sensitive to fibrinogen levels and function. Routine screening procedures such as the APTT and PT return variable results. Addition of reagent fibrinogen will correct these endpoints. Platelet counts in hypofibrinogenemia are within the reference range, as are the concentrations of other procoagulant factors. Prolonged Reptilase^R (venom) clotting times occur in dysfibrinogenemia. Tests measuring the activity of fibrinogen are relatively insensitive to structural changes and vary unpredictably with the defect.

Postcoagulation Stabilization Defects

Factor XIII (Fibrin-Stabilizing Factor) Deficiency
CLINICAL FINDINGS. A rare disorder, factor XIII deficiency is an autosomal recessive trait in which only homozygotes express the syndrome. The homozygous patient exhibits spontaneous bleeding and poor wound healing with unusual scar formation. General symptoms are similar to those of mild hemophilia. The syndrome is incompatible with pregnancy unless replacement therapy is provided throughout gestation. All patients should avoid aspirin products.

LABORATORY FINDINGS. Inadequate crosslinking of fibrin results in an unstable and friable clot with excessive red cell "fall out." Fibrin clots incubated with 5 M urea or 1% monochloracetic acid dissolve rapidly, and if adequate controls for excessive fibrinolysis are included, this test is relatively specific. The condition cannot be evaluated in the presence of heparin. Elaborate specific factor XIII assay procedures are available but are not suitable for routine clinical use. Immunologic procedures to measure quantities of factor XIII exist.

THERAPY. Therapy is accomplished with infusion of donor plasma or commercial purified, lyophilized placental factor XIII.

ACQUIRED DISORDERS OF COAGULATION AND FIBRINOLYSIS

Hepatic Disease

The liver is the principal site of synthesis of procoagulant, fibrinolytic, and coagulation inhibitory proteins. Liver disorders present two challenges: decreased synthesis of coagulation, lysis, and inhibitory proteins, and impaired clearance of activated hemostatic components.

The type of disorder differs in neonates and adults. Neonates display decreased levels of plasma contact factors secondary to hepatic immaturity. They also lack sufficient levels of plasminogen and antithrombin III. In addition, neonates express a unique fetal fibrinogen that does not behave in the same manner as adult fibrinogen, and they have decreased levels of fibrinogen (hypodysfibrinogenemia). Decreases of vitamin K-dependent factors in the neonate will be discussed later in this chapter.

In adults, parenchymal liver diseases, such as cirrhosis and hepatitis, and diseases that infiltrate liver tissue, such as neoplasm, affect the synthetic capacity of the organ. Hemostatic changes often are subtle. Prolongation of the PT is considered a sign of worsening disease because of depression of vitamin K-dependent factor synthesis, poor dietary intake, or malabsorption of vitamin K. Fibrinolytic events and thrombocytopenia may accompany liver disease.

Laboratory Findings
Screening tests such as the PT, APTT, TCT, bleeding time, platelet count, fibrinogen levels, and fibrin split products determinations are used to monitor hemostatic status in liver disease.

Therapy
Infusion of fresh plasma may bolster the circulating levels of procoagulants and minimize the hemorrhagic risk. Commercial prothrombin complex concentrates generally are not used in liver disease because of the depressed levels of inhibitory antithrombin III available.

Vitamin K Deficiency

Vitamin K is a necessary cofactor for the conversion of terminal glutamic acid residues to gamma-carboxyglutamic acid on factors II, VII, IX, and X as well as on protein C. This conversion takes place in the hepatocyte and is necessary for proper function. Vitamin K is produced by the normal flora of the gastrointestinal tract and absorbed. Deficiencies can occur if the normal flora is not present (because of broad-spectrum oral antibiotics), if absorption is decreased (obstructive jaundice), or if antagonistic drugs (coumarin family) are taken. Vitamin K may be a required dietary supplement for the neonate, because the supply through the placenta is minimal during gestation, and the gut is sterile for several days after birth. The less than 10% activity levels of prothrombin (II) in newborn plasma may result in hemorrhage, and premature infants are even more susceptible.

Breastfed babies are more prone to vitamin K deficiency than are babies on prepared formulas, because maternal milk provides less of the vitamin than babies require. Breast milk also is sterile; therefore, seeding of the newborn gut with bacteria is further retarded. Injections of vitamin K administered to neonates help overcome this temporary deficiency. Maternal drugs should be screened to ascertain that no antagonists to vitamin K are being ingested and transferred by way of milk to the baby.

The one-stage PT is used to assess levels of vitamin K-dependent coagulation factors in the newborn when clinically indicated.

Therapeutic Anticoagulation

Heparin

Heparin is the intravenous anticoagulant most frequently used in clinical medicine. It is used extensively in specimen collection for laboratory studies and in preventing fibrin deposition on intravenous tubing devices residing in vessels. Heparin is an acid mucopolysaccharide that acts in conjunction with antithrombin III to inhibit most of the serine proteases in the coagulation pathways. It is metabolized by the liver and has a half-life of approximately 3 hours.

Coumarin Drugs (Oral Anticoagulants)

The oral anticoagulants were discovered in Wisconsin during an investigation of hemorrhagic disease in cattle. The herds were consuming contaminated fodder containing spoiled sweet clover, which contains bishydroxycoumarin that caused the bleeding.

Warfarin is the most frequently used coumarin. It is water soluble and is administered orally. It is absorbed in the small bowel and circulates loosely bound to albumin in plasma. It can cross the placenta and appear in breast milk. Warfarin interferes with the carboxylation of the vitamin K-dependent plasma factors in the liver by interrupting the enzymatic phase of this reaction. This results in nonfunctional proteins circulating in plasma that are referred to as *proteins induced by vitamin K antagonist* (PIVKA).

Circulating Anticoagulant (Inhibitory) Substances

Substances produced by the body that inhibit coagulation are termed *circulating anticoagulants.* Such products are considered pathologic and are produced in response to a variety of stimuli. The majority of these substances are antibodies, and the existence of an antibody to each of the protein procoagulants has been demonstrated. Stimuli include infusion of blood or blood products, release of tumor substances into the circulation, and autoimmune disorders.

Inhibitory activity directed against factor VIII/vWF and factor IX have been discussed with the deficiency states. The laboratory results in the presence of such activity will mimic those seen in the hemophiliac states.

An inhibitor has been described in 5% to 10% of patients with systemic lupus erythematosus (SLE). Affected patients exhibit prolonged whole-blood clotting times and PTs.[28] This same circulating anticoagulant activity has since been documented in patients who have drug-induced lupus, other immune disorders or malignant tumors, as well as in persons exhibiting no primary disease. Patients treated with phenothiazines appear especially likely to produce this inhibitor.[5]

Increased levels of fibrin(ogen) split (degradation) products (FSP or FDP), as seen in disseminated intravascular coagulation and lytic disorders, exert an anticoagulant effect. The FSPs interfere with the polymerization of fibrin strands and combine with procoagulant molecules in plasma to form complexes incapable of normal coagulant reactivity. Control of fibrin formation to limit the quantities of FSP produced with component replacement therapy, if necessary, are used to manage this problem. Laboratory procedures utilized to evaluate this process include latex FSP agglutination tests, measurement of fibrin monomers, platelet counts, fibrinogen levels, APTT, and PT.[14]

Massive Transfusion Effects

Transfusion of large quantities of blood can jeopardize hemostatic competency for one or more of the following reasons: (1) excessive quantities of infused citrate; (2) a donor product incompatible with the recipient's system; and (3) deficient labile clotting factors or platelets in the stored blood.

As a powerful chelator, citrate can bind plasma Ca^{+2} needed for hemostasis; however, clinical bleeding does not occur secondary to citrate excess. The decrease in ionized calcium levels in the plasma is directly related to the rate of infusion of blood product[4,19,26] and may affect cardiac rhythm adversely. Citrate is cleared eventually from the body through the liver and kidneys. Hypotension, hepatic disease, hypothermia, and hypovolemia all limit citrate clearance.

The physiologic results of incompatibility between the donor red cells and recipient plasma or serum are well documented in texts of immunohematology. Screening coagulation studies should be obtained postreaction to ascertain hemostatic competence and document recovery.

Infusion of enormous quantities of blood implies tissue trauma or disease of extraordinary proportions. Platelets and factors V and VIII:C are especially vulnerable to storage. The *in vivo* effect of infusing decreased levels of all the procoagulants is cumulative. Alternating infusions of red cells, fresh plasma, and platelet components may be required to maintain adequate levels of procoagulants.

The bleeding time is considered a sensitive indicator of depressed platelet function in extensively transfused patients. The APTT and PT values are less sensitive but useful in deciding whether to supplement therapy with cryoprecipitate or fresh plasma.

Artificial Surface Effects

The demonstrated consequences of exposing blood to an artificial surface include the formation of thrombi and emboli, consumption of procoagulant proteins and platelets, alteration of the function of these proteins, and incitement of systemic syndromes (fever, vasoconstriction, and bronchial constriction) as a sequela of interactive reactions with surfaces.[31] When blood and artificial surface meet, plasma proteins, especially fibrinogen, coat the exposed area (Fig. 55-3). Platelets may or may not attach, spread, and degranulate. Antifibrinogen antibodies do not react with layered fibrinogen, giving support to the theory that the deposited protein has changed its antigenic properties. The protein coat may change its composition over time, becoming less thrombogenic as it ages.

In the presence of complement, neutrophils and macrophages are attracted to protein-coated artificial surfaces and may assist in debriding the surface of both platelets and

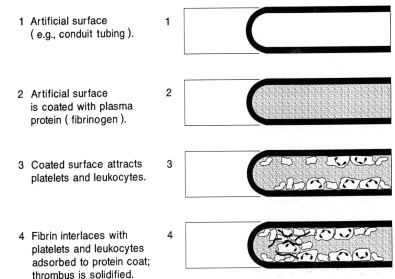

1 Artificial surface
(e.g., conduit tubing).

2 Artificial surface
is coated with plasma
protein (fibrinogen).

3 Coated surface attracts
platelets and leukocytes.

4 Fibrin interlaces with
platelets and leukocytes
adsorbed to protein coat;
thrombus is solidified.

FIG. 55-3   Interaction of blood components with artificial surface.

protein. Aggregates of leukocytes may form and be displaced into the circulation, forming microemboli as a result of complement activation.

The APTT, PT, platelet count, fibrinogen level, plasminogen level, antithrombin III assay, FSP determinations, and fibrin monomer titer may all be used to evaluate and monitor the effects of an artificial surface within a patient's vascular system.

Disseminated Intravascular Coagulation

Disseminated intravascular coagulation (DIC) is a complication of other primary disorders. It results in consumption of coagulation proteins and platelets into thrombi, which are deposited locally or widely in the circulation. Coagulation and fibrinolytic processes occur simultaneously, and either one may dominate at a given time.

There is no age group or gender preference for DIC, and much variation occurs in its clinical presentation. The single common thread connecting all versions of DIC is the liberation of a thromboplastic substance that subsequently results in coagulation. Plasmin is activated by the contact phase reactions or by tissue activators released by damaged cells (see Fig. 50-4). The progress of DIC may be controlled by plasmin or thrombin at any given moment which results in a dominant clinical exhibition of either hemorrhage or thrombosis.

Damage to tissue, with the resulting release of tissue fluid and the exposure of foreign surfaces to blood, brings about activation of coagulation. Endothelial cells may be damaged by bacterial toxins, hypoxic shock, acidosis, antigen-antibody reactions, overwhelming infections, and malignancies.[9] Thromboplastic substances also can be injected directly into the circulation through insect or snake bites or released along with plasminogen activators in complicated pregnancies and deliveries, malignant diseases, and syndromes involving severe tissue trauma (burns, heat strokes, surgery, or crush injuries).

Acute DIC develops in a matter of hours, hemorrhage nearly always occurs; and skin signs of purpura, gangrene, and bullae may appear. The mortality rate is estimated at 60% to 80% in these cases (CS Greenberg, unpublished data). Chronic DIC occurs in patients who have already exhibited a thrombotic tendency or event, and hemorrhage is much less frequent.

Laboratory evidence that DIC is in progress includes prolonged TCT, PT, and APTT; decreased platelets, fibrinogen, and AT-III levels; and elevated FSP and fibrin monomers. The D-dimer test (see Chap. 54) is positive in DIC as soon as 4 hours after onset. Fibrinogen levels may decrease in 4 to 24 hours; platelets decrease up to 48 hours post onset (CS Greenberg; unpublished data). Peripheral blood films may reveal erythrocyte fragments, as well as decreased numbers of platelets. Hemoglobin and hematocrit values reflect the severity of hemorrhage.

Use of heparin in the treatment of DIC is controversial. Heparin may be of benefit if thrombosis is damaging organ function, reversal of the damage is possible, and there are no contraindications to the use of heparin. It is most important to correct the disorder that invoked the DIC in the first place.

Replacement therapy with blood components may be necessary following acute DIC to control hemorrhaging. Fresh frozen plasma, platelet concentrates, and cryoprecipitates may be used. A complete profile of coagulation and lysis should be performed at clinically determined intervals to assess this syndrome during management.

Fibrinolysis

Often referred to as *primary fibrinolysis* (pathologic fibrinogenolysis or PF), the fibrinolysis syndrome in a pure form is unusual. The disease is a result of the release of excessive amounts of plasminogen activators into the circulation either from damaged cells or from malignant cells, as in prostatic carcinoma. These activators convert plasminogen into plasmin in the absence of fibrin formation. Plasmin is nonspecific in its action and will cleave fibrinogen, as well as factors V and VIII. As fibrinogen is broken down, FSP accumulate, which have an anticoagulant effect. The net result is the inability of the blood to clot and thus bleeding.

It is important to distinguish primary fibrinolysis from secondary fibrinolysis, such as occurs in DIC. The laboratory evidence for fibrinolysis is similar to that demonstrated in DIC. Nearly all tests are abnormal in both syndromes. Four tools may be applied to distinguish the two syndromes: (1) the euglobulin clot lysis time will be markedly shortened in primary fibrinolysis (PF) but normal to only slightly shortened in DIC; (2) the platelet count remains greater than $100 \times 10^9/L$ in PF, whereas it frequently drops below this level in DIC; (3) antithrombin III assays will demonstrate decreased levels in DIC and normal levels in PF; and (4) the D-dimer test, which is specific for the degradation of fibrin, will be positive in DIC and negative in PF.

In the absence of any evidence of thrombosis (DIC), antifibrinolytic drugs may be used to treat the condition.

These drugs include natural antiplasmins, bovine parotid extract (aprotinin), and synthetic lysine analogues epsilon-aminocaproic acid (EACA) or trans-p-aminomethyl-cyclohexanecarboxylic acid (AMCA). Often, however, DIC is assumed to be present and the patient managed accordingly. Prolonged cardiopulmonary bypass pump time in surgery and acute trauma to and hypoxia of tissues have precipitated the primary fibrinolytic state. Such cases are brief and self-limited. Prostatic carcinoma has produced a long-term lytic syndrome that necessitates therapy.

Drug Interactions with Coagulation Systems

Table 55-3 presents an abbreviated list of drugs with their known effects on hemostasis mechanisms. Drugs may directly enhance, retard, or inhibit reactions or indirectly stimulate the formation of inhibitory substances that neutralize reactants. Many of these drugs are in common use,

TABLE 55–3. Drug Interactions with Coagulation Systems

DRUG	HEMOSTATIC EFFECT
Penicillin G (carbenicillin and ticarcillin)	Impairs platelet function; increases bleeding time; impairs platelet aggregation; impairs interaction of vWF with platelets
DDAVP (1-desamino-8-D-arginine vasopressin)	Increases plasma levels of VIII:C by releasing endogenous protein from body storage sites; can shorten the APTT
Isoniazid (INH)	Can produce thrombocytopenia; increases bleeding time; stimulates production of inhibitors of factors I, V, and XIII after long-term exposure. APTT, PT, and lysis tests can reflect presence of inhibitors
Estrogen therapy (oral contraceptives)	Produces a slight decrease in platelet numbers; has potential to provoke deep vein thrombosis; can degranulate platelets; can shorten baseline coagulation tests
Aspirin products	Prolongs bleeding time by interfering with thromboxane A_2 synthesis in the platelets
Dextran, high-molecular-weight products	Increases the bleeding time by coating platelets; impairs aggregation reactions; lowers circulating levels of VIIIR:Ag and VIII:vWF
Cephalosporins	Prolongs the one-stage PT; can provoke a thrombocytopenia or a thrombocytosis
Phenothiazines	Stimulates the production of a "lupus anticoagulant" in circulation; prolongs the APTT; may affect the PT if the factor II levels are also affected
Cholestyramine	Impedes the pharmacologic effect of warfarin; can shorten the one-stage PT in patients also receiving warfarin
Phenylbutazone	Impairs platelet function and enhances the effect of warfarin; may prolong the bleeding time; may increase the PT in a patient on both drugs
Metronidazole	Enhances the effect of warfarin in a patient on both drugs; can prolong the PT
Barbituates	Accelerates the clearance of warfarin from the body; can shorten the PT
Oral hypoglycemic agents and phenytoin	Slows the clearance of warfarin; can prolong the PT
Procainamide	Stimulates formation of an antibody (inhibitor) directed against prothrombin and participants in the contact phase of coagulation
Streptomycin	Stimulates formation of inhibitors to factor V; can prolong the PT and possibly the APTT
Penicillin, sulfonamides, phenytoin	Stimulates formation of inhibitors to factor VIII; may prolong the APTT
Pentoxifylline	Decreases fibrinogen levels and platelet aggregation; may prolong PT

and it therefore behooves the coagulation laboratory to be aware of their potential influence on testing systems and the possibility of within-patient variation during therapy with these agents.

CHAPTER SUMMARY

Coagulation disorders are categorized by mode of acquisition into inherited or acquired types. Inherited disorders may be further divided by site of biochemical disturbance within the intrinsic, extrinsic, common, or stabilization pathways. Most inherited disorders involve only one procoagulant defect.

Multiple factor deficiencies and inhibitory substances may coexist in the acquired syndromes. The roles and effects of exogenous substances such as vitamins, drugs, transfusions, and introduction of artificial surfaces or prothrombotic or proteolytic substances into the circulation are considered.

The patient's history, demographic category, and clinical status are codeterminants in the interpretation and value of laboratory data in hemostatic disorders.

CASE STUDY 55-1

A 12-year-old boy of normal height but underweight was admitted to the hospital for evaluation of frequent epistaxis and easy bruising. Pertinent history features were hematuria at age 3 years at which time no evidence of renal disease was demonstrated. Periodic routine urinalysis reports revealed microhematuria. Tonsillectomy and adenoidectomy performed at 5 years of age resulted in exaggerated hemorrhage necessitating packing of the nose. A knee injury at age 7 years required a 14-day hospitalization to manage the hemarthrosis. Loss of the baby teeth resulted in exaggerated bleeding. To date, the patient has not received any blood or blood components to manage these episodes. He is the only child in the family, and no other family member reports such a history.

The laboratory data with the reference ranges were as follows: APTT 68 seconds (23–34 seconds) corrected with adsorbed normal plasma, PT 10.5 seconds (9.3–11.1 seconds), Simplate bleeding time 17 minutes (3–10 minutes), platelet count 289 × 10⁹/L (150–400 × 10⁹/L) with normal morphology; factor VIII:C 11% (50%–200%), factor VIIIR:Ag 30% (50%–150%), factor VIII:vWF multimer pattern low- and intermediate-molecular weight multimers (high- and low-molecular weight multimers), and factor VIIIR:RCo platelet aggregation 5% (50%–150%).

1. What common denominator is evident in this patient's history? Of what significance is the family history?
2. What disorder does this patient have? What laboratory data contributed to your decision?
3. What is the significance of the results of the VIII:vWF multimer pattern in this case? What "type" of disorder does this patient have?
4. Why is single-donor cryoprecipitate component therapy superior to use of commercial concentrates of factor VIII:C for this patient?

REFERENCES

1. Beck EA: Congenital disorders of fibrin formation and stabilization. In Colman RW, Hirsch J, Marder VJ et al (eds): Hemostasis and Thrombosis: Basic Principles and Clinical Practice, p 192. Philadelphia, JB Lippincott, 1982
2. Bezeaud A, Guillin MC, Olmeda F et al: Prothrombin Madrid: A new familial abnormality of prothrombin. Thromb Res 16:47, 1979
3. Braunstein KM, Blatt PM: Diagnosis and therapy of hemophilia B (Christmas disease). In Koepke JA (ed): Laboratory Hematology, vol 1, p 522. New York, Churchill Livingstone, 1984
4. Bunker JP, Stetson JB, Coe RC et al: Citric acid intoxication. JAMA 157:1361, 1955
5. Canoso RT, Hutton RA: A chlorpromazine-induced inhibitor of blood coagulation. Am J Hematol 2:183, 1977
6. Chediak J, Telfer M, Jaojaroenkul T et al: Lower factor VIII coagulant activity in daughters of subjects with hemophilia A compared to other obligate carriers. Blood 55:552, 1980
7. Colman RW: Formation of human plasma kinin. N Engl J Med 291:509, 1974
8. Colman RW: Deficiencies of factor XII and prekallikrein and high molecular weight kininogen. In Colman RW, Hirsch J, Marder VJ et al (eds): Hemostasis and Thrombosis: Basic Principles and Clinical Practice, p 3. Philadelphia, JB Lippincott, 1982
9. Colman RW, Marder VJ: Disseminated intravascular coagulation (DIC): Pathogenesis, pathophysiology, and laboratory abnormalities. In Colman RW, Hirsch J, Marder VJ et al (eds): Hemostasis and Thrombosis: Basic Principles and Clinical Practice, p 654. Philadelphia, JB Lippincott, 1982
10. Feinstein DI: Acquired inhibitors of factor V. Thromb Haemost 39:663, 1978
11. Feinstein DI: Acquired inhibitors against factor VIII and other clotting proteins. In Colman RW, Hirsch J, Marder VJ et al (eds): Hemostasis and Thrombosis: Basic Principles and Clinical Practice, p 564. Philadelphia, JB Lippincott, 1982
12. Giddings JC, Seligsohn U, Bloom AL: Immunological studies in combined factor V and factor VIII deficiency. Br J Haematol 37:257, 1977
13. Girolami A, Violante M, Cella G et al: Combined deficiency of factor V and Factor VIII: A report of another case. Blut 32:415, 1976
14. Greenberg CS, Pizzo S, McCann RL et al: DIC panel. In Coagulation Laboratory Manual, Duke University Medical Center, p 17. Durham, Duke University, 1987
15. Handin RI, Moloney WC: Antibody-induced von Willebrand's disease. Blood 44:933, 1974; 48:393, 1976
16. Hathaway WE, Belhanson LP, Hathaway HS: Evidence for a new plasma thromboplastin factor: Case report, coagulation studies, and physiochemical properties. Blood 26:521, 1965
17. Hirsh EF, Magajima T, Oshima G et al: Kinin-system responses in sepsis after trauma in man. J Surg Res 17:147, 1974
18. Hougie C: Hemophilia and related conditions-congenital deficiencies of prothrombin (factor II), factor V, and factors VII to XII. In Williams WJ, Beutler E, Erslev AJ et al (eds): Hematology, 2nd ed, p 1404. New York, McGraw-Hill, 1977
19. Howland WS, Bellville JW, Zucker MB et al: Massive blood replacement. V: Failure to observe citrate intoxication. Surg Gynecol Obstet 105:529, 1957
20. Ingram GIC, Kingston PJ, Leslie J et al: Four cases of acquired von Willebrand's syndrome. Br J Haematol 21:189, 1971
21. Iwanga S, Kato H, Maruyama I et al: Fluorogenic peptide substrates for proteases in blood coagulation, kallikrein-kinin, and fibrinolysis systems: Substrate for plasmin and factor XIₐ. Thromb Haemost 42:49, 1979
22. Josso F, Rio Y, Beguin S: Prothrombin Metz; A new variant of human prothrombin: Double heterozygosity for congenital hypoprothrombinemia and dysprothrombinemia. XVIIth Congress Int Soc Hematol II:800, 1978 (abstr)
23. Mannucci PM: Diagnosis and therapy of hemophilia A. In Koepke JA (ed): Laboratory Hematology, vol 1, p 522. New York, Churchill Livingstone, 1984
24. Mason EC: Thaw-siphon technique for production of cryoprecipitate concentrate of factor VIII. Lancet 2:15, 1978

25. Meyer D, Zimmerman TS: von Willebrand's disease. In Colman RW, Hirsch J, Marder VJ et al (eds): Hemostasis and Thrombosis: Basic Principles and Clinical Practice, p 69. Philadelphia, JB Lippincott, 1982

26. Nakasone N, Watkins E Jr, Janeway CA et al: Experimental studies of circulatory derangement following the massive transfusion of citrated blood: Comparison of blood treated with ACD solution and blood decalcified by ion exchange resin. J Lab Clin Med 43:184, 1954

27. Pavlovsky A: Contribution to the pathogenesis of hemophilia. Blood 2:185, 1947

28. Rapaport SI, Ames SB, Duvall BJ: A plasma coagulation defect in systemic lupus erythematosus arising from hypoprothrombinemia combined with antiprothrombinase activity. Blood 15:212, 1960

29. Roberts HR, Grizzle JE, McLester WD et al: Genetic variants of hemophilia B: detection by means of a specific PTC inhibitor. J Clin Invest 47:360, 1968

30. Saito H, Goldsmith AH Jr: Plasma thromboplastin antecedent (PTA; factor XI): A specific and sensitive radioimmunoassay. Blood 50:377, 1977

31. Salzman EW, Merrill EW: Interaction of blood with artificial surfaces. In Colman RW, Hirsch J, Marder VJ et al (eds): Hemostasis and Thrombosis: Basic Principles and Clinical Practice, p 931. Philadelphia, JB Lippincott, 1982

32. Shapiro SS: Antibodies to blood coagulation factors. Clin Haematol 9:207, 1979

33. Shapiro SS, McCord IS: Prothrombin. In Spaet TH: Hemostasis and Thrombosis, vol 4, p 177. New York, Grune & Stratton, 1978

34. Shapiro SS, Martinez J, Holburn RR: Congenital dysprothrombinemia: An inherited structural disorder of human prothrombin. J Clin Invest 48:2251, 1969

35. Silverberg M, Kaplan AD: Deficiency of factor XI. In Colman RW, Hirsch J, Marder VJ et al (eds): Hemostasis and Thrombosis: Basic Principles and Clinical Practice, p 24. Philadelphia, JB Lippincott, 1982

36. von Willebrand EA: Hereditare Pseudohamophili. Finska Lak Sallsk Handl 68:87, 1926

37. Weinger RS, Rudy C, Moake JL et al: Prothrombin Houston: A dysprothrombin identifiable by crossed immunoelectrofocusing and abnormal *Echis carinatus* venom activation. Blood 55:811, 1980

38. Zimmerman TS, Ratnoff OD, Powell AE: Immunologic differentiation of classic hemophilia (factor VIII deficiency) and von Willebrand's disease. J Clin Invest 50:244, 1971

SUGGESTED READING

Bloom A, Thomas D (eds): Haemostasis and Thrombosis. New York, Churchill Livingstone, 1981

Disorders

Leading

to

Thrombosis

Gordon E. Ens

PATHOPHYSIOLOGY

PRIMARY DISORDERS LEADING TO THROMBOSIS
    Antithrombin III Deficiency
    Protein C Deficiency
    Protein S Deficiency
    Fibrinolytic System Disorders
    Dysfibrinogenemia
    Homocystinuria

SECONDARY DISORDERS OF THROMBOSIS
    Lupus Anticoagulant
    Hemostatic Protein Abnormalities
    Platelet Abnormalities
    Blood Vessel and Flow Abnormalities

The expression "disorders of thrombosis" refers to an increased tendency to develop thrombi and emboli, sometimes called the *hypercoagulable state*.[5,36,54,91,100] Patients may present with laboratory abnormalities (such as antithrombin III or protein C deficiency) or with clinical conditions (such as the postoperative state or malignancy) that have been associated with an increased incidence of thrombosis or thromboembolic complications.

Thrombotic disorders have many etiologies that usually are divided into primary and secondary types. Primary disorders usually are inherited, and their number continues to increase as diagnostic laboratory techniques are developed. Secondary disorders are more common and usually are associated with more than one hemostatic abnormality.

PATHOPHYSIOLOGY

Hemostasis is the complex process of inhibition of blood loss through the combined action of platelets, coagulation factors, and blood vessel integrity. A critical balance between clot activating, inhibiting, and lysing factors is essential.[105] Thrombosis results when hemostasis occurs at an inappropriate time or place.

There are three natural anticoagulant mechanisms that control thrombus formation (Fig. 56-1).[28,53,86] The first, antithrombin III (AT-III), an α_2-globulin serine protease inhibitor, neutralizes thrombin and the other activated serine proteases in the coagulation cascade. Heparin accelerates the formation of antithrombin–thrombin complexes and neutralization of thrombin activity.[84] The second mechanism is the protein C pathway.[22] Protein C, a vitamin K-dependent glycoprotein, is converted by thrombin to activated protein C (pC_a), a serine protease. The rate of activation is greatly increased by thrombomodulin, a cofac-

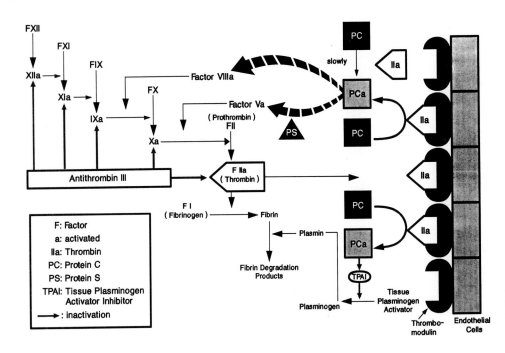

FIG. 56-1.   Interrelations among endothelial cells, protein C, protein S, antithrombin III, and coagulation scheme for regulation of thrombus formation.

tor found on endothelial cell surfaces.[37] The pC_a exerts its anticoagulant effect by inactivating factors V_a and VIII_a, with protein S, another vitamin K-dependent protein, serving as a cofactor.[112] In addition, pC_a facilitates fibrinolysis by neutralizing an inhibitor of plasminogen activator.[70]

The third mechanism is the fibrinolytic system, activation of which produces the serine protease plasmin, which lyses the fibrin clot into fibrin degradation products (FDP). The generation of plasmin from plasminogen is the result of plasminogen activators, which are found in various tissues (*e.g.*, prostate, uterus, kidney). Tissue plasminogen activator (tPA) has a high affinity for fibrin, making it specific for converting plasminogen to plasmin in the forming clot. Tissue plasminogen activator is probably the principal plasminogen activator in blood vessels.

PRIMARY DISORDERS LEADING TO THROMBOSIS

The primary thrombotic disorders are congenital conditions usually involving a single component of the hemostatic system, generally a protein of the coagulation or fibrinolytic system rather than a platelet abnormality. The list of recognized primary disorders (Table 56-1) continues to grow. Patients suffer recurrent thrombosis, often starting at an early age. Some patients are asymptomatic, the condition being discovered by laboratory testing as part of family studies. It is important to recognize risk factors such

TABLE 56-1. Primary Disorders of Thrombosis

Antithrombin III deficiency
Protein C deficiency
Protein S deficiency
Fibrinolytic system disorders
Dysfibrinogenemia
Homocystinuria

as malignancy, postoperative state, pregnancy, and lupus anticoagulant that make these patients more susceptible to thrombosis.

Antithrombin III Deficiency

Quantitative and qualitative defects of AT-III are the best defined and understood of the primary thrombotic disorders. The principal inhibitor of thrombin in plasma, AT-III functions by complexing with and inhibiting thrombin and other activated serine proteases such as factors XII_a, XI_a, X_a, IX_a, plasmin, and protein C. Heparin potentiates the action of AT-III *in vitro* and *in vivo*. Recent evidence indicates that a heparin-like substance (heparan) on the endothelial cell surface plays an important part in regulating thrombosis.[18]

Congenital AT-III deficiency was first reported in 1965 in a family with recurrent venous thromboembolism and approximately 40% of normal plasma AT-III levels.[34] Since then, numerous families have been reported having partial deficiencies of AT-III together with venous and arterial thrombotic disorders. The deficiency is more common than is generally realized, with the estimated incidence in the general population approaching 1 in 2000.[85] Two to three percent of patients hospitalized for deep venous thrombosis or pulmonary embolus have AT-III deficiency.[104] Typically, the defect is inherited as an autosomal dominant trait with males and females being affected equally.[77,114] Heterozygous persons have AT-III levels between 25% and 60% of normal. The homozygous state has not been reported.

Clinical Findings

The most frequent clinical characteristics of AT-III deficiency are recurrent lower-extremity thrombophlebitis and pulmonary embolism; however, thromboembolic events may occur at other anatomic sites.[113] Thrombosis may be seen from the neonatal period to late in life, although, the majority of affected persons manifest symptoms before the age of 35 years.[104] At least 85% of AT-III-deficient individuals will have a thrombotic event by the age of 60.[39] Most thrombotic events are initiated by factors that may also cause thrombosis in persons not deficient in AT-III, especially surgery, trauma, pregnancy, oral contraceptive use, and infection.[113]

Laboratory Findings

The deficiency is detected by measuring antigenic and functional levels of AT-III. Functional AT-III methods should be used to screen for the deficiency state, with an immunologic measurement, if necessary, to confirm a molecular defect or decreased protein level.[38] Immunologic assays (e.g., radioimmunodiffusion, radioimmunoassay) have been used to measure antigenic levels of the molecule, whereas functional activity is determined by measuring the ability of AT-III to inhibit thrombin. See Chapter 53 for details of these assays.

The normal range for functional AT-III in plasma is approximately 80% to 125% of the normal level. Levels of 60% to 80% indicate a moderate thrombotic risk, and levels below 50% to 60% indicate significant risk. Serum rather than plasma levels of functional AT-III are the preferred indicator of thrombotic risk, because serum reflects low plasma AT-III levels in addition to increased consumption of AT-III during the clotting process.[46] The normal range of serum AT-III is 70% to 125% of reference populations.

Effects of Treatment on Laboratory Results

Most patients with AT-III deficiency can be treated with heparin during the acute episodes, and with warfarin for maintenance therapy. Higher than the usual doses of heparin may be required for effective anticoagulation in patients with very low levels of AT-III. Treatment with heparin may temporarily lower the AT-III level by 10% to 15% in patients with active thrombosis. Conversely, treatment with warfarin has been reported to raise AT-III levels, the mechanism being unknown.[69] Concentrates of AT-III are becoming available and can be used to increase the levels during acute episodes of thrombosis or periods of extreme thrombotic risk. Clinical trials are being conducted to define the treatment protocol.

Protein C Deficiency

A more recently described cause of thrombotic disorders is a deficiency of another regulator of the hemostatic system, protein C. Protein C is a vitamin K-dependent glycoprotein that inactivates factors V_a and VIII_a, important cofactors in the generation of coagulation factors X_a and thrombin.[71]

Protein C was discovered in 1960; however, the initial report of a clinical deficiency was not made until 1981.[47] Two types of hereditary protein C deficiency have been reported. In Type I, both the antigen and the activity are below the normal range, whereas in Type II, only the activity is below normal.[22] The incidence of Type I protein C deficiency is about 5% in patients with venous thrombosis under age 40. Frequently, protein C deficiency is inherited as an autosomal dominant trait. Homozygous deficiencies have been reported in infants with severe

thrombosis who have almost no measurable plasma protein C.[22,95] The heterozygous state is associated with venous thrombotic disease and immunologic protein C levels of 40% to 50% of normal.[17]

Clinical Findings

Individuals with protein C deficiency present at an early age with recurrent superficial or deep vein thrombophlebitis and frequent pulmonary emboli. Approximately 50% experience a thromboembolic episode before 30 years of age.[11]

Laboratory Findings

Protein C levels are measured in the laboratory by immunologic and functional assays. Normal ranges for both assays are approximately 70% to 125% of reference levels. Both assays should be performed to distinguish type I from type II deficiency. Because protein C is a vitamin K-dependent protein, levels will be low in patients receiving warfarin. Deficiencies can be determined in anticoagulated patients by measuring immunologic levels of other vitamin K-dependent factors and comparing them with the protein C level. Congenitally deficient individuals will have a disproportionately low level of protein C.

Treatment

Long-term warfarin therapy has been effective in management.[47,95] Warfarin-induced skin necrosis occurs in some patients during the initiation of such therapy, suggesting the advisability of the concomitant use of heparin during this time.[72] Protein C supplementation appears to be useful. Factor IX concentrates are rich in protein C and have been effective in a number of cases.[94] With the development of monoclonal antibodies and genetic cloning, purified protein C may become available soon.[10]

Protein S Deficiency

In 1980, a cofactor was discovered that enhanced the in vitro inactivation of factor V_a by protein C_a. This cofactor was found to be identical to a vitamin K-dependent protein that had been described in 1977 and named protein S.[48]

Clinical Findings

Heterozygous deficient individuals have recurrent venous thrombosis together with immunologic protein S levels of 30% to 60% of reference levels. These persons are similar clinically to patients with heterozygous deficiencies of protein C and AT-III, having an increased tendency for recurrent venous thrombotic disorders that begin in early adulthood.[27,93]

Laboratory Findings

Measurement of protein S by immunologic and functional methods is similar to that of protein C; however, the functional method is not routinely available. Normal ranges are approximately 70% to 125% of reference plasma activity. Warfarin will lower protein S levels, because protein S is vitamin K dependent. Protein S is found free in plasma as well as bound to C4b-binding protein, an inhibitor of the complement system.[93] The C4b-binding protein must be removed from the plasma before measuring protein S, as only the free protein S serves as a cofactor for protein C.

Treatment

Warfarin appears to be the treatment of choice in those individuals with recurring venous thrombosis.

Fibrinolytic System Disorders

Plasminogen, the inactive precursor of plasmin, circulates in the blood in close association with fibrinogen and is trapped in the forming fibrin clot. Plasminogen is activated by tissue or plasma activators. Regulation of the activation to form plasmin is a complex process involving tPA release from the vessel wall, plasma plasminogen activated by factor XII$_a$, and the action of activated protein C to release tPA. Inhibitors such as α_2-antiplasmin retard or halt these processes.

Congenital and acquired disorders involving the fibrinolytic system can impair the breakdown of fibrin, resulting in the buildup of fibrin and thus thrombosis. Quantitative and functional abnormalities of plasminogen have been reported in individuals with recurrent thrombosis,[4,68] and several families with defective release of tPA from the vessel wall have been reported.[60,99] Deficiencies in factor XII may result in reduced activation of plasma plasminogen activator.[33] Circulating inhibitors of plasminogen activator may also reduce the activation of plasminogen.[76]

Functional (qualitative) and immunologic (quantitative) assays for plasminogen are available. Generally, the functional levels are decreased more than immunologic levels, indicating a qualitative defect in the plasminogen molecule.[65,88] Assays for tissue and plasma plasminogen activators and tPA inhibitor are just being introduced into the clinical laboratory.

Dysfibrinogenemia

Congenital disorders with clinically significant functional abnormalities of fibrinogen (dysfibrinogenemia) have been reported occasionally in conjunction with increased thrombosis.[2,19,35] The functionally abnormal fibrinogen molecule forms a rigid fibrin gel that is resistant to the fibrinolytic enzyme system.

Homocystinuria

A rare autosomal recessive disorder, homocystinuria is associated with a high incidence of arterial and venous thrombosis early in life, resulting in a high morbidity and mortality rate.[51] Endothelial cell injury apparently is responsible for the abnormal platelet–vessel wall interaction.

SECONDARY DISORDERS OF THROMBOSIS

The secondary disorders of thrombosis (Table 56-2) consist of a variety of clinical conditions associated with a high degree of thromboembolic complications. The exact pathophysiology leading to the thrombosis is not yet fully understood; however, several abnormalities of hemostasis

TABLE 56–2. Secondary Disorders of Thrombosis

Lupus anticoagulant
Hemostatic protein abnormalities
Postoperative state
Malignancy
Pregnancy
Oral contraceptives and estrogens
Other
Nephrotic syndrome
Coronary artery disease
Stroke
Platelet abnormalities
Diabetes mellitus
Hyperlipidemia
Myeloproliferative disorders
Heparin-induced thrombocytopenia
Blood vessel and flow abnormalities
Artificial surfaces
Damaged vessels
Abnormal blood flow

have been observed. Understanding these associations is important in selecting the most appropriate therapy or in eliminating the underlying cause. Many disorders have more than one mechanism affecting normal hemostasis, making classification difficult.

Lupus Anticoagulant

An acquired immunoglobulin directed against phospholipids, lupus anticoagulant, has been associated with an increased risk of thrombosis, possibly secondary to prostacyclin inhibition.[20,74] The immunoglobulin can be present in patients with systemic lupus erythematosus, other autoimmune disorders, or neoplasms; during certain drug therapy; or sometimes without apparent cause.

Inhibition of phospholipid by the lupus anticoagulant in in vitro clotting test systems results in a prolonged APTT and occasionally, a prolonged PT. The tissue thromboplastin inhibition test or the platelet neutralization procedure can be used to quantitate the circulating anticoagulant (see Chap. 53).

Hemostatic Protein Abnormalities

Several clinical conditions discussed below, such as postoperative states, malignancies, and pregnancy, have been associated with increased thrombosis. Laboratory findings are similar in that changes are observed in hemostatic proteins.

There may be increases in one or more coagulation factors (I, II, V, VII, VIII, IX, and X) or decreases in AT-III, protein C, or fibrinolytic activity. Increased thrombin generation may also be observed.[8] It should be noted, however, that hypercoagulability attributable solely to increased levels of coagulation factors is not a universally accepted cause of thrombosis. A mechanism of factor activation usually is present also.

Postoperative State

The postoperative state, particularly after orthopedic procedures, is a complex example of secondary hypercoagulability.[50,58] A contributor to the evolution of a thrombotic event is the exposure of blood to activating tissue substances released during surgery. This probably is exaggerated by the venous stasis accompanying patient immobility. The frequency of deep venous thrombosis in patients undergoing hip surgery is reported to be as high as 50% with a high incidence of pulmonary embolus.[62,98] Patients with primary hypercoagulable states are at increased risk. Contributing risk factors include immobilization, advanced age, obesity, malignancy, oral contraceptive use, pregnancy, and the increase in platelets that often follows surgical trauma.

Malignancy

Increased thrombosis in malignancy frequently is related to the release of coagulation activating factors by the neoplastic cells. This relation has been observed for years, beginning with Trousseau's report more than a century ago.[109] The incidence of thrombosis in cancer patients is approximately 5% to 15% generally and is as high as 50% in certain malignancies.[12,83] Patients with adenocarcinomas seem to be especially susceptible to thrombosis.[45,81,97,102]

Treatment of thrombosis in cancer patients is difficult because of resistance to anticoagulation and the potential for bleeding complications from necrotic tumor sites. Typically, the hemostatic abnormalities are corrected by elimination of the malignancy.

Pregnancy

The placenta is rich in tissue thromboplastin and may be one of the underlying factors causing thrombosis in pregnancy. Other potential etiologies are decreased blood flow (stasis), increased levels of coagulation proteins (especially factors VII, VIII, and fibrinogen), and decreased levels of AT-III.

There is a definite increase in the incidence of thromboembolic complications during the antepartum period.[1,40,57,106] The actual frequency of thrombosis during pregnancy may be underestimated because of failure to recognize subclinical events.[107] Antepartum subclinical events may become evident in the postpartum period as thrombophlebitis, venous insufficiency, pulmonary hypertension, or postphlebitic syndrome. During the first month after delivery, a 20- to 50-fold increase exists in the risk of phlebitis and thromboembolism. Thromboembolic risk during pregnancy increases with age, parity, hypertension, and nonvaginal delivery. The risk is much greater in women who have preeclampsia or eclampsia or who have cesarean section.[13,52]

Oral Contraceptive or Estrogen Use

Oral contraceptive use increases the risk of cardiovascular,[8,63,106] cerebrovascular,[24,29,32,101] and venous thromboembolic events[87,89,111] according to the results of most epidemiologic studies. Other thromboembolic complications that have been associated with oral contraceptive use include renal artery thrombosis,[43] peripheral artery occlusion,[79] mesenteric vascular insufficiency,[82] aorto-iliac arterial thrombosis,[30] and Budd-Chiari syndrome.[67]

Estrogen used to treat prostate cancer[14] or arterial disease[29] and to prevent lactation[31] has likewise been associated with an increase in thromboembolic disease. Estrogens

may increase the thrombotic risk by altering the rate of blood flow[44] and blood viscosity.[5,6]

Other Causes

Secondary hypercoagulable states may be found in patients with nephrotic syndrome,[41,66] coronary artery disease,[59,80] and stroke.[56,115] In addition to plasma protein abnormalities, these patients frequently exhibit hyperactive platelet function and elevated levels of von Willebrand factor.

Decreased levels of AT-III have been observed in individuals who are morbidly obese[7] or severely burned.[16]

Platelet Abnormalities

Platelet abnormalities typically observed in secondary thrombotic disorders include elevated numbers; increased aggregation response to ADP, collagen, and epinephrine; and increased levels of beta-thromboglobulin and platelet factor 4. Clinical conditions in which these abnormalities are frequently observed include diabetes mellitus,[26,75] hyperlipidemia,[21,108] myeloproliferative disorders,[90] and heparin-induced platelet agglutination and thrombocytopenia.[9,64]

Blood Vessel and Flow Abnormalities

Artificial Surfaces

Situations in which circulating blood is exposed to artificial surfaces create a substantial risk of thrombosis. The more common situations are vascular grafts, prosthetic heart valves, and hemodialysis or hemoperfusion procedures. The foreign surface activates platelets, causing increased adhesion and aggregation with activation of the coagulation system.

Abnormal Vascular Surfaces

Damaged blood vessels may contribute to thrombosis by disrupting the normal antithrombotic function of endothelium. This is seen in a variety of disease states such as vasculitis,[78] scleroderma,[61] systemic lupus erythematosus,[3,74] Kawasaki disease,[73] chronic occlusive arterial disease,[110] and Behçet's disease.[92] Increased levels of von Willebrand factor and decreased fibrinolytic activity are typical laboratory findings. The use of veins as coronary artery bypass grafts may create an environment that increases the risk of thrombosis.

Abnormal Blood Flow

Venous stasis, a risk factor for thrombosis, probably causes vascular endothelial damage through local hypoxia[49] and slow removal of activated clotting factors from a site of vascular injury.[96] Immobilization is an important contributor to venous stasis,[42,55] as is hyperviscosity, because of the elevated numbers of cells, increased cell rigidity, or elevated plasma protein concentrations.[15]

CHAPTER SUMMARY

This chapter has addressed laboratory and clinical recognition of disorders leading to thrombosis, as well as the pathophysiology of the primary thrombotic states and some of the clinical conditions associated secondarily with thrombotic states. Significant progress has been made in our understanding of thrombosis and thrombotic risk; however, much remains to be discovered. As new tests are developed and become more widely available, the diagnosis of the thrombotic disorders and management of affected patients will be easier.

REFERENCES

1. Aaro LA, Johnson TR, Juergens JL: Acute deep venous thrombosis associated with pregnancy. Obstet Gynecol 28:553, 1966
2. Al-Mondhiry HAB, Bilezikian SB, Nossel HL: Fibrinogen "New York," an abnormal fibrinogen associated with thromboembolism: Functional evaluation. Blood 45:607, 1975
3. Angles-Cano E, Sultan Y, Clauvel JP: Predisposing factors to thrombosis in systemic lupus erythematosus: Possible relation to endothelial cell damage. J Lab Clin Med 94:312, 1979
4. Aoki N, Moroi M, Sakata Y et al: Abnormal plasminogen: A hereditary molecular abnormality found in a patient with recurrent thrombosis. J Clin Invest 61:1186, 1978
5. Aronson HB, Magora F, Schenker JG: Effect of oral contraceptives on blood viscosity. Am J Obstet Gynecol 110:997, 1971
6. Ball AP, McKee PA: Fibrin formation and dissolution in women receiving oral contraceptive drugs. J Lab Clin Med 89:751, 1977
7. Batist G, Bothe A Jr, Bern M et al: Low antithrombin III in morbid obesity: Return to normal with weight reduction. JPEN 7:447, 1983
8. Bauer KA, Rosenberg RD: Assays for thrombin generation in humans with prethrombotic states. Thromb Haemost 50:159, 1983
9. Bell WR, Tomasulo PA, Alving BM et al: Thrombocytopenia occurring during the administration of heparin: A prospective study in 52 patients. Ann Intern Med 85:155, 1976
10. Bertina RM, Broekmans AW: Protein C concentrates for therapeutic use. Lancet 2:1348, 1982
11. Bertina RM, Broekmans AW: Congenital deficiency of protein C. Symposia by Diagnostica Stago, October 11, 1983
12. Bick RL: Alterations of hemostasis associated with malignancy. Semin Thromb Hemost 5:1, 1978
13. Biland L, Duckert F: Coagulation factors of the newborn and his mother. Thromb Diath Haemorrh 29:644, 1973
14. Blackard CE, Doe RP, Mellinger GT et al: Incidence of cardiovascular disease and death in patients receiving diethylstilbestrol for carcinoma of the prostate. Cancer 26:249, 1970
15. Bloch JD, Maki DD: Hypervisocosity syndromes associated with immunologulin abnormalities. Semin Hematol 10:113, 1973
16. Braunstein KM, Dodds KA, Steward G et al: Heparin cofactor activity following thermal injury. Am J Clin Pathol 70:632, 1978
17. Broekmans AW, Veltkamp JJ, Bertina RM: Congenital protein C deficiency and venous thromboembolism: A study of three Dutch families. N Engl J Med 309:340, 1983
18. Bussel JB: Circulating anticoagulants: Physiologic and pathologic. Hosp Pract 18:169, 1983
19. Carrel N, Gabrial DA, Blatt PM et al: Hereditary dysfibrinogenemia in a patient with thrombotic disease. Blood 62:439, 1983
20. Carreras LO, Vermylen JG: "Lupus" anticoagulant and thrombosis: Possible role of inhibition of prostacyclin formation. Thromb Haemost 48:33, 1982
21. Carvalho ACA, Colman RW, Lees RS: Platelet function in hyperlipoproteinemia. N Engl J Med 290:434, 1974
22. Clouse LH, Comp PC: The regulation of hemostasis: The protein C system. N Engl J Med 314:1298, 1986
23. Collaborative Group for the Study of Stroke in Young Women: Contraceptives and stroke in young women. JAMA 288:871, 1973
24. Collaborative Group for the Study of Stroke in Young Women: Oral contraception and increased risk of cerebral ischemia or thrombosis. JAMA 231:718, 1975
25. Collins GJ Jr, Ahr DJ, Rich NM et al: Detection and management of hypercoagulability. Am J Surg 132:767, 1976
26. Colwell JA, Halushka PV: Platelet function in diabetes mellitus. Br J Haematol 44:521, 1980
27. Comp PC, Esmon CT: Recurrent venous thromboembolism in patients with a partial deficiency of protein S. N Engl J Med 311:1525, 1984
28. Conard J, Samama MM: Inhibitors of coagulation, atherosclerosis and arterial thrombosis. Semin Thromb Hemost 12:87, 1986
29. Coronary Drug Project Research Group: The coronary drug project: Initial findings leading to modifications of its research protocol. JAMA 214:1303, 1970
30. Dahlback LD, Rais D: Aorto-iliac arterial thrombosis in young women: Report of 3 cases. Acta Chir Scand 143:127, 1977
31. Daniel DG, Campbell H, Turnbull AC: Puerperal thromboembolism and suppression of lactation. Lancet 2: 287, 1967
32. Durand JL, Bressler R: Clinical pharmacology of the steroidal oral contraceptives. Adv Intern Med 24:97, 1979
33. Dyerberg H, Stoffersen E: Recurrent thrombosis in a patient with factor XII deficiency. Acta Hematol 63:278, 1980
34. Egeberg O: Inherited antithrombin deficiency causing thrombophilia. Thromb Diath Haemorrh 13:516, 1965
35. Egeberg O: Inherited fibrinogen abnormality causing thrombophilia. Thromb Diath Haemorrh 17:176, 1967
36. Ens GE, Hamstra RD: Hypercoagulation. Monograph, 1981
37. Esmon CT: Protein-C: Biochemistry, physiology and clinical implications. Blood 62:1155, 1983
38. Fareed J, Messmore HL, Walenga JM et al: Laboratory evaluation of antithrombin III: A critical overview of currently available methods for antithrombin-III measurements. Semin Thromb Hemost 8:288, 1982
39. Filip DJ, Eckstein JD, Veltkamp JJ: Hereditary antithrombin III deficiency and thromboembolic disease. Am J Hematol 2:343, 1976
40. Fleischner FG: Recurrent pulmonary embolism and corpulmonale. N Engl J Med 276:1213, 1976
41. Francis RB, Sandler RM, Levitan D: Use of noninvasive laboratory testing in the prediction of thrombosis in the nephrotic syndrome. Am J Nephrol 4:43, 1984
42. Gallus AS: Venous thromboembolism: Incidence and clinical risk factors. In Madden JPL, Hume M (eds): Venous Thromboembolism: Prevention and Treatment. New York, Appleton-Century-Crofts, 1976
43. Golbus SM, Swerdlin AR, Mitas JA et al: Renal artery thrombosis in a young woman taking oral contraceptives. Ann Intern Med 90:939, 1979
44. Goodrich SM, Wood JE: Peripheral venous distensibility and velocity of venous blood flow during pregnancy or during oral contraceptive therapy. Am J Obstet Gynecol 90:740, 1964
45. Gordon SG, Cross BA: A factor X-activating cysteine protease from malignant tissue. J Clin Invest 67:1665, 1981
46. Gray AJ: Antithrombin III Check Sample: Thrombosis and Hemostasis No. TH 80-5 (TH-11). Chicago, American Society of Clinical Pathologists, 1981
47. Griffin JH, Evatt B, Zimmerman TS et al: Deficiency of protein C in congenital thrombotic disease. J Clin Invest 68:1370, 1981
48. Griffin JH, Mosher DF, Zimmerman TS et al: Protein C, an

antithrombotic protein, is reduced in hospitalized patients with intravascular coagulation. Blood 60:261, 1982

49. Hamer JD, Malone PC, Silver IA: The pO_2 in venous valve pockets: Its possible bearing on thrombogenesis. Br J Surg 68:166, 1981

50. Hampson WGJ, Harris FC, Lucas HK et al: Failure of low-dose heparin to prevent deep vein thrombosis after hip replacement arthroplasty. Lancet 1:795, 1974

51. Harker LA, Slichter SJ, Scott CR et al: Homocystinemia: Vascular injury and arterial thrombosis. N Engl J Med 291:537, 1974

52. Hathaway WE, Bonnar J: Perinatal Coagulation. New York, Grune & Stratton, 1978

53. Hill RJ, Ens GE: The protein C pathway. Clin Hemost Rev 1:1, 1987

54. Hirsch J: Hypercoagulability. Semin Hematol 14:409, 1977

55. Hirsch J, Genton E, Hull R: Venous Thromboembolism. New York, Grune & Stratton, 1981

56. Hossmann V, Heiss WD, Bewermeyer H: Antithrombin III deficiency in ischaemic stroke. Klin Wochensch 61:617, 1983

57. Howie PW: Thromboembolism. Clin Obstet Gynecol 4:397, 1977

58. Hume M, Turner RH, Kuriakose TX et al: Venous thrombosis after total hip replacement. J Bone Joint Surg 58:933, 1976

59. Innerfield I, Goldfischer JD, Reicher–Reiss H: Serum antithrombin in coronary-artery disease. Am J Clin Pathol 65:64, 1976

60. Johanson L, Hedner U, Nilsson IM: A family with thromboembolic disease associated with deficient fibrinolytic activity in vessel wall. Acta Med Scand 203:477, 1978

61. Kahaleh MB, Osborn I, LeRoy EC: Increased factor VIII/von Willebrand factor antigen and von Willebrand factor activity in scleroderma and in Raynaud's phenomenon. Ann Intern Med 94:482, 1981

62. Kakkar VV: The diagnosis of deep vein thrombosis using the ^{125}I fibrinogen test. Arch Surg 104:152, 1972

63. Kaplan NM: Cardiovascular complications of oral contraceptives. Annu Rev Med 29:31, 1978

64. Kappa JR, Fisher CA, Berkowitz HD et al: Heparin-induced platelet activation in sixteen surgical patients: Diagnosis and management. J Vasc Surg 5:101, 1987

65. Kazama M, Tahara C, Suzuki Z et al: Abnormal plasminogen, a cause of recurrent thrombosis. Thromb Res 21:517, 1981

66. Kendall AG, Lohmann RC, Dossetor JB: Nephrotic syndrome, a hypercoagulable state. Arch Intern Med 127:1021, 1971

67. Lewis JH, Tice HL, Zimmerman HJ: Budd-Chiari syndrome associated with oral contraceptive steroids: Review of treatment of 47 cases. Dig Dis Sci 28:673, 1983

68. Lottenberg R, Dolly FR, Kitchens CS: Pulmonary hypertension and recurrent thromboembolic phenomena associated with hypoplasminogenemia. Clin Res 31:318A, 1983 (abstr)

69. Marciniak E, Farley CH, DeSimone PA: Familial thrombosis due to antithrombin III deficiency. Blood 43:219, 1974

70. Marlar RA, Kleiss AJ, Griffin JH: Mechanism of action of human activated protein C, a thrombin-dependent anticoagulant enzyme. Blood 59:1067, 1982

71. Marlar RA, Kleiss AJ, Griffin JH: Human protein C: Inactivation of factors V and VIII by the activated molecule. Ann NY Acad Sci 370:303, 1981

72. McGehee WG, Klotz TA, Epstein DJ et al: Coumarin necrosis associated with hereditary protein C deficiency. Ann Intern Med 101:59, 1984

73. Mercer S: Kawasaki disease and its complications. Compr Ther 7:52, 1981

74. Mueh JR, Herbst KD, Rapaport SI: Thrombosis in patients with the lupus anticoagulant. Ann Intern Med 92:156, 1980

75. Mustard JF, Packham MA: Platelets and diabetes mellitus. N Engl J Med 311:665, 1984 (edit)

76. Nilsson IM, Krook H, Sternby NH et al: Severe thrombotic disease in a young man with bone marrow and skeletal changes and with a high content of an inhibitor in the fibrinolytic system. Acta Med Scand 169:323, 1961

77. Nossel HL, Yudelman I, Canfield et al: Measurement of fibrinopeptide A in human Blood. J Clin Invest 54:43, 1974

78. Nusinow SR, Federici AB, Zimmerman TS et al: Increased von Willebrand factor antigen in the plasma of patients with vasculitis. Arthritis Rheum 27:1405, 1984

79. O'Conner J, Pollock JG: Acute arterial occlusion and the contraceptive pill. J Cardiovasc Surg 16:176, 1975

80. Pickering NJ, Brody JI, Fink GB et al: The behavior of antithrombin III, alpha-2-macroglobulin and alpha-1 antitrypsin during cardiopulmonary bypass. Am J Clin Pathol 80:459, 1983

81. Pineo GF, Brzin MC, Gallus AS et al: Tumors, mucus production and hypercoagulability. Ann NY Acad Sci 230:262, 1974

82. Prust FW, Kuman GK: Massive colonic bleeding and oral contraceptive "pills." Am J Obstet Gynecol 125:695, 1976

83. Rickles FR, Edwards RL: Activation of blood coagulation in cancer: Trousseau's syndrome revisited. Blood 62:14, 1983

84. Rosenberg RD, Damus PS: The purification and mechanism of action of human antithrombin–heparin cofactor. J Biol Chem 248:6490, 1973

85. Rosenberg RD: Actions and interactions of antithrombin and heparin. N Engl J Med 292:146, 1975

86. Rosenberg RD, Rosenberg JS: Natural anticoagulant mechanisms. J Clin Invest 74:1, 1984

87. Sager S, Thomas DP, Stamatakis JD et al: Oral contraceptives, antithrombin III activity and postoperative deep-vein thrombosis. Lancet 1:509, 1976

88. Sakata Y, Aoki N: Molecular abnormality of plasminogen. J Biol Chem 255:5442, 1980

89. Sartwell PE: Oral contraceptives and thromboembolism: A further report. Am J Epidemiol 94:192, 1971

90. Schafer AI: Bleeding and thrombosis in the myeloproliferative disorders. Blood 64:1, 1984

91. Schafer AI: The hypercoagulable states. Ann Intern Med 102:814, 1985

92. Schmitz–Huebner U, Knop J: Evidence for endothelial cell dysfunction in association with Behçet's disease. Thromb Res 34:277, 1984

93. Schwarz HP, Fisher M, Hopmeier P et al: Plasma protein S deficiency in familial thrombotic disease. Blood 64:1297, 1984

94. Seghatchian MJ: Protein C in clinical factor IX concentrates. Lancet 1:1047, 1983

95. Seligsohn U, Berger A, Abend M et al: Homozygous protein C deficiency manifested by massive venous thrombosis in the newborn. N Engl J Med 310:559, 1984

96. Shattil SJ: Diagnosis and treatment of recurrent venous thromboembolism. Med Clin North Am 68:577, 1984

97. Slichter SJ, Harker LA: Hemostasis in malignancy. Ann NY Acad Sci 230:252, 1974

98. Smyrnis SA, Kolios AS: Deep vein thrombosis in surgical patients: A phlebographic study. Surgery 73:692, 1973

99. Stead NW, Bauer KA, Kinney TR et al: Venous thrombosis in a family with defective release of vascular plasminogen activator and elevated plasma factor VIII/von Willebrand's factor. Am J Med 74:33, 1983

100. Stead RB: The hypercoagulable state. In Goldhaver SZ (ed): Pulmonary Embolism and Deep Venous Thrombosis. Philadelphia. WB Saunders, 1985

101. Stolley PD, Tonascia JA, Tockman MS et al: Thrombosis with low-estrogen oral contraceptives. Am J Epidemiol 102:97, 1975

102. Sun NC, McAfee WM, Hum GJ et al: Hemostatic abnormalities in malignancy, a prospective study of one hundred eight patients. I: Coagulation studies. Am J Clin Pathol 71:10, 1979

103. Teitel JM, Bauer KA, Lau HK et al: Studies of the prothrombin activation pathway utilizing radioimmunoassays for the F_2/F_{1+2} fragment and thrombin:antithrombin complex. Blood 59:1086, 1982

104. Thaler E, Lechner K: Antithrombin-III deficiency and thromboembolism. Clin Haematol 10:369, 1981

105. Thompson AR, Harker LA: Manual of Thrombosis and Hemostasis, p 142. Philadelphia, FA Davis, 1983

106. Tooke JE, McNicol GP: Thrombotic disorders associated with pregnancy and the pill. Clin Haematol 10:613, 1981

107. Treffers PE, Huidekoper BL, Weenink GH et al: Epidemiological observations of thromboembolic disease during pregnancy and in the puerperium in 56,022 women. Int J Gynaecol Obstet 21:327, 1983

108. Tremoli E, Maderna P, Sirtori M et al: Platelet aggregation and malondialdehyde formation in type IIA hypercholesterolemic patients. Haemostasis 8:47, 1979

109. Trousseau A: Phelegmasia alba dolens. Clin Med Htel Dieu Paris 3:94, 1865

110. Verstraete M, Vermylen J, Verhaeghe RH: Peripheral arterial diseases. Clin Haematol 10:669, 1981

111. Vessey MP, Mann JI: Female sex hormones and thrombosis. Br Med Bull 34:157, 1978

112. Walker FJ: Regulation of activated protein C by protein S. J Biol Chem 256:1128, 1981

113. Winter JH, Fenech A, Ridley W et al: Familial antithrombin III deficiency. Q J Med 51:373, 1982

114. Yudelman I, Greenberg J: Factor affecting fibrinopeptide A levels during anticoagulant therapy. Blood 59:787, 1982

115. Zheng L: Increased factor VIII related antigen in cerebral thrombosis. Thromb Res 32:321, 1983

Laboratory Monitoring of Anticoagulant Therapy

Harlene S. Palkuti

The aim of anticoagulant therapy is the prevention of thrombus formation or extension. Thrombi usually begin in two ways: attached to an injured vessel wall or as unattached intravascular masses. The term *thrombosis* implies an abnormal mass that partially or totally obstructs a vein or artery.

The approaches to the treatment of thrombosis differ according to the differences between arterial and venous thrombus formation. Treatment with anticoagulant drugs tends to be effective when intravascular fibrin formation is the predominant pathologic process (*e.g.*, deep vein thrombosis), whereas such treatment is of limited value when platelet aggregation is the principal factor in thrombus formation (*e.g.*, coronary artery thrombosis). Antiplatelet drugs may be of value in these cases. The objectives of therapy in deep vein thrombosis are to prevent propagation and embolization of the thrombi and to minimize damage to the vessel itself. Two treatments that have historically been used to slow the formation of fibrin are parenteral heparin and oral anticoagulants. An important therapeutic treatment for arterial thrombosis and platelet emboli is inhibition of normal platelet function (adhesion and aggregation) by agents such as aspirin, sulfinpyrazone, and dipyridamole. A type of anti-clot therapy capable of producing direct clot lysis *in vivo*, such as the use of plasminogen activators, is considered in life-threatening conditions such as acute extensive occlusions of the coronary arteries, peripheral deep veins (leg or arm), or pulmonary arteries. Various laboratory procedures have been useful in demonstrating that an effective dose of plasminogen activator has been administered and that the potential for significant lysis of a thrombus exists.

HEPARIN THERAPY

Heparin was the first agent administered as an anticoagulant.[11] Heparin can be used to prevent the formation of thrombi in veins or to prevent the propagation of previously formed thrombi in veins and arteries. It is now used extensively throughout the world for the treatment of venous thrombosis and pulmonary embolism. It also remains the recommended treatment for active thrombophlebitis and arterial thrombosis.[19]

Anticoagulant Activity

Therapeutic heparin is a mixture of mucopolysaccharides of various chain lengths and molecular weights. Heparin interferes with hemostasis both *in vivo* and *in vitro* by inhibiting the action of factors XII_a, XI_a, X_a, IX_a, and II_a; the conversion of fibrinogen to fibrin; the aggregation of platelets by thrombin; and the activation of fibrin-stabilizing enzyme.[21] Heparin activity requires the presence of antithrombin III (AT III), which is an α_2-globulin produced in the liver. Heparin interacts with a lysine group on the AT III molecule, exposing a reactive arginine site. This exposed site then inhibits the active site of other serine proteases, including coagulation factors XII_a, XI_a, X_a, IX_a, and II_a.[28]

The molecular weights of different heparin molecules influence their anticoagulant activity. Low-molecular-weight heparin (derived from porcine mucosa) causes fewer hemorrhagic complications, because platelet function is altered to a lesser extent than when high-molecular-weight heparin is employed. High-molecular-weight fractions of heparin (derived from bovine lung) may prolong the bleeding time.[10]

Rarely, heparin results in a persistent and severe thrombocytopenia (below $10 \times 10^9/L$) that develops from the first to the 21st day after drug administration and necessitates monitoring of the platelet count every 2 days for the first 3 weeks of therapy. Once heparin is discontinued, platelet counts usually return to the reference range within 2 to 5 days.

The anticoagulant activity of heparin can be reversed immediately with protamine sulfate, which combines with heparin to form a nondissociable salt.[29] Other drugs that inhibit the anticoagulant properties of heparin include antihistamines, digitalis, nicotine, phenothiazines, penicillin administered intravenously, and tetracycline.[21]

Administration

The physician chooses one of three methods to administer heparin: intermittent bolus injection, continuous infusion, or minidose subcutaneous injection. The laboratory is required to monitor the effectiveness of heparin regardless of the method of administration. The most conventional method of administration of heparin in the past was the use of pulsed intravenous (IV) injections of 5000 U every 4 to 6 hours.[29] Immediately after injection, there is an excessive prolongation of the coagulation mechanism, followed by a rapid falloff in the effect because of the short (1- to 2-hour) half-life of heparin. Therefore, immediately before the next scheduled injection, the patient may no longer be anticoagulated. Laboratory tests to monitor the effects of this mode of therapy may be requested as many as four to six times daily.

Continuous IV infusion of heparin has now become the most popular method of administration. It can achieve a steady antithrombotic effect by using constant-rate pumps or conventional IV sets with heparin added to the bottles. A loading dose of 5000 U is given with the rate of administration then decreased to 1000 U hourly.[29] Laboratory monitoring is required once per day.

Low-dose heparin (also called "minidose heparin") administered by subcutaneous injection (5000 U every 12 hours) lowers the risk of hemorrhage, as well as the need to monitor the effects by laboratory testing. The circulating level of heparin seldom exceeds 0.1 U/mL of plasma.[19] Low-dose heparin is used *prophylactically* to protect against pulmonary embolism by preventing deep vein thrombosis. This particular approach to anticoagulant therapy has been useful in preventing thromboembolism when administered prior to, during, and after surgery. Concentrations as low as 0.02 U/mL of plasma have been effective in the prevention of venous thromboembolism after major surgery.[26] Minidose heparin also has been used in other high-risk groups such as patients of advanced age; those with leg fractures, cancer, or obesity; those undergoing hip surgery, varicose vein surgery, or estrogen therapy; those having disseminated intravascular coagulation (DIC) or congestive heart failure; and those with a history of venous thrombosis.[32]

Laboratory Monitoring and Therapeutic Range

The clinician strives to attain an optimal dose of heparin, one that will prevent the extension of thrombosis with a minimum of hemorrhage, generally termed the *therapeutic range*. Attainment of this range should correspond to a laboratory result that represents 0.2 to 0.5 U of heparin/mL of plasma.[10] Distinct differences in the sensitivity to heparin have been demonstrated for various laboratory procedures such as the Lee–White or whole blood clotting time (LWCT), the activated coagulation time (ACT), the activated partial thromboplastin time (APTT), the prothrombin time (PT), and the thrombin time (TT).[17]

The first method used to monitor the effect of heparin was the LWCT.[14] Studies have shown that prolongation of the result occurs with increasing concentrations of heparin; however, there may be considerable scatter in the clot times produced at each concentration of heparin (poor reproducibility), and typical coefficients of variation are 15% to 30%.[29] This test also lacks sensitivity in that doubling the circulating level of heparin may produce minimal change in the LWCT, whereas other procedures often demonstrate a twofold to threefold change. Finally, the test is time consuming to perform.

The ACT has been advocated for monitoring heparin,[9] but there appears to be poor correlation between the amount of heparin present and the clotting times produced.[17] Excess activation of contact-phase factors may mask the effect of heparin. In addition, problems may be encountered in developing a quality control program for the ACT because of the lack of adequate commercial controls.

The APTT is a useful sensitive procedure for monitoring heparin therapy, and the College of American Pathologists survey data indicate that the APTT has become the method of choice for this application.[3] Clinical studies have demonstrated that the risk of recurrent venous thromboembolism is low (3%) provided the APTT is maintained at 1.0 to 1.5 times the control time, corresponding to a heparin level of 0.3 to 0.5 U/mL of plasma.[10] The procedure is sensitive to relatively small amounts of heparin, but considerable variation is exhibited in the presence of higher concentrations. Relatively small scatter of the data for various concentrations of heparin and clotting times produced has been demonstrated.[17] Unfortunately, some phospholipid extracts, as well as activators in current commercial reagents for the APTT, may lack the sensitivity needed to demonstrate the presence of small concentrations of heparin and so may fail to detect therapeutic levels adequately.[2,5,18,26] Also, a recent study has demonstrated a marked variation in heparin sensitivity among different reagents, and the development of a national APTT standard reagent has been proposed.[4] Laboratories that use various types of clot detection instrumentation may discover the need to generate an *in vitro* heparin therapeutic range for each instrument, as demonstrated in Figure 57-1. It is recommended that each hospital choosing to monitor heparin therapy with the APTT determine its own therapeutic range to reflect the laboratory's specific reagents, instrumentation, and personnel.[12] Finally, if an expected prolongation of the APTT is not achieved, the possibility of decreased levels of AT III should be considered.[24]

The TT can be used to monitor any form of heparin administration, and it is not influenced by plasma factor deficiencies, as are the ACT and APTT tests. Although some authors view the fact that the TT measures only the effect of heparin on thrombin as a disadvantage,[29] this technique may be useful in monitoring heparin therapy for a patient with known coagulation factor deficiency. The TT

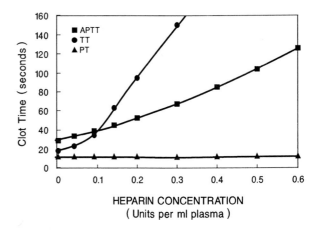

FIG. 57-2.   Sensitivity to heparin of various laboratory tests. Observe the sensitivity to small amounts achieved by recalcified thrombin time. Note also that PT test is insensitive to therapeutic concentrations of heparin.

is sensitive to heparin effects for several hours but may be subject to considerable inaccuracy and difficulty in obtaining good duplicate readings on the same test sample. Some authors claim that the recalcified TT technique has a slightly better sensitivity to low-dose heparin with a more easily detectable endpoint than the conventional test.[22,26] Clot times produced in the therapeutic range (0.2–0.5 U of heparin/mL) are long (94–150 seconds) and may be difficult to reproduce on current laboratory instrumentation. Figure 57-2 presents one study demonstrating the effect of heparin on the recalcified TT results, as well as those of the PT and the APTT.[17]

A laboratory may be asked to quantitate the heparin in a blood sample rather than to evaluate its effect on the hemostatic system. For example, it may be important to verify the presence of heparin in the circulation or to rule out an error in calculation of the dosage of heparin administered. The actual amount of heparin present in the test sample may be determined by two recently introduced methods: chromogenic and fluorogenic substrate assays.[1,29] The disadvantages of these techniques are that they are time-consuming, which makes them impractical on a day-to-day basis; that some methods are insensitive to clinically important small concentrations of heparin; and that they require special instrumentation not available in many routine coagulation laboratories.[26]

ORAL ANTICOAGULANTS

Oral anticoagulants include dicumarol and warfarin, both derivatives of 4-hydroxycoumarin. Warfarin is more popular because of the lower number of harmful side effects reported. These oral anticoagulants prevent the activation of the clotting sequence by altering hepatic synthesis of vitamin K-dependent procoagulant zymogens, clotting factors II, VII, IX, and X (also known as the prothrombin group factors). Oral anticoagulants have no direct effect on clot lysis.

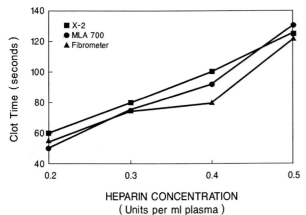

Instrument Sensitivity to Heparin Using the APTT Test

FIG. 57-1.   Differences in sensitivity to heparin levels demonstrated by various clot detection instruments.

Anticoagulant Activity

Therapy with warfarin-type compounds results in the inability of the liver to carboxylate the glutamyl residues of factors II, VII, IX, and X, leading to lower levels of normal vitamin K-dependent factors. The resultant nonfunctional proteins (formerly referred to as *proteins induced by vitamin K antagonists* or PIVKA; more recently called des-γ-carboxy proteins) do not have calcium-binding properties that allow them to bind to a phospholipid surface, a necessary step for activation of clotting.[32]

The rate of reduction in the prothrombin group factors after administration of oral anticoagulants is related to the normal metabolic turnover (half-life) of each individual factor. Factor VII has the shortest half-life and therefore decreases first: between 5 and 6 hours after the initiation of warfarin. Factor IX decreases within 28 to 40 hours, followed by factor X with a half-life of 40 to 50 hours and last, factor II, which has the longest half-life (48–60 hours). Consequently, the total anticoagulant effect is not reached until several days have elapsed and will require daily monitoring by the PT, APTT, or both.

In contrast to the immediate reversal of the anticoagulant activity of heparin by protamine sulfate, the inhibition of carboxylase activity requires injection of high concentrations of vitamin K. Thereafter, 6 to 24 hours is required for vitamin K-dependent factors to return to normal levels. If indicated, an immediate reversal of the clotting defect produced by oral anticoagulants can be achieved by transfusion of fresh frozen plasma or plasma concentrates rich in vitamin K-dependent clotting factors (prothrombin group).[32]

The effects of warfarin can be greatly affected by other drugs given concurrently. Agents that inhibit warfarin could result in thrombosis, whereas those that enhance its effects could lead to hemorrhage. Some of these drugs are various antibiotics, phenylbutazone, indomethacin, tolbutamide, salicylates, quinidine, steroids, barbituates, diuretics, and oral contraceptive agents. A complete listing of the many potential drug interactions can be found in several other publications.[21,23,28] An abbreviated list can be found in Chapter 55 of this text.

Administration

Patients with venous thrombosis usually are treated with heparin for a 7- to 10-day period and then by oral anticoagulants for weeks to months to prevent delayed recurrences. It is common practice to overlap heparin and oral anticoagulants for 4 or 5 days to provide maximum protection against recurrence during the initial stages of anticoagulant therapy.[10]

Laboratory Monitoring and Methods of Reporting Results

The monitoring of warfarin therapy has historically been achieved by the one-stage PT. Many variables affect the PT, but the two most important are the type of thromboplastin and the instrumentation used. In general, the thromboplastins used in North America are derived from rabbit brain and lung. These appear to be less sensitive to the reduction of vitamin K-dependent factors than are the thromboplastins derived from human brain that are used in the United Kingdom and other European countries.

The same depletion of clotting factors acceptable as therapeutic at one institution might be considered or interpreted as a dangerous overdose at another. The potential danger to patients caused by interlaboratory variations has led to a demand for standardization of the PT.

The optimal therapeutic range for laboratory control of oral anticoagulation has been debated for more than 30 years. Within an institution, the therapeutic range is determined according to the method being used to report PT. The recommended method is to report reference range values along with the patient time in seconds. It is felt that the reference range more accurately reflects the PT test system in use at that institution,[26] and it is suggested that an appropriate therapeutic window for most US thromboplastins by this method of reporting is 1.5 to 1.9 times the reference range in seconds.[25,32]

After many years of trial and error, an international system of standardization has been proposed by the World Health Organization (WHO), the International Committee for Standardization in Haematology, and the International Committee for Haemostasis and Thrombosis. Primary and secondary reference thromboplastin preparations have been prepared. In addition, a statistical model for calibration of local or commercial thromboplastins against these reference preparations has been suggested. Calibration of a thromboplastin against the international reference preparation results in the generation of an international sensitivity index (ISI) number for that lot of thromboplastin. Using the ISI, the observed ratio of the patient time to the reference range can be converted to the ratio that would have been obtained had the primary WHO reference thromboplastin been used to perform the test (the international normalized ratio or INR): $INR = (observed\ ratio)^{ISI}$.[20] See Chapter 62 for a detailed explanation of the ISI and INR.

ANTIPLATELET FUNCTION THERAPY

Studies in the 1970s suggested that recurrence of thrombotic episodes decreased when normal platelet function was curtailed by antiplatelet drugs. These drugs now are used in preventing arterial thrombosis, the pathologic counterpart of the beneficial role that normal platelets play in maintaining hemostasis.[8,26]

Anticoagulant Activity

Figure 57-3 demonstrates the effect that one substance (aspirin) has on normal platelet function. When platelets are stimulated with a variety of agents (ADP, collagen, thrombin), arachidonic acid is made available by hydrolysis of membrane phospholipids. Subsequently, arachidonic acid is converted by cyclooxygenase to intermediate cyclic endoperoxides, which are precursors of thromboxane A_2. Thromboxane A_2 is a potent stimulant of platelet aggregation and is also a powerful vasoconstrictor. Aspirin, probably the most common inhibitor of platelet function, acts by irreversibly acetylating cyclooxygenase.[12]

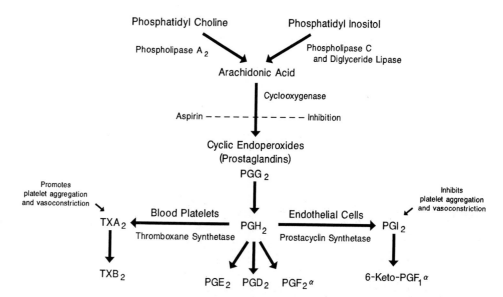

FIG. 57-3. Aspirin effect on platelet biochemical reactions: inhibition of cyclooxygenase and thus of thromboxane A_2 generation, resulting in decreased adhesion and aggregation.

Other agents that have demonstrated an ability to inhibit normal platelet function seem to be growing in number. A few are other nonsteroidal anti-inflammatory agents such as phenylbutazone and indomethacin, antibiotics (penicillins, cephalosporins), antidepressants and antipsychotics (chlorpromazine), propranolol and other beta-blockers, diuretics, sulfinpyrazone, dextran, and alcohol.[16]

Laboratory Monitoring

Although antiplatelet drugs are reported to be effective in decreasing platelet adhesion or aggregation, their use usually requires no laboratory management.[26] However, when the laboratory is asked to monitor the effectiveness of antiplatelet therapy, either the bleeding time or platelet aggregation studies may be helpful.

The bleeding time is one of the best tests of platelet function in general. The two most widely used tests today are the Ivy and the template methods.[12] Platelet aggregation procedures monitor the platelet release reaction. After ingestion of aspirin, aggregation studies reveal an absence of the secondary wave of aggregation in response to ADP and epinephrine. A reduced response also occurs with the use of collagen and arachidonic acid as aggregating agents.[12,27] See Chapter 59 for further discussion of tests for platelet function.

IN VIVO CLOT LYSIS

All previously discussed methods of anticoagulant therapy have no effect on already organized clots. Fibrin deposits, both intravascular and extravascular, are removed through fibrinolysis, the enzymatic dissolution of insoluble fibrin polymer. This phenomenon is regulated by the plasminogen–plasmin system, which can be enhanced by therapeutic infusions of plasminogen activators. Three agents used as plasminogen activators will be discussed: streptokinase, urokinase, and tissue plasminogen activator (tPA).

Fibrinolytic Activity

Streptokinase and urokinase impair hemostasis by at least three mechanisms: (1) direct lysis by plasmin of fibrin in hemostatic plugs; (2) production of a generalized coagulation abnormality characterized by hypofibrinogenemia, reduced levels of factors V and VIII, and an increase in FDP; and (3) the direct effect of plasmin on platelet membrane glycoproteins, which produces defective platelet function.[10,21] This condition is sometimes referred to as a *lytic state.*

Streptokinase and urokinase are administered by either systemic IV infusion or intra-arterial localized infusion. Streptokinase forms a 1:1 complex with plasminogen, which activates free plasminogen to plasmin. Urokinase directly cleaves plasminogen to form plasmin.[31] The advantage of urokinase over streptokinase is its lack of antigenicity.

Thrombolysis with streptokinase and urokinase is used for the treatment of venous thrombosis and pulmonary embolism, but it is being reevaluated for the treatment of acute myocardial infarction.[10] These plasminogen activators are effective in achieving early thrombolysis in patients with acute venous thrombosis, acute pulmonary embolism, and coronary artery thrombosis.[21] The principal side effect of thrombolytic therapy with streptokinase and urokinase is hemorrhage due to the fact that thrombolytic agents produce fibrinogenolysis as well as fibrinolysis.

A new plasminogen activator called tPA has been developed. This enzyme is a serine protease isolated from a human melanoma cell line and produced by recombinant DNA technology. It has theoretical advantages over streptokinase and urokinase because it induces fibrinolysis with a reported reduction in associated hemostatic defects caused by circulating plasmin.[10] High doses (>60 mg) may result in systemic fibrinogenolysis.[30]

Laboratory Monitoring

It is important to monitor fibrinolytic activity during treatment with these agents, because some conditions may prevent the conversion of plasminogen to plasmin. These conditions include: (1) high titers of antistreptococcal antibodies (when using streptokinase); (2) low plasminogen levels; (3) naturally occurring inhibitors; and (4) infiltration of the IV infusion. The laboratory may be called on to have monitoring procedures available on a 24-hour basis.

Although several tests are sensitive to the effects of thrombolytic drugs, many require lengthy assay procedures or special techniques. Of the laboratory procedures that have been recommended (such as PT, TT, APTT, quantitative fibrinogen, euglobulin clot lysis, and plasminogen levels), the TT has become widely accepted because it is fast, and practical, does not require special equipment,[17] and will detect the decrease in fibrinogen levels as well as the presence of fibrin and FDP.[12] See Chapter 54 for a discussion of the D-dimer test, which is also used to detect fibrin degradation.

CHAPTER SUMMARY

Anticoagulant therapy is an attempt to prevent the formation, or to promote the lysis, of a thrombus. The type and location of the thrombus usually determines the type of anticoagulant to be administered and the treatment protocol. For deep vein thrombosis, the usual protocol requires injection of heparin (monitored by the APTT), followed by long-term oral anticoagulants (monitored by the PT, APTT, or both). When thrombus formation is thought to be mediated by platelet activation, the patient frequently is given agents to interrupt normal platelet function, which may be monitored by bleeding times or platelet aggregation studies.

The newest treatment for life-threatening thrombus formation uses plasminogen activators to accelerate clot lysis. The action of some of these agents produces a lytic state that can be demonstrated in the laboratory.

CASE STUDY 57-1

A 28-year-old woman was admitted to the intensive care unit after a diagnosis was made of pulmonary embolism. Heparin (5000 U) was administered immediately by intravenous injection. Two hours later, the physician ordered an APTT. The laboratory reported an APTT of 40 seconds (reference range 25–36 seconds), and the physician called the laboratory to verify the results.
1. Identify any possible problems.
2. Identify possible solutions.

REFERENCES

1. Anido G, Freeman D: Heparin assay and protamine titration. Am J Clin Pathol 76:410, 1981
2. Bain S, Foster T, Sleigh B: Heparin and the activated partial thromboplastin time: A difference between *in-vitro* and *in-vivo* effects and implications of the therapeutic range. Am J Clin Pathol 74:668, 1980
3. Banez G, Triplett DA, Koepke JA: Laboratory monitoring of heparin therapy: The effect of different salts of heparin on the activated partial thromboplastin time: An analysis of the 1978 and 1979 CAP Hematology Survey. Am J Clin Pathol 74:569, 1980
4. Bjornsson TD, Nash PV: Variability in heparin sensitivity of APTT reagents. Am J Clin Pathol 86:199, 1986
5. Brandt J, Triplett DA: Laboratory monitoring of heparin: Effects of reagents and instruments on the activated partial thromboplastin time. Am J Clin Pathol 76(suppl):530, 1981
6. Carr JM, Kinney M, McDonagh J: Diagnosis of disseminated intravascular coagulation: Role of the D-dimer. Am J Clin Pharmacol 91:280, 1989
7. Deykin D, Miale J: Clinical Importance of the Bleeding Time Test. Durham, NC, Organon Teknika, 1979
8. Harker L: Hemostasis Manual, 2nd ed. Philadelphia, FA Davis, 1974
9. Hattersley PG: Activated coagulation time of whole blood. JAMA. 196:436, 1966
10. Hirsh J: Basis for the Therapeutic Range for Anticoagulant Therapy. Atlanta, Dade Company Thrombosis–Hemostasis Conference, 1984
11. Jorpes E: Heparin in the Treatment of Thrombosis: An Account of its Chemistry, Physiology and Application in Medicine, 2nd ed. New York, Oxford Press, 1946
12. Lenahan J, Smith K: Hemostasis Manual, 18th ed. Durham, NC, Organon Teknika, 1986
13. Koepke JA: Coagulation testing systems. In Koepke JA (ed): Laboratory Hematology, p 1137. New York, Churchill Livingstone, 1984
14. Lee RI, White PD: A clinical study of the coagulation time of blood. Am J Med Sci 145:495, 1913
15. McGann MA, Triplett DA: Interpretation of antithrombin III activity. Lab Med 13:742, 1982
16. Morgan C, Penner J: Bleeding complications during surgery. I: Defects of primary hemostasis and congenital coagulation. Lab Med 17:207, 1986
17. Palkuti H: Laboratory monitoring of anticoagulant therapy. J Med Techol 2:81, 1985
18. Palkuti H, Huang A, Kales A: APTT method for standardization in heparin therapy. Chicago, American Society of Clinical Pathologists Summary Report, March 1976
19. Penner J, Hiss R: Heparin therapy in the 70's. Univ Mich Med Center J 40:57, 1974
20. Poller L: Progress in standardization in anticoagulant control. Hematol Rev 1:225, 1987
21. Sherry S, Bell WR, Duckert FH et al: Thrombosis and Thrombolysis, 2nd ed. Somerville, NJ, Hoechst-Roussel Pharmaceuticals, 1979
22. Sirridge M: Laboratory Evaluation of Hemostasis. Philadelphia, Lea & Febiger, 1974
23. Soloway HB: Drug-induced bleeding. Am J Clin Pathol 61:622, 1974
24. Soloway HB, Christiansen T: Heparin anticoagulation during cardiopulmonary bypass in an antithrombin III deficient patient: Implications relative to the etiology of heparin rebound. Am J Clin Pathol 73:723, 1980
25. Tammes AR: Standardization of the prothrombin time. Rockford, IL, College of American Pathologists Computer Center, Quality Assurance Service, September 1985
26. Thomson J: Blood Coagulation and Haemostasis, 2nd ed. New York, Churchill Livingstone, 1980
27. Triplett DA: Platelet Function: Laboratory Evaluation and Clinical Application. Chicago, American Society of Clinical Pathologists Press, 1978
28. Triplett DA: Anticoagulant therapy: Monitoring techniques. Lab Manage 20:32, 1982
29. Triplett DA: Laboratory Evaluation of Coagulation. Chicago, American Society of Clinical Pathologists Press, 1982
30. Triplett DA: Tissue plasminogen activator (t-PA). Thromb Hemost No. TH86-4(TH-46). Chicago, American Society of Clinical Pathologists Press, 1986
31. Verstraete M, Vermylen J, Schetz J: Biochemical changes noted during intermittent administration of streptokinase. Thromb Haemost 39:61, 1978
32. Wessler S: A Guide to Anticoagulant Therapy, 3rd ed. Dallas, American Heart Association, 1984

58

The Megakaryocyte–Platelet System: Structures and Function

Michael R. Buchanan

Blood platelets either directly or indirectly influence blood coagulation, vessel wall tonicity and healing, and other aspects of hemostasis and thrombosis. This review will focus on three aspects of the platelet: (1) the maturation and structure of the cell from which it evolves, the megakaryocyte; (2) structure; and (3) function.

MEGAKARYOCYTE MATURATION AND STRUCTURE

The maturation of the cells of the megakaryocytic system has been divided into four stages. They are, from least to most mature, the megakaryoblast, the promegakaryocyte, the megakaryocyte, and the metamegakaryocyte. It is generally the metamegakaryocyte that ultimately produces thrombocytes or platelets. Some investigators consider the megakaryocyte to be the platelet-producing stage. Each stage is discussed below, and the features of each are summarized in Table 58-1.

The Megakaryoblast

At the turn of the century, James Wright provided evidence that platelets were derived from megakaryocytes within the bone marrow.[133] Since these initial observations, much work has been performed to understand better the life cycle of megakaryocytic cells and their offspring, platelets. Platelets evolve through a sequence of events. The primitive megakaryocyte or megakaryoblast differentiates, by some unknown mechanism, from a hematopoietic progenitor cell capable of evolving into any of the three cell lines: erythrocytes, granulocytes, or megakaryocytes (Chap. 6). A specific hormone, thrombopoietin, is responsible for the

TABLE 58–1. Morphologic Differentiation of Megakaryocytic Cell Series

MATURATION STAGE	CYTOPLASMIC GRANULES	CYTOPLASMIC TAGS	NUCLEAR FEATURES	THROMBOCYTES VISIBLE?
Megakaryoblast	Absent	Present	Single nucleus, fine chromatin structure, nucleoli	No
Promegakaryocyte	Few	Present	Double nucleus	No
Megakaryocyte	Numerous	Usually absent	Two or more nuclei	No
Metamegakaryocyte	Aggregated	Absent	Four or more nuclei	Yes

commitment of the megakaryoblast to differentiate further into more mature stages.

Megakaryocytic cells are unusual in that their nuclei are able to undergo multiple mitotic divisions without cytoplasmic division, generating giant multinucleated or polyploid cells. This is referred to as *endomitosis*. The multiple nuclei in these cells divide simultaneously and usually remain connected. Thus, megakaryocytic cells, including the megakaryoblast, can be seen to have 1, 2, 4, 8, and even 16 or 32 nuclei. After the first nuclear division, megakaryocytic cells always have an even number of nuclei.

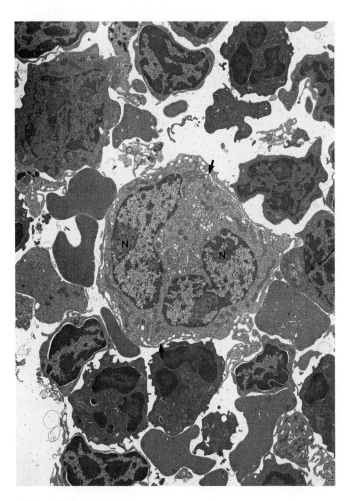

FIG. 58-1.   Immature mouse megakaryocyte. Some demarcation membranes are present at periphery (arrow). Nucleus (N) has two lobes, and Golgi complex, along with some alpha granules, mitochondria, and centrioles, are present in cytoplasm (see Fig. 58-6). (Original magnification × 4800. With permission of photographer, Dr. P. E. Stenberg, Veterans Administration Medical Center, San Francisco.)

The megakaryoblast is the earliest recognizable stage of maturation. This cell displays blunt protrusions from its cytoplasmic membrane and contains a multitude of polyribosomes and clear vacuoles with diameters as large as 0.2 μm as seen by electron microscopy (Fig. 58-1). The central area of the megakaryoblast contains mitochondria and a primitive endoplasmic reticulum. The nucleus, which occupies most of the cell volume, has prominant nucleoli and distinct but barely marginated chromatin characteristic of immature cells (see Fig. 58-1). The Golgi complex (vacuoles, lamellae, and vesicles) occupies the area surrounding the nucleus. Alpha-granules and centrioles are also found in the cytoplasm.

Most megakaryocytes at any stage of maturation and their precursors, the megakaryoblasts, normally are found only in bone marrow (1 to 4 per 1000 nucleated cells), not in the peripheral blood. A few may be found in the lungs. These cells constitute less than 1% of the nucleated cells within the bone marrow but are easily identified by their large size. Most of these cells in the marrow are in the third or fourth stage of maturation.

The megakaryoblast (Plate 62) is identified by light microscopy using a Romanowsky-stained marrow specimen by the following features. First, it has a diameter of 15 to 50 μm. There may be a single, centrally located nucleus or multiple round and oval nuclei containing several nucleoli and distinct but fine, delicate chromatin strands. The cytoplasm stains a diffuse blue, indicating absence of specific granules. The megakaryoblast is irregular in shape and has blunt protrusions of cytoplasm (cytoplasmic tags) extending into its external environment. These features are illustrated diagrammatically in Figure 58-2.

The Promegakaryocyte

The megakaryoblast, as it matures to the promegakaryocyte stage, increases in volume (see Fig. 58-2). Cell size ranges from 20 to 80 μm. The cell membrane retains its characteristic blunt protrusions, and the cytoplasm is rich in polyribosomes, as shown by electron microscopy (Fig. 58-3). The number of nuclear lobes begins to increase, but there is still only barely detectable margination of the chromatin around the nuclear membrane. Although the cell still appears somewhat immature, it is thought to be capable of protein synthesis, because, as seen by electron microscopy, there is a more developed network of membranes within the cytoplasm, a network known as the *demarcating membrane system* (DMS), which forms by invagination of the plasma membrane (see Fig. 58-3). Morphologic studies indicate that the outer cell membrane and the demarcating membranes have structural similarities, suggesting that the DMS functions as the future membrane system of the meta-

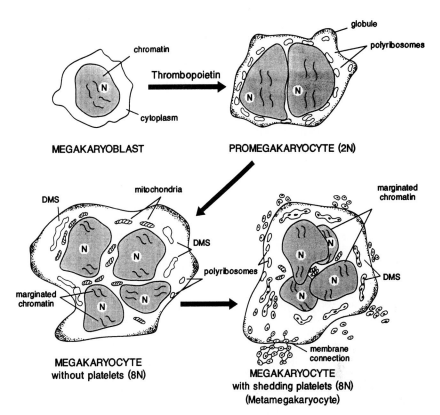

FIG. 58-2. Morphologic maturation of megakaryocyte system. DMS, demarcating membrane
system; N, nucleus.

megakaryocyte's new offspring, the platelet.[5,29,96] The development of the DMS also denotes individual platelet
areas that finally result in the fragmentation of the metamegakaryocyte cytoplasm into platelets and megakaryocytic fragments.

The promegakaryocyte differs from the megakaryoblast
in a number of ways when examined by light microscopy
using a Romanowsky stain (see Plate 62). These differences
are illustrated diagrammatically in Figure 58-2. The
promegakaryocyte is larger, and the nucleus has usually
undergone one or two divisions. Bluish-stained granules
(not present in the megakaryoblast) are apparent around the
periphery of the nuclei. One promegakaryocyte variant has
a distinct marginal zone with blunt cytoplasmic protrusions
that stain a dark blue and often contain small colorless
globules.

The Megakaryocyte

The megakaryocyte represents the maturation stage
following the promegakaryocyte. As viewed on
Romanowsky-stained marrow by light microscopy, this
cell is round and is expanded in volume, with multiple
nuclei and even, peripheral margins (Plate 62). The abundant cytoplasm contains numerous small, rather uniformly
distributed granules with a reddish-blue hue. The chromatin pattern is linear and coarse, with distinct spaces between
the strands (see Fig. 29-7).

As the megakaryocyte matures, it begins to contain all of
the structural constituents of a metamegakaryocyte; however, the organizational arrangement of these constituents
and their number within the megakaryocyte differ from
that of the metamegakaryocyte when viewed by electron

microscopy. The megakaryocyte cytoplasm is devoid of
specific organelles other than polyribosomes (see Fig. 58-2)
and numerous mitochondria located in the central area of
the cell. There is also an incomplete endoplasmic reticular
system.

The megakaryocyte is known as the stage that does not
ordinarily produce platelets. However, megakaryocytes
with at least four nuclei can produce platelets.[82]

The Metamegakaryocyte

The metamegakaryocyte is the fourth stage of maturation.
It is a very large cell, many times the size of the mature
granulocyte, with a decreased nuclear–cytoplasmic ratio
compared with the immature stages of development. By
light microscopy on Romanowsky-stained marrow, the
metamegakaryocyte nucleus is multilobed (see Fig. 58-2);
and ploidy (the number of sets of chromosomes in the cell,
with 23 chromosomes per set) ranges from 4N to 16N
when not stressed to produce more platelets.[54,82] For example, a four-lobed nucleus is termed 8N because it has eight
single sets (i.e., four paired sets) of chromosomes. Ploidy
levels can be as high as 64N under abnormal conditions.

In the cytoplasm, there is an aggregation of granular
material into masses that are separated by relatively clear
areas that represent the DMS or vesicles. These aggregates
of granular cytoplasm may be seen near the periphery of the
cell. Platelets may be seen adhering to the cell membrane as
they begin to break away from the metamegakaryocyte.

On electron microscopy, the metamegakaryocyte periphery is seen to contain predominantly polyribosomes,[83]
with occasional mitochondria (see Fig. 58-2). The remainder of the cytoplasm contains the extensive DMS, which

creates the future platelet fields (Fig. 58-4). Each future platelet contains mitochondria and cytoplasmic granules.

Problems in Identification of Maturation Stage

In differentiating the maturation stages of the megakaryocytic cells, emphasis should be placed on the cytoplasmic appearance rather than the number of nuclei or the chromatin structure, as is usually the rule in evaluating other hematologic cells. The reason is that occasionally, a megakaryocytic cell with only one or two nuclei forms platelets.

Problems in Identification of Cells in the Megakaryocytic Series

Megakaryocytes and metamegakaryocytes are usually identified easily by their large size in comparison with other bone marrow cells and their 4N or greater ploidy. However, it should be recognized that there are other cell types in the marrow, both normal and pathologic, with which the megakaryoblast, megakaryocyte, and metamegakaryocyte can be confused. These are the normal osteoclast (see Fig. 29-6), the osteoblast (see Fig. 29-5), and reticulum cells and the abnormal multinucleated erythroblast, multinucleated plasma cell and red cell, various tumor cells, and Reed-Sternberg cells. Tables 58-2 and 58-3 summarize the differentiating features of these cells. Plates

63A through F and 64A through H present examples of the megakaryocytic cells and the cells with which they may be confused.

Initiation of Platelet Formation

A number of explanations have been offered for the initiation of platelet formation within the mature megakaryocyte.[6,86] It has been suggested that the DMS becomes dilated, and the individual platelets become apparent.[89] The platelets, in turn, appear to be attached to the main mass of the megakaryocytic cytoplasm by connecting pieces of membrane. On completion of this demarcation, and following the appropriate stimulus, megakaryocytes extend portions of their cytoplasm through the basement membrane and between the endothelial cells of the marrow sinusoids. Megakaryocytes normally develop close to the venous sinusoids so that platelet shedding is facilitated. The platelets are shed into the bone marrow sinuses on their way to the circulation. It has been estimated that each megakaryocyte can shed 1000 to 4000 platelets. Once the mature megakaryocyte has released all of its platelet progeny, it is presumed that its nuclei and remaining cytoplasm and organelles are phagocytized by neighboring macrophages.

Platelet Shedding

To facilitate the release of platelets into the bone marrow sinus, cytoplasmic pseudopodia of the megakaryocytes

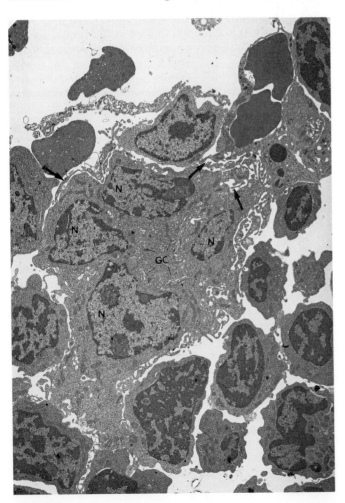

FIG. 58-3.   Maturing mouse megakaryocyte. Cell is more irregular in contour, and demarcation membranes (arrows) penetrate cytoplasm to greater extent than in immature cell. Also, nucleus (N) is more highly lobulated, and Golgi complex (GC) is enlarged. (Original magnification × 4800. With permission of photographer, Dr. P. E. Stenberg, Veterans Administration Medical Center, San Francisco.)

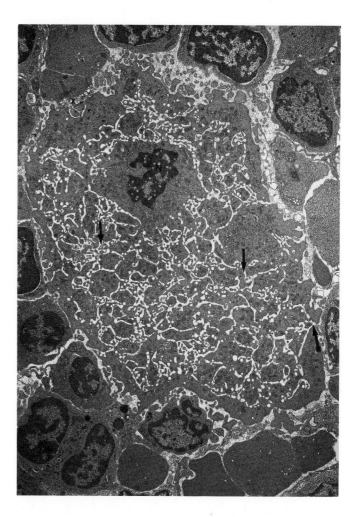

FIG. 58-4. Mature mouse megakaryocyte (metamegakaryocyte). Demarcation membrane system is well developed (arrows), and nucleus is pyknotic. Nuclear:cytoplasm ratio is decreased. (Original magnification × 4800. With permission of photographer, Dr. P. E. Stenberg, Veterans Administration Medical Center, San Francisco.)

protrude through the extravascular side of the endothelium, making an opening into the bone marrow sinus (see Figs. 5-4A and 5-4B). This opening facilitates the flow of more megakaryocytic cytoplasm containing new platelets into the sinus. Eventually, these cytoplasmic outflows separate from the body of the megakaryocyte, resulting in the release of an abundance of platelet fragments. These cytoplasmic fragments undergo further dissolution within the sinus from which individual platelets evolve.

Megakaryocytic Microtubular System

Within the megakaryoblast and megakaryocyte, there are a series of *microtubules* that converge on centrioles adjacent to the nucleus.[94] These microtubules function as the mitotic spindle. In contrast, within the metamegakaryocyte, there is a microtubule system dispersed throughout the cell that passes through the platelet fields and cytoplasm in a random pattern. This system is less developed than the more organized one seen in the circulating platelet.

Megakaryocytic Microfilaments

The microtubules in the immature megakaryocyte display a well-organized dispersement, whereas those of the mature megakaryocyte display a random dispersement. In con-

trast, the *microfilaments* in the immature megakaryocytes are abundant but disorganized, whereas in the mature megakaryocyte, they are organized, forming a pattern of microfilaments similar to that seen in the platelet. These microfilaments contain a significant amount of the contractile protein thrombosthenin (actomyosin), which comprises 15% of all proteins in platelets.[12,70] Thrombosthenin is composed of actin and myosin and may be involved in maintaining the discoid shape of the platelet and in regulating changes in platelet shape after activation.[9,10,88] Much as in the platelet response (discussed below), the megakaryocyte, when exposed to platelet-aggregating stimuli such as epinephrine and thrombin, reorganizes its peripheral rim of microfilaments, creating a tight, centrally located formation. This reorganization facilitates the expulsion of megakaryocyte constituents such as serotonin and megakaryocytic (platelet)-specific proteins.[28]

Megakaryocytic Protein Synthesis

A number of proteins common to both platelets and megakaryocytes have been identified. These include fibrinogen, factor VIIIR:Ag, myosin, actin, fibronectin, platelet factor 4, and the important platelet adhesive glycoprotein complex glycoprotein IIb-IIIa.[85,89] The significance of the apparent synthesis of these proteins by megakaryocytes is unclear. It is likewise unclear whether these proteins are

TABLE 58–2. Differentiating Features of Cells Confused with Megakaryoblasts

MEGAKARYOBLAST★	PLASMA CELL★	TISSUE NEUTROPHIL★ (FERRATA CELL)	OSTEOCLAST★	TUMOR CELLS	REED-STERNBERG CELL
See Plate 63A Single centrally located nucleus with one or more nucleoli; nuclear chromatin strands distinct; marginal cytoplasmic extensions represent early platelet formation; N:C = 10:1; cytoplasm is blue and nongranular.	See Plate 63B Single, round eccentric nucleus with nucleolus; cytoplasm is blue, "bubbly," and nongranular; cytoplasm is more abundant than megakaryoblast's; cytoplasm contains prominent light zone adjacent to nucleus. Generally smaller than osteoblast.	See Plate 63C Nuclear parachromatin more distinct than megakaryoblast's; nucleoli usually distinct; chromatin is more coarse and cytoplasm more abundant (N:C = 1:1) than megakaryoblast's; cytoplasm stains light blue; cytoplasmic granules vary in number and usually stain reddish-purple; cell is generally bizarre in shape with blunt cytoplasmic pseudopods.	See Plate 63D Very large cell; multinucleated; nuclei are separate and not visibly connected; number of nuclei may be uneven; cytoplasm has pink background with blue granules and frayed edges.	See Plate 63E Nuclei have variable color and chromatin clumping; nucleoli common; cells are variable in size and shape; cytoplasmic borders may be difficult to distinguish; cells tend to clump; cytoplasm color is variable.	See Plate 63F Nuclear lobes are often mirror images; nucleoli are more prominent than megakaryoblast's; cytoplasm color is variable.

★ From Diggs LW, Sturm D, Bell A: The Morphology of Human Blood Cells, 5th ed. Abbott Park, IL, Abbott Laboratories, 1985, with permission.

TABLE 58–3. Differentiating Features of Cells Confused with Promegakaryocytes, Megakaryocytes, and Metamegakaryocytes

PROMEGA-KARYOCYTE★	OSTEOBLAST★	MULTI-NUCLEATED RBC★	TUMOR CELL	MULTI-NUCLEATED PLASMA CELL★	OSTEOCLAST★	MEGA-KARYOCYTE★	METAMEGA-KARYOCYTE★
See Plate 64A Double centrally located nucleus; nuclei connected by strands or superimposed; cytoplasm is blue and scant but often has extensions that stain blue and have rounded contours with a homogeneous or bubbly appearance; bluish granules may appear near nucleus.	See Plate 64B Single, round eccentric nucleus with nucleolus; cytoplasm is blue, "bubbly," and nongranular; cytoplasm contains prominent light zone separated from nucleus. Generally larger than plasma cell.	See Plate 64C RBC cytoplasm polychromatophilic or pink and nongranular; nuclear chromatin clumpy; cell is smaller than pro- and meta-megakaryocyte.	See Plate 64D Nuclei have variable color and chromatin clumping; nucleoli are common; cells are variable in size and shape; cytoplasmic borders may be difficult to distinguish; cells tend to clump; cytoplasm color is variable.	See Plate 64E Foamy cytoplasm stains dark blue; nuclei may be double or triple but never more.	See Plate 64F Very large cell; multinucleated; nuclei separate and not visibly connected; number of nuclei may be uneven; cytoplasm has pink background with blue granules and frayed edges.	See Plate 64G Very large cell with 2 or more nuclei; number of nuclei is always even; nuclei connected by strands or superimposed; cytoplasm reddish-blue with granules; very similar to metamegakaryocyte except that platelet budding is not yet detectable.	See Plate 64H Very large cell with multiple (up to 32) nuclei; number of nuclei is always even; abundant granular cytoplasm (granules stain pinkish-red) with evident platelet budding.

★From Diggs LW, Sturm D, Bell A: The Morphology of Human Blood Cells, 5th ed. Abbott Park, IL, Abbott Laboratories, 1985, with permission.

synthesized by platelets, as the platelet is anucleate. It is possible that these proteins are simply released from platelets, and that platelets acquire these proteins either from the megakaryocyte or adsorption from the plasma once the platelets are released into circulation.

PLATELET STRUCTURE

The circulating platelet, although a minute fragment (1–4 μm in diameter) of the giant megakaryocyte, is a complex structure. By light microscopy, platelets appear as dense blue to purple particles with granules that stain with graded intensity during Romanowsky stain preparation. The detailed anatomy of the platelet is best seen by electron microscopy and can be subdivided into four major areas: (1) the *peripheral zone,* which consists of the platelet's outer membrane and related structures; (2) the *submembrane area,* which links the membrane and the inner cell body; (3) the *sol-gel zone,* which constitutes the matrix or muscle and skeletal portion of the platelet; and (4) the *organelle zone,* which consists of granules, dense bodies, lysosomes, and mitochrondria. The organelle zone serves as the metabolic center to influence platelet function in response to exogenous stimuli such as hypercoagulation, viruses, and foreign bodies.[126]

Peripheral Zone

The peripheral zone consists of the surface coat or *glycocalyx,* plasma membrane, and submembrane area (Figs. 58-5 and 58-6). Under homeostatic conditions, platelets circulate in the blood as discoid-shaped cells. The glycocalyx is relatively smooth and contains porelike indentations that open communication channels into the platelet cytoplasm, providing a distinct connection between the inside of the platelet and its surroundings. The glycocalyx is thicker and denser than that of most blood cells, ranging in thickness from 10 to 50 nm.[126] A number of glycoproteins are incorporated in this outer layer, including glycoproteins Ia, Ib, Ic, IIa, IIb, III, IV, and V, which play important roles in platelet adhesion and aggregation.[32,84] The glycocalyx also provides a surface to which some coagulation factors may adhere, including factors I, V, VIII, X, XI, XII, and XIII. All of these are absorbed selectively onto the platelet to facilitate assembly of the prothrombinase complex consisting of factors V_a, X_a, and calcium. This complex then acts on prothrombin to convert it to thrombin.

Underlying the glycocalyx is the plasma membrane, which serves as the physical and chemical barrier between the intracellular and extracellular constituents of the platelet. Within this membrane is the sodium/potassium ATPase ionic pump, which maintains a transmembrane ionic gradient.[130] The phospholipid constituents (phosphatidylserine, phosphatidylcholine, and phosphatidylinositol) and other fatty acid pools required for fatty acid metabolism are also located within this layer.[97] Finally, platelet factor VIII (*i.e.,* VIII:vWF), an important constituent for the acceleration of blood coagulation and for platelet adhesion, may also be located in the lipoprotein-rich plasma membrane.

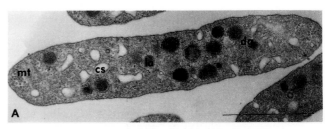

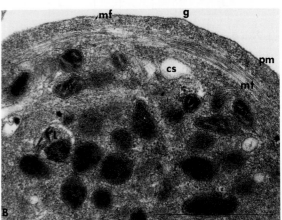

FIG. 58-5.   Transmission electron micrograph of normal human platelets in cross-section (A) and transverse section (B). Surface coat (glycocalyx, g) external to trilamellar plasma membrane (pm) is seen as faint electron-semidense coating. (Cationic dye, such as ruthenium red, is necessary to see this structure fully.) Microtubular system (mt) is shown in both cross-section and transverse section at periphery of platelet. Microfilaments (mf) are between microtubular system and plasma membrane. Light alpha granules (lα), dark alpha granules (dα), and dense granules (dg) are present in cytoplasm along with mitochondria (m) and lysosomal bodies (L). External canalicular system (cs) is seen as large empty spaces. (Bar = 1 μm. With permission of photographer, Dr M. Richardson, Department of Pathology, McMaster University, Ontario, Canada.)

Submembrane Area

The submembrane area underlies the plasma membrane. This region is identified as a specific area because the organelles within the inner matrix of unaltered platelets never come in contact with the internal side of the platelet cell wall, but appear instead to be separated from it by the submembrane area (see Figs. 58-5 and 58-6). This platelet region also contains an organized system of filaments, which are physically comparable to the microfilaments and submicrofilaments of the microtubule system.[123] They are distinct from the circumferential microfilaments and peripheral to them. They are usually obscured by the density of the sol-gel region matrix but can be made visible by special techniques.[135] These structures are thought to prevent contact between organelles and the cell membrane by their physical presence. The submembrane filaments may also contribute to the regulation of the normal platelet discoid shape, act as a base for pseudopod formation, and interact with other contractile proteins to modulate platelet adhesion and clot retraction after activation.

TRANSVERSE SECTION

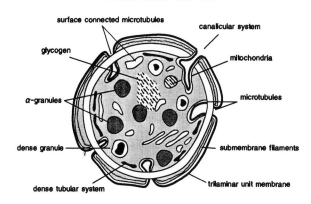

CROSS SECTION

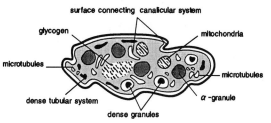

FIG. 58-6. Morphology of platelet as viewed in transverse (top) and cross-section (bottom).

Sol-Gel Zone

The sol-gel zone underlies the submembrane filaments. It consists of a circumferential microtubule system and randomly arranged microfilaments that form an intraplatelet matrix, both of which contribute to support of the platelet discoid shape. The microfilaments provide the contractile force after activation that directs the organelles toward the center of the cell with control and direction from the microtubules. The sol-gel zone serves as a stable gel component to regulate the arrangement of the internal organelles and microtubular system within the resting platelet body.[7] The sol-gel zone also influences communication of the organelles with the platelet's external surroundings.

Cross-section microscopic examination of unstimulated platelets reveals the circumferential microtubules, which extend around the platelet perimeter (see Figs. 58-5 and 58-6). Spaces in between the individual series of tubules contain submembrane filaments, which integrate one tubular system with another. In its position directly under the cell membrane, this microtubular system probably contributes significantly to the cytoskeletal support system. When platelets are stimulated and lose their discoid form, the circumferential band of microtubules disappears, but on reestablishment of the discoid shape of the platelets, such as by treatment with cooling or biochemical agents such as prostaglandin (PG) I_2, the microtubules reappear.[120,131]

It has been suggested that the microtubule system plays an important role in the contractile response of platelets to stimulation.[33,76,122] However, the microtubule system is not required for contraction;[121,134] rather, it most likely acts

as a governor and influences the extent of, rather than initiating, the platelet contractile response.

The microfilaments of a stimulated and spread platelet can be identified readily and are projected outward, forming pseudopodia. However, identification of microfilaments and their assembly within the sol-gel matrix of discoid-shaped platelets is difficult. Platelet filaments are approximately 50 nm in diameter and contain two proteins, actin and myosin. This suggests that the microfilaments (unlike microtubules) within the platelet sol-gel system are necessary for the contractile process. It also has been demonstrated that after secretion of platelet constituents in response to marked stimulation, platelets are able to recover their discoid form. When the stimulus is slight, aggregated platelets recover their discoid shape even more rapidly.[101] These observations suggest that microfilaments function in an organized and reversible manner.

Recently, an α-actinin- and actin-binding protein has been found in the platelet. This material is a transmembrane protein, linking the outer membrane to the microfilaments in the sol-gel area. This intracellular network may help to explain how the inner microfilaments influence platelet contraction by modulating the cytoskeleton of the outer layers of the platelet.[87] Thus, both circumferential and radial extensions of the microfilaments oriented in opposing directions may function as the platelet muscular system, which is able to facilitate, simultaneously, a centralized contraction of the platelet's granules and a reorganization of the platelet's shape in response to various stimuli.

Organelle Zone

Organelles constitute the major portion of the platelet cytoplasm. These structures include electron-dense granules, α-granules, peroxisomes, lysosomes, and mitochondria.

The *dense granules* are 250 to 350 nm in diameter and are classified as dense because of their appearance by electron microscopy. They contain adenosine, guanosine, diphosphates and triphosphates, calcium, magnesium, and serotonin.[24,62,130] The nucleotide ADP is probably the most important component secreted from the dense granules after platelet stimulation. When ADP is released, it binds to specific receptors and initiates platelet aggregation. However, this is a short-lived effect, because ADP is rapidly degraded to adenosine which, in turn, inhibits platelet function by enhancing cAMP levels (Fig. 58-7).

The importance of the minute amounts of calcium and magnesium ions released from the dense granules after platelet stimulation is not well understood. It is possible that the calcium concentration at the platelet surface or within the microtubule system is high and therefore influences the platelet microenvironment. Such a mechanism is thought to be important in the activation of membrane phospholipases, which are Ca^{+2} dependent and influence the subsequent liberation of arachidonic acid, the precursor of a number of metabolites required for platelet function (see Fig. 58-10, explained later in this chapter).

The *α-granule* is spherical and somewhat larger than the dense granule, with an overall diameter of 300 to 500 nm. The predominant constituents released from these granules are coagulation factors, a permeability factor, and cationic proteins such as the platelet-derived growth factor (PDGF)

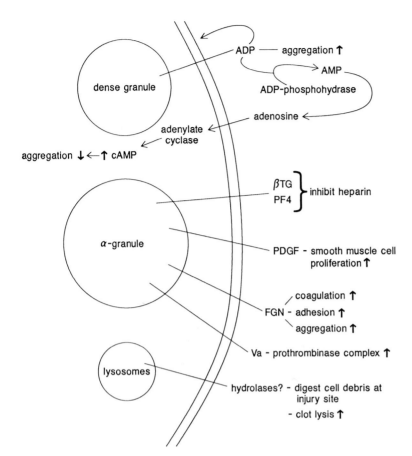

FIG. 58-7. Release products of platelet and their effects. FGN, fibrinogen.

(see Fig. 58-7). Two platelet-specific proteins are also released: platelet factor 4 (PF4) and β-thromboglobulin (βTG), both of which bind heparin.[13,92] It has been postulated that after platelet stimulation, PF4, in particular, binds endogenously released heparin and therefore neutralizes heparin's coagulation inhibitory effect. The mechanism for this effect remains to be elucidated.

The α-granule also contains fibrinogen and factor V (see Fig. 58-7). These two constituents are released after platelet stimulation and bind to the platelet surface at specific receptor sites, which in turn provide a base for the binding and assembly of other coagulant factors, including prothrombin and factor X_a, and the subsequent formation of the prothrombinase complex consisting of factors V_a and X_a with Ca^{+2} which together stimulate activation of prothrombin on the platelet surface. Fibrinogen acts as a bridge between ADP-stimulated platelets. It is likely that the release of fibrinogen from platelets within a hemostatic plug, rather than its recruitment from the plasma, better facilitates stabilization of the platelet plug. It is also possible that assembly of the fibrin matrix on the outer membrane of the platelet, in association with the contractile protein inside the platelet, acts synergistically to facilitate platelet-induced clot retraction, which is necessary for wound healing and vessel wall repair.

Because platelets are anucleate and therefore have finite metabolic capabilities, it is likely that the factor V or V_a released from platelet α-granules is not synthesized by the platelet. Most likely, these proteins are acquired by platelet absorption from the plasma or through pinocytosis by the megakaryocytes, as these proteins have been identified in both megakaryocytes and platelets.[85,89]

The relative importance of platelet-associated versus plasma coagulation proteins is not entirely clear. The sequestration of coagulation factors within α-granules allows for high local concentrations of these proteins when platelets are stimulated, thereby enhancing PF3 activity. Platelet factor 3 is not a discrete molecular species like PF4, but rather the catalytic ability of activated platelet membrane phospholipid to increase the reaction efficiency of the coagulation mechanism (Chap. 59).

The most important cationic protein released from platelets is the mitogenic factor PDGF. During platelet–vessel wall interactions after injury, PDGF is released from α-granules and stimulates smooth-muscle cell growth and proliferation.[91] For a number of years, it was thought that the hyperplastic response to vessel wall injury was mediated by platelet PDGF. However, more recent studies suggest that endothelial cells and other blood cells also can release "PDGF," indicating that PDGF is not specific to platelets.

Vessel wall permeability and tone are also influenced by a "permeability factor" released from platelet α-granules.[71] In thrombocytopenia, the vessel wall becomes "leaky," indicating the important contribution of platelets in keeping vessels intact. It would appear, therefore, that the circulating discoid (i.e, unstimulated) platelets, as well as factors released from stimulated platelets, contribute to vessel wall permeability (i.e, leakage prevention). Although this factor from unstimulated platelets has been recognized for years, its contribution to vascular hemostasis has not been elucidated.

Lysosomes are platelet vesicles that contain a number of acid hydrolases (see Fig. 58-7). These hydrolases are obtained from fractions of platelets rich in both mitochondria and light α-granules.[119] The significance of their release is unclear. Lysosomes may digest materials that the platelet endocytoses. However, platelets have limited ability to phagocytize any constituent. Therefore, the necessity for such an abundance of lysosomes remains puzzling. It is possible that lysosome acid hydrolases are released at the site of the forming thrombus or platelet plug to digest cellular debris and foreign material or that they contribute to clot lysis.

Platelet Membrane System

The platelet membrane system has two components, the *canalicular system* and the *dense tubular system*. The presence of an intracellular canalicular system that opens to the platelet's external environment is evidenced by the presence of indented pores on the platelet surface (see Fig. 58-6)[125] and by cross-sections illustrating interconnecting tubules reaching from the outer membrane to the intercytosol components of the cell (see Figs. 58-5 and 58-6). This is also known as the *surface-connecting canalicular system* and may serve as delivery routes for substances ingested by the platelet, as well as the route of extrusion of substances released from the stimulated platelet. These canalicular systems remain readily visible and clear throughout the sequences of platelet shape change, contraction, adhesion, and aggregation.[127,128]

Channels of the dense tubular system are randomly dispersed in the platelet cytosol and appear to be close to the circumferential band of microtubules (see Figs. 58-5 and 58-6).[8] This suggests that the dense tubular system has an important role in influencing the microtubules supporting the discoid platelet shape. This role seems likely because there is no evidence of any communication between the open canalicular and the dense tubular systems. It also has been suggested that platelets pump calcium out of the cytosol through the dense tubules and, perhaps, through the open canalicular system, influencing the metabolic activity in the platelet and contributing to the synthesis and release of various constituents such as arachidonic acid metabolites. The dense tubular system also contains specific peroxidase activity important for prostaglandin synthetase activity.[15] Therefore, the dense tubular system may, in fact, be the site of platelet prostaglandin synthesis (discussed below).

PLATELET LIFE SPAN AND TURNOVER RATE

Unlike erythrocytes, which circulate for approximately 120 days, platelets circulate for a short time. Under healthy steady-state conditions, the rate of platelet release from megakaryocytes is equivalent to the rate of platelet removal from the circulation. This net rate of production is expressed as platelet turnover, which has been estimated to be $35 \times 10^9/L \pm 4.3 \times 10^9/L$ per day.[39] When platelet life span

is studied using normal platelets injected into thrombocytopenic recipients, the life span ranges from 5 to 10 days and is, in part, dependent on the total number of platelets injected. In studies of "normal" recipients, the platelet life span ranged from 2 to 9 days.[2,40,41] These estimates unfortunately are influenced by the method of life span calculation.[68] Most studies have utilized radiolabels such as [111]indium and [51]chromium and have analyzed the radiolabel recovery curves by various statistical approaches. The question of which method is best is still debated.

Although the platelet life span is relatively short, the range in the "normal" population is great. The significance of this wide range is unclear. However, it has been suggested that the circulating platelets can be divided into two major populations: young and old.[98] Young platelets are hemostatically more effective. As they circulate, presumably they interact with minuscule stimuli throughout the cardiovascular system and collide randomly with one another, as a result of which, glycoproteins on their surfaces are destroyed. Hence, the old platelet is hemostatically less effective. The subsequent sequestration of old platelets from the circulation is also a matter of speculation; it may be attributable to a sufficiently altered membrane to render the platelet "foreign" to its surroundings, which results in sequestration by the reticuloendothelial system. In addition, at least 30% of the total circulating platelet population is normally sequestered in the spleen.[98] This platelet pool exchanges freely with the circulation; however, the significance of splenic sequestration is unclear, particularly because after splenectomy, platelet survival remains normal, and there is no apparent loss of hemostatic function.

PLATELET FUNCTION

Platelets interact with injured vascular wall structures, plasma proteins, and other circulating blood cells, all of which are fundamental in the regulation of hemostasis and the pathogenesis of thrombosis. When platelets are stimulated by way of these interactions, they release biologically active substances, which can interact with the vessel wall cells, including the endothelium, and influence plasma coagulation and the circulating cells that modulate hemostasis. In this section, the specific platelet response will be discussed, including adhesion, release, and aggregation and the effects of these responses on coagulation, hemostasis, and thrombosis.

Platelet Adhesion

Platelets do not adhere to the intact endothelial cell surface of blood vessels under homeostatic conditions; however, they do adhere to detached endothelial cells and the subendothelial network of collagen fibrils, fibrinectin, and basement membrane.[22,23,102,108] The degree of platelet response to such injury is, in part, influenced by the extent and depth of vessel wall injury (Fig. 58-8). Stimuli that cause endothelial cell desquamation only (*i.e.*, minor injury) expose platelets to the basement membrane, onto which they will adhere and spread. Under these conditions, the platelets do not release their constituents nor promote aggregation.[59] More recently, it has been demonstrated

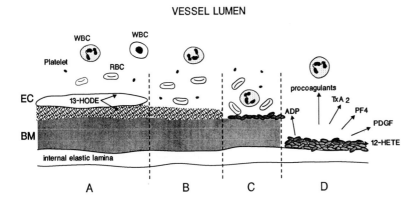

VESSEL LUMEN

FIG. 58-8. Platelet adhesion to vessel wall. Avidity of platelet adhesion is dependent on degree of injury. (A) With an intact endothelium (EC), there is no adhesion, which is regulated, in part, by 13-HODE inside EC. (B) With selective removal of EC and exposure of basement membrane (BM) lying immediately below, there is little platelet adhesion, also presumed to be attributable, in part, to presence of 13-HODE. (C) With exposure of deeper BM tissue, platelets adhere to BM but do not release their constituents. (D) When vessel wall is severely injured, platelets adhere to damaged site, and platelet aggregates form in response to constituents released from adherent platelets.

that an endothelial cell-derived chemorepellant,[18,19] 13-hydroxyoctadecadienoic acid (13-HODE), released from endothelial cells into the vascular tissues immediately underlying the endothelium, inhibits platelet adhesion to that surface,[16] indicating that even the basement membrane is not initially thrombogenic (prone to producing a clot). When the vessel is more severely injured, such as by rupture of an atherosclerotic plaque, exposing the deeper structures of the vessel wall, platelets not only adhere to that surface but also undergo the release reaction, facilitating further platelet aggregation and activating blood coagulation on their surfaces (see Fig. 58-8D).[4,118]

The differences in these platelet responses are likely to be attributable to differences in the vessel wall components to which the platelets are exposed.[107] For example, smooth muscle cells and endothelial cells both synthesize collagen but of different types. Collagen types I and III, which are synthesized by smooth muscle cells, are located in the deeper regions of the vessel wall[95,106] and promote platelet adhesion and facilitate aggregation and release.[3,4,118] Collagen types IV and V, which are synthesized by endothelial cells, are located immediately below the endothelium[45,93] and promote platelet adhesion but do not cause platelet aggregation except under specific conditions.[4,23,118]

Platelet adhesion to these collagens requires the plasma protein von Willebrand factor (abbreviated VIII:vWF), which acts as a link between the specific platelet glycoprotein receptor Ib and the subendothelial cell connective tissue.[109] The Ib receptor is absent in the rare inherited platelet abnormality known as Bernard-Soulier syndrome,[25] among other conditions (Chap. 61). The vWF glycoprotein is absent or defective in patients with von Willebrand's disease (Chap. 55).[21] Platelet adhesion is defective in both of these conditions.

Other plasma proteins likewise influence the interaction of platelets with artificial surfaces.[30,31,63,110,111] For example, when certain materials such as prosthetic valves or vessel wall grafts are implanted in the body, the surfaces rapidly become coated with plasma proteins such as albumin and fibrinogen. Thus, the biocompatibility of a prosthetic surface is influenced not only by its inherent physical properties but also by the effects of various plasma proteins bound to it, which, in turn, influence platelet adhesion.

Platelet Release Reaction

The two morphologically distinct platelet α-granules and dense granules, as well as lysosomes, contain an abundance of constituents that influence platelet function, vessel wall tonicity, and coagulation.[20,42-44,48,131] A number of biologic materials, such as collagen, thrombin, epinephrine, thromboxane A_2 (TxA$_2$), and other arachidonic acid metabolites, cause platelets to release their granular contents. With relatively weak stimuli, only the contents of the α-granules are released, but with increased stimuli from higher concentrations of these agents, the contents of the dense granules also are released.[51,69,80,81] Constituents released from the α-granules also contribute to platelet aggregation and activate the coagulation system by as yet unknown mechanisms. The importance of α-granules is evidenced by the abnormal platelet function in two patients with gray platelet syndrome (so named because the platelets appear gray on Romanowsky-stained blood films).[33] In this syndrome, the dense granules and lysosomes are normal, but there is a deficiency of α-granules.

On adhesion and subsequent platelet release, the cationic protein PDGF (discussed earlier) is released from the α-granules and influences smooth muscle cell proliferation and vessel wall hyperplasia after platelet–vessel wall interactions.[91] Platelets also appear to release a permeability factor following adhesion,[71] but its exact mechanism of influence on the vessel wall is unclear.

Platelet Aggregation

Platelet aggregation is induced by stimuli such as ADP, thrombin, TxA$_2$, collagen, and epinephrine. The aggregation reaction is preceded by a change in platelet shape, which is mediated by the direction of the microtubular system and contraction of the microfilament system within the platelet. This response is also characterized morphologically by pseudopod formation attributable in part to the outward projection of the microfilaments. There appear to be three independent mediators of platelet aggregation: ADP, thrombin, and TxA$_2$ (Fig. 58-9).

The *ADP* is released from the dense granules in response to collagen, epinephrine, or TxA$_2$ stimulation. It then acts on a specific receptor site and causes secondary, irreversible

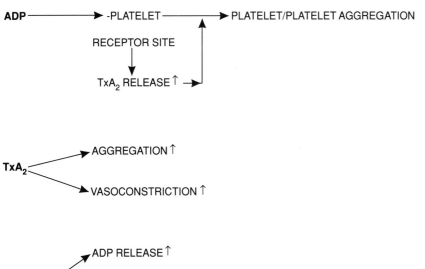

FIG. 58-9. Platelet aggregation induced by *in vitro* and *in vivo* ADP, TxA$_2$, and thrombin stimulation.

platelet aggregation. It may also recruit more platelets to participate in the thrombotic response at the site of injury.[42,43,48] The mechanism for ADP-induced aggregation appears to be dependent on the presence of a specific platelet glycoprotein receptor known as IIb-IIIa. The ADP-induced aggregation causes a change in the conformation of the IIb-IIIa complex on the platelet surface that allows binding of fibrinogen to the complex. The glycoprotein receptor IIb-IIIa is absent in the rare congenital platelet disorder thrombasthenia (Chap. 61). Thrombasthenic platelets do not aggregate with ADP, thrombin, collagen, epinephrine, or arachidonic acid as normal platelets do. When thrombin and collagen are used together, however, thrombasthenic platelets will undergo the release reaction.[76]

Thrombin induces platelet aggregation by at least three mechanisms. First, thrombin stimulates platelets to release ADP, mediating the ADP-induced secondary, irreversible aggregation.[43] Second, thrombin activates the platelet membrane phospholipases, initiating the formation of TxA$_2$.[55] Third, thrombin can induce platelet aggregation independently of the first two mechanisms, but this is poorly understood.[81]

Thromboxane A$_2$, an arachidonic acid metabolite (Fig. 58-10), also induces platelet aggregation. When the platelet is activated by any of a number of stimuli, including thrombin, endotoxin, and epinephrine, membrane phospholipases are activated, which, in turn, liberate arachidonic acid from the platelet phospholipid stores (see Fig. 58-10). The free arachidonic acid is then oxidized to the unstable endoperoxides PGG$_2$ and PGH$_2$ by a reaction that utilizes molecular oxygen and is catalyzed by the enzyme cyclooxygenase. This is the step that is inhibited by aspirin. The endoperoxides are subsequently converted into TxA$_2$ (the principal metabolite) by the enzyme thromboxane synthetase and then by the peroxidases into a number of other prostaglandins (PGD$_2$, PGE$_2$, and PGF$_2$). The TxA$_2$ promotes platelet aggregation directly and may also act synergistically with ADP and other stimuli (thrombin and collagen) to augment the platelet release reaction.[50] The endoperoxides PGG$_2$ and PGH$_2$ also are thought to induce platelet aggregation.[72] The TxA$_2$ is also a potent vasoconstrictor and thus can assist hemostasis and coagulation indirectly.

The same stimuli that activate arachidonic acid metabolism in the platelet also activate arachidonic acid metabolism in the vessel wall endothelium (see Fig. 58-10). As a result, endothelial cells metabolize arachidonic acid, through the cyclooxygenase pathway, into prostacyclin or PGI$_2$. This substance increases cAMP levels in platelets and in so doing inhibits platelet aggregation. The PGI$_2$ also causes vasodilation. These observations have led to the hypothesis that the relative amounts of TxA$_2$ and PGI$_2$ released from platelets and endothelial cells, respectively, modulate the hemostatic response at a site of vessel wall injury, thus ensuring adequate but not excessive coagulation activity.[67]

Free arachidonic acid also is metabolized in the platelet by the cytosol-located lipoxygenase into 12-hydroxyeicosatetraenoic acid (12-HETE), which appears to be important for platelet adhesion. Studies of the role of lipoxygenase metabolites in platelet adhesion and aggregation demonstrated that when TxA$_2$-mediated platelet aggregation is inhibited completely, and the platelets still are able to synthesize 12-HETE, the platelets adhere normally, if not better.[17] Conversely, when 12-HETE production is inhibited and platelet adhesion is impaired, the platelets still are able to synthesize TxA$_2$ and to aggregate normally. The hemorrhagic defect seen in a patient with primary thrombocythemia was also associated with a lipoxygenase deficiency and decreased adhesion, even though the patient's platelets aggregated normally.[35] These studies indicate that platelet adhesion is modulated, in part, by mechanisms regulated by lipoxygenase-derived arachidonic acid metabolites independent of the platelet aggregation phenomenon.

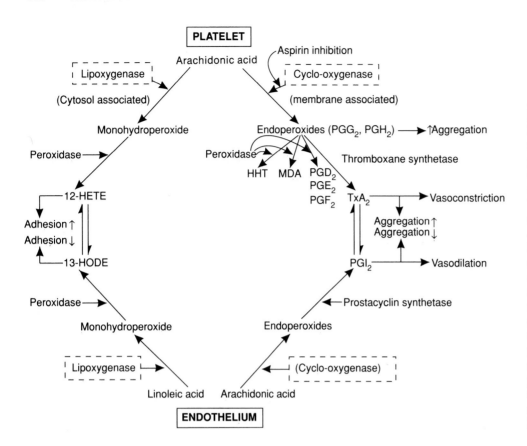

FIG. 58-10. Arachidonic and linoleic acid metabolism by platelets and endothelium. Antagonistic prostanoids TxA₂ and PGI₂ are produced by platelets and endothelial cells, respectively, in cyclooxygenase pathway (right). TxA₂ and PGI₂ modulate platelet aggregation and vasoconstriction. Antagonistic monohydroxides 12-HETE and 13-HODE are produced by platelets and endothelial cells in lipoxygenase pathway (left). Note that 13-HODE is derived from linoleic acid. 12-HETE and 13-HODE are thought to modulate membrane fluidity of platelets and vessel endothelium and in so doing to influence expression of adhesive moieties on surface of cells.[17,18] MDA, malonyldialdehyde; HHT, 17-hydroxyheptadecatetraenoic acid.

These results are relatively new, and their significance requires further study.

Influence of Platelets in Contact Activation

When platelet-poor plasma is recalcified, the plasma clotting time (or recalcification time; see Chap. 52) is much longer than the clotting time of recalcified platelet-rich plasma. The plasma clotting time of platelet-rich plasma is further shortened when ADP is added in a concentration that itself does not facilitate platelet aggregation.[115] This ADP effect has been termed *platelet contact-product forming activity* and represents the ability of platelets to initiate intrinsic coagulation in the presence of ADP by activating factor XII absorbed on the platelet surface. Collagen-induced activation of platelets (in concentrations that do not themselves aggregate platelets) also shortens the plasma clotting time by a mechanism that bypasses the requirements of factor XII.[115,116] Thus, there appear to be two independent but related mechanisms by which platelets can influence contact activation of blood clotting.

Coagulant Activities of Platelets

Platelets participate not only in the initiation of blood coagulation but also in thrombin generation in plasma.[105] Platelets provide a membrane surface on which several clotting factors can bind in order to activate factors X and II (Fig. 58-11).[99] In addition, stimulated platelets secrete a number of clotting factors such as fibrinogen, factor Vₐ, factor VIII (VIII:vWF), factor XI, and factor XII.[14,36,48,49,56–58,64,78,100,112,134] As a result of these ac-

tivities, the prothrombinase complex (see Fig. 58-11) is formed, leading to fibrin clot formation.

Interaction of Platelets with Coagulation Factors

Binding of VIII:vWF to platelets by a specific protein receptor is a prerequisite for *in vitro* platelet aggregation induced by a substance called ristocetin, which is used routinely to evaluate platelet function (Chap. 59).[46,47] This interaction is similar to that involved in the adherence of platelets to the subendothelium *in vivo*. It is unknown if the von Willebrand factor also serves as the platelet receptor site for the subsequent binding of the coagulant portion of factor VIII (Chaps. 50 and 55), which is required for intrinsic system activation of factor X (see below).

Platelet factor V and plasma factor V appear to be immunologically identical.[105] Factor V is most likely acquired by the platelet in the circulation. Factor V and Factor Vₐ bind avidly to the platelet, and this binding does not require platelet activation.[105] In contrast, factor X cannot bind to the unactivated platelet, and factor Xₐ binds avidly only after platelet stimulation.[66] Factor X activation by platelets may permit a more rapid formation of thrombin than conventional coagulation pathways.

Interaction of Platelets with Vitamin K-Dependent Clotting Factors

All vitamin K-dependent factors—II, IX, X, and VII—interact with platelets. Although factors II, IX, and X can bind to negatively charged phospholipids,[74] their ability to bind with high affinity to platelets in the absence of factor V

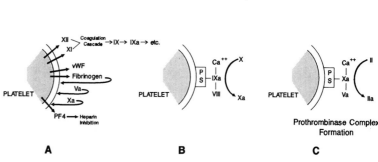

FIG. 58-11. Role of platelets in coagulation. (A) Factors released by platelet α-granule secretion and their interactions. (B) Surface interactions that activate factor X. PS, phosphatidylserine. (C) Conversion of prothrombin to thrombin by stimulation from prothrombinase complex (factors X_a and V_a with calcium).

has not been demonstrated.[66] It appears that factors II_a and X_a are the only vitamin K-dependent factors that can bind specifically to platelets.[66,103] Specific receptor sites for thrombin have been identified. The platelet-bound cofactor V_a appears to be the receptor site for factor X_a. When the calcium-dependent factor X_a is bound to the activated platelet surface, a prothombinase complex is formed (see Fig. 58-11), which, when bound, appears to be stabilized and less susceptible to inactivation by circulating inhibitors.[60,117] Preliminary studies suggest that factors VII and VII_a bind to platelets, facilitating their delivery to the site of hemostatic plug formation.[79]

In plasma, the activation of factor X by factor IX_a and cofactor VIII_a is dependent on the availability of platelet coagulant phospholipids.[61,73,113] The phospholipid reduces the concentration of factor X required to enable its activation by factors VIII and IX.[113]

The participation of platelets in the activation of prothrombin by the prothrombinase complex on the platelet surface has been well defined. The prothrombinase complex consists of factor X_a bound to its receptor (cofactor V_a) in the presence of calcium on the platelet surface.[37,117] The assembly of the prothrombinase complex does not appear to require the presence of prothrombin.[73] Binding of prothrombin to the prothrombinase complex is calcium dependent.[60,103] The relative rate of conversion of prothrombin to thrombin by the prothrombinase complex on the platelet surface is 300,000 times the rate achieved by factor X_a alone.[74]

Role of Platelets in Conversion of Prothrombin to Thrombin

When platelets are activated *in vitro* with suboptimal concentrations of collagen or thrombin, there is an increase in both the rate and the amount of thrombin generated compared with using gel-filtered, unstimulated platelets as a surface for the activation of prothrombin to thrombin by factor X_a.[136] Platelet activation with either collagen or thrombin causes the appearance of phosphatidylserine on the platelet surface.[136] Phosphatidylserine increases the interaction of factor V/V_a and prothrombin with platelets (see Fig. 58-11).[27,37,136] During this platelet activation, the surface changes initially favor the binding and activation of

factor X in preference to the other coagulant factors.[58] However, it is unlikely that surface phosphatidylserine by itself accounts for the ability of activated platelets to enhance the conversion of prothrombin to thrombin by factor X_a. Possibly, intact activated platelets provide a second component that facilitates the receptor-site binding of factor X_a more efficiently than the binding of factor X_a to phospholipids alone.[13,114]

Platelets release other granular constituents that indirectly influence thrombin generation. In particular, PF4 is released, which has specific antiheparinlike activity, thus promoting coagulation.[13,92] On the contrary, vessel wall–derived glycosaminoglycans, such as heparin sulfate and dermatan sulfate, inhibit thrombin generation[38,92] and act as regulators of the events at the site of injury. Therefore, the effects of these constituents released from the vessel wall may be neutralized by PF4, thus blocking their potential anticoagulant activity at the site of injury.

CHAPTER SUMMARY

Circulating blood platelets are formed from megakaryocytes within the bone marrow. Megakaryocytes initially evolve from undifferentiated stem cells. A specific hormone, thrombopoietin, is responsible for commitment of the stem cell to the megakaryocytic cell line. The megakaryoblast matures through three stages: (1) the promegakaryocyte, in which the network of the demarcating membrane begins to form; (2) the megakaryocyte, in which the various organelles and a more developed demarcating membrane system (DMS) are formed, making possible the identification of forming platelets; and (3) the metamegakaryocyte, in which an extensive DMS functions as platelet fields. These platelet fields or cytoplasmic fragments are shed from the metamegakaryocyte into the bone marrow sinuses, where they undergo further dissolution, forming individual anucleated platelets that are released into the circulation.

In the circulation, platelets perform a number of functions. Intact, unstimulated platelets contribute a "factor" (as yet unnamed) that influences vessel wall permeability. Platelets interact with numerous stimuli, such as coagulation factors and sites on the injured vessel wall, influencing various aspects of the hemostatic process. Adherence of platelets to the injured vessel wall provides a physical barrier to further blood loss. Specific constituents released from adhering platelets influence vessel wall tone (the vasoconstrictor TxA_2), vessel wall repair

(PDGF), and coagulation (factors V$_a$, VIII: vWF, XI, XII, PF4, and fibrinogen). Coagulation influence is achieved by the platelet providing a surface phospholipid on which the assembly of these coagulant factors takes place, facilitating the catalysis of prothrombin to thrombin, leading to the formation of a stable platelet–fibrin clot.

REFERENCES

1. Andersson LP, Brown JE: Interaction of factor VIII–von Willebrand factor with phospholipid vesicles. Biochem J 200:161, 1981

2. Aster RH, Jandl JH: Platelet sequestration in man. 1: Methods. J Clin Invest 43:843, 1964

3. Balleisen L, Gay S, Marx R et al: Comparative investigations on the influence of human bovine collagens type I, II, III on the aggregation of human platelets. Klin Wochenschr 53:903, 1975

4. Barnes MJ, Bailey AJ, Gordon JL et al: Platelet aggregation by basement membrane-associated collagens. Thromb Res 18:375, 1980

5. Behnke O: Electron microscope study of the megakaryocyte of the rat bone marrow. J Ultrastruct Res 24:412, 1968

6. Behnke O: An electron microscope study of the megakaryocyte. II: Some aspects of platelet release and microtubules. J Ultrastruct Res 26:111, 1969

7. Behnke O: Microtubules in disc-shaped blood cells. Int Rev Exp Pathol 9:1, 1970

8. Behnke O: The morphology of blood platelet membrane systems. Ser Haematol 3:3, 1970

9. Behnke O, Emmersen J: Structural identification of thrombosthenin in rat megakaryocytes. Scand J Haematol 9:130, 1972

10. Behnke O, Kristensen B, Nielson L: Electron microscopical observations on actinoid and myosinoid filaments in blood platelets. J Ultrastruct Res 37:351, 1971

11. Bensusan HB, Koh TL, Henry KG et al: Evidence that fibronectin is the collagen receptor on platelet membranes. Proc Natl Acad Sci USA 75:5864, 1978

12. Bettex–Galland M, Lüscher E: Thrombosthenin, the contractile protein from blood platelets and its relation to other contractile proteins. Adv Protein Chem 20:1, 1965

13. Bevers EM, Comforius P, van Rijn JLM et al: Generation of prothrombin converting activity at the outer surface of platelets. Eur J Biochem 122:429, 1982

14. Breederveld K, Giddings JC, tenCate JW et al: The localization of factor V within normal human platelets and a demonstration of a platelet-factor V antigen in congenital factor V deficiency. Br J Haematol 29:405, 1975

15. Breton–Gorius J, Guichard J: Ultrastructural localization of peroxidase activity in human platelets and megakaryocytes. Am J Pathol 66:277, 1972

16. Buchanan MR, Richardson M, Vallee E: Basement membrane underlying the vascular endothelium is not thrombogenic. Clin Invest Med 8(suppl B):B27, 1985

17. Buchanan MR, Butt RW, Markham B et al: Effects of aspirin and salicylate on platelet function. Prostaglandins Leukotrienes Med 21:157, 1986

18. Buchanan MR, Haas TA, Lagarde M et al: 13-Hydroxyoctadecadienoic acid is the vessel wall chemorepellant factor, LOX. J Biol Chem 260:16056, 1985

19. Buchanan MR, Butt RW, Magas J et al: Endothelial cells produce a lipoxygenase derived chemorepellant which influences platelet/endothelial cell interactions: Effect of aspirin and salicylate. Thromb Haemost 53:306, 1985

20. Buckingham S, Maynert EW: The release of 5-hydroxytryptamine, potassium and amino acids from platelets. J Pharmacol Exp Ther 143:332, 1964

21. Caen JP, Michel H, Tobelem G et al: Adhesion and aggregation of human platelets to rabbit subendothelium. A new approach for investigation: Specific antibodies. Experientia 33:91, 1976

22. Cazenave JP, Blondowska D, Richardson M et al: Quantitative radio-isotopic measurement and scanning electron microscopic study of platelet adherence to a collagen coated surface and to subendothelium with a rotating probe device. J Lab Clin Med 93:60, 1979

23. Cazenave JP, Packham MA, Kinlough–Rathbone RL et al: Platelet adherence to the vessel wall and to collagen coated surfaces. Adv Exp Med Biol 102:31, 1978

24. Davis RB, White JG: Localization of 5 hydroxytryptamine in blood platelets: A radioautographic and ultrastructural study. Br J Haematol 15:93, 1968

25. Degos L, Tobelem G, Lethielluex P et al: Molecular defect in platelets from patients with Bernard-Soulier syndrome. Blood 50:899, 1977

26. Dutilh CE, Haddeman E, Don JA et al: The role of arachidonic lipo-oxygenase and fatty acids during irreversible blood platelet aggregation in vitro. Prostaglandins Med 6:111, 1981

27. Esmon CT: The subunit structure of thrombin activated factor V: Isolation of factor V, separation of subunits and reconstitution of biological activity. J Biol Chem 254:964, 1979

28. Fedorko M: The functional capacity of guinea pig megakaryocytes. 1: Uptake of ^{3}H-serotonin by megakaryocytes and their physiology and morphologic response to stimuli for the platelet release reaction. Lab Invest 36:310, 1977

29. Fedorko M, Levine R: Tannic acid effect on membrane of cell surface origin in guinea pig megakaryocytes and platelets. J Histochem Cytochem 24:601, 1976

30. Feuerstein IA, Brophy JM, Brash JL: Platelet transport and adhesion to reconstituted collagen and artificial surfaces. Trans Am Soc Artif Intern Organs 21:427, 1975

31. Friedman LI, Liem H, Grabowski EF et al: Inconsequentiality of surface properties for initial platelet adhesion. Trans Am Soc Artif Intern Organs 16:63, 1970

32. George JN: Studies on platelet plasma membranes. IV: Quantitative analysis of platelet membrane glycoproteins by ^{125}I-diazotized diiodosulfanilic acid labelling and SDS-polyacrylamide gel electrophoresis. J Lab Clin Med 92:430, 1978

33. Gerrard JM, Philips DR, Rao GHR et al: Biochemical studies of two patients with the gray platelet syndrome. J Clin Invest 66:102, 1980

34. Gerrard JM, White JG: The structure and formation of platelets with emphasis on their contractile nature. In Ioachim HL (ed): Pathobiology Annual, p 31. New York, Appleton–Century–Crofts, 1976

35. Gibson BES, Buchanan MR, Barr RD et al: Primary thrombocythemia in childhood: Symptomatic episodes and their relationship to thromboxane A$_2$, 6-keto-PGE$_1$ and 12 hydroxyeicosatetraenoic acid production: A case report. Prostaglandins Leukotrienes Med 26:221, 1987

36. Giddings JC, Shearn SAM, Bloom AL: Platelet associated coagulation factors: Immunochemical detection and the effects of calcium. Br J Haematol 39:569, 1978

37. Guinto ER, Esmon CT: Formation of a calcium-binding site on bovine activated factor V following reconstitution of the isolated subunits. J Biol Chem 257:10038, 1982

38. Handin RI, Cohen HJ: Purification and binding properties of platelet factor 4. J Biol Chem 251:4273, 1976

39. Harker LA: Platelet survival time: Its measurement and use. Prog Hemost Thromb 4:321, 1978

40. Heaton WA, Davis HH, Welch MJ et al: Indium-III: A new radionuclide label for studying human platelet kinetics. Br J Haematol 42:613, 1979

41. Hirsch ED, Favre–Gilly J, Dameshek W: Thrombopathic thrombocytopenia: Successful transfusion of blood platelets. Blood 5:568, 1950

42. Holmsen H, Day HJ: The selectivity of the thrombin-induced

platelet release reaction: Subcellular localization of released and retained substances. J Lab Clin Med 75:840, 1970

43. Holmsen H, Day HJ, Storm E: Adenine nucleotide metabolism of blood platelets. VI: Subcellular localization of nucleotide pools with different functions in the platelet release reaction. Biochim Biophys Acta 186:254, 1969

44. Hovig T: The ultrastructure of rabbit blood platelet aggregates. Thromb Diath Haemorrh 8:455, 1962

45. Howard BV, Macarak EJ, Gunson D et al: Characterization of the collagen synthesized by endothelial cells in culture. Proc Natl Acad Sci USA 73:2361, 1976

46. Kao KJ, Pizzo SV, McKee PA: Demonstration and characterization of specific binding sites for factor VIII/von Willebrand factor on human platelets. J Clin Invest 63:656, 1979

47. Kao KJ, Pizzo SV, McKee PA: Platelet receptors for factor VIII/von Willebrand protein: Functional correlation of receptor occupancy and ristocetin-induced platelet aggregation. Proc Natl Acad Sci USA 76:5317, 1979

48. Kaplan KL, Broekman MJ, Chernoff A et al: Platelet alpha-granule proteins: Studies on release and subcellular localization. Blood 53:604, 1979

49. Keenan JP, Solum NO: Quantitative studies on the release of platelet fibrinogen by thrombin. Br J Haematol 23:461, 1972

50. Kinlough–Rathbone RL, Packham MA, Mustard JF: Synergism between platelet-aggregating agents: The role of the arachidonate pathway. Thromb Res 11:567, 1977

51. Kinlough–Rathbone RL, Reimers JJ, Mustard JF: Sodium arachidonate can induce platelet shape change and aggregation which are independent of the release reaction. Science 192:1011, 1976

52. Lajmanovich A, Hudry–Clergeon G, Freyssinet J-M et al: Human factor VIII procoagulant activity and phospholipid interaction. Biochim Biophys Acta 678:132, 1981

53. Levin J, Evatt BL: Humoral control of thrombopoiesis. Blood Cells 5:105, 1979

54. Levin J, Levin FC, Penington DG et al: Measurement of ploidy distribution in megakaryocyte colonies obtained from culture: With studies of the effects of thrombocytopenia. Blood 57:284, 1981

55. Lewis N, Majerus PW: Lipid metabolism in human platelets. II: De novo phospholipid synthesis and the effect of thrombin on the pattern of synthesis. J Clin Invest 48:2114, 1969

56. Lipscomb MS, Walsh PN: Human platelet factor XI: Localization in platelet membranes of factor XI-like activity and its functional distinction from plasma factor XI. J Clin Invest 63:1006, 1979

57. Lopaciuk S, Lovette KM, McDonagh J et al: Subcellular distribution of fibrinogen and factor XIII in human platelets. Thromb Res 8:453, 1976

58. Luscher EF: Ein fibrinstabilisierender Faktor aus Thrombocyten. Schweiz Med Wochenschr 87:1220, 1957

59. Madri JA, Dreyer B, Pitlick FA et al: The collagenase components of the subendothelium: Correlation of structure and function. Lab Invest 43:303, 1980

60. Mann KG, Prendergast FG, Bloom JW: The metal ion and phospholipid interactions of the vitamin-K dependent factors. In Mann KG, Taylor FB Jr (eds): The Regulation of Coagulation, p 3. New York, Elsevier, 1980

61. Marcus AJ, Zucker–Franklin D, Safier LB et al: Studies on human platelet granules and membranes. J Clin Invest 45:14, 1966

62. Martin JH, Carson FL, Race GJ: Calcium containing platelet granules. J Cell Biol 60:775, 1976

63. Mason RG, Mohammad SF, Chuang HY et al: The adhesion of platelets to subendothelium, collagen and artificial surfaces. Semin Thromb Hemostas 3:98, 1976

64. McDonagh J, Kiesselbach TH, Wagner RH: Factor XIII and antiplasmin activity in human platelets. Am J Physiol 216:508, 1969

65. Miale JB: Hemostasis and blood coagulation. In Miale JB: Laboratory Medicine Hematology, 6th ed, p 772. St. Louis, CV Mosby, 1982

66. Miletich JP, Jackson CM, Majerus PW: Properties of the factor X_a binding site on human platelets. J Biol Chem 253:6908, 1978

67. Moncada S, Vane JR: Arachidonic acid metabolites and the interactions between platelets and blood-vessel walls. N Engl J Med 300:1142, 1979

68. Murphy EA, Robinson GA, Rowsell HC et al: The pattern of platelet disappearance. Blood 30:26, 1967

69. Mustard JF, Perry DW, Kinlough–Rathbone RL et al: Factors responsible for ADP-induced release reaction of human platelets. Am J Physiol 228:1757, 1975

70. Nachman RL, Marcus A, Safier L: Platelet thrombosthenin: Subcellular localization and function. J Clin Invest 46:1380, 1967

71. Nachman RL, Weksler B, Ferris B: Increased vascular permeability produced by human platelet granule cationic extract. J Clin Invest 49:274, 1970

72. Needleman P, Whitaker MO, Wyche A et al: Manipulation of platelet aggregation by prostaglandins and their fatty acid precursors: Pharmacological basis for a therapeutic approach. Prostaglandins 19:165, 1980

73. Nesheim ME, Eid S, Mann KG: Assembly of the prothrombinase complex in the absence of prothrombin. J Biol Chem 256:9874, 1981

74. Nesheim ME, Taswell JB, Mann KG: The contribution of bovine factor V and factor V_a to the activity of prothrombinase. J Biol Chem 254:10952, 1979

75. Nurden AT, Caen JP: Specific roles for platelet surface glycoproteins in platelet function. Nature 255:720, 1975

76. O'Brien JR, Woodhouse MA: Platelets: Their size, shape and stickiness in vitro: Degranulation and propinquity. Exp Biol Med 3:90, 1968

77. Okuma M, Uchina H: Altered arachidonate metabolism by platelets in patients with myeloproliferative disorders. Blood 13:1258, 1979

78. Østerud B, Rapaport SI, Lavine KK: Factor V activity of platelets: Evidence for an activated factor V molecule and for a platelet activator. Blood 49:819, 1977

79. Ozge–Anwar AH, Ofosu FA, Blajchman MA: Evidence that intact human platelets provide factor VII-like activity for the activation of factor X by the extrinsic coagulation pathway. Thromb Haemost 54:176, 1985

80. Packham MA: Stages in the interaction of platelets with collagen. Thromb Haemost 36:269, 1976

81. Packham MA, Kinlough–Rathbone RL, Reimers H-J et al: Mechanisms of platelet aggregation independent of adenosine diphosphate. In Silver MJ, Smith JB, Kocsis JJ (eds): Prostaglandins in Hematology, p 247. New York, Spectrum Publishing, 1977

82. Paulus JM: DNA metabolism and the development of organelles in guinea pig megakaryocytes: A combined ultrastructural, autoradiographic and cytophotometric study. Blood 35:298, 1970

83. Paulus JM: Platelet size in man. Blood 46:321, 1975

84. Phillips DR, Agin PP: Platelet plasma membrane glycoproteins. Evidence for the presence of nonequivalent disulfide bonds using nonreduced–reduced two-dimensional gel electrophoresis. J Biol Chem 252:2121, 1977

85. Piovella F, Ascaari E, Sofar GM et al: Immunofluorescent detection of factor VIII-related antigen in human platelets and megakaryocytes. Haemostasis 3:288, 1974

86. Pisciotta A, Stefanini M, Dameshek W: Studies on platelets. X: Morphologic characteristics of megakaryocytes by phase contrast microscopy in normal patients and in patients with idiopathic thrombocytopenia purpura. Blood 8:703, 1953

87. Pollard TD: Functional implications of the biochemical and structural properties of cytoplasmic contractile proteins. In

Inoise S, Stephens RF (eds): Molecules and Cell Movement, p 259. New York, Raven Press, 1978

88. Puszkin E, Maldonado R, Spaet TH et al: Platelet myosin: Localization of the rod myosin fragment and effect of its antibodies on platelet function. J Biol Chem 252:4371, 1977

89. Rabellino EM, Nachman RL, Williams N et al: Human megakaryocytes. 1: Characterization of the membrane and cytoplasmic components of isolated marrow megakaryocytes. J Exp Med 149:1273, 1979

90. Rak K: Effect of vincristine on platelet production in mice. Br J Haematol 22:617, 1972

91. Ross R, Glomset J, Kariya B et al: A platelet-dependent serum factor that stimulates the proliferation of arterial smooth muscle cells in vitro. Proc Natl Acad Sci USA 71:1207, 1974

92. Rucinski B, Niewiarowski S, James P et al: Antiheparin proteins secreted by human platelets: Purification, characterization and radioimmunoassays. Blood 53:47, 1979

93. Sage H, Crouch E, Bornstein P: Collagen synthesis by bovine aortic endothelial cells in culture. Biochemistry 18:5433, 1979

94. Schulz H, Schiller K: Microtubuli and Filamente in prospektiven Plattachenfeldern der Megakaryocyten. Z Zellforsch 87:309, 1968

95. Scott DM, Horwood R, Grant ME et al: Characterization of the major collagen species present in porcine aorta and the synthesis of their precursors by smooth muscle cells in culture. Connect Tissue Res 5:7, 1977

96. Shaklai M, Tavassoli M: Demarcation membrane system in rat megakaryocytes and the mechanism of platelet formation: A membrane reorganization process. J Ultrastruct Res 62:270, 1978

97. Shick PK, Kurica KB, Chacko GK: Location of phosphatidylethanolamine and phosphatidylserine in human platelet plasma membrane. J Clin Invest 57:1221, 1976

98. Shulman NR, Watkins JP, Hscoitz SB et al: Evidence that the spleen retains the youngest and hemostatically most effective platelets. Trans Assoc Am Phys 81:312, 1968

99. Sixma JJ: Platelet coagulant activities. Thromb Haemost 40:163, 1978

100. Slot JW, Bouma BN, Montgomery R et al: Platelet factor VIII-related antigen: Immunofluorescent localization. Thromb Res 13:871, 1978

101. Steiner M, Ikeda Y: Quantitative assessment of polymerized and depolymerized platelet microtubules: Changes caused by aggregating agents. J Clin Invest 63:443, 1979

102. Stemerman MB, Spaet TH: The subendothelium and thrombogenesis. Bull NY Acad Med 48:289, 1972

103. Stenflo J, Dahlback B: Activation of prothrombin by factor X_a on the surface of platelets. In Mann KG, Taylor FB (eds): The Regulation of Coagulation, p 225. New York, Elsevier, 1980

104. Tobb–Smith AHT: Why the platelets were discovered. Br J Haematol 13:618, 1967

105. Tracy PB, Paterson JM, Nesheim ME et al: Interaction of coagulation factor V and factor V_a with platelets. J Biol Chem 254:10354, 1979

106. Trelstad RL: Human aorta collagens: Evidence for three distinct species. Biochem Biophys Res Commun 57:717, 1974

107. Trelstad RL: Special state of the fibril end: Site of growth, point of cell surface attachment, and possible site for platelet interaction. In Gastpar H (ed): Collagen-Platelet Interactions, p 153. New York, Schattauer Verlag, 1978

108. Tschopp TB, Baumgartner HR, Silbergauer K et al: Platelet adhesion and platelet thrombus formation on subendothelium of human arteries and veins exposed to flowing blood in vitro: A comparison with rabbit aorta. Haemostasis 8:19, 1979

109. Turritto VT, Baumgartner HR: Platelet interaction with subendothelium in flowing rabbit blood. Effect of blood shear rate. Microvasc Res 17:38, 1979

110. Turritto VT, Leonard EF: Platelet adhesion to a spinning disc. Trans Am Soc Artif Intern Organs 18:348, 1972

111. Turritto VT, Muggli R, Baumgartner HR: Platelet adhesion and thrombus formation on subendothelium, Epon, gelatin, and collagen under artificial flow conditions. Trans Am Soc Artif Intern Organs 24:568, 1978

112. Tuszynski GP, Bevacona SJ, Schmaier AH et al: Factor XI antigen and activity in platelets. Blood 59:1148, 1982

113. van Dieijen G, Tans G, Rosing J et al: The role of phospholipid and factor VIII_a in the activation of bovine factor X. Biochemistry 256:3433, 1981

114. van Zutphen H, Bevers EM, Hemker HC et al: Contribution of platelet factor V content to platelet factor 3 activity. Br J Haematol 45:119, 1980

115. Walsh PN: The role of platelets in the contact phase of blood coagulation. Br J Haematol 22:237, 1972

116. Walsh PN: The effects of collagen and kaolin on the intrinsic coagulant activity of platelets: Evidence for an alternate pathway not requiring factor XII. Br J Haematol 22:393, 1972

117. Walsh PN, Biggs R: The role of platelets in intrinsic factor X_a formation. Br J Haematol 22:743, 1972

118. Wang CL, Miyata T, Weksler B et al: Collagen induced platelet aggregation and release: Critical size and structural requirements of collagen. Biochim Biophys Acta 544:468, 1978

119. Weiss HJ, deWitte L, Kaplan KL et al: Heterogeneity in storage pool deficiency: Studies in granule-bound substances in 18 patients including variants deficient in α-granules, platelet factor 4, β-thromboglobulin and platelet-derived growth factor. Blood 54:1296, 1979

120. White JG: Effects of colchicine and vinca alkaloids on human platelets. 1: Influence on platelet microtubules and contractile function. Am J Pathol 53:281, 1968

121. White JG: Effects of colchicine and vinca alkaloids on human platelets. II: Changes in the dense tubular system and formation of an unusual inclusion in incubated cells. Am J Pathol 53:447, 1968

122. White JG: Fine structural alterations induced in platelets by adenosine diphosphate. Blood 31:604, 1968

123. White JG: The submembrane filaments of blood platelets. Am J Pathol 56:267, 1969

124. White JG: Effects of colchicine and vinca alkaloids on human platelets. III: Influence on primary internal contraction and secondary aggregation. Am J Pathol 54:467, 1969

125. White JG: Platelet morphology. In Johnson SA (ed): The Circulating Platelet, p 45. New York, Academic Press, 1971

126. White JG: Ultrastructural physiology and cytochemistry of blood platelets. In Brinkhous KM, Shermer RW, Mostofi FK (eds): The Platelet, p 85. Baltimore, Williams & Wilkins, 1971

127. White JG: Identification of platelet secretion in the electron microscope. Ser Haematol 6:429, 1973

128. White JG: Electron microscopic studies of platelet secretion. Prog Hemost Thromb 2:49, 1974

129. White JG: Physiochemical dissection of platelet structural physiology. In Baldini MG, Ebbe S (eds): Platelets: Production, Function, Transfusion and Storage, p 235. New York, Grune & Stratton, 1974

130. White JG, Conrad WJ: The fine structure of freeze-fractured blood platelets. Am J Pathol 70:45, 1973

131. White JG, Krivet W: An ultrastructural basis for the shape changes induced by chilling. Blood 30:625, 1967

132. Wood JG: Electron microscopic localization of 5-hydroxytryptamine (5-HT). Texas Rep Biol Med 23:828, 1965

133. Wright JH: The origin and nature of blood plates. Boston Med Surg J 154:643, 1906

134. Zucker MB, Broekman MJ, Kaplan KL: Factor VIII-related antigen in human blood platelets: Localization and release by thrombin and collagen. J Lab Clin Med 94:675, 1979

135. Zucker–Franklin D: The submembranous fibrils of human platelets. J Cell Biol 47:293, 1970

136. Zwaal RFA, Hemker HC: Blood cell membranes and haemostasis. Haemostasis 11:12, 1982

59

Laboratory Evaluation of Platelets

Charles E. Manner

The laboratory investigation of a disorder of hemostasis may center on the evaluation of platelet number and function. These two aspects are interrelated in that abnormalities of either or both will result in a hemostatic defect; however, tests of platelet function usually are indicated only if platelet numbers are adequate.

The evaluation of platelet number is a relatively straightforward matter and will not be covered in detail. Evaluation of platelet function is much more complex, and the majority of this chapter is devoted to this subject. Although von Willebrand's disease is not a disorder of platelet function *per se*, the deficiency of plasma von Willebrand factor (vWF) prevents normal platelet adhesion. Thus key tests for this disease utilize platelet aggregometry and consequently are included in the discussion of platelet function testing.

In light of the various roles played by the platelet in hemostasis, the laboratory evaluation of platelet function involves not only quantitation of their numbers but also tests that provide a measure of adhesion, aggregation, release, or clot retraction, either separately or in their sum.

ENUMERATION OF PLATELETS

Platelet numbers must be sufficient for them to play their supportive role in hemostasis. When evaluating a bleeding problem that may be traceable to platelets, the counting of platelets is an important and logical starting point. This may be done simply by estimating the number of platelets on a peripheral blood film or by using various manual or automated techniques.[19,23,24]

Estimates from Peripheral Blood Films

The procedure for peripheral blood film platelet estimates is detailed in Chapter 25 in the section on manual differentials. A general reference range for platelets is 140 to 440×10^9/L, meaning that there are approximately 10 to 40 red cells per platelet in normal peripheral blood. Thus, an oil-immersion field containing 100 red cells should have between 3 and 10 platelets, whereas a field containing 200 red cells should have between 5 and 20 platelets. Review of peripheral films is advantageous in detecting causes of artifactually low counts secondary to platelet clumping caused by anticoagulant-dependent platelet agglutinins or clots from poorly collected specimens. Giant platelets seen in some congenital platelet function defects and certain myeloproliferative disorders will also be appreciated by this method.

MANUAL PLATELET COUNTS

The two most commonly employed methods of manual platelet counts utilize a 1:100 or 1:200 dilution of blood applied to a Neubauer hemocytometer chamber. The two methods differ in the way the platelets are made visible. The Tocantins method using Rees-Ecker diluent employs a citrate-formaldehyde buffer with brilliant cresyl blue as a platelet stain for light microscopy.[21] This diluent fixes and preserves red blood cells as well as platelets to prevent their disintegration.

The more popular phase-contrast microscopy method uses a phase microscope and 1% ammonium oxalate diluting fluid, which lyses red cells and allows platelets to form pseudopods.[5] In other respects, the mechanics of handling the blood sample are similar.

Specimen Requirements

When possible, venous blood collected with EDTA is preferable, as capillary puncture samples can yield low counts secondary to platelet adhesion to the wound. If venipuncture is not possible, capillary puncture should be performed with a larger blade so that a deep wound with freely flowing blood is obtained, and the specimen should be taken off immediately to avoid significant platelet adhesion to the wound.

Reagents and Equipment

A Neubauer hemocytometer and coverslip is required for the Rees-Ecker method or a special thin, flat-bottom counting chamber for the phase method. Red blood cell diluting pipets or the Unopette platelet-counting system is used. Unopette systems may be purchased with premeasured diluent ready for use.

To make diluent for the Rees-Ecker method, combine 3.8 g of sodium citrate, 0.22 mL of neutral formaldehyde (38%), and 0.05 g of brilliant cresyl blue in approximately 50 mL of distilled water. Bring to 100 mL with distilled water and filter. The diluent for the phase-contrast method is filtered 1% ammonium oxalate in distilled water.

A standard light microscope or phase microscope with a long working distance phase condenser and phase objective is needed.

Procedure

Depending on laboratory preference, platelets may be counted either in 1/5 of a mm^2 or 1 mm^2 in the center of the chamber. Both sides of the chamber should be mounted and counted and the results averaged. With the Rees-Ecker method, platelets appear as highly refractile, round bodies that are approximately 1/10 the size of the surrounding red cells. With the phase-contrast method, red cells are lysed, leaving only platelets and leukocytes, which can be distinguished easily. See Chapter 25 for a detailed description of hemocytometer cell counts.

Calculations

Platelets are preferably reported per L but may be reported per μL (equivalent to mm^3). The number of platelets counted is multiplied by the dilution factor (100 or 200), by a chamber depth-correction factor (10) because the depth of the chamber is 0.1 mm, and by an area correction factor depending on whether 1 mm^2 or 1/5 mm^2 was counted (1 or 5). For example, if 1 mm^2 is counted and the dilution is 1:100, the number of platelets counted is multiplied by 1000 ($100 \times 10 \times 1$) to find the number of platelets per mm^3 or μL. Multiplying this result by 10^6 gives the result per liter (L).

Reference Range

The reference range is 140 to 440×10^9/L.

Comments and Sources of Error

Rigid standardization of technique and quality control is extremely important in manual platelet counting. Results should be checked periodically against peripheral blood estimates, automated counts, or both.

The phase microscope must be checked periodically according to manufacturer recommendations to ensure that the phase objective and annulus condenser are aligned correctly (Chap. 4).

Special care should be taken to keep the chambers free of dirt or debris that might be mistaken for platelets. It is useful to check the chamber microscopically with a coverslip in place for such dirt or debris before adding the diluted platelet suspension. Ethyl alcohol (95% v/v) and a lint-free cloth or lens paper are recommended for cleaning.

Platelet clumping or discrepancies between the two chambers of 20% or more necessitates repeat counts. A fresh specimen may be necessary.

When the platelet count is low, a larger volume on each side may need to be counted to improve accuracy and precision. For very low counts (i.e., less than 50×10^9/L), a 1:20 dilution should be made in a white cell diluting pipet and a new dilution factor used in the calculation. This allows more platelets to be counted. The coefficient of variation (discrepancies in duplicate counts on the same patient) for this method typically is 10% for the phase-contrast method and 16% to 25% for the Rees-Ecker method.

AUTOMATED PLATELET COUNTS

Automated counters employ either optical methods (detection of the degree of light scattering) or electrical methods (change in the electrical resistance or capacitance across a circuit) to detect particles as they stream through an aperture tube or flow cell. Varying the suspending diluent or the threshold settings of the circuitry allows separate counting of blood cells of different sizes. (Chaps. 41 through 43 provide a detailed discussion of the principles of automated cell counting.) Briefly, various instruments exist for counting platelets, including multiparameter instruments (Chap. 43) and a few instruments dedicated solely to platelet counts. Automatic platelet counters may sample whole blood and discriminate platelets from red cells on the basis of their size; sample whole blood, lyse the red cells, and discriminate between platelets and leukocytes on the basis of their size; or sample platelet-rich plasma (PRP) and calculate platelet counts on the basis of sample dilution, volume counted, and hematocrit of original sample. The last-named method is more prone to errors caused by the manipulation of blood samples to procure PRP.

Quality Control

Regardless of the instrument, it must be standardized against reference methods such as the phase-contrast method or against a single-channel instrument that has been calibrated by means of platelet threshold curves. Once an instrument has been standardized or calibrated, suspensions of fixed human platelets, which are available from several suppliers, may be used as day-to-day controls. Controls are usually run at the beginning of each batch of platelet counts and may be interspersed between patient samples when batches of more than 15 samples are run. Records of quality control data must be examined periodically to detect subtle instrumental or reagent problems.

Samples from each batch should be screened for accuracy by quick estimates from the peripheral blood film. Where the estimates and automated counts do not agree, results should be obtained by the phase-contrast method. Histograms of platelet populations provide a further means of quality control.

Comments and Sources of Error

The greatest advantage of automated platelet counts is their precision. Depending on the particular instrument, the coefficient of variation is 1% to 5%.

The key to reliable platelet counts by these methods is good quality control. There are several sources of error. Falsely high platelet counts may result from contamination of reagents with particles or bacteria; carry over from a prior sample with a high platelet count; or particles that should not be counted but are registered as platelets, such as fragments of red or white blood cells, insufficiently lysed red cells, or red cells with inclusion bodies (with methods that lyse red cells). Falsely low counts may result from platelet agglutinins or platelet satellitism. Exceptionally large platelets may not be counted if upper as well as lower thresholds are used. Each of these sources of error can be eliminated with a good quality control regime, including careful review of histograms generated by automated instruments and review of the peripheral blood film.

Reference Range

The reference range is 140 to 440 $\times$ 10^9/L

PLATELET ADHESION

Platelet adhesion to a vessel wound with exposed subendothelial collagen or to glass beads *in vitro* requires the presence of plasma von Willebrand factor (VIII:vWF), platelets capable of interacting with vWF (platelets with glycoprotein Ib receptors), and platelet capacity to aggregate. Several tests measure these aspects of platelet function. The preferred test is the bleeding time. Two other tests have been in clinical use: one utilizes a glass bead column; the other is an *in vivo* test that measures the number of platelets that have adhered to a standardized skin wound. However, these tests are seldom performed in the routine hematology laboratory today, because the bleeding time and aggregation studies provide more valuable information. Details of these procedures may be found in other textbooks of hematology. For academic purposes, only the principles and reference ranges of these two tests are presented below.

THE BLEEDING TIME
Principle

The bleeding time is the time it takes for a standard wound to stop bleeding. It is a comprehensive test of platelet action *in vivo* and is sensitive to abnormalities of platelet numbers and function, to plasma VIII:vWF deficiencies, and to abnormalities of vessel wall composition that interfere with platelet function.[9,11,15,16] The key to precision in the bleeding time is standardization of the wound. This standardization was a problem

with the tests described earlier by Duke and Ivy.[11] Modifications of the Ivy method using a template such as described by Mielke et al[16] or the commercially available devices that make a standard wound[15] are attempts to solve this problem. These tests require standardization of venous and capillary pressure with the use of a blood pressure cuff inflated to 40 mm Hg for the duration of the test. This application of constant venous pressure also increases the sensitivity of the test.

Procedure
1. Inspect the volar surface of forearm carefully for a site that is free of visible vessels (*e.g.*, veins or capillary beds) and hair. Clean the site with alcohol sponges and allow it to dry thoroughly.
2. Position the sphygmomanometer about the upper arm (do not place over clothing), and inflate it to 40 mm Hg. Maintain this pressure throughout the procedure.
3. Hold the template or commercial device firmly and position it on the skin without exerting excessive pressure: avoid indenting skin surface. Incisions should be made parallel to the elbow crease. Start the stopwatch as soon as blood appears in the wound. Blot the blood from the wound at 30-second intervals with the edge of filter paper. Care must be taken not to touch the incision. The test is complete when blood ceases to stain the filter paper. If a device with two blades is used for duplicate testing, the times for the two incisions to stop bleeding should agree within 1 minute and are averaged for the final result.

Reference Range

Two to nine minutes is a general reference range. However, each laboratory should establish its own range.

Comments and Sources of Error

The bleeding time test requires care and skill on the part of the operator. The volar skin must be absolutely dry before proceeding, and the template device must be held firmly so an adequate incision of the proper depth is made. The incision site should not be touched directly by the filter paper. The arm must not be held such that traction is put on the skin about the incision site.

Some normal individuals are more susceptible to the effects of aspirin-containing medication. Patients should be questioned regarding medications they are taking. They should not have taken any aspirin or aspirin-containing products during the week preceding testing. Medications of the nonsteroidal anti-inflammatory class, such as ibuprofen, tolmetin sodium, and naproxen, should be discontinued 24 hours before the test.

Patients with mild qualitative platelet disorders and a significant bleeding history may manifest variability in their bleeding times and occasionally will have a normal result.[8] Sometimes, it is necessary to perform several bleeding time tests before a diagnosis can be made.

To ensure consistency in test performance and results, the procedure should be reviewed periodically with all personnel who perform it.

The bleeding time is prolonged in thrombocytopenia, von Willebrand disease, acquired and inherited platelet disorders, afibrinogenemia, severe hypofibrinogenemia, and some vascular disorders.

GLASS BEAD RETENTION TEST
Principle

When blood is passed through a glass bead column, normal platelets that have access to normal vWF will adhere and aggregate to the beads such that the effluent from the column will have a much lower platelet count than the starting sample.[4,12]

Reference Range

The percentage of platelets retained in the glass bead column should be approximately 70% or greater. Each laboratory should establish its own reference range with the equipment used.

PLATELET ADHESIVENESS IN VIVO

The *in vivo* adhesiveness test involves serial platelet counts on blood exuding from a forearm incision. Normally, the platelet counts decrease because of platelet adhesion to the wound. These counts are compared with a venous blood platelet count as a control to calculate percent platelet adhesiveness.[2,18] This test is seldom performed today, because the results are no better or more specific than those of the bleeding time test.

The literature range for the percentage of platelet adhesiveness is 15% to 45%. Each laboratory should establish its own reference range.

CLOT RETRACTION

The clot retraction test was popular before sophisticated tests of platelet function were available. It is seldom performed today. The detailed procedure is available in some other textbooks of hematology.[6] For academic purposes, it will be discussed only briefly.

The principle of the test is that within 1 hour after whole blood is allowed to clot in a clean glass tube at 37°C, the clot will begin to shrink and retract from the walls of the tube. This retraction process is maximal at 24 hours, by which time the clot occupies about half of the original blood volume. This process depends on normal numbers of contractile platelets, the presence of calcium and ATP, and a normal concentration of fibrinogen. The interaction of platelets with fibrinogen and fibrin must also be normal for clot retraction to occur.

Clot retraction is abnormal with thrombocytopenia, low or abnormal fibrinogens, paraproteinemias (multiple myeloma, macroglobulinemia) that interfere with fibrin formation, and Glanzmann's thrombasthenia in which the platelet is incapable of interacting with fibrin.

PLATELET FACTOR ASSAYS

PLATELET FACTOR 3 AVAILABILITY
Principle

Platelets facilitate the ability of plasma to clot by providing a surface to which certain clotting factors bind, thereby enhancing their reaction rates. This facilitative platelet capacity in clot formation is synonymous with platelet factor 3 (PF3). Platelet factor 3 is a functional concept rather than a discrete molecular substance, as is usually implied by the word "factor."[10] When platelets are incubated with kaolin and epinephrine, they are stimulated to provide PF3 activity. Thus, the clotting time of PRP incubated with kaolin and epinephrine is considerably shorter than that of platelet-poor plasma (PPP). The test compares the clotting time of the patient's PRP with that obtained for a group of normal individuals.

Specimen Requirements

Blood collected in 3.2% sodium citrate (3.2% to 3.8% is acceptable) as for coagulation is used.

Reagents and Equipment

0.030 M $CaCl_2$.

Kaolin, 1.5% suspension (1.5 g/100 mL) in Owren's veronal buffer, pH 7.35 (11.75 g of sodium diethylbarbituate and 14.67 g of NaCl in 1570 mL distilled water to which 430 mL of 0.1 N HCl is added).

Epinephrine (109 μM): a 1:1000 vial of epinephrine for injection (1 mg/mL) is diluted 50-fold in Tris saline buffer pH 7.4. This solution contains 20 μg/mL of 109 μM epinephrine (Note: this is the same stock solution of epinephrine used for platelet aggregometry).

Commercially available normal control plasma or pooled PPP (minimum 20 donors).

Procedure and Quality Control

1. Platelet-rich and platelet-poor plasma are prepared as described for platelet aggregometry later in this chapter. Plasmas should be kept at room temperature in plastic tubes.
2. Perform a platelet count on patient's PRP and dilute with patient PPP to a final concentration of 50×10^9/L. (Note: if patient has a prolonged PTT because of a factor deficiency, dilute PRP with normal control PPP).
3. Prepare the following in duplicate:
   a. 0.1 mL of control PPP + 0.1 mL of kaolin suspension + 0.01 mL of epinephrine stock.
   b. 0.1 mL of patient PPP + 0.1 mL of kaolin suspension + 0.01 mL of epinephrine stock.
   c. 0.1 mL of patient plasma with platelets (50×10^9/L) + 0.1 mL of kaolin suspension + 0.01 mL of epinephrine stock.
4. Incubate these three mixtures at 37°C for 10 minutes with occasional shaking.
5. Add 0.1 mL of $CaCl_2$ solution, and measure the clotting time with a stopwatch. The endpoint is the first visible clumping of the kaolin.
6. The clotting time of mixture c should be considerably shorter than that of mixtures a or b and is a reflection of PF3 availability. The clotting times of mixtures a and b should be close; these results serve as controls for a patient coagulation factor defect. If b is longer than a by 10 seconds or greater, or if the PTT of the patient is abnormal, patient's PRP should be diluted with normal control PPP (see step 2). The clotting time of each is noted.

Reference Range

Each laboratory should establish its own reference range. The range in our laboratory is 37 to 51 seconds for PRP adjusted to 50×10^9/L. Clotting times longer than the reference range are reported semiquantitatively as reduced PF3 availability.

Comments

Platelet factor 3 availability is decreased in acquired or congenital defects of platelet secretion or release. In some cases, impaired function of factors V and X_a has been demonstrated.

ASSAYS OF PLATELET FACTOR 4
AND BETA-THROMBOGLOBULIN

Platelet factor 4 (PF4) and beta-thromboglobulin are heparin-binding proteins found in platelet alpha-granules.[14] As such, their levels *in vivo* are an indicator of the presence of ongoing platelet activation in a variety of disease states such as myocardial infarction, venous thrombosis, diabetes, inflammatory states, and myeloproliferative disorders.[17] Alternatively, release of these proteins from aggregating platelets in PRP can be examined for patients suspected of having storage pool disease or a release defect.

Procedure

There are several commercial RIA kits available for PF4 and beta-thromboglobulin measurement in plasma or from alpha-granule release.

Comments

The clinical value of PF4 and beta-thromboglobulin assays is still under investigation. At present, they are considered research procedures.

PLATELET AGGREGATION

Studies of platelet aggregation *in vitro* are now commonly performed to assist in the diagnosis of hereditary and acquired platelet disorders.

PLATELET AGGREGOMETRY
Principle

Aggregating agents added to a stirred suspension of PRP induce a shape change and aggregation of platelets. As a result, the PRP changes from a turbid suspension to one that transmits more light as the aggregates are formed (Fig. 59-1). Thus, the process of platelet aggregation can be followed by a platelet aggregometer (Fig. 59-2) that measures and records a change in light transmission.[3,7,20]

Special Patient Requirements

Preferably, the patient and the normal control should be fasting. Otherwise, they should have had a relatively fat-free meal; this eliminates the optical problems of lipemic plasma. The patient should not be taking aspirin or nonsteroidal anti-inflammatory drugs.

Specimen Requirements

Venous blood is drawn from the patient and from a normal control into plastic syringes. Nine parts of blood is added to a plastic tube containing one part 3.8% trisodium citrate. Platelet-rich plasma is obtained from both patient and control

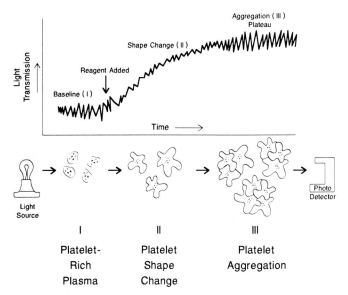

FIG. 59-1. Principles of aggregometry. (Modified from Penner JA: Manual of Blood Coagulation: Blood Coagulation Course. East Lansing, MI, Michigan State University College of Human Medicine, 1982, with permission.)

specimens by centrifuging at room temperature at 200 × g for 10 minutes. The supernatant PRP is withdrawn gently, taking care not to aspirate any red cells, and transferred to another plastic tube, stoppered, and kept at room temperature. Testing must be completed within 2 hours. Platelet-poor plasma is obtained from both specimens by further centrifuging the remaining PRP and red cells in the tubes at 2500 to 3000 × g for 30 minutes. The PPPs should be kept at room temperature until use. As a consequence of processing of the PRP, platelets sometimes exhibit a "platelet shock" phenomenon and will be poorly or not responsive to ADP, collagen, and epinephrine for as long as 30 minutes. If a poor response is obtained with one of these reagents, the test is repeated 30 minutes later. This problem may also be avoided by either waiting 30 minutes before initiating testing or by performing tests with these agents well into the testing session after recording the results with other stimuli, such as ristocetin.

Aggregating Agents

There are many acceptable methods of maintaining stock solutions of aggregation agents. Stock concentrations and the volumes of aggregating agents added should be modified to suit the cuvette volumes of a particular aggregometer model. The following procedures utilize concentrations and volumes that are convenient for a 0.5-mL sample size.

ADP (125 μM). Ten milligrams is diluted with 196 mL of saline and stored frozen in 1.0-mL aliquots. Twenty microliters of 125 μM ADP added to 0.5 mL of PRP will result in a final concentration of 5 μM ADP. A 20-μL sample of a 1:2 dilution of the stock solution (125 μM ADP added to 0.5 mL of PRP) will result in 2.5 μM ADP. Other appropriate dilutions may be made for lower concentrations of ADP.

Epinephrine (109 μM). A 1:1000 vial of epinephrine for injection is diluted 50-fold in Tris saline buffer pH 7.4 for a stock solution. This is stored frozen in 1.0-mL aliquots. A 50-μL sample of stock solution in 0.5 mL of PRP gives a final concentration of 10 μM epinephrine; 25 μL in 0.5 mL of PRP yields a 5 μM final concentration of epinephrine.

Collagen. Acid-soluble collagen reagent is reconstituted with distilled water to yield a stock solution of 50 μg/mL. A 50-μL sample of stock solution added to 0.5 mL of PRP gives a final concentration of 5 μg of collagen/mL.

Thrombin (human). Lyophilized human thrombin is reconstituted in saline to a final concentration of 7.8 units/mL and stored frozen in 1.0-mL aliquots until use. A 20-μL aliquot of the stock solution added to 0.5 mL of PRP results in a final concentration of 0.3 units of thrombin/mL.

Ristocetin. Ristocetin reagent is diluted in saline to a final concentration of 20 mg/mL. This is stable at 4°C for 2 weeks. A 40-μL sample of stock solution added to 0.5 mL of PRP results in a final concentration of 1.5 mg of ristocetin/mL; 25 μL in 0.5 mL of PRP produces a concentration of 1.0 mg/mL.

Arachidonic acid is a clear viscous oil at room temperature and is not readily soluble in concentrated aqueous solvents. A 50 mM stock is made by thoroughly mixing 657 μL of 70% ethanol with the contents of a 10-mg vial of arachidonic acid. This stock is stable for 2 to 3 weeks if kept at −20°C in a sealed vial under N$_2$ atmosphere entered only with a Hamilton micropipette. If these conditions are not available, the stock solution should be made fresh each day. A 10-μL portion of stock solution added to 0.49 mL of PRP results in a final concentration of 1.0 mM. Lower concentrations can be made with a predilution in ethanol.

Procedure

1. Perform platelet counts on patient and control PRP; adjust the platelet counts to 200 to 300 × 10^9/L by diluting with

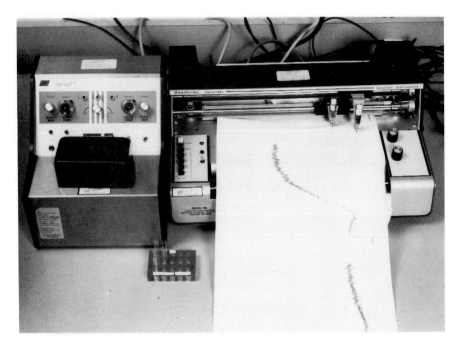

FIG. 59-2. Platelet aggregometer and recorder. One aggregation curve is plotted by recorder for each aggregating agent used in platelet aggregation test procedure. (Courtesy of Section of Laboratory Hematology, Division of Laboratory Medicine, The University of Texas at Houston, M.D. Anderson Hospital and Tumor Institute, Houston, TX.)

their respective aliquots of PPP. Keep samples stoppered at room temperature.

2. Warm 0.5-mL aliquots of PRP in appropriate cuvettes to 37°C for several minutes as needed for testing.

3. Adjust the 100% transmittance of the platelet aggregometer using patient PPP.

4. Place warmed PRP samples in the aggregometer and adjust the baseline reading after at least 1 minute.

5. After stirring PRP for 2 minutes with small magnetic stir bars, forcefully add the appropriate volume of aggregating agent to ensure adequate mixing.

6. Record the aggregation curve for 3 to 5 minutes or until no further change is noted.

7. Repeat steps 2 through 6 for each aggregating agent with patient and control PRP.

Comments

To ensure platelet viability during the procedure, all testing should be completed within 2 hours of blood collection.

Specimens for platelet aggregation studies should not come in contact with any type of glassware. Glass will prematurely activate platelets and thus result in a less-than-optimal response to aggregating agents. Nor should such specimens be refrigerated, as platelets kept cold do not respond optimally to aggregating agents.

While awaiting testing, platelets are viable longer if they are kept at room temperature; however, aggregation occurs best at 37°C. Temperature monitoring should be run with a tube of plasma in the instrument heating block to determine the optimal warming time for samples.

Because stirring affects reagent mixing and platelet aggregate collisions, it has a significant effect on platelet aggregation. Most aggregation instruments rotate the stir bars at 1200 rpm. Multichannel instruments are synchronized to ensure comparability. Instruments should be checked periodically with a strobe light to determine the actual stirring rate. Stir bar characteristics can also be a source of variability; if two bars are used, they should be identical.

Extremes of hematocrit will affect the concentration of citrate anticoagulant in the plasma. A 9-mL blood sample requires more anticoagulant if the hematocrit is low and less if the hematocrit is high. Nomograms for these adjustments are available[20] and should be consulted if one is working with samples in which this is a problem. Low levels of calcium are necessary for platelet aggregation; therefore, if a sample is over-anticoagulated with citrate (which binds calcium), it will appear less responsive and will require higher agent concentrations to produce a response.

The issue of pH is complex. The pH optima of the various aggregating agents are different: ADP and epinephrine responses are best between pH 7.7 and 8.0, whereas ristocetin responses are best at pH 7.3 and decline sharply above pH 7.7. Collagen has a broad optimal range, between 7.0 and 8.0; pH 7.7 therefore is a reasonable compromise. Unfortunately, PRP has weak buffering capacity, and CO_2 will diffuse out, causing a rise in PRP pH. Such a rise increases the chelation of calcium by citrate, and the responsiveness to aggregating agents will decline as discussed above. Stoppering PRP tubes will retard the CO_2 loss, as will keeping the PRP under an oil layer or in a 5% CO_2-filled chamber. Attention to and monitoring of these pH effects will improve test reliability.

Typical aggregation response curves are seen in Figure 59-3. At low concentrations of ADP or epinephrine, an initial (primary) response is seen, followed by disaggregation and a return of the reading to baseline (Fig. 59-3A; lower curve). At optimal reagent concentrations, two aggregation waves are seen; the primary response is followed by a brief plateau, and then a much larger secondary response occurs during which platelets aggregate irreversibly (Fig. 59-3A; middle curve, and Fig. 59-3B). At higher concentrations of ADP and epinephrine, the stimulus is strong enough to obliterate the primary response, and a single wave of aggregation is seen (Fig. 59-3A; upper curve). For the majority of normal samples, there is an optimal concentration of these aggregating agents that results in a two-wave response. This concentration should be sought and used in testing to increase the sensitivity of the procedure to subtle defects in secretion or storage pools, where there is an absence of the secondary aggregation wave. Using a concentration of ADP or epinephrine that is too high will cause a single large primary wave to be seen, leading to a mistaken interpretation of normality. Because of the many variables that affect platelet aggregation (discussed above), the optimal concentrations of

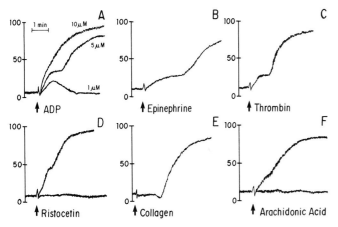

FIG. 59-3. Typical platelet aggregation patterns in response to various platelet agonists. X-axis reflects time in minutes, y-axis is percent transmittance. (A) Dose response to ADP. There is a primary wave only to 1 μM ADP, followed by disaggregation, whereas there is a single large wave with 10 μM ADP, and 5 μM ADP gives the optimal two-wave response. (B) Normal response to 10 μM epinephrine. Note subtle, shallow primary wave. (C) Normal response to thrombin 0.3 units/mL. (D) Responses to ristocetin 1.5 mg/mL; lower curve is an absent response from patient with severe von Willebrand's disease. Upper curve is a normal response; note slight shoulder of primary wave occasionally seen with this agent. (E) Normal response to collagen 5 μg/mL; note lag phase preceding single-wave response. (F) Responses to arachidonic acid 1.0 mM; upper curve is normal; lower curve is an absent response in patient who had taken aspirin the day before.

ADP and epinephrine that give this important two-wave response will differ from laboratory to laboratory. The concentrations suggested in the reagent section are simply guidelines. It is also important to note that approximately 30% of the normal population does not respond to epinephrine, presumably because of a lack of surface membrane receptors responsible for platelet sensitivity to epinephrine. Another 30% of normal subjects have only a single wave of aggregation in response to ADP regardless of concentration.

Thrombin and ristocetin aggregation curves also may yield a two-wave response, depending on the concentration of the stimulus (Fig. 59-3C and D). It is a good idea to test both patient and control PRP at several concentrations of each agent before drawing conclusions. For example, some individuals with normal levels of vWF and otherwise-normal platelets will respond to ristocetin, 1.0 mg/mL, whereas other normal subjects require 1.5 mg of the aggregating agent per milliliter. Reliance on only one concentration of aggregating agent can lead to mistaken conclusions and further expensive and time-consuming workups.

Collagen produces a single wave of aggregation after a lag phase (Fig. 59-3E). The factors responsible for this response involve the polymerization of acid-soluble collagen to the fibrillar form in plasma, adhesion of platelets to the collagen fibril, platelet release of ADP, and the response of other platelets to released ADP. An abnormal response can be secondary to Glanzmann's thrombasthenia or to a defect in platelet release or storage pool ADP. As is the case with ADP and epinephrine, using a concentration of collagen that is too high can cover up a subtle release or storage pool defect. Only thrombasthenic platelets will not respond to excessively high concentrations of collagen. Thus, to increase the sensitivity of collagen aggregation, each laboratory should determine and use the lowest concentration of collagen that still stimulates aggregation in a large number of normals. The concentration should be verified if lots or suppliers of acid-soluble collagen change.

The response to arachidonic acid is typically a two-wave response. Abnormal responses are most commonly a perfect flat line and are easy to detect (Fig. 59-3F). A problem with the platelet cyclooxygenase enzyme, thromboxane A_2 production, or thrombasthenia are rare causes of an abnormal response. The most common cause of an abnormal response is aspirin. Other medications discussed in the bleeding time section will also cause an abnormal response to arachidonic acid.

Interpretation of platelet aggregation tests first involves comparison of the patient's curves with the corresponding curves of a normal control. Minor differences in the slope (rate) of aggregation and in the extent (plateau) of aggregation of as much as 25% are not significant. In distinguishing normal from abnormal, however, it is not sufficient to compare a single control with the patient. One must keep in mind the many variables in the aggregation response and appreciate the variability of the curves of a large number of normal individuals. Thus, the interpretation of aggregometry is somewhat subjective and is best left to one who does interpretations daily and appreciates the variability of normal responses. A file of normal results and plotting of the upper and lower limits of a large number of normal controls is helpful. In no way does this diminish the value of the daily normal control, which is a check on reagent stability, a guide to agent concentration adjustments, and a check on platelet viability during the testing session.

ASSAY OF VON WILLEBRAND FACTOR

Von Willebrand factor circulates in plasma as a noncovalent complex with factor VIII coagulant (Chap. 55).[13] This circulating complex of two proteins has five measurable aspects as shown in Table 55-1. The assay described here is used to measure VIIIR:RCo, the factor VIII-related activity required for platelet aggregation with ristocetin.

Historically, von Willebrand's disease was thought to be a combined defect of the factor VIII molecules and platelets. We now know this is not true. The defect leading to a prolonged bleeding time, a decrease in platelet adhesiveness, and reduced glass bead retention in this disease is a quantitative or qualitative disorder of the vWF molecule circulating in the plasma; the platelets are normal. Although this disease is not a platelet disorder, the function of the vWF may be assayed by using platelet aggregometry[1,22] and is appropriately discussed here. The platelet response to ristocetin requires the presence of vWF and a platelet receptor for that factor (glycoprotein Ib). This response does not require active platelet metabolism; hence, formalin-fixed platelets have come to be the preferred reagent for vWF assays because of their convenience. Because aggregation is a function of viable platelets, and because the test described below uses fixed platelets, we will use the term "platelet agglutination" with respect to this particular test.

VON WILLEBRAND FACTOR ASSAY
Principle

Agglutination of fixed platelets in response to ristocetin depends on the presence of vWF in plasma. The rate or percentage

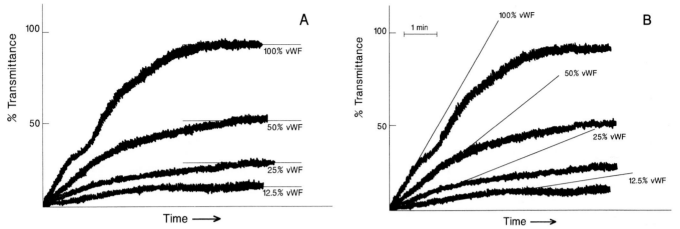

FIG. 59-4.   Construction of standard curves for von Willebrand factor. Identical series of curves are shown analyzed two ways. In panel A, final percentage of agglutination (plateau of percent light transmittance) is measured for each curve corresponding to reference plasma dilutions. Thus, standard curve relates a change in percent transmittance or agglutination to percent of von Willebrand factor. In panel B, initial rates of agglutination (change in percent transmittance per minute) are represented by slopes drawn through aggregation curves. Standard curve constructed from these data relates slopes to percent von Willebrand factor. Note that when agglutination curves are biphasic, only slope of first wave is used. Whether data are analyzed using plateau method (A) or slope method (B), results obtained for an unknown are the same.

of agglutination is proportional to the amount of vWF present. Thus, a standard curve of the amount of vWF versus platelet agglutination can be constructed, and the amount of VWF in an unknown can be determined by reference to this standard curve.

Specimen Requirements

Blood is collected in 3.2% sodium citrate, as for coagulation tests.

Reagents and Equipment

A platelet aggregometer is needed that allows continuous comparison between the test sample and a blank and resetting of the baseline for deflections when ristocetin is added.

Ristocetin, 20 mg/mL in saline

Phosphate-buffered saline (PBS), pH 7.3

Bovine serum albumin (BSA), 4 g/100 mL of PBS

Pooled normal PPP or commercial lyophilized control plasma assayed for vWF

Commercial formalin-fixed platelet suspension adjusted to 400 to $500 \times 10^9/L$

Plastic tubes and pipets

Procedure

1. Platelet poor plasma is prepared from the patient specimen by centrifugation at $2500 \times g$ for 20 to 30 minutes. Normal PPP is diluted in twofold series from 1:2 to 1:16 using BSA. Patient PPP is diluted 1:2 and 1:4 with BSA.
2. A 100% transmittance blank is prepared with PPP.
3. To aggregometer cuvette is added 0.4 mL of fixed platelet suspension and 0.1 mL of normal PPP with stir bar.
4. The sample is placed in the aggregometer (no incubation necessary with fixed platelets), the setting is adjusted to the baseline, and readings are recorded for at least 1 minute.
5. Ristocetin (50 μL) is added; if necessary, the baseline is read-justed after maximum deflection. Generally, a transient decrease in light transmission occurs after ristocetin is added. If it is not possible to rezero the aggregometer after adding ristocetin to the sample, one should start again at step 3 with a fresh sample of fixed platelets and PPP. The 0% baseline is adjusted to 15% or 20% to ensure that the ristocetin-induced

trough can be seen on the recorder. When the curve appears to have returned to original baseline, this is adjusted to read 0% transmittance.

6. The change in the percent transmittance is recorded until no further agglutination occurs.
7. Steps 3 through 6 are repeated for each normal PPP dilution to construct a standard curve.
8. Steps 3 through 6 are repeated for patient PPP samples: undiluted and diluted 1:2 and 1:4.

Calculations

A standard curve of the percent of vWF versus either the slope of agglutination or the percent agglutination (curve plateau) is constructed (Fig. 59-4). Undiluted normal PPP or lyophilized control plasma is considered 100% vWF, the 1:2 dilution 50%, and so forth. The results from the patient samples are converted to percentages of vWF according to where they fall within the standard curve and are corrected for the dilution factor. Results falling along the standard curve are averaged. If commercial standard plasma is used for the standard curve, the patient results can be corrected relative to the standard. For example, if the reference plasma contains 105% vWF, the standard curve is constructed using 100% as the maximum. The final results of the patient from the standard curve are then multiplied by 1.05 to relate them to the reference plasma. Another acceptable practice is to use normal pooled PPP for the standard curve and to test dilutions of reference (standard) plasma just as the patient samples are tested. Patient results can then be corrected with regard to the reference plasma. For example, if our 105% vWF reference plasma is 115% in our assay, the patient results would be adjusted by a factor of $105/115 = 0.91$ in order to relate them to the reference plasma.

Reference Range

The reference range is 45% to 140%.

Comments

Once reconstituted, the lyophilized formalin-fixed platelets are not stable indefinitely. They can give satisfactory results the next day if refrigerated, but generally, they should not be used after 24 hours. There are protocols for inhouse fixation of platelets, but the commercial preparations are easier to use and give consistent results.

Patients with severe von Willebrand's disease will have essentially no vWF. Those with variants of the disease have typically low values, but these differ greatly and, depending on the testing circumstances, may be normal (*e.g.*, in pregnancy, during estrogen use, after trauma or surgery).

Patients with Bernard-Soulier disease and those with von Willebrand's disease both have PRP that does not respond to ristocetin in the platelet aggregometry profile. In the vWF assay, Bernard-Soulier patients have normal results, and those with von Willebrand's disease will have abnormal findings.

CHAPTER SUMMARY

Platelets must be present in the peripheral blood in sufficient numbers to be effective in their hemostatic role. Methods to enumerate platelets have been discussed in this chapter, both manual (Tocantins method using Rees-Ecker diluent and light microscopy or phase methods) and automated. Provided numbers are adequate, the laboratory evaluation of platelets may also involve various tests of how well they function.

Some tests of function are comprehensive and nonspecific. What they measure is a composite of several functions such as adhesion, release, aggregation, and interaction with the coagulation system. The most popular screening test is the bleeding time. Abnormalities of this test simply confirm that a problem with platelet function exists. Other tests are more discriminating, such as platelet factor 3 availability and platelet aggregometry. Abnormalities of these tests may identify a deficiency in a particular aspect of platelet function.

Von Willebrand factor plays an important role in platelet adhesion. The technique of platelet aggregometry is used to measure the function of this factor.

REFERENCES

1. Allain JP, Cooper HA, Wagner RM et al: Platelets fixed with paraformaldehyde: A new reagent for assay for von Willebrand factor and platelet aggregating factor. J Lab Clin Med 85:318, 1975

2. Borchgrevink CF: A method for measuring platelet adhesiveness *in vivo*. Acta Med Scand 168:157, 1960

3. Born GRV, Cross J: The aggregation of blood platelets. J Physiol 168:178, 1963

4. Bowie EJW, Owen CA: The value of measuring platelet "adhesiveness" in the diagnosis of bleeding diseases. Am J Clin Pathol 60:302, 1973

5. Brecher G, Cronkite EP: Morphology and enumeration of human blood platelets. J Appl Physiol 3:356, 1950

6. Budtz-Olsen OE: Clot Retraction. London, Blackwell Scientific, 1951

7. Coller BS: Platelet aggregation by ADP, collagen and ristocetin: A critical review of methodology and analysis. In Schmidt RM (ed): Hematology, vol I: Handbook Series in Clinical Laboratory Science, p 381. Boca Raton FL, CRC Press, 1979

8. Czapek EE, Deykin D, Salzman E et al: Intermediate syndrome of platelet dysfunction. Blood 52:103, 1978

9. Feusner JH: Normal and abnormal bleeding times in neonates and young children utilizing a fully standardized template technic. Am J Clin Pathol 74:73, 1980

10. Hardisty RM, Hutton RA: Kaolin clotting time of platelet-rich plasma: A test of platelet factor 3 availability. Br J Haematol 11:258, 1965

11. Harker LA, Slichter SJ: The bleeding time as a screening test for evaluation of platelet function. N Engl J Med 287:155, 1972

12. Helem AJ: Platelet adhesiveness in von Willebrand's disease. Scand J Haematol 7:374, 1970

13. Hoyer LW: The factor VIII complex: Structure and function. Blood 58:1, 1981

14. Kaplan KL, Nossel HL, Drillings M et al: Radioimmunoassay of platelet factor 4 and beta-thromboglobulin: Development of application to studies of platelet release in relation to fibrinopeptide A generation. Br J Haematol 39:129, 1978

15. Kumar R, Ansell JHE, Canoso RT et al: Clinical trial of a new bleeding time device. Am J Clin Pathol 70:642, 1978

16. Mielke CH, Kaneshiro NM, Maher JA et al: The standard normal Ivy bleeding time and its prolongation by aspirin. Blood 34:204, 1969

17. Niewiarowski S, Varma KG: Biochemistry and physiology of secreted platelet proteins. In Colman RW, Hirsh J, Marder VJ et al (eds): Hemostasis and Thrombosis: Basic Principles and Clinical Practice, p 427. Philadelphia, JB Lippincott, 1982

18. Owen C, Bowie E, Didisheim P et al: The Diagnosis of Bleeding Disorders, p 80. Boston, Little Brown, 1969

19. Ross DW, Ayscue L, Gulley M: Automated platelet counts. Am J Clin Pathol 74:151, 1980

20. Triplett DA (ed): Platelet Function: Laboratory Evaluation and Clinical Application. Chicago, American Society of Clinical Pathologists, 1978

21. Tocantins LM: Technical methods for the study of blood platelets. Arch Pathol 23:850, 1937

22. Weiss HJ, Hoyer LW, Rickles FR et al: Quantitative assay of a plasma factor deficient in von Willebrand's disease that is necessary for platelet aggregation: Relationship to factor VIII procoagulant activity and antigen content. J Clin Invest 52:2708, 1973

23. Wertz RK: Cell counting—the platelet. In Schmidt RM (ed): Hematology, vol I: Handbook Series in Clinical Laboratory Science, p 361. Boca Raton, FL, CRC Press, 1979

24. Wertz RK, Triplett DA: A review of platelet counting performance in the United States. Am J Clin Pathol 74:575, 1980

Quantitative

Platelet

Disorders

Judith K. Fincher

The reference range for platelets generally is considered to be between 140 and 440×10^9/L. Quantitative platelet disorders are conditions resulting in decreased (thrombocytopenia) or increased (thrombocytosis and thrombocythemia) platelet counts. Classifications of the quantitative platelet disorders are presented in Tables 60-1 and 60-2.

THROMBOCYTOPENIA

Thrombocytopenia is a common clinical disorder and results from one or any combination of mechanisms, including production defects, accelerated loss or destruction, and splenic sequestration.

Decreased Production

Pathophysiology

Thrombocytopenia diminishes the effectiveness of hemostasis, and bleeding may result. The severity of bleeding is related to the degree of thrombocytopenia. Hemostatic defects are said to be more severe when the platelet count falls rapidly rather than gradually.[43]

Clinical Presentation

Small-vessel bleeding attributed to thrombocytopenia results in petechiae, purpura, or ecchymoses (hemorrhages into the skin of different sizes: < 3 mm, 1 cm, and > 3 cm, respectively). The skin and mucous membranes of the nose and mouth and the gastrointestinal, urinary, and respiratory tracts are common sites. Significant bleeding usually does not occur until the platelet count is less than 60×10^9/L; however, the level of circulating platelets at which bleeding occurs differs among patients. Minor bruising,

TABLE 60–1. Classification of Thrombocytopenia

DECREASED PRODUCTION
Megakaryocyte hypoproliferation
Aplastic anemia
Drug toxicity
Alcohol toxicity
Viral infection
Congenital states
Ineffective thrombopoiesis
Megaloblastic anemia
Paroxysmal nocturnal hemoglobinuria (PNH)
Thrombopoietin deficiency
Ethanol abuse without malnutrition
Severe iron-deficiency anemia
Viral infection
Marrow replacement
Leukemia
Plasma-cell dyscrasia
Metastatic carcinoma
Myelofibrosis
Lymphoma
Granulomatous infections
INCREASED LOSS OR DESTRUCTION
Nonimmunologic
Loss
Severe hemorrhage
Extensive transfusion
Consumption
Diffuse intravascular coagulation (DIC)
Thrombotic thrombocytopenic purpura (TTP)
Hemolytic uremic syndrome (HUS)
Foreign surfaces
Thermal injury
Sepsis without DIC
Immunologic
Isoimmune
Neonatal purpura
Post-transfusion purpura
Refractory to platelet transfusions
Autoimmune
Immune thrombocytopenic purpura (ITP)
Disease associated
Drug induced
Viral infection
SPLENIC SEQUESTRATION

TABLE 60–2. Classification of Thrombocytosis

PRIMARY–CHRONIC MYELOPROLIFERATIVE DISORDERS
Essential thrombocythemia
Polycythemia vera
Chronic granulocytic leukemia
Myelofibrosis with myeloid metaplasia
REACTIVE
Physiologic
Iron deficiency anemia
Rapid blood regeneration
Acute blood loss
Hemolytic anemia
Rebound
Postoperative
Infections and inflammatory diseases
Chronic disorders
Tuberculosis
Ulcerative colitis
Sprue
Rheumatoid arthritis
Osteomyelitis
Acute infections
Neoplasms
Carcinoma
Hodgkin's disease

menorrhagia, and postoperative or post-traumatic bleeding are common manifestations of platelet counts ranging from 20 to 60 × 10⁹/L, whereas spontaneous bleeding into the skin and mucous membranes is common when platelet counts fall below 20 × 10⁹/L. The central nervous system (CNS) is the most serious site of spontaneous bleeding, which may be fatal.

Laboratory Findings

By definition, the platelet count is decreased. As long as platelet function is normal, the template bleeding time is not increased when platelet counts are greater than 100 × 10⁹/L. When the count falls below this, the degree to which the bleeding time is prolonged is inversely proportional to the decrease in the platelet count.[32] Clot retraction usually is abnormal when the platelet count is below 60 × 10⁹/L.[18] Platelet aggregation studies require platelet-rich plasma (PRP), which is difficult to prepare from the blood of thrombocytopenic patients; however, reproducible results are possible on PRP suspensions containing at least 50 × 10⁹/L.

Etiologies

Generalized bone marrow suppression leading to a decrease in all cell types is characteristic of aplastic anemia. Acquired aplastic anemia may be the consequence of toxic chemical or physical agents. Ionizing radiation and chemotherapeutic agents produce a dose-dependent suppression of cells at the stem cell level. Patients with Fanconi syndrome, a congenital form of aplastic anemia, present with chromosome abnormalities, skeletal defects, and pancytopenia. Viral infections also have been implicated in bone marrow hypoplasia. Invasion of the multipotential stem cell by viral agents produces direct damage, the severity of which depends on the virulence of the virus.[13]

Selective suppression of the megakaryocyte is associated with chlorothiazide (a diuretic) and other drugs. Although the mechanism by which thiazides and related compounds induce thrombocytopenia is unclear, it is not considered to be immunologic but rather related to drug toxicity.[51]

Thrombocytopenia with absent radius (TAR) syndrome is an inherited disorder of megakaryocyte production that is characterized by episodes of thrombocytopenia in the neonate, absent or decreased and abnormal bone-marrow megakaryocytes, congenital deformities of the arm, and early death usually secondary to hemorrhage.[28]

Thrombopoietin, analogous to erythropoietin, stimulates megakaryocyte maturation and platelet production.[52] Infusion of normal plasma results in megakaryocyte maturation, platelet proliferation, and a rise in the platelet count to at least normal levels in a patient deficient in thrombopoietin.[75,76]

A *myelophthisic process* is a space-occupying lesion in the bone marrow such as metastatic tumor, fibrosis, or leukemia. The thrombocytopenia is related to abnormal cells crowding out or replacing normal bone marrow elements. There is a poor correlation between the number of bone marrow megakaryocytes and the platelet count in myelophthisic processes; hence, the thrombocytopenia may be caused by multiple factors.

Ineffective thrombopoiesis is associated with ethanol abuse with and without malnutrition, megaloblastic states, severe iron-deficiency anemia, paroxysmal nocturnal hemoglobinuria (PNH), some viral infections, and certain inherited anomalies. Alcohol-related thrombocytopenia without malnutrition may develop secondary to ethanol interruption of megakaryocyte differentiation. Megaloblastic states are characterized by thrombocytopenia that is presumably secondary to impaired DNA synthesis caused by folate or vitamin B_{12} deficiency. The consequent limitation in nuclear endoduplication results in decreased platelet production.[70] In severe iron deficiency, thrombocytopenia is thought to develop because iron is essential for the enzyme systems involved in platelet protein synthesis.[21] Platelets in PNH possess a membrane defect that results in abnormal sensitivity to complement and various antibodies.[5] However, platelet survival is normal, and the observed thrombocytopenia is more likely the result of ineffective thrombopoiesis.[30] Megakaryocyte invasion by viral agents also may interfere with platelet production.[14,67,85,87]

The thrombocytopenia associated with May-Hegglin anomaly is thought to result from ineffective thrombopoiesis and increased platelet destruction.[15] A defect in the production or release of platelets is thought to be the cause of thrombocytopenia in the Wiskott-Aldrich syndrome (WAS), a condition characterized by immune deficiencies, hemorrhage, eczema, and extreme susceptibility to infections.[49] Bernard-Soulier syndrome is characterized by thrombocytopenia and giant platelets with impaired function (Chap. 61).

Dilutional Loss

Extensive blood transfusion often is accompanied by thrombocytopenia, the degree of which is directly proportional to the number of units transfused.[3,81] The viability and survival of platelets from blood stored at 4°C for more than a few days is essentially nil. Thus, patients requiring extensive transfusions develop thrombocytopenia by two mechanisms: acute blood loss and dilution of their own platelet pool.

Nonimmune Destruction

Nonimmune platelet destruction may result from exposure of platelets to nonendothelial surfaces, activation of the coagulation process, or platelet consumption by endovascular injury with no measurable depletion of coagulation factors.

Artificial surfaces such as cardiovascular prosthetic devices,[31] prosthetic vascular grafts,[33] and dialysis membranes[27] may induce platelet adherence as well as formation of platelet microaggregates. During the early period after extensive thermal injury, thrombocytopenia and decreased platelet survival are observed, possibly because of the effects of exposure of platelets to subendothelial surfaces.[20] Occasionally, drugs unexpectedly affect platelets. For example, ristocetin, an antibiotic, was discontinued in clinical use because it causes thrombocytopenia by inducing plate-

let aggregation and agglutination *in vivo*.[22] During IgE-induced systemic anaphylaxis, a platelet-activating factor, now recognized as a potent lipid mediator,[29] is released from IgE-sensitized mast cells and other inflammatory cells. This factor may produce acute thrombocytopenia, intravascular platelet aggregation, and platelet sequestration in the microvasculature during allergic reactions.[56] In some cases, sepsis-induced thrombocytopenia may be the result of direct interaction between the organism and platelets, resulting in lysis or phagocytosis by the reticuloendothelial system.

Activation of the coagulation system, such as is seen in disseminated intravascular coagulation (DIC), leads to intravascular thrombin generation, platelet aggregation, and consumption of factors I, V, VIII, and XIII. In addition to consuming platelets through aggregation, the thrombin-mediated reaction traps platelets in fibrin networks within the microvasculature and prematurely destroys circulating thrombin-activated platelets.[9] (See Chap. 55 for a detailed discussion of DIC.)

Hemolytic uremic syndrome (HUS) and *thrombotic thrombocytopenic purpura* (TTP) are clinically and pathologically similar disorders characterized by microangiopathic hemolytic anemia secondary to platelet aggregates or platelet-fibrin thrombi in small blood vessels. There is no evidence of coagulation.[35]

Pathophysiology

Thrombus formation in TTP affects many organs,[71] whereas in HUS, it predominantly involves the afferent arterioles and glomeruli of the kidneys.[23] Two mechanisms are offered for the platelet thrombus formation: intravascular aggregation, and endothelial injury.[34] A plasma factor or factors may act on circulating platelets and lead to their aggregation as platelet thrombi and subsequent lodging in the microvasculature. Platelet thrombi injure or modify the endothelium, drawing additional platelets to the site. In the second mechanism, endothelial injury occurs first.[8,54] It is possible that causative agents act on both the platelet and the endothelial surface. A summary of specific etiologies for platelet thrombus formation in HUS and TTP is presented in Table 60-3.

Clinical Presentation

Vomiting and diarrhea are the most common symptoms preceding the anemia and renal failure characteristic of HUS. In some patients, a brief febrile disease may be the antecedent symptom. The patient frequently is pale and slightly jaundiced and may present with purpura and bleeding from the mucous membranes. Platelet thrombi in the kidneys lead to renal failure. Hemolytic uremic syndrome is seen most frequently in children under 8 years of age but has been reported in renal transplant recipients,[39] postpartum women, and women taking oral contraceptives.[74] Some families may possess an inherited predisposition to HUS.[38]

Thrombotic thrombocytopenic purpura is diagnosed most frequently in patients between the ages of 10 and 40, with a peak incidence in the third decade of life, women being affected more frequently than men. Fever, pallor, petechiae, neurologic manifestations, and renal disease are the chief clinical features. Neurologic manifestations,

TABLE 60–3. Mechanisms of Platelet Thrombus Formation in TTP and HUS

ENDOTHELIAL INJURY
  Endotoxins
  Soluble immune complexes
  Antiendothelial antibody
  Infectious agents
INTRAVASCULAR PLATELET AGGREGATION
  Platelet-bound immunoglobulin
  Endothelial prostacyclin deficiency
  Plasma platelet-aggregating factor
  Plasma platelet-aggregation–inhibitor deficiency

which are remittent and subject to sudden change, include headache, delirium, and altered states of consciousness. The distribution of platelet thrombi in the brain accounts for the neurologic problems. The mortality rate for TTP is approximately 25%; for HUS, it is approximately 5%.

Laboratory Findings

Analysis of the peripheral blood reveals anemia, reticulocytosis, polymorphonuclear leukocytosis, thrombocytopenia, and numerous fragmented erythrocytes. There is increased variation of red cell size (*i.e.*, marked anisocytosis).[7]

Hemoglobinemia, decreased haptoglobin levels, markedly increased lactate dehydrogenase (LD), mildly elevated bilirubin levels, hemosiderinuria, and hemoglobinuria result from the intravascular hemolysis. The urine contains casts, erythrocytes, leukocytes, and large quantities of albumin because of the lesions in the kidney. Serum levels of creatinine and urea nitrogen are increased because of reduced glomerular filtration.

Fibrinogen levels, prothrombin time, and activated partial thromboplastin time usually are normal; however, fibrin degradation products may be increased slightly. These test results may be helpful in differentiating HUS or TTP from DIC, in which the blood film morphology may be similar.

Current tests for circulating soluble immune complexes or platelet-associated immunoglobulin (PAIg) are inconclusive, and yield various results. They are not readily available in the routine clinical laboratory.[72]

Treatment

The cause of the thrombotic microangiopathy remains uncertain; therefore, treatment tends to be based on the practical experience of the clinician. In addition, no single therapeutic approach is likely to be effective in all patients because of the heterogeneity of pathogenesis in these disorders.[8] Glucocorticoids and inhibitors of platelet function are administered to reduce platelet aggregation. Exchange plasmapheresis, whole-blood exchange transfusion, or plasma infusion are undertaken to remove, reduce, or modify the effects of soluble immune complexes and to replace plasma factors. Platelet transfusions are avoided because rapid clinical deterioration and life threatening hemorrhaging are likely to result. The response to therapy usually is monitored by serum LD assays and platelet counts. An increase in the platelet count and a decrease in the serum LD

level within 24 to 48 hours are considered favorable responses.

Immune Platelet Destruction

Increased platelet destruction by immune mechanisms is associated with increased levels of immunoglobulins (usually IgG) or complement on the platelet surface.[45] Antigenic determinants associated with immune platelet destruction include the major histocompatibility complex (HLA), the ABH(O) blood group system, and platelet-specific alloantigens such as Pl^{A1}. Immune thrombocytopenias may be caused by alloantibodies (*isoimmune*), autoantibodies (*autoimmune*), or drugs. Immune thrombocytopenia purpura (ITP) is grouped with the autoimmune disorders, although the etiology of its platelet-associated immunoglobulin is unknown.

Post-transfusion (Isoimmune) Purpura

Post-transfusion (isoimmune) purpura (PTP) is a rare complication characterized by sudden, profound, and self-limited thrombocytopenia (less than 20×10^9/L). Bleeding occurs 2 to 12 days after the transfusion of products containing platelet antigens, with the time of recovery ranging from 5 to 60 days.[65] Most cases have been reported in women who lacked the platelet-specific antigen Pl^{A1} and who had been sensitized by pregnancy or transfusions. This antigen is located on platelet membrane glycoprotein III and is present in 97% of the general population.[59] The antibody produced shows Pl^{A1} specificity and fixes complement in some cases, although not in others.[24] The mechanism responsible for the destruction of the patient's Pl^{A1}-negative platelets is unknown. After recovery, transfusion with blood containing the antigen does not always restimulate antibody production or cause thrombocytopenia, but recurrences have been reported years after the initial episode. Plasmapheresis appears to be most effective in resolving bleeding complications, with an increase in the platelet count within 48 hours.[10]

Neonatal Isoimmune Thrombocytopenia

Neonatal isoimmune thrombocytopenia is caused by transplacental passage of maternal IgG antibodies directed against fetal platelet antigens inherited from the father and absent on the mother's platelets.[69] Sensitization to the platelet antigen by previous pregnancies or transfusions appears unimportant. The disorder is analogous to Rh hemolytic disease. The infants, born of hematologically normal women, may have a severe generalized petechial rash or may appear normal at birth and develop symptoms of thrombocytopenia within 2 or 3 days. Usually, all hematologic parameters are normal except the platelet count, which may be 30×10^9/L or less. Because maternal IgG antibodies can be transferred across the placenta and produce neonatal thrombocytopenia, it is important to differentiate alloimmune and autoimmune IgG antibodies to select the proper treatment. Assays for maternal platelet antigen IgG (PA IgG) and serum platelet-bindable IgG are useful for this purpose.[44] The treatment of choice is transfusion with maternal platelets[2] washed with ABO-compatible plasma to reduce the likelihood of further transfer of maternal alloantibody to the infant.[44] In the maternal platelets, the infant receives platelets that are nonreactive with the alloantibody, regardless of antigen specificity.

Patients Refractory to Platelet Transfusion

Patients refractory to platelet transfusion, such as those with aplastic anemia or acute leukemia who have received long-term platelet support, may have developed platelet alloimmunization. This condition is characterized by failure to achieve adequate increments in the circulating platelet count after transfusion.[78] The alloantibodies produced in about two-thirds of the cases are directed against HLA antigens. Because of the polymorphic nature of the HLA system, it may be difficult to find suitable random donors. Family members often are used[19] unless subsequent bone marrow transplantation from these individuals is contemplated.[79] Leukocyte-poor platelet concentrates may alleviate the problem for some recipients.[36]

For life threatening situations, two additional treatments are proposed: extensive platelet infusion and plasmapheresis.[47] Extensive platelet infusion temporarily reduces the level of offending alloantibody by adsorption, allowing the excess platelets to halt bleeding. Plasmapheresis reduces the alloantibody level prior to platelet transfusion.

Primary Autoimmune Thrombocytopenia

Primary autoimmune thrombocytopenia includes immune thrombocytopenic purpura (ITP), which may run either an acute or a chronic course. In the past, ITP was the acronym for idiopathic (i.e., unknown etiology) thrombocytopenic purpura. The illness is no longer considered strictly idiopathic but rather immune. It is too early to rename the condition "autoimmune thrombocytopenic purpura;" however, because it is not known whether the platelet-associated immunoglobulin is an autoantibody directed against the platelet, an immune complex bound to the platelet surface, or an antibody directed against a nonautologous antigen adsorbed to the platelet.[45]

Acute ITP, the most common cause of thrombocytopenia in children, is a self-limited disorder affecting boys and girls equally, most frequently those between the ages of 2 and 6 years.[60] This acquired disorder occurs predominantly in the winter and spring months after a viral illness such as measles, chickenpox, rubella, or infectious mononucleosis. The platelet count usually returns to normal spontaneously within 6 months,[53] but approximately 10% of the cases become chronic.

Chronic ITP occurs primarily in adults, and women are affected more frequently than men at a ratio of 2 to 4:1.[41] The onset is insidious, and the disease may last for years, almost never remitting spontaneously.

Pathophysiology

Because acute ITP frequently follows a viral illness, the immune system may be responding to viral antigen adsorbed onto the platelet surface or to immune complexes bound to the platelet.[57] The increased PA IgG levels are consistent with either hypothesis.

The PA IgG of chronic ITP is thought to be an antiplatelet antibody produced by splenic cells.[58] Studies suggest an abnormality of suppressor T cells.[80] The antibody binds to both autologous and homologous normal platelets, as well as to megakaryocytes but not to platelets from

patients with Glanzmann thrombasthenia, which lack glycoproteins IIb and IIIa.[82] The antiplatelet antibody present in the serum of about 95% of patients with chronic ITP is IgG, either alone or in combination with IgA or IgM. Serum from the remaining 5% of patients only demonstrates IgM antibodies.[83]

Clinical Presentation

Symptoms of thrombocytopenia, including petechiae, ecchymoses, and mucosal bleeding, usually appear abruptly in patients with acute ITP. The clinical history of chronic ITP is longer and includes easy bruising and abnormal menstrual bleeding. If mucosal bleeding occurs over long periods, iron deficiency may develop. Blood blisters in the mouth, hematuria, epistaxis, hematemesis, and melena are associated with more severe cases of chronic ITP.[55]

Laboratory Findings

The peripheral blood displays isolated thrombocytopenia, with platelet counts generally less than $50 \times 10^9/L$ and an increased percentage of megathrombocytes, whereas bone marrow megakaryocytes are normal or increased in number. Thrombocytopenia causes a prolonged bleeding time and abnormal clot retraction. Megathrombocytes represent young, metabolically active platelets and may explain why some patients with ITP have less bleeding than would be expected for the degree of thrombocytopenia.[32] Antibody bound to platelets is demonstrable in more than 90% of the cases of ITP.

Treatment

The purpose of therapy is to raise the platelet count to a level that will maintain hemostasis.[45] Patients with acute ITP often recover spontaneously. Chronic ITP may be treated with splenectomy to remove a major site of platelet storage and destruction and antibody synthesis or with immunosuppressants such as corticosteroids.

The management of ITP in pregnancy requires special consideration, because the IgG antibody from the mother is transported across the placenta to the fetus, causing neonatal thrombocytopenia. Postnatal thrombocytopenia created by this mechanism usually is self-limited, with platelet counts returning to normal within 1 to 2 months.[68] Intracranial hemorrhage may occur in the thrombocytopenic infant secondary to trauma to the head during vaginal delivery; therefore, low platelet counts on blood obtained from a fetal scalp vein early in labor may indicate need for a caesarean section.[77]

Secondary Autoimmune Thrombocytopenia

About 5% to 10% of patients with chronic lymphocytic leukemia and a smaller percentage of patients with other lymphoproliferative disorders develop immune thrombocytopenia.[37] Thrombocytopenia also is noted in 14% to 26% of patients with systemic lupus erythematosus (SLE).[11] Splenomegaly is usual, the bone marrow has a larger than normal number of megakaryocytes, and increased levels of PA IgG frequently are demonstrated.[57]

Immune thrombocytopenia appears to be a manifestation of the acquired immunodeficiency syndrome (AIDS).[63]

Bone marrow megakaryocytes are adequate to increased, PA IgG is increased, and patients are seropositive for antibodies to the causative retrovirus, human immunodeficiency virus (HIV).[1] Unexplained thrombocytopenia in otherwise healthy homosexual men may be an early manifestation of AIDS.[25]

Drug-Induced Immune Thrombocytopenia

The great majority of cases of immune thrombocytopenia are caused by a few drugs, notably quinidine, quinine, gold salts, sulfonamides and their derivatives, chloroquine, and rifampicin.[64] The role of the immune system in some drug-associated thrombocytopenias, such as that involving heparin, is debatable.[46]

The diagnosis of drug-induced immune thrombocytopenia is based primarily on the clinical history of drug ingestion and the exclusion of other causes. The clinical history should document thrombocytopenia while the patient is receiving the drug and normalization of the platelet count after the drug is discontinued. Reproducible, sensitive, and specific *in vitro* tests for drug-induced thrombocytopenia are not widely available.

Pathophysiology

Drug-induced immune thrombocytopenias appear to be analogous to the drug-induced immune hemolytic anemias. The antibody is directed against either a drug-platelet complex or a drug-plasma protein complex that then binds to the platelet.[62] Drug-induced synthesis of platelet autoantibody is a third possible mechanism, similar to that of methyldopa (Aldomet)-induced autoimmune hemolytic anemia (Chap. 19), but there is no direct evidence for this.[57] The drug may bind to the platelet membrane, with the antibody then attaching to the drug alone, or the drug may expose neoantigenic sites on the platelet membrane, with antibody binding to these sites. The altered platelets are then removed from the circulation by the reticuloendothelial system.

Drugs may also act as haptens, binding to a plasma protein and inducing antibodies that bind to the drug, forming an immune complex. The complexes settle on the platelets ("innocent by-standers"), which are then removed by the reticuloendothelial system.

Clinical Presentation

Most patients with drug-induced immune thrombocytopenia seek medical attention because of the sudden onset of petechiae, ecchymoses, blood-filled blisters in the mouth, and mucosal bleeding. The severity of the purpura may be disproportionate to the degree of thrombocytopenia, suggesting that the antibody also damages endothelium or induces a platelet function defect.[26] Most patients experience spontaneous recovery, with the platelet count returning to normal limits 7 to 10 days after the drug is discontinued, although in some patients, thrombocytopenia persists for 3 to 4 weeks.

Laboratory Findings

Laboratory results are similar to those described for other immune thrombocytopenias.

Therapy

The most important aspect of treatment is to discontinue the drug suspected of triggering the immune thrombocytopenia. Corticosteroids may be administered because of their positive effects on vascular integrity.

Sequestration

The spleen may be responsible for thrombocytopenia either by increased phagocytosis and destruction of damaged platelets or by increased sequestration of normal, undamaged platelets. Normally, 30% to 45% of the total circulating platelet pool is sequestered by the spleen from which it may be mobilized readily when needed.[4] In some conditions associated with splenomegaly, 50% to 90% of the platelets may be sequestered. The splenic pool consists of a larger proportion of megathrombocytes, which are younger and possibly more effective in hemostasis than the remainder of the circulating platelets.[40] Hypersplenism may be the chief mechanism of thrombocytopenia in Gaucher disease,[61] sarcoidosis,[17] and Felty syndrome.[6] Therapy usually is directed at correcting the primary disorder.

THROMBOCYTOSIS

Thrombocytosis is an abnormal increase in the number of circulating platelets as a result of physiologic or pathologic processes. A transient increase in the platelet count occurs with mobilization of the splenic platelet pool during physiologic stress such as vigorous exercise[16] or epinephrine infusion.[4] Increased platelet production may be classified as either primary or secondary.

Primary

Primary thrombocytosis (uncontrolled proliferation of platelets) is characteristic of the myeloproliferative disorders, particularly polycythemia vera (PV), essential thrombocythemia (ET), and some cases of chronic granulocytic leukemia (CGL). Megakaryocyte number and volume are increased in these disorders in spite of the high circulating numbers, suggesting autonomous proliferation. These disorders are described in detail in Chapter 35.

Secondary (Reactive)

A broad spectrum of acute and chronic illnesses elicit an increase in platelet production. However, the platelet count usually is not as great as that seen in primary thrombocytosis. Hemorrhage or thrombotic episodes are less likely to occur because the thrombocytosis usually is transient.

Iron deficiency may be associated with thrombocytosis. It is believed that iron normally is involved in regulating thrombopoiesis by inhibiting thrombopoietin, thereby inhibiting platelet production.[42] When iron deficiency develops, this control mechanism is decreased, and thrombocytosis occurs.

An increased platelet count is a common feature of rapid blood regeneration; therefore, thrombocytosis is observed with hemolytic anemias and acute blood loss.[66] In addition, increased platelet counts may be seen after cessation of cytotoxic drugs, withdrawal from alcohol, treatment of megaloblastic anemia, or recovery from postoperative thrombocytopenia.[12]

A modest elevation in the platelet count usually follows any major surgical procedure and is secondary to tissue damage.[66] Splenectomy is followed by thrombocytosis, with platelet counts of 1000 to 2000 $\times$ 10^9/L not uncommon.[73] An increase in the platelet count is noted 1 to 10 days after splenectomy and peaks 1 to 3 weeks later. Normally, the thrombocytosis subsides over weeks to months without ill effects.

The mechanism by which thrombocytosis occurs in a variety of acute and chronic infections, inflammatory disorders, and neoplasms remains obscure.

CHAPTER SUMMARY

Alterations in the number of circulating platelets are a frequent finding. Thrombocytopenia may result from a variety of causes, with mucosal bleeding being a common symptom. The clinical history and the peripheral blood film findings, bone marrow evaluation, coagulation studies, PA IgG levels, and other routine studies may provide helpful data to elucidate the cause. Thrombocytosis may be a benign, reactive process or a manifestation of a myeloproliferative disorder. Patients with reactive thrombocytosis usually do not have any bleeding tendencies, whereas those with primary thrombocytosis may present with hemorrhaging or a thrombotic episode.

CASE STUDY 60-1

A 36-year-old black woman was admitted through the emergency room with chief complaints of headache, dizziness, lethargy, nausea, vomiting, and weakness. Three months earlier, she underwent a subtotal gastrectomy for adenocarcinoma of the stomach. She was placed on mitomycin therapy, a cancer chemotherapeutic agent. Diagnostic procedures indicated recurrence of the carcinoma.

Repeated manual platelet counts ranged from 10 to 50 $\times$ 10^9/L except for brief increases that followed platelet transfusions. The APTT and fibrinogen concentrations remained within the normal range throughout most of the patient's hospitalization. The PT was slightly prolonged (13-17 seconds; reference range 10.5 to 13.0 seconds) until her death from respiratory failure on day 19.

The admission CBC showed:

		REFERENCE RANGE
WBC ($\times$ 10^9/L)	17.1	4.8–10.8
RBC ($\times$ 10^{12}/L)	2.29	3.80–5.50
Hb (g/dL)	8.1	12.0–15.2
HCT (L/L)	0.23	0.37–0.46
MCV (fL)	95.7	79–101
MCH (pg)	35.4	27–33
MCHC (g/dL)	35.0	31–34
RDW	18.5	11.5–14.5
Plt ($\times$ 10^9/L)	48.0	140–440
MPV (fL)	11.2	7.4–9.4
DIFFERENTIAL COUNT (%)		
Polys	79	30–70
Bands	3	0–10
Lymphs	11	20–50
Monos	6	2–12
Baso	1	0–2
NRBC (/100 WBC)	3	0
Marked anisocytosis		
Marked RBC fragmentation		

Additional laboratory data were:

		REFERENCE RANGE
URINALYSIS		
pH	5	5–7
Protein	< 300 mg/dL	Nondetectable
RBC	60–100	Nondetectable
Casts	Granular and hyaline	Nondetectable
SERUM CHEMISTRY		
LD (U/L)	1288	
Creatinine (mg/dL)	3.1	0.7–1.3
BUN (mg/dL)	39	8–22
Haptoglobin (mg/dL)	Nondetectable	50–150

1. Why was the patient's platelet count monitored by manual rather than automated methods?
2. What are the possible diagnoses and why?
3. What may have triggered the acute onset?
4. What other laboratory data may be of value in determining the pathogenesis of the thrombocytopenia?

REFERENCES

1. Abrams DI, Kiprov DD, Goedart JJ et al: Antibodies to human T-lymphotropic virus type III and development of the acquired immunodeficiency syndrome in homosexual men presenting with immune thrombocytopenia. Ann Intern Med 104:47, 1986
2. Adner MM, Fisch GR, Starobin SG et al: Use of "compatible" platelet transfusions in treatment of congenital isoimmune thrombocytopenic purpura. N Engl J Med 280:244, 1969
3. American Association of Blood Banks Technical Manual, 9th ed, p 252. Washington DC, AABB, 1985
4. Aster RH: Pooling of platelets in the spleen: Role in the pathogenesis of "hypersplenic" thrombocytopenia. J Clin Invest 45:645, 1955
5. Aster RH, Enright SE: A platelet and granulocyte membrane defect in paroxysmal nocturnal hemoglobinuria: Usefulness for the detection of platelet antibodies. J Clin Invest 48:1199, 1969
6. Barnes CG, Turnbull AL, Vernon-Roberts B: Felty's syndrome: A clinical and pathologic survey of 21 patients and their response to treatment. Ann Rheum Dis 30:359, 1971
7. Bessman JD, Gilmer PJ, Gardner FH: Improved classification of anemias by MCV and RDW. Am J Clin Pathol 80:322, 1983
8. Brain MC, Neame PB: Thrombotic thrombocytopenic purpura and the hemolytic uremic syndrome. Semin Thromb Hemost 8:186, 1982
9. Buchanan MR, Carter CJ, Hirsh J: Decreased platelet thrombogenicity in association with increased platelet turnover and vascular damage. Blood 54:1369, 1979
10. Budd JL, Wiegers SE, O'Hara JM: Relapsing post-transfusion purpura: A preventable disease. Am J Med 78:361, 1985
11. Budman DR, Steinberg AD: Hematologic aspects of systemic lupus erythematosus. Ann Intern Med 86:220, 1977
12. Burstein SA, Harker LA: Control of platelet production. Clin Haematol 12:3, 1983
13. Camitta BM, Nathan DG, Forman EN et al: Posthepatic severe aplastic anemia: An indication for early bone marrow transplantation. Blood 43:473, 1974
14. Chesney PJ, Taher A, Gilbert EMF et al: Intranuclear inclusions in megakaryocytes in congenital cytomegalovirus infection. J Pediatr 92:957, 1978
15. Davis JW, Wilson SJ: Platelet survival in the May-Hegglin anomaly. Br J Haematol 12:61, 1966
16. Dawson AA, Ogston D: Exercise-induced thrombocytosis. Acta Haematol 42:241, 1969

17. Dickerman JD, Holbrook PR, Zinkham WH: Etiology and therapy of thrombocytopenia associated with sarcoidosis. J Pediatr 81:758, 1972

18. Didisheim P: Screening tests for bleeding disorders. Am J Clin Pathol 47:622, 1967

19. Duquesnoy RJ: Donor selection in platelet transfusion therapy of alloimmunized thrombocytopenic patients. Prog Clin Biol Res 28:229, 1978

20. Eurenius K, Mortensen RF, Meserol PM et al: Platelet and megakaryocyte kinetics following thermal injury. J Lab Clin Med 79:247, 1972

21. Freedman ML, Karpatkin S: Requirement of iron for platelet protein synthesis. Biochem Biophys Res Comm 54:475, 1973

22. Gangarosa EJ, Johnson TR, Ramos HS: Ristocetin-induced thrombocytopenia: Site and mechanism of action. Arch Intern Med 105:83, 1960

23. Gianantonio C, Vitacco M, Mendilaharzu F et al: The hemolytic-uremic syndrome. J Pediatr 64:478, 1964

24. Gockerman JP, Shulman NR: Isoantibody specificity in post-transfusion purpura. Blood 41:817, 1973

25. Goldsweig HG, Grossman R, William D: Thrombocytopenia in homosexual men. Am J Hematol 21:243, 1986

26. Hackett T, Kelton JG, Powers P: Drug-induced platelet destruction. Semin Thromb Hemost 8:116, 1982

27. Hakim RM, Schafer AI: Hemodialysis-associated platelet activation and thrombocytopenia. Am J Med 78:575, 1985

28. Hall JG, Levin J, Kuhn JP et al: Thrombocytopenia with absent radius. Medicine 48:411, 1969

29. Hanahan DJ, Demopoulos CA, Liehr J et al: Identification of platelet activating factor isolated from rabbit basophils as acetyl glyceryl ether phosphorylcholine. J Biol Chem 255:5514, 1980

30. Harker LA, Finch CA: Thrombokinetics in man. J Clin Invest 48:963, 1969

31. Harker LA, Slichter SJ: Studies of platelet and fibrinogen kinetics in patients with prosthetic heart valves. N Engl J Med 283:1302, 1970

32. Harker LA, Slichter SJ: The bleeding time as a screening test for evaluation of platelet function. N Engl J Med 287:155, 1972

33. Harker LA, Slichter SJ: Platelet and fibrinogen consumption in man. N Engl J Med 287:999, 1972

34. Harlan JM: Thrombocytopenia due to non-immune platelet destruction. Clin Haematol 12:39, 1983

35. Hayasaka T, Yoshiki T, Shiral T et al: Comparative immuno-pathologic studies of thrombotic thrombocytopenic purpura, hemolytic-uremic syndrome and disseminated intravascular coagulation. Acta Pathol Jpn 31:569, 1981

36. Herzig RH, Herzig GP, Bull MI et al: Correction of poor platelet transfusion responses with leukocyte-poor HLA-matched platelet concentrates. Blood 46:743, 1975

37. Kaden BR, Rosse WF, Hauch TW: Immune thrombocytopenia in lymphoproliferative diseases. Blood 53:545, 1979

38. Kaplan BS, Chesney RW, Drummond KN: Hemolytic uremic syndrome in families. N Engl J Med 292:1090, 1975

39. Kaplan BS, Drummond KN: The hemolytic-uremic syndrome is a syndrome. N Engl J Med 298:964, 1978

40. Karpatkin S: Heterogeneity of human platelets. VI: Correlation of platelet function with platelet volume. Blood 51:307, 1978

41. Karpatkin S: Autoimmune thrombocytopenic purpura. Blood 56:329, 1980

42. Karpatkin S, Garg SK, Freedman ML: Role of iron as a regulator of thrombopoiesis. Am J Med 57:521, 1974

43. Kelton JG, Ali AM: Platelet transfusions: A critical appraisal. Clin Oncol 2:549, 1983

44. Kelton JG, Blanchette VS, Wilson WE et al: Neonatal thrombocytopenia due to passive immunization: Prenatal diagnosis and distinction between maternal platelet alloantibodies and autoantibodies. N Engl J Med 302:1401, 1980

45. Kelton JG, Gibbons S: Autoimmune platelet destruction: Idio-pathic thrombocytopenic purpura. Semin Thromb Hemost 8:83, 1982

46. King DJ, Kelton JG: Heparin-associated thrombocytopenia. Ann Intern Med 100:535, 1984

47. Klein CA, Blajchman MA: Alloantibodies and platelet destruction. Semin Thromb Hemost 8:105, 1982

48. Kressel BR, Ryan KP, Duong AT et al: Microangiopathic hemolytic anemia, thrombocytopenia, and renal failure in patients treated for adenocarcinoma. Cancer 48:1738, 1981

49. Krivit W, Yunis E, White JG: Platelet survival studies in Aldrich syndrome. Pediatrics 37:339, 1966

50. Kunicki TJ, Johnson MM, Aster RH: Absence of the platelet receptor for drug-dependent antibodies in the Bernard-Soulier syndrome. J Clin Invest 62:716, 1978

51. Kutti J, Weinfeld A: The frequency of thrombocytopenia in patients with heart disease treated with oral diuretics. Acta Med Scand 183:245, 1968

52. Levin J, Evatt BL: Humoral control of thrombopoiesis. Blood Cells 5:105, 1979

53. Lightsey AL, Koenig HM, McMillan R et al: Platelet-associated immunoglobulin G in childhood idiopathic thrombocytopenic purpura. J Pediatr 94:201, 1979

54. Machin S: Thrombotic thrombocytopaenic purpura. Br J Haematol 56:191, 1984

55. Martin JN, Morrison JC, Files JC: Autoimmune thrombocytopenic purpura: Current concepts and recommended practices. Am J Obstet Gynecol 150:86, 1984

56. McManus LM, Morley CA, Levine SP et al: Platelet activating factor (PAF) induced release of platelet factor 4 (PF4) in vitro during IgE anaphylaxis in the rabbit. J Immunol 123:2835, 1979

57. McMillan R: Immune thrombocytopenia. Clin Haematol 12:69, 1983

58. McMillan R, Martin M: Fixation of C3 to platelets in vitro by antiplatelet antibody from patients with immune thrombocytopaenic purpura. Br J Haematol 47:251, 1981

59. McMillan R, Mason D, Tani P et al: Evaluation of platelet surface antigens: Localisation of the Pl^{A1} alloantigen. Br J Haematol 51:297, 1982

60. McWilliams NB, Maurer HM: Acute idiopathic thrombocytopenic purpura in children. Am J Hematol 7:87, 1979

61. Medoff AS, Bayrd ED: Gaucher's disease in 29 cases: Hematologic complications and effect of splenectomy. Ann Intern Med 40:481, 1954

62. Miescher PA: Drug-induced thrombocytopenia. Semin Hematol 10:311, 1973

63. Morris L, Distenfeld A, Amorosi E et al: Autoimmune thrombocytopenic purpura in homosexual men. Ann Intern Med 96:714, 1982

64. Moss RA: Drug induced immune thrombocytopenia. Am J Hematol 9:439, 1980

65. Mueller-Eckhardt C, Lechner K, Heinrich D et al: Post transfusion thrombocytopaenia purpura: Immunological and clinical studies in two cases and review of the literature. Blut 40:249, 1980

66. Murphy S: Thrombocytosis and thrombocythaemia. Clin Haematol 12:89, 1983

67. Oski FA, Naiman JL: Effect of live measles vaccine on the platelet count. N Engl J Med 275:352, 1966

68. Pearson HA, McIntosh S: Neonatal thrombocytopenia. Clin Haematol 7:111, 1978

69. Pearson HA, Shulman NR, Marder VJ et al: Isoimmune neonatal thrombocytopenic purpura: Clinical and therapeutic considerations. Blood 23:154, 1964

70. Queisser U, Queisser W, Spiertz B: Polyploidization of megakaryocytes in normal humans, in patients with idiopathic thrombocytopaenia and with pernicious anaemia. Br J Haematol 20:489, 1971

71. Ridolfi RL, Bell WR: Thrombotic thrombocytopenic purpura:

Report of 25 cases and review of the literature. Medicine 60:413, 1981

72. Rote NS, Lau RJ: Immunologic thrombocytopenic purpura. Clin Obstet Gynecol 28:84, 1985

73. Salter PP, Sherlock EC: Splenectomy, thrombocytosis and venous thrombosis. Am Surg 23:549, 1957

74. Schoolwerth AC, Sandler RS, Klahr S et al: Nephrosclerosis postpartum and in women taking oral contraceptives. Arch Intern Med 136:178, 1976

75. Schulman I, Abildgaard CF, Cornet J et al: Studies on thrombopoiesis. II: Assay of human plasma thrombopoietic activity. J Pediatr 66:604, 1965

76. Schulman I, Pierce M, Lukens A et al: Studies on thrombopoiesis. I: A factor in normal human plasma required for platelet production: Chronic thrombocytopenia due to its deficiency. Blood 16:943, 1960

77. Scott JR, Cruikshank DP, Kochenour NK et al: Fetal platelet counts in the obstetric management of immunologic thrombocytopenic purpura. Am J Obstet Gynecol 136:495, 1980

78. Sintnicolaas K, Vriesendorp HM, Sizoo W et al: Delayed alloimmunisation by random single donor platelet transfusions: A randomised study to compare single donor and multiple donor platelet transfusions in cancer patients with severe thrombocytopenia. Lancet 1:750, 1981

79. Slichter SJ: Controversies in platelet transfusion therapy. Annu Rev Med 31:509, 1980

80. Trent RJ, Clancy RL, Danis V et al: Disordered immune homeostasis in chronic idiopathic thrombocytopenic purpura. Clin Exper Immunol 45:9, 1981

81. Urbaniak SS, Cash JD: Blood replacement therapy. Br Med Bull 33:273, 1977

82. van Leeuwen EF, van der Ven JTM, Engelfriet CP et al: Specificity of autoantibodies in autoimmune thrombocytopenia. Blood 59:23, 1982

83. von dem Borne AEG, Helmerhorst FM, van Leeuwen EF et al: Autoimmune thrombocytopaenia: Detection of platelet autoantibodies with the suspension immunofluorescence test. Br J Haematol 45:319, 1980

84. Weisbrot IM, Hollenberg LM: Platelet counting methods. Lab Med 11:307, 1980

85. Yeager AM, Zinkham WH: Varicella-associated thrombocytopenia: Clues to the etiology of childhood idiopathic thrombocytopenic purpura. Johns Hopkins Med J 146:270, 1980

86. Zimmerman SE, Smith FP, Phillips TM et al: Gastric carcinoma and thrombotic thrombocytopenic purpura: Association with plasma immune complex concentrations. Br Med J 284:1432, 1982 (abstr)

87. Zinkham WH, Medearis DN, Osborn JE et al: Blood and bone marrow findings in congenital rubella. J Pediatr 71:512, 1967

Gerald L. Davis

INHERITED DEFECTS
    Adhesion Defects
    Aggregation Defects
    Release Disorders

ACQUIRED DEFECTS
    Drugs
    Diet
    Diseases

CASE STUDY 61-1

Thrombocytopathy designates platelets that are qualitatively abnormal. This defective platelet function can be caused by a large variety of conditions (Table 61-1). Occasionally, qualitative and quantitative platelet disorders are present simultaneously.

Qualitative platelet disorders can be either inherited or acquired. They may be attributable to a primary defect in the platelet or secondary to another condition where the products of the disease affect platelet function. Table 61-2 lists the qualitative platelet disorders according to whether they are inherited or acquired.

The clinical picture of a qualitative platelet disorder resembles that of thrombocytopenia; however, the platelet count is normal. Epistaxis, menorrhagia, easy bruising, and postoperative bleeding are the most common presenting features.

INHERITED DEFECTS

Adhesion Defects

Platelet adhesion refers to the sticking of platelets to any surface except that of other platelets. Disruption of the endothelial vascular lining exposes subendothelial components such as collagen and basement membrane. When normal platelets come in contact with these surfaces, they undergo a shape change, expose certain membrane-bound glycoprotein receptors, and adhere to the exposed foreign surface. The glycoprotein receptor required for adhesion has been referred to as glycoprotein Ib (Gp Ib). This substance is a receptor for von Willebrand factor (vWF) and is required for platelet adhesion in small vessels.[18]

In the smaller vessels, wall shear rates are much higher than in large arteries. Platelet adhesion in the smaller ves-

TABLE 61-1. Qualitative Platelet Abnormalities

DEFECTS OF ADHESION	DEFECTS OF PRIMARY AGGREGATION	DEFECTS OF RELEASE
Bernard-Soulier syndrome	Glanzmann's thrombasthenia	Storage pool disease
Uremia	Afibrinogenemia	Gray platelet syndrome
Disseminated intravascular coagulation		Wiskott-Aldrich syndrome
		Hermansky-Pudlak syndrome
Paraproteinemias		Chédiak-Higashi anomaly
		Thrombocytopenia with absent radius (TAR)
		Uremia
		Aspirin
		Cyclooxygenase deficiency
		Ethanol

sels, where wall shear rates exceed 1000 sec^{-1}, requires availability of Gp Ib and vWF. In the large arteries, where the wall shear rates are less, Gp Ib and vWF are not required for platelet adhesion to the subendothelium.[9]

Bernard-Soulier Syndrome

In 1948, Bernard and Soulier first described the condition that now bears their names.[2] To date, only a few additional cases have been reported. A prolonged bleeding time, abnormal prothrombin consumption, and giant platelets are characteristic. The condition is inherited as an autosomal recessive disorder, usually involving consanguinity. For some unexplained reason, the severity of the hemorrhagic problems, which usually are first observed during infancy or early childhood, tend to decrease with age.

PATHOPHYSIOLOGY.   The platelets lack the membrane receptor Gp Ib that is necessary for them to bind with vWF. The deficiency of this membrane receptor results in platelets that are unable to adhere to surfaces such as collagen.

LABORATORY FINDINGS.   Mild to moderate thrombocytopenia is a frequent but inconsistent finding. Platelet anisocytosis on a blood film is marked. The majority of the platelets are large (2.5–8 μm in diameter), with some of them being as big as lymphocytes.[10] Other than size, the appearance of the large platelets generally is normal, although occasionally, there is a central clustering of granules referred to as a pseudonucleus. The granular contents and the

TABLE 61-2. Hereditary and Acquired Platelet Disorders

HEREDITARY	ACQUIRED
Bernard-Soulier syndrome	Myeloproliferative disorders
Glanzmann's thrombasthenia	Uremia
von Willebrand's disease	Aspirin
Afibrinogenemia	Penicillin-type antibiotics
Gray platelet syndrome	Ethanol exposure
Wiskott-Aldrich syndrome	Dextran
Hermansky-Pudlak syndrome	C$_{19}$ and C$_{21}$ fatty acids
Chédiak-Higashi anomaly	Onions, garlic, etc.
Thrombocytopenia with absent radius (TAR)	Disseminated intravascular coagulation
Aspirin-like deficiency	Paraproteinemias
Cyclooxygenase deficiency	

amount of vWF in these platelets are higher than in normal platelets.[7]

A bleeding time in excess of 20 minutes is a common finding. Clot retraction is normal. Platelet factor 3 (PF3) availability is normal, as determined by the kaolin method (Chap. 59). Platelet retention by glass bead columns is decreased. Ristocetin platelet agglutination studies are abnormal, and the addition of normal plasma, which contains vWF, does not correct the abnormal response. Both plasma and platelet factor VIII antigen levels are normal to increased.[7]

Platelet aggregation studies using ADP, epinephrine, and arachidonic acid produce normal results, but the results of aggregation studies with collagen and thrombin are variable. Platelet aggregation studies are difficult on platelets from these patients, because it is hard to separate the large platelets from the red blood cells and lymphocytes, especially when using centrifugation for obtaining platelet-rich plasma. The influence of the large platelets may also affect the light scattering and size of the platelet aggregates, resulting in altered aggregation curves. The variable findings for the aggregation response to collagen and thrombin may be a consequence of these technical problems.

The findings of normal clot retraction, normal ADP and epinephrine aggregation, decreased platelet retention, and abnormal ristocetin agglutination are important criteria for distinguishing Bernard-Soulier syndrome from other giant platelet abnormalities and from Glanzmann's thrombasthenia.

Von Willebrand's Disease

Patients with von Willebrand's disease lack the plasma protein that appears to link the platelet with the damaged vessel. The interaction of vWF with the platelet is primarily through the Gp Ib receptor, and, as noted earlier, both the vWF and the Gp Ib must be present for normal platelet adhesion. In von Willebrand's disease, it is the plasma component that is defective, whereas in Bernard-Soulier syndrome, it is the platelet. Von Willebrand's disease, a plasma factor (VIII:vWF or VIII:Ag) deficiency, is discussed in Chapter 55.

Aggregation Defects

Platelet aggregation is the sticking of platelets to platelets. Aggregation is a dynamic and metabolically active process that should not be confused with agglutination, which refers to platelet clumping that is not dependent on metabolic processes such as the release of ADP. Dead platelets, such as formalin-fixed or freeze-dried platelets used in the ristocetin test, will agglutinate, but they cannot aggregate. The ability of platelets to aggregate requires Gp IIb and Gp IIIa, which together form the fibrinogen receptor. This receptor, GPIIb–IIIa, as well as fibrinogen, are necessary for normal aggregation.

Glanzmann's Thrombasthenia

The autosomal recessive disorder known as Glanzmann's thrombasthenia, which has been associated with consanguinity, affects the two sexes equally. Only homozygotes have a clinically recognizable hemorrhagic disorder. Glanzmann's thrombasthenia appears to occur most frequently among Iraqi Jews, Jordanian Arabs, Indians, and French gypsies.[5,15]

PATHOPHYSIOLOGY.   Fibrinogen is a necessary cofactor for the aggregation of human platelets by ADP. During ADP-induced shape change and aggregation, fibrinogen becomes associated with the Gp IIb–IIIa complex on the platelet membrane. Glanzmann's thrombasthenia has been divided into: Type I and Type II.[8] The former is the more severe, with the platelets lacking Gp IIb–IIIa as well as intraplatelet fibrinogen. Clot retraction is absent. In Type II, platelets contain subnormal levels of fibrinogen, and the amount of Gp IIb–IIIa complexes is around 15% of normal. Clot retraction is observable.

CLINICAL PICTURE.   The hemorrhagic symptoms of bruising, epistaxis, bleeding from mucous membranes, gastrointestinal bleeding, and menorrhagia are typical. Ecchymoses frequently are seen at birth or early in life, but the severity of the hemorrhagic complications tends to decrease with age. In some individuals, the bleeding is severe enough to necessitate blood transfusions.

LABORATORY FINDINGS.   The platelets are normal in size and morphology and have a normal life span. However, these platelets do not support clot retraction adequately, and PF3 availability is deficient, as demonstrated by an abnormal prothrombin consumption test using the patient's platelets. When placed on a wettable surface such as a glass slide, the platelets fail to spread and form pseudopods; consequently, they will not form clumps on blood films made from capillary blood as normal platelets do. These platelets do not aggregate with ADP, epinephrine, collagen, or thrombin but will agglutinate on the addition of ristocetin.[9] The ability of the platelets to secrete the contents of their granules is not impaired. Normal amounts of platelet factor 4 (PF4), serotonin, and ADP secretion can be induced by exposure to thrombin.[19] Platelet retention in a glass bead column that requires both adhesion and aggregation is reduced markedly in most cases. Adhesion to vascular subendothelium is normal. With few exceptions, the lack of clot retraction in the presence of a normal platelet count is diagnostic of Glanzmann's thrombasthenia.[5]

The platelet Gp IIb–IIIa content is about 50% of normal in patients who are heterozygous for Glanzmann's thrombasthenia. However, these persons have normal clot retraction, aggregation studies, and bleeding times.

Multitransfused patients with Type I thrombasthenia may develop an IgG alloantibody to Gp IIb-IIIa complex. The addition of this antibody to normal platelets will cause them to exhibit the same laboratory abnormalities as Glanzmann's thrombasthenia platelets.

TREATMENT.   Type I thrombasthenic platelets lack the platelet-specific alloantigen P1^{A1}. Because 98% of the normal population has platelets that contain the P1^{A1} antigen, platelet transfusions for the treatment of Glanzmann's thrombasthenia must be used with caution to reduce the chance of alloantibody formation. Other forms of treatment include the use of hormones in menorrhagia and oral iron supplements for the anemia associated with chronic bleeding. Recently, an allogeneic bone marrow transplant was successful in correcting Type I Glanzmann's thrombasthenia in a 4-year-old boy. Steroids have not proved to be beneficial.

Afibrinogenemia

Just as von Willebrand's disease represents a plasma defect that will mimic the abnormalities seen in Bernard-Soulier syndrome, afibrinogenemia is a plasma defect that will cause a platelet aggregation disorder similar to Glanzmann's thrombasthenia. Afibrinogenemia is a rare disorder. The condition usually is treated by fibrinogen replacement using cryoprecipitate.

Release Disorders

Abnormal release of ADP may be secondary to a lack of granules or a deficient quantity of ADP stored in the granules, in which case, the condition is classified as storage pool disease. A second type of release disorder is caused by impaired secretion of normal granule contents. In platelet storage pool and release disorders, the primary wave of aggregation usually is normal (Chap. 59). The platelets undergo a shape change, expose various membrane-related glycoproteins, and clump. However, the secondary wave of aggregation, being dependent on the release of endogenous ADP from the beta (dense) granules in response to exogenous ADP and epinephrine, is abnormal.

Storage Pool Defects

Platelet storage pool deficiencies (SPD) can involve defects or lack of alpha granules, beta granules, or both. This is a heterogeneous group of disorders. Beta-granule deficiencies are much more common and are more likely to be associated with severe bleeding than are alpha-granule deficiencies. Possible explanations for the increased incidence of beta-granule deficiencies and the greater severity of bleeding are that alpha granules are present in excess of need, the ratio being about 800 alpha granules to 1 beta granule, and that the contents of the beta granules are more critical for platelet plug formation.

The *gray platelet syndrome* is an example of an SPD in which alpha granules are lacking. A Wright-stained blood film shows the platelets to be larger than normal and to be gray or blue-gray, in contrast to the lavender-purple granular appearance of normal platelets, probably because of the lack of granules or an increase in vacuoles. Tests for constituents of the alpha granule, such as PF4, beta-thromboglobulin, and fibrinogen, are abnormal. Decreases in PF3 also have been reported.[12] Tests for beta-granule contents (*e.g.*, uptake and storage of serotonin, ADP, and the ATP:ADP ratio) are normal. The dense tubular system (DTS), which is thought to be the storage site of calcium and cyclooxygenase, is abnormal in this syndrome and may be associated with abnormal release and variable aggregation findings.[13]

The gray platelet syndrome is rare, and for this reason, the method of genetic transmission is not certain, although it appears to be autosomal dominant.[12] Except for mild bleeding, moderate thrombocytopenia, abnormal platelet morphology, and modestly impaired aggregation, these patients appear to be hemostatically normal. In a few cases, the bleeding is serious. In one case involving a 4-year-old girl, the bleeding was controlled with platelet infusions and fibrinolytic therapy.[6]

Wiskott-Aldrich syndrome is characterized by the triad of thrombocytopenia, recurrent infections, and eczema. It is a sex-linked immunodeficiency, and affected boys rarely survive childhood because of the high risk of hemorrhage and infection.

The thrombocytopenia in these patients has been attributed to both rapid platelet turnover and ineffective production.[14] The platelets are small, measuring about two-thirds of the normal size, and they have abnormal cellular membranes because of the lack of a surface protein. This membrane defect also is present in the lymphocytes.[14] Wiskott-Aldrich platelets have been reported to be lacking in storage pool nucleotides. In addition, decreases in the number of alpha granules and mitochondria have been reported by several investigators, but these changes do not appear to be present in all cases. Being qualitatively defective, the platelets are subject to rapid sequestration in the spleen. Splenectomy has been effective in increasing the number of circulating platelets, but, because of the associated risk of infection, this treatment is not universal. Bone marrow transplantation may alleviate the symptoms.

Hermansky-Pudlak syndrome is characterized by a triad of tyrosinase-positive oculocutaneous albinism, accumulation of ceroid-like pigment in macrophages, and a bleeding tendency associated with abnormal platelet function. This is an extremely rare autosomal recessive condition associated with a striking lack of beta (dense) granules. Numbers of alpha granules are normal.

Chédiak-Higashi anomaly is characterized by albinism, recurrent infections, and giant lysosomes in all granule-containing cells. Chapter 28 describes this disorder in detail. Hemorrhage is a prominent feature, and although thrombocytopenia does occur, the prolongation of the bleeding time exceeds what would be expected on the basis of the platelet count, suggesting defective platelet function. The ratio of ATP to ADP in these platelets is consistent with a beta-granule deficiency.[16] The platelet response to ADP, epinephrine, collagen, arachidonic acid, and the calcium ionophore A231987, although variable, usually is deficient.[1] Typically, it is the secondary wave of aggregation that is abnormal or absent.

Granule Release Defects

The clinical picture and laboratory findings in the heterogeneous group of granule-release defects (also known as aspirin-like defects) are similar to those for SPD except that the stored contents of the alpha and beta granules are normal. The absence of the secondary wave of aggregation with ADP and epinephrine and the abnormal collagen-induced platelet aggregation are attributable to impaired release or secretion of ADP from the beta granules.

Deficiencies of platelet prostaglandin (PG) enzymes include defects in cyclooxygenase and abnormal thromboxane A_2 (TxA_2) activity. The abnormal platelet aggregation curve obtained by the addition of arachidonic acid to platelets deficient in cyclooxygenase will be corrected by the addition of prostaglandin G_2. Prostaglandin G_2 will not correct the abnormal aggregation caused by deficient TxA_2 or impaired calcium mobilization.

Patients with *cyclooxygenase deficiency* have a mild bleeding disorder, and treatment usually consists of avoiding antiplatelet drugs and use of hormonal therapy to control menorrhagia. Because thrombin will cause platelet release by way of a mechanism other than prostaglandins, the release of normal platelet contents in the presence of thrombin will differentiate this condition from an SPD.

Only two families have been reported with TxA_2 deficiency, and little is known about the clinical and laboratory features.

ACQUIRED DEFECTS

Platelet function may be affected by many drugs, diets, and diseases. The effects may be biochemical, mechanical, or both.

Drugs

There is a long list of drugs reported to affect platelet function, with aspirin, the penicillins, and alcohol being reported to cause clinical bleeding problems.[4] Patients taking aspirin have an abnormal secondary aggregation wave attributable to the inhibition of cyclooxygenase by irreversible acetylation of the enzyme's active site. Because platelets do not synthesize cyclooxygenase, the inhibitory effect lasts the life of the platelet (approximately 10 days). The prolongation of the bleeding time after aspirin ingestion is variable. Two hours after taking aspirin, most people show a 2- to 9-minute prolongation. About 10% to 15% of the population will have less than a 2-minute prolongation, and about 10% to 15% of the population will show greater than a 9-minute increase. The extent of prolongation of the bleeding time cannot be predicted by the bleeding time before aspirin ingestion. Marked prolongation of the bleeding time can be secondary to a variety of conditions, including vascular disorders, thrombocytopenia, vWF deficiency, and circulating anticoagulants. As in the SPD, the prolongation of the bleeding time is increased in proportion to the decrease in the ADP released from the beta granules. Other drugs that similarly affect platelets are indomethacin, ibuprofen, and butazolidine. Collectively, this group of drugs is referred to as *nonsteroidal anti-inflammatory agents*.

Carbenicillin is the most potent of the penicillin group of antibiotics capable of affecting platelet function. The mechanism of action is not clear, but it has been postulated that these drugs interact with glycoproteins on the surface of the platelet, causing a reduced response to most aggregating agents.

Prolonged exposure to alcohol, in addition to causing thrombocytopenia, impairs PF3 release and reduces secondary aggregation.[11] One possible mechanism is the direct impairment of prostaglandin synthesis by ethanol. Thromboxane A_2 release has been reported to be inhibited in alcoholic patients on hospital admission. During abstinence, the platelet count, bleeding time, and TxA_2 release return to normal.[11] The reduced platelet count and impaired platelet function may contribute to the increased incidence of gastrointestinal hemorrhage associated with excessive alcohol intake.

Finally, patients given significant amounts of intravenous dextran (*e.g.*, as prophylaxis against deep venous thrombosis during surgery), exhibit reduced platelet function, probably as a result of interaction between dextran and the platelet membrane.

Diet

Populations whose diet contains significant amounts of fish have decreased platelet function, as demonstrated in aggregation studies. It is believed that the C_{19} or C_{21} chain fatty acids or eicopentoic acids present in fish oils result in the replacement of arachidonic acid and production of inactive prostaglandins.[4] Another ethnic dietary component—an herb used in Szechwan cooking—decreases the platelet release reaction. Finally, onions, garlic, and related plants have an extractable substance capable of inhibiting platelet aggregation.

A deficiency in vitamin B_{12} or folate may lead to a qualitative platelet defect, as well as to thrombocytopenia. Large amounts of vitamin E can also affect platelet lipids through peroxidation, with resulting defects in prostaglandin synthesis.

Diseases

Myeloproliferative disorders frequently are associated with large, hypogranular platelets, which may be defective in any or all functions (adhesion, aggregation, release, or contraction). These abnormalities reflect a fundamental defect in megakaryocyte maturation.

Uremia is associated with qualitative platelet defects that can be corrected with dialysis. Various platelet defects have been described in conjunction with uremia, including decreased adhesion and aggregation and defective release. It is believed that these defects are a result of high concentrations of metabolites of urea such as guanidinosuccinic acid and hydroxyphenylacetic acid. Some patients with uremia also exhibit defective factor VIII:vWF complexes, especially the high-molecular-weight polymers necessary for adequate platelet adhesion.

Disseminated intravascular coagulation affects platelets in many ways other than by overt destruction. Prematurely activated platelets may release granules, causing an acquired platelet SPD. In addition, the fibrin(ogen) degradation products that circulate in this disorder are believed to interact with platelet membranes and inhibit adhesion or aggregation.

SUMMARY

The inability of platelets to function properly is characterized by symptoms that are identical to those seen in thrombocytopenias; however, the platelet count is normal or even increased. Disorders of platelet function can be classified according to the specific affected function (Table 61-1) or according to whether they are hereditary or acquired (Table 61-2).

Hereditary defects in adhesion and aggregation may be caused by platelet membrane abnormalities or plasma abnormalities. Hereditary defects in the platelet's ability to release granule contents are either caused by a decreased number of granules or an impaired release mechanism. Acquired platelet defects are more common and are discussed according to the primary cause: drugs, diet, or disease.

CASE STUDY 61-1

The patient was a 6-year-old boy whose aunt—a medical technologist—became concerned over his repeated nosebleeds and tendency to bruise. She examined a blood film made from a fingerstick and noted that the boy's platelet count appeared normal but that, contrary to expectation, his platelets were not clumped on the blood film. She persuaded her sister to take the boy to a physician. The patient's CBC was normal, with a platelet count of $380 \times 10^9/L$. His bleeding time was reported to exceed 15 minutes. The PT, APTT, TT, and fibrinogen were normal. Platelet aggregation studies revealed a total lack of response to ADP, a partial response to collagen, and a normal response to ristocetin.

1. What is a likely cause for the patient's bleeding history, and what other laboratory tests might be helpful?
2. What is the basic defect in this condition?
3. What information was supplied by the original fingerstick blood film?

REFERENCES

1. Apitz-Castro R, Cruz MR, Ledezma E et al: The storage pool deficiency in platelets from humans with the Chédiak–Higashi syndrome: Study of six patients. Br J Haematol 59:471, 1985
2. Bernard J, Soulier JP: Sur une nouvelle variété de dystrophie thrombocytaire hémorrhagipare congénitale. Sem Hôp Paris 24:3217, 1948
3. Coller BS: Disorders of platelets. In Ratnoff OD, Forbes CD (eds): Disorders of Hemostasis, p 73. New York, Grune & Stratton, 1984
4. Firkin BG: The Platelet and its Disorders. Boston, MTP Press, 1984
5. George JN, Reimann TA: Inherited disorders of the platelet membrane: Glanzmann's thrombasthenia and Bernard Soulier disease. In Colman RW, Hirsch J, Marder VJ et al (eds): Hemostasis and Thrombosis: Basic Principles and Clinical Practice, p 496. Philadelphia, JB Lippincott, 1982
6. Gootenberg JE, Buchanan GR, Holtkamp CA et al: Severe hemorrhage in a patient with gray platelet syndrome. J Pediatr 109:1017, 1986
7. Howard MA, Montgomery DC, Hardisty RM: Factor VIII-related antigen in platelets. Thromb Res 4:617, 1974
8. Lee H, Nurden AT, Thomaidis A et al: Relationship between fibrinogen binding and the platelet glycoprotein deficiencies in Glanzmann's thrombasthenia Type I and Type II. Br J Haematol 48:47, 1981
9. Legrand YJ, Karniguiah A, Lefrancier P et al: Interaction of platelets with a nonpeptide derived from type III collagen. Blood 58:198a, 1981
10. Lusher JM, Barnhart MI: Congenital disorders affecting platelets. Semin Thromb Hemos 4:123, 1977
11. Mikhailidis DP, Jenkins WJ, Barradas MA et al: Platelet function defects in chronic alcoholism. Br Med J 293:715, 1986
12. Mori K, Suzki S, Sugai K: Electron microscope and functional

studies on platelets in gray platelet syndrome. Tohoku J Exp Med 143:261, 1984

13. Mori K, Suzki S, Sugai K et al: Morphological changes of platelets during the process of platelet aggregation in gray platelet syndrome. Tohoku J Exp Med 149:425, 1986

14. Ochs HD, Slichter SJ, Harker LA et al: The Wiskott-Aldrich syndrome: Studies of lymphocytes, granulocytes and platelets. Blood 55:243, 1980

15. Reichert N, Seligsohn U, Ramot B: Clinical and genetic aspects of Glanzmann's thrombasthenia in Israel. Thromb Diath Haemorrh 34:806, 1975

16. Rendu F, Breton-Gorius J, Lebret M et al: Evidence that abnormal platelet functions in human Chédiak-Higashi syndrome are the result of a lack of dense bodies. Am J Pathol 111:307, 1983

17. Stuart MJ, McKenna R: Diseases of coagulation: The platelet and vasculature. In Nathan DG, Oski FA (eds): Hematology of Infancy and Childhood, 2nd ed, p 123. Philadelphia, WB Saunders, 1981

18. Weiss HJ, Tschopp TB, Baumgartner HR et al: Decreased adhesion of giant (Bernard-Soulier) platelets in subendothelium: Further implications of the role of the von Willebrand factor in hemostasis. Am J Med 57:920, 1974

19. White GC II, Workman EF, Lundblad RL: Thrombin binding to thrombasthenic platelets. J Lab Clin Med 91:76, 1978

Instrumentation and Quality Control in Hemostasis

Ruth Ann Henriksen

In this chapter, practical considerations for obtaining consistent and reliable results in the clinical coagulation laboratory are presented. The development of instrumentation, beginning with manual techniques and extending to modern instruments controlled by microprocessors and designed for computer interfacing, is reviewed, along with considerations in selecting instrumentation. Because of the complex enzymatic nature of the coagulation process and the usual use of the biologic phenomenon of fibrin clot formation as an endpoint in many coagulation tests, the results of these tests may have a larger coefficient of variation than do many tests in the clinical laboratory. Nevertheless, careful adherence to principles of quality control (QC) in instrument maintenance, specimen collection and handling, use of controls, preparation of standards, and selection of reagents will yield results that provide information essential to physicians in meeting the diagnostic and therapeutic needs of patients.

INSTRUMENTATION FOR TESTS OF HEMOSTASIS

Historical Development

The blood coagulation process and its associated disorders have been investigated for nearly two centuries. As early as 1911, the length of time required for a fibrin clot to form in glass tubes was used to study the characteristics of normal and hemophilic plasmas.[1] This manual technique for clotting time determination was used in the clinical laboratory for many years to identify patients with disorders of blood coagulation.[2,9,14,15] Later, the need to monitor anticoagulant therapy used in the treatment of thrombotic disorders brought additional demands for coagulation testing.

To increase the efficiency and precision of the determination of plasma clotting times, semiautomated instruments were introduced in the 1950s. Although these instruments generally required the manual addition of specimen and reagents, they provided an automatic clotting time determination. In general, the clotting time is inversely proportional to the rate of thrombin generation or fibrinopeptide A release from fibrinogen and is detected by a change in a physical property associated with conversion of the soluble fibrinogen molecule to insoluble polymerized fibrin.

During the 1970s, instruments were designed that automatically add reagents to a plasma sample and determine the clotting time. Such instrumentation now is used extensively and usually incorporates photo-optical sensing of fibrin clot formation.

Visual Detection of Fibrin Clot Formation

The use of glass tubes, a water bath for temperature regulation, a timing device, and visual observation for determination of clotting time continues to find limited application. This method, also known as the *tilt tube method*, is described in Chapter 52. Variables that must be controlled include the temperature, pipetor calibration, and the accuracy of the timing devices. It is difficult to control temperature in this method because the tube is repeatedly removed from the water bath to tilt it and check for clot formation. However, the most difficult and least controllable aspect is the visual detection of the clotting endpoint. As a result, there may be significant variability in the results obtained by different staff members. Nevertheless, with a little practice, it is possible to develop considerable skill and obtain much useful information.

Because manual methods are less precise, are very time-consuming, and require careful observer concentration to obtain reproducible results, nearly all manual methods have been replaced with more precise automated or semiautomated instruments. However, in situations where plasma fibrinogen levels are severely decreased, it may be possible to detect an endpoint in the prothrombin time (PT) or partial thromboplastin time (PTT) tests visually by the tilt tube method when automated methods fail.

When instruments are not available, coagulation disorders may be diagnosed and anticoagulant therapy monitored using manual procedures. Laboratories may rely on these techniques when the expense of instrumentation cannot be justified, such as when the number of determinations needed is relatively small, or in research where the experimental protocol is not adapted easily to available instrumentation. In smaller laboratories, manual techniques may serve as backup methods when instruments fail.

Electromechanical Detection of Fibrin Clot Formation

Principle of Operation

A modification of the manual technique, in which fibrin strand formation is detected by using a wire loop or hook, has been incorporated into a semiautomated electromechanical instrument. Electromechanical systems detect fully formed fibrin. These instruments (*e.g.*, the Fibrometer; BBL Microbiology Systems, Division of Becton Dickinson, Cockeysville, MD) require the operator to add all the reagents to a reaction cup (Fig. 62-1), but temperature control and a timing device for clot detection are provided by the instruments. Timing is initiated either automatically through activation by the pipetor (see Fig. 62-1) or manually by depressing the timer bar. When the timer is started, the probe arm, which consists of two metal electrodes (Fig. 62-2) with electrical contact through the timing device, drops so that the electrodes dip into the reaction mixture. One of the electrodes remains stationary, while the other moves out of the reaction mixture every 0.5 second. When a fibrin strand is formed and engaged by the moving electrode, which has a small hook at the end, electrical contact with the stationary electrode is maintained as the moving electrode rises out of the reaction mixture, causing the timer to shut off.

Accuracy and Sensitivity

Even though the timer is calibrated to the nearest 0.1 second, the mechanical nature of the Fibrometer results in detection of clot formation at only 0.5-second intervals. Thus, precision cannot be better than ±0.5 seconds on multiple tests of any given specimen. This instrument is somewhat more sensitive to low fibrinogen levels (<50 mg/dL) than are optical instruments.

Sources of Error

Satisfactory use of electromechanical devices requires that activated coagulation factors not be transferred by the probes from one sample to the next, as such contamination will result in shortened clotting times. To prevent contamination, the probes must be cleaned carefully between each test. This may be achieved by dipping the probes into a dilute acid solution, such as 2% acetic acid, and rinsing them with distilled water. Proper system operation also requires that the total volume of the reaction mixture be maintained so that the moving probe rises out of the liquid on the upward stroke. To meet the requirements of different test procedures, the manufacturer supplies two types of probes: one for a 0.3-mL reaction volume and another for 0.4 mL. It is important that the reaction cups be manufactured to exact specifications so that the cup has the correct diameter and may be seated properly in the reaction well.

Comments

Use of the Fibrometer is less labor intensive than manual techniques, and operator-dependent variability is reduced considerably. In 1981, nearly one third of the laboratories participating in College of American Pathologists (CAP) surveys reported that their results for PT and PTT were obtained using a Fibrometer.[7] This instrument continues to serve as a backup for photo-optical instruments. Also, because of differences in sensitivity, the Fibrometer frequently is used to recheck suspected aberrant results (*e.g.*, PT and PTT) obtained from optical instruments. Because it is relatively inexpensive, it may be well suited to situations where test volume is low.

Helena Laboratories (Beaumont, TX) has incorporated the capabilities of the Fibrometer into an instrument marketed as the Dataclot 2. This instrument has a heating block and the equivalent of two Fibrometer units. It features

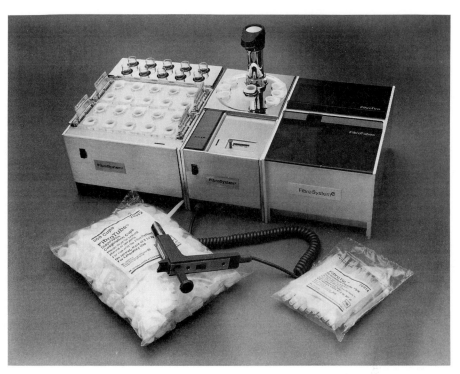

FIG. 62-1. Complete FibroSystem Fibrometer. Left back section provides incubation wells for 12 × 75-mm test tubes containing reagent that requires warming. Left front section provides incubation wells for coagulation cups containing reagent or patient specimen. Center section is electromechanical device for detection of fibrin clot formation (see Fig. 62-2). Note coagulation cup placed in reaction well ready for testing. Right front section provides storage for FibroTube coagulation cups. Right back section is used to store Fibrotips, which are disposable pipets that attach to automatic pipet shown attached to Fibrometer by electrical cord in front of instrument. (Courtesy of BBL [Baltimore Biological Laboratory] Microbiology Systems, Division of Becton Dickinson, Cockeysville, MD 21030.)

continuous temperature monitoring and display, timers with automatic reset, and two additional built-in stop watches for timing the incubation steps.

Photo-Optical Detection of Fibrin Clot Formation

Principle of Operation

Another method for detecting fibrin clot formation depends on the increase in light scattering associated with the conversion of soluble fibrinogen molecules to the insoluble polymerized fibrin clot. In general, visible light passes through the reaction mixture, and in most instruments of this type, the transmitted light is detected by a photocell. As the fibrin clot forms, more light is scattered, and the amount of light transmitted decreases. The signal generated by the photocell is analyzed by algorithms that determine the point at which clot formation occurs in each sample. These instruments also include a timer to determine the interval between the addition of the final reagent, which initiates the clotting reaction, and the point of clot formation.

Instruments

Semiautomated photo-optical instruments include the Electra 750 and 750A (Medical Laboratory Automation, Inc, Pleasantville, NY) the Fibrintimer series of instruments (LAbor Fibrintimer, Hamburg, Germany), and the FP 910 Coagulation Analyzer (Lab Systems, Inc, Chicago, IL). These instruments have from one to as many as ten channels for clot detection.

Instruments designated as automated will automatically add reagents to a sample supplied to the instrument in a disposable cuvette. These instruments include the Ortho Koagulab 16S (Fig. 62-3) and 40A (Ortho Diagnostic Systems, Inc, Raritan, NJ), the Coag-A-Mate X2 and XC

(Organon Teknika Corp, Durham, NC), and the MLA Electra 700 and 800 (Medical Laboratory Automation, Inc, Pleasantville, NY). The ACL Automated Coagulation Laboratory System (Instrumentation Laboratory, Lexington, MA) (Fig. 62-4) and the Microsample Coagulation Analyzer (Bio/Data Corp, Hatboro, PA) use smaller

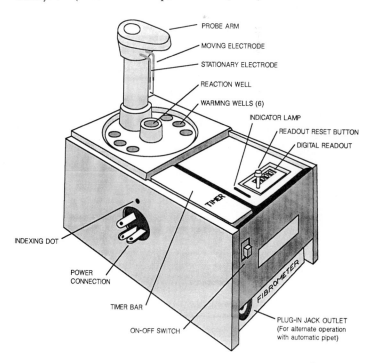

FIG. 62-2. Fibrometer, indicating essential features. Instrument uses electromechanical principle for detection of fibrin clot formation. (Courtesy of BBL Microbiology Systems, Division of Becton Dickinson, Cockeysville, MD 21030.)

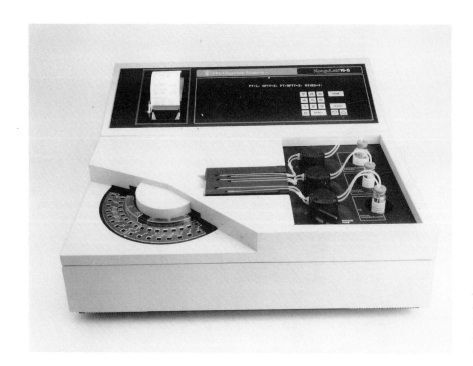

FIG. 62-3.   Ortho Koagulab Model 16S is an automated photo-optical instrument used for performing most coagulation tests with a fibrin clot endpoint. (Courtesy of Ortho Diagnostic Systems Inc, Raritan, NJ.)

sample volumes than other instruments. The instruments generally feature control by microprocessors and data storage and may be interfaced with a computer. They differ in flexibility for accepting different tests, compatibility with single or duplicate testing, and rate of test throughput.

Sources of Error

To allow for specimen variability and to avoid false endpoint detection secondary to the optical rippling that typically follows the addition of reagents to a sample, all instruments delay endpoint detection for a set time after reagent addition. During this "guard interval," a baseline is established for the transmitted light intensity of each sample. Therefore, a specimen with a clotting time shorter than the guard interval may be reported erroneously as having the maximum clotting time.

Photo-optical systems detect a rapid and substantial decrease in light transmission. Therefore, optical instruments may fail to detect the clotting endpoint in certain abnormal specimens. Extremely icteric, lipemic, or hemolyzed specimens may yield erroneous clotting times if the instrument cannot compensate sufficiently for the light absorbance by

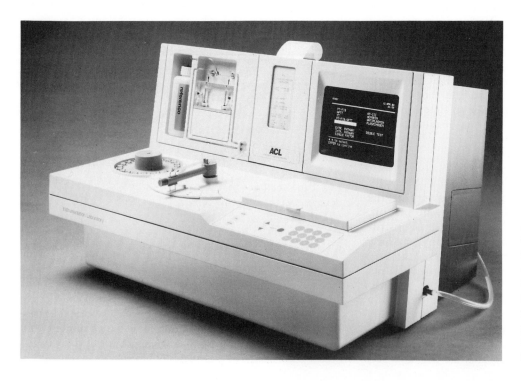

FIG. 62-4.   ACL Automated Coagulation Laboratory System, a centrifugal analyzer dedicated to coagulation testing. It may be used for tests where fibrin clot formation is detected photo-optically or to monitor hydrolysis of chromogenic substrates. (Courtesy of Instrumentation Laboratory, Lexington, MA 02173.)

the abnormal specimen itself, which prevents detection of decreased light transmission associated with clot formation. Samples with low levels of fibrinogen or high levels of heparin may also yield erroneous results, perhaps because (1) clot formation is too slow for detection of an endpoint by the instrument or (2) the formation of weak or fragmented fibrin occurs with little or no change in light transmission.

Occasionally, proteins precipitate in plasma samples, resulting in apparently short clotting times. This could occur if there is a large amount of cryoglobulin and the plasma is prepared by centrifugation at room temperature. Protein may also precipitate in some macroglobulinemias, where the addition of reagents for coagulation testing decreases the ionic strength of the test mixture. Difficulty in obtaining acceptable clotting time results also may be associated with disseminated intravascular coagulation (DIC) or improper specimen collection and processing. When any of these problems is present, the sample should be tested again using another method, preferably manual, to assure accurate results.

Some instruments require the light transmission to continue to increase for a full second for a valid result. This feature prevents acceptance of false endpoints that can be caused by delayed rippling in the sample. The 1-second observation period is subtracted from the instrument clock automatically before the results are reported. Other possible sources of error in photo-optical instrument operation are discussed under Quality Control for Instrument Operation.

Comments

Reproducibility of clotting times determined by photo-optical instruments is expected to be ±0.1 seconds, which is better than that for electromechanical instruments. Photo-optical clot detection is the basis of most automated and semiautomated instruments used in large clinical laboratories today, being the method used for more than 90% of PT and PTT results reported in the 1987 CAP surveys.[5] As new instruments are introduced, improvements in optics permit more accurate detection of clot formation. Many instruments now feature sophisticated data handling capabilities for both patient results and QC.

Selecting an Instrument for the Laboratory

Instrument and Operational Costs

A number of factors need to be considered in selecting a coagulation testing instrument. A prime consideration is the initial cost. Manufacturers of coagulation reagents may make instruments available as a part of a purchase agreement for reagents, but even though such agreements may be attractive because no capital equipment expenditure is required, it may be informative to determine what the cost would be for purchase of reagents and equipment separately.

Both the cost of the equipment and the labor cost for instrument operation should be considered in purchase decisions. In small laboratories performing only a few tests, it may not be possible to recover the cost of expensive instrumentation; therefore, semiautomated equipment may be the best choice. Additional considerations are the performance record of similar equipment, the cost and accessibility of repairs, and the cost of maintenance contracts.

Finally, the cost of disposables associated with instrument operation must be considered. Because the reaction cuvettes usually are unique to each instrument, it may be necessary to buy the cuvettes from the equipment manufacturer, allowing little possibility for competitive pricing. Reagent tubing may need to be replaced regularly. Other disposables are the reagent vessels, stir bars, pipet tips for handling reagents and specimens, and printer paper or report forms.

Matching the Instrument with Laboratory Needs

It is important to consider what tests the laboratory wishes to perform and which of these can be done on a given instrument. Instruments currently being marketed generally have a number of testing possibilities. Although this feature may be useful in small- to medium-sized operations, in laboratories where the test volume is large and peak periods require a high throughput of specimens, it may be preferable to devote one instrument to the PT test, another to the PTT test, and yet another to other tests with a lower request volume. Therefore, in a large laboratory, an instrument's ability to perform numerous tests may not be utilized. In some cases, it may be preferable to have two or more small instruments that provide additional backup in case of equipment failure.

Other features to be considered are instrument flexibility for adding new tests, varying test parameters, and compatibility with the reagents used currently. Adaptability to the desired testing pattern is also important. In other words, it may be helpful to be able to perform more than one test (e.g., PT and PTT) in a single run rather than being limited to performing a single test on each batch of samples. Laboratories that use single test results rather than duplicate testing should determine whether the instrument performs tests in one or both of these configurations. Decreasing the plasma volume required for testing may be particularly attractive to laboratories where there is a need to minimize specimen volume. In addition, decreasing specimen size reduces the required reagent volume, which results in considerable cost savings. The instrument software that is used to report results should be compatible with the laboratory data handling needs, whether this involves a computer interface or manual result reporting. Finally, to enhance laboratory efficiency, the instrument should be simple to operate and maintain in order to minimize the requirements for operator supervision.

QUALITY CONTROL FOR INSTRUMENT OPERATION

The QC checks selected to monitor instrument operation will depend on the instrument in use. Many modern automated instruments have internal system operation detection circuits. The laboratory should regularly (at least daily or every shift) monitor and record the temperatures for all temperature-regulated equipment, including refrigerators, freezers, and water baths. For instruments without a self-contained system for monitoring hemostature, care must be exercised in determining temperatures. Test and reagent wells may be filled with water and a calibrated thermometer used. In this method, thermometer bulbs must be small enough to be immersed in the liquid, and sufficient time must be allowed for equilibration. If these precautions are not observed, inaccurate and irreproducible temperatures and test results will be observed. Surface temperature probes may permit faster and more accurate monitoring.

Inconsistent reagent delivery may cause erratic problems in automated instruments. Although some newer instruments have a system for detecting reagent delivery or reaction volume, older instruments generally do not. Awareness of potential problems such as crimped tubing, insufficient reagent, or other causes of erratic delivery is important. In the extreme case, these problems appear as a series of results with the maximum clotting time. Such an occurrence always demands further investigation.

Personnel also must know how to operate all instruments properly. Consider, for example, the selection of an incorrect testing mode. If PT testing is selected accidentally instead of PTT, the instrument may not be able to detect the error. In this situation, the wrong reagent volume may be dispensed to the reaction cuvette, among other instrument "errors," causing all specimen results to be erroneous. This scenario is a particular problem when it is necessary to change instrument settings continually because the same instrument is used for several tests.

Instrument operation manuals contain general guidelines for maintenance and QC. Some important variables are listed in Table 62–1. No program for monitoring and recording variables will detect all possible sources of error in a testing system, and there is no substitute for careful attention to system operation. Consider, for example, an acute failure in instrument temperature regulation. If this is not detected before the next scheduled temperature check, many inaccurate results could be reported, whereas the alert operator may quickly detect inconsistencies in patient or control results or both and avoid a larger problem ultimately affecting patient care. The need for careful attention to changes in performance becomes even more critical as

laboratories become increasingly computerized and results are reported with minimal review by personnel.

QUALITY CONTROL FOR HEMOSTASIS TESTING

Specimen Quality Control

Quality control in hemostasis begins with proper specimen collection, handling, and processing, as presented in Chapter 51. Table 62-1 lists specimen variables affecting coagulation test results. When blood is removed from the vessel, small amounts of thrombin are generated quickly, and in the absence of anticoagulant, a clot is formed within a few minutes. In some disease states, the delicate balance of the coagulation pathway is disturbed so that the rate of thrombin generation in the absence of anticoagulant is even faster. In these situations, it is even more important that the QC procedures associated with specimen collection be followed carefully.

Reagent Quality Control

In this section, the focus is on the quality control procedures for ensuring satisfactory reagents for performing routine coagulation tests, including the PT, PTT, functional fibrinogen level, and thrombin time.

Commercially available thromboplastin reagents for the PT are derived principally from bovine and rabbit brain or lung. Activated PTT reagents contain one of several types of activators. In the past, activators for the PTT test generally were regarded as particulate or soluble. Particulate activators included (and still include) kaolin, silica, or diatomaceous earth (Celite) which provide a surface for the activation of factor XII. Soluble activators were defined as those reagents containing ellagic acid. However, additional study has shown that even for "soluble" ellagic acid activators, activation of the intrinsic pathway is dependent on a particulate (insoluble) complex between ellagic acid and metal ions,[3] consistent with the observation that a surface is needed for the activation of factor XII.

Test results are dependent on the specific reagents and instrumentation used. Therefore, reference ranges and sensitivity to individual factor deficiencies will differ according to the test system used. (A "system" is defined as any reagent-instrument combination.) Data from CAP survey samples or other QC programs may help identify differences in results obtained for the various reagents and instruments.

Reagent Selection for Prothrombin Time and Partial Thromboplastin Time Testing

In selecting reagents for use in laboratory testing, several factors should be considered, as outlined below.

PURPOSES FOR PERFORMING THE TESTS.   Although the PT and PTT may be used as routine screening tests for coagulation disorders, these tests may be used even more frequently to monitor anticoagulant therapy (Chap. 57). Therefore, reagent performance in producing reliable results for both types of testing must be considered.

TABLE 62–1. Some Variables Affecting Coagulation Testing and Quality Control.

Instrument
    Temperature
    Light source
    Detector
    Timer
    Disposables
    Reagent delivery
Specimen
    Collection system
    Anticoagulant
    Phlebotomy technique
    Centrifugation
    Delays in handling
    Storage conditions
Reagents and controls
    Shipping conditions
    Storage conditions
    Reconstitution
    Contamination
    Deterioration
    Lot changes

REAGENT-INSTRUMENT COMPATIBILITY. It is important that the reagents selected be compatible with available instrumentation. This may be readily achieved by selecting reagents and equipment marketed by the same vendor. However, this kind of package may be more costly and may not always best satisfy laboratory needs.

REAGENT COST. Cost must be considered in light of budgetary constraints. When more than one reagent will perform satisfactorily, a cost savings may be realized by requesting competitive bids from suppliers.

REPRODUCIBILITY. Reproducibility of the results obtained with a given reagent may be determined by the laboratory or from examination of the results obtained by many laboratories on survey samples.

REAGENT SENSITIVITY. In evaluating a reagent, the laboratory needs information regarding test system sensitivity to specific factor deficiencies, sensitivity of the PTT to therapeutic levels of heparin, and the expected results for the PT in patients receiving coumarin derivatives. Because of its possible association with an increased incidence of thrombosis, there is considerable interest in the sensitivity of PTT reagents to the lupus anticoagulant.

An important feature of a satisfactory reagent is its sensitivity to changes in coagulation factors of interest at the normal-abnormal interface. Adequate information regarding reagent sensitivity often is not available from the manufacturer or literature sources. To determine sensitivities, the concentration of the component in question must be varied by mixing a factor-deficient plasma and the plasma reference pool obtained from 20 normal donors who are taking no medications and have no known illnesses. For coagulation factor VIII, for example, this is achieved by mixing plasma severely deficient only in factor VIII (commercially available) with the reference pool (in which factor VIII is defined as 100%) in various proportions. The percentage of the plasma reference pool contained in each mixture corresponds to the percentage of factor VIII present. Using semilogarithmic graph paper, a plot of factor concentration in percent is made on the logarithmic scale against the PTT in seconds on the linear scale (Fig. 62-5). The straight line that best fits all points indicates reagent sensitivity. Using this graph, the percent of factor VIII at which the PTT becomes abnormal, according to the reference range established by the laboratory for this reagent, may be determined. To screen adequately for mild factor VIII deficiency, an abnormal PTT should be obtained at no less than 35% factor VIII if the population reference range has been determined correctly. If this criterion is not met, further investigation of the situation is required. This may include attention to proper handling of all plasma specimens and evaluation of alternative reagents or different lots of the same reagent.

As an example, the graph in Figure 62-5 indicates that for this instrument-reagent system, a 35% factor VIII level corresponds to a PTT of 32.5 seconds. Therefore, this laboratory's population reference range upper limit should be no higher than 32.5 seconds; otherwise, patients with a mild factor VIII deficiency would go unidentified using this

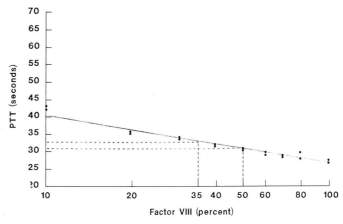

FIG. 62-5. Sensitivity of PTT reagent to factor VIII level. The PTT was determined for plasma containing various concentrations of factor VIII. Plasma samples were mixtures prepared from a reference pool and plasma severely deficient in factor VIII (obtainable commercially). Using this particular reagent and instrument combination, graph indicates that 50% factor VIII activity corresponds to PTT of 30.5 seconds, whereas 35% factor VIII activity corresponds to 32.5 seconds. To detect deficiency conditions adequately, a reagent–instrument system should detect an abnormal PTT at a minimum of 35% factor activity. To achieve this goal, this laboratory should set its PTT upper normal limit at 31 or 32 seconds. This finding should correspond to the upper limit of laboratory's population reference range for PTT. If the two are not almost identical, population range may need to be determined again. Sensitivity of reagent to each intrinsic pathway factor should be checked using this technique. (Every laboratory must determine its own sensitivity curve using its reagents and instrumentation. This graph is presented as an example from one laboratory. Data supplied by Special Hematology Laboratory, Department of Pathology, University of Iowa Hospitals and Clinics, Iowa City, IA.)

system. Refer to Figure 62-5 for further details. Sensitivities to other factors may be determined similarly.

Once a reagent has been selected, the laboratory should secure enough from a single lot to permit use for at least 1 year. Most reagents will have some lot-to-lot variability, and as a result, reference ranges and sensitivities need to be checked for each new lot even though the reagent is obtained from the same manufacturer.

Reagent Selection for Fibrinogen Determination
As with the PT and PTT, the results of fibrinogen determination by the Clauss method[4] are dependent on the reagent and equipment manufacturer.[5] This is unfortunate, because fibrinogen is a well-characterized and readily isolated plasma protein. It should, therefore, be possible to prepare a standard fibrinogen plasma, which, when used to establish a standard curve, would allow determination of fibrinogen in patient specimens without dependence on the source of thrombin. This is not the present situation, and as a consequence, the reference range for fibrinogen is somewhat system dependent. Whatever reagent is selected, it must be used both to establish the reference range and to determine patient values.

The laboratory selection of reagents depends on a combination of reagent cost and the equipment available. Fibrinogen commonly is determined by semiautomated electromechanical detection of fibrin clot formation, although photo-optical instruments may be used also. Generally, photo-optical instruments use the same methodology and reagents as the electromechanical ones. Alternative methods for evaluating fibrinogen are available on two instruments. The Koagulab (Ortho Diagnostic Systems, Inc) detects the maximum light scattering attained on fibrin clot formation in the PT test and reports a qualitative or relative measure of fibrinogen level. Another instrument, the ACL System (Instrumentation Laboratory; see Fig. 62-4), likewise monitors fibrin formation in the PT test. However, in this case, a quantitative fibrinogen level is reported. For this procedure, the PT reagent (Fisher Diagnostics) contains an antiheparin agent to prevent heparin in the undiluted plasma from interfering with the test.

Sources of Error in Coagulation Reagent Use

Once reagents are selected for the laboratory, it is important that they be shipped, stored, and reconstituted as appropriate and handled in accordance with the manufacturer's recommendations. If these guidelines are not followed, erroneous test results may be obtained.

Several possible sources of error are associated with coagulation reagents. Deterioration will prolong clotting times. Evaporation from opened vials of reagent also must be avoided. If not attributable to a change in reagent lot number, short times usually result from reagent contamination. Shipping or storage problems related to excessive exposure of reagents to either heat or cold, especially temperatures around 0°C, where liquid reagents may freeze and later thaw, can cause deterioration of reagents.

Lyophilized reagents are far less susceptible to damage caused by excessive heat or cold. They must be reconstituted, using a volumetric pipet, with the volume of distilled or deionized water specified by the manufacturer. Erroneous clotting times may result from too little or too much diluent.

Expiration dates and stability guidelines for reconstituted reagents are provided by the manufacturers and must be heeded. The laboratory regulatory and licensing agencies do not approve of using reagents beyond their expiration date. All manufacturers' reagents and controls are different and have different claims; all package literature should be filed with the procedures and posted with QC guidelines.

Apparent problems may arise with changes in reagent lots. These changes are to be expected and may necessitate reevaluation of the laboratory's control and population reference ranges when switching to a new reagent lot. The change in the control range may be more noticeable in abnormal than in normal control ranges.

Control Materials

Prothrombin Time and Partial Thromboplastin Time

In the discussion below, it should be remembered that a control plasma is intended only for use by the laboratory in QC to monitor the performance of the testing system: the control is not a standard. Control values do not in any way define a reference range. Further, it should be remembered that the use of control plasmas in the laboratory does not detect problems associated with specimen collection, handling, processing, or storage. Most laboratories use commercially prepared and lyophilized plasmas as normal and abnormal controls to verify the performance of reagents and equipment. Because these materials are intended only for use as coagulation controls, they are not a satisfactory substitute for normal human plasma in other procedures, such as factor assays or mixing studies.

Commercially available controls generally perform as specified by the manufacturer and provide both convenience and a method of monitoring precision to ensure reliable results. In many instances, reagent manufacturers will assist in interlaboratory comparison of results, which may be particularly helpful for smaller laboratories. If this type of interlaboratory comparison is not needed, a large volume of normal plasma may be obtained by the laboratory, aliquoted, and stored at −70°C for use as a control.

The CAP hematology inspection checklist suggests that controls for coagulation tests be run once each shift, or after every 20 samples, whichever occurs more frequently. A troubleshooting guide for unacceptable control results is given in Table 62-2. Besides monitoring the testing system, repeated performance of a given test on the same lot of control plasma permits determination of the standard deviation of the clotting time for the particular reagent and instrumentation being used. This information may be helpful in interpreting patient results, particularly those at the borderline between normal and abnormal. Long-term monitoring of the mean and standard deviation for control results may indicate subtle shifts or trends in the testing system attributable, for example, to one of the variables listed in Table 62-1.

Because of the nature of coagulation test systems, these tests generally do not have the precision seen in clinical chemistry tests. As a result, the National Committee for Clinical Laboratory Standards (NCCLS) guidelines covering the performance of coagulation assays specifies that coagulation tests should be performed in duplicate.[12] If manual or semiautomated coagulation tests are being used, these tests are almost uniformly performed in duplicate. However, in an effort to decrease testing time and the expense of reagents and supplies when using automated equipment, some laboratories perform only single tests for

TABLE 62–2. Troubleshooting Unacceptable Prothrombin Time and Partial Thromboplastin Time Controls

PROBLEM	POSSIBLE CAUSE*
Unacceptable normal and abnormal control results in only one test system (PT or PTT)	Test reagents
Unacceptable normal and abnormal control results in both PT and PTT	Instrumentation variables
Unacceptable results only on normal control in both PT and PTT	Normal control
Unacceptable results only on abnormal control in both PT and PTT	Abnormal control
Mixed pattern of longer and shorter results	Lot changes of reagents or controls; instrument variables

* See Table 62-1 for additional details.

routine procedures such as PT and PTT. To make the change to the single-test mode legitimately, the laboratory should demonstrate that not more than 1% of the results determined in this mode would have a statistically significant difference from the average result obtained in the duplicate mode. The use of on-line delta checks (comparison of current result with the most recently reported result for any given patient) also can assist the laboratory in detecting occasional aberrant test results that warrant verification.[11]

Fibrinogen and Thrombin Time

Fibrinogen values usually are available for commercially prepared control plasmas supplied for PT and PTT testing. However, the laboratory may expect to obtain this stated result only if the reagent and instrument system is the same as that specified by the manufacturer.

Because the thrombin time test is very sensitive to small changes in thrombin concentration, the control clotting time obtained on a normal plasma prepared and handled similarly to patient plasma should be reported with the patient result. If the laboratory wishes to use a commercially prepared normal control plasma in this test, it must be established that the control plasma yields the same clotting time as fresh normal plasma.

Establishing the Population Reference Range

To establish a population reference range, coagulation results for the normal population should be determined by each laboratory.[16] Commercial controls are not acceptable for use in determining a population reference range. Controls are designed only to check assay system precision and to allow for observation of shifts and trends indicating system malfunction. Therefore, each laboratory should establish a population reference range by testing plasma specimens from a group of normal individuals to provide an objective means of deciding whether patient specimen results are normal or abnormal. The procedure for establishing population reference ranges is detailed in Chapter 46.

The sensitivity of the PTT reagent, particularly to factor VIII and IX levels, also should be considered (see Reagent Selection for Prothrombin Time and Partial Thromboplastin Time Testing) in arriving at the best estimate for the laboratory's population reference range. Once established, the reference range should not vary unless there is a change in the test system. System changes that might influence the reference range include changes in the sample collection system (e.g., changing the concentration of sodium citrate used as sample anticoagulant); changes in testing methodology (e.g., from manual to automated); a change in instrumentation (manufacturer or model with the same manufacturer); a change in reagents; or repair or replacement of instrument parts.

Reference (Activity) Curve Generation for Factor Assays

The fundamental point of reference in blood coagulation is a plasma pool obtained from 20 normal donors. Generation of factor assay reference curves (also called "standard" or "factor activity" curves) requires the use of either a reference pool collected from 20 normal donors or a commercial reference plasma with assayed factor concentrations.

For laboratories choosing to prepare and store their own reference pool, special care must be taken to assure the quality of the pooled plasma and its stability during long-term storage. Samples from all 20 donors must be drawn within a short time (30–60 minutes) into the same anticoagulant used in routine testing. These samples are then processed rapidly by centrifugation to separate the plasma and cells followed by high-speed recentrifugation of the pooled plasma to remove residual platelets. The platelet-free plasma is aliquoted quickly and frozen at −70°C. This procedure must be completed rapidly to prevent denaturation of the labile coagulation factors. Obtaining a reference pool requires attention to detail and a commitment by both laboratory personnel and donors to the task at hand. For smaller laboratories, it may not be feasible to collect such a pool.

By definition, the level of coagulation factors and other coagulation-related proteins in the reference pool is 100% of normal or 1 unit/mL. For fibrinogen, the concentration (mg/dL) is based on a determination of the clottable protein. Further details on the generation and use of the reference or standard curve for factor assays may be found in Chapter 53. A sample reference curve is shown in Figure 53-3.

Lyophilized reference plasmas with stated assay values for the various coagulation proteins are available commercially. Following lyophilization, it generally is not possible to recover all the activity. Therefore, the assay values for the lyophilized material are determined by repeated assay of the reconstituted material against a 20-donor plasma pool. A frozen reference plasma is available with the stated values of about 100% for all coagulation proteins. Variability in handling the reference plasma as well as patient specimens contributes to wide variations in factor assay results, as may be seen in CAP coagulation survey results.

The commercial pooled reference plasma cannot be used to determine the population reference range or expected normal values for the PT or PTT. Rather, it is used specifically for establishing reference curves in assays for specific coagulation factors.

There are only a few primary reference materials available with known activity for a single coagulation factor. To facilitate comparison of results, principally among research laboratories, there are standards for thrombin and factor X_a. A standard for factor VIII is available from the CAP, Skokie, Illinois. In the United States, this reference material should assist in standardizing factor VIII assays.

Proficiency Testing

The use of single lots of plasma for interlaboratory comparison of coagulation test results assists individual laboratories in identifying and assessing their performance relative to that of other laboratories. Such interlaboratory comparison should increase the reliability of coagulation tests performed in all laboratories. However, the results obtained for PT and PTT are dependent on the reagent system used and the method of endpoint detection. Therefore, in CAP surveys, results are compared only with those of other laboratories that use the same testing system. Unfortunately, as new instruments and reagents are marketed, a particular method may not be used by enough laboratories to allow a statistically valid comparison of results. In general, clotting times are more dependent on the reagents used than on the instrumentation.

INTERNATIONAL NORMALIZED RATIO FOR PROTHROMBIN TIME REPORTING

The PT and PTT results are routinely reported to the nearest one-tenth second along with the population reference range. For the PT, another method of reporting has been proposed to facilitate interlaboratory comparison and more importantly, to assist physicians in prescribing more consistent warfarin therapy.[13] The international normalized ratio (INR) is a PT result that is calculated by comparing the patient value with the "normal" value and the result is normalized to an international reference preparation (IRP) of thromboplastin. Normalization is achieved by use of the international sensitivity index (ISI), which is determined for each reagent used in PT testing. Because of the complex mathematical manipulations and extensive comparative testing necessary to establish the ISI, it is expected that the manufacturers of commercial reagents will supply this value.[8] The INR is obtained from the equation INR = (patient PT/normal PT)^{ISI} or the observed ratio of the patient PT to the reference (normal) PT raised to the power of ISI. With the computerization of instrumentation and reporting, the laboratory should be able to calculate and report INR values routinely. Alternatively, the ISI could be used by the laboratory to calculate a PT therapeutic range (determined from INR values) for warfarin therapy.[12] For example, if the PT of the plasma reference pool is 12.0, the ISI for the reagent being used is 2, and a therapeutic range of 2.0 to 3.0 is selected for the INR, the PT therapeutic range in seconds is determined as follows:

$$2.0 = (x/12.0)^2 \qquad 3.0 = (x/12.0)^2$$
$$288.0 = x^2 \qquad 432.0 = x^2$$
$$17.0 = x \qquad 20.8 = x$$

The appropriate therapeutic range for warfarin therapy would then be 17.0 to 20.8 seconds.

The importance of this method of reporting arises from observations that most PT reagents available in the United States are less sensitive to depressed factor levels than are the reagents typically used in Europe. As a result, it has been observed that when warfarin therapy is regulated by the PT, patients generally receive higher doses of anticoagulant in the United States and Canada than in Europe.[6,10] Therefore, the results of clinical trials may not be directly comparable (Chap. 57).

Standardization in reporting PTT results, as described above for the PT, has not been achieved. It should be noted, however, that PTT reagents have variable sensitivities to heparin and that therapeutic ranges are reagent dependent.

AGGREGOMETRY QUALITY CONTROL

A platelet aggregometer measures the decrease in light scattering or the increase in light transmission as a function of time as platelets aggregate or clump in response to an added stimulus (see Fig. 59-1). Several companies market instruments for measuring platelet aggregation, and manufacturer's recommendations for operation and maintenance should be followed. Proper operation requires correct function of the light source, photodetector, temperature regulation, the motor that operates the small magnetic specimen stir bars, and the recording device for data output.

Release of platelet granule contents is associated with normal platelet aggregation, but each component released may be monitored independently. Stimulation of platelets results in the release of both ATP and ADP from the dense granules. The release of ATP may be monitored with the firefly luciferase assay, in which ATP supplies energy for visible light production that may be detected by a sensitive photocell. The ATP release and platelet aggregation may be detected simultaneously if two photocells are positioned at a 90° angle, one to measure the increase in light transmission as the stirred platelets aggregate and the other to measure light emission secondary to ATP release. By using compounds that fluoresce in the presence of ionized calcium, it is possible, in a similar manner, to determine the release of Ca^{+2} from platelets in response to various stimuli.

To interpret results of platelet aggregation studies properly, it is important that reproducible procedures be followed. Citrated platelet-rich plasma (PRP) should be prepared by a standard reproducible centrifugation procedure. The preservatives in commercial specimen collection tubes may affect platelet function, and for this reason, caution should be exercised in the use of such tubes.

Reagents used in stimulating platelet aggregation need to be stored under conditions that will maintain maximum stability. Reagents in solution generally may be stored for 1 year at −70°C. Because of its susceptibility to oxidation, arachidonic acid is particularly difficult to handle. A concentrated solution of arachidonic acid prepared in dimethylsulfoxide that has been purged with nitrogen is stable for several months at −70°C when stored in polypropylene microcentrifuge tubes that have been swept with nitrogen before filling and closing.

Although maintaining the quality of reagents is the best assurance of satisfactory platelet aggregation results, a further QC measure may include performing aggregation studies on a normal specimen in parallel with the patient specimen. Because of individual variability in platelet aggregation responses and the frequent presence of aspirin or other antiplatelet drugs in either patient or control specimens, the occurrence of abnormal responses should be confirmed by repeat testing in the absence of all medication.

SYNTHETIC SUBSTRATES IN TESTS OF HEMOSTASIS

Basis for Coagulation Assays with Synthetic Substrates

Because the blood coagulation cascade consists of a series of enzymatic reactions catalyzed by serine proteases, the activity of these enzymes may be measured by methods and instrumentation more familiar to clinical chemists. Application of synthetic substrate technology to coagulation (Chap. 53) is presenting new and exciting opportunities to test specific constituents not testable with conventional "global" clotting tests. These constituents include the natural inhibitors, plasminogen, and individual clotting factors. At this time, the principal drawback of the technology is the expense of the reagents and instrumentation. Substrates are not yet available to measure all coagulation constituents directly.

Generally, these assays of enzymatic activity use a synthetic peptide substrate in which the free carboxyl group is blocked by an alcohol or amine leaving group. Enzymatic hydrolysis of the substrate results either in measurable fluorescence changes or in a change in light absorption, either of which may be converted to a quantitative measure of enzyme activity. Figure 62-6 illustrates the spectral change resulting from hydrolysis by thrombin of a tripeptide-p-nitroanilide to yield p-nitroaniline and the tripeptide. The change in molar absorptivity per 1 cm at 405 nm (the wavelength at which the change in absorbance is measured to determine thrombin activity; see Fig. 62-6 for explanation) is 10^4 (*i.e.*, for every mole of substrate hydrolyzed, the absorbance at 405 nm increases by 10,000 for

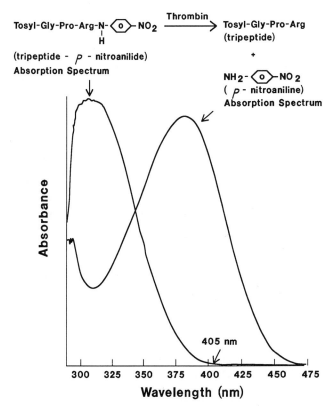

FIG. 62-6. Spectral shift resulting from enzymatic hydrolysis of chromogenic substrate p-nitroanilide by coagulation enzyme thrombin. The spectrum of tripeptide–p-nitroanilide (Tosyl-Gly-Pro-Arg-p-nitroanilide) is shown before enzymatic hydrolysis by thrombin at pH 8.3. Wavelength of maximum absorbance for p-nitroanilide is 316 nm. After enzymatic hydrolysis, maximum absorption of product p-nitroaniline occurs at 381 nm. Note that absorbance by substrate becomes negligible at approximately 405 nm, whereas product has significant absorbance at 405 nm. Thus, by monitoring change in absorbance at 405 nm, thrombin activity may be quantitatively measured with minimal interference from substrate absorbance.

a sample path length of 1 cm). As a result of such a large change in molar absorptivity, assays with this type of substrate are sensitive to low levels of enzyme.

Instrumentation

Improved methods of peptide synthesis have provided substrates with various degrees of specificity for activated coagulation factors. Numerous methods have been developed in which assays of coagulation-related proteins are performed on clinical chemistry analyzers. In general, these analyzers provide automatic addition of a plasma specimen, reagents, and substrate to a reaction cuvette. The extent of substrate hydrolysis is then determined from the change in light absorbance or, in a few cases, a change in fluorescence. Through the use of a calibration curve, a quantitative measure of a particular protein may be obtained.

Coagulation assays using synthetic substrates have been described for a number of centrifugal analyzers (*e.g.*, the CetrifiChem, Cobas-Bio, Flexigem, Gemeni, and Multistat). Numerous automated kinetic analyzers also have been used for chromogenic substrate assays of coagulation proteins. Du Pont has several assays available on the aca instrument, and equipment manufactured by Abbott, Technicon, Gilford, and LKB as well as other manufacturers has been used for chromogenic substrate assays.

In a small laboratory where it is not feasible for an instrument to be dedicated to this type of coagulation testing, it may be well to consider whether the desired assays might be performed on an available clinical chemistry instrument. It is not necessary that the equipment be fully automated, as most of these assays are readily performed on a visible-range spectrophotometer with a temperature-controlled cell compartment and a means of recording the change in light absorbance as a function of time.

The ACL System (Instrumentation Laboratory) and the Protopath (Baxter Dade Division) are two instruments intended for use in coagulation assays with chromogenic or fluorogenic substrates. The ACL System (see Fig. 62-4) is an adaptation of its manufacturer's Multistat System centrifugal analyzer. The ACL System is dedicated to coagulation testing, including both chromogenic substrate assays and tests relying on photo-optical detection of fibrin clot formation. The Protopath is a fluorimeter dedicated to specific coagulation assays, including heparin, antithrombin III, plasminogen, and α_2-antiplasmin. This instrument measures the changes in fluorescence associated with the hydrolysis of a fluorescent group blocking the carboxyl terminus of a synthetic peptide. The accurate measurement of fluorescence requires careful attention to technique to obtain reliable results and may be more suitable for specialized laboratories.

Applications

Of the chromogenic substrate assays available, the most widely accepted are those in which an enzyme inhibitor is determined by the addition of purified enzyme to a plasma specimen or those assays in which a protein not involved in clot formation is determined. These assays include antithrombin III, α_2-antiplasmin, plasminogen, and more recently, plasminogen activators and plasminogen activator inhibitors. Quantitation of heparin and heparinoids (low-molecular-weight heparin) likewise is readily achieved by this type of assay.

Two special considerations arise with respect to coagulation factor assays. First, some coagulation factors, such as factor VIII, do not catalyze a biochemical reaction but are instead cofactors for an enzymatic reaction. Therefore, factor VIII concentration cannot be measured *directly* using chromogenic substrates, and a coupled assay must be used. A coupled assay that is commercially available for factor VIII depends on the hydrolysis of a chromogenic substrate by factor X_a generated in the presence of factor IX_a and the cofactor, factor VIII_a. Second, the serine protease coagulation factors have limited biologic specificities, and the low-molecular-weight synthetic substrates may not allow discrimination among the various enzyme activities. To overcome this difficulty, a coupled assay needs to be designed in which the component of interest acts on its biologic substrate. Specificity may be introduced by using specific activators or inhibitors and by careful selection of substrates and assay conditions to maximize the activity of the enzyme of interest. Because the specificity determinants for low-molecular-weight synthetic substrates are different from those of biologic substrates, it is particularly important that chromogenic substrate assays be carefully selected and interpreted when they are being used to evaluate congenital coagulation factor deficiency states or acquired deficiencies in response to warfarin therapy. Similar considerations pertain to the use of immunologic assays for the detection of deficiency states, as a cross-reactive protein may be present that reacts in the immunologic assay but lacks functional activity.

Many tests of coagulation proteins are now available. In selecting which tests the laboratory should offer, it is important to consider not only the costs for labor and reagents and the availability of required instrumentation, but more significantly, the need for a particular test in making clinical decisions. In general, tests will most frequently be needed to diagnose congenital or acquired deficiency states that may result in excessive bleeding or to monitor factor replacement or anticoagulant therapy.

CHAPTER SUMMARY

Testing in the clinical coagulation laboratory relies heavily on photo-optical instrumentation in which the change in light scattering associated with fibrin clot formation is detected as a decrease in visible light transmission through reaction mixtures containing the test plasma. In selecting instruments for purchase, laboratory needs should be matched with the available instrumentation with consideration for providing adequate backup during instrument failure. Careful and consistent adherence to QC procedures in specimen collection, handling, and processing, as well as in the performance of tests and maintenance of equipment, is essential to obtaining reliable results.

For the PT and PTT, the test results are system dependent, differing with both the instrumentation and the reagents used. Therefore, it is important for each laboratory to establish a population reference range using its own test systems to permit identification of coagulation abnormalities.

For coagulation factor assays, the primary standard is a reference plasma pool obtained from at least 20 donors within 30 to 60 minutes, processed quickly, and frozen. The enzymatic nature of the coagulation pathway makes factor assays sensitive to differences in handling of the factor-deficient plasma, commercial standards, or the reference plasma pool, as well as specimens. As a consequence, large laboratory-to-laboratory variability in results is seen.

As understanding of the biochemical features of the coagulation pathway has increased, enzymatic methods for detecting and quantitating proteins of the coagulation and fibrinolytic pathway have been developed that use synthetic substrates. Although these methods may be particularly valuable additions to the research laboratory, some caution, in terms of both assay specificity and utility for patient management, needs to be exercised in applying these generally costly assays in the clinical laboratory.

CASE STUDY 62-1

An 8-year-old boy was seen in the emergency room for uncontrollable bleeding from a wound to the knee. The parents reported no known bleeding disorder in this child; however, they had heard of relatives who had had "bleeding problems." The clinician ordered a PTT to screen for factor VIII deficiency before deciding on any further, more expensive, testing. The patient's PTT was 32.0 seconds, the control PTT value was 31.5 seconds, the commercial control range for PTTs was 31.0 to 33.0 seconds, and the population reference range established for this laboratory was 22.0 to 29.0 seconds.

1. What bearing do the control range and population reference range have on the interpretation of the patient result?
2. Is there any indication for follow-up testing? If so, what might be recommended?

CASE STUDY 62-2

In the coagulation laboratory, PT and PTT results on controls run at the beginning of the evening shift were within acceptable limits. During the following 2 hours, it was noticed that there were an excessive number of PT and PTT results shorter than the reference range. The short times generally did not occur on the same patient (*i.e.*, if the PT for any patient was short, the PTT for that patient was within the reference range or vice versa). There were occasional discrepancies between duplicates. When specimens with discrepant duplicate results were retested, the results agreed with the longer clotting time of the discrepant pair. A physician called the laboratory requesting to speak with the supervisor because the PTT on a patient receiving heparin was reported as normal, and the physician believed this could not possibly be correct.

1. Is there cause for concern in this situation? Why or why not?
2. Did the controls at the beginning of the shift indicate any problem?
3. Do the erratic, discrepant results indicate any particular problem (*i.e.*, instrument, reagent, or specimen abnormalities)? Why or why not? Must all variables listed in Table 62-1 be reviewed as possible sources of the problem?
4. Should the physician be told that the specimen result is definitely correct because the controls were within acceptable limits prior to running that specimen? If not, what should be done?
5. Should the controls be repeated at this point?
6. Would a check of system precision be useful at this time? If so, how could this be performed? Should control material be used?
7. If the problem is not detected after reviewing all possibilities and erratic results persist, is it necessary to switch to a backup instrument if one is available? Should the manufacturer's technical service be contacted, or should the laboratory continue to investigate the problem on its own?
8. In any situation where a problem is suspected, should the PT and PTT be performed in duplicate until the problem is resolved, even if the laboratory normally uses a single determination for these tests? Why or why not?

REFERENCES

1. Addis T: The pathogenesis of hereditary hemophilia. J Pathol Bacteriol 15:427, 1911

2. Biggs R, Douglas AS: The thromboplastin generation test. J Clin Pathol 6:23, 1953

3. Bock PE, Srinivasan KR, Shore JD: Activation of intrinsic blood coagulation by ellagic acid: Insoluble ellagic acid-metal ion complexes are the activating species. Biochemistry 20:7258, 1981

4. Clauss A: Gerinnungs physiologische schnell Methode zur Bestimmung des Fibrinogens. Acta Haematol 17:237, 1957

5. College of American Pathologists: Comprehensive Coagulation Module 1987 Survey, Set H2-A. Skokie, IL, CAP, 1987

6. Hull R, Hirsh J, Jay R et al: Different intensities of anticoagulation in the long-term treatment of proximal venous thrombosis. N Engl J Med 307:1676, 1982

7. Koepke JA: Coagulation testing systems. In Koepke JA (ed): Laboratory Hematology, vol 2, p 1113. New York, Churchill Livingstone, 1984

8. Koepke JA, Triplett DA: Standardization of the prothrombin time—finally. Arch Pathol Lab Med 109:800, 1985

9. Langdell RD, Wagner RH, Brinkhous KM: Effect of antihemophilic factor on one-stage clotting tests: A presumptive test for hemophilia and a simple one-stage antihemophilic factor assay procedure. J Lab Clin Med 4:637, 1953

10. Loeliger EA, Lewis SM: Progress in laboratory control of oral anticoagulants. Lancet 2:318, 1982

11. Morris MW, Brooker DW, Miller JL et al: Single versus duplicate prothrombin time assays. Lab Med 18:524, 1987

12. National Committee for Clinical Laboratory Standards: Collection, transport, and preparation of blood specimens for coagulation testing and performance of coagulation assays; Approved guidelines. NCCLS Document H21-A. Villanova, PA, NCCLS, 1986

13. Poller L: Progress in standardization in anticoagulation control. Hematol Rev 1:225, 1987

14. Proctor RR, Rapaport SI: The partial thromboplastin time with kaolin: A simple screening test for first stage plasma clotting factor deficiencies. Am J Clin Pathol 36:212, 1961

15. Quick AJ, Stanley-Brown M, Bancroft FW: A study of the coagulation defect in hemophilia and in jaundice. Am J Med Soc 190:501, 1935

16. Triplett DA, VanderSluys C: The importance of establishing the normal population range in coagulation testing. The Texan, Texas J Med Technol 3(4):8, 1986

Part XII

MANAGEMENT

Each day, the hematology supervisor faces a challenge—accomplishing the day's work and making the best possible use of available resources. In many ways, the job is no different from that of a manager in any business undertaking, and the hematology supervisor can gain valuable help from general management texts and guides. However, there are some important differences that make the laboratorian's job more interesting and more challenging.

Laboratory employees differ from the general workforce. They have specific technical training and expert knowledge in various areas, and they expect to use that knowledge. They are part of a complex health care delivery system and have a need to feel involved in patient care. The services they provide have a direct effect on peoples' health and well-being.

The hematology supervisor's job also is different; it requires interaction with other experts in health care. Some of these share an expertise in the area of laboratory hematology; others do not. Supervisors must deal with an increasingly complex regulatory environment. They must balance the conflicting demands of improving service while reducing operating costs. Applying general management techniques to this environment requires adaptation and innovation.

Managers accomplish their tasks using three tools: people, money, and time. This chapter provides a review of ways to use the first two, because they are controlled most easily.

MANAGING PEOPLE

Analyzing the Current Staff

The first step in managing people is to hire the best. However, few supervisors get the chance to build a team from the ground up. They must work instead with a staff that is already in place by surveying the current situation and determining how the staff functions. Next, the supervisor must determine which areas are working well and which need help, and look for the reasons in both cases. Effective performers should be identified so that the supervisor can begin to control the laboratory activities through them and identify a future leadership pool.

The supervisor should be involved in setting the schedules, placing orders, and solving problems but should not displace the people who are doing an effective job. Instead, he or she should help while learning from them. The long-term goal of any supervisor is to build an independent staff that can work toward the goals set by management and the laboratory director.

Delegating Responsibility

Because the supervisor's job is to lead, he or she needs to have a support team for assistance. Members of this team need to have authority and responsibility so that they can learn to handle both. By training the support team, the supervisor becomes a mentor. The best training tool a supervisor has is delegation.

The process of delegating begins with a review of the staff, matching their skills with the jobs to be done. The supervisor should be prepared to help the staff correct mistakes but should resist the temptation to do the job for them. They will do things differently and will work more slowly while they are learning. Giving them new responsibility teaches them to function independently. There must still be control mechanisms to catch errors and to determine when staff members begin to work beyond the bounds of their skills or authority.

Hiring Personnel

Methods

While a supervisor is working with current staff, plans must be developed for replacements and growth. The personnel office can help the supervisor learn the rules and techniques of interviewing and hiring.

A standard hiring protocol should be followed. A list of the tasks associated with the job should be compiled, with a list of the training, experience, and qualities necessary to perform each one. This protocol makes the job of choosing easier, and it helps to avoid problems with regulatory agencies because it ensures that everyone is judged by the same criteria.

The supervisor must also follow the institution's procedures for checking references. Personnel offices usually have guidelines for making reference checks that meet legal requirements. Failure to check references may prove costly. It is easier to avoid hiring a potentially poorly performing employee than to remove one who is already hired.

Identifying Appropriate Skills

Hematology requires people with two seemingly disparate skills: mechanical and analytical. To achieve this, the common characteristics of people with these skills must be identified. Experience or attitudes that show interest and ability to analyze data and solve problems should be sought in potential employees. Good microscopists and instru-

ment technologists must be able to assimilate data from a variety of sources and come to a rational conclusion.

Another predictive factor is the ability to teach. The willingness to learn enough about something to be able to teach it to others is a good predictor of the ability to learn a skill well enough to apply it in daily work.

Developing Training Programs

Hematology technologists work with two kinds of data: objective (numeric data) and subjective (e.g., relative size, color, and granularity of stained cells). Technologists must understand how to turn raw data into valuable information. The leukocyte differential cell count, for example, is an interpreted test in which an enormous amount of data is collected to generate the final results. When the differential cell count is performed manually, technologists must perform this assimilation and analysis rapidly, because the hematology laboratory usually is a high-production operation with a large workload.

Training with Procedure Manuals

A procedure manual is an excellent training tool. It must teach more than stepwise performance of tests, including examples of data interpretation and of errors that may occur. It should also include references such as College of American Pathologists (CAP) and National Committee for Clinical Laboratory Standards (NCCLS) recommended procedures.

Training by the Team Approach

Another effective training method is teaming new employees with experienced technologists who will serve as mentors. New employees can learn to meet the accuracy standards of the laboratory by working with others. Analytical skill and speed come only from experience. New technologists can be placed in critical positions on slower days, with support from their mentors. New employees need the confidence that comes from handling difficult situations successfully.

Continuing Education Programs

Whereas new employees need intensive training, current staff technologists need continuing education and expanded training. The supervisor is responsible for finding the means and time to do both. A regular continuing education (CE) program is a way to ensure that all technologists are using the same criteria for subjective data analysis. Reviewing definitions of cell types, especially through CAP surveys and teaching slide sets, can point out discrepancies and trends that diverge from the preferred definitions and practice.

New ways to provide education must be sought because of the loss of funding for traditional methods, particularly off-site training. Continuing education must be supported by the laboratory and hospital or corporate management.

The best and least expensive source of CE is the staff itself. Case studies from the laboratory's own patient population can be used to review the role of laboratory information in diagnosis and treatment. They also can be used to teach the staff to handle quality assurance, quality control, and management problems. Vendors often are willing to provide demonstrations of new instruments or kits for CE.

Other possible sources of material are CAP teleconferences and videotape presentations from industry sources.

Another technique that helps both the laboratory and the staff is cross-training. If each person is trained to cover several sections, the staff becomes more versatile, and their daily routine can be more varied.

Motivating Personnel

The most difficult part of a supervisor's job is motivating people. It is difficult, not because people do not want to work, but because of misconceptions about the meaning of motivation. Motivation is not trying to excite people about their job. Rather, it is persuading people that the job is worth doing and that they can attain their individual goals through the job. People have a variety of goals in life. Their talents should be matched to assigned tasks whenever possible. The supervisor's job is to find out what each person needs, then show him or her how the job can help meet those needs. Some people respond to having more responsibility, and others like interacting with people. Some need to feel secure in the job, and some respond to money. Few laboratory supervisors can provide frequent salary increases or promotions, but the organization can relate performance to future salary increases and opportunities for promotion. Praising good work and criticizing and correcting work that does not meet standards help employees learn how to perform.

Most important in a job is recognition of a person's value. Telling someone that the job he or she has done, especially a performance that meets expectations, is recognized and appreciated, is a potent motivator. It is neither belittling nor hypocritical to praise average performance. Average, after all, is the level of performance that a person should be able to meet daily. Willie Mays once noted that it is not hard to be great occasionally: the difficult job is being good every day.

MANAGING MONEY

Managing Under DRGs

Laboratories generally are adept at controlling costs. Under the cost reimbursement payment system that was in place in past years, hospitals were paid for every laboratory test performed. The system changed under a new governmental program known as diagnosis-related groups (DRGs). The DRGs are a set of defined diagnoses that Medicare, and now many insurance companies, recognize as valid reasons for reimbursement. Each DRG has a reimbursement figure, which is assumed by the payor to cover all costs related to the patient's hospital stay. The hospital can keep the difference between the DRG payment and the actual cost of care (if there is one) but cannot recover any cost overruns. Under this scheme, the laboratory is no longer a revenue generator. Rather, it has become a cost center, similar to nursing or payroll. Under DRGs, performing more tests than necessary reduces the profit margin available to the hospital.

Reducing Operating Costs

The DRG payment systems are making hospital management look for ways to reduce costs in all departments.

Under current reimbursement schemes, a dollar saved is a dollar earned. There are three general approaches that a laboratory can use to reduce costs: change technology, use less expensive materials, or change management techniques. In hematology, some specific cost-reduction measures are available, as outlined below.

Reducing the Number of Differentials Performed

The most labor-intensive test performed in the hematology laboratory is the differential cell count. The complete blood count (CBC) is widely defined as an instrument cell count combined with a manual differential. Several studies[1,7] have shown that the laboratory can reduce the frequency of this expensive test without reducing the quality of patient care. Changing the ordering habits of physicians requires cooperation between the medical staff and the laboratory director. The laboratory must develop procedures to ensure that those who need the information from a manual differential will have it. For example, the laboratory could supplement the automated differential with a manual film review without specific orders when the sample is from an oncology patient or when the results are above or below defined values. Reducing the number of manual differentials frees technologist time to perform other tests as the workload increases.

Reducing Duplicate Coagulation Testing

Reviewing expenses in the area of coagulation testing can demonstrate opportunities for savings. Duplicate testing is unnecessary for good patient care.[5] Running prothrombin times and partial thromboplastin times as single determinations will result in immediate cost savings. The coagulation laboratory also can act as a consultant for the clinician. Appropriate recommendations concerning the sequence and series of tests needed to investigate a given diagnosis permit the clinician to order diagnostic tests that are likely to yield useful data. By providing such a panel with guidelines for its appropriate use, the laboratory can save the costs of multiple specimen collections and reduce excessive use of controls and reagents. Panels can help to avoid the shotgun approach to diagnosis.

Cost Reduction Through New Technology

New technology may offer a chance to reduce future costs. One example is the use of a screening or partial differential, available on many cell counters. The screening differential is especially useful in outpatient clinics and for patients who need repeat differentials to monitor granulocyte levels, such as oncology patients. One possible cost-saving technique is to perform a screening differential and a film review on all new admissions.[2,4,6] This study establishes a baseline value for the patient. Subsequent orders for differentials may then be met with the screening differential, the results of which can be monitored for significant changes from the baseline values that indicate shifts in the leukocyte population and necessitate a manual review—in other words, a classic differential cell count. This technique can reduce the number of expensive differentials, reducing the per-test cost of operation.

Cost Reduction Through Outpatient Laboratories

Outpatient and satellite laboratories can use smaller, less expensive instruments. Several manufacturers are introducing new analyzers for physician offices. By using these instruments in satellite laboratories, the number of large analyzers in the main laboratory may be reduced. Placing instruments in satellite laboratories also can save the cost of sample transport and result reporting. Quality control (QC) procedures must be devised to ensure that the results in satellite laboratories are comparable to those in the central laboratory; the cost of such a QC program is small compared with the savings in transportation costs and the improvement in services.

Analyzing Costs and Benefits of Existing Equipment versus Replacement

The cost of acquiring capital equipment to replace older technology often prevents a laboratory from instituting new methods. The supervisor must be able to determine the real cost of operating older instrumentation so that upper management can see the benefits of the investment. Older technology often requires more manual labor. Recent federal government figures show that in the cost mix of providing health care, 51.8% is labor and 7.3% is capital, and of that, only 2.4% is equipment.[3] New technology rarely replaces people. However, it does provide a means of reducing the rate of growth of the laboratory staff. It also allows for the shift of employees to new tasks, introduction of new income-producing tests, and improvement of services in labor-intensive sections.

Cost Reduction Through Reducing Length of Patient Hospital Stay

The laboratory's part in reducing health care costs by reducing patient hospital stay requires a staff commitment to providing rapid but reliable service. It must be combined with the support of the pathologist or hematologist directing the laboratory. The director must be involved in the definition of panels that provide the clinician with a suggested sequence and series of tests to investigate a given diagnosis. Appropriate testing algorithms help the physician to make the diagnosis and begin patient treatment more quickly, thereby reducing hospital operating costs by reducing the length of the patient's hospital stay.

Cost Control Through Budgeting

The budgeting process appears to be set in concrete in many organizations, but there are some budget techniques that can make the procedure a useful control measure. Textbooks of management and accounting describe such budgeting techniques.

COMMON PROBLEMS IN HEMATOLOGY LABORATORY MANAGEMENT

Hematology laboratories share certain common management problems. This section will review some of these problems and examine possible solutions.

Staffing for Fluctuating Workloads

A recurring problem is staffing for widely fluctuating workloads. The supervisor must plan for handling loads that vary hourly and daily. Plans must also be in place for periods of staff shortages during vacations, illnesses, and holidays. Centralized laboratories have to deal with large workloads that come simultaneously, resulting in long queues. The linear workflow system (log in, make slides, count cells, etc.) causes turnaround times to degrade during the peak work hours.

There are several tactics that may help to improve turnaround time, spread the work, and improve the total efficiency. First, the supervisor must hire multitalented people who can cover more than one or two work stations. The staff must be trained to be flexible in their assignments. Second, the supervisor can look for ways to incorporate part-time people to help during peak periods. It is possible to hire qualified people who want only part-time work, and such hiring can help to control the size of more expensive full-time staff. Full time people must be made to feel appreciated and motivated to stay, because these people are the foundation of the laboratory, and a loss of one is more critical. Third, the supervisor should reward productivity during peak periods by providing interesting alternatives during off-peak hours. The schedule should provide some slack time for other activities such as CE or developmental projects.

Determining the Most Efficient Laboratory Layout

A busy laboratory is filled with noise, vibration, and other distractions. In hematology, these are critical problems because of the requirement for a quiet, vibration-free area for microscopy. This special need must be considered when designing a hematology laboratory or modifying the layout of an existing one.

A supervisor must analyze the workload in the laboratory and determine the most efficient physical layout. Many laboratories have outgrown their layout but have not made significant changes except for the addition of large analyzers. Bottlenecks or multiple crosspoints should be removed to improve workflow. Using a floor plan, the supervisor can examine the path that specimens and reports take as they move through the laboratory. The goal is to relocate work stations to minimize walking and reduce specimen transport. The analyzer often is the focal point. One may consider placing it in the middle of the room, ringing other stations around it. Stations that share the specimen should be close together. The flow should be arranged so that the final patient report is created in a logical, stepwise manner. If the staff is small or the late-shift staff is limited, all work stations used frequently should be arranged in one area. This is especially useful if the late-shift must cover more than one area. Having the most frequently used stations in an island makes it possible for them to handle the work with minimum travel.

Handling Large Workloads with Parallel Processing

Laboratories that handle large batches of samples at discrete intervals may benefit by handling the workload using the parallel processing technique. First, samples are separated into similar groups (e.g., routine, urgent, and specials). Urgent samples are those that can be processed quickly but are not STAT, such as those that do not require reticulocyte counts or sedimentation rates. These samples can go immediately to the analyzer. If the laboratory is using screening differentials, these samples may not require any further processing.

Routines include those tests that require a film review or tests in addition to an analyzer count. They can be routed to the blood film preparation area first and reach the analyzer after the urgent samples have been completed. Special tests can go to a "specials bench," where the tests can be performed. The samples then can go to the film preparation area or the analyzer after the other samples are complete.

SUPERVISING LABORATORY INSPECTIONS

One event that is often of serious concern, particularly to new supervisors, is the laboratory inspection. Whether the inspectors are from a state or federal agency or from the CAP, there is natural concern over exposing the laboratory's shortcomings. The embarrassment of having these revealed to employees may be even greater than the fear of failure. Both attitudes are mistaken.

The inspection is a valuable chance to have the laboratory reviewed by competent professional consultants who have faced the same problems and found ways to solve them. The first step is a review of the laboratory prior to the inspection to detect variances from required practice. This is a chance to compare the laboratory operation with an objective standard. If the staff finds correctable variances, they can fix them. If they cannot fix them, the supervisor should document the efforts and the results. This is necessary both for the inspection and to send to the director for further action.

During the inspection, the supervisor should ask questions about requirements that were not clear in the inspection guidelines, and find out what the inspectors would suggest to correct a condition, or what they would have accepted as meeting the standard. The CAP inspectors are pathologists and laboratory professionals who come from CAP-approved laboratories. State and federal inspectors may not be laboratory professionals, but they too are interested in correcting deficiencies and improving the laboratory operation.

After inspection, the administration will receive a list of deficiencies. The laboratory will have a chance to refute a finding. If the inspecting agency still feels there are deficiencies, then the laboratory supervisor can send a list of needed corrections to the administration for action. This becomes objective evidence to support requests for improvements, evidence that might not have been available without the inspection.

WORKLOAD MANAGEMENT

Control of the laboratory's workload may seem beyond possibility. However, by taking an active role, the supervisor can affect many of the factors that determine workload. The number of tests ordered, time of day, and types and intensity of patient care are subject to some control.

Past practice may have merged all patients into one workflow, putting STATS at the head of the line, but otherwise making no adjustments. If the laboratory has a large STAT workload, management can consider opening a separate STAT laboratory, even within the hematology laboratory. The physicians might agree to having a longer turnaround time for certain tests. For example, they may accept a WBC and hemoglobin done STAT, with the remaining results following. Screening differentials may replace manual differentials in STATs. An active medical director can influence clinical colleagues positively to make beneficial changes.

If the laboratory serves many outpatients, one may consider separating them from the workload to be run as a group. A separate outpatient laboratory may also be a possibility. Outpatients often have a demand for turnaround time that approaches STAT. The laboratory can hire additional part-time staff for the peak outpatient hours. The in-patients who are having routine repetitive studies done may be able to tolerate slower turnaround. These tests can be moved to the end of the run.

When looking at the in-patient workload, a supervisor has to consider the level of care that the hospital provides. For example, the impact of transplant technology on the hematology laboratory is tremendous. The coagulation problems are complex. The surgical staff requests frequent and rapid platelet counts and acts on small changes that strain the precision of the analyzer. The supervisor must develop methods to handle these demands.

COMPUTERS IN LABORATORY MANAGEMENT

Computers have become a valuable asset to the hematology supervisor in the daily operation and control of a busy laboratory. Several vendors of quality control (QC) products provide personal computers and software to support their QC programs. These computers can be used to support management functions when they are not being used for QC.

Laboratory and Hospital Information Systems

Mainframe Computer Applications

Laboratories generally have access to two types of computers: mainframe and personal. The mainframe system is a fully implemented laboratory information system (LIS) that may provide some of the following applications: order entry by patient care units, work lists for the laboratory and phlebotomy staff, data entry (manual or direct from the analyzer), and on-line result reporting. It may also collect statistics on workload, handle QC data collection and plotting, and provide billing information. The LIS may be tied to the hospital information system (HIS), which contains nonlaboratory patient data.

Supervisors may use the daily workload figures to watch trends and plan staffing. The ability to monitor daily trends allows supervisors to use part-time people more effectively. Work lists allow monitoring workload stations, even planning for variations in the coming hours by looking to see what orders are still pending. On-line QC data give management or the QC technologist immediate information on instrument performance. If the LIS or HIS handle billing, management can get accurate revenue data by service, dates, types of patients, and even individual physicians.

This information helps in planning budgets and predicting levels of service that the laboratory will need to provide.

Personal Computer Applications

The LIS-based systems usually do not give the supervisor a way to manipulate data; rather, the information comes in predesigned printed reports. However, a laboratory system that includes personal computers (PCs) provides the opportunity to analyze data in a variety of ways. If the data can be obtained from the mainframe system ("downloaded," in the language of computer systems), the supervisor can view it and manipulate it using a PC to print ad hoc reports. Once the data are available, the supervisor has a powerful tool for analyzing laboratory performance.

Personal computers are valuable tools in QC. If the laboratory has several sites performing hematology tests, the QC technologist may want to implement an interlaboratory QC program. Patient samples can be split and run on each analyzer. The data can then be entered in a program that performs the necessary calculations to see if each instrument meets expected performance limits. This is an effective tool for immediate QC in a multi-instrument system.

There are programs supplied by vendors of QC materials that test the QC data against a selection of Westgard's rules and plot the results on the screen. The technologist can see immediately if the run is acceptable. This is an improvement over the time-consuming process of manually plotting QC data, then finding patterns that indicate problems *after* patient data have been released.

The laboratory budget is one of the first management jobs to be tackled on a PC. By using a spreadsheet program, supervisors can test the effects of proposed expenditures, program changes, and inflation factors on the laboratory.

The PC also is useful for instrument evaluation. There are statistical programs that will, for example, help the staff analyze method comparison data, calculate linear regression, and identify outliers (Chap. 46). The ease of data handling makes it feasible to compare several methods before making a selection and easier to follow NCCLS recommendations for method evaluation. Reference range studies for the laboratory's own patient population can be performed on a PC.

CHAPTER SUMMARY

The supervisor of the hematology laboratory has to balance two demanding jobs: being a technical expert in hematology and being a skilled manager of a professional staff. Despite the temptation to try to be both all the time, the supervisor has to give most of his or her attention to managing people. A supervisor must lean on the technical skill of the technologists. Supervisors need to use their technical knowledge instead to identify laboratory problems. However, the implementation of solutions and the prevention of problems must come from the full staff. Supervisors must become skilled in coordinating the efforts of their staffs. It will require all the talent available to deal with the challenges of new tests, DRGs, and ever-increasing demands for service on ever-tighter budgets. The supervisors' rewards will be in knowing that they make a positive difference in the laboratory and in the quality of patient care.

REFERENCES

1. Brecher G, Anderson RE, McMullen PD: When to do diffs: How often should differential counts be reported? In Ross DW, Brecher G, Bessis M (eds): Automation in Hematology: What to Measure and Why? p 263. Berlin, Springer International, 1981
2. Dutcher TF: Automated differentials: A strategy. Blood Cells 11:49, 1985
3. Health Care Financing Administration (HCFA): Changes to the inpatient hospital prospective payment system and fiscal year 1987 rates: Proposed rule. Fed Reg 51:19, 986, June 3, 1986
4. Koepke JA, Dotson MA, Shifman MA et al: A flagging system for multichannel hematology analyzers. Blood Cells 11:113, 1985
5. Koepke JA: Coagulation testing systems. In Koepke JA (ed): Laboratory Hematology, p 1113. New York, Churchill Livingstone, 1984
6. Korpman RA, Bull B: Whither the WBC differential? Some alternatives. In Ross DW, Brecher G, Bessis M (eds): Automation in Hematology: What to Measure and Why? p 253. Berlin, Springer International, 1981
7. Rich EC, Crowson TW, Connelly DP: Effectiveness of differential leukocyte count in case finding in the ambulatory care setting. JAMA 249:633, 1983

SUGGESTED READING

Barbieri LA: Choosing a personal computer for your laboratory. J Med Technol 2:643, 1985

Berman HJ, Weeks LE: Operational planning. In The Financial Management of Hospitals, 5th ed, p 457. Ann Arbor, Hospital Administration Press, 1982

Cannon WG: Lab budgeting and cost accounting under DRGs. Med Lab Observer 17(2):47, 1985

Griswold DJ, Champagne VD: Evaluation of Coulter S-Plus IV three-part differential in an acute care hospital. Am J Clin Pathol 84:49, 1985

Hershey P, Blanchard KH: Life cycle theory and leadership. In Richards MD, Neilander WA (eds): Readings in Management, 4th ed, p 476. Cincinnati, South-Western Publishing, 1974

Koepke JA, Dotson MA, Shifman MA et al: Streamlining blood counts with a microcomputer. Med Lab Observ 16(11):53, 1985

Mayer K: Presence of abnormal cells. Blood Cells 11:25, 1985

Morris MW, Martin BG, Winkelman JW: Modifications for expense reduction. 2: Hematology. Lab Med 15: 670, 1984

Pierre RV: The routine differential leukocyte count vs automated differential counts. Blood Cells 11:11, 1985

Ross DW, Watson JS, Davis PH et al: Evaluation of Coulter three-part differential screen. Am J Clin Pathol 84:481, 1985

Rue LW: Breaking the delegation barrier. Lab Med 18:173, 1987

Sharp JW: A DRG survival plan for the laboratory budget. Med Lab Observ 16(7):38, 1984

Special report: Microcomputers in the lab. Med Lab Observ 16(5):May, 1984

Yapit MK: An in-house proficiency survey for WBC differentials. Med Lab Observ 16(11):77, 1984

Appendices

APPENDIX A   ANSWERS TO CASE STUDIES

CHAPTER 9
CASE STUDY 9-1

1. The discrepancy in these results relates to the Rule of Three, which states that $3 \times Hb = HCT \pm 3$. In this sample, $3 \times 15 = 45$, which is not equal to 36 ± 3.
2. The four possible sources of this discrepancy are an elevated leukocyte count, a lipemic specimen, abnormal globulins in the specimen, or Hbs S or C.
3. To correct for an elevated leukocyte count, centrifuge the Hb mixture and determine Hb on the supernatant fluid; to correct for lipemia, add 0.02 mL of patient plasma to 5.0 mL of the cyanmethemoglobin reagent and use this as the patient blank. Abnormal globulins should not be a problem with modified Drabkin's reagent. If using the original Drabkin's, correct for globulin presence by adding 0.1 g of potassium carbonate to 1 L of Drabkin's before use to keep the globulins in solution. If Hb S or Hb C is present, correct for the cells' resistance to hemolysis by diluting the specimen 1:1 with distilled water and multiplying the result by 2.

CASE STUDY 9-2

1. No. The Hb and HCT are not normal for an adult female, because normally, the Hb does not exceed approximately 16.0 g/dL and the HCT does not exceed 0.46 L/L. These values are "falsely" elevated in this case by the extreme dehydration (fluid loss) associated with the burn.
2. The Hb and HCT are technically accurate and comply with the Rule of Three. However, there is a physiologic error inherent here, because this is a burn victim. Burn victims normally lose a significant amount of fluid at the burn sites, causing plasma volume to drop. This causes the temporary appearance of a high Hb and HCT. When fluids lost because of the burn are replaced in treatment, the Hb and HCT will fall sharply. In addition, erythrocytes damaged by the heat are expected to lyse, causing an even further decrease in the Hb and HCT (see Chap. 18).

CASE STUDY 9-3

Two possible explanations for the Hbs being lower than expected compared with the HCTs are:

1. Adequate time may not have been allowed for conversion of the Hb to cyanmethemoglobin, causing the Hb to be falsely decreased.
2. The technologist may not have centrifuged the HCT specimens long enough to achieve maximum packing time, thus causing falsely increased values.

CASE STUDY 9-4

Setting the rack of sedimentation rate tubes on top of the refrigerator could lead to the following:

1. A falsely decreased ESR because of lower temperatures from air rushing out on opening the refrigerator or freezer;
2. A falsely increased ESR attributable to vibrations from opening and closing the refrigerator and freezer doors; or
3. A falsely increased ESR because of heat released from the refrigerator motor.

CASE STUDY 9-5

A technologist could consistently read HCTs higher than coworkers because of the following:

1. Incorrect reading of the HCT scale on the reader wheel;
2. Incorrect use of the reader wheel; or
3. Including buffy coats in the HCT reading when the leukocyte count is elevated.

CASE STUDY 9-6

1. The RBC, Hb, and HCT are all suspect in this case, because they do not meet the criteria of the Rule of Three.
2. The most likely reason for the abnormal results is the markedly elevated leukocyte count.
3. Because the abnormality seems to relate to the elevated leukocyte count, one should investigate whether the Hb was erroneously determined before or correctly determined after centrifugation of the mixture to remove the leukocytes. For the HCT, it should be verified that the buffy coat was not included. Any procedural errors should be corrected and the results rechecked, which will most likely remove the discrepancies. The RBC count probably is correct, because this value would be unaffected by a leukocyte count at this level.

CHAPTER 11
CASE STUDY 11-1

1. Aplastic anemia is the most likely diagnosis, based on the hypocellular bone marrow with mostly fat cells and the biopsy demonstrating less than 5% cellularity. The marrows in acute leukemia, megaloblastic anemia, and most myelodysplastic syndromes are hypercellular. The diagnosis cannot be Fanconi anemia, because the disorder appeared at age 25 in this man.
2. Bone marrow transplantation is the preferred method of treatment for aplastic anemia if a suitable donor can be found.

3. The marrow aspirate results are NOT sufficient to make the diagnosis. A marrow biopsy is critical to verify aplastic anemia, as sampling error may give the impression of a hypoplastic marrow by aspirate alone.
4. Helpful questions about the patient's history would include inquiry concerning his possible exposure to chemicals, drugs (both prescribed and over-the-counter), and radiation. Inquiry concerning recent infections, particularly viral (e.g., viral hepatitis), should also be made.
5. To support an immune etiology for this disorder, a response to antithymocyte globulin with improving peripheral blood cell counts would be expected. Because this patient did not respond, an immune etiology is unlikely; however, it cannot be ruled out entirely.

CASE STUDY 11-2

1. The most likely diagnosis is Fanconi anemia, because the onset of symptoms was at age 10, and cytogenetic abnormalities were found.
2. Fanconi anemia is believed to be an autosomal recessive disorder.
3. Other body systems expected to be abnormal include renal, skeletal, brain, genital, and skin.
4. Prognosis with Fanconi anemia is poor, with most patients not surviving many years after the onset of hematologic abnormalities. Progression to acute leukemia is common and believed to be related to the multiple chromosomal abnormalities in these patients.

CHAPTER 12
CASE STUDY 12-1

1. Several of the blood count results are abnormal. The RBC, Hb, and HCT values are all decreased; the MCV and MCH are elevated. They indicate macrocytic anemia, the cause of which must be sought through additional tests, patient history, and physical examination. The increased MCH value is common in megaloblastic anemia.
2. Serum B_{12} is markedly decreased since the approximate reference range is 140 to 700 ng/L. Serum folate is within the approximate reference range of 3 to 16 μg/L.
3. Yes. The Schilling test is appropriate in this case to try to identify the cause of the vitamin B_{12} deficiency. The test results after administration of B_{12} alone indicate that the patient is not absorbing B_{12}, since the 24-hour urine ^{57}Co B_{12} is less than 7%. After administration of B_{12} with IF the test results indicate correction of the B_{12} absorption problem. Figure 12-6 shows the possible causes of the malabsorption, including pernicious anemia, inert IF, gastric resection, and ingestion of corrosives.
4. Yes. There is a possible relation between the patient's diabetes mellitus and his anemia. This is suggested by research that has shown that autoimmune disorders, including diabetes, occur with greater frequency among patients with PA than among people in the "normal" population.

5. IF-blocking antibodies bind with IF and block its vitamin B_{12} binding site, rendering IF unable to bind and protect B_{12} during its transit through the GI tract. The positive result of the IF-blocking antibodies text indicates a strong possibility that the patient has pernicious anemia, since it is the immunologic test of choice for diagnosis of PA.
6. No. Macroovalocytes and hypersegmentation of the nucleus of neutrophils do not differentiate between vitamin B_{12} and folate deficiency. Together they indicate the possibility of a megaloblastic anemia, but they do not allow identification of the specific cause. This morphology is not specific for megaloblastic anemia; nuclear hypersegmentation of neutrophils and macroovalocytes can also be found in the myelodysplastic syndromes. To be considered hypersegmented a neutrophil should have at least five nuclear lobes.
7. The most likely diagnosis is pernicious anemia, based on the decreased serum B_{12} value, positive IF-blocking antibodies, Schilling test results, increased MCV, macroovalocytes, hypersegmentation, and the patient's age and diabetic condition.

CHAPTER 13
CASE STUDY 13-1

1. From the patient's history, nutritional anemia might be expected. Because iron deficiency anemia is the most common form of anemia and occurs with high frequency in premenopausal women, it is the most likely cause for anemia in this case.
2. The CBC shows that the patient has microcytic (MCV 70 fL), hypochromic (MCHC 31.2 g/dL) erythrocytes. Morphologically, there is significant anisocytosis and poikilocytosis with hypochromia. These features rule out certain nutritional deficiencies that typically produce macrocytosis (e.g., folate deficiency) and further suggest iron deficiency anemia.
3. Yes, the chemistry findings do confirm the suspected diagnosis. The absence of ferritin indicates that iron stores are totally depleted. Serum iron is also extremely low, as is transferrin saturation. These features are indicative of iron deficiency.
4. The patient is expected to show a significant reticulocyte response to a therapeutic trial of iron. If reticulocytosis does not occur within 2 weeks of the beginning of therapy, the iron should be discontinued, and the patient should be reevaluated.
5. Most likely, a sound diagnosis of iron deficiency could have been made on the basis of the CBC results and the serum ferritin alone. If the diagnosis were incorrect, this would become obvious if the patient did not respond to iron therapy with an increase in her reticulocyte count within 1 to 2 weeks.
6. On initial diagnosis, a bone marrow examination is not appropriate, because the laboratory tests and patient history point to the most common type of anemia, iron deficiency, for which treatment is simple and patient response easily monitored without a bone marrow examination.

CHAPTER 14
CASE STUDY 14-1

1. The most probable diagnosis is sickle cell disease, owing to (1) the severity of the anemia, (2) the recurring chronic ulcers in the lower tibial region, and (3) the elongated red cells and target cells on the peripheral blood film.
2. To verify the diagnosis, a sickle solubility test (dithionite tube test) should be performed first as a quick method of screening for Hb S before further laboratory testing decisions are made.
3. If the sickle solubility screening test is positive, cellulose acetate hemoglobin electrophoresis (pH 8.4) should be performed next to confirm Hb S. If Hb S is present, it will migrate between Hb A_2 and Hb F (see Fig. 14-4).
4. The elevated leukocyte count is indicative of an infection, as is the fever. The most common infections associated with Hb S disease are pneumonia and *Salmonella*.

CASE STUDY 14-2

1. The first laboratory procedure performed should be the sickle solubility tube test as a screening measure. For Hb S, the results should be positive.
2. The hemoglobins that could be indicated on cellulose acetate electrophoresis include Hb S, Hb D, Hb C, Hb C-Harlem, Hb E, and Hb O-Arab.
3. To confirm the diagnosis in this case and determine exactly which hemoglobins are present on cellulose acetate, citrate agar electrophoresis at acid pH should be performed. Hb C would migrate farthest toward the anode, with Hb S behind it. Hb C-Harlem would migrate in the same position as Hb S. Hb E would migrate in the same position as Hb A (which migrates slowly toward the cathode), whereas Hb O-Arab would migrate just slightly behind the Hb A position toward the cathode (see Fig. 14-4).

CASE STUDY 14-3

1. The abnormalities shown by electrophoresis are due to the decreased percentage of Hb A and the presence of Hb S. Alkali denaturation indicates an increase in Hb F (for adults normal is less than 2%), and microchromatography indicates an increase in Hb A_2 (normal is 2.5% to 3.5%).
2. For the hemoglobinopathies listed, increased levels of Hb F are associated with sickle cell disease and Hb S–thalassemia, while increased A_2 usually occurs only in Hb S–thalassemia.
3. Based on the rationale in answer 2, the most likely diagnosis is Hb S–β^+ thalassemia. β^+ thalassemia is indicated by the presence of some Hb A, which requires some production of β chains.
4. The MCV of 84 fL and the severe anemia are not generally consistent with a diagnosis of Hb S–β^+ thalassemia. This disorder usually causes a decreased MCV, whereas 84 fL is within the reference range for adults.
5. If no Hb A had been found on cellulose acetate electrophoresis of this patient's specimen while hemoglobins S,

F, and A_2 were increased, the most likely diagnosis would be Hb S–β° thalassemia. In β° thalassemia, no Hb A is produced because no β chains are produced.

CHAPTER 15
CASE STUDY 15-1

1. Heterozygous β thalassemia. The increased RBC count, Hb F, and Hb A_2, the decreased MCV and MCH, and the borderline-normal packed cell volume suggest heterozygous β thalassemia. The increased Hb A_2 and Hb F exclude α thalassemia. The lack of clinical findings in this 22-year-old patient exclude β thalassemia major, and most likely thalassemia intermedia, since there is essentially no anemia. Silent thalassemia is excluded because hemoglobin electrophoresis is normal in this condition, but this patient's electrophoresis pattern is slightly abnormal.
2. The blood film evaluation for red cell morphology was expected to and did show the following: microcytosis, slight hypochromia, slight poikilocytosis, and basophilic stippling.
3. Heterozygous β thalassemia usually is not associated with any clinical disability in men, therefore, treatment is not necessary.
4. Affected persons have a normal life span.
5. The thalassemias follow simple Mendelian segregation. Assuming, for example, that both parents had the heterozygous genotype β/β°, possible outcomes for offspring are: 25% chance of being homozygous β thalassemia (β°/β°); 50% chance of being heterozygous for β thalassemia (β/β° or β°/β); and 25% chance of being normal (β/β).

		Mother	
		β°	β
Father	β°	β°/β°	β°/β
	β	β/β°	β/β

CASE STUDY 15-2

1. A hemoglobinopathy or thalassemia would be likely in this case because the disorder appears to be hereditary and these abnormalities are common in Southeast Asians. Hemoglobin electrophoresis at alkaline pH on cellulose acetate is a reasonable test to perform, since this is an initial screening procedure that can be helpful in identifying many of the hemoglobinopathies and thalassemias.
2. Alpha thalassemia in Southeast Asians may be associated with a one– (-α/$\alpha\alpha$), two– (--/$\alpha\alpha$ or -α/-α), three– (--/-α), or four– (--/--) α gene deletion. The four-gene deletion, Barts hydrops fetalis, is ruled out since the patient is 17 years old. Little or no anemia is associated with one– and two– α gene deletions. Most likely, this

patient has Hb H disease ($--/-\alpha$), since her anemia is moderate.

3. Because the mother has mild anemia, her genotype is most likely heterozygous α° thalassemia ($--/\alpha\alpha$). The father is not anemic, but the daughter is believed to have Hb H disease ($--/-\alpha$), so he may be heterozygous ($-\alpha/\alpha\alpha$) for α^+ thalassemia.

4. If this patient does in fact have Hb H disease, Hb H (2 to 40%) should appear on cellulose acetate electrophoresis (alkaline pH) along with Hb A and decreased A_2. A trace amount of Hb Barts might also be seen.

CHAPTER 16
CASE STUDY 16-1

1. The normal MCV represents the average cell volume of a mixture of small and large erythrocytes as seen on the blood film. Therefore, the RDW would be increased. The reticulocyte count should be elevated if the patient's bone marrow is able to respond to the anemia. The presence of moderate polychromasia suggests that the reticulocyte count is elevated.

2. The presence of schistocytes, microspherocytes, and echinocytes suggests hemolysis due to mechanical damage. This patient's anemia was due to both erythrocyte destruction by the prosthesis and blood loss in the lungs.

3. Red cell fragmentation due to prosthetic valves can occur in the immediate postoperative period as a result of poor valve design or placement. Later, if the valve becomes infected, local clotting may occur. Deposition of fibrin strands in the area injures red cells as they pass through the vessels. Also the infection and clotting may cause the valve to function poorly, forcing red cells to pass through an irregular opening with more turbulence than is normal in the heart.

4. The prolonged PT and PTT, along with the decreased platelet count and the abnormal red cell morphology, suggest intravascular coagulation, though it may be local rather than disseminated in this case (Chap. 55). The presence of fibrin split products or decreased fibrinogen would support the diagnosis, although the patient's liver disease may affect the reliability of those results. Chemistry laboratory results would probably show increased serum unconjugated bilirubin and LD and decreased serum haptoglobin. Urinalysis would probably reveal increased urobilinogen.

CHAPTER 17
CASE STUDY 17-1

1. The most likely diagnosis is hereditary spherocytosis. The peripheral blood film and other laboratory data indicate a spherocytic hemolytic anemia and a positive family history indicates a familial disorder.

2. An osmotic fragility test is necessary for diagnosis, and results should reveal increased susceptibility of the patient's red cells to osmotic lysis.

3. The patient is suffering from aplastic crisis. The viral infection associated with influenza has temporarily halted erythropoiesis while hemolysis continues.

4. The patient's mother and brother most likely suffer from the same disorder. Both should have increased numbers of microspherocytes on the peripheral blood film with mild anemia. Although it would be costly and probably unnecessary to check, both most likely have an increased erythrocyte osmotic fragility.

CASE STUDY 17-2

1. The ascorbate-cyanide test is positive as the brown color indicates that methemoglobin formed due to G6PD deficiency in the patient's specimen. This test is less specific but more sensitive than the G6PD fluorescent spot test. On the contrary, the fluorescent spot test probably indicates a normal G6PD due to the suspected hemolytic episode. Hemolytic episodes cause increased levels of reticulocytes and some younger cells in the circulation, which temporarily may elevate G6PD levels to the normal range in G6PD deficient individuals.

2. The fluorescent spot test can be repeated using a centrifuged specimen from which the top portion of the erythrocyte population, which contains reticulocytes, has been removed. This procedure lessens the effect of higher levels of G6PD in reticulocytes and younger red cells and would be expected to yield no fluorescence in the G6PD fluorescent spot test, indicating a G6PD deficiency.

3. The RPI calculation is:

$$\frac{22 \times \dfrac{0.19}{0.45}}{2.5} = 3.7$$

Since the general rule for adequate response to anemia is >3.0 (Chap. 10), it appears that the bone marrow in this case is mounting a good erythropoietic response to anemia.

CHAPTER 18
CASE STUDY 18-1

1. Without laboratory data, there are probably many possible diagnoses. "Kidney trouble" could indicate several kidney disorders. Ecchymoses, pallor, listlessness, and pale mucous membranes indicate a bleeding disorder and some degree of anemia that requires laboratory tests. Fever, sore throat, and palpable cervical nodes indicate an infection, which also can be identified only through laboratory tests.

2. The CBC and RBC morphology in part support the diagnosis of hemolytic uremic syndrome (HUS) owing to the fact that anemia is present, and the burr cells are particularly diagnostic in this case. These factors, together with the boy's age and the infectious process, led to the initial diagnosis of HUS, and further laboratory tests were ordered to corroborate this.

3. To confirm the diagnosis of HUS, urinalysis, and measurements of blood urea nitrogen, creatinine, bilirubin, and electrolytes should be performed.
4. If HUS is the correct diagnosis, prognosis is good if the renal damage can be arrested.
5. The finding of β-hemolytic *S. pyogenes* in the throat culture does relate to the HUS condition. Often in HUS there is an inciting event such as infection or trauma, which may have been the case for this child. Treating the infection might go a long way toward correcting both the renal damage and the hemolytic process.
6. The variable red cell morphology may be due to a combination of hemolysis due to the HUS and incipient iron deficiency, both of which could produce the population of microcytic cells and the slight hypochromia. Iron deficiency may be due to inadequate dietary intake, since the child's appetite has been poor and he is at an age when iron requirements are increased because of growth.

CHAPTER 19
CASE STUDY 19-1

1. Yes. The hemoglobin and hematocrit match according to the Rule of Three, since the hemoglobin is 8.0 g/dL and 3 × 8.0 = 24.0. By definition, the hematocrit must fall within 24 ±3%, which it does at 22% or 0.22 L/L.
2. Red urine can be caused by some drugs, some dyes (e.g., phenolsulfonphthalein), and congenital erythropoietic porphyria. Red urine also may be caused by hemoglobin, red cells, or myoglobin (muscle hemoglobin).
3. Since ingestion of drugs or other toxic material was denied, hemoglobinopathy, red cell metabolic deficiency, hemolytic anemia, or PNH should be considered.
4. Additional tests that could be diagnostically helpful include urinalysis with microscopic, DAT and antibody identification if result of DAT is positive, bilirubin, Donath-Landsteiner test, and haptoglobin. In this case study, urinalysis revealed the presence of hemoglobin; the result of the DAT was positive, with polyspecific sera and with anticomplement sera. The blood film review showed some rouleaux. The haptoglobin value was decreased. Results of the Donath-Landsteiner test were positive; the antibody showed anti-P specificity.
5. Reticulocyte counts began to rise significantly within a week, as expected in response to the hemolytic episode. The boy's problem was diagnosed as paroxysmal cold hemoglobinuria; the hemolytic episode was apparently precipitated by the previous viral infection and exposure to cold. This hemoglobinuria is self-limited, and the boy recovered spontaneously.

CASE STUDY 19-2

1. No. The hemoglobin and hematocrit values do not match according to the Rule of Three, since the hemoglobin is 13.5 g/dL and 3 × 13.5 = 40.5. By definition in this case, the hematocrit must fall within 40.5 ±3%, which, at 36% or 0.36 L/L, it does not. The technologist should not expect the hemoglobin and hematocrit values to match, since the indices indicate macrocytic and hyperchromic cells, whereas the Rule of Three applies only to normal cells.
2. All indices are above the usual reference range, and the MCH is particularly suspicious because it is grossly abnormal.
3. After the technologist reviewed these results, the sample was inspected and was seen to contain some small clumps of red cells. The patient, indeed, had a significant amount of cold agglutinins. At room temperature, the sample red cells began to clump producing the erroneous low red count and elevated MCV (each clump is seen as one large cell by the automated cell counter). The automated hematocrit value appears lower than it should be and should therefore be performed again using the microhematocrit method. The MCH and MCHC values are also abnormal owing to the agglutinating cells. The hemoglobin is correct, since all cells, single or clumped, are hemolyzed in the procedure, and the leukocyte count is also unaffected.
4. The specimen should be warmed to 37°C for at least 15 minutes, mixed while warm, and sampled immediately in order to produce reliable results in these cases.

CHAPTER 20
CASE STUDY 20-1

1. Iron deficiency anemia is the most common of all microcytic, hypochromic anemias. The slightly elevated RDW corroborates the possible diagnosis of iron deficiency, although alone it is not specific for iron deficiency.
2. Gastrointestinal bleeding is the most likely cause of anemia in a 40-year-old man who is not complaining of ill health.
3. An analysis of stool for occult blood would quickly confirm a diagnosis of gastrointestinal bleeding.

CHAPTER 25

EXERCISES

1. $(250 + 265)/2 = 257.5 = $ Average no. cells counted

$$\frac{257.5 \times 2.0}{4 \times 0.1} \times 10^6/L = 12.9 \times 10^9/L$$

2. A. Based on the peripheral blood findings, the leukocyte count estimate is $(70 \times 1.5 \times 10^9/L) = 105.0 \times 10^9/L$.
   B. Based on Table 24-1, a 1:200 dilution should be made for manual WBC counting. An RBC Thoma pipet should be used.
   C. $(170 + 184)/2 = 177 = $ Average no. cells counted

$$\frac{177 \times 200}{4 \times 0.1} \times 10^6/L = 88.5 \times 10^9/L$$

3. Yes, all differential counts that reveal more than five nucleated RBCs per 100 leukocytes indicate the need for a leukocyte count correction.

$$\frac{20.0 \times 10^9/L \times 100}{20 + 100} = 16.7 \times 10^9/L$$

4 A. $\dfrac{194 \times 10}{4 \times 0.1} \times 10^6 = 4.9 \times 10^9/L$

   B. $\dfrac{383 \times 20}{4 \times 0.1} \times 10^6 = 19.2 \times 10^9/L$

   C. $\dfrac{273 \times 10}{8 \times 0.1} \times 10^6 = 3.4 \times 10^9/L$

   D. $\dfrac{207 \times 200}{8 \times 0.1} \times 10^6 = 51.8 \times 10^9/L$

   E. $\dfrac{50 \times 32}{40 \times 0.2} \times 10^6 = 0.2 \times 10^9/L$

5. $\dfrac{40 \times 32}{6.4} \times 10^6 = 160 \times 10^6/L = 0.2 \times 10^9/L$

6. $(0.08 \times 8.4 \times 10^9/L) = 0.7 \times 10^9/L$. This result is *not* within the usual reference range: it indicates eosinophilia.

CASE STUDY 25-1

1. No. Tech number 3's results do not fall within the 95% confidence limits. According to Table 25-7, the 95% confidence limits for a 100-cell differential count for the observed automated value of 10% should be 4% to 18% monocytes. All other technologists' results are within the expected range.

CHAPTER 26
CASE STUDY 26-1

1. The findings that are compatible with CML include the markedly increased white cell count, severe left shift, including blast forms and the presence of nucleated red cells, which might indicate marrow replacement by leukemia cells. The findings that are unusual for CML are the lack of increased eosinophils and basophils and the lack of circulating immature forms of eosinophils and basophils.

   Note: the toxic morphology is not helpful, since patients with CML and a superimposed infection and those receiving chemotherapy may exhibit toxic morphology, such as toxic granulation, in their neutrophils.
2. The toxic granulation is most likely real for two reasons: (1) only 60% of neutrophils are affected and (2) the presence of Döhle bodies supports the toxic morphology.
3. There is an absolute monocytosis. Two percent multiplied by the total leukocyte count equals increased numbers per liter.
4. An NAP of 316 is increased and indicates reactive rather than malignant leukocytosis. Further investigation revealed that this patient had a brain abcess; the infection was subsequently controlled with antibiotics. It should be noted that occasionally a patient with CML may experience bacterial infection or another stressful condition that causes the normal granulocytes to react with an increased amount of alkaline phosphatase. For example, a patient with CML and an NAP score of 2 contracted a bacterial infection. The patient's NAP score rose to 98, which is within the normal range.

CHAPTER 27
CASE STUDY 27-1

1. Probable diagnosis: sepsis, possible toxic shock syndrome. Cause of thrombocytopenia could be bone marrow depression, or possibly peripheral destruction of platelets. Cause of the leftward shift, a toxic reaction to foreign antigens.
2. A viral infection, possibly CMV acquired through the transfusions. Confirmation: CMV antibody titers and heterophil antibody test.

CHAPTER 28
CASE STUDY 28-1

1. Both red cells and platelets were being sequestered and possibly destroyed by the enlarged spleen.
2. Thrombocytopenia, abnormal platelet function, and liver dysfunction all could have contributed to the bleeding problem.
3. The increased bilirubin, increased liver enzymes, and the prolonged prothrombin time reflect liver dysfunction.

CHAPTER 31
CASE STUDY 31-1

1. The CSF cell count reference range for a 5-week-old infant is WBC $0–30 \times 10^6/L$ and RBC $0 \times 10^6/L$. Therefore, the WBC count is normal, but the RBC count is markedly elevated.
2. No, the data are not sufficient to determine whether there was a traumatic tap or actual CNS disease. The peripheral blood RBC count is needed but not available here.
3. The peripheral blood RBC count must be obtained. In this patient, it was $2.5 \times 10^{12}/L$, which must be translated for comparison with WBCs (reported in units of $10^9/L$): $2500 \times 10^9/L$.
4. The RBC:WBC ratio in the peripheral blood must be compared with that in the CSF. If these two ratios are approximately the same or the ratio is higher in the CSF, it cannot be determined whether the patient actually has CNS disease, because a traumatic lumbar puncture has occurred. In this case study, the RBC:WBC ratios in the peripheral blood and CSF are calculated as follows:

   Peripheral blood:

$$\frac{RBC}{WBC} = \frac{2500 \times 10^9/L}{283 \times 10^9/L} = 8.8$$

   Cerebrospinal fluid:

$$\frac{RBC}{WBC} = \frac{5180 \times 10^6/L}{2 \times 10^6/L} = 2590$$

Because the ratio in the CSF is much higher than that in the peripheral blood, a traumatic lumbar puncture did occur in this patient, and CNS disease cannot be diagnosed using this specimen.

5. Yes. Acute lymphocytic leukemia is the most common leukemia to infiltrate the CNS.

CASE STUDY 31-2

1. No. The normal cell count does not rule out CNS infection.
2. Yes. The cytocentrifuge will concentrate the organisms so more are available for observation.
3. The organism will stain with Wright stain, but the capsule will not.
4. Other tests to assist in the diagnosis include fungal stains and cultures and the India ink preparation.

CHAPTER 33
CASE STUDY 33-1

1. A dysmyelopoietic disorder seems likely in this case because of the two cytopenias (red cells and leukocytes), the macrocytic red cell population with a dimorphic picture, and the marrow evidence of both dyserythropoiesis (megaloblastoid morphology and ringed sideroblasts) as well as dysmegakaryopoiesis (round nuclei).
2. This patient was most likely classified as refractory anemia with ringed sideroblasts (RARS) because of the large number of ringed sideroblasts found in the marrow. Other DMPS subgroups may have ringed sideroblasts but they generally comprise less than 15% of the red cell precursors.

CHAPTER 34
CASE STUDY 34-1

1. The most likely FAB classification in this case is M5. Based on the description of the marrow, it appears to be M5a (predominance of monoblasts).
2. The abnormal cells appear to be monocytic in nature; therefore, the cells should be strongly positive for nonspecific or butyrate esterase staining.
3. Finding megaloblastoid red cell precursors in the marrow is not surprising because ara-C inhibits DNA synthesis (see Table 34–6).

CHAPTER 35
CASE STUDY 35-1

1. The sudden appearance of a marked basophilia is one of the signs of impending blast transformation. Other signs may be: (1) the appearance of dysplastic myelogenesis; (2) a sudden onset of thrombocytopenia coupled with a rise in the blast count; (3) a rise in the leukocyte count, decrease in the platelet count, and increase in the blast count; and (4) appearance of lymphoblasts.

2. Plate 53A contains a single micromegakaryocyte. Plate 53B contains three micromegakaryocytes, as evidenced by platelet blebs on the cytoplasm; there is also a neutrophil, and the other two cells are blasts. Plate 53D contains two micromegakaryocytes, a blast (upper left), and an early promyelocyte (lower left).
3. The final diagnosis is megakaryocytic blast transformation of CML. The prognosis is grave. Most treatment at this point is supportive only, with transfusions and antibiotics. Standard chemotherapy appears insufficient for treatment of nonlymphocytic blast transformation of any of the MPDs.

CASE STUDY 35-2

1. The finding of $Ph^1(-)$ cells is unusual in CML. Rather, cells from the malignant proliferating clone in most patients are $Ph^1(+)$. Because $Ph^1(+)$ cells usually are paramount in the diagnosis of CML, one must speculate on the possibility that $Ph^1(-)$ CMLs are truly myelodysplastic syndromes rather than MPDs.
2. Patient survival in CML is approximately 42 months, and these patients often respond to standard chemotherapy and enter remission for a period of time. The fact that four patients in this study did not respond to chemotherapy suggests misdiagnosis. Because the myelodysplastic syndromes do not respond to conventional therapy for MPDs, one may speculate that the poor response of the patients with the $Ph^1(-)$ disorder to conventional therapy indicates misdiagnosis.
3. The prognosis is less favorable for $Ph^1(-)$ (8–15 months survival) than for $Ph^1(+)$ (40–42 months survival) patients. The possibility that these patients are myelodysplastic could be part of the explanation for the less favorable prognosis.

CASE STUDY 35-3

1. The most likely diagnosis is polycythemia vera (PV). The patient's age is typical for a MPD. The laboratory values indicate PV, because by definition for a female patient, Hb should be greater than 15.5 g/dL, and HCT should be greater than 0.47 L/L for a tentative diagnosis of PV. This patient's Hb and HCT far exceed these criteria in their marked abnormality. The RBC count is also markedly increased over the diagnostic criterion of $>5.9 \times 10^{12}/L$. The MCV indicates a microcytic population of red cells, also typical of PV. Another key finding is the RCM of 43.6 mL/kg, which far exceeds the diagnostic criterion of >32 mL/kg for females. It also is common in PV to find a low normal MCHC and leukocytosis, which this patient displayed, and a thrombocytosis, which was not quite definitive on her first blood count but was on the second.
2. Her itching of the eyes is one of the many possible symptoms in patients with PV. The purple color of her skin is a classic physical finding: these patients may have a ruddy (reddish purple) complexion, also known as "ruddy cyanosis."
3. Serum iron, serum B_{12}, and arterial O_2 saturation are useful in differentiating PV and secondary polycythemia

(see Table 35-2). If these indicators are not definitive, a serum EPO measurement may help, because the value usually is decreased in PV but normal or increased in secondary polycythemias. An LAP test could also be useful; however, it probably is the least reliable test because of its susceptibility to technical error in staining and interpretation.

4. Usually, the plasma volume is elevated in PV, whereas, this patient's was decreased for some unknown reason.
5. Treatment with ^{32}P and therapeutic phlebotomy were routine treatment regimens for PV patients in the early 1980s when this patient was treated. In the late 1980s and 1990s, hydroxyurea provides an alternative to ^{32}P and may be the drug of choice for myelosuppression, because it has been reported to be less leukemogenic than other myelosuppressive drugs.

CHAPTER 36
CASE STUDY 36-1

1. The blasts must have been small and homogeneous with scanty cytoplasm and indistinct nucleoli.
2. The anemia and thrombocytopenia probably were caused by marrow replacement by the malignant cells.
3. Yes. L1 ALL is most frequently seen in children between the ages of 2 and 10.
4. They are not B cells, because SIg is less than 10%. They are not T cells, because E rosettes were less than 10%. The presence of cytoplasmic immunoglobulins shows that these cells are most likely pre-B ALL.

CASE STUDY 36-2

1. The cases have similar features: a high leukocyte count with a predominance of blasts along with anemia and thrombocytopenia. Cytochemical stains and immunologic markers show similar results, although PAS reactivity frequently is not as positive in L2 as it is in L1. Morphologically, the blasts in Case Study 36-2 showed more variability in size. Also, the cytoplasm was more abundant and nucleoli more visible. The patient was a young adult. These are features consistent with ALL Type 2.
2. Type L1 carries a better prognosis than L2. The use of cranial irradiation and intrathecal chemotherapy have decreased the incidence of CNS involvement and greatly improved survival. Bone marrow transplantation also is being used to increase survival.

CHAPTER 37
CASE STUDY 37-1

1. Chronic lymphocytic leukemia (CLL).
2. Autoimmune hemolytic anemia.
3. Because the HCT and Hb are decreased, whereas the reticulocyte count and the serum bilirubin are increased.
4. The prednisone helps suppress the activity of the immune system, thus decreasing hemolysis. As long as the

marrow is not replaced by lymphocytes and retains its ability to make erythroid precursors, the red cell destruction is compensated for by new production.

CHAPTER 38
CASE STUDY 38-1

1. No. This patient is not anemic; the reference range for Hb in females is approximately 12.0 to 16.0 g/dL. It is not unusual for a patient with Hodgkin disease to have a normal Hb and HCT.
2. An elevated granulocyte count might be expected, because the patient's disease was staged as mixed cellularity and IVB, although granulocytosis generally is seen in only 25% of Hodgkin disease patients.
3. Yes. It is common to find a normal bone marrow aspirate but an abnormal biopsy core in patients with Hodgkin disease. In Stage IV disease in particular, there usually is an associated fibrosis such that the neoplastic cells are retained in the biopsy but are not aspirated and therefore are not found free in bone marrow films.
4. Chemotherapy may cause a decrease in erythrocyte, leukocyte, and platelet counts.
5. No. A platelet count of 35×10^9/L is not an indication for platelet transfusion unless there are signs of bleeding. The usual platelet count that signals the need for platelet transfusion is 20×10^9/L, at which point there is a significant danger of spontaneous hemorrhaging.
6. A relative increase in monocytes usually heralds the coming increase of peripheral blood granulocytes. This usually precedes the granulocyte increase by 3 to 5 days.

CHAPTER 39
CASE STUDY 39-1

1. Both were to confirm or rule out meningitis that was suggested by the neck stiffness and pain.
2. The ESR, rouleaux, and plasma cells on the blood film and the increased total protein all indicate the need for further testing.
3. Plasma cell leukemia can be ruled out because abnormal cells in the peripheral blood did not number more than 2.0×10^9/L. Neither do heavy chain diseases fit the data, as there is no hypogammaglobulinemia with an increased total protein and decreased albumin.

CHAPTER 49
CASE STUDY 49-1

1. Vitamin C (ascorbic acid) deficiency is the most likely cause of the abnormal findings.
2. The disorder is called scurvy. It affects the vascular system by preventing the formation of an intact vascular basement membrane and decreases the synthesis of both collagen and the substance that holds endothelial cells and small vessels together.
3. The tourniquet test could easily be performed, because it

requires only a blood pressure cuff, which the team probably would have among its supplies. The expected results are positive (*i.e.*, formation of petechiae).

4. The tourniquet test is only qualitative (positive or negative). It is a simple screening test for capillary fragility.

5. A blood pressure cuff is required for the test. It is inflated on the arm to between 70 to 90 mm Hg and left in place for 5 minutes. However, in severely vitamin C-deficient patients, petechiae may be extensive and severe, and shorter times for cuff placement probably are indicated to avoid such problems.

6. Positive results are indicated by petechiae formation on the arm, wrist, or hand. Negative or normal results are indicated by the formation of few or no petechiae.

7. Coagulation tests and the bleeding time of these patients would be expected to be normal, as vitamin C deficiency affects the vessels, not coagulation factors or platelets.

8. The treatment of choice would be ascorbic acid (vitamin C).

CHAPTER 54
CASE STUDY 54-1

1. The FDP level is elevated because the streptokinase resulted in fibrin(ogen) lysis. This process generated many FDP (X, Y, D, and E). The latex particles in this test are sensitive to the latter two products (D and E).

2. The decreased plasminogen level is a result of the conversion of plasminogen to plasmin by the streptokinase.

3. The D-dimer assay is not greatly elevated, because the thrombolytic therapy did not lyse the clot. In order for this test to be positive, degradation products arising from crosslinked fibrin must be present. In this case, the streptokinase caused lysis of the fibrinogen in the plasma but very little lysis of the fibrin clot.

CHAPTER 55
CASE STUDY 55-1

1. This patient demonstrates a continuous hemorrhagic history throughout his short life span. The family history is significant in that no known close relative is similarly afflicted; therefore, the problem could be acquired.

2. This patient has von Willebrand's disease, as revealed by the results of the factor VIIIC:Ag assay, the VIIIR:RCo platelet aggregation results, the factor VIII multimer pattern, Simplate bleeding time, the APTT, and the factor VIII assay. The absence of a transfusion history is significant in that the bleeding events were managed without replacement therapy, an unlikely pattern if this patient were suffering from hemophilia A.

3. The presence of intermediate-sized multimers of von Willebrand factor and an absence of high-molecular-weight forms of multimers confirms the presence of one form (variant) of von Willebrand's disease (Type II).

4. Single-donor cryoprecipitate contains all the multimer forms of the factor VIII/vWF complex necessary to correct the platelet problem in von Willebrand's disease.

Commercial concentrates of factor VIII do not contain all these forms and will not correct the platelet defect.

CHAPTER 57
CASE STUDY 57-1

1. The APTT should be prolonged considerably over the normal range because heparin acts immediately, and the test was requested only 2 hours after administration. Possible causes for the unexpected result are: (1) laboratory error; (2) a low level of AT-III, which is a cofactor for heparin; (3) excessively high numbers of platelets that were activated during specimen collection and released platelet factor 4 (antiheparin); (4) the presence of a drug that is inhibiting the effects of heparin (*e.g.*, digitalis, antihistamines).

2. Possible solutions: (1) eliminate discrepancies attributable to laboratory error by checking the procedures used for specimen collection and processing, checking quality control results, and reviewing reagents and instrumentation. Then repeat the APTT; (2) assuming no laboratory error, inquire about any underlying diseases or conditions that decrease the level of AT-III, such as cirrhosis, nephrotic syndrome, or, in this patient, the use of oral contraceptives. Suggest the determination of AT-III levels; (3) review the patient's drug history, as the anticoagulant properties of heparin can be inhibited by synergistic effects of other drugs.

CHAPTER 60
CASE STUDY 60-1

1. Platelet counts performed by automated particle counters may be spuriously increased in the presence of microcytic or fragmented erythrocytes (see Chap. 60, ref 84). The original CBC reported a platelet count of 48×10^9/L; however, the phase platelet count was 25×10^9/L and correlated much better with the peripheral smear.

2. The CBC results, differential cell count, and erythrocyte fragmentation are consistent with a microangiopathic hemolytic anemia (MHA). The increased LD and decreased haptoglobin are characteristic of intravascular erythrocyte destruction associated with MHA such as DIC, TTP, or HUS. In both HUS and TTP, platelets are consumed and deposited in the microvasculature without consumption of coagulation factors. Symptoms and data supporting renal disease are characteristic of these conditions. Thrombotic thrombocytopenic purpura is more common in women, and neurologic problems, including headaches, are frequently associated with this disorder.

3. The acute onset of symptoms probably is related to several factors. Mitomycin has been implicated as the etiologic factor in a number of patients who developed fragmentation hemolysis, thrombocytopenia, and renal failure concomitantly (see Chap. 60, ref 48). In addition, immune complexes have been demonstrated in patients with gastric carcinoma and TTP-like syndromes (see Chap. 60, ref 86). One of the immune complexes iden-

tified reacted with tumor cells and a glycoprotein from autologous platelets, producing platelet aggregation.
4. Detection of circulating immune complexes or PAIg. However, this is an inconsistent feature, the test is not readily available, and the role of immune complexes in TTP remains unclear.

CHAPTER 61
CASE STUDY 61-1

1. This is a typical example of Glanzmann's thrombasthenia. Other helpful laboratory tests include clot retraction, which should be abnormal, abnormal platelet retention on glass beads, and normal vWF assay.
2. The basic defect is decreased or defective membrane glycoproteins IIb and IIIa, which are responsible for the platelet's ability to bind fibrinogen.
3. A blood film taken from a capillary puncture has sometimes been referred to as the "poor man's aggregation study." The fact that the patient's platelets were normal in number but did not form small clumps (*i.e.*, looked more like blood from an EDTA specimen) points to a platelet function abnormality.

CHAPTER 62
CASE STUDY 62-1

1. The commercial control range for the PTTs in this laboratory has no bearing on the interpretation of the patient's test results except to ensure that the test system is functioning properly. The narrow range of 31 to 33 seconds for the control is used only to check for system performance and to determine shifts and trends in control results indicating a possible system failure (see Table 62-2). Patient results must be compared with the laboratory's established PTT population reference range based on a sample of "healthy" subjects. In this laboratory the patient's PTT of 32 seconds appears prolonged in comparison with the normal population, for which the upper limit of the reference range was 29 seconds.
2. Further testing is warranted because the PTT is prolonged. The tests to assist in diagnosis would most likely include a prothrombin time, thrombin time, and fibrinogen, with factor assays to follow, as indicated by other test results and the patient's history.

CASE STUDY 62-2

1. The unexpected occurrence of erratic PT and PTT results should definitely raise suspicion as this causes doubt about precision and accuracy. Further investigation is warranted.
2. The controls at the beginning of the shift indicated that

the system was in control. Therefore, at the time, there was no cause for concern.
3. Erratic, discrepant results do not point specifically to a problem with the instrument, reagent, or specimens, which makes problem identification difficult. Therefore, all variables listed in Table 62-1 should be reviewed as possible problem sources. Possible instrument problems include malfunction of the light source, detector, clotting timer, electrical circuitry, or some combination. Incorrect reagent delivery is not a likely cause of the problem, because this error usually results in excessively long clotting times. Reagents do not appear to be a source of trouble in this case; however, it is well to be certain that they are being used in accordance with established guidelines for stability. Reagents should be in homogeneous suspension without large particles or aggregates. The erratic pattern of discrepant results most likely does not indicate a specimen-handling problem either, because the short results generally do not occur on the same patient. However, it would be well to verify that specimens are being drawn properly, delivered to the laboratory promptly, and processed and tested with minimal delay.
4. No. The physician should not be told that the specimen result is definitely correct. If the system problem has not yet been resolved, it would be best to review the procedure for obtaining and delivering coagulation specimens with the personnel involved and request another specimen for repeat testing. Until the source of the problem is known, repeat testing should be done on a backup instrument if available.
5. Yes. The controls should be repeated at this point to be certain they are still within acceptable limits.
6. Yes. A check of system precision would be useful. A series of 15 tests for the PT and PTT should be run on the same normal plasma to check for precision and reproducibility. It is unnecessary to use commercial control material, which is expensive, to check system precision when running each test 15 times. A normal plasma serves the same function.
7. Yes, if the problem is not detected and corrected, a backup instrument should be used if available until the malfunction can be evaluated by a service technician. Technical service definitely should be called. Alternatively, if, after running the controls again and checking system precision, no problem with the instrument is found, the laboratory should continue to monitor the results carefully on this instrument with an increased use of controls to try to identify any pattern of discrepant results.
8. Yes, when a problem is suspected, all tests should be performed in duplicate (even if the laboratory normally performs only single tests) and the average result reported to assist in identifying the problem and verifying patient results. Duplicate testing should be continued until the problem is resolved.

APPENDIX B   PERCENT TRANSMITTANCE–ABSORBANCE CONVERSION TABLE

% T	ABSORBANCE* 0.00	0.25	0.50	0.75	% T	ABSORBANCE* 0.00	0.25	0.50	0.75	% T	ABSORBANCE* 0.00	0.25	0.50	0.75	% T	ABSORBANCE* 0.00	0.25	0.50	0.75
1	2.000	1.903	1.824	1.757	26	0.585	0.581	0.577	0.573	51	0.292	0.290	0.288	0.286	76	0.119	0.118	0.116	0.115
2	1.690	1.648	1.602	1.561	27	0.569	0.565	0.561	0.557	52	0.284	0.282	0.280	0.278	77	0.114	0.112	0.111	0.100
3	1.523	1.488	1.456	1.426	28	0.553	0.549	0.545	0.542	53	0.276	0.274	0.272	0.270	78	0.108	0.107	0.105	0.104
4	1.398	1.372	1.347	1.323	29	0.538	0.534	0.530	0.527	54	0.268	0.266	0.264	0.262	79	0.102	0.101	0.100	0.098
5	1.301	1.280	1.260	1.240	30	0.523	0.520	0.516	0.512	55	0.260	0.258	0.256	0.254	80	0.097	0.096	0.094	0.093
6	1.222	1.204	1.187	1.171	31	0.509	0.505	0.502	0.498	56	0.252	0.250	0.248	0.246	81	0.092	0.090	0.089	0.088
7	1.155	1.140	1.126	1.112	32	0.495	0.491	0.488	0.485	57	0.244	0.242	0.240	0.238	82	0.086	0.085	0.084	0.082
8	1.097	1.083	1.071	1.059	33	0.482	0.478	0.475	0.472	58	0.237	0.235	0.233	0.231	83	0.081	0.080	0.078	0.077
9	1.046	1.034	1.022	1.011	34	0.469	0.465	0.462	0.459	59	0.229	0.227	0.226	0.224	84	0.076	0.074	0.073	0.072
10	1.000	0.989	0.979	0.969	35	0.456	0.453	0.450	0.447	60	0.222	0.220	0.218	0.216	85	0.071	0.069	0.068	0.067
11	0.959	0.949	0.939	0.930	36	0.444	0.441	0.438	0.435	61	0.215	0.213	0.211	0.209	86	0.066	0.064	0.063	0.062
12	0.921	0.912	0.903	0.894	37	0.432	0.429	0.426	0.423	62	0.208	0.206	0.204	0.202	87	0.061	0.059	0.058	0.057
13	0.886	0.878	0.870	0.862	38	0.420	0.417	0.414	0.412	63	0.201	0.199	0.197	0.196	88	0.056	0.054	0.053	0.052
14	0.854	0.846	0.838	0.831	39	0.409	0.406	0.403	0.401	64	0.194	0.192	0.191	0.189	89	0.051	0.049	0.048	0.047
15	0.824	0.817	0.810	0.803	40	0.398	0.395	0.392	0.390	65	0.187	0.186	0.184	0.182	90	0.046	0.045	0.043	0.042
16	0.796	0.789	0.782	0.776	41	0.387	0.385	0.382	0.380	66	0.181	0.179	0.177	0.176	91	0.041	0.040	0.039	0.037
17	0.770	0.763	0.757	0.751	42	0.377	0.374	0.372	0.369	67	0.174	0.172	0.171	0.169	92	0.036	0.035	0.034	0.033
18	0.745	0.739	0.733	0.727	43	0.367	0.364	0.362	0.359	68	0.168	0.166	0.164	0.163	93	0.032	0.030	0.029	0.028
19	0.721	0.716	0.710	0.704	44	0.357	0.354	0.352	0.349	69	0.161	0.160	0.158	0.157	94	0.027	0.026	0.025	0.024
20	0.699	0.694	0.688	0.683	45	0.347	0.344	0.342	0.340	70	0.155	0.153	0.152	0.150	95	0.022	0.021	0.020	0.019
21	0.678	0.673	0.668	0.663	46	0.337	0.335	0.332	0.330	71	0.149	0.147	0.146	0.144	96	0.018	0.017	0.016	0.014
22	0.658	0.653	0.648	0.643	47	0.328	0.325	0.323	0.321	72	0.143	0.141	0.140	0.138	97	0.013	0.012	0.011	0.010
23	0.638	0.634	0.629	0.624	48	0.319	0.317	0.314	0.312	73	0.137	0.135	0.134	0.132	98	0.009	0.008	0.007	0.006
24	0.620	0.615	0.611	0.606	49	0.310	0.308	0.305	0.303	74	0.131	0.129	0.128	0.126	99	0.004	0.003	0.002	0.001
25	0.602	0.598	0.594	0.589	50	0.301	0.299	0.297	0.295	75	0.125	0.124	0.122	0.121	100	0.000	0.0000	0.0000	0.000

* Absorbance = 2 − log % T

Relative Centrifugal Force Nomograph

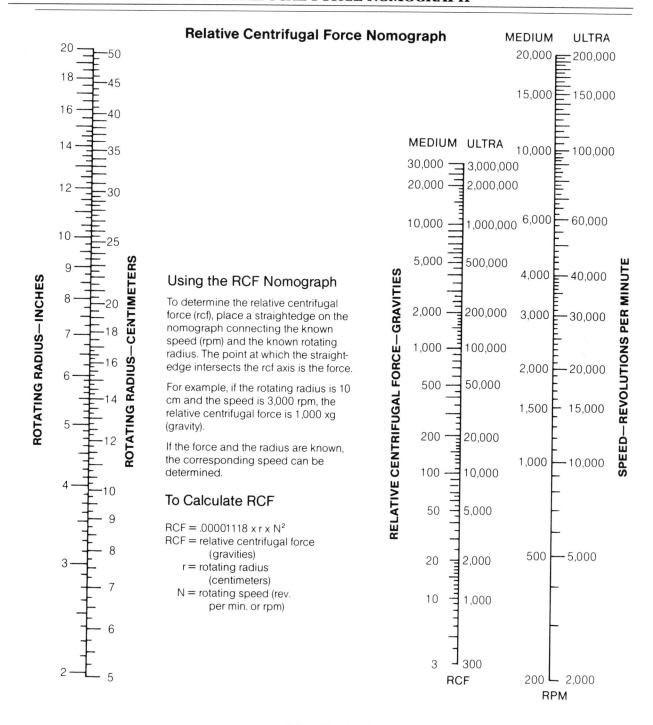

Using the RCF Nomograph

To determine the relative centrifugal force (rcf), place a straightedge on the nomograph connecting the known speed (rpm) and the known rotating radius. The point at which the straight-edge intersects the rcf axis is the force.

For example, if the rotating radius is 10 cm and the speed is 3,000 rpm, the relative centrifugal force is 1,000 xg (gravity).

If the force and the radius are known, the corresponding speed can be determined.

To Calculate RCF

$$RCF = .00001118 \times r \times N^2$$

RCF = relative centrifugal force (gravities)

r = rotating radius (centimeters)

N = rotating speed (rev. per min. or rpm)

ROTATING TIP RADIUS

The distance measured from the rotor axis to the tip of the liquid inside the tubes at the greatest horizontal distance from the rotor axis is the rotating tip radius.

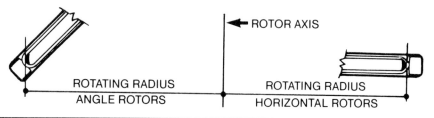

(Reprinted by permission from International Equipment Co., Damon Corporation)

INDEX

Numbers followed by an *f* indicate a figure, *cf* indicates a color figure, and *t* indicates tabular material.